KT-176-208

A TEXTBOOK OF RADIOLOGY AND IMAGING

A TEXTBOOK OF RADIOLOGY AND IMAGING

EDITED BY

DAVID SUTTON

M.D., F.R.C.P., F.R.C.R., D.M.R.D., M.C.A.R.(Hon.)
Director, Radiological Department, St Mary's Hospital and Director of Radiology, St Mary's Hospital Medical School, London.
Consultant Radiologist to the National Hospitals for Nervous Diseases (Queen Square and Maida Vale), London.

THIRD EDITION

VOLUME TWO

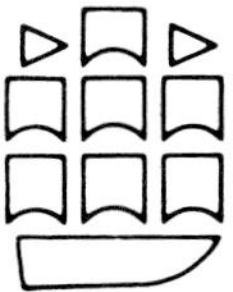

CHURCHILL LIVINGSTONE
EDINBURGH LONDON MELBOURNE AND NEW YORK 1980

CHURCHILL LIVINGSTONE
Medical Division of the Longman Group Limited

Distributed in the United States of America by
Churchill Livingstone Inc., 19 West 44th Street,
New York, N.Y. 10036, and by associated companies,
branches and representatives throughout the world.

First edition 1969
Second edition 1975
Third edition 1980

ISBN 0 443 02371 9 (Two-volume edition)

British Library Cataloguing in Publication Data
A textbook of radiology and imaging.
3rd ed.
1. Radiology, Medical
I. Sutton, David, *b. 1917*
616.07′57 R895 80–40679

Printed in Great Britain by Wm. Clowes (Beccles) Ltd, Beccles

PREFACE TO THE THIRD EDITION

When the last edition of this book was published in 1975 Radio-isotope Scanning was well established and Ultrasound had already made a major impact on radiology, particularly obstetric radiology. News of Hounsfield's remarkable new invention of Computed Tomography (C.T.) was first published in 1973 but we were able to include only a preliminary report in the second edition.

In the last six years progress in C.T. scanning has been remarkable, and exploration of the new fields opened up continues apace. Further important advances have also been made in Ultrasound, and Nuclear Medicine has also steadily progressed.

Imaging, as these new disciplines are usually called, is now a major force which has profoundly influenced the practice of radiology. It has become commonplace to refer to a 'Department of Radiology and Diagnostic Imaging'. These major advances have been incorporated in this third edition of the Textbook and to signal this the title has been changed to *A Textbook of Radiology and Imaging*.

Conventional radiology has not remained static in this period and we have attempted to update all sections of the book to take account of changing views and recent work. We hope that this new edition will provide an accurate picture of the present state of the art despite the time lag between writing and publication which is inevitable in a major work like this. To cope with the increased material the format and size of the book have been changed. Another new feature in response to many requests from students is the inclusion of an increased number of References and Suggestions for Further Reading at the end of individual chapters.

London, 1980 David Sutton

LIST OF CONTRIBUTORS

PART 1: BONES AND JOINTS

Philip Jacobs
T.D., D.M.R.D., F.R.C.P., F.R.C.R.
Consultant Radiologist, Royal Orthopaedic Hospital, Birmingham, Birmingham General Hospital, Birmingham Accident Hospital and Warwickshire Orthopaedic Hospital for Children. Clinical Lecturer in Radiology, University of Birmingham

R. O. Murray
M.B.E., M.D.(Cantab.), F.R.C.P.(Edin.), F.R.C.R., D.M.R.(Lond.), F.A.C.R.(Hon.), F.R.A.C.R.(Hon.)
Consultant Radiologist, Royal National Orthopaedic Hospital and Institute of Orthopaedics, London W.1. Formerly Senior Lecturer in Orthopaedic Radiology, University of London.

Denis J. Stoker
M.B., F.R.C.P., F.R.C.R.
Consultant Radiologist, Royal National Orthopaedic Hospital, London W.1 and St George's Hospital, London SW.17. Director of Radiological Studies, Institute of Orthopaedics, University of London.

PART 2: THE CHEST

Ronald G. Grainger
M.D., F.R.C.P., D.M.R.D., F.R.C.R., F.A.C.R.(Hon.), F.R.A.C.R.(Hon.)
Consultant Radiologist, Royal Hallamshire Hospital, Sheffield and Cardio-thoracic Centre, Northern General Hospital, Sheffield. Clinical Teacher, University of Sheffield.

J. W. Pierce
M.D., F.R.C.P., F.R.C.R.
Honorary Consultant Radiologist, St Thomas' Hospital, London SE.1 and Brompton Hospital for Diseases of the Chest, London SW.3.

PART 3: CARDIOVASCULAR SYSTEM

R. E. Steiner
C.B.E., M.D., F.R.C.R., F.R.C.P.
Professor of Diagnostic Radiology, University of London at the Royal Postgraduate Medical School and Hammersmith Hospital.

John Dow
M.C., F.R.C.P.E., B.Sc., F.R.C.R.
Consultant Radiologist, Guy's Hospital, London SE1 and the Evelina Children's Hospital, London SE1. Teacher in Radiology, University of London.

Michael Pearson
M.A., M.B., B.Chir., M.R.C.P., F.R.C.R.
Consultant Radiologist, Brompton Hospital, London SW.3 and London Chest Hospital, London E.2. Honorary Consultant Radiologist, South West Thames RHA. Honorary Senior Lecturer, Cardiothoracic Institute, University of London.

David Sutton
M.D., F.R.C.P., F.R.C.R., D.M.R.D., M.C.A.R.(Hon.)
Director, Radiological Department, St Mary's Hospital, London W.2 and Director of Radiology, St Mary's Hospital Medical School. Consultant Radiologist to the National Hospitals for Nervous Diseases (Queen Square and Maida Vale).

J. O. M. C. Craig
F.R.C.S.(I), D.M.R.D., F.R.C.R.
Consultant Radiologist, St Mary's Hospital, London W.2 and Bolingbroke Hospital, London SW.11. Teacher in Radiology, University of London.

PART 4: THE GASTRO-INTESTINAL TRACT AND ABDOMEN

Eric Samuel
C.B.E., B.Sc., M.D., F.R.C.S., F.R.C.S.E., F.R.C.P.E., F.R.C.R., F.R.C.R.I.(Hon.), F.A.C.R.(Hon.)
Professor Emeritus, University of Edinburgh and Professor, Department of Radiology, University of Pretoria, South Africa.

J. W. Laws
M.B., F.R.C.P., F.R.C.R., F.A.C.R.(Hon.), F.R.A.C.R.(Hon.)
Director of Radiology, King's College Hospital, London SE.5. Director of Radiological Studies, King's College Hospital Medical School.

C. G. Whiteside
B.M., B.Ch.(Oxon.), F.R.C.R., D.M.R.D.
Consultant Radiologist, Middlesex Hospital, London W.1, Royal Masonic Hospital, London W.6, Royal National Throat, Nose and Ear Hospital, London WC.1. Teacher in Diagnostic Radiology, University of London.

David Sutton
M.D., F.R.C.P., F.R.C.R., D.M.R.D., M.C.A.R.(Hon.)
Director Radiological Department, St Mary's Hospital and Director of Radiology, St Mary's Hospital Medical School. Consultant Radiologist to the National Hospitals for Nervous Diseases (Queen Square and Maida Vale).

PART 5: THE UROGENITAL TRACTS

David Edwards
M.B., F.R.C.P., F.R.C.R.
Director, Department of Radiology, University College Hospital, London WC.1. Teacher in Diagnostic Radiology, University of London.

J. H. Highman
M.B., F.R.C.P., D.M.R.D., F.R.C.R.
Consultant Radiologist, St Mary's Hospital, London W.2. Teacher in Radiology, University of London.

PART 6: E.N.T.; EYES; TEETH SOFT TISSUES

Eric Samuel
C.B.E., B.Sc., M.D., F.R.C.S., F.R.C.S.E., F.R.C.P.E., F.R.C.R., F.R.C.R.I.(Hon.), F.A.C.R.(Hon.)
Professor Emeritus, University of Edinburgh and Professor, Department of Radiology, University of Pretoria, South Africa.

Glyn A. S. Lloyd
M.A., D.M., D.M.R.D., F.R.C.R.
Director, Department of Radiology, The Royal National Throat, Nose and Ear Hospital, London WC.1 and Institute of Laryngology and Otology. Consultant Radiologist, Moorfields Eye Hospital, London EC.1 and Institute of Opthalmology.

Frank L. Ingram
D.M.R.D., L.D.S., M.R.C.S., L.R.C.P.
Consultant Radiologist to the Dental Department, Guy's Hospital, to the Eastman Dental Hospital and to the Canterbury and Isle of Thanet Hospital Groups. Teacher of Dental Radiology at Guy's Hospital Medical School and at the Institute of Dental Surgery in the Eastman Dental Hospital.

F. Starer
F.R.C.P.(Edin.), F.R.C.R.
Consultant Radiologist, Westminster Hospital Group, Teacher in Radiology, University of London.

I. H. Gravelle
B.Sc., M.B., Ch.B., F.R.C.P.(Edin.), F.R.C.R., D.M.R.D.
Consultant Radiologist, University Hospital of Wales, Cardiff. Clinical Teacher, Welsh National School of Medicine.

PART 7: THE CENTRAL NERVOUS SYSTEM

David Sutton
M.D., F.R.C.P., F.R.C.R., D.M.R.D., M.C.A.R.(Hon.)
Director, Radiological Department, St Mary's Hospital and Director of Radiology, St Mary's Hospital Medical School. Consultant Radiologist to the National Hospitals for Nervous Diseases (Queen Square and Maida Vale).

N. A. Lewtas
M.B., F.R.C.P., F.R.C.R.
Consultant Radiologist, Sheffield Area Health Authority (T). Honorary Clinical Lecturer in Radiodiagnosis, University of Sheffield.

PART 8: IMAGING

David Sutton
M.D., F.R.C.P., F.R.C.R., D.M.R.D., M.C.A.R.(Hon.)
Director, Radiological Department, St Mary's Hospital and Director of Radiology, St Mary's Hospital Medical School. Consultant Radiologist to the National Hospitals for Nervous Diseases (Queen Square and Maida Vale). Teacher in Radiology, University of London.

Ivan Moseley
B.Sc., M.D., M.R.C.P., F.R.C.R., D.M.R.D.
Consultant Radiologist, National Hospital for Nervous Diseases, Queen Square. Teacher in Radiology, University of London.

Ian Isherwood
M.B., Ch.B., D.M.R.D., M.R.C.P., F.R.C.R.
Professor of Diagnostic Radiology, University of Manchester. Consultant Radiologist, Manchester Royal Infirmary.

W. St Clair Forbes
M.A., M.B., B.Ch., D.R.C.O.G., D.M.R.D., F.R.C.R.
Consultant Radiologist, Salford Royal Hospital and Hope Hospital, Salford (University of Manchester School of Medicine) and Department of Diagnostic Radiology, University of Manchester.

E. Rhys Davies
F.R.C.P.E., F.R.C.R., F.F.R.R.C.S.I.(Hon.)
Consultant Radiologist, Bristol District (Teaching). Clinical Lecturer, University of Bristol.

Frank G. M. Ross
M.B., B.Ch., F.R.C.R., D.M.R.D.
Consultant Radiologist, Bristol Royal Infirmary Clinical Lecturer in Radiology, University of Bristol.

J. H. Highman
M.B., F.R.C.P., D.M.R.D., F.R.C.R.
Consultant Radiologist, St Mary's Hospital, London W.2. Teacher in Radiology, University of London.

CONTENTS
VOLUME ONE

CONTENTS
VOLUME TWO

PART 4

THE GASTRO-INTESTINAL TRACT AND ABDOMEN

CHAPTER 32

THE SALIVARY GLANDS, PHARYNX AND OESOPHAGUS

The parotid, submandibular and sublingual glands are the three paired salivary glands and are placed symmetrically on either side of the buccal cavity. They are situated in relationship to the posterior aspect of the angle (parotid gland), the medial aspect of the body (submandibular) and the posterior aspect of the symphysis (sublingual) of the mandible. The parotid and submandibular glands empty via relatively large single ducts. These open respectively on papillae on the buccal mucosa opposite the second upper molar tooth, and on either side of the frenulum beneath the tongue. The sublingual glands empty by smaller, multiple ducts near the sublingual papilla and sometimes directly into the submandibular duct.

The salivary glands are all alveolo-racemose glands but differ in the nature of their secretions, that from the parotid being serous, from the submandibular mucous and serous, and from the sublingual mucous only. These differences probably determine the different patterns of ductular branching within the glands and to some extent the differing susceptibility to inflammatory processes and to stone formation.

Radiological investigation

Pathological changes in the salivary glands can be investigated by plain radiography or after the injection of oily or watery contrast medium into the parotid or submandibular ducts. The sublingual glands because of their duct system cannot be demonstrated by the injection of contrast material.

Plain films. The anatomical sites of the salivary glands necessitate special radiographic views so that the glands can be thrown clear of overlapping shadows of the mandible and maxilla.

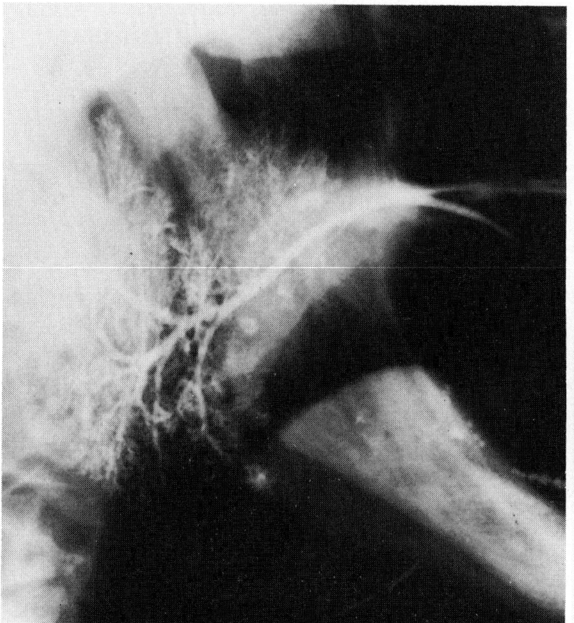

Fig. 32.1 Normal parotid sialogram showing the outline of the parotid duct and the accessory duct arising from its upper end.

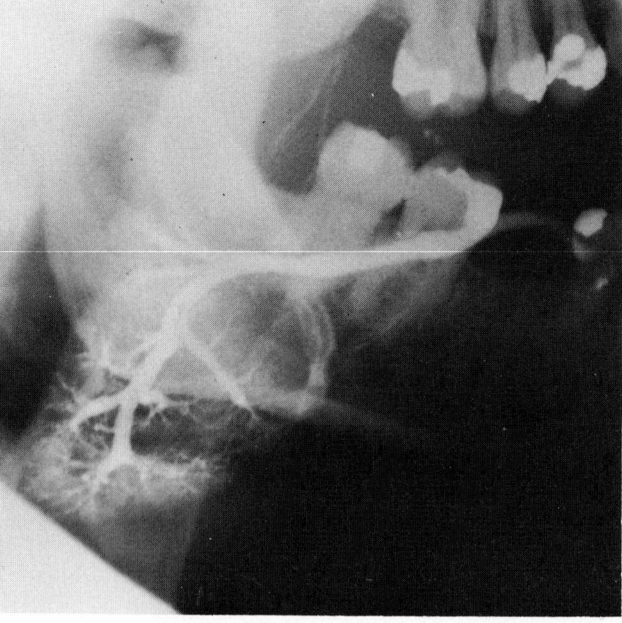

Fig. 32.2 Normal submandibular sialogram showing the branching of the duct within the gland to be less fine than that of the parotid duct.

The parotid gland lodged behind the angle of the mandible can be visualized free of overlapping bone shadows by a tangential anteroposterior film. The submandibular gland lying below the mandible can best be seen in a lateral oblique view of the mandible supplemented by a second view taken while the tongue, and hence the submandibular gland, is being depressed by the patient's finger.

The submandibular duct and, to a lesser extent, the parotid duct, have considerable submucosal segments within the mouth. Consequently occlusal films should be used to demonstrate changes in these parts of the ducts.

Sialography. Catheterization of the parotid and submaxillary duct using a blunt angled 18 gauge needle or a fine polythene catheter, can be performed after preliminary dilatation of the duct orifice. No anaesthesia is required. The injection of 1–2 cc of a viscous contrast medium (Neohydriol or Lipiodol) is usually sufficient to outline the main duct and all its branches, and overdistension is avoided by completing the injection when a feeling of fullness is noted by the patient.

In the parotid sialogram the accessory parotid, with its duct and frequently a further second accessory duct, is frequently seen as an anatomical variation (Fig. 32.1). The submandibular duct on the other hand is less liable to anatomical variations (Fig. 32.2).

PATHOLOGICAL CONDITIONS

Salivary calculi. Because of the high radio-opacity (in virtue of a high calcium carbonate content) relatively small salivary calculi can be demonstrated. This is especially so when bone-free films of the submandibular duct and parotid ducts are used (Fig. 32.3). About 20 per cent of salivary calculi are not opaque and cannot be seen. Large calculi tend to be oval in shape, homogeneous in consistency and lie along the line of the duct. Such large stones are most frequently seen in the submandibular duct. Parotid calculi are less common and usually occur at the gland hilum or in the gland substance itself.

Salivary stones, because of their high calcium content, seldom appear as negative shadows in a sialogram, but obstruction of the duct results in dilatation of the duct system (sialectasis) behind the stone (Fig. 32.4).

Differential diagnosis. Submandibular and parotid calculi must be differentiated from calcified tuberculous glands, and arterial calcification, by their site and homogeneous consistency. A sialogram will confirm the diagnosis in cases of doubt.

Infections. Acute non-suppurative parotitis is most frequently due to mumps and radiological examination is only required to exclude parotitis due to other causes or calculus formation. In instances where a sialogram has been inadvertently performed in mumps a normal pattern is found or slight beading of the smaller ducts is the only change noted (Fig. 32.6 A and B).

Chronic non-suppurative conditions such as Sjögren's syndrome produce sialographic changes with thin thread-like ducts which may show beading along their course (Fig. 32.5 A and B). Reflux of contrast medium into the gland structure is probably the result of rupture of minute ducts and can also be seen in non-suppurative parotitis.

Suppurative parotitis usually follows an obstruction of the duct or occurs post-operatively. Sialograms in this condition show the ducts to be dilated and saccular, and

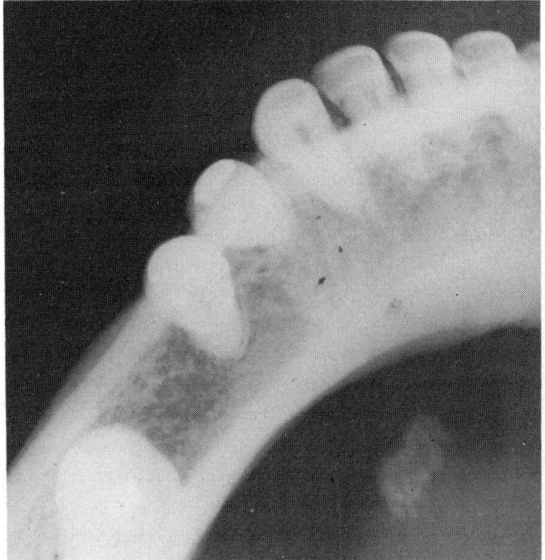

Fig. 32.3 Intra-oral view of submandibular duct showing a large irregular salivary calculus lodged in the anterior end of the duct.

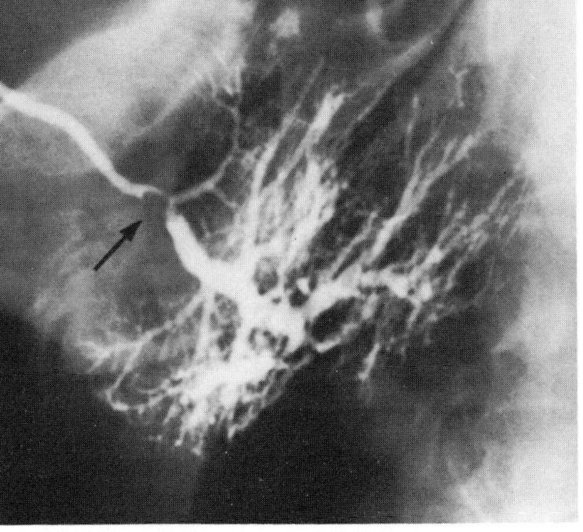

Fig. 32.4 Sialogram showing non-opaque calculus lodged near the hilus of the gland and associated with distension of the duct (sialectasis) behind the stone.

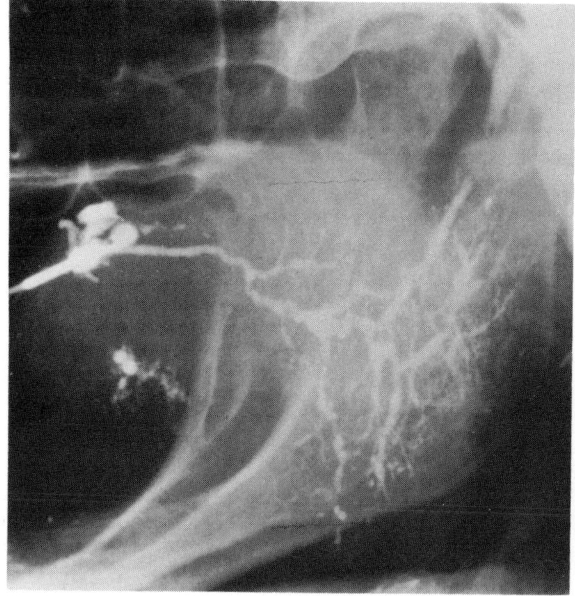

A

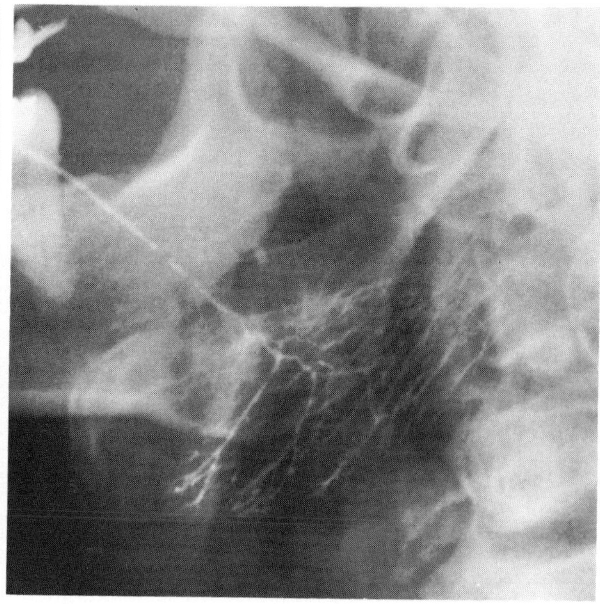

B

Fig. 32.5 A Sialogram showing cylindrical dilation of the duct system in Sjögren's syndrome. B Sjögren's syndrome. Sialogram showing the hypoplastic ducts evenly involved throughout the whole of the gland.

an irregular cavity full of contrast medium indicates breakdown of the gland with abscess cavity formation.

Overdistension of the duct system during injection, especially in cases of non-suppurative parotitis, will produce small bead-like appearances on the duct system. These represent minute intraglandular duct ruptures, with spread of the contrast medium into the gland substance. This appearance must not be mistaken for true sialectasis.

Pin-hole meatus. Trauma to the parotid papilla, most frequently the result of ill-fitting dentures, results in a fibrous stenosis of the duct orifice with swelling and pain in the parotid gland after eating. Catheterization of the duct may only be achieved with difficulty, and after dilatation of the duct orifice with lachrymal probes. This manoeuvre usually temporarily relieves the condition. Sialography demonstrates a dilation of the duct as far as the gland hilum, but without any intraglandular dilation of the duct system.

Tumours. The commonest tumours of the salivary glands are the mixed salivary tumours, less commonly frank carcinoma occurs. Benign tumours, adenoma and fibromata, are rarities and involvement by lymphomas (Mikulicz's disease) is usually part of a generalized syndrome.

Mixed salivary tumours. A mixed salivary tumour is histologically an adnexal cell tumour and the variable

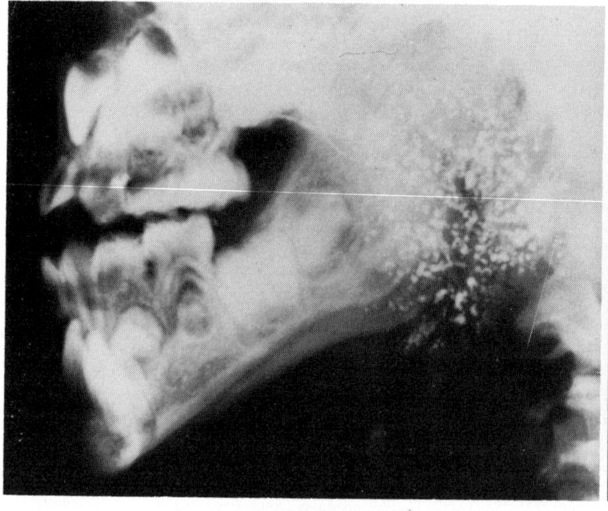

Fig. 32.6A

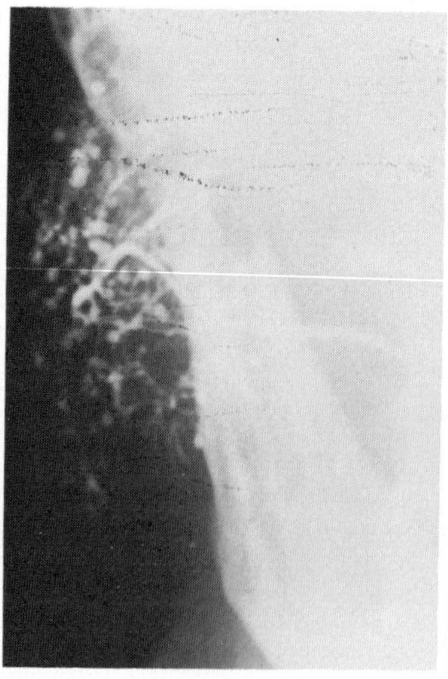

Fig. 32.6B

Fig. 32.6 A Sialectasis—parotid sialogram showing the punctate dilatations of the duct system filled with contrast medium. B Oblique view of the parotid gland showing severe sialectasis.

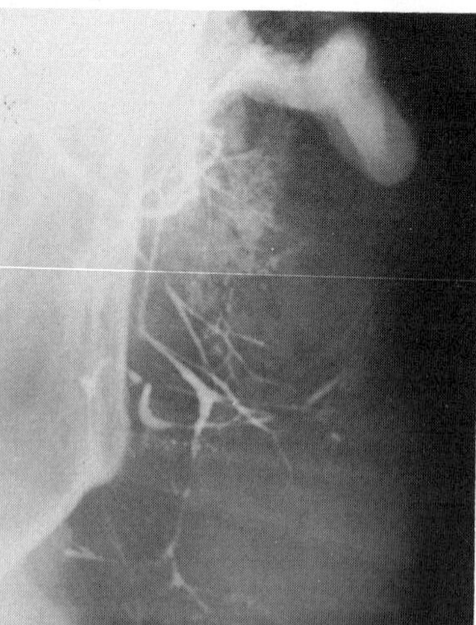

Fig. 32.7

Fig. 32.7 Mixed salivary tumour—sialogram of parotid gland showing the distortion and the irregular narrowing of the branches and the general expansion of the duct system.

histological structure is readily appreciated when the growth potentialities of that cell are considered.

Radiologically there is soft-tissue swelling, but mixed salivary tumours do not erode the mandible unless surgical attempts at removal have been made. However, if such tumours occur in the hard palate, bone erosion may occur.

Sialograms demonstrate a displacement and expansion of the intraglandular branches of the duct system without any true invasion or destruction of the ducts such as characterize a frank carcinoma of the salivary gland (Fig. 32.7).

Carcinoma. Adenocarcinoma is most commonly seen in the parotid gland. Inadequate surgical removal frequently confers a frank invasive tendency on a mixed salivary tumour, and as a sequel of surgery carcinomata may occur in any salivary gland.

The sialogram demonstrates a gross distortion of the intraglandular duct system associated with invasion of the duct system rather than simple displacement of the ducts.

PHARYNX AND OESOPHAGUS

Radiological investigation

The aim is to demonstrate in two projections, preferably at right angles, each part of the pharynx and oesophagus when fully distended and when collapsed. In the pharynx and cervical oesophagus, antero-posterior and lateral projections are the easiest to interpret, while in the thoracic oesophagus oblique projections are the best for demonstration of intrinsic lesions since the oesophagus is then projected clear of the spine. When the thoracic oesophagus is displaced or directly involved by some extrinsic lesion, this is often most easily appreciated in the antero-posterior or lateral projection.

Soft tissue radiographs. A lateral film of the nasopharynx taken at a 6-foot tube film distance without a grid is an essential preliminary to any radiographic examination of the nasopharynx. Radio-opaque foreign bodies and soft tissue tumours as well as erosion and destruction of adjoining bony structures can be seen in this film. A lateral view taken during a Valsalva manoeuvre may help to distinguish between a calcification in thyroid cartilage, which moves forward, and one in an embedded foreign body, which does not.

The lateral film shows anteriorly from above downwards, the posterior border of the tongue, the soft tissue shadow of the vallecula, the epiglottis and larynx. Posteriorly the soft tissue of the muscular wall of the pharynx and the pre-vertebral soft tissues in the adult are usually not more than 0.5 cm thick but widen slightly in the nasopharynx where they curve forward to reach the base of the skull.

Barium studies. Full distension of the upper oesophagus occurs only momentarily during the swallowing of a bolus so that cine radiography or video-tape recording may be needed in order to study such lesions as a post-cricoid web or small diverticulum and for the analysis of functional or neuro-muscular disorders of the oesophagus.

The thoracic oesophagus may be fully distended only when the abdominal pressure is raised as when the patient lies prone over a bolster or some form of 'anti-gravity' swallow is employed.

In the oesophagus the primary peristaltic wave begins with the act of swallowing and proceeds along the oesophagus to the cardia. The main secondary propulsive waves start at the level of the aortic knuckle and proceed rhythmically to the cardia and are followed by a wave of relaxation. Tertiary contractions which are non-propulsive contractions of circular muscle are not seen in the normal young adult but occur in the elderly and in a number of conditions associated with neuro-muscular disorders.

All patients complaining of dysphagia in whom the cause is not readily demonstrated should have a careful examination of the lower oesophagus, cardia and fundus of the stomach. The investigation of the competence of the cardia should always be carefully undertaken in the examination of the lower end of the oesophagus. Raising intra-abdominal pressure by various movements such as leg raising, use of abdominal pressure pad or by lying the patient prone over a bolster may all cause reflux of barium from the stomach into the oesophagus.

In the newborn, congenital strictures and atresias of the oesophagus should be examined initially by plain films to see if there is any gas in the abdominal cavity (Fig. 32.10A), followed by the passage of a soft catheter into the oesophagus to demonstrate the site of any major obstruction (Fig. 32.9). One ml of Lipiodol may be injected down the tube under screening control to demonstrate the anatomy more clearly (Fig. 32.10B). The Lipiodol may then be aspirated. Water-soluble contrast medium such as Gastrografin should not be used because it has five times the osmolarity of plasma and any aspirated into the lung would have a dangerous effect.

Small tracheo-oesophageal fistulae may be very difficult to demonstrate and some can be shown only by cine radiography in the prone position using a horizontal ray. It is best to introduce a tube into the lower oesophagus and inject contrast medium as the tube is slowly withdrawn so that the exact site of the fistula may be seen and any confusion with possible aspiration of contrast through the larynx avoided.

PATHOLOGICAL CONDITIONS

Congenital abnormalities. Congenital atresia, oesophageal stricture and tracheo-oesophageal fistulae prob-

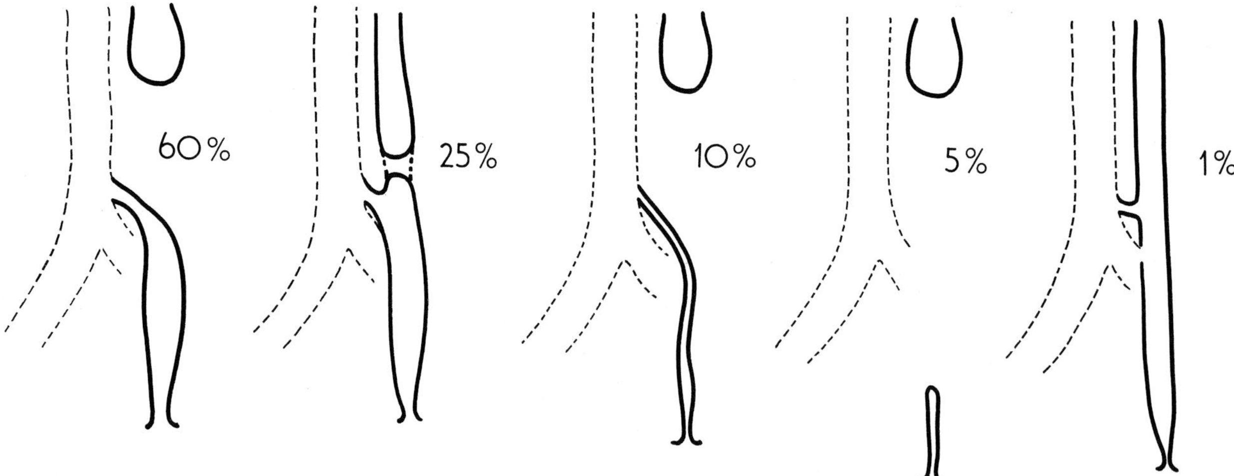

Fig. 32.8 Drawing showing the types of tracheo-oesophageal atresia. The relationship of the trachea to the lower segment of the oesophagus is important in determining the presence of air in the stomach.

ably represent varying degrees of failure of separation of the primitive tracheo-oesophageal tube. The tracheal stricture may be complete or partial and likewise the communication with the oesophagus may be of the same order. The variations of tracheo-oesophageal atresia and strictures are shown diagrammatically in Figure 32.8.

In the newborn a plain film of the abdomen may, by the absence of air in the stomach and intestines, indicate a complete oesophageal atresia. If, however, the lower oesophageal segment communicates with the trachea, gas may be present in the stomach (Figs. 32.9 and 32.10A).

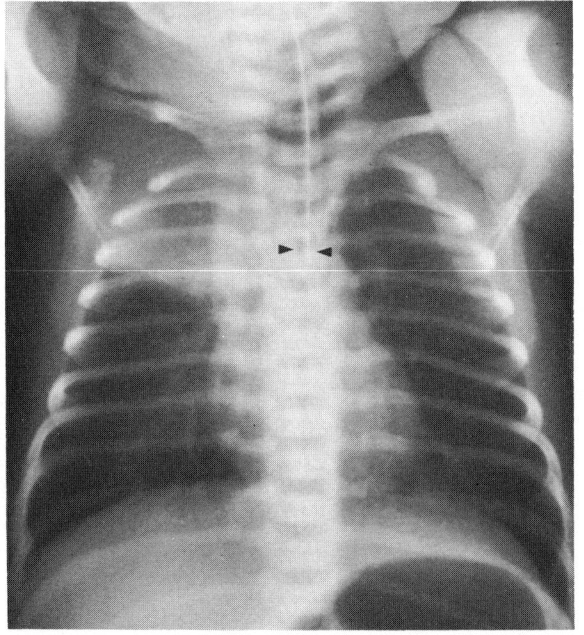

Fig. 32.9 Soft opaque catheter in the oesophagus demonstrating the site of the oesophageal atresia (*arrows*).

Radiological demonstration of the oesophageal atresia is performed by passing a soft rubber catheter as far as the site of obstruction and instilling 1–2 cc Lipiodol; in this way the blind outline of the upper pouch can be demonstrated (Fig. 32.10B). In older infants where partial atresia is present the infant may swallow Lipiodol or barium sulphate mixed with a feed in sufficient amount of demonstrate the outline of the area of the atresia.

In some instances only a tiny fistulous communication may be present between the anterior wall of the oesophagus and the trachea. These children may suffer from repeated attacks of pulmonary infection. The fistula may be shown only by cine radiography in the lateral projection, with the child prone.

Pouches and diverticula

Pouches or diverticula of the oesophagus may be classified according to their anatomical site.

Lateral pharyngeal diverticula. Lateral pharyngeal diverticula are vestigial remnants of the second branchial cleft, and as they have wide mouths and do not retain barium they are only readily seen during swallowing in the recumbent position. Less frequently they can be seen filled with air when the pharynx is distended by the Valsalva manoeuvre.

Pharyngeal diverticula. A pulsion diverticulum of the pharynx is a protrusion of the pharyngeal mucosa through the dehiscence between the oblique and transverse fibres of the inferior constrictor of the pharynx. Pharyngeal pouches usually manifest themselves in the elderly, presenting with local discomfort on swallowing and regurgitation of undigested food.

Disturbance of swallowing associated with the diverticulum frequently results in aspiration of contents into the lungs. This causes low grade infective changes usually affecting the right but frequently both bases. Cough may be the presenting symptom of an oesophageal pouch.

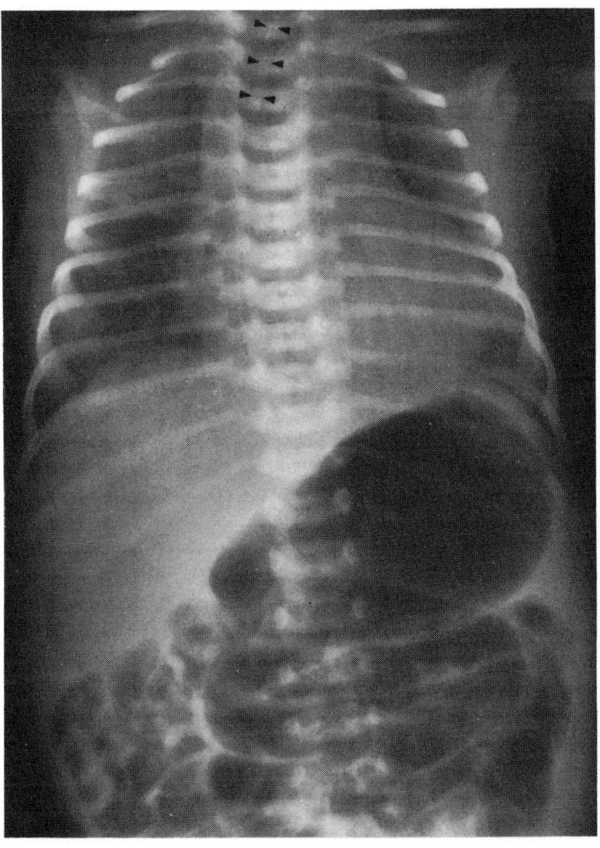

A

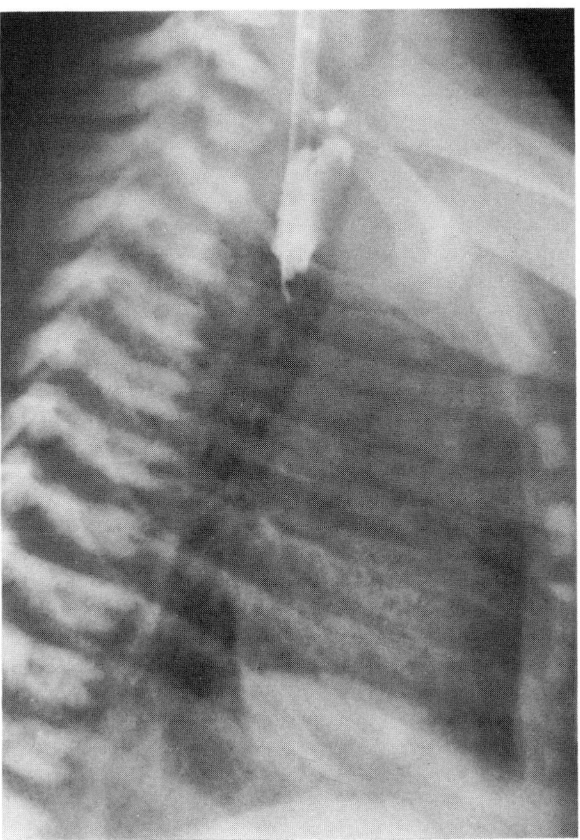

B

Fig. 32.10 A Atresia of the oesophagus. Plain film demonstrates gas in a distended stomach indicating that there is a communication between the lower portion of the oesophagus and the stomach. B Atresia of the oesophagus. Lateral view of the chest after installation of 1 ml of Lipiodol showing the blind upper end of the oesophagus filled with Lipiodol.

Plain films of the cervical region in the erect position may show a fluid level in the pouch (Fig. 32.11). Larger sized diverticula may extend into the superior mediastinum and present radiographically as a rounded dense shadow mimicking an upper mediastinal mass.

The barium swallow shows that the pouch projects posteriorly and usually to the left, displacing the oesophagus forward (Figs. 32.12 and 32.13). In consequence of the oesophageal displacement anteriorly the diverticulum comes to lie in the line of the swallowed foodstuff. The pharyngeal pouch tends to grow rapidly in size as the swallowed food first fills the pouch. Only when the pouch is full does it spill over fowards into the oesophagus.

Food remnants remaining in the oesophageal pouch produce filling defects when the pouch is filled with barium, which may suggest carcinomatous changes. The two conditions can be differentiated by the site and constancy of the filling defects. These tend to occur around the neck of the pouch when carcinomatous changes develop, whereas filling defects due to food remnants tend to occur in the fundus of the pouch and are inconstant.

Mid-portion diverticula. Diverticula in the mid-portion of the oesophagus are usually traction diverticula and are associated with tuberculous glands at the bifurcation of the trachea (Fig. 32.14). Some of these diverticula may, however, represent developmental defects associated with failure of complete closure of the last portion of the tracheo-oesophageal communication. Such diverticula are most easily demonstrated in the prone or supine barium swallow (Fig. 32.15) and in the erect position they may not be visible. Intramural diverticulosis is exceedingly rare; the diverticula do not pass completely through the wall of the oesophagus (Fig. 32.16). Multiple intramural diverticula may produce an irregular outline to the barium-filled oesophagus and mimic oesophageal moniliasis. The cause is not known but some cases are associated with lower oesophageal obstruction. They usually disappear spontaneously.

Epiphrenic diverticula. Diverticula at the lower end of the oesophagus occur far less frequently than diverticula in other parts of the oesophagus.

Aetiologically they are probably varieties of intestinal duplication. They have to be distinguished from a para-

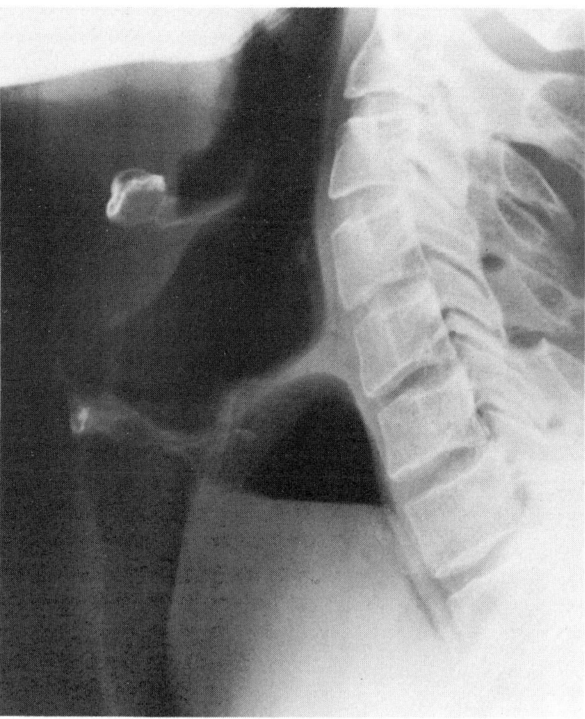

Fig. 32.11

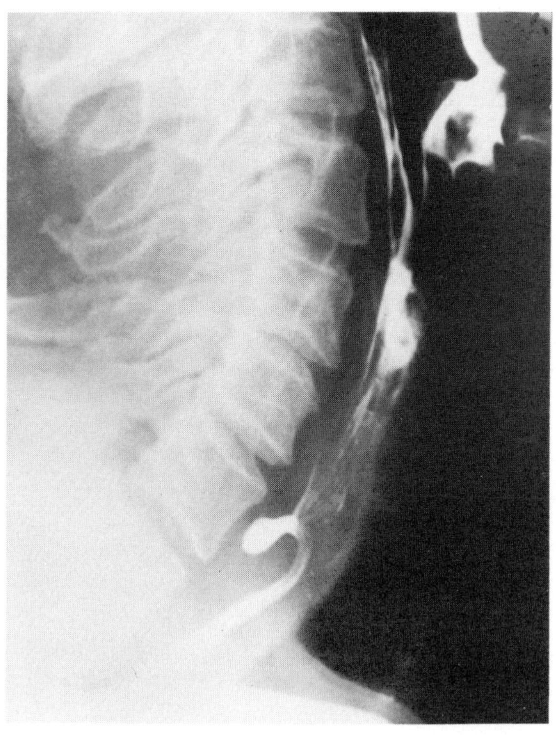

Fig. 32.12

Fig. 32.11 Lateral view of a large pharyngeal diverticulum demonstrating a fluid level and forward displacement of the air filled trachea.

Fig. 32.12 Pharyngeal diverticulum. Lateral view of the barium swallow showing a small pharyngeal diverticulum. Note that the oesophagus is displaced forwards.

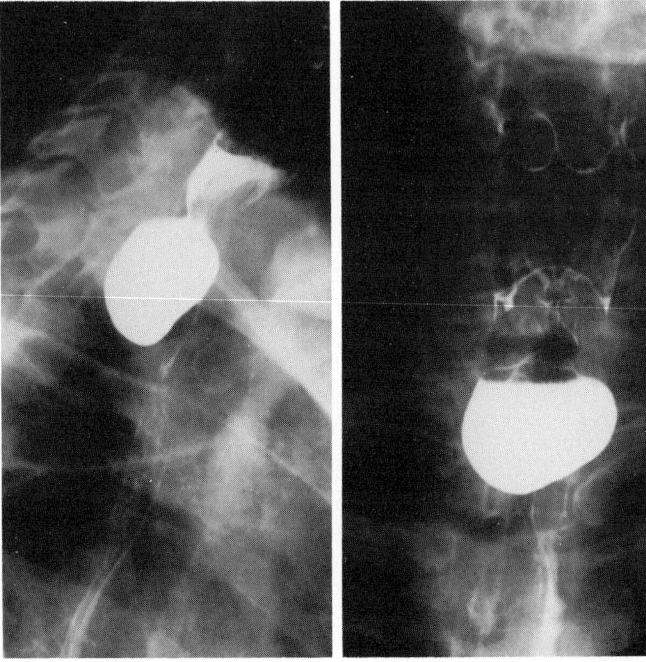

Fig. 32.13 Pharyngeal diverticulum. Oblique and antero-posterior views of the diverticulum.

oesophageal pouch of stomach herniated through the diaphragmatic oesophageal hiatus.

Epiphrenic diverticula are again best seen in the supine position and may not fill at all in the erect position. They usually attain a considerable size before they cause symptoms of dysphagia or dyspepsia (Fig. 32.17). They may be associated with altered motility of the oesophagus such as tertiary oesophageal contraction.

Cricopharyngeal impression. The cricopharyngeus muscle consists of oblique and transverse fibres with a relatively thin triangular area posteriorly between the confluence of the oblique and transverse fibres. Rarely the transverse portion of the cricopharyngeus muscle may become thickened and produce a smooth, rounded impression in the posterior wall of the barium filled oesophagus. Many authorities believe that hypertrophy of this segment of muscle is the initiating cause of pharyngeal pouch and certainly in cases with pharyngeal pouches the defect caused by the cricopharyngeus can be seen. Whether hypertrophy of the cricopharyngeus itself without a concomitant pharyngeal pouch is a cause of symptoms has not yet been established. Demonstration of the cricopharyngeal impression is best seen in cine radiographic or video-tape studies of the barium swallow (Fig. 32.18). Rarely, patients with laryngeal speech following laryngectomy may develop dysphagia due to gross hypertrophy of the cricopharyngeal muscle (Fig. 32.19).

Retropharyngeal abscess. Retropharyngeal abscess

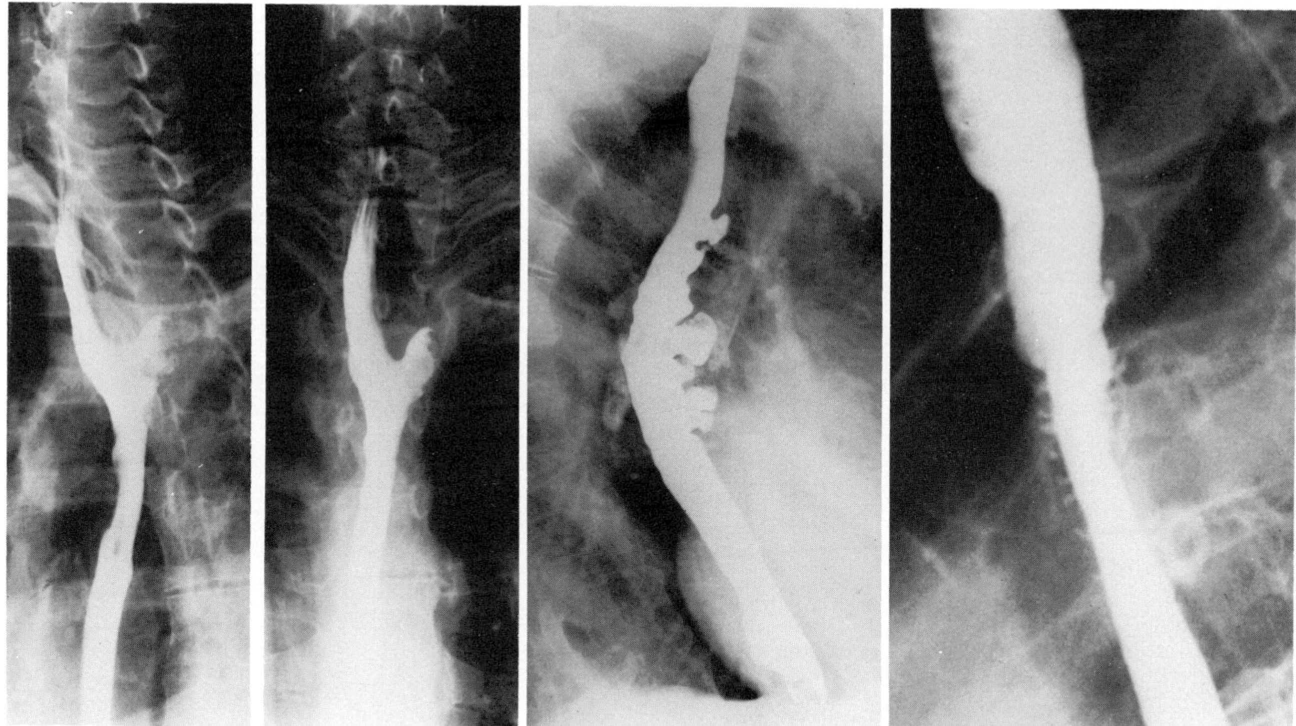

Fig. 32.14 *Fig. 32.15* *Fig. 32.16*

Fig. 32.14 Traction diverticulum of the oesophagus. The upward direction of the diverticulum with the irregularity of its base indicate the aetiology.

Fig. 32.15 Multiple diverticula arising from the anterior wall of the oesophagus. Diverticula in these sites are usually considered to be the sequel of traction, but from the shape of the diverticulum many are more likely to be congenital in origin.

Fig. 32.16 Intramural diverticulosis of the oesophagus. A middle-aged woman with dysphagia localized to the upper oesophagus. A repeat examination after a month showed the oesophagus to be normal.

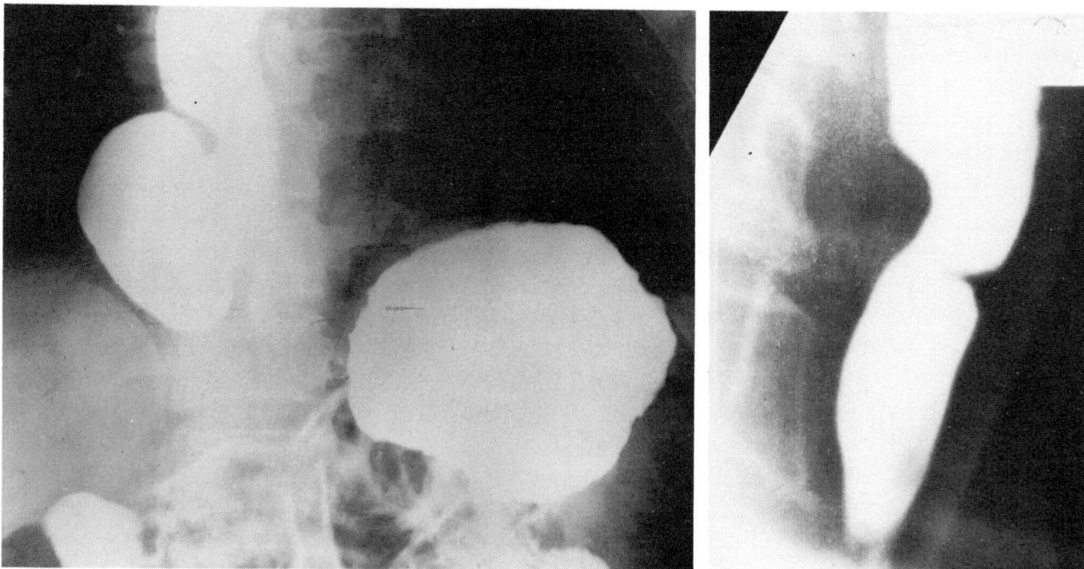

Fig. 32.17 *Fig. 32.18*

Fig. 32.17 Epiphrenic diverticulum—the large smooth diverticulum arising from the right side of the lower oesophagus may be mistaken for a hiatus hernia unless careful fluoroscopy is undertaken.

Fig. 32.18 Cricopharyngeal impression. Lateral view of the oesophagus showing the smooth rounded defect in the posterior wall of the oesophagus caused by the horizontal portion of the cricopharyngeus muscle. The linear defect in the anterior wall of the oesophagus is caused by an oesophageal web.

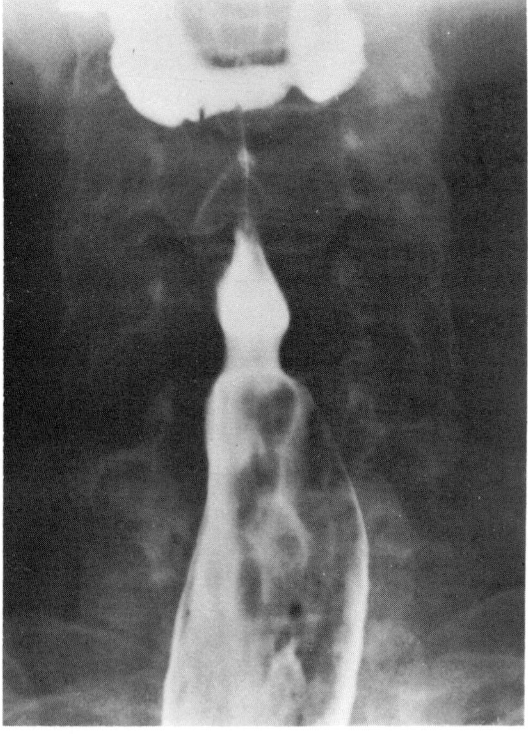

A

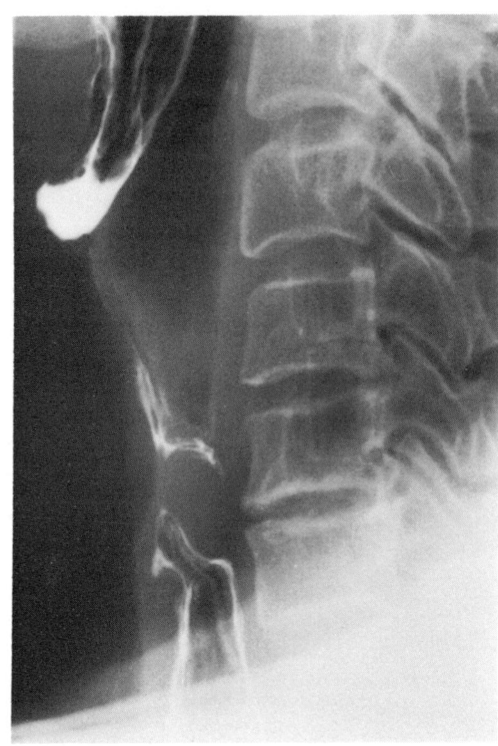

B

Fig. 32.19 A Anterior and B lateral view of a barium swallow in a patient with dysphagia following laryngectomy. There is a grossly hypertrophied cricopharyngeus muscle indenting the oesophagus posteriorly. This hypertrophy followed several years of oesophageal speech.

is usually a sequel of spread of infection to the retropharyngeal space either from a tonsillar infection, less frequently from the pharynx itself as a result of perforation, and even more infrequently as a consequence of forward spread of infection from a vertebral body. The last type of infection is usually tuberculous or staphylococcal. Perforation of the pharynx or oesophagus may follow a swallowed foreign body or after instrumentation.

Radiologically the features are widening of the retropharyngeal soft tissues with forward displacement of the oesophagus and air filled trachea (Fig. 32.20). Gas may be seen in the abscess.

Sideropenic web (cricopharyngeal web); Paterson-Brown-Kelly syndrome; Plummer-Vinson syndrome. An iron deficiency anaemia occuring in middle-aged females is frequently associated with dysphagia and radiologically demonstrable web formation in the post-cricoid region. These webs, however, may occur without associated anaemia, although a degree of iron deficiency may be present.

The sinister significance of the web formation is that it sometimes precedes the development of a post-cricoid carcinoma. Recognition of the web formation by endoscopic examination is difficult and histological reports on the nature of the web are indefinite.

Web formation is best demonstrated with the patient in the lateral position. The webs appear as thin filling defects arising from the anterior wall of the cervical oesophagus immediately below the cricopharyngeus. They are seen only when the oesophagus is distended

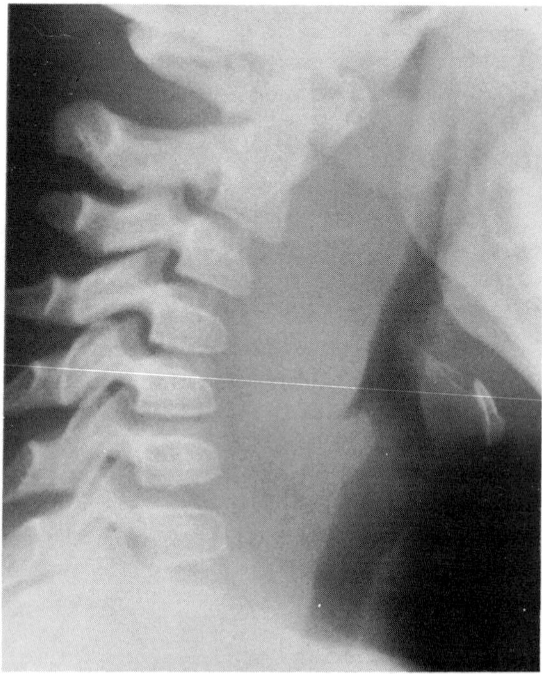

Fig. 32.20 Retropharyngeal abscess. Lateral view of the neck showing forward displacement of the trachea by an abscess which followed tonsillitis.

with barium and, since no hold up of the barium is noted, are best shown by rapid cine or video-tape examination (Figs. 32.18 and 32.21).

Enterogenous cysts. Failure to produce complete vacuolation of the primitive gut results in the development of enterogenous cysts. These present as smooth, round or oval homogenous shadows in the upper or the posterior mediastinum and may distort the oesophagus by pressure. There are no specific radiological features, but the intimate relation to the oesophagus usually suggests the diagnosis. They do not normally communicate with the oesophagus.

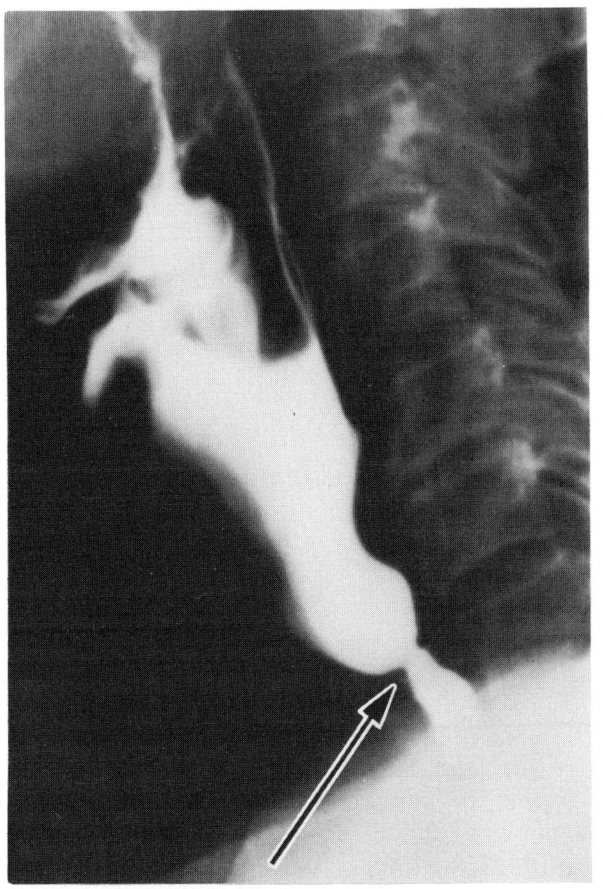

Fig. 32.21 A sideropenic post-cricoid web in an anaemic man 5 years after a Polya gastrectomy.

Corrosive poisoning. Ingestion of corrosive poisons may occur accidentally in children or be associated with suicidal attempts in adults. Caustic soda solution is a common household commodity and is the poison accidentally ingested most frequently. Alkaline poisons tend to produce burns at the sites of temporary hold-up in the oesophagus; at the crossing of the left main bronchus (Fig. 32.22) or more frequently at its lower end (Fig. 32.23).

During the acute phase immediately after the ingestion of the alkali the radiological features are those of spasm of the oesophagus with loss of the mucosal pattern. Narrowing of the oesophagus at these levels is usually associated with spasm and oedematous swelling of the mucosal wall.

The onset of stricture formation at the site of corrosion usually depends on the severity of the burn. In some instances a period of months or years may elapse before the progressive narrowing of the oesophagus produces symptoms of dysphagia; in others these symptoms may appear immediately after the acute stage.

Radiologically the features of a caustic stricture are (Fig. 32.23):

1. The stricture is usually long, often several inches in length.
2. The upper end of the stricture is funnel-shaped and its upper limits gradually taper off into normal oesophagus.
3. The mucosal pattern within the strictured area is lost and the outline of the stricture is smooth.

Acid poisons are not a common cause of oesophageal strictures, but if a stricture develops as a sequel of ingestion of acid poison, it may be indistinguishable from that produced by alkaline poisons.

Caustic strictures of the oesophagus have to be differentiated from (1) strictures associated with peptic (reflux) oesophagitis; such strictures, although also funnelled in outline, generally show a more irregular mucosal outline and are usually associated with a hiatus hernia and oesophageal reflux; (2) traumatic oesophageal stricture, which may follow an in-dwelling gastric tube or other trauma; such strictures may be elongated and show a smooth mucosa, making differentiation difficult; and (3) malignant strictures which are usually much shorter in length and associated with mucosal destruction, although in the squamous type carcinoma the stricture outline may be relatively smooth.

Oesophageal varices. Obstruction to the venous return from the portal system opens up venous anastomotic channels along the lower end of the oesophagus via the left gastric and oesophageal veins. Some of these collateral vessels may be submucosal varices which may bleed, while others may lie in the deeper layer of the oesophagus and do not distort the oesophageal mucosa or bleed. Varicosities have also been demonstrated at the upper end of the oesophagus associated with superior vena caval obstruction.

Oesophageal varices can be demonstrated by careful barium swallow examination in the vast majority of cases. They are best demonstrated on mucosal pattern films of a relaxed oesophagus (Fig. 32.24). Whereas one film may be sufficient to demonstrate gross varices, at least six films of the relaxed oesophagus should be taken in an effort to exclude them. The patient should

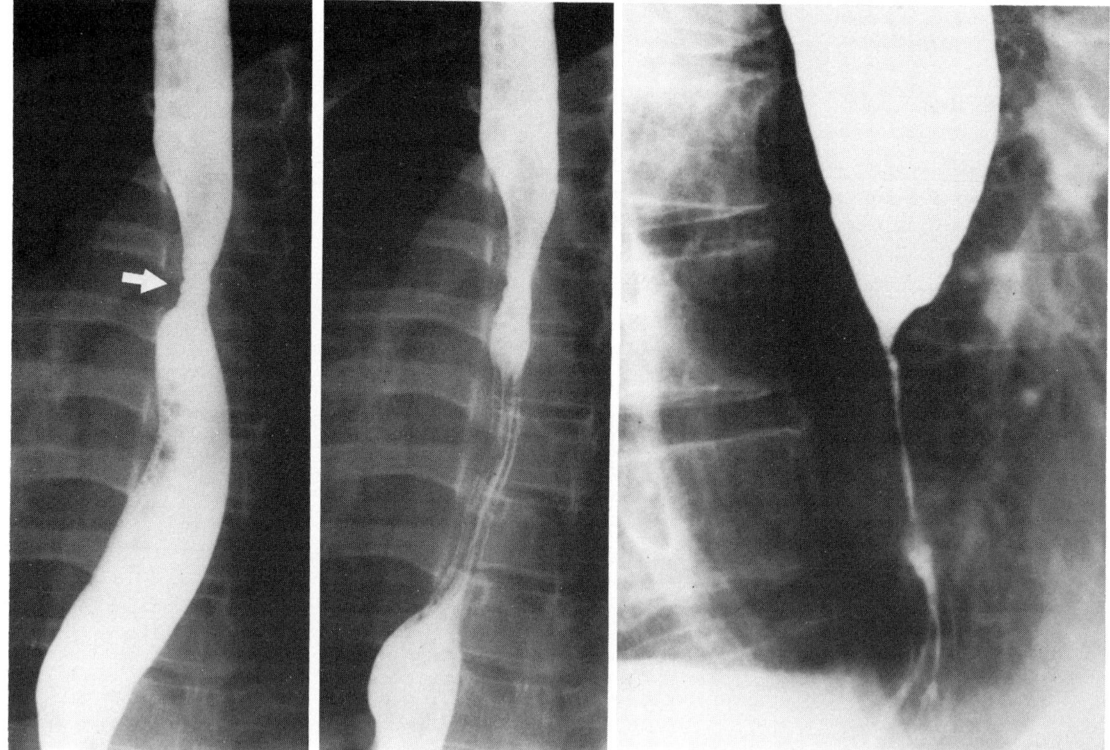

Fig. 32.22A Fig. 32.22B Fig. 32.33

Fig. 32.22 Corrosive stricture in the middle third of the oesophagus at the level of the carina in a diabetic patient who accidentally swallowed a Clinitest tablet.

Fig. 32.23 Corrosive stricture of the oesophagus following ingestion of caustic soda. Oesophagitis has developed which has produced fibrosis with subsequent shortening of the oesophagus. There is gross dilatation of the oesophagus above the stricture.

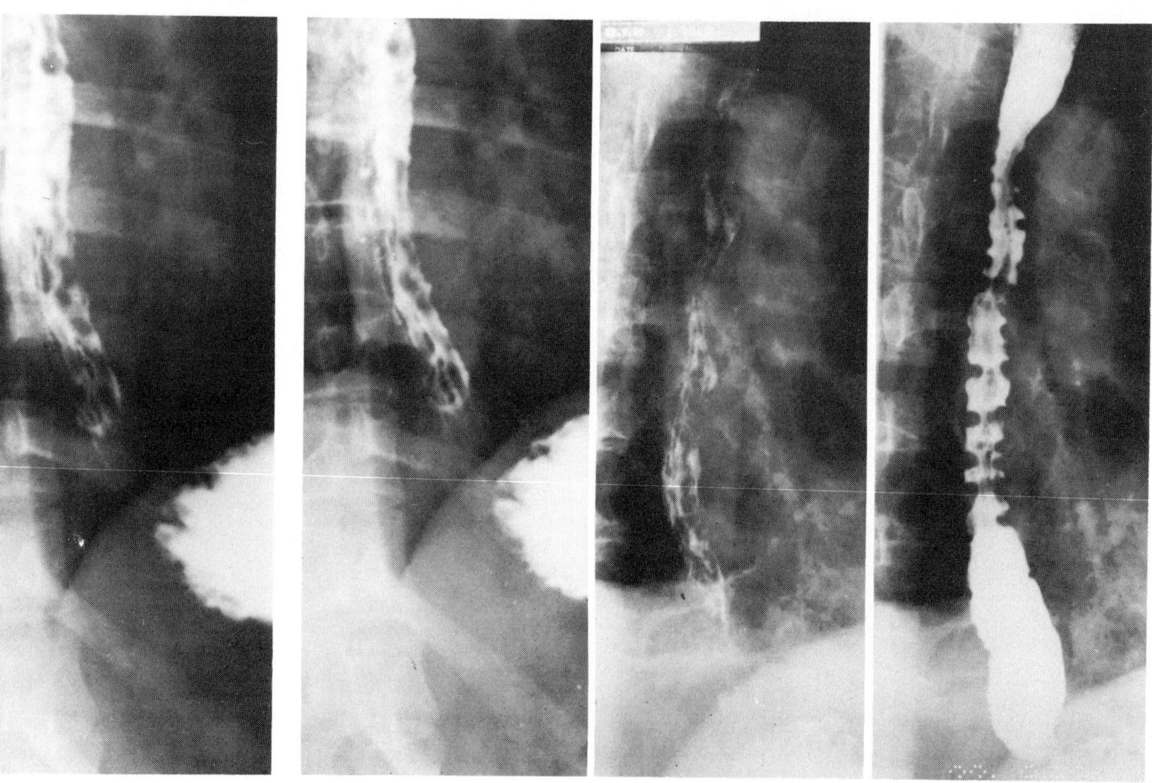

Fig. 32.24A Fig. 32.24B Fig. 32.25A Fig. 32.25B

Fig. 32.24 Oesophageal varices. Barium swallow showing the tortuous appearance of the lower oesophageal folds associated with oesophageal varices. The alteration of the appearances with inspiration A and expiration B is characteristic of oesophageal varices.

Fig. 32.25 Oesophageal varices. A Well seen when the oesophagus is coated with barium and relaxed. B Obscured by 'tertiary contractions' and too much barium.

be examined in the erect and supine positions. Small varices are easily obscured when the oesophagus is filled with barium or in the contracted state (Fig. 32.25). Hyoscine-N-butylbromide (Buscopan) 20 mg i.v. or i.m. may enhance the demonstration in borderline cases by causing complete relaxation of the oesophagus. Normally three or four continuous folds are seen. Small varices interrupt these folds and larger ones give rise to a serpiginous outline. When large varices are present the oesophagus is usually dilated.

The extent to which the varices spread up the oesophagus varies but they seldom extend above the level of the azygos vein. Oesophageal varices as well as para-oesophageal veins in the deeper layers may be demonstrated by portal venography, but even this method does not invariably fill the varices, and in rare instances the varices may be shown by the barium examination and yet not be visualized on splenoportography. Prone instead of supine splenoportography may show such varices.

Equally well, it must be remembered that oesophagoscopy itself is not infallible in the detection of varices, although the end-viewing fibre-optic endoscopes together with the use of muscle relaxants are making this method more reliable and less disturbing for the patient.

When examining patients with cirrhosis of the liver, portal hypertension and varices, a careful examination should be made for peptic ulceration, since about 30 per cent of patients with cirrhosis who have a haematemesis or melaena bleed from some cause other than varices, usually a peptic ulcer or a gastric erosion.

Moniliasis. Infection of the oesophagus with yeast fungus (monilia) frequently occurs as a complication in debilitated states or after antibiotic or immunosuppressive therapy. The infection may be the terminal event in the debilitated subjects.

The radiological appearances of moniliasis are those of irregularity of outline of the barium filled oesophagus giving rise to a shaggy outline of the oesophagus. The lesion is diffuse and the whole of the oesophagus is involved.

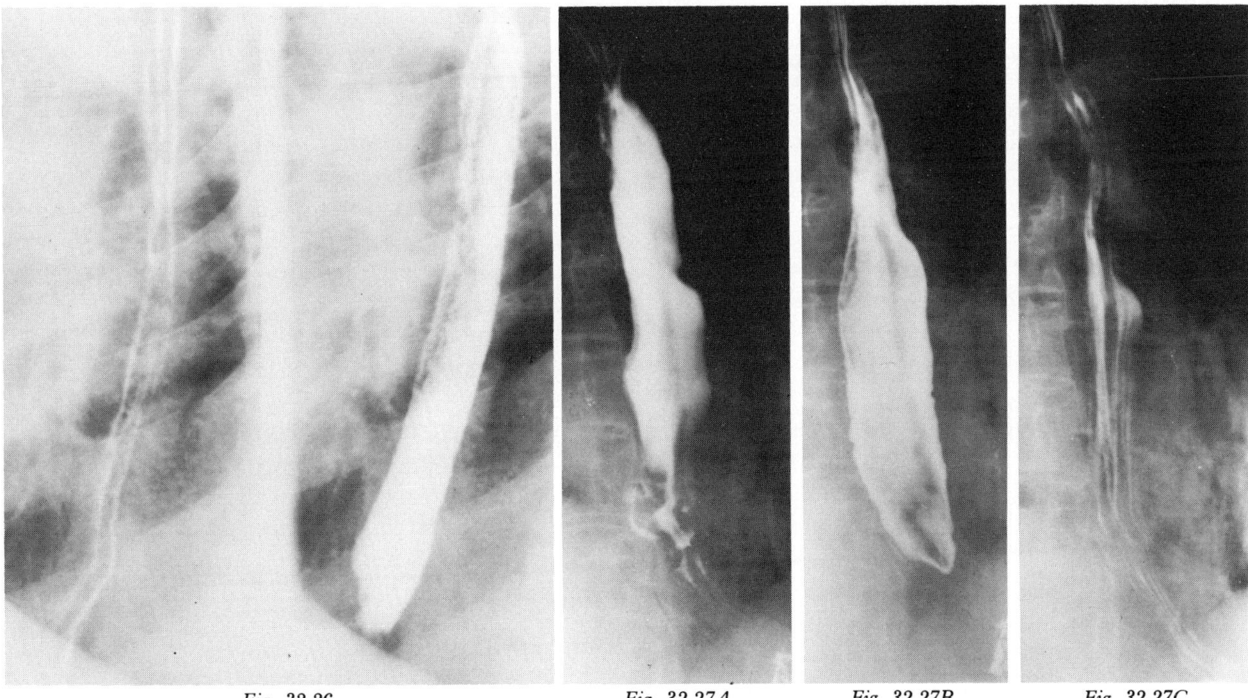

Fig. 32.26 *Fig. 32.27A* *Fig. 32.27B* *Fig. 32.27C*

Fig. 32.26 Moniliasis of the oesophagus. There is a fine irregularity throughout the length of the oesophagus due partly to fine ulceration and to the presence of colonies of monilia.

Fig. 32.27 Scleroderma of the oesophagus. Three views of the oesophagus showing a moderately dilated oesophagus with no peristalsis and no stripping wave.

Moniliasis has to be differentiated from chemical poisoning, which in the early stages after the ingestion of poison may give rise to a ragged mucosal outline due to ulceration of the mucosa (Fig. 32.26). Intramucosal diverticulosis of the oesophagus has also to be differentiated as it causes an irregularity of the oesophageal outline suggesting a ragged mucosa. It is, however, excessively rare (Fig. 32.16).

Scleroderma. The oesophagus is certainly the most easily recognized and probably the most common part of the gut to be involved in scleroderma (diffuse sclerosis). In the early stages of the condition no abnormality may be seen if the patient is examined in the upright position. Barium passes down the oesophagus and into the stomach under the influence of gravity. Even at this stage, however, the oesophagus may not contract normally, there may be no stripping wave and there may be air in the oesophagus even at rest. When the patient is examined in the horizontal position, however, the oesophagus will show diminished and ineffective peristalsis, most of the barium remaining within the oesophagus until the patient is brought upright again. There is commonly air visible in the oesophagus at all times.

At a later stage the oesophagus dilates further and becomes aperistaltic (Fig. 32.27). The cardia may become wide, open and allow free reflux, a form of secondary chalasia. Strictures may occur within the oesophagus, probably as a result of gastro-oesophageal reflux, and dysphagia may become extreme. The slow emptying of the oesophagus and the gastro-oesophageal reflux may give rise to aspiration of fluid into the lung and contribute to the pulmonary fibrosis seen in some patients with diffuse sclerosis. The association of calcinosis circumscripta, Raynaud's phenomenon, scleroderma involving the oesophagus and telangectasia is sometimes referred to as the C.R.S.T. syndrome.

TUMOURS

Benign tumours of the oesophagus.

Benign tumours of the oesophagus are of two main types, epithelial tumours arising from the mucosa and non-epithelial tumours arising from the wall. Tumours of mucosal origin, usually papillomas or adenomas, tend to be smooth and intraluminal and may be either pedunculated or sessile (Fig. 32.28). Tumours of non-epithelial origin, usually leiomyomas, fibromas or lipomas, arise in the wall and may grow either inwards or outwards. Although both types of benign tumours may produce symptoms of dysphagia, they are frequently found by chance—on barium swallow in the case of the intraluminal tumours and on a plain chest film in the case of extraluminal tumours.

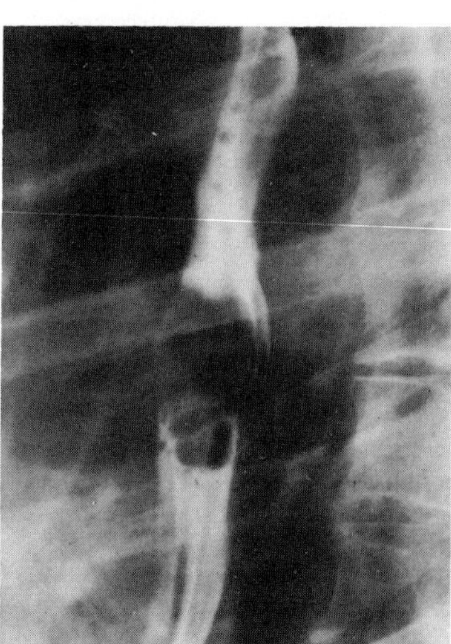

Fig. 32.28 Benign adenoma of the oesophagus. There is a smooth polypoid filling defect in the middle third of the oesophagus with normal adjacent mucosal folds.

Polypoid intraluminal mucosal tumours cause a smooth, round filling defect in the oesophagus which may be distended around the tumour. Peristalsis is unaffected by the tumour and the overlying mucosa is smooth. Such tumours may prolapse into the stomach. Large tumours may show ulceration of the free pole. The differential diagnosis is from a foreign body impacted above a stricture, an air bubble or solitary oesophageal or gastric varix. Air bubbles are inconstant and varices change in size with the state of contraction and relaxation of the oesophagus.

Although some tumours of submucosal origin may grow into the lumen and give an appearance similar to mucosal tumours, they more frequently grow outwards and give rise to a smooth indentation similar to that caused by extrinsic pressure. The wall may be rigid so that the primary peristaltic wave stops at the level of the tumour. The mucosal folds may be smoothed out over the tumour. The extraluminal extent of the tumour can sometimes be seen outlined by air in the lungs. When a benign tumour is irregular and ulcerated, it may be impossible to differentiate it from a malignant tumour.

Carcinoma of the oesophagus

Carcinoma of the oesophagus occurs more commonly in men than in women. The tumour, which starts in the mucosa, spreads both around and along the length of the oesophagus. Spread of the tumour into the remaining lymphatic lymph nodes may accentuate the deformity of the oesophagus.

The main symptoms are dysphagia, pain and loss of weight. Since patients with dysphagia do not locate the true site of the obstruction accurately (they commonly feel it to be at too high a level), they should be prepared as for a barium meal examination and have the stomach examined if no lesion is found in the oesophagus. Cine or video-tape may be of value in detecting small lesions. If there is doubt about the possibility of malignancy after a full radiological examination, immediate endoscopy is indicated rather than repeating the examination after an interval (Fig. 32.31).

Radiological investigation. In the plain lateral films of the neck a widened post-cricoid space due to soft-tissue tumour is seen in post-cricoid carcinoma (Fig. 32.29). Estimation of what constitutes an increase in the width of the post-cricoid space may be difficult, but in 6-foot films if the width exceeds the width of the adjacent cervical vertebral body, it may be regarded as abnormal.

Carcinoma of the oesophagus may be of three main

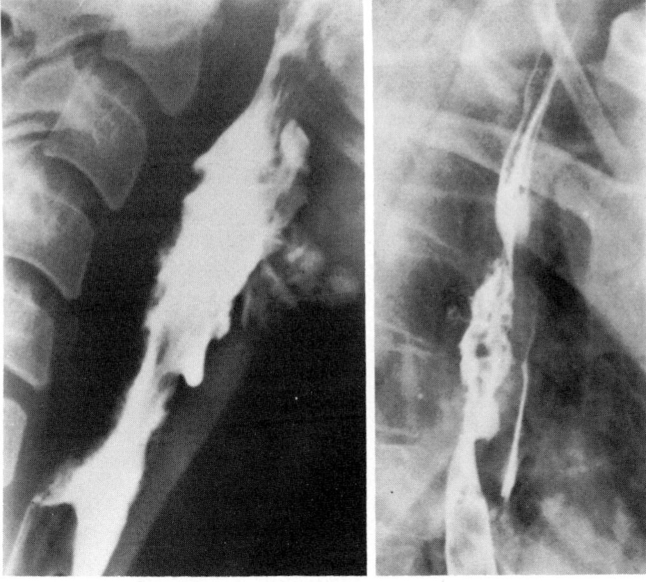

Fig. 32.29 *Fig. 32.30*

Fig. 32.29 Post-cricoid carcinoma of the oesophagus. There is irregularity of the posterior wall of the oesophagus with increase in the amount of soft tissue between the cervical spine and the posterior wall of the oesophagus.

Fig. 32.30 Carcinoma of the middle third of the oesophagus. There is extensive mucosal destruction with very little dilatation of the oesophagus above the quite extensive carcinoma. Some barium has been aspirated into the trachea.

types—fungating, ulcerative or stenotic. The fungating papillary tumour forms an irregular mass with a rolled edge which projects into the lumen of the oesophagus and destroys the mucosa at first on one wall but later the whole circumference of the oesophagus is involved (Figs. 32.32 and 32.33). The mass may become quite large before causing dysphagia (Fig. 32.29). Barium examination shows an abrupt change between normal and abnormal parts of the oesophagus with irregular polypoid masses projecting into the lumen through which the barium permeates. There may be little dilation above the lesion (Fig. 32.30) since onstruction may not occur until the mass is quite large.

The ulcerative type, which is less common, appears as a marginal mass jutting into the lumen of the oesophagus, with a central ulcer crater. Since the opposite wall may be normal, the lesion is best demonstrated in profile and may be easily missed unless the oesophagus is examined in both oblique projections. An ulcer niche may be seen projecting either into or beyond the general outline of the oesophagus. The oesophagus above and below is rigid and peristalsis does not pass through. The degree of rigidity is best demonstrated when the oesophagus is fully distended.

The stenotic or infiltrative type of carcinoma forms a short rigid structure often with a tapering transition to the normal oesophagus above and below. The overlying

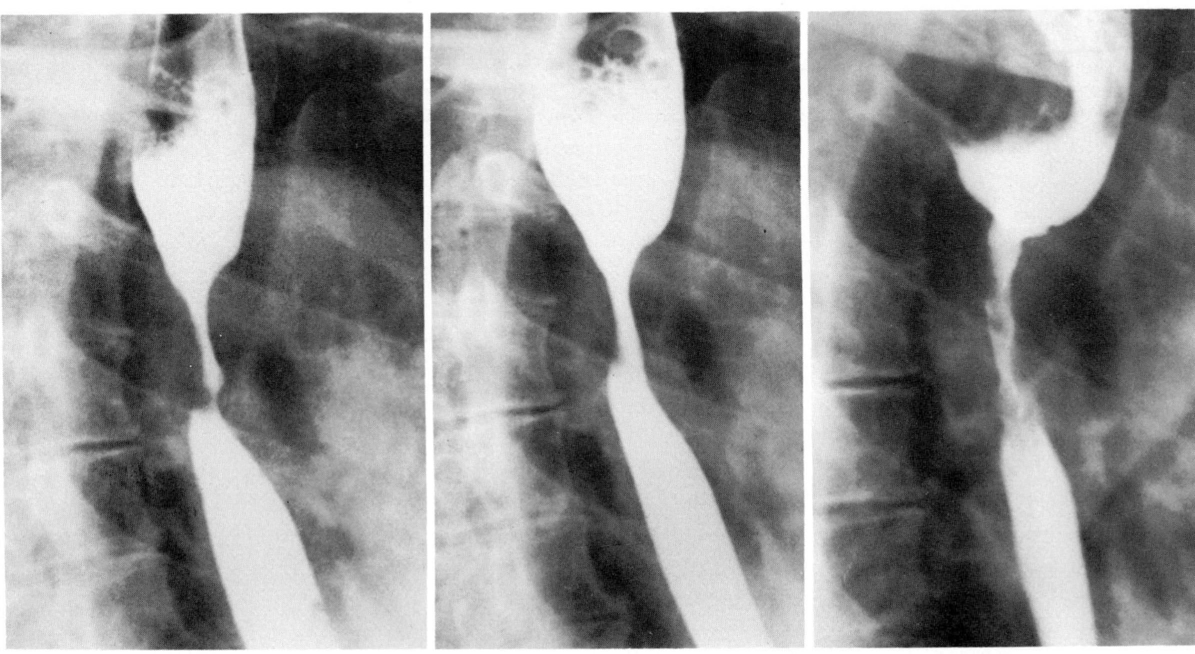

Fig. 32.31A *Fig. 32.31B*

Fig. 32.31 A Stricture in the middle third of the oesophagus with smooth tapering margins and proximal dilitation. Oesophagoscopy and biopsy at this stage showed no evidence of malignancy. B Same patient 2 months later showing extensive mucosal destruction and considerable proximal dilatation. An obvious carcinoma of the middle third of the oesophagus.

mucosa may be smooth and intact (Fig. 32.31A). The appearances may be indistinguishable from a benign stricture secondary to reflux oesophagitis. It is not uncommon for a small infiltrating carcinoma of the lower end of the oesophagus to be associated with a small hiatus hernia and gastro-oesophageal reflux, possibly because the rigidity of the oesophagus adjacent to the cardia interferes with the anti-reflux mechanism. This association of carcinoma and hiatus hernia makes the differential diagnosis difficult. Not uncommonly endoscopy and biopsy are negative also at an early stage of this disease. Since the progression of infiltrating carcinoma is slow, in cases of doubt repeated endoscopy and repeated biopsy may be necessary to establish a diagnosis (Fig. 32.31).

Carcinoma at different sites in the oesophagus have their own special features. Post-cricoid carcinoma occur more commonly in women than in men and may occasionally be associated with the Plummer-Vinson syndrome. Symptoms occur early in this disease and a mass may be visible on the soft tissue lateral film of the neck. Aspiration of fluid including barium, may occur into the lungs.

Carcinoma of the middle third of the oesophagus, particularly when at the level of bifurcation of the trachea, may involve the trachea and bronchi by direct extension. A tracheo-bronchial fistula may occur with passage of barium into the bronchial tree. Some dilatation of the oesophagus above the level of the tumour, almost invariably present, may be associated with some degree of tracheo-bronchial spill of barium.

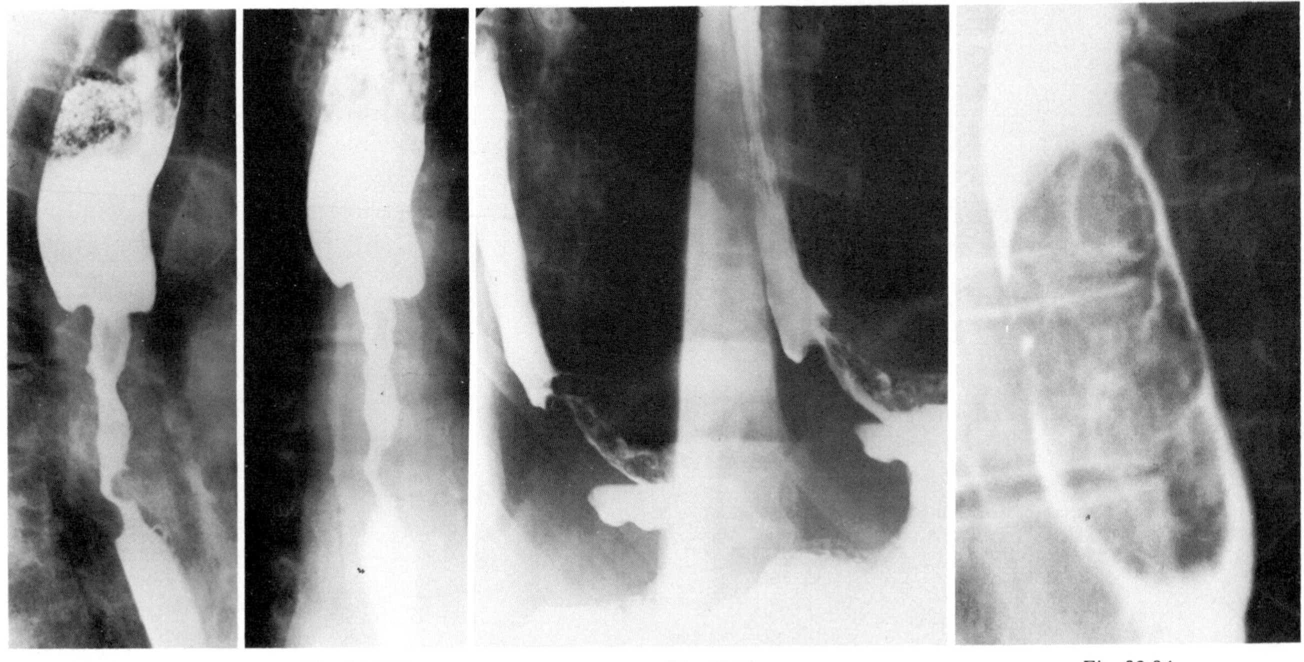

Fig. 32.32A *Fig. 32.32B* *Fig. 32.33* *Fig. 32.34*

Fig. 32.32 A and B Carcinoma of the middle third of the oesophagus. The barium swallow shows extensive mucosal destruction, narrowing of the lumen and shouldering at each end of the tumour.

Fig. 32.33 Carcinoma of the lower end of the oesophagus. The tumour has spread into the fundus of the stomach and there is a typical shoulder at the other end of the growth.

Fig. 32.34 Carcinosarcoma of the oesophagus. There is a large irregular intraluminal polypoid defect in the middle third of the oesophagus, attached over a small area to the right posterior margin of the oesophagus.

Squamous cell carcinoma occurring at the lower end of the oesophagus may give rise to dilatation of the oesophagus with very little disruption of the mucosal pattern. Differentiation of this kind of tumour from achalasia of the cardia may be very difficult and biopsy is essential.

Sarcomatous tumours of the oesophagus are usually leiomyosarcoma. They are usually very cellular and polypoid tumours some producing rounded filling defects with regular outlines resembling benign tumours (Fig. 32.34).

In summary, a carcinoma of the oesophagus may show one or more of the following features:

(*a*) An irregular filling defect in the barium filled oesophagus. The growth may occupy only one side of the oesophageal wall but usually the growth circumvents the whole oesophageal lumen.

(*b*) The edges of the filling defect are usually sharp and clear cut. This re-entrant angle corresponds to the rolled edge of an epithelioma on the skin (Figs. 32.32 and 32.33).

(*c*) In the oblique position, when the oesophagus is

thrown clear of the cardiac shadow, the outline of the soft tissue shadow of the growth may be visible contrasting with air in the adjacent lung.

(*d*) Whilst the encircling character of the oesophageal growth is most readily appreciated, the spread of the tumour along the long axis of the oesophagus should not be overlooked. The tumour is usually more extensive than is apparent on the films.

(*e*) Ulceration of the oesophagus into the mediastinum may be seen as a deep ulcer crater with an irregular base and outlines. In later stages fixation to the trachea may lead to the development of a tracheo-bronchial fistula with the passage of barium into the bronchial tree.

(*f*) A degree of dilatation of the oesophagus above the level of the growth is almost invariably present and may be associated with some degree of tracheo-bronchial spill of barium.

(*g*) Squamous cell growths occurring at the lower end of the oesophagus may be associated with considerable dilatation of the oesophagus and if there is no ulceration, differentiation from achalasia of the cardia may be impossible.

(*h*) Adenocarcinoma at the lower end of the oesophagus may be of gastric origin and occur in association with a hiatus hernia.

Differential diagnosis

1. Ulcerative forms of carcinoma of the oesophagus have to be differentiated from peptic ulcer of the oesophagus occuring in columnar epithelium. This might be at the oesophago-gastric junction when it is commonly in association with a hiatus hernia and peptic stricture or in heterotopic gastric tissue (Barrett's ulcer). These ulcers tend to be small, very well defined and are not associated with a soft tissue mass or much surrounding irregularity.

2. Submucosal carcinoma and tumours giving rise to stricture formation without significant ulceration have to be differentiated from the strictures in squamous epithelium associated with hiatus hernia and reflux. The presence of a hiatus hernia and the absence of any soft tissue mass help to distinguish the two conditions, but it should be remembered that carcinoma arising around the cardia may predispose to reflux and give rise to hiatus hernia with stricture formation.

3. Malignant lesions in the mediastinum either bronchial carcinoma or malignant lymph nodes around the carina may secondarily involve the oesophagus, giving rise to obstruction and ulceration of the oesophagus. Such lesions will commonly give rise to localized displacement of the oesophagus and the soft tissue mass is usually clearly visible on the plain film.

4. Benign tumours of the oesophagus are usually smooth and polypoid and only the larger tumours ulcerate on their free pole.

FUNCTIONAL DISTURBANCES OF THE OESOPHAGUS

The physiological processes involved in the passage of a bolus of food or barium along the oesophagus are complex. A wave of relaxation affecting the oesophageal wall precedes a contractile wave which propels the bolus along the oesophagus. To what degree changes in the intrathoracic pressure initiate the first wave of relaxation is not understood. Alterations in the normal contraction waves in the oesophagus may cause considerable functional disturbances.

Tertiary contractions. These non-propulsive uncoordinated contractions of circular muscle of the oesophagus are seen not uncommonly in the elderly, in early achalasia and sometimes in association with hiatus hernia and gastro-oesophageal reflux. They cause the outline of the oesophagus to be indented on each side equally by a series of ring contractions, which may last a few seconds (Fig. 32.25) before relaxation occurs, to be followed by contraction at other sites. They may be transitory and may be precipitated by swallowing. The patient has no symptoms referable to this radiological appearance.

Corkscrew oesophagus. This motility disorder is similar to tertiary contractions but may occur at any stage and is often associated with retrosternal discomfort or pain during swallowing. The contracted segments are usually in the retro-cardiac oesophagus, sparing the upper third and extreme lower end. The contractions may be extremely severe and obliterate the lumen. Smooth pouches or pseudo-diverticula appear between the contracted areas (Fig. 32.35A). These irregular pouches, usually between three and five, may completely disappear between spasms, but more commonly the oesophagus remains dilated and the bulges persist forming wide-necked pulsion diverticula. Commonly the oesophagus does not empty completely and there is no effective stripping wave. There may be an associated hiatus hernia with gastro-oesophageal reflux (Fig. 32.35B).

Achalasia of the oesophagus (cardiospasm). Achalasia of the cardia is due to a defect in the myenteric plexus as a consequence of which the cardio-oesophageal sphincter fails to relax when the contractile wave arrives. The oesophagus retains much of its content and becomes progressively dilated.

The radiological appearances vary according to the severity of the condition. In the early stage the oesophagus may be only slightly but uniformly dilated throughout its length. Peristalsis is weak or absent and ineffectual tertiary contractions are seen. The patient can sustain a large collection of barium in the oesophagus before a critical pressure is arrived at, when barium may enter the stomach in small spurts. The patient may have learnt to swallow air to raise oesophageal pressure in order to hasten this process. The lower end of the oesophagus tapers smoothly to a beak-like narrowing (Fig. 32.36A). There is little or no air in the stomach since fluid in the oesophagus forms a waterseal and prevents air getting in when the patient is in the erect position. At the early stage the diagnosis may be difficult and at times the appearances may be indistinguishable from those seen in early submucosal carcinoma or in extrinsic pressure from enlarged peri-oesophageal lymph nodes secondary to carcinoma of the pancreas or other abdominal malignancy. Moreover, the restricted flow of barium into the stomach makes a thorough examination of the fundus of the stomach and the exclusion of a small gastric carcinoma difficult.

In cases of uncertainty the acetyl-beta-methylcholine ('Mecholim') test may be helpful. Five to 10 mg of the drug is injected subcutaneously with the patient lying down to avoid sudden fainting. In patients with achalasia the middle third of the oesophagus undergoes a strong contraction and the patient experiences retrosternal pain.

Endoscopy and biopsy are essential if there is any doubt about the diagnosis of early achalasia. As the oesophagus dilates further it becomes elongated and redundant at its lower end (Fig. 32.36B). At this stage the absence of air from the gastric fundus and the smooth beak-like lower end of the barium-filled oesophagus associated with the dilated oesophagus readily allows the diagnosis to be made. Later fibrotic changes occur in the lower end with the formation of a true fibrous stricture.

In the postero-anterior chest films the dilated oesophagus shows a characteristic linear shadow extending along the right side of the mediastinum and blending with the heart shadow (Fig. 32.37). In the superior mediastinum a mottled appearance may be seen due to the mixture of air and retained food in the dilated oesophagus. Less frequently a fluid level due to the separation of fluid and air contents in the dilated oesophagus may give a ready explanation for the enlarged mediastinal shadow. Spillage of the oesophageal contents into the lungs gives rise to a pneumonitis and basal fibrosis, whilst liquid paraffin misguidedly taken or administered may give rise to a lipoid pneumonia or a paraffinoma of the lungs.

Although dilatation of the lower end of the oesophagus by mercury bougie may give symptomatic relief, it seldom makes any material difference to the radiological appearances. Likewise after surgical treatment by

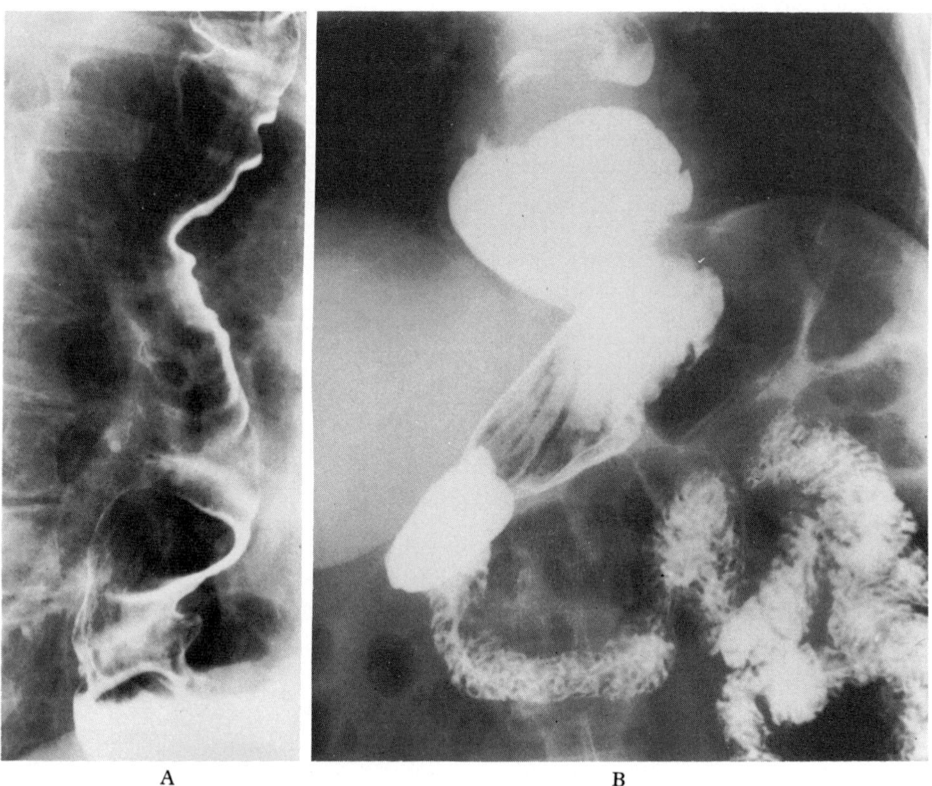

Fig. 32.35 Corkscrew oesophagus with diaphragmatic hernia. A There is gross dilatation and sacculation of the oesophagus with completely irregular and non-propulsive peristalsis. B There is a large diaphragmatic hernia with gastro-oesophageal reflux.

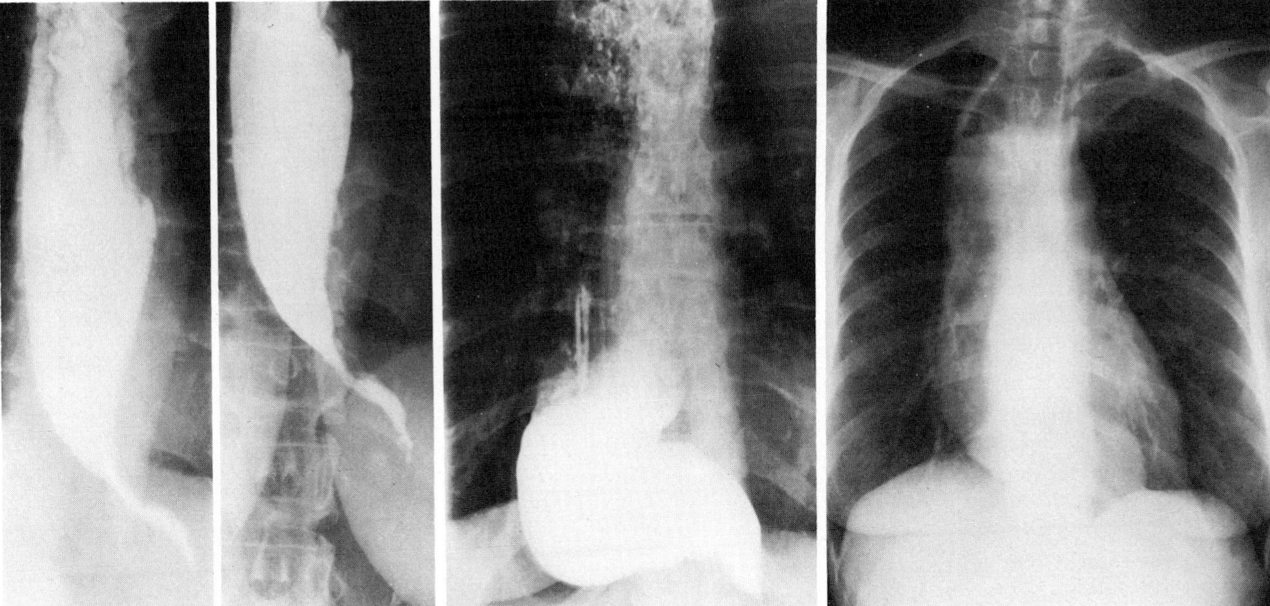

Fig. 32.36A *Fig. 32.36B* *Fig. 32.37*

Fig. 32.36 A and B Achalasia of the cardia showing a smooth cigar-shaped lower end of the oesophagus. The absence of gas in the fundus of the stomach is a diagnostic feature.

Fig. 32.37 Chest film in achalasia of the oesophagus showing widening of the mediastinum associated with the dilated oesophagus. There is a fluid level in the oesophagus in the upper mediastinum.

Heller's operation the dilated oesophagus may remain unchanged in appearance despite clinical improvement. The emptying of the barium from the oesophagus into the stomach is, however, much improved.

Carcinoma of the oesophagus, not necessarily at the lower end, is a complication of achalasia. The constant filling defect of the tumour must be distinguished from the inconstant filling defects of retained food debris. Rarely inspissated food may become adherent to the wall of the oesophagus giving a bizarre appearance and closely simulating malignancy.

CHALASIA

Chalasia of the cardia usually presents in the first 3 months of life with a complaint that the infant regurgitates part of its food and that it is failing to thrive. On barium examination the oesophagus is found to be moderately dilated. The peristalsis within it is quite effective in carrying barium into the stomach when the infant is horizontal but the stripping wave must be ineffective since residual barium commonly remains within the oesophagus. The oesophago-gastric junction is lax and widely patent. Reflux from a fully distended stomach usually occurs easily but herniation of the stomach through the wide hiatus may not be demonstrated (Fig. 32.38A).

If at this stage the infant is kept upright by postural nursing the condition may improve (Fig. 32.38B) and by 9 to 12 months the cardia may appear normal and the child may have a competent anti-reflux mechanism. Although the cause of this condition is not known, it appears that in some infants at least there is a delay in the development of a competent oesophago-gastric sphincter mechanism. Other infants develop oesophagitis with stricture formation, shortening of the oesophagus and a hiatus hernia. Once this occurs, the reflux tends to continue and eventually surgical correction may be necessary.

In adults, chalasia of the cardia may develop as a complication of scleroderma of the oesophagus, usually at quite a late stage when the oesophagus is considerably dilated and peristalsis within it either absent or totally ineffective. Sometimes chalasia is seen without any underlying condition. The oesophagus is usually distensible and forms a continuous tube through a wide hiatus into the stomach. Reflux occurs easily. It is impossible to exclude the presence of a hiatus hernia since the exact position of the mucosal junction cannot be determined radiologically, but there is no demonstrable loculus of the stomach to be seen above the diaphragm.

DIAPHRAGMATIC HERNIA

Herniation of abdominal viscera into the thoracic cavity may occur through any of the normal anatomical orifices in the diaphragm, through abnormal openings, which are the result of failure of closure of congenital foramina, or as the result of actual tears in the diaphragm.

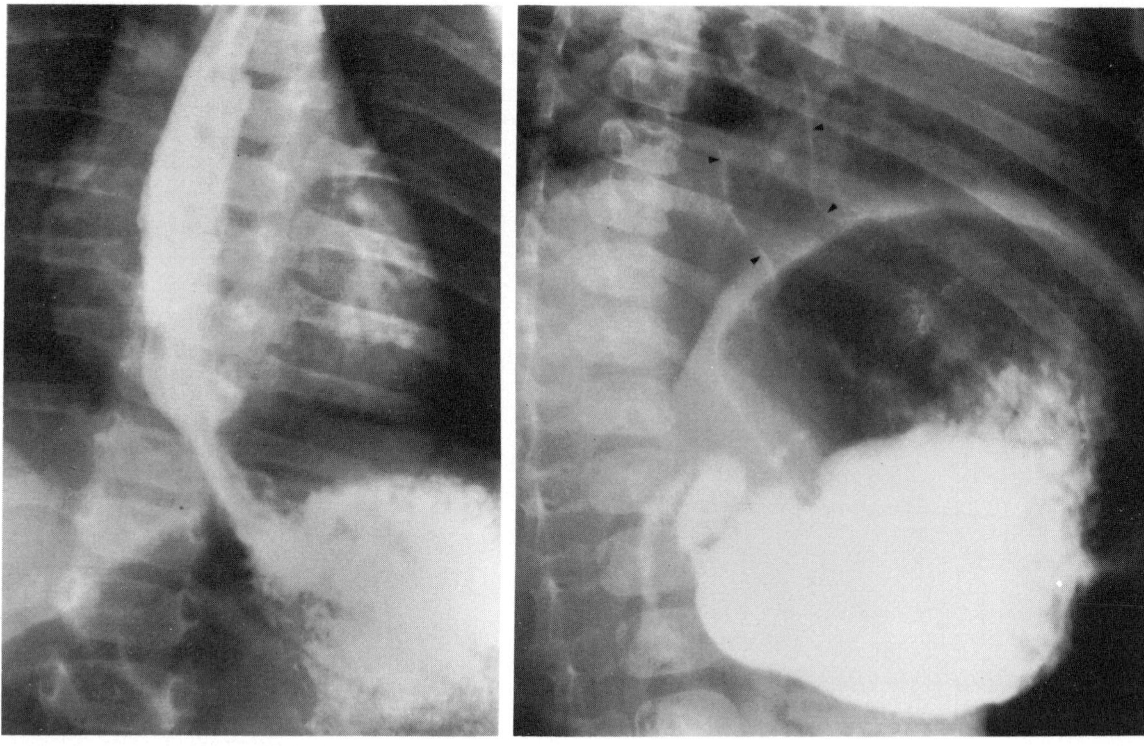

Fig. 32.38 Chalasia of the oesophagus. A Supine view. Dilated oesophagus with free reflux but no evidence of hernia. B Prone view showing very wide hiatus and gas filled distended oesophagus.

Developmental hernias

The diaphragm is developed in the fetus as a transverse septum which divides the primitive coelomic cavity into thoracic and abdominal cavities. The last portion of the diaphragm to close and seal off the thoracic from the abdominal cavity is the pleuroperitoneal canal, and persistence of this canal gives rise to a defect in the diaphragm through which abdominal contents may herniate into the thoracic cavity. It is obvious that in this type of hernia the thoracic and abdominal cavities are in direct communication and the herniated viscera are not surrounded by a hernial sac. Herniation of abdominal viscera most frequently occurs in the left side, and the defect, when it occurs in the right leaf of the diaphragm, is protected by the liver and herniation of bowel is consequently less likely.

Pleuroperitoneal Hernia. Herniation of abdominal contents through this hiatus (Bochdalek's foramen) may present as a respiratory emergency immediately after birth when the extent of the hernia imperils the infant's life by respiratory obstruction. Immediate diagnosis is important, the erect film of the chest will reveal the gas-filled loops lying in the pleural cavity, and in cases where there is any doubt, water-soluble contrast medium should be given to outline the intestinal coils. Immediate operation with reduction of the hernia may be life-saving, although other congenital defects are frequently associated with deformity and in consequence the outcome of surgery may be less successful than anticipated (Fig. 32.39).

In other instances, the herniation may not be noticed until adult life, when it may be difficult to differentiate from traumatic diaphragmatic hernia.

If the subject reaches adult life the herniated coils of gut can be seen lying in the thoracic cavity and a lateral film reveals that they lie posterior to the lung. A barium meal and follow-through examination usually allows the herniated coils of bowel to be identified. On the left side the spleen or kidney may herniate through the pleuroperitoneal foramen and in the absence of an associated herniation of bowel, the nature of the solid opacity in the chest may cause difficulties in diagnosis. Both herniated spleen and kidney lie posteriorly to the lung in the paravertebral sulcus and the presence of an opacity with clear-cut outlines in this region always raises the possibility of such a herniation. Plain films of the abdomen and isotope scans will assist by demonstrating the absence of the herniated viscus from its normal intra-abdominal site.

Anterior diaphragmatic hernia. Anteriorly the diaphragm is attached by muscular slips to the xiphisternum. A failure of complete closure in this portion of the diaphragm results in a persistent foramen (Morgagni's foramen, Larrey's space).

Abdominal contents may herniate through this space and may give rise to clinical symptoms or remain completely asymptomatic.

Extraperitoneal fat is the commonest structure to herniate through this opening and it presents as a triangular opacity in the postero-anterior chest film obscuring the right cardiophrenic angle. It has to be differentiated from atelectatic, right paracardiac or middle-lobe collapse, which may cast a shadow obscuring the right cardiophrenic angle. A lateral film usually demonstrates a triangular nature of the collapsed lobe and also the convex border of the herniated fat. The low density of the herniated fat as well as the convex border also indicates the true nature of the opacity.

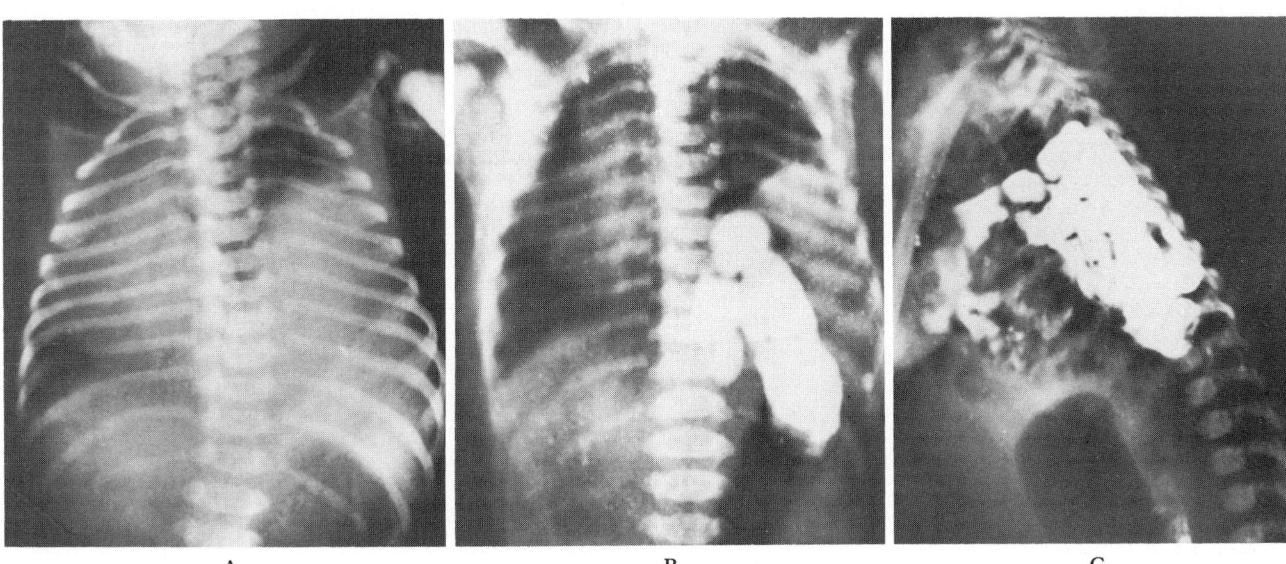

Fig. 32.39 A Pleuroperitoneal hiatus. Film of a newborn infant showing almost complete opacity of the left hemithorax and displacement of the mediastinum and heart towards the right side. B Same case after the administration of a barium swallow showing the stomach and bowel contents lying in the left pleural cavity. C Lateral view of the same case showing the small bowel lying in the left pleural cavity.

In other instances omentum may herniate through Morgagni's foramen and still less frequently the transverse colon. Obstruction of the colon seldom occurs in this type of hernia but a barium meal follow-through demonstrates the transverse colon ascending in front of the liver and lying in the hernial sac. Herniation of omentum can be recognized even when there is no bowel in the sac; in these cases the barium filled transverse colon, instead of looping down into the abdomen, is kinked upwards in a reverse V appearance.

Hiatus hernia

The mechanism of the oesophageal closure and the prevention of reflux of gastric contents into the oesophagus is still incompletely understood. The acuteness of the gastro-oesophageal angle, the pressure of the right crus of the diaphragm and an intrinsic muscle sphincter have all been credited with some part in this mechanism. One fact is certain, namely that when the fundus or a portion of the fundus of the stomach herniates through the oesophageal orifice, this mechanism is disturbed and reflux of gastric contents usually occurs. Provided some of the oesophagus remains below the diaphragm and subject to normal abdominal pressure, reflux is unlikely to occur. Any shortening of the oesophagus due to spasm of longitudinal muscle fibrosis, infiltration with neoplasm, or even retching, tends to remove the intra-abdominal part of the oesophagus and predisposes to reflux.

The term hiatus hernia covers the herniation of a portion of the stomach through the oesophageal hiatus. Two main types of hernia occur. In one the cardio-oesophageal orifice slides upwards into the thorax—the so-called hiatus hernia (sliding hernia) (Fig. 32.40). This gives rise to gastro-oesophageal reflux and oesophagitis. In the second and less common type, a hernia of the fundus of the stomach occurs and the cardio-oesophageal junction remains in its normal anatomical position (para-oesophageal hernia, rolling hernia). The herniated portion of the stomach in these cases passes by the side of the oesophagus and the cardio-oesophageal junction remains in its normal intra-abdominal position (Fig. 32.41). In this type, gastro-oesophageal reflux does not occur, there are frequently no symptoms and the lesion is first diagnosed by the air-fluid level being seen on a chest film. As the hernia orifice widens the para-oesophageal hernia may become a third 'mixed' type and show both hiatal and para-oesophageal components.

Incarcerated hiatus hernia. The presence of a fluid level in a hiatus hernia implies that the herniated portion of the stomach is irreducible. The presence of two fluid levels in the herniated sac usually implies that a volvulus is present in the herniated stomach.

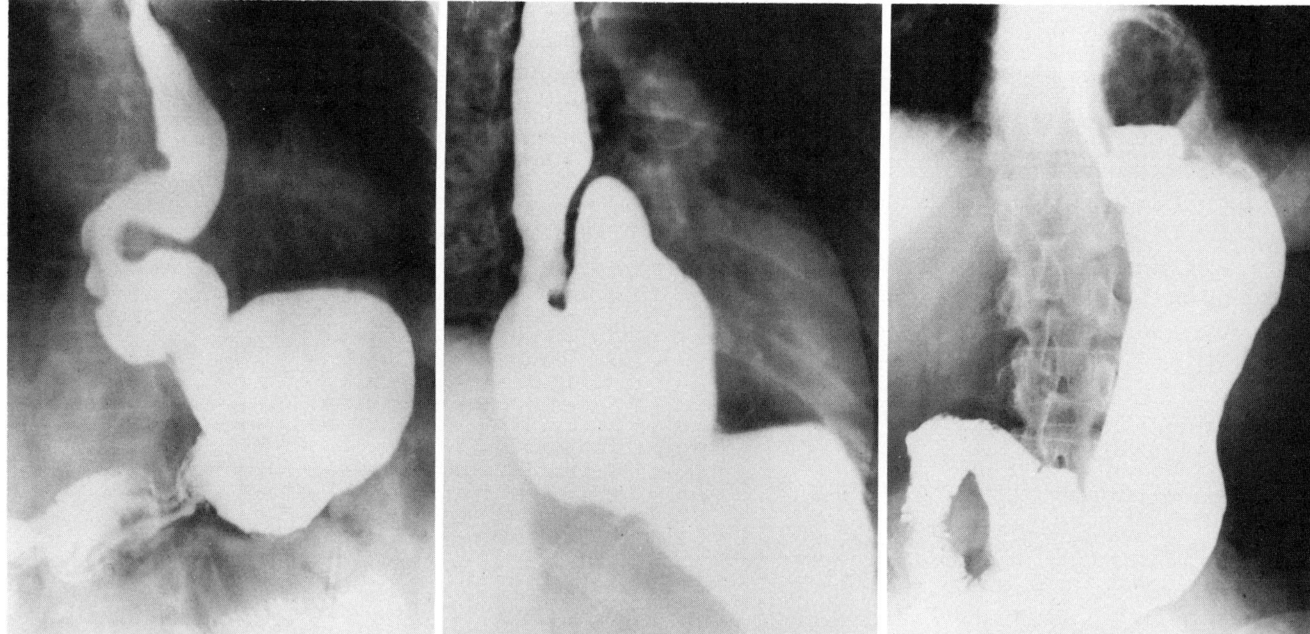

Fig. 32.40 *Fig. 32.41A* *Fig. 32.41B*

Fig. 32.40 Sliding hiatus hernia.

Fig. 32.41 Para-oesophageal hernia.

The absence of any gas and fluid levels from the small bowel in a case presenting clinically as intestinal onstruction may indicate an incarceration of a coil of small bowel within a diaphragmatic hernia.

Radiological technique

In the erect position many hiatus hernias spontaneously reduce, but in others the herniated portion of the stomach remains irreductible. It is important by examining the patients in the Trendelenburg position to demonstrate the full extent of herniation and the ease with which any gastro-oesophageal reflux occurs. Reflux is episodic and may occur more easily on one day than another. A large volume (300–500 ml) of dilute barium may be used to distend the fundus.

The examination of a hiatus hernia should attempt to determine the following features:

(*a*) the presence of gastro-oesophageal reflux and the ease with which it occura.

(*b*) the presence of ulceration in the oesophagus or in the herniated portion of stomach.

(*c*) the degree of any narrowing in the lower end of the oesophagus.

(*d*) the extent of gastric herniation.

(*e*) the appearance of the mucosal pattern in the herniated portion of the stomach.

Patients suspected of having a hiatus hernia with reflux should be examined in the upright and horizontal positions. The patient first swallows barium while in the erect position and is asked to take a full inspiration just as the barium is reaching the lower end of the oesophagus. The normal patient can sustain a column of barium approximately 10 cm high within the oesophagus during full inspiration, the barium passing into the stomach on expiration. If the hiatus is wide the flow of barium is not checked in this way and passes directly into the stomach. When the stomach has been filled with barium and it is seen that there is no residual barium in the oesophagus, the patient is placed in the supine position. If barium then appears in the oesophagus, reflux must have occurred. Herniation of the cardia through the hiatus can also be recognized. Increasing intra-abdomial pressure by raising the legs or using a pressure balloon on the abdomen may increase the size of the hernia, but under these circumstances the degree of herniation is hardly comparable to that occurring in normal conditions. Careful fluoroscopy with the patient supine and turning from side to side unaided raises abdominal pressure levels in a manner more akin to what occurs normally and is a better estimate of what is likely to occur. The right posterior oblique position with the patient turned slightly towards his right side is probably the best single position to elicit reflux and demonstrate a hernia. The act of swallowing saliva may precipitate reflux, probably because of contraction of the longitudinal muscles of the oesophagus, which consequently shortens slightly with elevation of the cardia and loss of the abdominal segment of the oesophagus. Occasionally reflux is demonstrated only in the lateral position with the patient stooping down to touch his toes.

After testing for reflux and herniation it is necessary

to look for complications of reflux within the oesophagus, notably ulceration and stricture formation. For this part of the examination, the patient may be placed prone in a slight Trendelenburg position with a bolster under the abdomen. He then drinks barium through a straw and as the barium reaches the lower oesophagus, takes a full inspiration. This fully distends the lower oesophagus and the maximum size and length of any stricture will be demonstrated. Careful fluoroscopy and films taken in several different projections while the oesophagus is fully dilated with air will be necessary to exclude ulceration.

The presence of a bolus of barium in the lower end of the oesophagus has to be assessed as to whether it is part of the barium ingested and lying in a phrenic ampulla or whether it represents true reflux from the stomach. If the stomach is filled with the patient upright and the oesophagus is shown to be empty before the patient is put in the supine position, this difficulty need not arise. To test for reflux the patient subsequently need only swallow saliva or perhaps a mouthful of water. The herniated portion of the fundus of the stomach may look identical to the ballooned lower end of the oesophagus comprising the phrenic ampulla. Usually, however, there are not more than three longitudinal folds of mucosa in the oesophagus while in cases of hiatus hernia more gastric folds may be seen in the hernia. However, identification of the mucosal pattern, whether oesophageal or gastric, which would enable gastric identification is not always possible, but the swallowing of a mouthful of water in the Trendelenburg position will often enable swallowed barium to be differentiated from regurgitated barium. The phrenic ampulla is probably formed by the arrival of the swallowed bolus of barium at the lower end of the oesophagus coinciding with a contraction of the diaphragmatic pinch-cock, which normally occurs on full inspiration, the oesophagus ballooning out to form a round barium filled pouch in front of the propulsive oesophageal wave. On expiration the barium passes into the stomach and the phrenic ampulla disappears.

COMPLICATIONS OF HIATUS HERNIA

a. Peptic (reflux) oesophagitis. The regurgitation of the acid/pepsin contents of the stomach produces an irritation of the lower oesophagus leading to a localized oesophagitis. Oesophagitis is followed by a superficial ulceration of the squamous epithelium which may lead to both stricture formation and shortening of the oesophagus. This shortening of the oesophagus predisposes to further reflux since it destroys one of the main anti-reflux mechanisms—that is the presence of a short segment of oesophagus below the diaphragm and at abdominal pressure. Thus a vicious circle is set up and progressive stenosis and shortening of the oesophagus may occur. In infancy and childhood this shortening may occur with alarming rapidity and stricture formation is very common. If it is allowed to persist the oesophago-gastric junction may rise within the thorax to the level of the tracheal bifurcation or even higher giving rise to what was formerly thought to be a 'congenital short oesophagus'. In many instances, however, with correct postural nursing the oesophagus lengthens and the oesophago-gastric junction may return to within the abdomen. It thus appears that in the earlier stages at least this shortening is not due to true fibrosis.

The shortening which occurs as a sequel of oesophagitis results in a segment of the stomach being drawn up tightly into the thorax so that, particularly when the patient is upright, it has a similar diameter to the normal oesophagus. In order to demonstrate the true nature of this loculus of stump, it is necessary to place the patient horizontally, distend it fully with either barium or air and to demonstrate the gastric folds within it and the large number of gastric folds passing through the diaphragmatic hiatus. Provided one can get enough barium past the stricture into the stomach to distend the lower segment, it should not be difficult to demonstrate the loculus of intrathoracic stump from below (Fig. 32.43A and B).

In the adult, particularly when there is a short history, it should be remembered that infiltrating carcinoma around the cardia may predispose to gastro-oesophageal reflux, shortening of the oesophagus and hiatus hernia. In any case of doubt, endoscopy and multiple biopsies are essential.

b. Ulceration. Two types of ulceration may be seen in association with a hiatus hernia and reflux. There may be superficial ulceration in metaplastic squamous squamous mucosa, which commonly is circumferential and gives rise to stricture formation and shortening of the oesophagus, as described above (Fig. 32.42). There may also be ulceration of the peptic type in columnar epithelium. This appears as a niche in the same way as peptic ulcers are demonstrated in the stomach (Fig. 32.43A). This latter type of ulceration may occur near the oesophago-gastric junction but is also seen in the para-oesophageal type of hernia, where it appears along the lesser curve of the herniated portion of the stomach. This type of ulcer is prone to bleed and is probably traumatic in origin since it occurs in the neck of the hernia as it passes through the diaphragm.

c. Malignant degeneration. A malignant tumour, usually an adenocarcinoma, may occur within a hernia and give rise to iron deficiency anaemia without any gastro-intestinal symptoms. The tumour has the same radiological appearances as a carcinoma occurring in a normally sited stomach but may be more difficult to demonstrate because of the distortion due to the presence of the para-oesophageal hernia. Rigidity of the cardia due

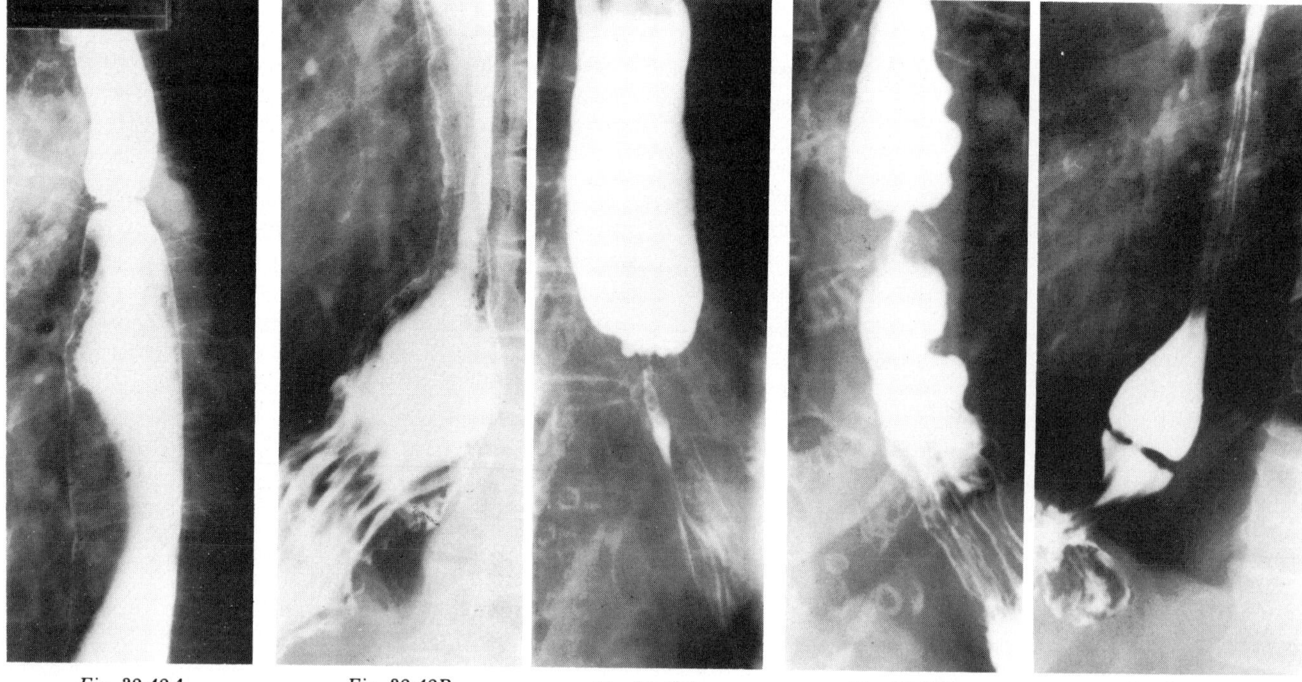

Fig. 32.42A *Fig. 32.42B* *Fig. 32.43A* *Fig. 32.43B* *Fig. 32.44*

Fig. 32.42 A Stricture at the level of the aortic knuckle shown on endoscopy to be at the junction of squamous and columnar epithelium. B Large diaphragmatic hernia with free reflux.

Fig. 32.43 Oesophageal stricture due to gastro-oesophageal reflux. A Erect film showing dilatation of the oesophagus above the stricture. There is a small ulcer just above the stricture. B Supine film showing gastro-oesophageal regurgitation and a fixed hiatus hernia with shortening of the oesophagus.

Fig. 32.44 Schatzki's ring at lower end of the oesophagus showing a well-defined classical indentation with narrow central lumen (diameter 9 mm).

to an infiltrating carcinoma either of the oesophagus or stomach may predispose to gastro-oesophageal reflux, oesophagitis, shortening of the oesophagus and the formation of a hiatus hernia.

Lower oesophageal ring (Schatzki ring).

The clinical presentation is usually that of bolus obstruction sometimes referred to as the 'steak house syndrome'. An extra large piece of food becomes impacted temporarily in the lower oesophagus and causes a complete obstruction. After a short time the food is either vomited or passes into the stomach.

The Schatzki ring represents the oesophago-gastric junction and since this lies above the diaphragm, indicates the presence of a hiatus hernia. It is best demonstrated in the Trendelenburg position or with the patient prone over a bolster. The patient swallows a large bolus of barium and as the barium nears the lower end of the oesophagus, is told to hold his breath on deep inspiration. The ring is seen as a narrow indentation 2–3 mm deep extending inwards from both sides of the fully distended oesophagus (Fig. 32.44). Below the ring the lumen narrows where the stomach passes through the diaphragmatic hiatus. Unless the lower oesophagus is fully distended, the Schatzki ring will not be demonstrated. It is said that a narrow ring (diameter less than 12 mm) causes episodes of bolus obstruction while a large ring (greater than 18 mm) causes no symptoms unless associated with gastro-oesophageal reflux.

Table 32.1 *Lesions causing deviation of the oesophagus*

1. Cervical spondylosis.		
2. Enlargement of the thyroid and parathyroid glands.		
3. Pulmonary fibrosis.		
4. Mediastinal tumours and lymph nodes.		
5. Cardio-vascular lesions.		
a. Infants	— vascular rings and anomalies (see Appendix C).	
b. Adults	— aberrant right subclavian artery	— right-sided aortic arch.
	— coarction of the aorta	— unfolded and tortuous aorta.
	— enlarged left atrium	— aortic aneurysm.

EXTRINSIC LESIONS AFFECTING THE OESOPHAGUS

Cervical spondylosis. Although large anterior osteophytes in the lower cervical spine commonly indent the posterior wall of the oesophagus when it is fully distended, it is uncommon for them to give rise to dysphagia. The oesophagus appears to slide freely over the pre-vertebral fascia in spite of this deformity. Occasionally, however, when there are adhesions between the oesophagus and the pre-vertebral tissues, dysphagia may arise.

Thyroid and parathyroid enlargement. Enlargement of the thyroid gland frequently displaces the oesophagus and trachea, usually laterally, and both oesophagus and trachea to a similar degree. Both the oesophagus and trachea may be compressed. Occasionally there may be a localized enlargement of the thyroid gland between the spine and the oesophagus when the oesophagus may be displaced forwards. On fluoroscopy even large benign goitres will be seen to rise upwards on swallowing. Occasionally if the neck is hyper-extended a partially retrosternal thyroid will move upwards into the neck when the patient swallows—the so-called 'plunging goitre'. Failure of an enlarged thyroid to move upwards on swallowing should raise the possibility of a carcinoma or Hashimoto's disease.

Although functional parathyroid adenoma are usually small, about 1 in 10 is big enough to cause a lateral indentation on the wall of the oesophagus seen on the anterior view.

Pulmonary fibrosis. Fibrosis in the apex of the lung frequently causes traction of the oesophagus, which is deviated to the side of the lesion. The oesophagus is usually dilated and has a pseudo-diverticular appearance. Peristalsis in that segment may be disturbed so that food residue collects in it. There may be overall shortening of the oesophagus with a hiatus hernia and reflux.

Mediastinal tumours and lymph nodes. Displacement of the middle third of the oesophagus by mediastinal tumours or lymph nodes is best recognized on antero-posterior and lateral views of the barium filled oesophagus, which must be taken in the supine and prone position. Enlarged lymph nodes from carcinoma of the bronchus, stomach or other malignant tumours such as a seminoma frequently displace the oesophagus in the subcarinal area. The walls of the oesophagus remain parallel to each other and peristalsis is unaffected unless the oesophagus is directly infiltrated by the lymph nodes. The mass of lymph nodes can sometimes be seen outlined by air in the adjacent lung.

Primary tumours and cysts of the mediastinum usually cause a smooth displacement of the oesophagus without any sign of direct invasion.

Cardio-vascular lesions. Abnormalities of the great vessels (see Appendix C) commonly give rise to symptoms of dysphagia either in infancy or in the elderly with arteriosclerotic vessels. The *aberrant right subclavian artery* arises from the aortic arch distal to the left subclavian artery and passes upwards and to the right behind the oesophagus giving rise to a characteristic smooth oblique indentation on the posterior wall of the barium filled oesophagus, best seen on the left anterior oblique view. The presence of a *right-sided aorta* can be confirmed by the demonstration of the indentation of the right side of the oesophagus at the level of the aortic arch. Acquired abnormalities of the aorta, including aneurysms of the aortic arch and descending aorta, frequently give rise to dysphagia and cause considerable localized displacement of the oesophagus.

Left atrium. Enlargement of the left atrium causes a characteristic localized posterior displacement of the oesophagus. When the left atrium is very large the oesophagus may slip off the back of the heart and be displaced to the right as well as slightly posteriorly. It is uncommon for a large left atrium to give rise to dysphagia but a localized oesophagitis with stricture formation may occur in patients in heart failure who are taking tablets such as Slow K which stick in the oesophagus at the upper level of the enlarged left atrium (Fig. 32.45). Oesophageal intramural haematoma after surgical repair or displacement of the cardiac valves occasionally produces dysphagia in the post-operative period and the barium swallow shows a smooth filling defect similar to a benign tumour. The haematoma resolves spontaneously with disappearance of the clinical symptoms and cardiological appearances.

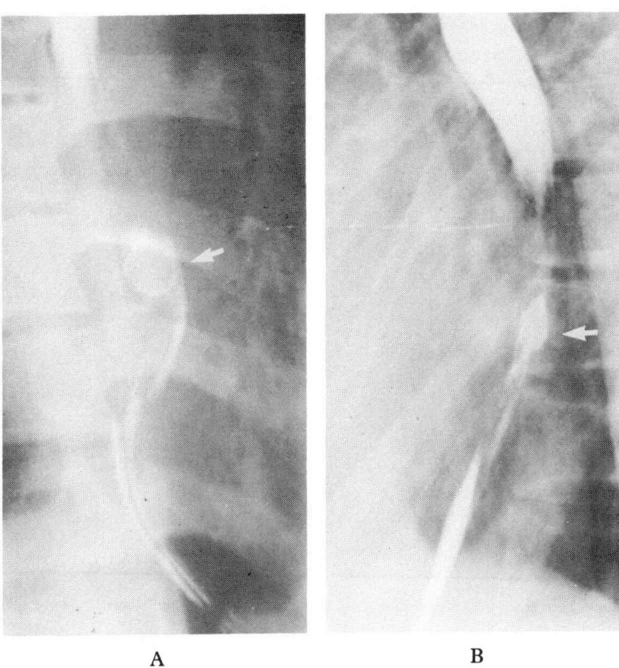

Fig. 32.45 A and B Ulcer in the middle third of the oesophagus in a patient who was being treated with diuretics and Slow K capsules, one of which stuck in the oesophagus due to enlargement of the left atrium and gave rise to a superficial ulcer (*Courtesy of Dr. S. Meyer, Cape Town University.*)

Unfolding and tortuosity of the aorta. As the aorta becomes atheromatous, it dilates, elongates and becomes tortuous. The diameter of the aorta at the level of the aortic arch can be assessed from the displacement of the oesophagus at that level. As the descending aorta becomes tortuous, the oesophagus usually becomes similarly displaced, following the posterior sweep of the aorta in its middle third. Although the displacement may be considerable it seldom gives rise to dysphagia. On the other hand, when the lower third of the oesophagus is displaced by a dilated and tortuous aorta the patient frequently experiences discomfort on swallowing. Transmitted pulsation may be seen on fluoroscopy at the site of the local displacement of the oesophagus. The lumen may be narrowed from side to side by stretching and extrinsic pressure.

REFERENCES AND SUGGESTIONS FOR FURTHER READING

ATKINSON, M. (1962) Mechanisms protecting against gastro-oesophageal reflux; a review. *Gut*, **3**, 1–15.

ATKINSON, M. & SUMMERLING, M. D. (1966) Oesophageal changes in systemic sclerosis. *Gut*, **7**, 402–408.

BARRETT, N. R. (1957) The oesophagus lined with gastric mucous membrane. *Surgery St. Louis*, **41**, 881.

EDWARDS, D. A. W., THOMPSON, H., SHAW, D. G., MISIEWICZ, J. J., BENNETT, J. R. & TORRANCE, B. (1973) Symposium on gastro-oesophageal reflux and its complications. *Gut*, **14**, 233–237.

JOHNSON, H. D. (1966) The fluid mechanics of the control of reflux. *Lancet*, **2**, 1267–1268.

JOHNSON, H. D. & LAWS, J. W. (1966) The cardia in swallowing, eructation and vomiting. *Lancet*, **2**, 1268–1273.

KOEHLER, R. E., MOSS, A. A. & MARGULIS, A. R. (1976) Early radiographic manifestations of carcinoma of the oesophagus. *Radiology*, **119**, 1–5.

PIERCE, J. W. & CREAMER, B. (1963) The diagnosis of the columnar lined oesophagus. *Clinical Radiology*, **14**, 64–69.

SCHATZKI, R. & GRAY, J. E. (1953) Dysphagia due to a diaphragm-like localised narrowing in the lower oesophagus ('lower oesophageal ring'). *American Journal of Roentgenology*, **70**, 911.

SEAMAN, W. B. (1969) Functional disorders of the pharyngo-oesophageal junction: achalasia and chalasia. *Radiologic Clinics of North America*, **7**, 113–119.

STEINER, G. M. (1977) Gastro-oesophageal reflux, hiatus hernia and the radiologist, with special reference to children. *British Journal of Radiology*, **50**, 164–174.

TEDESCO, F. J. & MORTON, W. J. (1975) Lower oesophageal webs. *American Journal of Digestive Diseases*, **20(4)**, 381–383.

WALDRAM, R., NUNNERLEY, H. B., DAVIS, M., LAWS, J. W. & WILLIAMS, R. (1977) Detection and grading of oesophageal varices by fibreoptic endoscopy and barium swallow with and without buscopan. *Clinical Radiology*, **28**, 137–141.

WIGHTMAN, A. J. A. & WRIGHT, E. A. (1974) Intramural oesophageal diverticulosis: a correlation of radiological and pathological findings. *British Journal of Radiology*, **47**, 496–498.

ZBORALSKE, F. F. (1965) The oesophagus in the geriatric patient. *Radiologic Clinics of North America*, **3**, 321–330.

ZBORALSKE, F. F. & DODDS, W. J. (1969) Roentgenographic diagnosis of primary disorders of oesophageal motility. *Radiologic Clinics of North America*, **7**, 147–162.

CHAPTER 33

THE STOMACH AND DUODENUM

TECHNIQUE OF EXAMINATION

Contrast media. A barium sulphate suspension in water is the universal contrast medium used for examination of the upper gastrointestinal tract. A simple barium sulphate/water mixture has several undesirable properties such as a tendency to sediment and unpalatability. Consequently many commercial barium meal preparations have been developed to obviate these unfavourable features.

The barium sulphate must of course be chemically pure, as the contaminant barium carbonate is extremely poisonous. The ideal barium sulphate/water mixture has yet to be developed, but the following properties are of utmost importance.

(a) Particle size. Ordinary barium sulphate particles are coarse, measuring several millimetres in size, but ultrafine milling of the crude barium sulphate results in 50 per cent of the particles having a size of between 5 μm and 15μm. As rate of sedimentation is proportional to particle size, the smaller the barium sulphate particle the more stable the suspension.

(b) Non-ionic medium. The charge on the barium sulphate particle influences the rate of aggregation of the particles. Charged particles attract each other and thus form larger particles which sediment more readily. They tend to do this even more in the gastric contents and consequently sediment more readily in the stomach.

(c) pH of the solution. The pH of the barium sulphate solution should be around 5·3, as more acid solutions tend to become more so in the gastric contents and consequently precipitate more readily in the stomach.

(d) Palatability. Undoubtedly ultrafine milling reduces much of the chalky taste inherent in any barium sulphate/water mixture, but many commercial preparations contain a flavouring agent which further disguises the unpleasant taste. The barium sulphate/water mixture is usually 1/4 weight/volume, and has a viscosity of 15–20 cp, but thicker or thinner suspensions may be used. Many commercial preparations contain carboxymethyl cellulose (Raybar, Barosperse), which retains fluid and prevents precipitation of the barium suspension in the normal small bowel.

The development of the double contrast technique has stressed the need for adequate mucosal coating and much of the present manufacturing efforts are devoted to achieving this. An excess of mucus and undue collection of fluid in the stomach greatly inhibit adequate coating of the gastric mucosa, as does hypermotility of the stomach.

To achieve double contrast examination of the stomach, air or carbon dioxide gas must be introduced and there is no doubt that introduction of air or gas via a nasogastric tube is the best means of obtaining a controlled degree of gastric distension. However, the passage of a gastric tube is an unpleasant procedure and is not acceptable to all patients. Consequently most radiologists use effervescent tablets (sodium bicarbonate 35 mg, tartaric acid 35 mg, calcium carbonate 5·0 mg) to react with the gastric contents to produce carbon dioxide. The amount of gas produced by these methods is variable and over-distension of the stomach in the double contrast technique associated with poor coating can be, from a diagnostic viewpoint, as disastrous as inadequate distension. Some commercial preparations contain carbon dioxide gas under pressure in the barium mixture, but usually the quantity of gas is not adequate to produce good double contrast meals. An anti-foaming agent may need to be added to some barium preparations to avoid the formation of bubbles.

Water soluble iodine-containing contrast media (e.g. Gastrografin) are of value when there is a suspected perforation or leakage of an anastomosis after operation. The low radio-opacity of the iodine compared with the barium, and the high osmolarity which results in dilution within the small bowel, make it of little value for routine use in investigation of the small bowel. Water soluble contrast media are contraindicated if there is any danger of aspiration into the lungs. It also should not be used in dehydrated infants in whom a dangerous hypovolaemia may occur due to the hygroscopic effect of the Gastrografin in the small bowel.

A successful double contrast barium meal with adequate coating of the mucosa should outline the *areae gastricae* of the mucosa (Fig. 33.1), a pattern which must be distinguished from the mucosal fold pattern (Fig. 33.2). The mucosal fold pattern is governed by the state and tonus of the muscularis mucosa and to some extent by the size of the longitudinal, oblique and transverse muscle coats of the stomach. The areae gastricae have an irregular pavement-like appearance peculiar to the gastric mucosa. They are best seen in the body of the stomach and pyloric antrum but less clearly seen in the fundus of the stomach. The demonstration of this pattern is essential in the diagnosis of mucosal changes, e.g. in erosive gastritis, and can only be seen on double contrast meals of good quality.

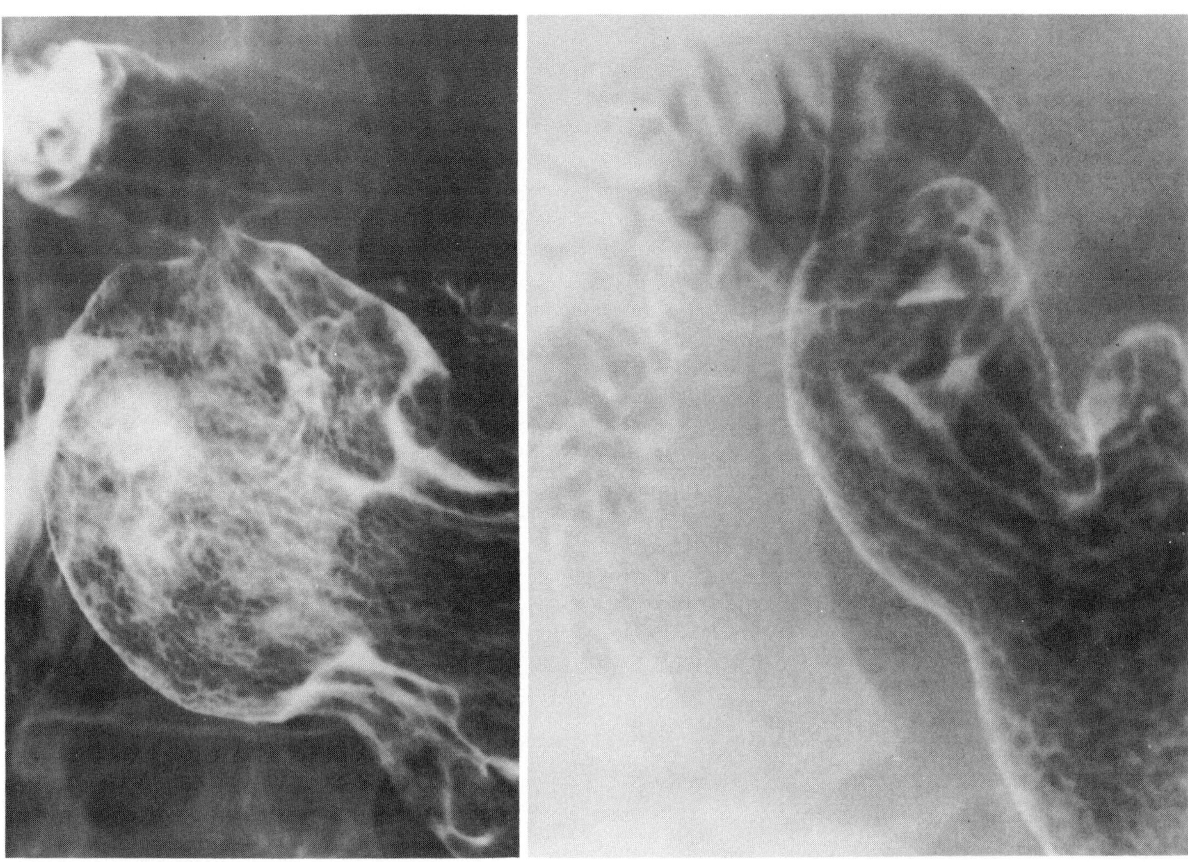

Fig. 33.1 *Fig. 33.2*

Fig. 33.1 The areae gastricae pattern in the pyloric antrum is demonstrated as a fine lace-like pattern throughout the antrum.

Fig. 33.2 Mucosal fold pattern of stomach showing the folds running through the pyloric antrum of stomach and the areae gastricae pattern still retained over the folds.

The normal gastric folds (rugae) consist of two longitudinal folds on the anterior and posterior walls adjoining the lesser curvature. These prominent longitudinal folds run along the length of the stomach through the pyloric antrum and pylorus into the duodenum. Other smaller and thicker folds run horizontally in the mid-portion of the body of the stomach and may result in a gross irregularity of the greater curvature. There may be considerable difficulty in separating these normal appearances from those produced by infiltration by disease processes, e.g. lymphoma.

An inconstant oblique mucosal fold running from the cardio-oesophageal junction to the greater curvature corresponds to the oblique muscle of the stomach.

The cardio-oesophageal junction lies on the posterior gastric wall towards the lesser curvature about 5 cm down from the highest point of the fundus. It may have a stellate appearance due to mucosal puckering when viewed *en face* and frequently a curved mucosal fold forms a 'hood' over the orifice of the oesophagus. This hood-like appearance has been likened to a Burnous and must not be mistaken for pathological changes (Fig. 33.3).

At the junction of the vertical portion of the body of the stomach with the pyloric antrum, a sharp indentation on the lesser curve constitutes the normal membrana angularis defect which must be differentiated from a congenital pyloric diaphragm.

Radiographic technique. High kilovoltage (100–115 KVP) are usually used with conventional barium meal examinations. However, when double contrast examination is undertaken a lower KV with a corresponding increase in the milliamperage improves contrast and allows a clearer demonstration of the areae gastricae. The size of the anode focal spot should not exceed 0·6 mm.

The administration of glucagon 0·1–0·5 mg or Buscopan 10–20 mg by intravenous or intramuscular injection greatly improves the film quality with double contrast. Glucagon probably produces better relaxation than Buscopan with a consequent improvement in visualization of the areae gastricae. It is however, considerably more expensive to use.

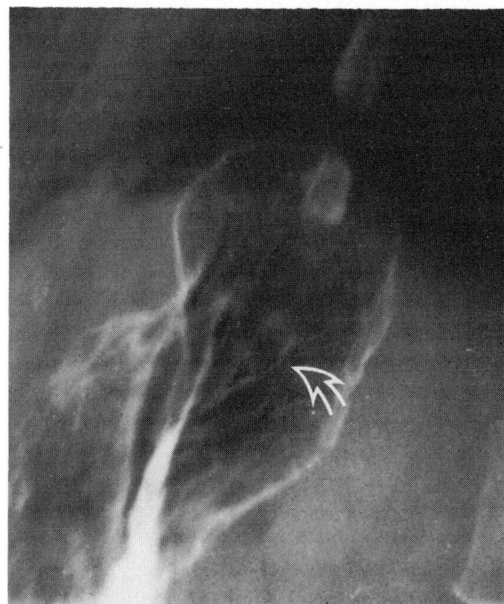

Fig. 33.3 Gastric folds in the fundus of the stomach. The hood-like fold over the cardio-oesophageal junction is seen (*arrow*) (Burnous Sign).

Using these drugs the areae gastricae are so well shown that quite frequently in the profile view of the filled stomach a fine serrated outline is seen. This is considered to be barium between the step-like plates of the areae gastricae, and this serrated appearance should not be mistaken for changes in the stomach wall associated with gastritis.

Whilst the double contrast examination is essential for the diagnosis of early malignancy, mucosal erosions or gastritis, there is no doubt that examination of the duodenal cap by this method may be more difficult for the less experienced observer. In the younger patient with a dyspeptic history suggestive of duodenal ulceration the older method of barium examination (compression technique) may prove easier and more effective in diagnosis.

Method of examination. There are many variations in the method of radiological examination of the stomach and duodenum, but essential features of a barium meal examination should include the assessment of the competence of the cardio-oesophageal junction; the demonstration of the gastric and duodenal mucosal pattern; the visualization of the stomach and duodenum filled with barium to assess any abnormalities of peristalsis and gastric emptying as well as deformities due to extrinsic pressure, and the demonstration of the duodenal cap.

The examination commences with the patient in the erect right anterior oblique position. The first and second mouthfuls of barium are followed under fluoroscopic control along the oesophagus into the stomach. The barium can then be palpated around the stomach with the gloved hand to coat the gastric mucosa. If insufficient barium has been taken a third mouthful of barium will assist in further coating the stomach. Care must be taken at this stage not to introduce an excessive amount of barium and 100–200 ml of the mixture is usually sufficient.

Ten to 20 mg of Buscopan or 0·1–0·5 mg glucagon are now injected intravenously and gas introduced into the stomach to produce the necessary ingredient for a double contrast study. The gas accumulates in the fundus of the stomach and when this is distended the table is tilted and the patient turns into the prone position. When the patient then turns into the supine right oblique position gas rises to the body and allows double contrast studies of the pyloric antrum and the lower part of the body of the stomach to be seen. It is usually necessary to roll the patient briskly from side to side in order to remove a surface coating of mucus and demonstrate the areae gastricae. By rotating the patient to the left anterior oblique position the mucosal pattern in the body of the stomach may be seen and the excess barium in the fundus of the stomach will pass into the pyloric antrum through the pylorus into the duodenum and distend the duodenal cap. Deformities in outline of the filled cap can be readily seen in this position.

The table is then tilted into the Trendelenburg position and the patient rotated back into the right oblique position and instructed to swallow a few more mouthfuls of barium and the presence of any gastro-oesophageal reflux noted. Raising the intra-abdominal pressure by manual abdominal palpation or asking the patient to raise the legs may produce reflux into the oesophagus which is not present in the resting phase. Serial films of any abnormality noted during the preceding fluoroscopic manoeuvres are taken but for the double contrast films fine focus tubes (0.6 mm) capable of heavy loading to minimize motional blur are essential to show the detail required in good double contrast studies.

The patient is then brought back to the erect position and a further 300 to 400 ml of barium sulphate mixture are swallowed to allow the filled stomach to be examined. Rigidity and lack of peristalsis are best appreciated in the filled stomach. The duodenal cap should be examined in the right and left oblique position to demonstrate the anterior and posterior walls of the duodenal cap and

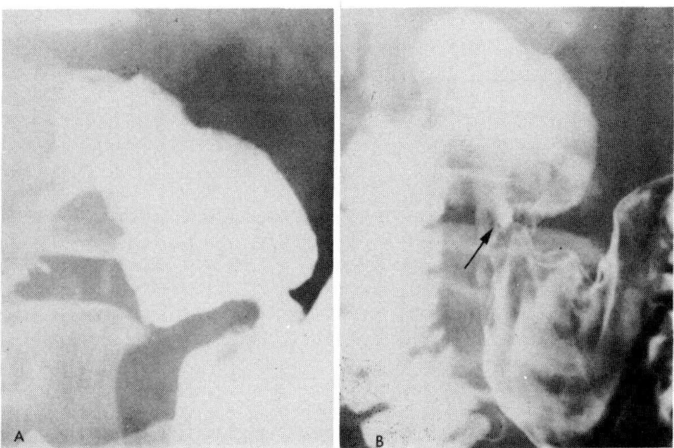

Fig. 33.4 A Right anterior oblique views of the filled duodenal cap demonstrating the fact that a filled cap does not exclude ulceration. B The compressed cap showing the ulcer crater filled with barium (*arrow*).

any deformities of the cap can be noted and compression studies will demonstrate ulcer craters (Fig. 33.4).

It must be appreciated that this suggested technique is a compromise between the conventional compression method and the double contrast method, and it may be that like any compromise the best of each method used alone is not realized. It may be that conventional or full double contrast method should be employed related to the clinical condition being investigated. It must be appreciated that the appearances of lesions in the conventional and double contrast meal are radically different and many of the errors arise because the signs (e.g. of ulceration) in a conventional meal are looked for in the double contrast meal.

The modern remote control screening units do not allow palpation and consequently with some units more reliance has to be placed on positioning the patient to achieve double contrast studies of the mucosa as a means of detecting early lesions.

The minimum films obtained should include:

1. Right and left anterior oblique views of the filled oesophagus. A split film usually allows the two views to be taken on a 35×45 cm film.
2. Supine and supine oblique double contrast films of the stomach showing the duodenal cap and loop.
3. Prone films demonstrating the fundus, body and lower end of the oesophagus.
4. Supine right anterior oblique view of the filled stomach.
5. Erect right anterior oblique view of the filled stomach.
6. Serial views of the duodenal cap in the erect and supine positions both in the filled and double contrast state.

The technique of examination of the stomach and duodenum in cases of active bleeding from the stomach

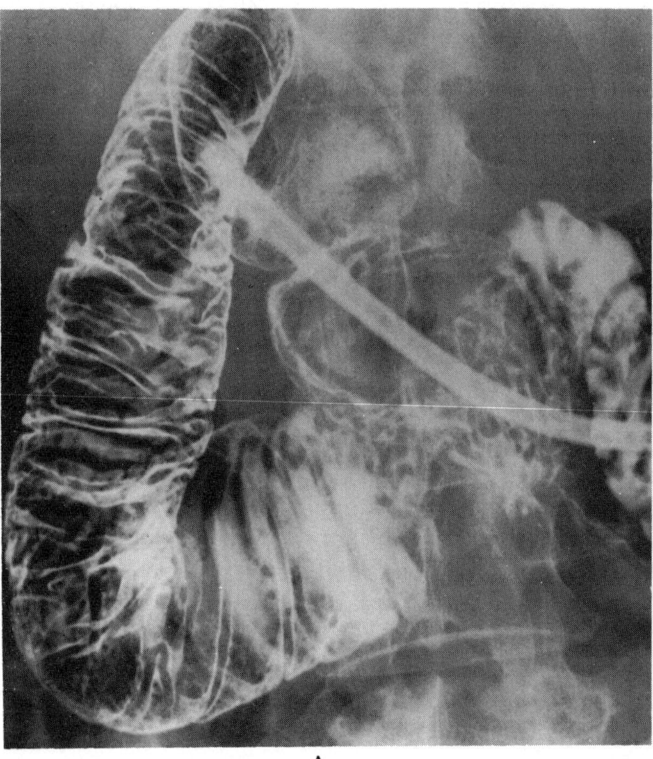

A

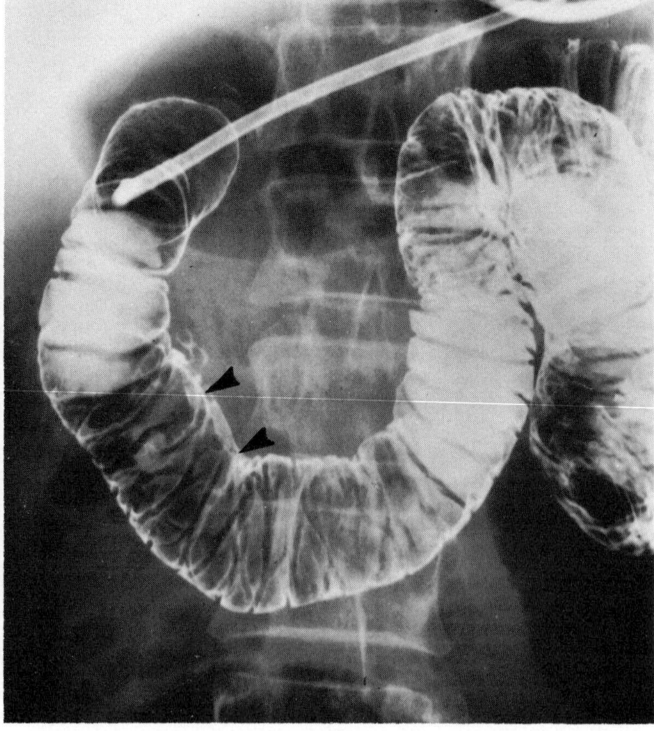

B

Fig. 33.5 A Normal hypotonic duodenogram. B Normal hypotonic duodenogram. Note the straight fold, the frenulum, on the medial aspect of the second part covering the duodenal papilla (*arrows*).

(haematemesis and melaena) is described in Chapter 36.

Pharmacological methods. *Buscopan* or *glucagon* have been used to produce relaxation of the gastric wall and outline the stomach by double contrast methods. *Metoclopramide* (*Maxolon*), 20 mg intravenously, may also be of value in increasing peristaltic activity in the stomach and in highlighting areas of mucosal or gastric rigidity, important points in the early diagnosis of malignancy. Metoclopramide has additional value in that it speeds the passage of the barium through the small bowel and allows the small bowel and terminal ileum to be completely investigated within 30 minutes.

Hypotonic duodenography. Lesions of the duodenum are best demonstrated when the duodenal mucosa is coated with barium and the loop distended with gas and aperistaltic. This can be done without intubation using a double contrast technique and glucagon; or to obtain relaxation a duodenal tube is introduced into the duodenum and 20–30 ml barium sulphate mixture is injected through the tube and allowed to coat the duodenum. Twenty to 30 mg Buscopan is then given intravenously and as soon as peristalsis has ceased air is introduced through the tube and under fluoroscopic control the duodenum is distended. Serial views of the double contrast duodenum in both oblique positions can be readily achieved and indentations and early infiltrations can be recognized.

Buscopan is contraindicated in patients suffering from glaucoma or prostatism. Massive dilatation of the stomach may also be a complication of hypotonic duodenography.

The mucosal pattern in the duodenum consists of short transverse folds. The papilla of the ampulla of Vater (duodenal papilla), the most important structure in the second part of the duodenum, cannot be recognized with any degree of constancy. A longitudinal fold (plica longitudinalis) extends down to the papilla and often forms a signpost to the site of the duodenal papilla (Fig. 33.5).

CONGENITAL ABNORMALITIES

Congenital lesions affecting the stomach may be classified as:

1. Abnormalities of site
   - (i) dextroposition
   - (ii) eventration and herniation of the diaphragm
2. Intrinsic abnormalities
   - (i) duplication of the stomach
   - (ii) gastric diverticuli
   - (iii) enterogenous cysts
   - (iv) congenital gastric septa
3. Infantile hypertrophic pyloric stenosis

Abnormalities of site. Complete transposition of the viscera is associated with dextroposition of the stomach. Isolated dextroposition of the stomach is extremely rare.

Congenital diaphragmatic hernia through the pleuroperitoneal hiatus may be associated with the stomach lying in the left pleural cavity and may be a rare cause of respiratory distress in the newborn.

Duplication of the stomach. Duplication of the stomach is very rare but probably represents the extreme stage of failure of subdivision of the embryonic coelonic tube. Gastric diverticula and enterogenous cysts probably represent minor degrees of abnormality of the same subdivision process.

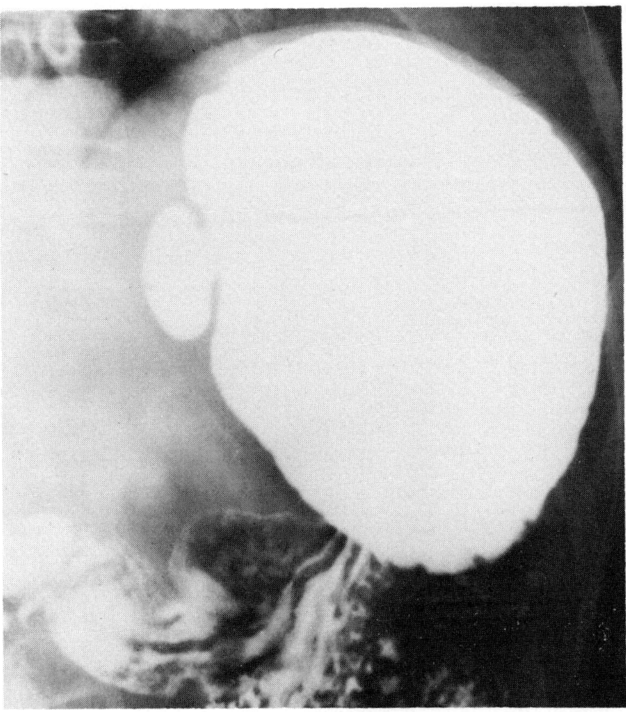

Fig. 33.6 Gastric diverticulum. Supine oblique film of barium-filled stomach demonstrating the smooth contours and narrow neck of the diverticulum arising just below the cardio-oesophageal junction.

In duplication of the stomach the accessory stomach lies along the greater curvature and usually communicates with the stomach in the region of the pyloric antrum. In the only case seen by the authors, ulceration (with haematemesis) had occurred at the junction of the abnormal stomach with the normal stomach.

Gastric diverticula. Congenital gastric diverticula are usually in the fundus and tend to occur near the cardio-oesophageal orifice (Fig. 33.6). They are usually small, have a narrow neck and a flask-like outline with mucosal folds radiating into the diverticulum—features which enable the diverticulum to be differentiated from a gastric ulcer.

A less common form of congenital diverticulum is the intramural variety which is small and is not visible on the

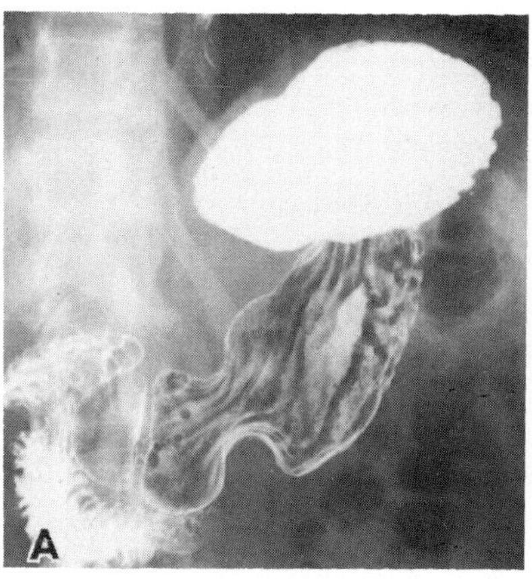

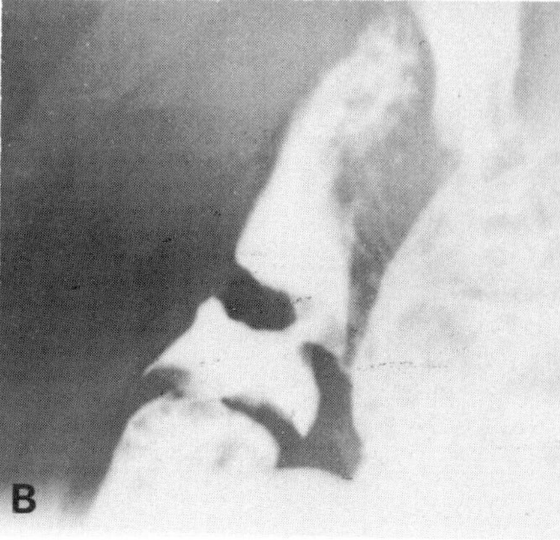

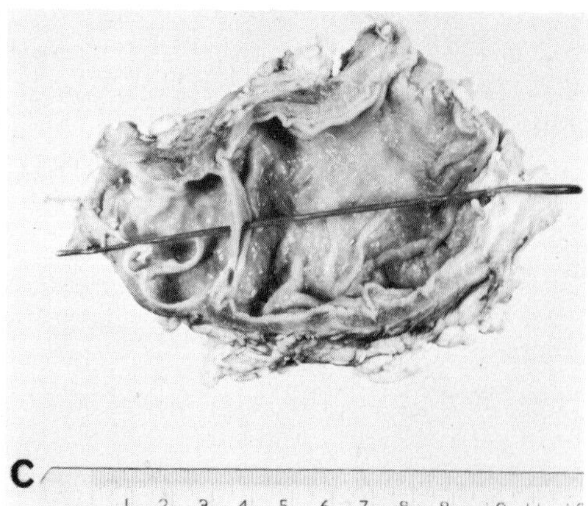

Fig. 33.7 (A and B) Pyloric antrum demonstrating an antral membrane. C Resected specimen showing small central channel through the membrane (*Courtesy of Dr. G. de B. Hinde.*)

serosal surface. This type of diverticulum has to be differentiated from a dilated pancreatic duct system which may occur in a congenital pancreatic rest in this area. The embryological basis of these intramural diverticula is not understood.

Other gastric diverticula not of congenital origin are those which arise following penetration or local perforation of a gastric ulcer. These are not lined by mucosa nor do they show a muscular coat, features found in the truly congenital variety. Furthermore the outlines of such diverticula tend to be irregular. Shortening of the lesser curvature of the stomach in association with a penetrating ulcer may result in the cavity of the stomach appearing as a large diverticulum.

Small diverticula are frequently found around the anastomotic line after surgical resection of the stomach. Such diverticula may be produced by surgical oversewing and must not be mistaken for anastomotic ulceration. They are frequently multiple and almost invariably have a flask-like outline with a narrow neck.

Enterogenous cysts. These probably represent a minor form of intestinal duplication. They are only rarely seen in the stomach but should always be considered in the differential diagnosis of any apparently benign tumour occurring in an infant or young child. They have the classic appearance of an intramural tumour with the mucosa stretched and smoothed over the tumour.

Gastric diaphragms. Pyloric antral diaphragms consist of a thin diaphragm crossing the pyloric antrum with the passage through the diaphragm often reduced to a small pinhole. The clinical features are those of pyloric obstruction often without pain. Careful radiological examination particularly with the double contrast method will reveal the thin mucosal diaphragm and the true pylorus lying distal to the diaphragm (Fig. 33.7).

Infantile hypertrophic pyloric stenosis. The presence of a palpable muscle mass associated with projectile vomiting allows a fairly confident clinical diagnosis, but in other instances where a mass is impalpable the differentiation of pylorospasm from hypertrophic pyloric stenosis may be difficult. It is in these cases that radiological examination is called for.

The administration of small quantities of a barium sulphate mixed with water or the infant's food and fluoroscopic examination in the right lateral position will allow the pyloric antrum and frequently the elongated pyloric canal to be outlined. There is delay in the commencement of gastric emptying. (Small quantities of water-soluble contrast medium may also be mixed with the barium mixture and on occasions may show the elongated pyloric canal more readily.)

The radiological signs (Fig. 33.8) are:

(a) *String sign.* This is a thin track of barium extending between the pyloric antrum and duodenal cap representing the narrowed pyloric canal. This usually shows a slight upward curve to the left.

(b) *Shoulder sign.* An indentation into the barium filled pyloric antrum is caused by the thickened pyloric muscle.

(c) *Beak sign.* This occurs where the barium column extending into the narrowed pyloric canal is cut off, giving the appearance of a small beak.

(d) *Double track*—parallel folds of mucosa extend through the elongated pyloric canal.

The duodenal cap also frequently shows an enlargement of its base caused by the symmetrical indentation of the cap by the hypertrophied pyloric muscle.

After surgical myotomy the radiological features may still persist and some of these signs may be visible in adult life. Long-term follow-up of patients who had suffered from hypertrophic pyloric stenosis in infancy shows an increased susceptibility to gastric and duodenal ulcer in adult life.

Adult hypertrophic pyloric stenosis. Certain adults show thickened hypertrophied pyloric muscle.

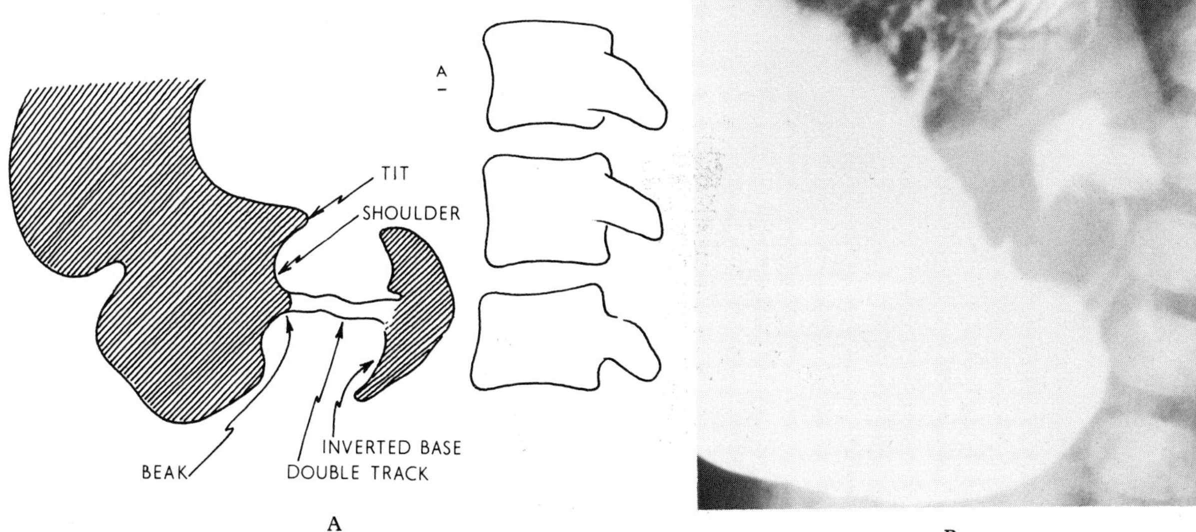

Fig. 33.8 A Line drawing showing the radiological signs of pyloric stenosis. B Barium meal of a case of pyloric stenosis showing the signs illustrated in Diagram A.

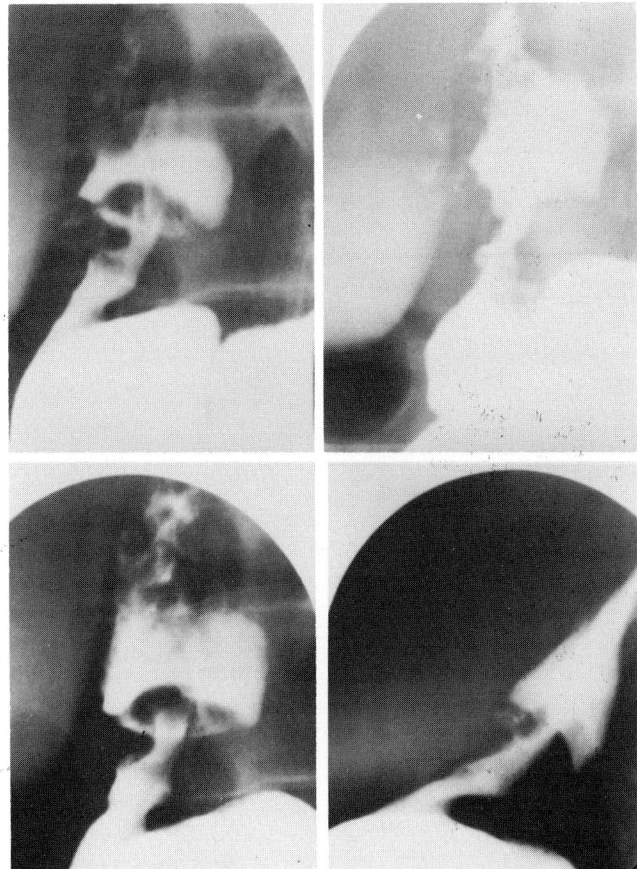

Fig. 33.9 Adult hypertrophic pyloric stenosis. Note the narrowed pyloric and prepyloric segment with the intervening fold thought to be characteristic of adult hypertrophic pyloric stenosis.

This is recognized radiologically by a narrowed pyloric canal with an altered prepyloric segment and a niche between the two segments.

It is difficult to determine what proportion of adult hypertrophic pyloric stenosis is secondary to pyloric ulceration. Certainly some cases of pyloric ulceration cause thickening and hypertrophy of the pylorus, but in some resected specimens of the pylorus no ulceration can be detected and the hypertrophy must be regarded as primary (Fig. 33.9) (pyloric torus defect) (Brebner, 1968, Keet, 1957, 1958).

ACQUIRED GASTRIC LESIONS

Foreign bodies in the stomach. The onward passage of ingested foreign bodies is governed by their ability to pass through the pyloric canal. Foreign bodies may be accidentally ingested, or in children and mental defectives bizarre foreign bodies may be swallowed and be retained in the stomach.

Such foreign bodies may become surrounded by food material and may occupy almost the whole of the stomach lumen (*bezoars*) (Fig. 33.10). The foreign bodies may also be wholly made up of swallowed material such as hair (*trichobezoar*), or may be composed of vegetable fibres giving rise to a *phytobezoar*.

Bezoars which in themselves are not radio-opaque present as smooth or lobulated filling defects in the barium-filled stomach and have a characteristic mobility on fluoroscopic palpation. This free mobility associated with the fact that the mass is wholly surrounded with barium, enables a bezoar to be differentiated from leiomyoma, polypoid adenoma and even encephaloid carcinoma of the stomach.

Hypertrophied gastric rugae. Along the greater curvature of the stomach the horizontal mucosal folds

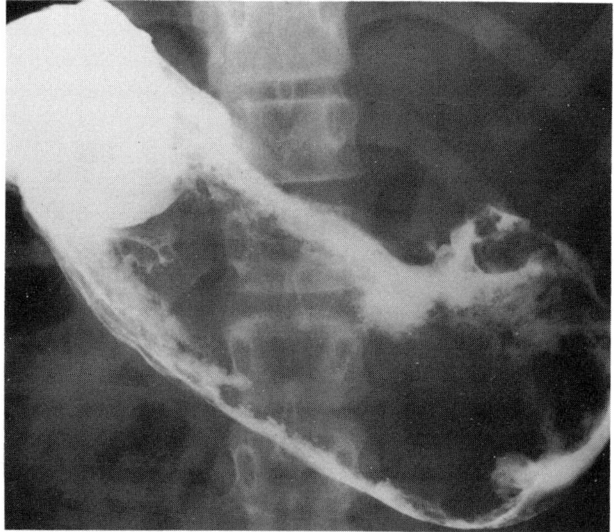

Fig. 33.10 Trichobezoar. Prone film showing large filling defect following the outline of the stomach with mottling produced by barium projecting into the interstices of the mass. On palpation bezoars show free mobility in the stomach unless they are large as illustrated.

form a distinctive pattern and are a necessary part of the physiological ability of the gastric organ to distend after a meal. Differentiation between prominent but normal folds and pathologically thickened folds can be extremely difficult.

Prominence of these folds presenting as polypoid thickening is seen in *Ménétrier's disease,* which is associated with a protein-losing enteropathy. Thickening and prominence of these folds has also to be differentiated from *lymphomatous infiltration* of the gastric wall and less commonly from *eosinophilic infiltration.*

Pliability of the gastric wall under fluoroscopic palpation is an important diagnostic feature in separating normal from infiltrated folds.

The advent of endoscopy with biopsy has rendered *parietography* obsolete as a method of determining the significance of these thickened mucosal folds. Parietography involved inducing a penumoperitoneum and simultaneous distension of the gastric lumen by effervescent powder. Features which allow differentiation by simple X-ray examination are listed in Table 33.1.

Table 33.1

Hypertrophic gastric rugae
1. Most marked over greater curvature
2. No rigidity of gastric wall
3. Normal peristalsis in affected area
4. No extragastric mass

Lymphomatous infiltration
1. May occur in any part
2. Stiffness of gastric wall
3. Absent peristalsis
4. May show extragastric mass and fixity to other organs

Crohn's disease of the stomach. Granulomatous infiltration of the gastric wall may occur in association with granulomatous lesions in other parts of the alimentary canal.

Occasionally, however, involvement of the stomach may present as an isolated lesion when differentiation from malignant disease may be difficult or impossible. As in other parts of the alimentary canal, the lesion is a transmural one with the stomach assuming a 'J' shaped appearance as the lesion most frequently commences in the pylorus. This is associated with loss of peristalsis and lack of distensibility in that portion of the stomach, and with rapid gastric emptying.

The changes in the mucosal pattern depend on the stage of the disease and the degree of healing, the normal complex mucosal pattern becoming replaced by a smooth pattern as healing occurs.

Volvulus of the stomach. Classically volvulus of the stomach is classified according to the plane around

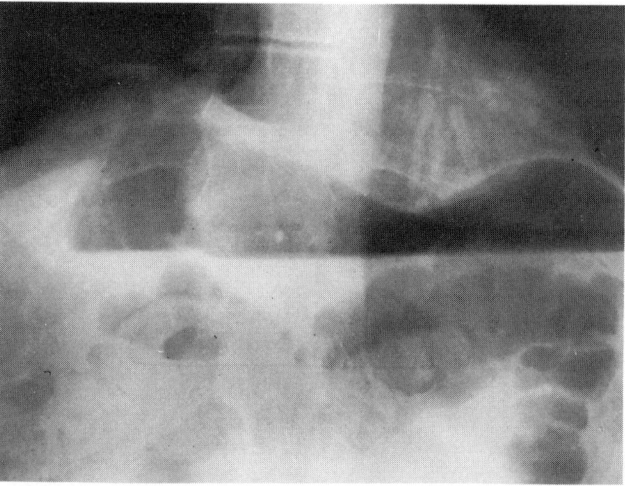

A

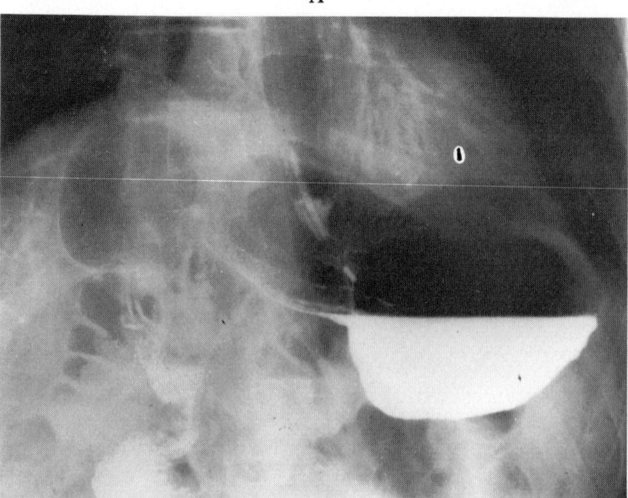

B

Fig. 33.11 Volvulus of stomach. A Simple erect film. B Erect film with barium.

which rotation occurs—the *organo-axial* which occurs around an axis through the cardio-oesophageal junction and pyloric canal, and the *axial* which occurs around a vertical *axis* through the cardio-oesophageal junction (Figs. 33.11 and 33.12).

In the vast majority of cases the twist occurs along the organo-axial line, the greater curvature of the stomach riding upwards. Consequent on this rotation the pylorus and pyloric antrum are directed downwards, and the presence of a duodenal cap and pyloric antrum constantly

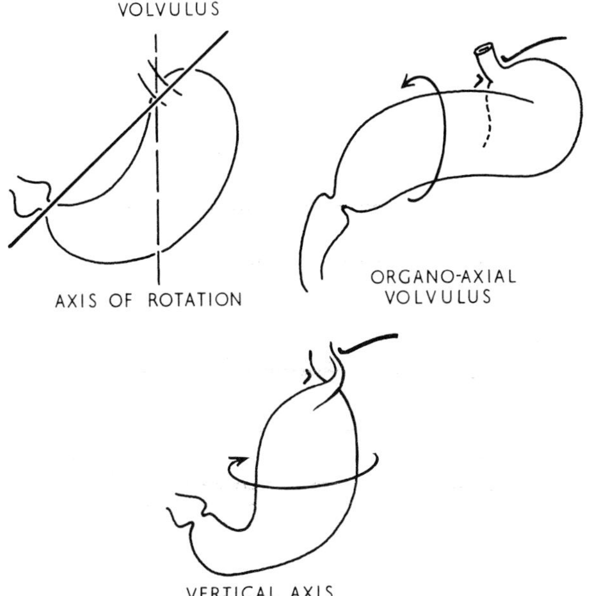

Fig. 33.12 Line drawing of the different types of volvulus. Organo-axial volvulus is most commonly seen in a hiatus hernia (rolling hiatus hernia).

directed downwards and backwards should suggest the possibility of a volvulus. Volvulus of the stomach is particularly liable to occur when the stomach is in a diaphragmatic hernia, and the presence of two fluid levels in a hiatus hernia should suggest a volvulus of the stomach within the hernial sac.

Organo-axial volvulus of the stomach has to be differentiated from many conditions especially a *'cup and spill'* (cascade) stomach, deformities due to external adhesions, and from displacements of the stomach. These latter conditions may be associated with some degree of rotation of the stomach.

A *'cup and spill'* stomach can be readily appreciated on lateral views of the stomach when the upper segment of the cascade stomach is seen to lie posterior to the main body of the stomach. Deformities due to perigastric adhesions are best excluded by careful palpation of the barium-filled stomach under fluoroscopic control. Mucosal relief studies in such cases show that there is no torsion of mucosal folds as seen in a true volvulus.

Gastric displacements. Enlargement of any one of the structures forming the gastric bed readily produces changes in the barium-filled stomach and the manner in which the shape and position of the stomach is altered gives a ready assessment of which organ is enlarged.

Variations in the position of the organs forming the gastric bed may cause difficulties in diagnosis. Thus, the normal spleen which usually lies along the long axis of the 10th left rib may lie above or even medial to the fundus of the stomach, creating the impression of a fundal tumour.

More usually enlargement of the spleen causes a forward and medial displacement of the stomach whilst masses originating in the left kidney usually displace the stomach forwards.

Lesions causing enlargement of the left lobe of the liver, however, lie anterior to the stomach and cause backward displacement of the fundus and body of the stomach.

Tumours of the body and tail of the pancreas causing enlargement of that organ produce forward displacement of the stomach. To detect such displacement it is essential that the horizontal ray films should be taken with the patient supine so that the filled stomach can fall backwards on the enlarged organ. Pancreatic cysts arising in the gastric bed usually present through the lesser omentum displacing the stomach forwards and stretching the lesser curvature around the cyst (Fig. 33.13). More rarely cystadenomas, especially affecting the distal half of the body of the pancreas, may present below the stomach causing an upward indentation of the greater curvature.

Smaller and more solid tumours may not present above or below the stomach but merely by forward displacement show a half shadow in the mid-part of the stomach, the mucosa being smooth and stretched in this portion of the stomach.

Prolapsed gastric mucosa. A polypoid appearance in the base of the duodenal cap may be due to herniation of the thickened mucosal folds into the duodenal cap. Prolapse of the gastric mucosa into the duodenal cap is less likely to be a cause of symptoms than the conditions sometimes associated with it, such as duodenal or gastric ulceration.

The prolapsed mucosa appears as a polypoid defect at the base of the duodenal cap and is most readily seen in compression studies of the duodenal cap. It has to be differentiated from the polypoid appearance of the mucosa caused by *Brunner's glands* and the cobblestone pattern of the *oedematous duodenal mucosa* often associated with duodenal ulceration or high gastric acidity. These defects, unlike prolapsed mucosa, are not localized to the base of the cap.

Gastritis. Inflammatory changes in the gastric mucosa are known as gastritis. The aetiological causes

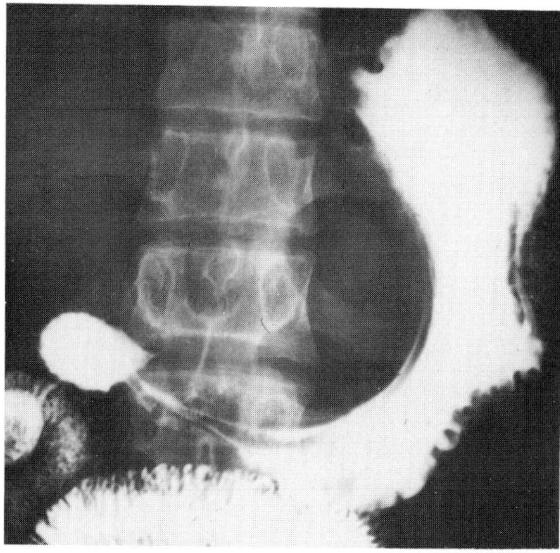
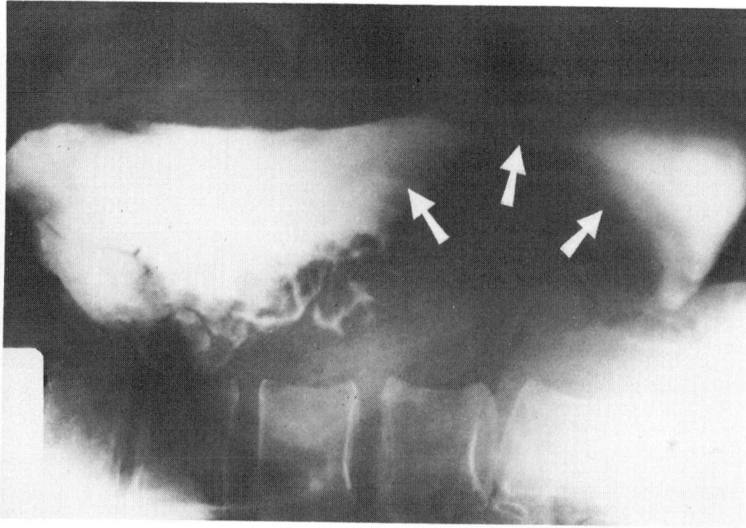

A B

Fig. 33.13 A Pancreatic cyst projecting above the lesser curvature showing characteristic displacement. B Pancreatic cyst. Lateral view of same case demonstrating the forward displacement of the stomach.

are numerous. They include alcohol and irritant foods and spices, and auto-immune and immune states leading to atrophy of the mucosa.

The double contrast technique has correctly focused attention on the changes in the areae gastricae as the only radiological evidence of gastritis (Fig. 33.14). Changes in the tone of the muscularis mucosa which may grossly alter the mucosal fold pattern in the stomach, do not in themselves constitute signs indicative of gastritis.

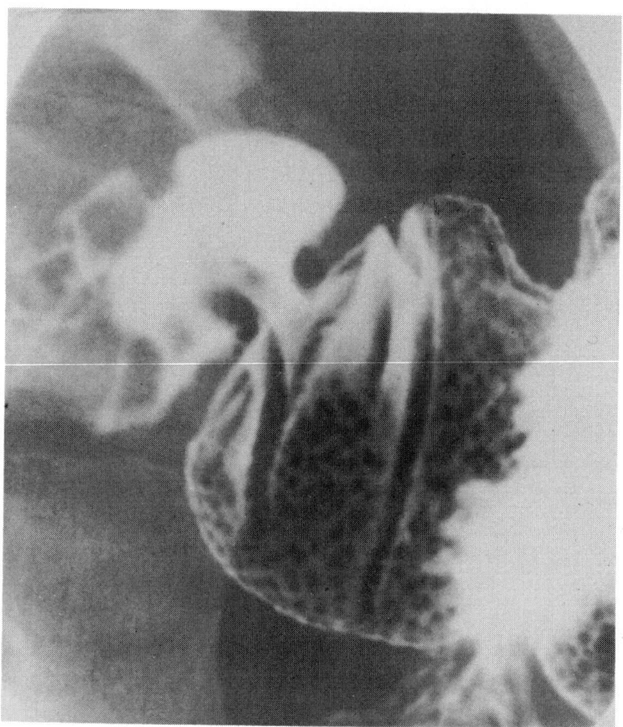

Fig. 33.14 Gastritis showing mammillary appearance. An associated duodenal ulcer is present.

Modern endoscopy has shown what marked changes can occur in the gastric mucosa without any apparent change in the radiological appearances.

Gastric atrophy and atrophic gastritis. In pernicious anaemia there is atrophy of the mucosa in the body and fundus of the stomach whilst that in the pyloric antrum appears relatively normal. Histological sections show there is atrophy of all coats of the stomach with a loss of the normal glands and relatively little cellular infiltration.

In atrophic gastritis the changes are usually less marked than seen in pernicious anaemia and tend to be more patchy in distribution. Histologically in this type of atrophic gastritis there is usually a greater degree of cellular infiltration of the mucosa and the atrophy may not involve the whole thickness of the wall as in pernicious anaemia. Patients with atrophic gastritis may have other auto-immune disease, e.g. Hashimoto's thyroiditis.

The radiological features of gastric atrophy and atrophic gastritis are similar although the former changes are more marked. The areae gastricae pattern is lost, and there is a dimunition in the size and number of mucosal folds, particularly well seen in the fundus and body of the stomach. The signs are best recognized in the conventional barium meal without paralysis and full distension. In the erect film the greater and lesser curvatures of the stomach tend to be parallel and the fundus of the stomach may have no mucosal pattern ('bald' fundus) (Fig. 33.15A and B). Sometimes the mucosal pattern may have a crumpled tissue paper appearance with thin folds running in a complete haphazard pattern (Fig. 33.16).

The pyloric antrum on the other hand is normal and shows normal peristalsis. Serial follow-up studies of

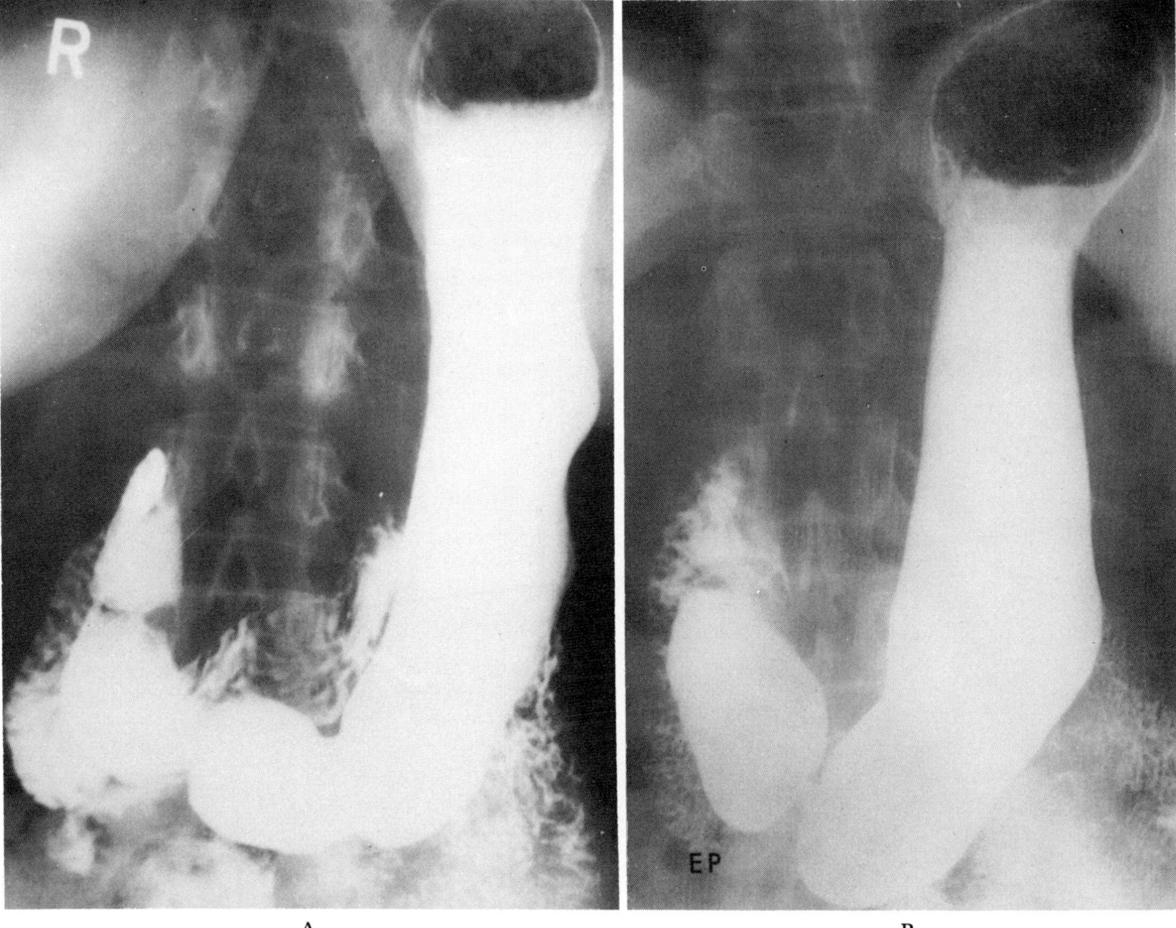

A B

Fig. 33.15 Radiological gastric atrophy in A pernicious anaemia and B atrophic gastritis. In each case the fundus of the stomach is smooth and devoid of folds as is the greater curve. The general shape of the stomach is tubular. There is active peristalsis in the antrum and the duodenal cap is normal.

cases of gastric atrophy are important as gastric polypi or adenocarcinoma may develop (Fig. 33.17). Whether follow-up examination should be by endoscopy or serial barium meals is not yet agreed. Any patient with Addisonian (pernicious) anaemia who develops iron deficiency or any form of dyspepsia should have a barium examination or endoscopy as a matter of urgency.

Hyperchlorhydria. There is overall correlation between the gastric parietal cell mass, maximum acid output of the stomach and the size of the gastric folds as demonstrated radiologically. At one extreme is the radiological gastric atrophy seen in pernicious anaemia and associated with total achlorhydria; at the other is the giant gastric rugae in the body and fundus and extending right down the greater curve seen in the **Zollinger-Ellison Syndrome.** In between these extremes lie the patients with high acid output and duodenal ulcer who have gastric folds of above average size. When gastric acid output is high the duodenal folds are also coarser than normal. In the Zollinger-Ellison syndrome these thickened folds may extend well down the jejunum, and miltiple peptic ulcers may occur (Fig. 33.18).

There may be giant gastric rugae in *protein-losing gastroenteropathy* but here the folds weep protein and not acid. In fact achlorhydria is frequently present.

Infiltration of the mucosa may be produced by *inflammatory changes, leukaemia, granulomata* or by *malignant deposits.* All these conditions cause enlargement and thickening of gastric rugae by infiltration of the mucosa with cells typical of the various conditions.

As noted above the interpretation of the significance of prominent gastric rugae which particularly affect the folds on the greater curvature of the stomach is difficult. Sometimes they are associated with a protein-losing enteropathy whilst in other instances they are apparently asymptomatic and unassociated with any disease.

Lymphomatous deposits and *lymphosarcoma* may be associated with prominent gastric rugae but these rugae are generally less pliable on fluoroscopic palpation than normal folds.

Interstitial emphysema. Gas formation in the wall of the stomach may result from a variety of causes but is an exceedingly rare occurrence. As with interstitial gas

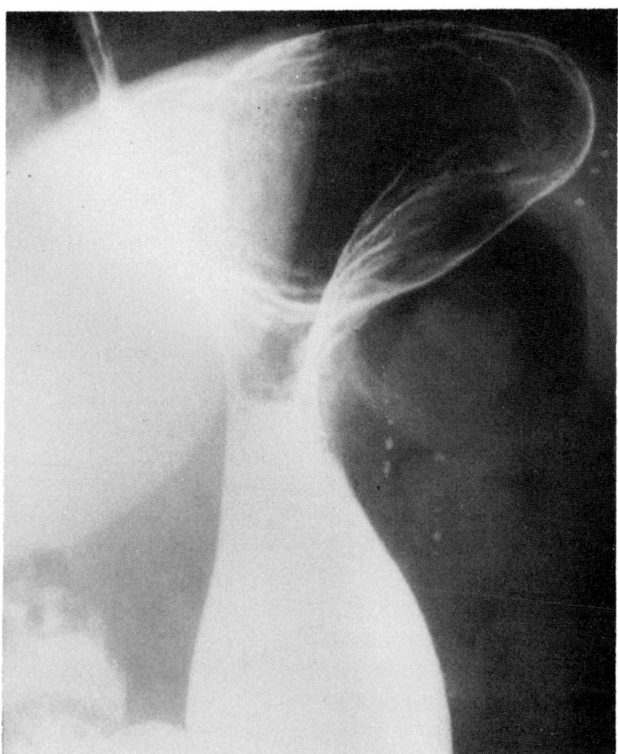

Fig. 33.16 Atrophic gastritis. The thin mucosal folds over the fundus and upper part of the greater curvature are shown.

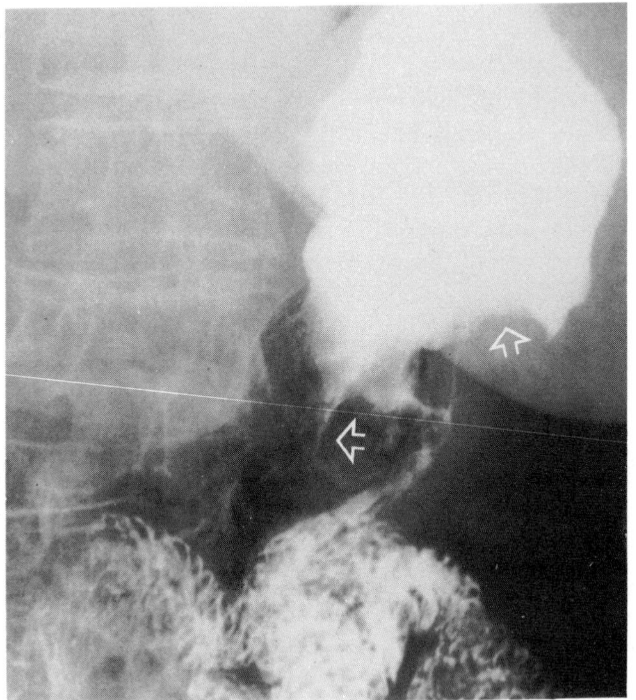

Fig. 33.17 Malignant change following atrophic gastritis in pernicious anaemia. The atrophic mucosa is shown by the absence of folds, and the cancer is in the mid-portion of the body of the stomach (*arrows*). (*Courtesy of Dr. T. Philp.*)

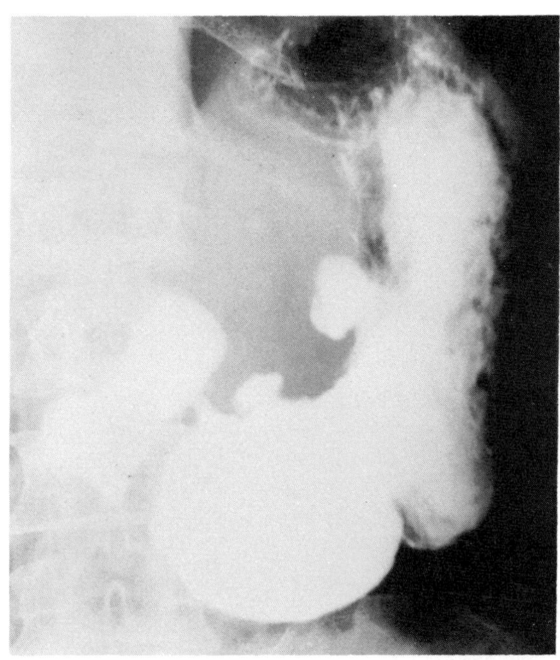

Fig. 33.18 Multiple gastric ulcers. A feature which is frequently noted in association with a delta-celled tumour of the pancreas (Zollinger-Ellison syndrome).

formation in other parts of the alimentary tract the commonest causes are *mechanical* (after gastroscopy), *inflammatory* (phlegmonous gastritis or enterocolitis) and *ischaemic* (infarction). It may also be associated with a raised intragastric pressure, with or without vomiting.

The radiological features are characteristic, a fine linear radiolucent shadow outlines the gastric wall on the plain radiograph of the abdomen.

GASTRIC ULCER

Apart from ulceration occurring in the stomach caused by the ingestion of *drugs* (e.g. aspirin, Butazolidin, steroids, etc.) and ulcers associated with *trauma* or *burns* (Curling's ulcer) the cause of the spontaneously developing peptic ulcer is unknown. Certainly peptic ulceration only occurs in those parts of the alimentary canal which are bathed in the acid/pepsin secretions.

Our knowledge of peptic ulceration has been greatly increased as a result of the development of fibreoptic endoscopy, and although it had been known for many years that the vast majority of gastric ulcers occur along the lesser curvature of the stomach, the natural history of the acute gastric erosions and the chronic gastric ulcer (with its phases of development and healing) has only recently been appreciated.

The radiological features of the acute mucosal erosion are vastly different from those seen in the established or chronic ulcer, and an appreciation of the type of lesion

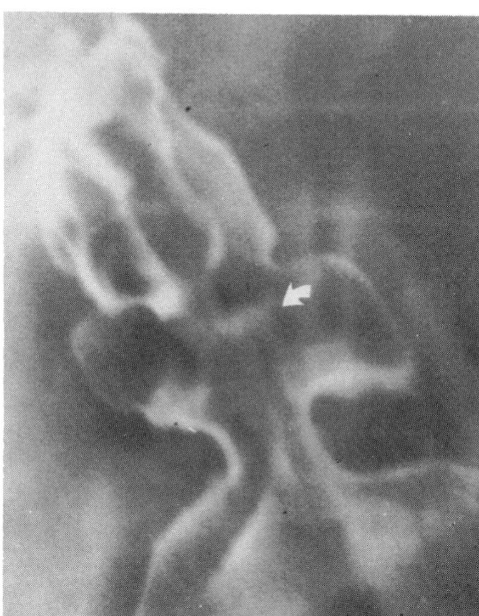

Fig. 33.19 Acute peptic ulcer in the duodenal cap showing fleck of barium surrounded by oedema (cf Fig. 36.23, p. 774) and disturbance of the longitudinal folds.

likely to be met in any clinical situation has considerable influence on the accuracy of radiological diagnosis.

Probably all ulcers commence as mucosal erosions and the established ulcer develops by penetration of the erosion into the submucosa and through the muscularis mucosa, giving rise to a chronic ulcer. The whole thickness of the gastric wall may be breached giving rise to a perforation of the ulcer into the peritoneal cavity or penetration into an adjoining viscus.

Perforation of the ulcer into the general peritoneal cavity gives rise to peritonitis and an 'acute abdomen' erosion into a major gastric artery causes haematemesis or melaena.

Healing of a gastric ulcer may cause fibrosis, giving rise to pyloric stenosis if the ulcer is situated near the pyloric canal, or less frequently to an hour-glass deformity of the stomach if the ulcer lies in the body of the stomach.

Gastric erosions and mucosal ulcers. Small gastric erosions which are frequently multiple may present with haematemesis. Small erosions can only be recognized by gastroscopy but larger erosions causing loss of mucosal thickness may be seen with double contrast barium meal examination. Patients presenting with a history of melaena or haematemesis or a recent acute history of dyspepsia are likely candidates for acute gastric erosions and a careful search for such erosions should be undertaken.

As the erosion does not penetrate through the mucosa and consequently has little depth, profile views are less informative than *en face* views. It is important to realize that quite large areas of mucosal loss may occur without any great depth of penetration of the crater (Figs. 33.19 and 33.20). This is particularly so in the elderly patient.

The radiological signs which may be seen in mucosal erosions are:

(a) *Ring sign.* The undercut edge of the ulcer may remain filled with barium whilst the centre of the crater may remain free of barium, giving a 'ring' appearance. Gas bubbles trapped between the mucosal folds can be recognized by the blurred outline of the barium ring being outside the clear-cut inner margin whilst the reverse holds in ulcers.

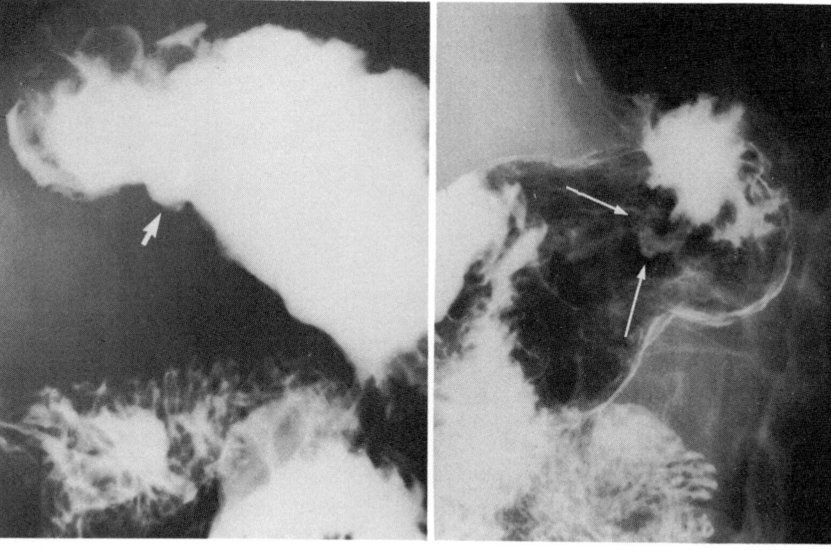

A B

Fig. 33.20 High gastric ulcer A in the barium filled stomach, B with double contrast. The ulcer crater is viewed *en face* in the double contrast studies and the irregular nature of the ulcer crater can be appreciated.

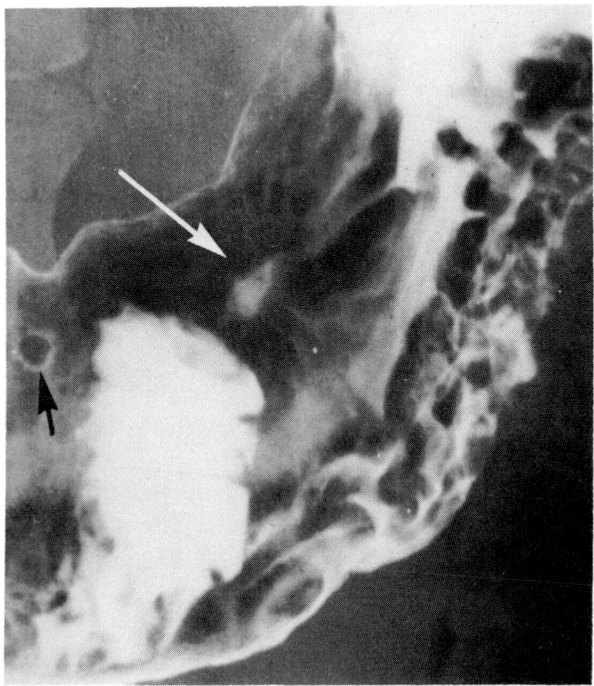

Fig. 33.21 Gastric ulcer seen in double contrast with the folds extending into the ulcer crater (*white arrow*). Black arrow shows the characteristic appearance of an air bubble. Note that the inner margin of the air bubble is sharply defined while the outer edge of the barium surrounding the air bubble is indistinct. This is the complete reverse of the appearances in acute gastric erosion.

(b) *Arc sign.* If the mucosal edge is less undercut in parts of the ulcer crater only a fragment of the barium ring may appear giving rise to an arc sign.

(c) *Smudge sign.* Occasionally the whole crater may be filled with a shallow barium trough giving rise to a localized smudge of barium, and this may be difficult to differentiate from a residuum of barium trapped between mucosal folds (Fig. 33.21).

In mucosal ulcers and indeed in chronic gastric ulcers too much emphasis should not be placed on the circular nature of the ulcer. Many peptic ulcer craters are linear and acute erosions equally may have a linear character (Fig. 33.22).

Chronic peptic ulcer. When the ulcerative process has broken through the mucosa into the submucosa, the muscularis mucosa is irritated and various spastic deformities of the stomach wall occur. Infiltration of the gastric wall with inflammatory cells and oedema produces swelling around the ulcer crater, thus apparently increasing the depth of penetration of the ulcer (Figs. 33.23 and 33.24). The ulcer may actually erode through the gastric wall and its base be formed by pancreas, liver or omentum. In such cases an accessory pocket is formed outside the stomach wall and may show a fluid level in the erect position. The demonstration on the erect film of a fluid level in a gastric ulcer almost invariably means that the ulcer has penetrated through the gastric wall (Fig. 33.24). The oedematous collar around a simple ulcer crater forms a half-shadow on the radiograph lying outside the line of the wall of the stomach. This can be differentiated from a similar appearance produced by a malignant collar around an ulcerating carcinoma (Carman's sign) when the half shadow lies within the line of the wall of the stomach.

During the development of the ulcer crater the ulcer crater is triangular in shape, as viewed in profile, and often in the greater curvature of the stomach spasm of the muscularis mucosa produces an indrawing of that curvature (the incisura) (Fig. 33.24).

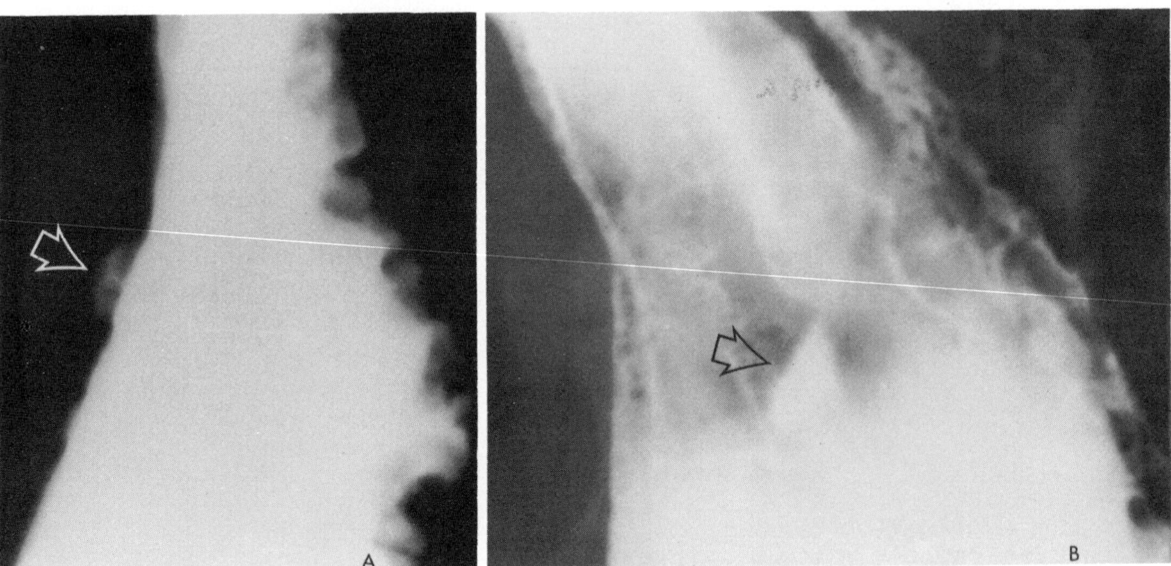

Fig. 33.22 A Filled views of the lesser curvature of the stomach showing an ulcer crater. B *En face* view demonstrating the linear margins of the ulcer.

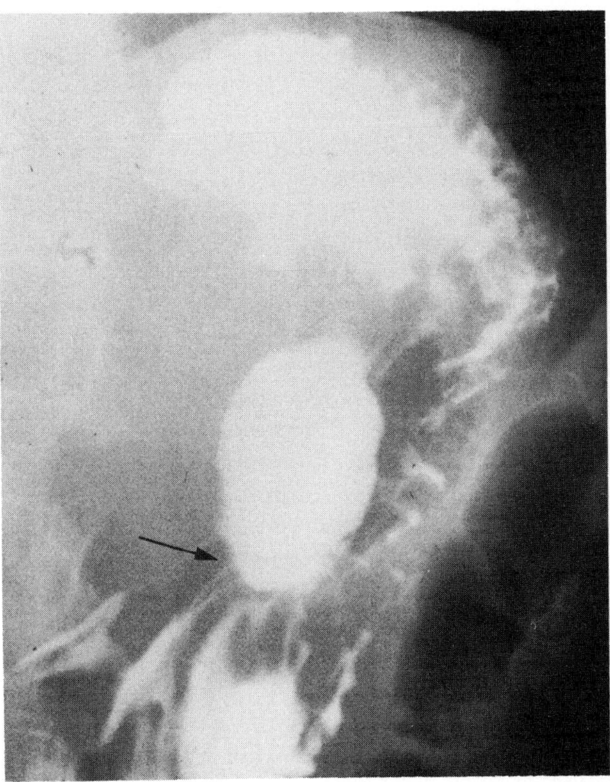

Fig. 33.23

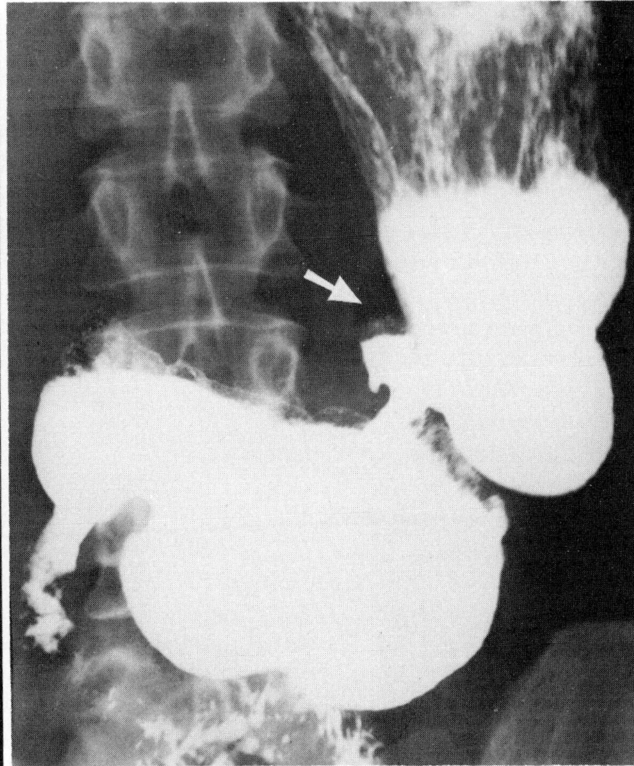

Fig. 33.24

Fig. 33.23 Giant gastric ulcer on the lesser curvature of the stomach showing the cavity filled with barium. Arrow at the lower part of the illustration indicates the gastric folds extending into the ulcer crater—a feature diagnostic of benign ulceration.

Fig. 33.24 Penetrating gastric ulcer. The gas cap above the ulcer crater indicates that total penetration of the gastric wall has occurred (*arrow*).

A less common site for ulcers is the pyloric antrum but here again ulcers tend to occur along the lesser curvature. Eccentric spasm of the greater curvature results in a gross distortion of the antrum mimicking a pyloric cancer. In such cases examination after the administration of 0·1–0·5 mg of intravenous glucagon or 20 mg Buscopan will usually relax the spastic muscle and allow the ulcer crater to be seen. Frequently the ulcer crater lies astride the lesser curvature (saddle ulcer) and is relatively shallow.

Ulcers situated in the pyloric canal produce a degree of gastric stasis due either to spasm or fibrotic pyloric stenosis. Examination of cases of pyloric stenosis should only be undertaken after adequate gastric aspiration if any information as to the nature of the obstruction is to be obtained from the radiograph.

When an ulcer crater is demonstrated in profile view it shows a characteristic square appearance, whilst double contrast studies of a barium-filled crater appear as a rounded irregular opacity seen to be surrounded by a transparent halo representing the oedematous collar. The gastric folds, however, are seen to extend into the crater, a feature which is of diagnostic importance in differentiating the simple ulcer from a cancer (Figs. 33.21 and 33.23).

At this stage the base of the ulcer crater is covered by a slough and healing occurs by epithelialization of the base by ingrowth from the edges of the crater. In large ulcers complete epithelialization of the ulcer may not be achieved and this probably accounts for the frequency with which the ulcers tend to relapse. During healing the ulcer crater becomes shallower, more triangular and gradually disappears in the profile view. A flat plaque of barium frequently remains in the site of the ulcer crater and it is often difficult to differentiate such a scar from a shallow unhealed crater.

Complications of peptic ulcer. (a) *Perforation.* A gastric ulcer may rupture through the gastric wall and allow the escape of gastric contents into the peritoneum (see Ch. 36, p. 760).

(b) *Haematemesis and melaena.* Bleeding may occur from either a gastric erosion or in a chronic ulcer when a vessel is involved in the base (see Ch. 36, p. 773).

(c) *Penetration.* Ulcers on the posterior gastric wall are more prone to penetration and they readily become adherent to the structures forming the gastric bed.

(d) *Fibrosis.* Fibrotic deformities of the stomach consequent on healing of a gastric ulcer are not now commonly seen. Earlier treatment has avoided the deep ulcers which healed with grotesque deformities of hour-glass and pseudodiverticulum of the stomach. Shortening of the lesser curve of the stomach may follow penetration of an ulcer crater into the lesser omentum with approximation of the cardio-oesophageal and pyloric orifices; when this occurs the body of the stomach becomes dilated and may suggest a large diverticulum.

RADIOLOGY OF THE POST-OPERATIVE STOMACH

The varied and numerous surgical operations that have been undertaken for the treatment of peptic ulceration may be classified as follows.

(a) Local excision—
1. Sleeve resection, local resection
2. Pyloroplasty
3. Vagotomy (truncal and selective)

(b) Partial excision—
1. Antrectomy plus restitution of normal passage (Bilroth I, Schumaker, etc.) (Fig. 33.25).
2. Antrectomy plus gastro-jejunal anastomosis (Polya I and Bilroth II) (Fig. 33.26).
3. Antrectomy with valve formation and gastro-jejunal anastomosis (Polya II, Lane, Finstere, Hoffmeister, etc.) (Fig. 33.27).

(c) Total excision of stomach—
1. Oesophago-jejunostomy
2. Colonic replacement of stomach

(d) Short circuit operations—
1. Anterior and posterior gastro-enterostomy
2. Gastro-enterostomy with vagotomy

Radiological technique. It is essential that in the examination of a stomach which has been resected or where a short circuit has been performed, only a small quantity (2 oz) of barium sulphate/water mixture be used to demonstrate the mucosal pattern in the gastric stump and in the afferent and efferent jejunal loops. Until these structures have been examined and localised films taken, no attempt should be made to distend the gastric remnant with barium.

Since the site of surgical anastomosis as determined by the surgeon frequently migrates as the gastric stump dilates post-operatively, no single position can be advocated as the best for visualisation of the stoma. However, the rapidity with which the gastric stump empties demands that the major part of the examination be conducted in the recumbent position. Rotation into the supine right and left oblique position will allow double contrast views of the stoma line to be seen in full face view and in profile (Fig. 33.28).

Profile views of the niche alone can be misleading as the surgical oversewing along the lesser curvature of the stomach often gives rise to pocketing of barium and simulates niche formation.

The stomach is then filled with barium and the rate of emptying of the gastric stump varies considerably.

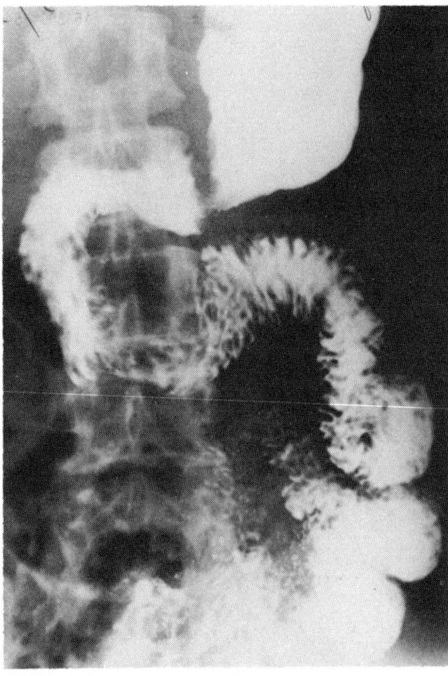

Fig. 33.25

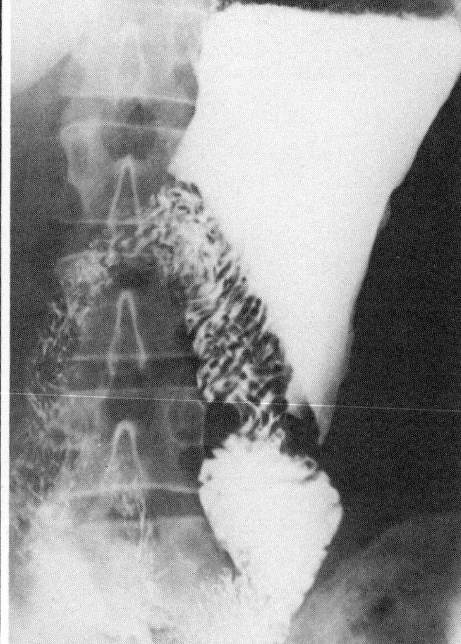

Fig. 33.26

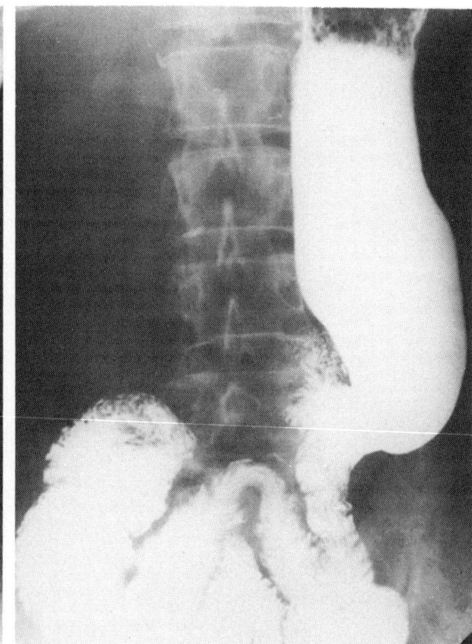

Fig. 33.27

Fig. 33.25 Billroth I gastrectomy. Barium filled stomach demonstrating the similarity to the normal appearances, with the duodenal loop filled in continuity.

Fig. 33.26 Billroth II showing the absence of any valve at the site of anastomosis and afferent and efferent loops filled.

Fig. 33.27 Polya gastrectomy—with the valve formation. Compare with Fig. 33.26. No filling of afferent loop has occurred.

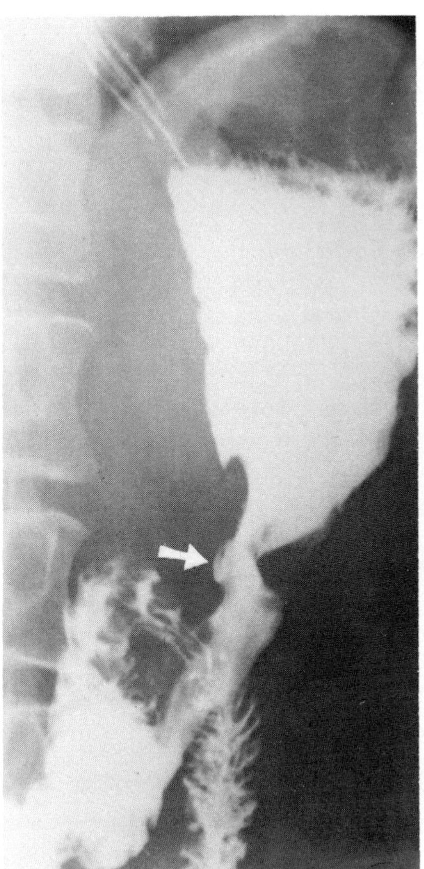

A

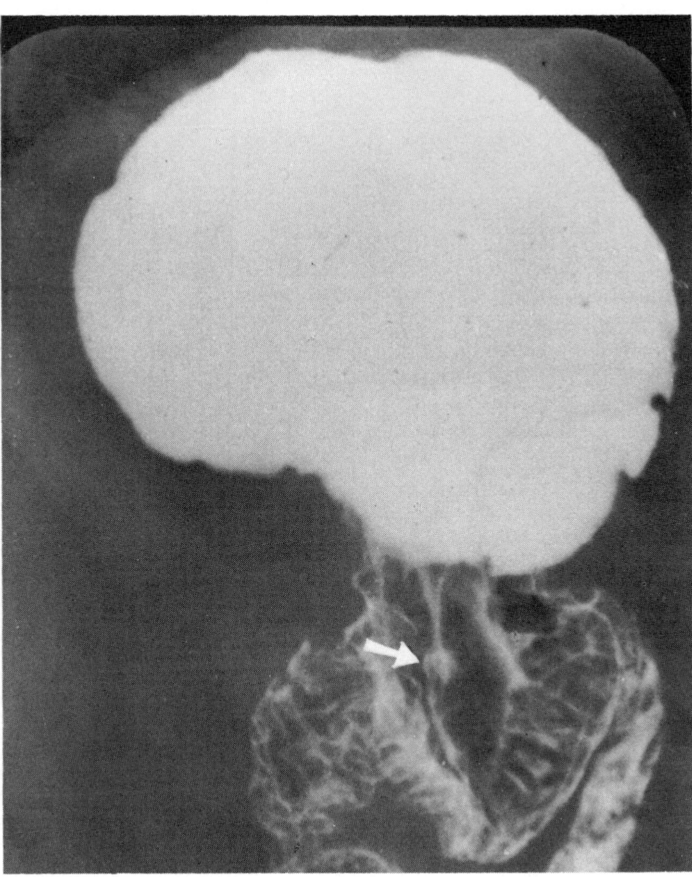

B

Fig. 33.28 A Anastomotic ulcer after Polya gastrectomy demonstrating the ulcer in the efferent loop. Note that the afferent loop has not filled proximal to the ulcer. B Recurrent anastomotic ulcer demonstrating the ulcer crater shown *en face* through the double contrast study of the efferent loop.

The valves which are carefully fashioned by the surgeon at operation frequently seem to have little effect on the rate of gastric emptying. Deductions of clinical implications from the rate of gastric emptying should also be made with great care as there is a wide variation in the rate of emptying.

In short-circuit operations, e.g. gastroenterostomies, attempts should be made to decide on the relative amount of barium emptying via the pylorus and via the stoma, and examination should attempt to outline both these routes. When gastroenterostomy is associated with vagotomy there may be a considerable decrease in the gastric tone associated with hypomotility and delay in the gastric emptying.

The commonly used method of pyloroplasty consists in a longitudinal incision in the line of the pyloric antrum 2–5 cm on either side of the pylorus and then sewing the edges of the horizontal incision transversely. The result is a pouch at the level of the suture and a constriction proximal and distal to it.

In patients who have suffered from chronic duodenal ulceration the duodenal aspect of the pyloroplasty may be altered. Asymmetrical pouching frequently occurs as a result of scarring and fixation of the posterior wall of the duodenal cap. The lines of traction of the pylorus also result in flattening of the mucosal pattern with the folds running parallel. The anterior wall folds may be drawn into a transverse pattern and the superimposition of both patterns may superficially mimic radiating folds in ulcer.

The sphincteric action of the pylorus is lost so that the stomach empties rapidly and no gastric resting juice is seen.

COMPLICATIONS OF GASTRIC SURGERY

Anastomotic ulcers. Following gastroenterostomy or gastrectomy the upper jejunal loops become exposed to the direct action of gastric juices and peptic ulceration may develop.

Peptic ulcers most commonly occur in the efferent loop within two inches of the anastomosis to the stomach, less commonly they occur astride the anastomotic line and still less frequently in the gastric stump or in the afferent jejunal loop. The frequency of recurrent ulceration after surgical operation varies considerably with

Table 33.2 Distribution of recurrent ulcer, 1947–1957 (After Small, 1964)

Type of recurrent ulcer	No. of patients
Jejunal	56
Gastric	11
Suture line	4
Recurrent or reactive duodenal ulcer	4
TOTAL	75

published reports. The sites of occurrence in one series are shown in Table 33.2.

As with peptic ulcers occurring elsewhere the firm radiological diagnosis should rest on the demonstration of the ulcer crater, but in its absence associated spasm of the jejunum and the coarseness and widening of the mucosal folds frequently indicate the presence of an ulcer.

Recurrent ulceration after a gastroenterostomy may occur in the duodenal cap at the site of the original ulcer but anastomotic ulceration is more common. The accuracy rate of radiological diagnosis is approximately 80 per cent.

Radiological features. The radiological features of anastomotic ulceration are:

(a) Demonstration of the ulcer niche—this is best demonstrated as a round barium filled opacity in full face view (Figs. 33.29 and 33.30). It is important that only small quantities of barium sulphate should be used as ingestion of larger quantities obscures the loops. The ulcer niche must not be confused with surgically produced diverticula which are caused by oversewing of the mucosa around the anastomotic line.

(b) Associated spasm. This especially affects the efferent loop, where a niche with an incisura or multiple spastic areas may be seen.

(c) Irregularity and thickening of the jejunal folds due to oedema or jejunitis. The fine feathery pattern of the mucosa in the jejunum is replaced by thickened, coarse, transverse folds.

Functional disturbances

Dysphagia. Truncal vagotomy may be followed by dysphagia occurring 7 to 10 days after operation. Its causation is not fully understood and its frequency varies in different series. It usually lasts from one to several weeks and resolves spontaneously.

The barium swallow shows a tapering smooth lower end of the oesophagus similar to that seen in achalasia of the cardia. The radiological signs disappear when the clinical symptoms clear.

Other changes in the alimentary tract after vagotomy consist in hypotonia and delayed emptying of the stomach and also a transient hypotonia of the small bowel.

Hypotonia of the gall bladder with delayed emptying and stone formation has also been reported to occur after vagotomy.

Far less frequently dysphagia is due to a peptic oesophagitis or a stricture may occur after gastric operations. In some instances the peptic oesophagitis may be part of the original condition demanding surgery or it may be associated with a prolonged use of the indwelling gastric tube.

Dumping syndrome. Following resection or short-circuit operations on the stomach the patient may suffer from an epigastric bloating and distension followed by nausea, faintness, sweating and hypotonia. These may be

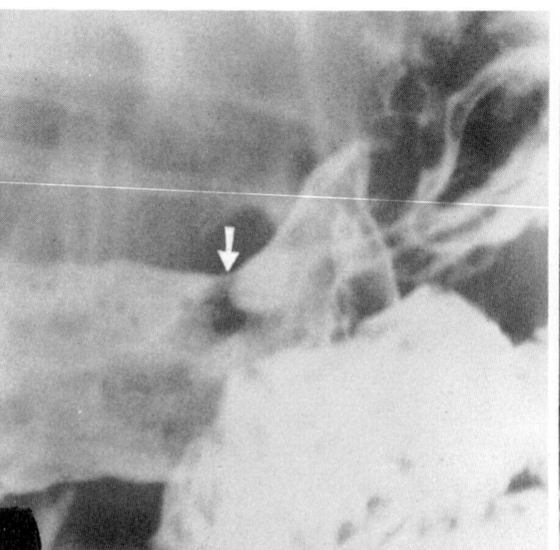

Fig. 33.29A

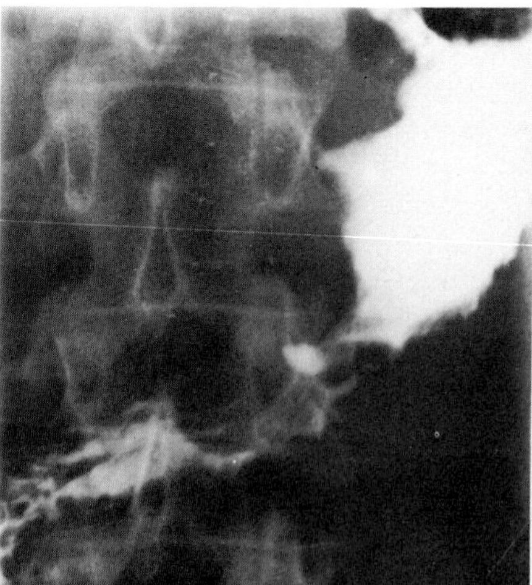

Fig. 33.29B

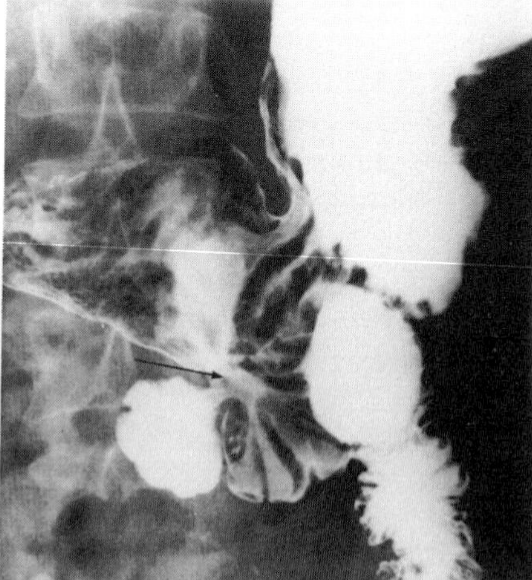

Fig. 33.30

Fig. 33.29 (A and B) Anastomotic ulcers developing after a Billroth I gastrectomy. The ulcer crater has occurred in the duodenum just beyond the suture line.

Fig. 33.30 Anastomotic ulcer developing in the efferent loop after gastroenterostomy. Ulcer crater filled with barium (*arrow*).

aggravated by a meal rich in starch. Many hypotheses have been put forward to account for this distressing syndrome—vasomotor collapse, hypoglycaemia and other causes associated with the rapid passage of the meal into the upper jejunum.

Great care must be taken in assessing the radiological findings as rapid emptying of the gastric stump with some degree of dilatation of the upper coils of jejunum may be a normal finding and not associated with symptoms.

The transit time of the barium meal through the small bowel is also more rapid than in the normal patient.

Afferent loop syndrome. Vomiting of bile unmixed with food may occur after gastrectomy or gastroenterostomy and is the result of regurgitation of bile and pancreatic secretions back into the stomach after the meal has left the stomach.

Food in the stomach is the normal stimulus to the appearance of these secretions in the second part of the duodenum. They normally mix with the ingested meal. As a result of kinking or malposition of the afferent loop or stoma these secretions remain in the duodenum and spill over into the stomach after the meal has left. Bile and pancreatic secretion not only cause gastric irritation and vomiting but may cause oesophagitis with stricture formation.

Radiologically after a gastrectomy or gastroenterostomy the meal is seen to pass into both afferent and efferent loops although most will enter the efferent loop. Failure of any barium to enter the afferent loop should suggest that some kinking or other abnormality is present and that the patient may be a candidate for the 'afferent loop syndrome'.

Obstruction of the efferent loop gives rise to vomiting after eating but the vomitus consists of food and bile. Usually obstruction of the efferent loop occurs as it passes through the mesocolon.

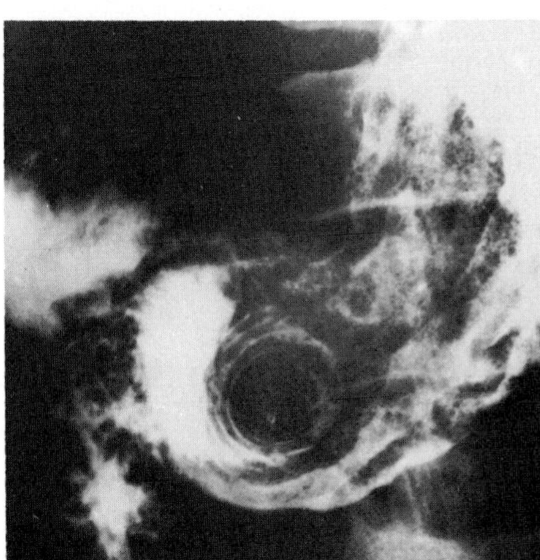

Fig. 33.31 Retrograde intussusception showing the appearances of intussusception after a gastroenterostomy with the characteristic circular appearance of the mucosal folds around the defect.

Retrograde jejunal intussesception. A delayed complication of gastroenterostomy is a retrograde intussusception of the efferent loop into the stomach. The clinical manifestations are those of vomiting and colicky abdominal pain suggesting obstruction, although some patients have relatively few symptoms.

Radiologically the herniated loop appears as a rounded filling defect in the stomach and the coiled appearance of the mucosal folds clearly indicates the nature of the filling defect (Fig. 33.31). Herniation of the afferent loop into the stomach is an extreme rarity. In the immediate post-operative period invagination of the oedematous enterostomy stoma into the stomach may give rise to an acute obstructive syndrome with vomiting. Radiologically an obstruction at the stoma is all that is usually seen.

A complication in the immediate post-operative period after gastroenterostomy is a herniation of coils of small bowel into the lesser sac. These constitute a grave emergency as the loops become quickly strangulated and plain films are frequently negative (no-gas obstruction, see Ch. 36). The value of 'negative' plain films under these conditions must be recognised if mistaken diagnosis is to be avoided.

GASTRIC NEOPLASMS

Benign tumours

Benign tumours of the stomach may arise from any of the constituent layers of the gastric wall. The commonest are those arising from the mucosal glands (*adenoma*) and from the muscle coats (*leiomyoma*). Less common benign tumours are *lipoma* derived from fat cells and *Schwannoma* originating from nerve sheaths.

All tumours arising from the connective tissue components of the gastric wall (leiomyoma, Schwannoma and lipoma) present as smooth, well-demarcated defects protruding into the barium filled stomach. Mucosal examination shows that the mucosa is stretched over the tumour but not invaded and the edges of the mass are sharply defined (acute angled) from the remainder of the gastric wall. Leiomyoma may grow to a considerable size and the stretched mucosa may ulcerate due to ischaemic changes giving rise to a characteristic ulcer crater over the apex of the mass (Figs. 33.32 and 33.33). Massive haematemesis may be the presenting symptom of a leiomyoma. A sarcomatous change may develop in a leiomyoma and this change should be suspected when there is a large portion of the leiomyoma lying outside the gastric wall as well as projecting into the stomach.

Gastric lipoma are difficult to distinguish from leiomyoma but these radiological features are helpful in diagnosis.

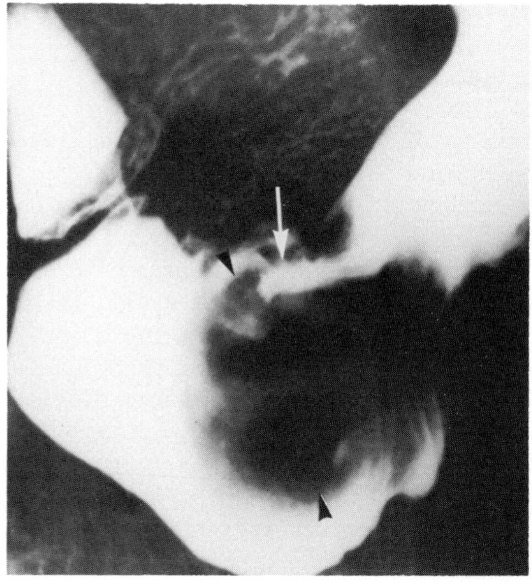

Fig. 33.32

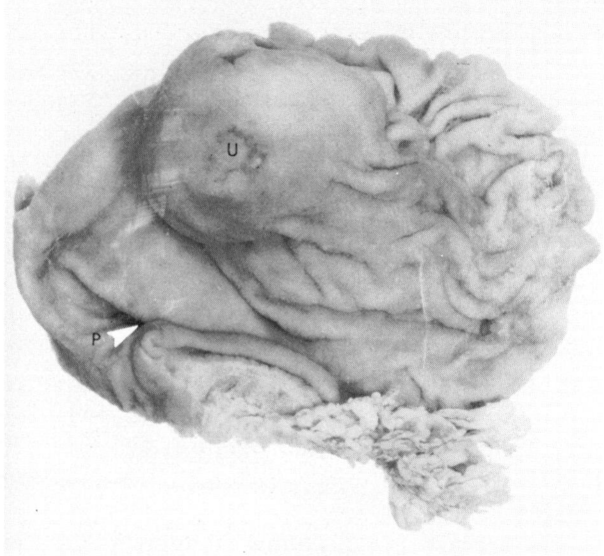

Fig. 33.33

Fig. 33.32 Leiomyoma. Barium examination showing well-marked filling defect with clear-cut outlines (*black arrows*) and large white arrow indicates site of ulceration on superficial aspect of mass.

Fig. 33.33 Pathological specimen after resection. P—indicates pyloric canal. U—superficial ulceration over tumour mass.

(a) The tumour readily changes its shape depending on gastric pressure and peristalsis.

(b) The tumour adapts to fill the gastric lumen with peristalsis.

(c) On palpation considerable mobility and compression of the mass can be recognised.

Gastric polyps. The common types of gastric polyp are hyperplastic with no malignant potential or an adenomatous polyp which is a true tumour and often becomes malignant. Hamartoma and retention polyps are far rarer types of polyp and are usually seen in diffuse gastro-intestinal polyposis. The gross and radiological appearances of the hyperplastic and adenomatous polyps are shown in Table 33.3.

The term 'gastric polyposis' applied when multiple polyps are seen in the stomach (Fig. 33.34) is meaningless as both adenomatous and hyperplastic polyps may co-exist in this condition. The frequency of malignant change is probably more related to the associated chronic gastritis as much as to the likelihood of malignant change in the polyp itself (Si-Chun Ming, 1976).

Benign tumours arising from the gastric mucosa may be villous papilloma or polypoid adenoma, both types

Table 33.3

	Hyperplastic polyps		Adenoma	
Characteristics	Gross pathology	Radiology	Gross pathology	Radiology
Multiplicity	Common	—	Occasionally	—
Location	Random	Random	Antral	Antral
Average size	1 cm	1–4 cm	Papillary type up to 4 cm and flat less than 2 cm	Same
Shape	Oval or nipple-shaped	Round or oval filling defect	Papillary or villous	Irregular outline
Contour	Smooth	Smooth	Irregular	Sessile irregular outline
Crevices	Absent	No barium within the filling defect	Present	Flecks of barium within the mass (soap bubbles)
Base	Sharply defined	Clear outline	Ill-defined	Blurred
Pedicle	Slender	May be long and thin	Broad	None seen

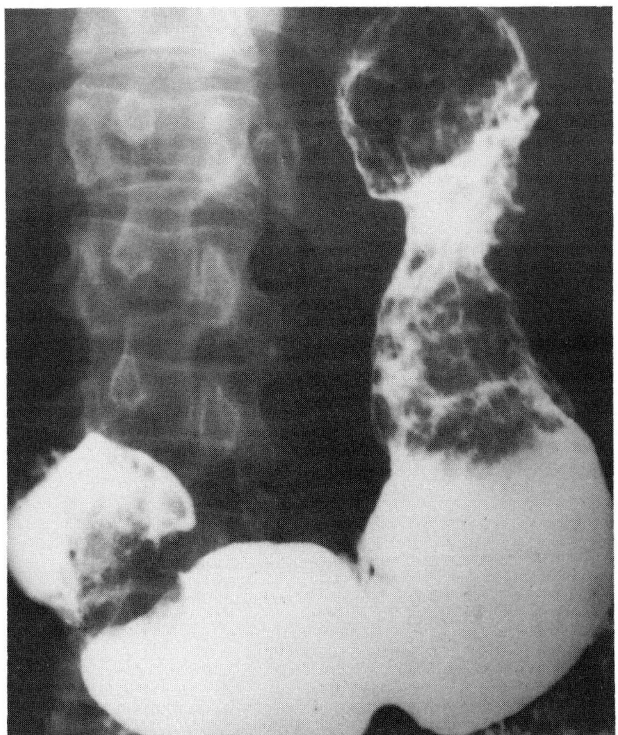

Fig. 33.34 Gastric polyposis. Note the large number of smooth outlined filling defects present in the body of the stomach and also in the pyloric antrum. Their constancy permits differentiation from food defects.

frequently being classed as gastric polypi. True polypoid adenomas of the stomach contains glandular elements within the polypi and many are pre-cancerous. Polypoid adenoma frequently occurs in pernicious anaemia and may precede the development of gastric cancer (Fig. 33.35). Polypoid adenomas need careful surveillance as malignant change may occur and radiological features which may help to differentiate them from the more benign are shown in Table 33.3.

A broad base with some rigidity of the gastric wall usually implies malignant change but when these changes are present the disease is usually advanced. Multiple polyps in the stomach may be mistaken for ingested food particles (Fig. 33.34) but careful palpation will reveal the fixed nature of the filling defects with polypi. Pancreatic rests are occasionally found in the stomach presenting as small submucosal polyps (Fig. 33.36).

Malignant tumours

Gastric cancer accounts for 20 per cent of all deaths from gastro-intestinal malignant disease and in certain areas of the world, e.g. Japan and Iceland, it may account for 50 per cent. Other malignant tumours such as lymphoma and sarcoma are relatively rare but their differentiation, particularly lymphoma, is important as the prognosis is so much better than that of gastric cancer.

The double contrast examination of the gastric mucosa popularized by Japanese workers has resulted in the detection of gastric cancer at an early stage when the tumour is located to the gastric mucosa. Detection of the tumour at this stage results in a marked improvement in the five-year survivals after surgical resection. These results have only been achieved after extensive mass screening surveys, and it is regrettable that in hospital practice in most countries the tumour has spread well

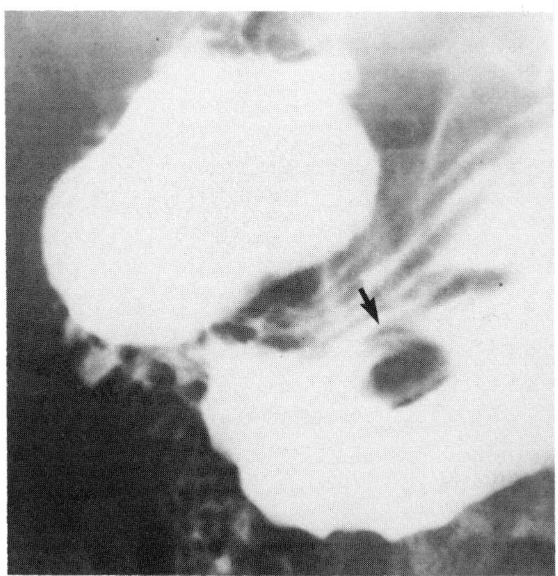

A

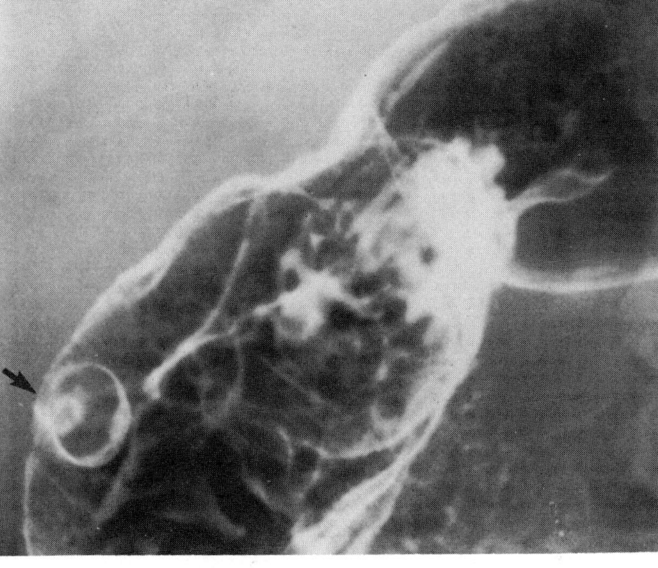

B

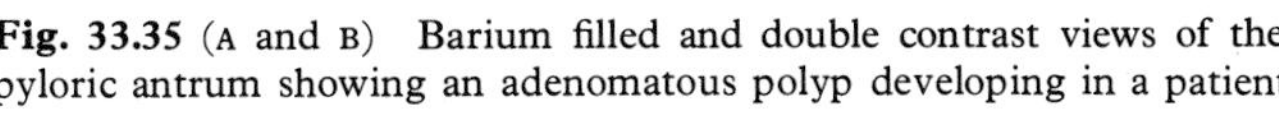

Fig. 33.35 (A and B) Barium filled and double contrast views of the pyloric antrum showing an adenomatous polyp developing in a patient with pernicious anaemia.

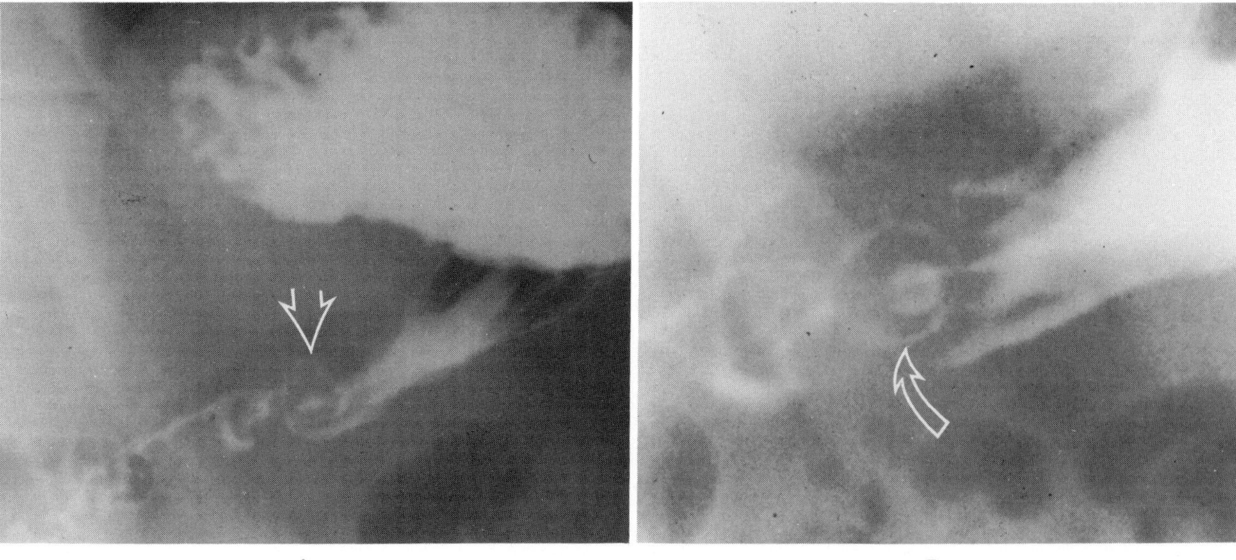

Fig. 33.36 (A and B) Pancreatic rest. Filled and double contrast views of the pyloric antrum showing a smooth round filling defect on the posterior wall caused by a pancreatic rest. The mucosal folds on the anterior wall appear as linear markings through the defect. Occasionally a small dimple of barium indicates the remnants of a rudimentary pancreatic duct system, and even more rarely branching of a rudimentary duct system filled with barium is seen, giving a pathognomonic appearance.

beyond the mucosa when it is first seen. The Japanese experience also suggests that many tumours may remain and spread in the mucosa for some time before infiltration of the submucosa occurs.

The radiological features of mucosal cancer are only seen in good quality double contrast studies, when the mucosal folds can be seen to terminate abruptly at some distance from a shallow ulcer or a raised plaque. The sharp cut-off of the folds (the spaces between the barium filled streaks) are an important differentiating point from the radiation of the folds towards a healing benign ulcer crater (Figs. 33.37 and 33.38).

When the tumour has extended beyond the mucosa it may present macroscopically as a polypoid mass projecting into the stomach (encephaloid type) (Fig. 33.39); a deep ulcer crater with a marked overhanging lip (ulcerative); or a variety in which submucosal spread is associated with marked contraction of the stomach wall (scirrhous type) (Fig. 33.40). Extensive infiltration of the

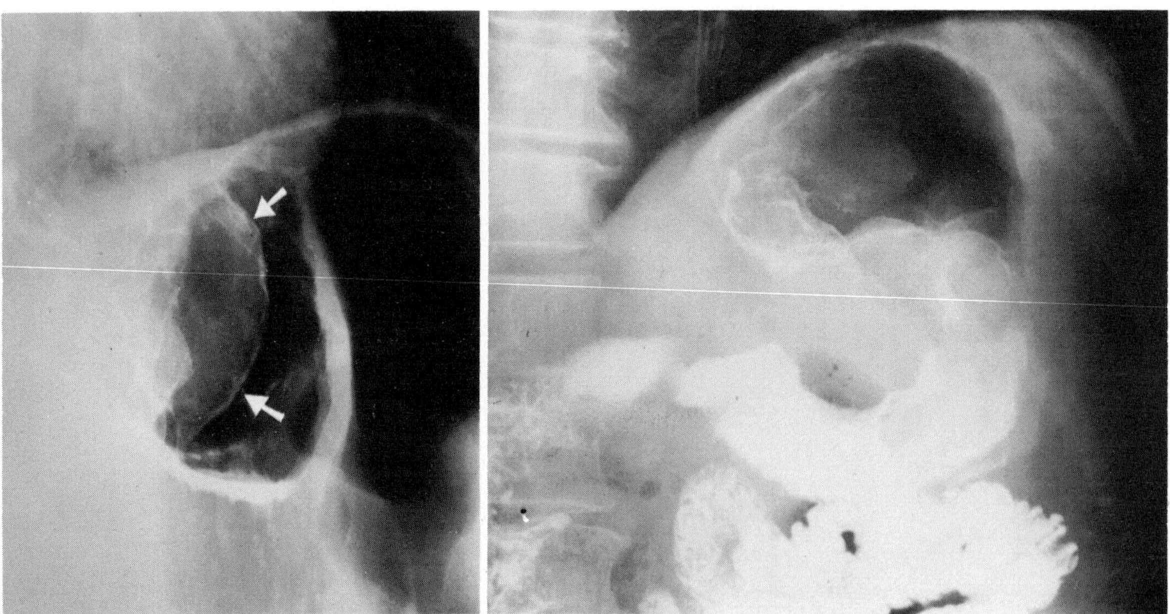

Fig. 33.37 Gastric carcinoma. Tumour projecting into the gas bubble in the fundus of the stomach and outlined by double contrast.

Fig. 33.38 Encephaloid growth of stomach extending from fundus through the body and showing extensive filling defects.

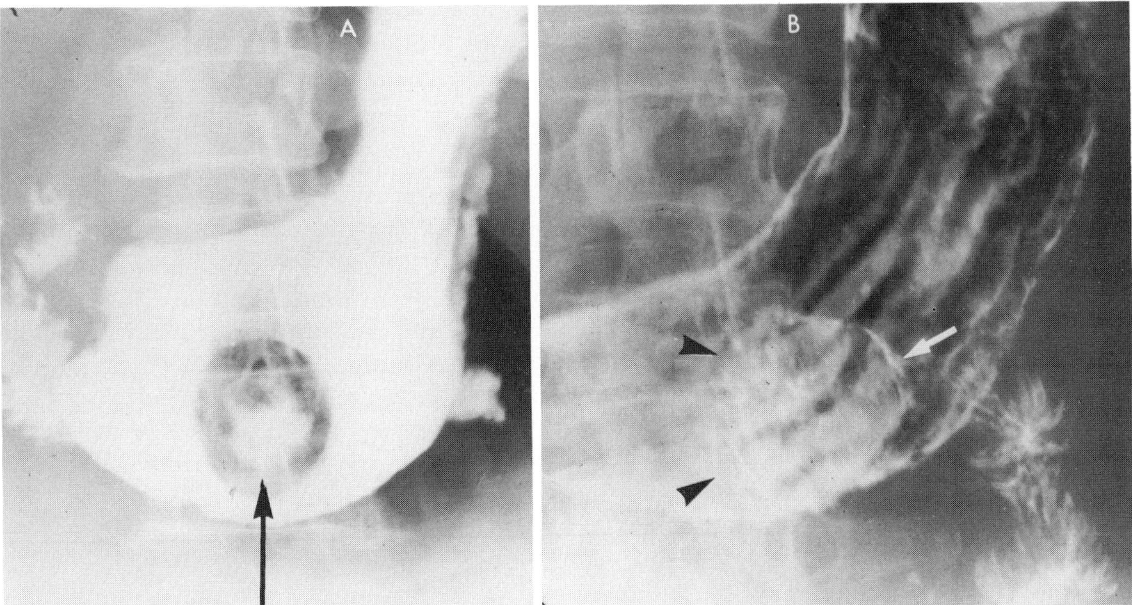

Fig. 33.39 A Encephaloid tumour with central ulceration mimicking leiomyoma. B Supine oblique view demonstrating the disruption of the mucosa by the tumour.

submucosa of the stomach produces a small rigid stomach with a considerable diminished capacity and lack of distensibility (linitis plastica) which has been likened to a leather bottle.

Ulceration in a gastric cancer may result from necrosis of the tumour mass and the extent of necrosis may be such that little tumour remains and ulceration is the main feature. Malignant change in a peptic ulcer is now considered to be a rare finding although the histological difficulties of differentiating infiltration from distortion of normal mucosal glands by fibrosis may be considerable.

Although these macroscopic appearances of gastric cancer differ considerably there is little evidence that prognosis is influenced by the type of growth. In all types spread occurs by lymphatics to the regional glands and via the portal blood stream to the liver and distally.

Radiological features. The radiological features of *mucosal* cancer have already been described. The *encephaloid* tumour produces a mass with fingerprint

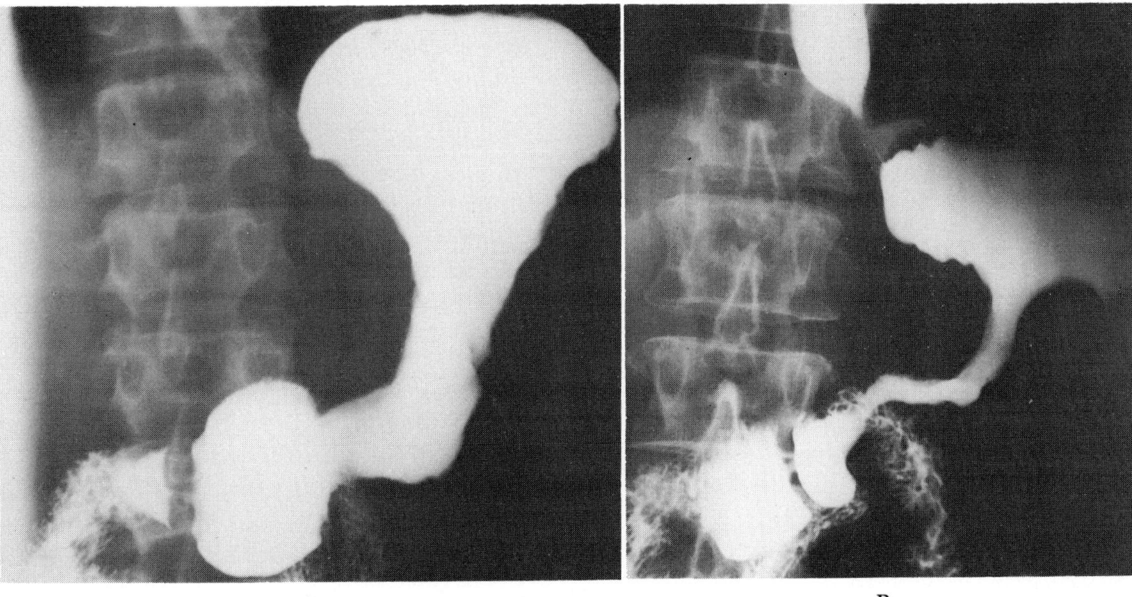

A B

Fig. 33.40 A Scirrhous carcinoma of the stomach demonstrating the narrowed, rigid segment in the middle third of the stomach with little evidence of ulceration. B Same case 6 months later showing the extensive infiltration of the tumour and the narrowed segment present in the mid-portion of the stomach.

deformities in the barium filled stomach and in double contrast studies the destruction of the mucosal pattern and the imperceptible blending of the mass with the normal mucosa is readily appreciated. Rigidity of the gastric wall and decreased peristalsis imply submucosal spread of the tumour.

Ulcerating growths of the stomach show an irregular crater with the rolled edges of the growth forming a half shadow around the crater (Carman's sign). The crater usually lies within the lumen of the stomach differentiating it from the giant peptic ulcer whose base lies beyond the line of the gastric wall. Likewise the halo of oedematous mucosa surrounding a simple peptic ulcer lies in the line of the gastric wall as opposed to the rolled edge of the malignant tumour which lies within the line of the stomach wall.

Scirrhous tumours of the stomach present with rigidity of the gastric wall, loss of peristalsis and destruction of the mucosal pattern. Advanced tumours produce lack of distensibility of the stomach and if the pylorus is involved may produce pyloric obstruction. In other instances the infiltrative process may keep the pylorus open with the consequent rapid emptying of the stomach.

GASTRIC INFILTRATION

The stomach wall may be infiltrated by several pathological lesions. Mention has already been made of *granulomatous* infiltration (Crohn's disease, p. 688) but the stomach may also be infiltrated by eosinophilic processes giving rise to *eosinophilic gastritis* and also be *lymphoma*.

Eosinophilic gastritis presents as a finely spiculated appearance in the pyloric antrum and the diagnosis from other types of gastritis is largely a histological one.

Lymphomatous infiltration may occur as part of a generalized disease or may present as a solitary manifestation. The radiological features of lymphomatous infiltration may be:

(1) A large superficial ulcer usually on the posterior wall of the stomach or the lesser curvature with thickened mucosal folds around the ulcer crater. When lymphoma presents as thickened folds the condition may be difficult to differentiate from hypertrophied gastric folds associated with Ménétrier's disease.

(2) A large tumour with little change in the contour or capacity of the stomach.

(3) Multiple polypoidal masses in the gastric mucosa often with central ulceration (target sign).

(4) Extension of the growth into the duodenum.

Metastatic tumour deposits may also occur in the gastric wall. The commonest site of the primary growth is melanotic carcinoma. The deposits show central ulceration (target appearance) and are very similar to the deposits seen in lymphoma.

MALIGNANT RECURRENCE AFTER GASTRECTOMY

The radiological study of the patient suspected of suffering from recurrent carcinoma demands special attention to the common sites of recurrence.

Consideration of the site of the original growth and the area of lymphatic drainage surgically removed to some extent determines the site of recurrence.

Local spread of the growth may involve adjoining viscera, e.g. pancreas or colon, and it should be appreciated that in such cases invasion of the stomach or jejunal loops is from the serosal side and consequently mucosal ulceration may be a relatively late sign.

The radiological findings may be grouped into (a) local recurrence (Figs. 33.41 and 33.42), (b) lymphatic node recurrence and (c) spread to adjoining viscera.

(a) *Local recurrence*

(i) Loss of distensibility of the lesser curve indicating infiltration.

(ii) Narrowing and elongation of the gastric stoma, often over a considerable distance.

(iii) Later, irregularity of the gastric mucosa with superficial ulceration.

(b) *Lymphatic node recurrence*

(i) The superior gastric and pancreatico-lienal are usually the only remaining lymph nodes—enlargement of these nodes will produce pressure indentation defects around the cardio-oesophageal area.

(ii) Later invasion of the gastric remnant from the involved nodes will result in stiffening of the gastric wall—later the infiltration may lead to a linitis plastica type of appearance.

(c) *Recurrence in local viscera*

(i) Opacification of the afferent loop is essential to demonstrate recurrence in the pancreatic bed and in the pancreatico-lienal group of lymphatic glands, and this is shown by segmental areas of narrowing and later dilations of the afferent loop. Complete narrowing of the afferent loop indicates diffuse involvement of the pancreatic bed.

(ii) Recurrence in the adjacent small bowel is shown by dilated and angulated loops containing stretched mucosal folds, often with atypical small bowel gas shadows on the plain films.

(iii) Recurrence in the transverse colon is a sequel of spread to the serosal surface and appears as small imprints on the transverse colon.

(iv) Recurrence in the mesentery and distal small intestine is shown by coarsening of the mucosal

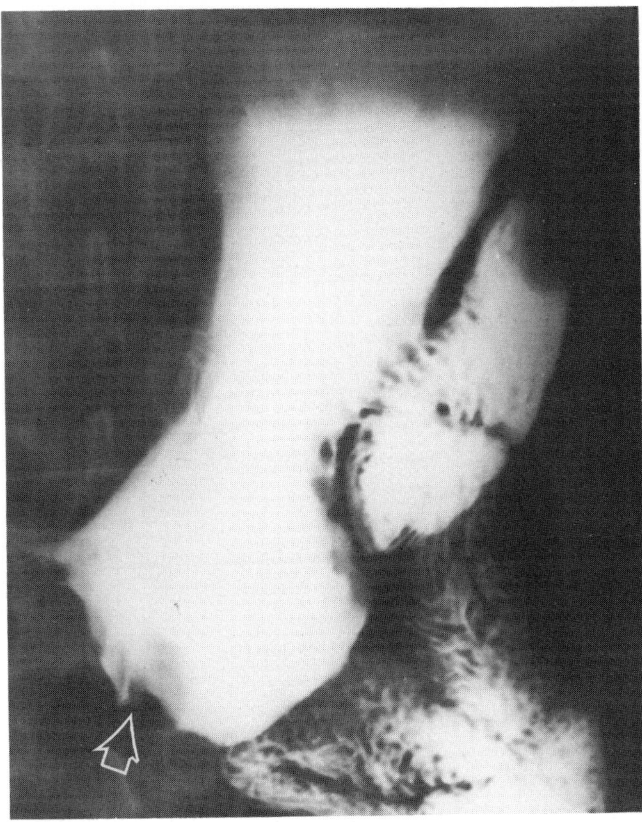

Fig. 33.41

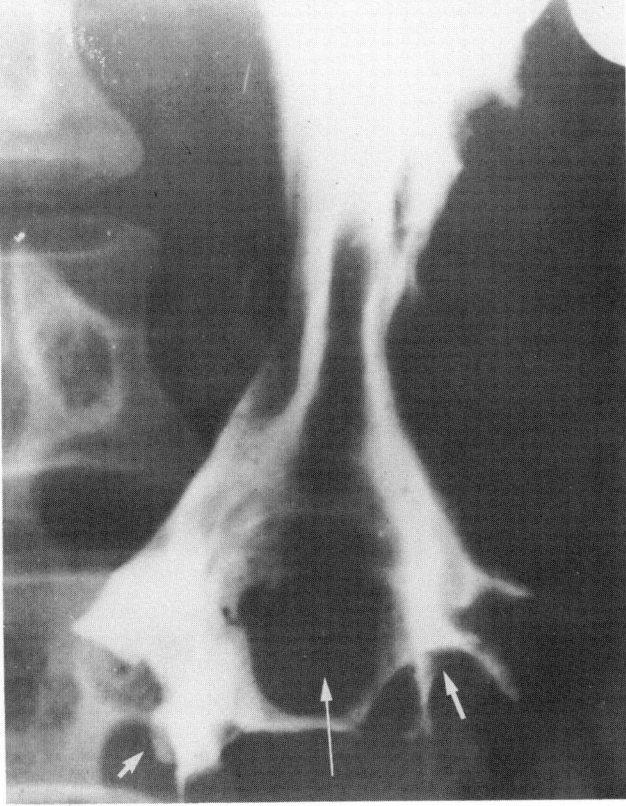

Fig. 33.42

Fig. 33.41 Carcinoma developing in pyloric antrum after a gastroenterostomy. Atrophy and lack of distensibility of the pyloric antrum frequently occurs after a gastroenterostomy. The malignant change in such antra has to be differentiated from simple atrophy of the antrum.

Fig. 33.42 Recurrent carcinoma developing after a partial gastrectomy, demonstrating the extrinsic fingerprint deformities and involvement and destruction of the gastric wall (*arrows*).

pattern associated with slight dilatation and narrowing of the gut lumen.

(v) Metastatic recurrence in the liver may be associated with enlargement of that viscus. Such enlargement is not frequently demonstrated even when considerable in size. Crescentic impression on the gastric remnant indicates enlargement of the liver.

THE DUODENUM

Anatomy. The duodenum consists of the bulb and pars superior constituting the first part of the duodenum. The bulb of the duodenum represents the first inch or so of the duodenum and has a triangular appearance—in the cadaver it is not a recognizable separate anatomical part of the duodenum.

The second or descending portion of the duodenum lies to the right of the spine and contains the duodenal papilla with the important opening of the bile and pancreatic ducts at the ampulla of Vater.

The third or horizontal portion of the duodenum crosses the spine and extends horizontally to the arteriomesenteric bundle and then upwards to the duodenojejunal flexure.

Technique of investigation. The duodenum is investigated as part of an upper gastro-intestinal examination and the two examination methods of compression study and double contrast, are equally important.

Lateral films with an over-couch tube are particularly useful to demonstrate the descending part of the duodenum and lesions occurring in the pars superior (post bulbar).

For a more detailed examination hypotonic duodenography (as described on p. 685) is used.

CONGENITAL ABNORMALITIES

Stenosis or narrowing of the second part of the duodenum may occur as a congenital abnormality. The site of narrowing is usually in the second part of the duodenum and varies from a thin membrane crossing the duodenum to an atretic segment with complete discontinuity of the bowel. The thin membrane associated with stenosis may lead to ballooning of one part of the diaphragm forming a localized sac and probably accounts for one type of so-called intraluminary diverticulum.

Sixty per cent of cases of duodenal stenosis are associated with other congenital anomalies and one third of the patients have Down's syndrome. A significant number also suffer from oesophageal atresia and microcolon.

When the stenosis is marked or complete, symptoms of vomiting occur with the first feeds immediately after birth. Plain films of the abdomen in the erect position demonstrate two fluid levels, one in the distended stomach and a second level in the distended duodenum proximal to the stricture. The supine film demonstrates the distension of the stomach and first part of the duodenum.

The possibility of other sites of stenosis in the colon must be looked for in all cases of duodenal stenosis and a barium enema should be performed to exclude colonic lesions.

When the obstruction is less severe symptoms may be mild and adult life may be reached before the lesion presents. Long-standing incomplete obstruction results in dilation of the duodenum above the site of obstruction.

Duodenum inversum and para-duodenal hernia. The normal 'C' curve of the duodenum may be reversed and the third part of the duodenum passes across the abdomen above the first part.

This malrotation of the bowel may be associated with the development of minor paraduodenal fossae on both sides of the spine. These fossae are peritoneal sacs formed by the incomplete fusion of the four peritoneal layers of the primitive colon. Their importance lies in the fact that herniation of small bowel may occur into these sacs forming an internal hernia and while they almost never cause obstruction they can nevertheless cause abdominal symptoms (Fig. 33.43).

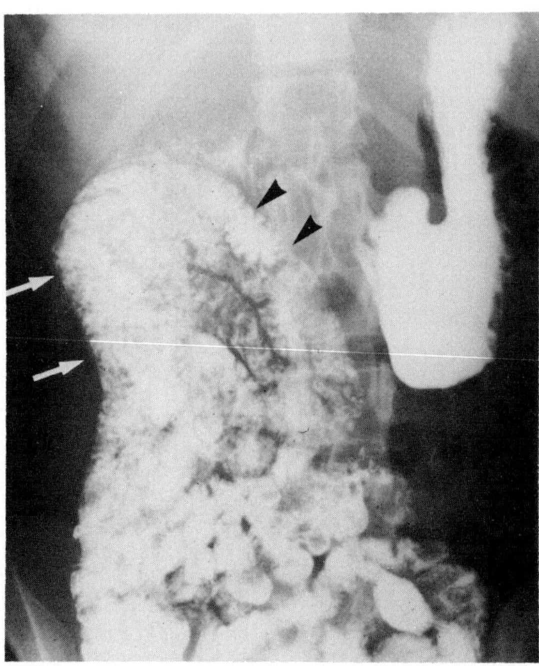

Fig. 33.43 Barium meal follow-through examination showing localization of coils of small bowel (arrowed) in the right hypochondrium in a paraduodenal fossa. (*From* Stuart, A. E., Smith, A. N. & Samuel, E. (Eds.) (1975) *Applied Surgical Pathology*. Oxford: Blackwell.)

Radiological diagnosis is made by a study of the follow-through films when the fixed coils of small bowel are seen to be immobile although their mucosal pattern is hardly altered.

Diverticula. Congenital duodenal diverticula differ from colonic diverticula in the fact that they contain all the muscular coats of the duodenum and are not herniations of the mucosa.

They most frequently arise on the medial wall of the duodenum from the second or third part. They may have quite narrow necks and food residues may be seen in the sac (Fig. 33.44). They may be associated with jejunal diverticula but frequently occur alone. They may be multiple and grow to quite large size. Duodenal diverticula occurring around the ampulla of Vater (periampullar diverticula) may obstruct the common bile duct or in rare instances the duct may actually open into the diverticulum.

Annular pancreas. Over-development of the uncinate process of the head of the pancreas leads to the development of a ring of pancreatic tissue surrounding the second part of the duodenum, the annular pancreas. The surrounding ring of tissue may sometimes be largely fibrous in nature and contain little pancreatic tissue.

Obstructive symptoms due to an annular pancreas may occur in infancy but in other less marked cases adult life may be reached before symptoms are noted.

Barium meal examination will reveal the dilated duodenum with the filling defect appearing as a major indentation on the lateral aspect of the descending portion of the duodenum.

Annular pancreas has to be differentiated from extrinsic pressure from abdominal lymph glands. In these the major deformities are on the medial aspect of the duodenum and the deformities are exaggerated in the prone position.

Duodenal ileus. A to-and-fro movement of barium frequently occurs in a normal patient in the supine position. Such physiological movements are, however, not associated with any dilation of the duodenum or any real stasis.

Stasis in the duodenum with dilatation may occur in association with arterio-mesenteric pressure (Fig. 33.45), although this entity is not wholly accepted by some clinicians. Typically the symptoms are relieved by the patient adopting a hands/knees position and radiologically the distended duodenum is seen to end at the level of the arterio-mesenteric bundle. The obstruction is associated with considerable peristaltic activity but in

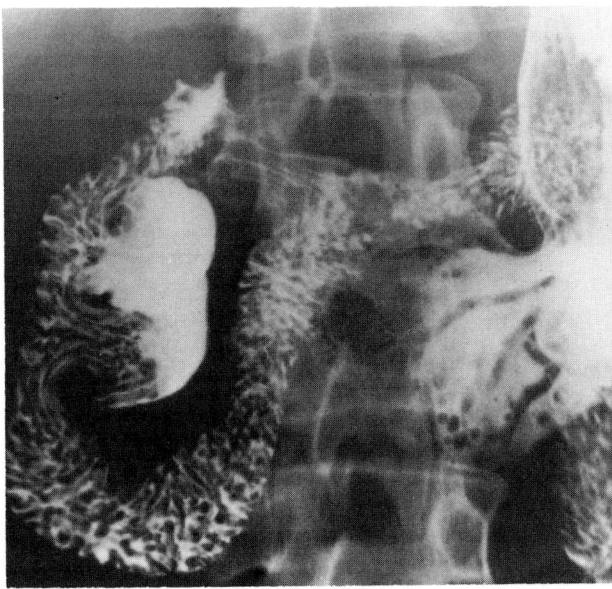

A

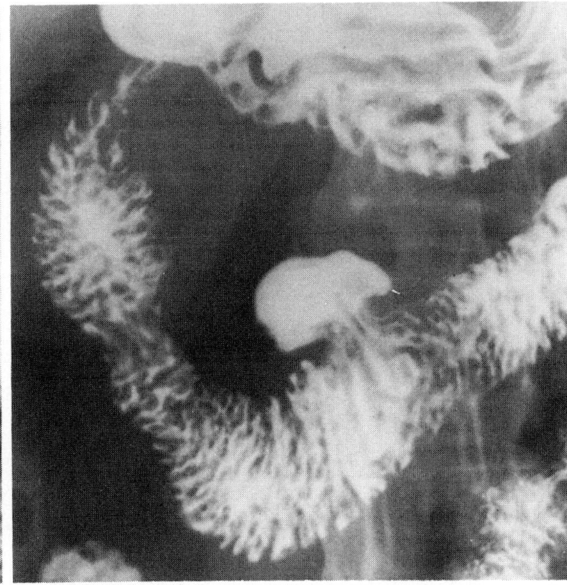

B

Fig. 33.44 A Duodenal diverticulum arising from the second part of the duodenum and showing the mucosal folds radiating into the diverticulum. B Duodenal diverticulum arising from the third part of the duodenum again showing the folds radiating into the diverticulum.

some instances the distended duodenum is completely atonic. The condition may occur as a complication of prolonged supine bed rest in elderly patients.

Hypertrophy of Brunner's glands. The normal fine linear mucosal folds of the duodenal cap are sometimes replaced by a 'cobblestone' appearance. The most frequent cause of this change is oedema of the mucosa associated with a duodenal ulcer and it usually disappears rapidly with treatment.

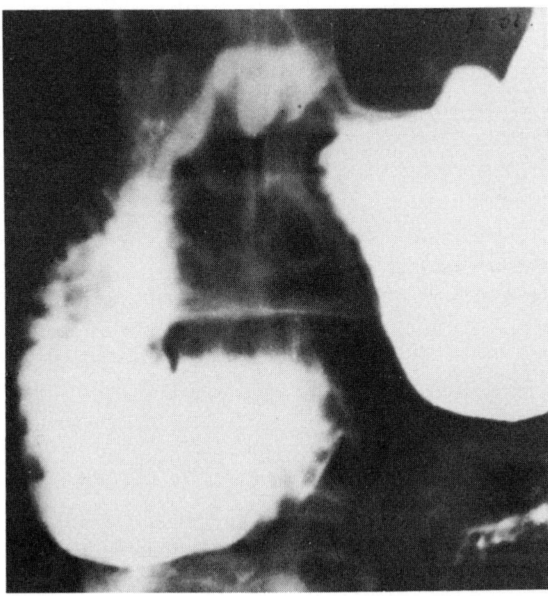

Fig. 33.45 Duodenal ileus at arterio-mesenteric border demonstrating the distended second and third portions of the duodenum.

When, however, these appearances persist the possibility of the polypoid defects being caused by hypertrophy of Brunner's glands must be considered.

Occasionally a polypoid defect in the duodenal cap (Fig. 33.46) may be caused by an aberrant pancreatic tissue and more rarely such deformities may be caused by a primary carcinoma of the duodenum. Involvement or pressure deformities of the duodenum may be also caused by enlarged glands around the head of the pancreas but the variability of the pressure defects associated with altered position of the patient is sufficient to enable these conditions to be recognized.

Varices of the duodenal cap. These appear in established portal hypertension and are particularly

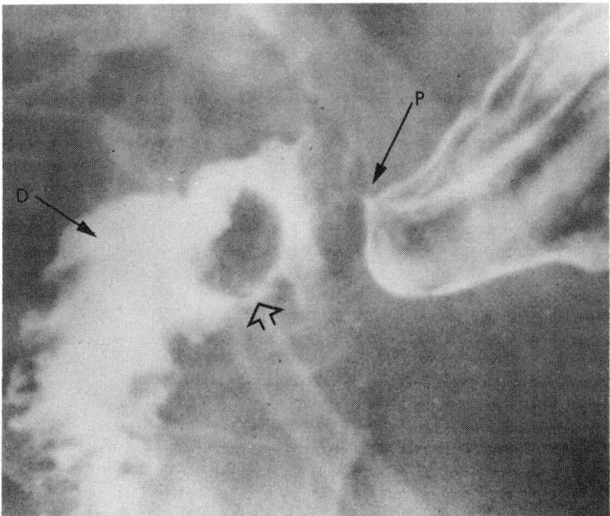

Fig. 33.46 Adenomatous polyp showing a filling defect in the duodenal cap (*hollow arrow*). Such polyps have to be differentiated from pancreatic rests (cf. Fig. 33.36). P—pylorus. D—duodenum.

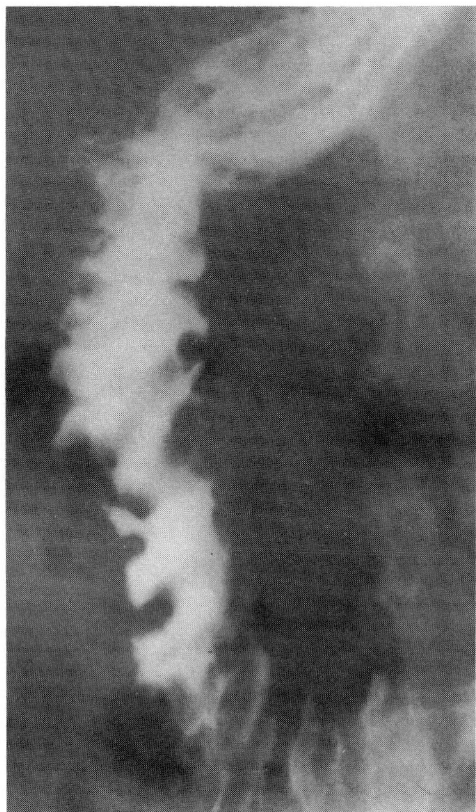

Fig. 33.47 Coarse duodenal folds associated with high gastric acidity. The normal fine parallel folds are replaced by coarse thickened folds.

liable to appear when the pancreatico-duodenal and right gastric veins are involved.

Radiologically they appear as smooth rounded defects in the base of the duodenal cap and are especially well seen in the prone position. Characteristically they tend to disappear in the erect position. They are almost invariably associated with varices in the oesophagus.

They have to be differentiated from other smooth filling defects in the cap; these include retained food, polypi and hypertrophy of Brunner's glands. Extrinsic pressure defects due to surrounding glands are more difficult to differentiate as they, like varices, tend to produce radiological appearances which vary with posture, being well defined in the prone position yet disappearing completely when erect.

Filling defects in the second part of the duodenum may be caused by coeliac artery stenosis with a consequent enlargement of the arteries in the pancreatico-duodenal arcade. This may be so marked as to cause impressions to appear in the barium-filled duodenum. Similar arterial impressions may occur with a tortuous hepatic artery.

Coarse mucosal folds. 'Coarse mucosal folds in the duodenum' was the term used by Fraser *et al.* (1964) to include both *duodenitis* and *hyperplasia of Brunner's glands.*

Radiologically the mucosal folds appear thickened and prominent and biopsy specimens show either inflammatory cells (duodenitis) or nodular hyperplasia (Brunner's glands).

These patients have a dyspeptic syndrome relieved by alkalis, and they also have a high acid output (Fig. 33.47). It is claimed that they respond to measures that reduce acid secretion, e.g. vagotomy, and that the radiological appearances then return to normal. In a series described by the above authors some patients ultimately developed frank duodenal ulcers.

Many of these patients have a gastric type epithelium lining the duodenum.

DUODENAL ULCER

It is estimated that 5 to 8 per cent of all males and 1 per cent of all females at some stage in their lives suffer from duodenal ulceration. As with gastric ulcers the acid pepsin secretion appears to be a necessary factor in their production.

The commonest site for duodenal ulceration is in the duodenal cap (i.e. the first inch or so of duodenum) and they may occur on either the anterior or posterior walls of the cap. Less frequently they occur more distally in the duodenum in the pars superior or second part of the duodenum (*post-bulbar ulcers*). Following surgical anastomosis of the small bowel to the stomach peptic ulceration may develop at the anastomotic line or in the adjoining part of the jejunum.

The natural history of duodenal ulcer is similar to gastric ulcer and it almost certainly begins as an erosion —frequently acute, which may either resolve completely or become recurrent or chronic. Acute duodenal ulcers may follow trauma, burns or intracranial operations and are sometimes associated with neurological lesions around the third ventricle. Like acute gastric erosions duodenal ulcers may occur following the ingestion of drugs but frequently these are really exacerbations of established ulcers.

The two main techniques are used to demonstrate duodenal ulcers, namely the standard *compression* method and more recently the *double contrast* method. As acute duodenal ulcers are relatively superficial the double contrast method is superior for demonstrating the acute ulcer. The ring, arc and smudge signs noted for acute gastric erosion may all be clearly seen in the duodenal cap and occasionally in the acute stage there may be little deformity of the cap due to local stiffening of the duodenal wall by the oedema. It is important to recognize that acute duodenal ulcers may occur in conjunction with a chronic duodenal ulcer and as these frequently occur in the anterior wall of the duodenal cap they may perforate. Lateral views of the cap are thus

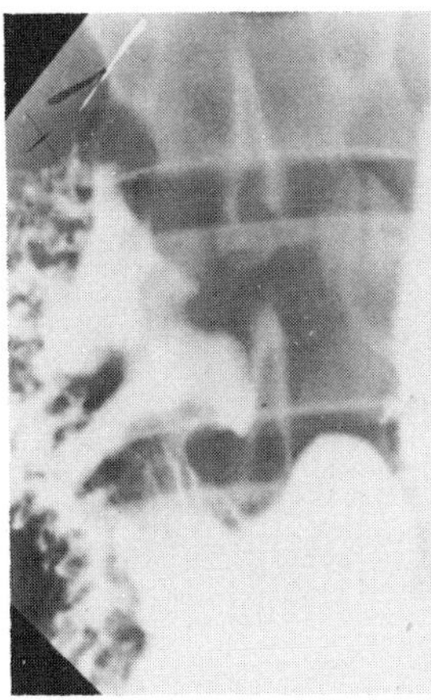
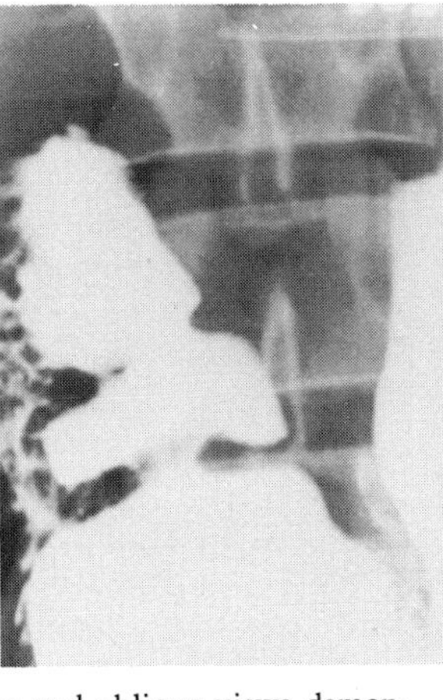
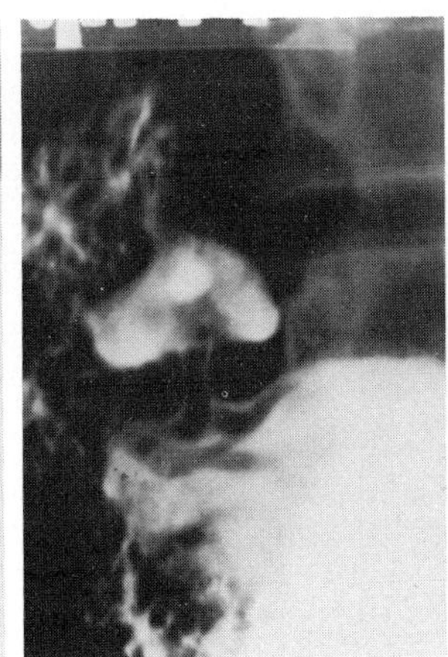
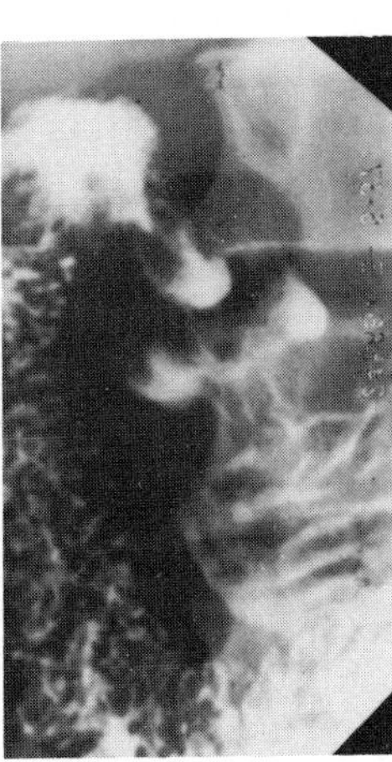

Fig. 33.48 Duodenal ulcer. Erect, supine and oblique views demonstrating the filled duodenal cap, and with increasing compression the barium filled ulcer crater on the posterior wall of the cap becomes visible.

essential in the investigation of established duodenal ulcers so that anterior wall ulcers are not overlooked.

In some cases of acute duodenal ulcers the degree of associated spasm of the cap may be such as to make recognition of the ulcer crater difficult. In such cases examination after the intravenous injection of Glucagon or Buscopan will relax the muscle spasm and allow the crater to be demonstrated.

The established or chronic duodenal ulcer crater is usually easier to demonstrate and the associated spastic deformities of the cap alert the examiner to the possibility of the presence of a duodenal ulcer. The rather fanciful names of 'pine tree', 'trefoil' etc. are really only of historic interest and refer to spastic deformities of the cap. The main aim of radiological examination must be the demonstration of the crater itself (Figs. 33.48 and 33.49).

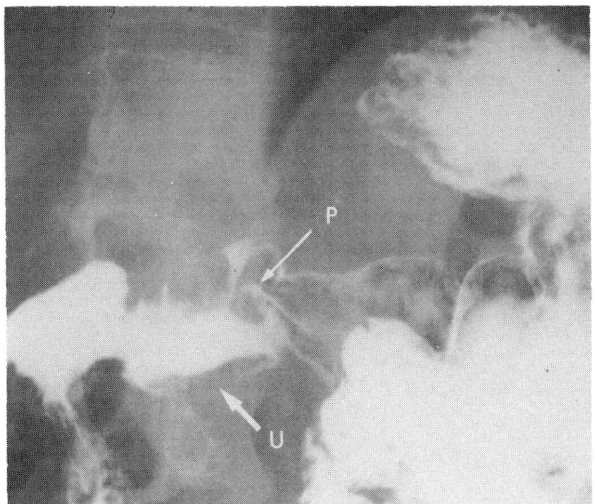

Fig. 33.49 Giant duodenal ulcer. Large ulcers may ulcerate almost the whole of the duodenal cap and in such cases may simulate a normal cap when the whole mucosa has actually been destroyed. P—indicates pylorus. U—ulcer crater with the base shown involving the pancreatic head.

Most of the duodenal deformities are spastic in nature as intravenous injection of an antispasmodic drug will show; but some deformities may be due to fibrosis in the duodenal wall or surrounding the cap as a sequel of healing or local perforation. It is important that only in these cases where the deformity persists after antispasmodics should the term 'scarred and deformed duodenal cap' be used in the report.

Healing of a duodenal ulcer follows the same pattern as in gastric ulcer; the crater becomes progressively shallower and the mucosal folds radiate towards the crater. Ultimately a small smudge of barium is all that remains and as such it may be difficult to distinguish from a healed scar.

Healing of the ulcer, particularly if there has been some degree of penetration or local perforation, may result in stenosis and if the pylorus is involved a pyloric stenosis may develop.

Penetration of the ulcer may occur through the posterior wall and a localized pocket formation may occur. A fluid level may be noted in the ulcer crater in the erect position and the surrounding oedema frequently presents an impression on the duodenum mimicking a tumour (Fig. 33.50).

Post-bulbar duodenal ulcer. Peptic ulcers occurring in the pars superior of the duodenum beyond the bulb and in the second part of the duodenum are classed as post-bulbar ulcers. They are especially prone to bleed, usually presenting as melaena or less frequently haematemesis. They also tend to penetrate the posterior abdominal wall causing local back pain. Ulcers in the second part of the duodenum are most frequently found on the posterior wall and consequently, when penetration occurs, the ulcer craters may attain a large size and may be mistaken for a duodenal diverticulum. The presence of associated spasm of the duodenal wall opposite the ulcer should allow differentiation to be made with reasonable certainty. Occasionally the degree of spasm associated

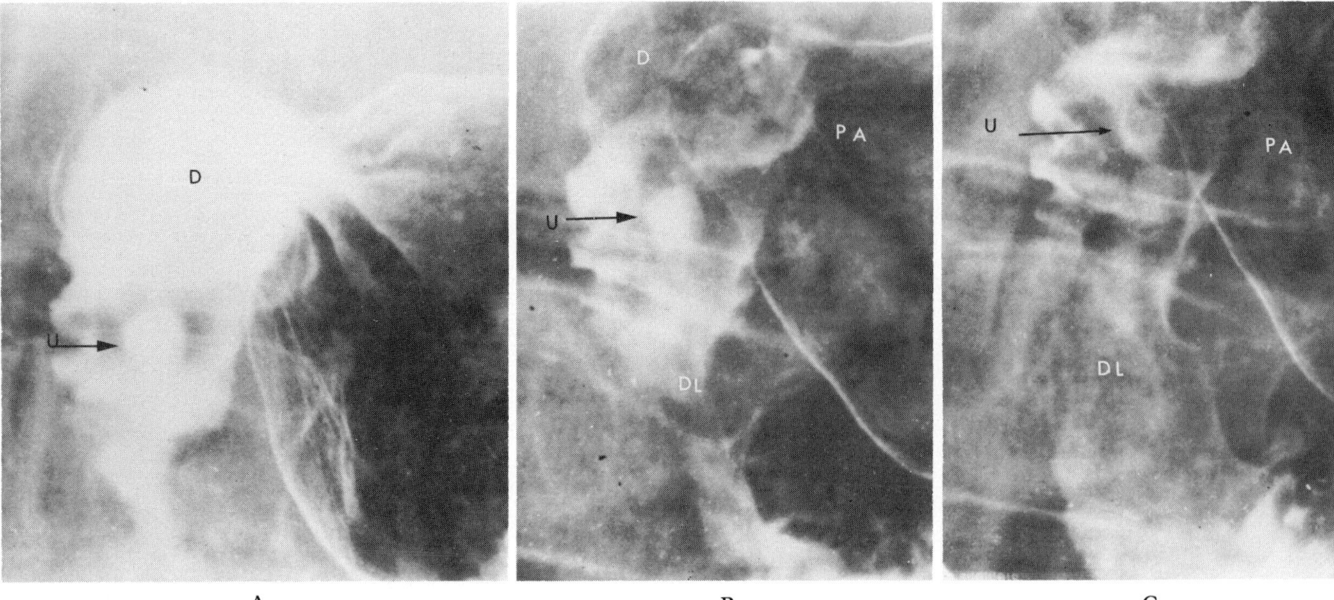

Fig. 33.50 A Double contrast features of a post bulbar ulcer. D—duodenal cap. U—ulcer crater filled with barium surrounded by a halo in the descending duodenum.

B PA view of pyloric antrum with mucosal pattern shown. D—duodenal cap. DL—descending loop of duodenum. PA—pyloric antrum. U—ulcer crater.

C Note that the ulcer crater has partly emptied of barium and a ring shadow remains.

with an ulcer of the second part may be so gross that the deformity mimics a carcinoma of the duodenum.

Ulcers of the pars superior and second part of the duodenum are best seen in films taken with the patient lying in the right lateral position.

Tumours

Benign tumours of the duodenal cap which are extremely uncommon are usually *adenomatous polypi* arising from Brunner's glands. Frequently polypi demonstrated in the duodenal cap are of gastric origin having prolapsed from the stomach, and the classical appearance of a polyp that can be displaced by palpation back into the stomach gives an unmistakable radiological appearance.

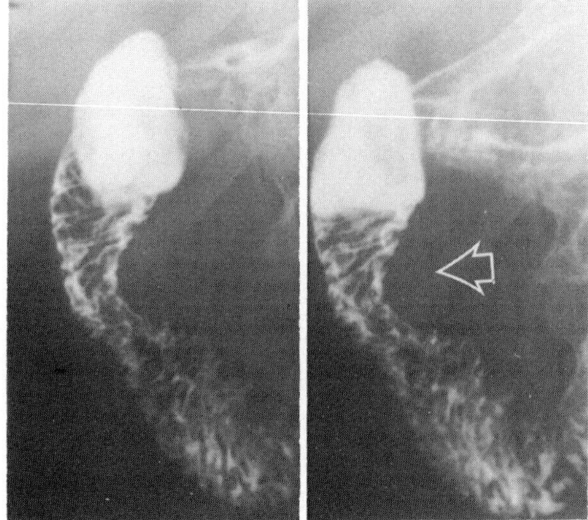

Fig. 33.51 Carcinoma of the pancreas showing infiltration and involvement of the medial wall of the duodenum by the malignant growth (*arrow*).

Malignant tumours of the duodenum are usually *adenocarcinoma* and rarely occur in the first part. They are more frequently seen in the second part, where they have to be distinguished from carcinoma of the ampulla of Vater, or secondary involvement of the duodenum by carcinoma of the head of the pancreas (Fig. 33.51). Radiological differentiation of these three types of tumour may be difficult as each may present with the classical features of a malignant tumour—fingerprint deformities, destruction of the duodenal mucosa, and varying degrees of obstruction of the duodenum. Non-malignant lesions may also cause difficulties in diagnosis (Figs. 33.52 and 33.53). Less commonly annular carcinoma of the duodenum is associated with a narrow stricture and the defect due to the growth is largely obscured by distended duodenum (Fig. 33.54).

Growths of the head of the pancreas may invade the duodenum and in the later stages the origin of the tumour may be difficult to determine. The sign of Frostberg (a reverse 3 appearance—Epsilon sign) caused by the central limb of the 3 being fixed by the pancreatic and bile ducts whilst the duodenal wall above and below are invaginated by the growth, is a valuable sign in the diagnosis of carcinoma of the pancreas (Fig. 33.51).

Ultrasound and computerized axial tomographic scans may be invaluable in the diagnosis of pancreatic tumours. Isotope scanning has not proved itself of great value in the diagnosis of pancreatic cancer.

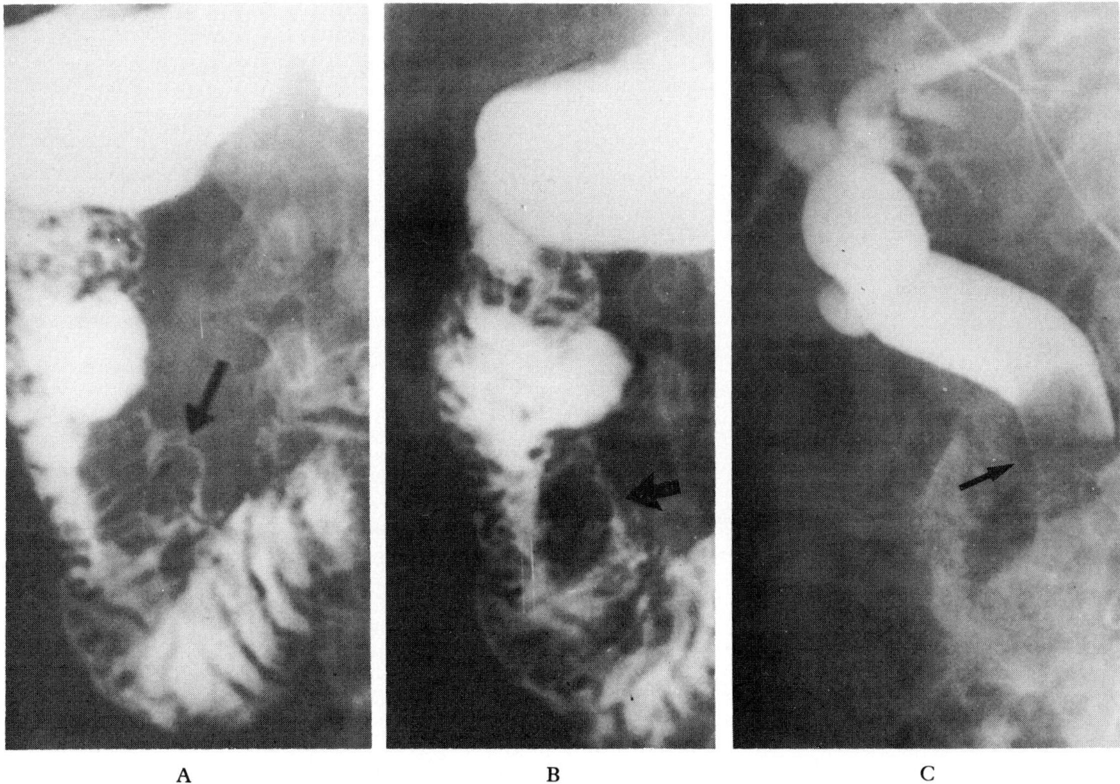

Fig. 33.52 Benign lesion of duodenum mimicking a carcinoma. A and B Filling defect in descending loop of duodenum suggesting a tumour at the ampulla. C Transhepatic cholangiogram showing that the defect in the duodenum is caused by a dilated common bile duct with a stone lodged in the lower end.

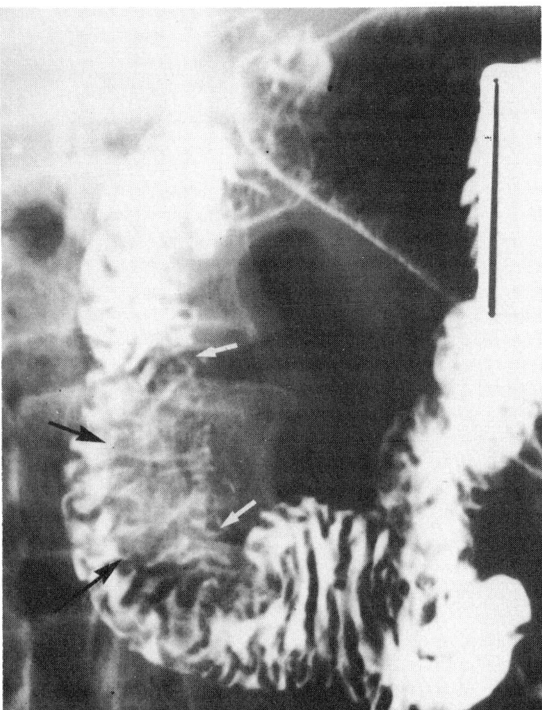

Fig. 33.53 Chronic pancreatitis showing an indefinite impression (*black arrows*) on the duodenum caused by an enlarged head of the pancreas and loss of mucosal wall over the medial aspect of the duodenum (*white arrows*).

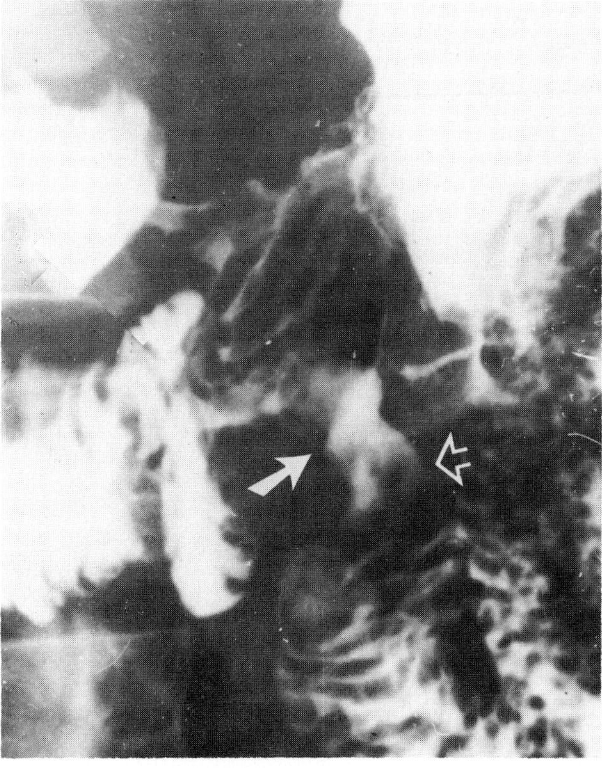

Fig. 33.54 Carcinoma at the duodeno-jejunal flexure showing narrowing of the lumen with obliteration and destruction of mucosal pattern.

Duodenal fistulae. Fistulae from the duodenum may be classified into:

(a) *External*—
  (i) Traumatic following stab wounds
  (ii) Post-operative
    —into subphrenic spaces
    —through abdominal incision
    —following bursting duodenal stump

(b) *Internal*
  (i) Into bile ducts
    —from penetrating ulcers
  (ii) Into gall bladder
    —cholecysto-duodenal following ulcerating gallstones or growths
  (iii) Into colon
    —usually neoplastic

If the fistula is external, i.e. post-operative or following an abdominal operation, a contrast injection of the fistula (sinogram) is usually the most rapid method of showing the origin of the fistula and its side-tracks.

Internal biliary fistulae are more difficult to detect, but careful barium meal follow-through studies usually enable the site of the fistula to be seen.

Internal fistulae into the bile ducts are recognizable by air in the bile ducts and in those involving the gall bladder the outline of the gall bladder may be seen on the plain films. Gas in the bile ducts does not invariably indicate a fistula as it may follow sphincterectomy, duodenal diverticulum, and other lesions which affect the ampulla of Vater.

Fistulae into the colon are best evaluated by means of a barium enema examination.

REFERENCES AND SUGGESTIONS FOR FURTHER READING

ATHEY, P. A., GOLDSTEIN, H. M. & DODD, G. W. (1977) Radiologic spectrum of opportunistic infections of the upper gastrointestinal tract. *American Journal of Roentgenology*, **129**, 419.

AUERBACH, R. C. & KOEHLER, P. R. (1973) The many faces of islet cell tumours. *American Journal of Roentgenology*, **119**, 133–140.

BREMNER, C. G. (1968) The lesser curve pyloric niche. *British Journal of Radiology*, **41**, 291–295.

COCKERILL, E. M. *et al.* (1976) Optimum visualisation of the oesophageal varices. *American Journal of Roentgenology*, **126**, 512–523.

GOLDSMITH, M. R. *et al.* (1976) Evaluation of routine double contrast views of the anterior wall of the stomach. *American Journal of Roentgenology*, **126**, 1159–1163.

GOLDSTEIN, H. M. & DODD, G. D. (1976) Double contrast examination of the oesophagus. *Gastrointestinal Radiology*, **1**, 3.

HERLINGER, H., GLANVILLE, J. N. & KREEL, L. (1977) An evaluation of the double contrast barium meal against endoscopy. *Clinical Radiology*, **28**, 307–314.

HUNT, J. H. & ANDERSON, I. F. (1976) Double contrast upper gastrointestinal studies. *Clinical Radiology*, **27**, 87–97.

HYSON, E. A., BURRELL, M. & TOFFLER, R. (1977) Drug induced gastrointestinal disease. *Gastrointestinal Radiology*, **2**, 183.

KEET, A. D. Jr. (1957) The prepyloric contractions in the normal stomach. *Acta Radiologica*, **48**, 413–424.

KEET, A. D., Jr. (1958) The prepyloric contractions in certain abnormal conditions. *Acta Radiologica*, **50**, 413–429.

KIHARA, T., OHTA, A., ISHIHARA, Y. & MORITA, M. (1971) Hypotonic duodenography. *Clinical Radiology*, **22**, 251–256.

KREEL, L. (1975) Pharmaco-radiology in barium examinations with special reference to glucagon. *British Journal of Radiology*, **48**, 691.

LAUFER, I. (1979) *Double Contrast Gastrointestinal Radiology with Endoscopic Correlation*. London: Saunders.

LINTOTT, D. J., SIMPKINS, K. C., DE DOMBAL, F. T. & NOAKES, M. J. (1979) Assessment of the double contrast barium meal. *Clinical Radiology*, **29**, 313–321.

MACKINTOSH, C. E. & KREEL, L. (1977) Anatomy and radiology of the areae gastricae. *Gut*, **18**, 855–864.

MARTELL, W., ABELL, M. A. & ALLAN, T. N. K. (1976) Lymphoreticular hyperplasia of the stomach (pseudolymphoma). *American Journal of Roentgenology*, **127**, 261–265.

MENUCK, L. & COEL, M. (1976) Vascular impressions of the gut secondary to chronic vascular occlusive disease. *American Journal of Roentgenology*, **126**, 970–973.

NUGENT, F. W., RICHMOND, M. & PARK, S. K. (1977) Crohn's disease of the duodenum. *Gut*, **18**, 115–120.

MEYERS, M. A. (1970) Paraduodenal hernias. *Radiology*, **95**, 199–201.

PEAVY, P. W. *et al.* (1975) Gastric pseudo-ulcers. Membrana angularis and pyloric tonus defects. *Radiology*, **114**, 591–595.

PICAZO, J. (Ed.) (1979) *Glucagon in Gastroenterology*. Lancaster: M. T. P. Press.

PULVERTAFT, C. N. (1974) Complications of gastric resection. In: *Recent Advances in Radiology*, 4th edition. Lodge, T. Edinburgh: Churchill Livingstone.

ROGERS, I. M., MOULE, B. *et al.* (1976) Endoscopy and routine and double-contrast barium meal in diagnosis of gastric and duodenal disorders. *Lancet*, **1**, 901–902.

SAXTON, H. M. (1977) Radiology now: starting the double contrast barium meal. *British Journal of Radiology*, **50**, 610–612.

SCHULMAN, A. (1971) Anastomotic, gastrojejunal ulcer: accuracy of radiological diagnosis in surgically proven cases. *British Journal of Radiology*, **44**, 422–433.

SHIMKIN, P. M. & PEARSON, K. D. (1972) Unusual arterial impressions upon the duodenum. *Radiology*, **103**, 295–297.

SHIRAKABE, H. (1966) *Atlas of X-Ray Diagnosis of Early Gastric Cancer*. Tokyo: Igaku Shoin.

SI-CHAN MING (1976) *Gastrointestinal Radiology*, **1**, 121.

STEVENSON, G. (1977) The distribution of gastric ulcers; double contrast barium meal and endoscopy findings. *Clinical Radiology*, **28**, 617–624.

WILLIAMS, J. H. & TOYE, D. K. M. (1970) Recurrent ulcer after vagotomy and pyloroplasty: the X-ray appearances and their value in diagnosis. *Gut*, **11**, 405–408.

WOLF, B. S. (1977) Observations on roentgen features of benign and malignant gastric ulcers. *Seminars in Roentgenology*, **6(2)**, 140–150.

ZOLLINGER, R. M. (1976) Islet cell tumours and the alimentary tract. *American Journal of Roentgenology*, **126**, 933–940.

CHAPTER 34

THE SMALL BOWEL

The mucosal pattern of the small intestine cannot normally be seen without the introduction of positive contrast media, usually barium sulphate mixture. Air swallowed during speech and eating may enter the small bowel and outline parts of it. This is commonly seen in patients lying supine during intravenous pyelography, when it may interfere with the examination by obscuring parts of the renal tract. In the absence of obstruction the swallowed air rapidly traverses the small bowel, usually in 5 to 20 minutes, but may remain in the colon for longer periods, before being expelled. There is so little gas in the normal small intestine and fluid is extracted so rapidly from the intestinal contents, that it is exceptional to see more than an occasional fluid level on erect films taken with a horizontal X-ray beam.

Pathological conditions which prevent the onward passage of the gas, such as obstruction or ileus, when the motility of the small or large bowel is inhibited, result in the accumulation of gas which outlines the mucosal pattern of the small bowel. When jejunum is distended the secondary folds are smoothed out and the soft tissue rings of the primary folds (*valvulae conniventes*) are outlined by gas. The distended ileum appears as a featureless tube devoid of folds.

The accumulation of gas and fluid above an obstruction enables the diagnosis to be made on plain radiographs. A film taken with a horizontal ray, with the patient in the erect or lateral decubitus position, demonstrates the presence and distribution of fluid levels separating the gas and fluid contents of the bowel. The supine film enables the bowel wall and its mucosal pattern to be outlined by virtue of its air contrast and by this means the individual segment of bowel can often be recognized. Jejunal coils are identified by the valvulae conniventes crossing the bowel, ileal coils on the other hand have a smooth outline and show no mucosal pattern. Colonic gas shadows are recognized by the haustrations and sacculations of the colon.

Accumulation of gas and fluid above a complete mechanical obstruction of the small bowel occurs quickly after the onset of obstruction and at 6 hours fluid levels can be demonstrated.

Adequate demonstration of the lumen of the small bowel and its mucosal pattern can usually be obtained by ingestion of a barium sulphate mixture. Since the radiological examination of the small bowel is time-consuming and involves the patient in considerable X-irradiation it should never become a routine addendum to a barium meal examination. The exact indications for the examination, together with details of any previous abdominal surgery, should be known before the examination is begun. There are many different ways of examining the small bowel, each having enthusiastic advocates. The method of choice often depends on the reason for the examination. Since each method has a different appearance in the normal, as well as in disease, it is essential that the radiologist should be thoroughly familiar with the method he is using. Although the techniques vary in detail the following principles are common to them all:

(*a*) The small intestine should be demonstrated in continuity by a continuous column of barium sulphate mixture.

(*b*) When any abnormality is seen on a supine film an erect horizontal ray film should be taken at the same time and the two films examined and diagnosed together; that is, just as paired erect and supine films are taken routinely in investigating an acute abdomen.

(*c*) Whenever possible the small bowel should be examined when distended as well as when collapsed.

(*d*) Overlapping coils should be separated by taking prone or oblique projections and by applying general or local abdominal compression.

Contrast media. The exact composition of commercial barium sulphate preparations is a trade secret and may be changed by the manufacturers without reference to the radiologists who use them. Since the radiological appearance and the interpretation of the findings depend to some extent upon the composition of the preparation this is not a desirable situation. Two of the major variables are the ease with which clumping and flocculation occur in the presence of mucus, and the osmolarity of the preparation when in the small bowel. Micropaque (Nickolas) and Baritop (Saka Chemicals) are barium sulphate suspensions which resist flocculation in most normal adults, but usually flocculate in infants and children. They coat mucosal surfaces well, demonstrate mucosal pattern well, and become concentrated by the extraction of water when in the small intestine, since they contain no hydroscopic agent (Fig. 34.1). Raybar and Barasperse are examples of barium sulphate preparation which contain carboxymethyl cellulose which acts as a hygroscopic agent and retains water within the lumen of the small intestine, giving a more bulky appearance and tending to distend the small bowel more than Micropaque. These preparations tend not to mix easily with mucus and so resist flocculation to a greater extent than Micropaque, but for the same reason, do not show the mucosal pattern quite so clearly.

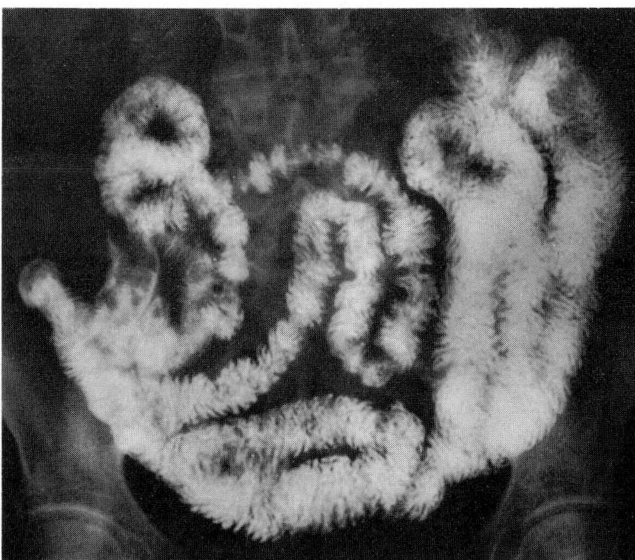

Fig. 34.1 Normal small bowel examination showed the normal feathery pattern of concentrated barium in the small intestine.

Water-soluble contrast media such as Gastrografin have been advocated particularly in suspected incomplete small bowel obstruction. However, its high osmolarity and consequent dilution in the small bowel makes it quite unsuitable. The resulting large volume of dilute contrast medium shows neither the site of the obstruction nor any detail of the mucosal pattern. A small volume (e.g. 10 ml) of Gastrografin may be added to barium sulphate preparation in order to increase the bulk of the contrast meal and to hasten transit into the colon. Magnesium sulphate 10–15 g will have a similar effect and will also prevent the barium becoming inspissated in the colon. This can be helpful, particularly in bedridden or elderly patients.

Most barium preparations are approximately isotonic and may give useful information in patients with subacute small bowel obstruction. They will never complete an incomplete obstruction of the small bowel, but should be used with caution if large bowel obstruction is suspected.

Conventional follow-through examination. The aim is to outline the small intestine throughout its length by a continuous column of barium in the shortest possible time with the least upset to patient and radiologist. There is a wide variation in transit time in the normal small bowel. The following principles are worth observing:

1. Enough barium sulphate preparation should be given for there to be some in the stomach throughout the examination. The presence of barium in the antrum acts as a stimulus to peristalsis, helping to propel the barium along the small intestine and shorten the examination time. If the stomach is found to be empty when most of the small bowel has been outlined and the barium has not yet reached the caecum, a dry meal (e.g. a sandwich and small cup of coffee) may be given instead of more barium sulphate in order to propel the barium on its way. If very dilute barium is used the excess added water will soon be removed in the jejunum and passed from the body as urine, unless a hydroscopic agent is present in or added to the barium preparation. Either neat or slightly diluted barium preparation should be used: 8–20 oz is an average volume needed to outline the small bowel.

2. During the whole of the examination, except during fluoroscopy, the patient should lie in the right lateral position. This ensures that barium leaves the stomach in a continuous column, as no air can leave until all the barium has left, and care is taken to ensure that there is always barium in the stomach throughout the examination. It also reduces the time of the examination by ensuring a constant stimulus to peristaltic activity being present in the proximal jejunum. In the upright or supine position gas and barium leave the stomach intermittently being governed by pyloric opening and giving rise to an interrupted column of barium in the small bowel which makes interpretation difficult.

3. The rate of gastric emptying can be assessed during preliminary fluoroscopy and films taken at intervals determined by this and by the particular reason for the examination. Films taken supine with a fine-focus undercouch tube and well coned are sufficient if the appearances are normal, but should be supplemented by erect films if any abnormality is seen on fluoroscopy. Localized views, using compression, are invaluable, particularly in showing the terminal ileum. The examination in most cases should be completed in $1\frac{1}{2}$ to 2 hours. Some normal patients fill their terminal ileum within 20 minutes. Others take up to 4 hours. Slow transit is found in some patients on anti-depressant and anti-spasmodic drugs (e.g. Propanthaline bromide or Buscopan).

Pharmacologically controlled follow-through examination. Various methods have been used to hasten the transit of barium through the small bowel, and so shorten the examination. Iced water or saline and Sorbital have been used as a 'chaser' to propel the barium already in the small bowel. But their action has been too unreliable to be of much use. Iced water tends to dilute the barium preparation and make interpretation difficult.

Probably the most reliable method of shortening the examination is by using Metoclopramide which acts by increasing peristaltic activity in the stomach and proximal small bowel, causing rapid gastric emptying and small bowel filling. Its action is most reliable when given intravenously (20 mg) but it may be given intramuscularly or by mouth, when 20 mg are given 20 minutes before the barium meal is begun. This oral route is less reliable than the intravenous route. Provided sufficient barium preparation is given to fill the whole of the small bowel and the patient lies on his right side, the examination should be completed within 75 minutes, barium often reaching the terminal ileum much sooner than this. The fact that Metoclopramide has been given should be recorded in the report and preferably on the films, as its administration modifies the radiological appearance. Patients who are hypokalaemic, on certain drugs, or who have had a vagotomy, may show no hastening effect from Metaclopramide.

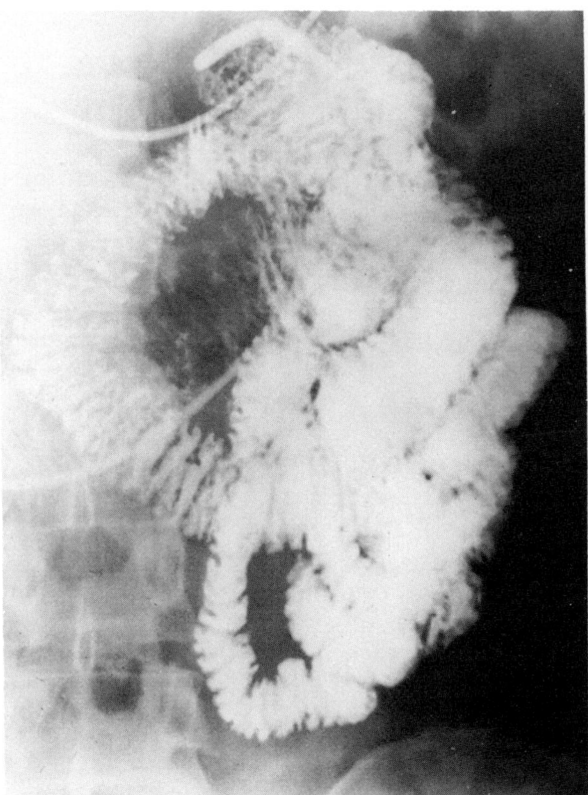

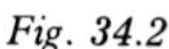

Fig. 34.2

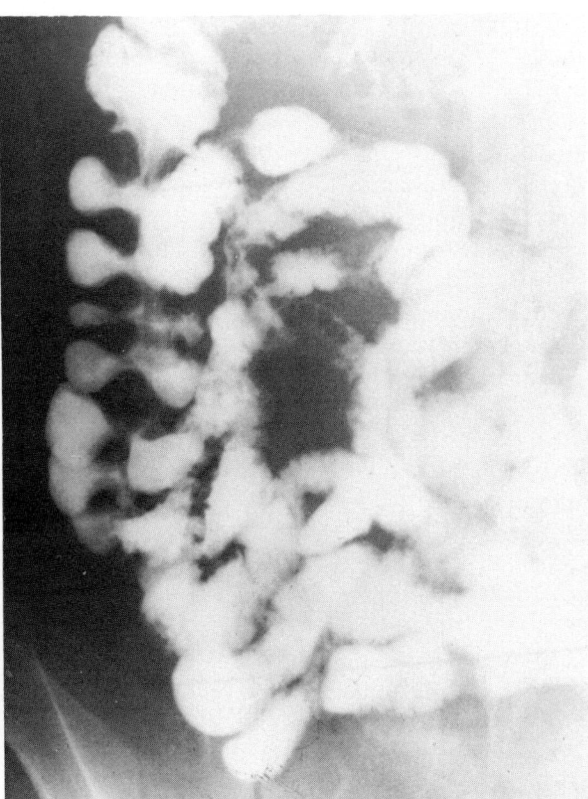

Fig. 34.3

Fig. 34.2 Small bowel enema showing filling of the upper coils of small bowel. The tip of the intestinal tube is lying near the duodeno-jejunal flexure.

Fig. 34.3 Small bowel enema demonstrating filling of the terminal loops of ileum and caecum.

Neostigmine 0.5 m subcutaneously has been used in order to shorten the time of small bowel examinations. It has more side effects than Metoclopramide and should be used with care in the elderly and in patients with hypertension and angina.

Small bowel enema. The small bowel enema is performed by the introduction of barium sulphate preparation directly into the small bowel through a naso-gastric tube passed through the pylorus into the duodenum (Figs. 34.2, 34.3 and 34.8). A Bilbao-Dotter duodenal tube is suitable since it has a guide wire of the correct rigidity. The tube may be introduced through the mouth or nostril into the stomach when the guide wire is passed down its lumen to within a few centimetres of the tip. Gentle but continuous pressure by the tip of the tube on the pylorus usually results in the pylorus relaxing and the tip passing into the duodenum. Firm manual pressure on the epigastrium may help at this stage. The guide wire is then removed and the tube, now more flexible, is manoeuvred into the third part of the duodenum. It may be difficult to get the tube beyond the descending limb of the duodenum sometimes because of the presence of a lax duodenum or duodenal diverticulum. The examination may still be carried out but reflux into the stomach is more likely to occur and this tends to spoil the examination.

Three hundred to 800 ml Barium sulphate of S.G.1.25 (approx.) is introduced down the tube at a rate of 100 ml per minute from a polythene bag under the influence of gravity. Infusion at a rate faster than this tends to cause nausea and reflux of contrast into the stomach. When the head of the contrast column has reached the ileum, a more dilute barium sulphate suspension containing 10–20 mg Metoclopramide may be substituted to a total volume of 1000 ml. This dilute barium results in less obscuring of detail if coils of bowel overlap each other. Finally, water may be infused rapidly through the small bowel to propel the barium into the caecum and distend the coils of small bowel giving a double contrast effect. Serial films of the distended bowel are supplemented by local films of suspected areas. This method allows a beautiful demonstration of the proximal small bowel, which is well seen by other methods, but it may still be difficult at times to demonstrate the distal loops of ileum. The examination can frequently be completed in 10 to 20 minutes. The chief disadvantage, apart from the discomfort of the intubation, is the feeling of nausea during the examination and the remote risk of perforation of the gut by the tube or guide wire. This latter risk is minimal if the guide wire is kept shorter than the tube and cannot protrude from it. For a more detailed description of the small bowel enema the reader is referred to monographs by G. Scott-Harden and J. L. Sellink.

Air or oxygen may be introduced rapidly into the small bowel after the initial barium bolus, in order to propel the barium onwards and give a double contrast examination, the bowel being coated with barium and distended with gas. Further distension and relaxation of the small bowel may be obtained by the intravenous injection of Probanthine 30 mg.

In many centres the small bowel is examined by the conventional method with or without Metoclopramide, and the small bowel enema is reserved for patients with specific problems in whom the simpler technique has not provided sufficient information.

Retrograde small bowel examination. Reflux of barium from the caecum into the terminal ileum frequently occurs during barium enema examinations. It is possible to examine the whole of the small bowel by this method. Barium sulphate preparation (20 per cent w/v) is introduced per rectum until the splenic flexure has been outlined, when water is used to push the barium round to the caecum and at the same time clear the barium from rectum and sigmoid colon. In most patients if the pressure is raised sufficiently reflux will occur into the ileum. The administration of atropine and meperidine hydrochloride (Demerol) is said to make the ileocaecal valve relax and allow reflux to occur more readily. The introduction of further water into the rectum will clear the sigmoid of opaque contrast medium and cause all coils of small bowel to fill with barium. Serial films of the distended small bowel are taken, supplemented with spot films as necessary. This method of examination is apt to be painful and unpleasant for the patient and has not received wide acceptance.

CONGENITAL ABNORMALITIES

Malrotation of the small bowel may be (a) complete with the colon lying on the left side of the abdominal cavity (this may occur in association with a complete situs inversus) or (b) partial malrotation where the caecum and ascending colon only are displaced to the left side. Both these congenital variants can be readily recognized on follow-through barium meal examination (Fig. 34.4).

Internal herniations into paraduodenal fossae and other peritoneal pockets are recognized by an immobility and relative fixity of a coil or several coils of small bowel. These internal herniations are usually seen on the right side in the region of the descending portion of the duodenum or near the ligament of Treitz on the left. Occasionally almost the whole of the small bowel may lie within an internal hernia. The fixed position of the coils in serial follow-through films or on fluoroscopy enables the herniation to be identified. Unless mechanical obstruction develops in an internal hernia they are usually completely asymptomatic.

Meckel's diverticulum occurs in .001 per cent of subjects but it is seldom recognized by radiological methods. Clinically the diverticulum may present with a melaena due to ulceration within ectopic gastric mucosa in its wall, or as an acute intra-abdominal inflammatory condition.

They may be recognized in follow-through barium examination, but this is uncommon as there is no significant hold up of the barium meal and the barium residue remaining in the Meckel's diverticulum is insignificant (Fig. 34.5).

Extremely rarely it may appear as a large gas-filled viscus, and a fluid level in the erect position may be present in the distended loop. Occasionally the Meckel's diverticulum may form an enormous gas-filled loop which may fill a large part of the abdominal cavity.

TRAUMATIC LESIONS OF THE SMALL BOWEL

The increasing use of safety belts in cars has resulted in closed injuries of the abdomen caused by acute flexion over the restraining strap. The duodenum is usually damaged because of its relative fixity to the posterior

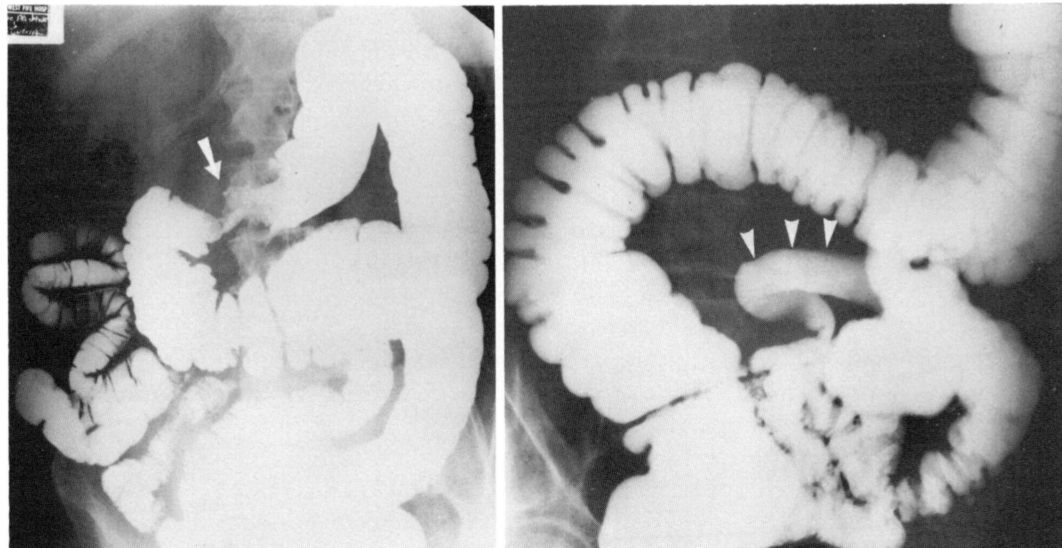

Fig. 34.4

Fig. 34.5

Fig. 34.4 Partial malrotation. Small bowel is lying to the right of the ascending colon in the right iliac fossa. There is also a carcinoma of the transverse colon (*arrow*).

Fig. 34.5 Meckel's diverticulum (*arrows*) shown by barium enema with reflux of barium into the terminal ileum.

abdominal wall. An intramural haematoma may cause complete obstruction at the level of the second part of the duodenum. This usually resolves in the course of a few days. There may be a compression fracture of an adjacent lumbar vertebral body.

Laceration of the mesentery or bowel may give rise to mucosal or extramucosal haematoma. Rupture of the small bowel resulting in the radiological features of perforation and peritonitis may occur in severe cases.

SPONTANEOUS INTRAMURAL BLEEDING

Intramural haematoma may occur in patients on anti-coagulant therapy or as a consequence of a coagulation defect due to some underlying disease such as haemophilia, leukaemia or thrombocytopenia. Bleeding of this type may occur anywhere in the small bowel and tends to be diffuse and include a long segment of bowel rather than give rise to a localized haematoma as is commonly seen in healthy persons following trauma (Fig. 34.6).

PARASITIC INFECTION OF SMALL BOWEL

Parasitic infection of the small bowel is due either to a flat worm infestation of the duodenum (*Taenia saginata*, *Taenia solium*) or a round worm infestation of the small bowel. Hookworm infestation (*ankylostoma duodenale*)

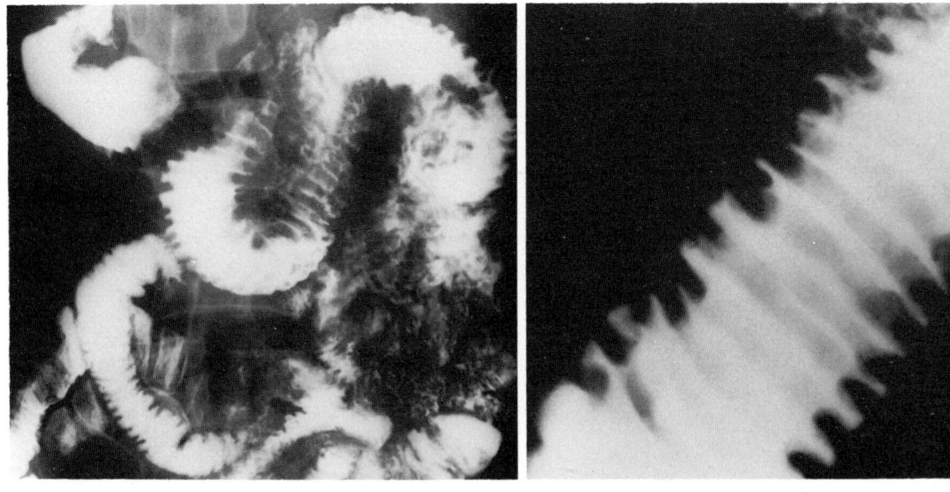

A

B

Fig. 34.6A Spontaneous intramural haematoma of the jejunum in a male of 45 years who was a known haemophiliac since childhood. Sudden onset of colicky abdominal pain followed by melaena.

B. Dilated loop of proximal jejunum with broad, coarse transverse folds resembling a 'picket fence'.

of the duodenum is also a common finding in some tropical areas.

Taenia or hookworm infestation causes irritability and irregularity of the mucosal pattern in the second part of the duodenum where the head of the worm is attached. The head is the only part of the worm which causes radiological signs and this merely from the irritability it produces. The flat segments forming the body of the worm lying in the small bowel are seldom recognized.

Round worm infestation (*Ascaris lumbricoides*) is a frequent infestation in tropical areas. In children the worms may multiply to such an extent as to form conglomerate masses which may cause intestinal obstruction. Trapping of intestinal gas between the masses of worms may give rise to appearances suggesting coiled locks of hair, the so-called 'Medusa locks' which can sometimes be seen on plain films of the abdomen.

In the adult the degree of worm infestation is seldom of such a degree as to produce any appearances on the plain film, but the worms can usually be seen on a barium meal follow-through examination of the small bowel. The adult worm casts a negative shadow in the barium-filled intestine which closely follows the anatomical configuration of the worm. Less frequently a central thin thread of barium indicates that the worm has ingested some of the barium and its own alimentary canal is outlined.

ULCERS OF THE SMALL BOWEL

Ulceration of the small bowel is usually part of a generalized enteritis, e.g. paratyphoid or typhoid fever, but a solitary ulcer may result as a sequel of the enteric coated potassium tablets administered in the treatment of hypertension. It has been suggested that the liberation of potassium locally in the small bowel results in local venous thrombosis, which may give rise to necrosis and solitary ulceration. Such ulcers develop circumferentially around the bowel wall and can be demonstrated on barium films. They may perforate and present as an acute abdomen, or as a more slowly developing granulomatous lesion around the ulcer giving rise to small bowel obstruction. In other cases healing of the ulcer may result in a fibrous stricture which may give rise to small bowel obstruction.

INFLAMMATORY LESIONS

Acute inflammatory lesions of the small bowel, when due to specific infections, e.g. typhoid or paratyphoid infection, or non-specific infections are investigated radiologically only when the diagnosis has not been established. The radiological signs are those of intestinal hurry and increased motility of the small bowel. Erect films may reveal isolated small fluid levels dispersed in a disorderly pattern all over the abdomen, but there is no proportionate gas distension of the bowel such as seen in true mechanical obstruction.

GRANULOMA

Chronic inflammatory granulomata of the small bowel usually affect the terminal ileum often accompanied by caecal changes. Regional ileitis (Crohn's disease) and specific granulomata such as tuberculosis or actinomycosis may all affect the terminal ileum.

The terminal ileum may also be involved (by reflux ileitis) in association with ulcerative colitis.

REGIONAL ENTERITIS (CROHN'S DISEASE)

Regional enteritis (Crohn's disease) is a chronic granulomatous condition which may affect any part of the gut from the stomach to the anus but is most commonly seen in the terminal ileum and colon. Its cause is unknown. The affected bowel is sharply demarcated from the normal. Several separate areas of disease (skip lesions) may be present in the bowel separated by lengths of normal intestine. The bowel wall is thickened, congested and rigid, its lumen usually narrowed and ulcerated. The attached mesentery is thickened and mesenteric lymph nodes enlarged. Affected loops become matted together so that perforation into the peritoneal cavity is rare but fistulae between loops and to adjacent viscera are common. Sinuses form in the skin of the abdominal wall. Abscesses often form between affected loops.

Histologically there is a chronic granulomatous inflammatory reaction with oedema and fibrosis affecting all coats of the intestinal wall. Deep fissured ulcers may extend into the submucosa and muscular layers. Non-caseating granulomas containing multinucleated giant cells, epitheloid and mononuclear cells may be seen in most resected specimens, but the ease with which they are found varies and they are not essential for diagnosis.

Regional enteritis may present at any age but is most commonly seen in the second and third decade. The onset may be acute, resembling acute appendicitis, or insidious leading to chronic ill health. Diarrhoea, colic, low-grade fever, anaemia, anorexia and loss of weight are common in the less acute cases. Subacute obstruction is very common but complete obstruction requiring immediate surgery is rare. Malnutrition may be severe especially in complicated cases following multiple resections or exclusion operations.

Radiological findings. The radiological appearance of the small bowel reflects various pathological lesions. Oedema of the mucosa and submucosa result in thickening and blunting of the mucosal folds with a smoothing out or effacement of the primary folds, the valvulae

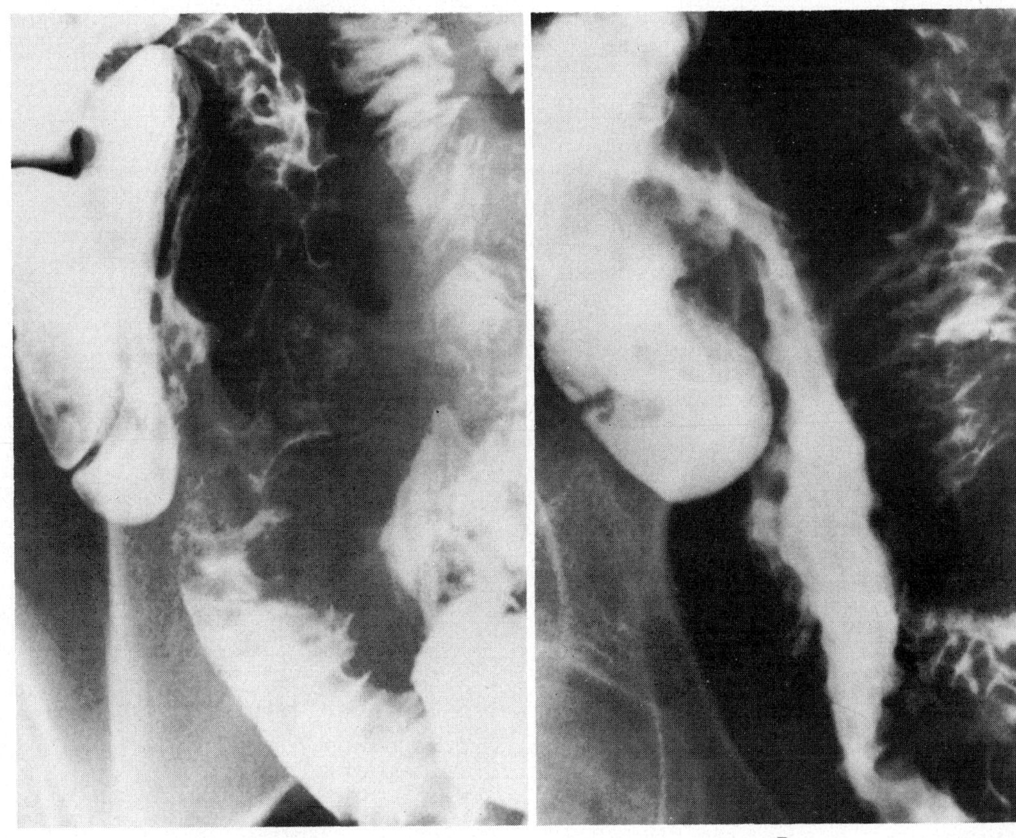

Fig. 34.7 A Crohn's disease of terminal ileum showing oedematous mucosa and deep ulceration.

Fig. 34.7 B Crohn's disease of terminal ileum showing deep ulceration. The affected loop is slightly dilated and has thickened wall.

conniventes, as well as the secondary folds. Congestion and oedema of the muscular layers cause rigidity and thickening of the walls so that the lumen of affected loops appears separated from neighbouring loops, whether normal or abnormal (Fig. 34.7A and B). Thus the abnormal loops stand out from the rest especially if all intestinal loops are filled by a continuous column of barium.

Ulceration when seen *en face* appears as longitudinal or transverse streaks of barium in deep fissured crevices, giving rise to a cobblestone appearance which is best seen in the jejunum. When seen in profile, these ulcers appear deep and fissured, so-called rose-thorn ulcers. Stenotic areas are common and are often multiple giving rise to subacute obstruction. Complete obstruction is surprisingly uncommon considering the length and narrowness of the strictures sometimes demonstrated. As fibrosis continues the ulceration may become less severe so that the intestine becomes a long thick walled rigid tube with a central lumen and devoid of peristalsis. Partially obstructed small bowel becomes dilated.

Adjacent loops often become matted together and fistulae develop between them. Ileo-ileal fistulae are difficult to demonstrate but ileo-colic fistulae may be easily shown by barium enema examination. Fistulae may form between the gut and the urinary bladder and sinuses may lead to the vagina or abdominal wall. Sinography is usually better than small bowel examination for demonstrating the source of the leak from the small intestine.

Dilatation of loops of bowel may be a particularly prominent feature of jejunal involvement. The duodenum is rarely involved unless there is widespread disease elsewhere in the bowel. Involvement of the stomach is extremely uncommon.

The acuteness of the pathological process to some extent parallel the clinical presentation, which can be grouped into:

(a) **Acute.** Symptoms and signs mimic those of an acute appendicitis and the radiological examination usually does not involve contrast studies but is confined to plain films of the acute abdomen. At this stage plain films show a single or a few small isolated fluid levels in the terminal ileum. This is a non-specific pattern indistinguishable from that seen in acute appendicitis or acute enteritis.

(b) **Subacute.** The commoner clinical presentation is one of a tender mass in the right iliac fossa sometimes associated with a low grade fever, general malaise, leucocytosis and frequently with colicky abdominal pain and diarrhoea. The radiological appearances may be seen either on a small bowel examination or on a barium enema examination when the terminal ileum is filled by reflux from the colon. The appearances may vary considerably from patient to patient and in the same patient from time to time. The radiological abnormalities include:

1. *Ulceration without narrowing.* Deep ulceration giving a *cobblestone* appearance when seen *en face* and *rose-thorn* ulcers when seen tangentially may occur without significant narrowing of the lumen (Fig. 34.7). In some instances there may be a little dilatation of the affected loop (Fig. 34.8). Commonly the wall is thickened and the loop is tender to palpation.

2. *Stenosis.* The lumen at some stage usually becomes narrowed sometimes for a few centimetres and at other times for 25 cm or more. The narrow lumen and thick wall separating it from other loops, together with the deep fissured ulcers, give rise to a long continuous thin column of barium with irregular edges resembling a frayed piece of string (*Kantor's string sign*) (Figs. 34.8 and 34.9).

3. *Failure of the caecum to fill.* The caecum may fail to fill as a result of spasm; later actual fibrosis may cause the caecum to become contracted (Fig. 34.10). Extreme contraction of the caecum is more common in tuberculous infection than in Crohn's disease.

4. *Multiple lesions.* Although Crohn's disease is usually most easily demonstrated when it involves the terminal ileum, it is common for multiple sites to be affected in the jejunum and ileum (Fig. 34.11A). Multiple local views taken with compression to avoid the confusion of overlying loops of bowel are necessary in order to

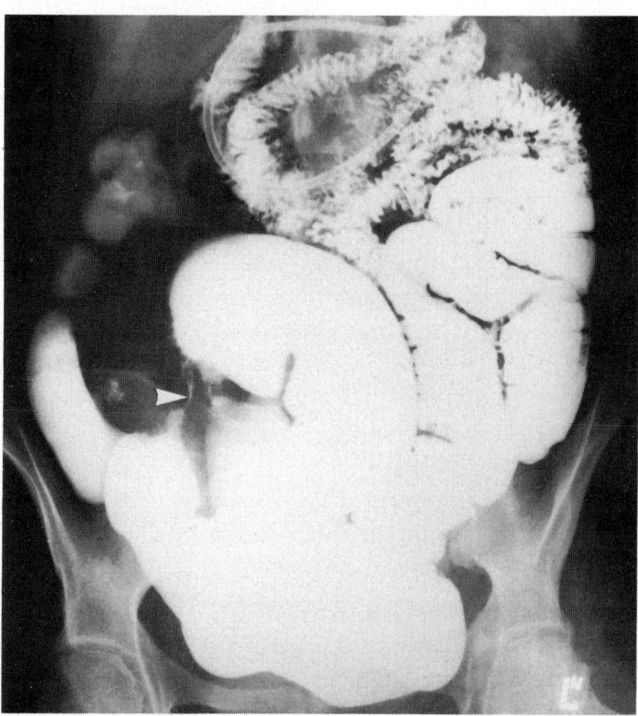

Fig. 34.8 Crohn's disease. Small bowel enema showing dilated loops and stricture (*arrow*).

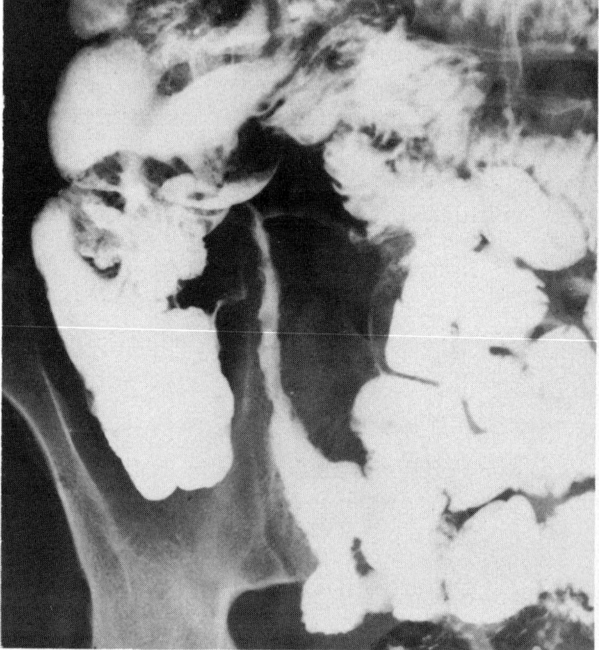

Fig. 34.9

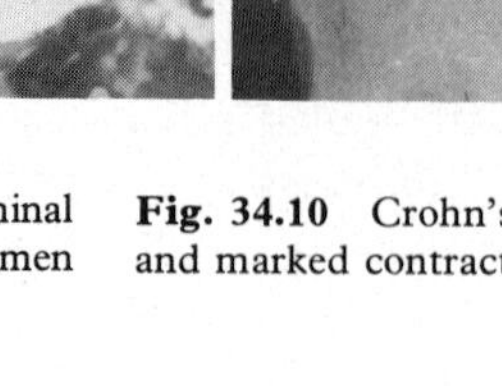

Fig. 34.10

Fig. 34.9 Crohn's disease showing marked narrowing of the terminal ileum. The wall of the affected loop is very thickened so that the lumen appears separated from the adjacent loops of bowel.

Fig. 34.10 Crohn's disease showing narrowing of the terminal ileum and marked contraction of the caecum and ascending colon.

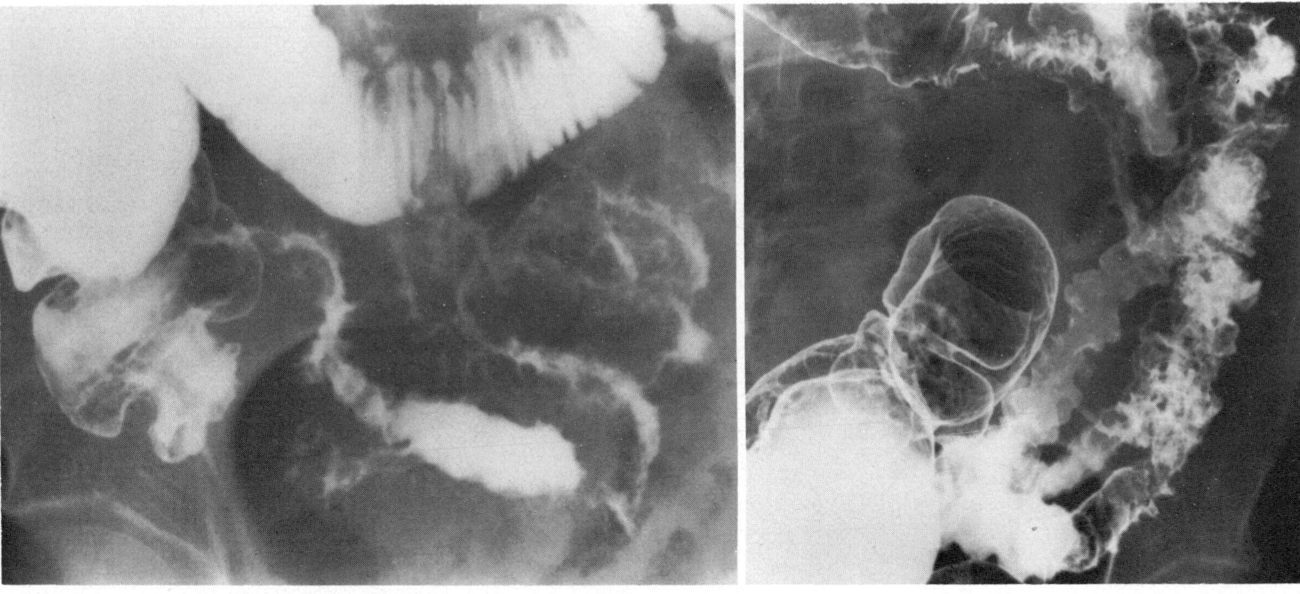

Fig. 34.11 Crohn's disease affecting the ileum and colon. A There is extensive involvement of distal loops of ileum with dilatation of proximal loops. B Same patient showing Crohn's disease affecting part of the transverse colon and the descending colon.

demonstrate the multiple lesions of Crohn's disease and these will materially affect clinical management.

(*c*) **Chronic.** In the later stages of Crohn's disease the clinical presentation is one of a fixed inflammatory mass, often with external sinus formation or internal fistulae. These fistulae usually pass into adjoining loops of ileum but may involve the sigmoid colon, bladder or vagina. Ureteric obstruction with hydronephrosis may occur. Fistulae between small bowel and colon are best demonstrated by a barium enema examination. Those between loops of small intestine may be very difficult or impossible to demonstrate. In some instances they are short and result in a length of the small bowel being short circuited and becoming a stagnant loop in which pockets of barium may be left behind when most of the contrast medium has left the small intestine. Sinus tracks on to the abdominal wall are best investigated by sinography when the exact site of leak from the gut can usually be demonstrated.

Colonic involvement. It is becoming increasingly recognized that Crohn's disease may affect the colon and in some clinics colonic Crohn's disease is seen more frequently than ulcerative colitis. The radiological examination of any patient suspected of having Crohn's disease is incomplete without a double contrast barium enema.

When Crohn's disease occurs in the large bowel it tends to involve the proximal rather than the distal colon. The lesions are often not in continuity so that normal lengths of colon are demonstrated between the abnormal areas (Fig. 34.11B). The lesions may also be discontinuous circumferentially so that one side of the wall of the colon may show deep ulceration whilst the opposite wall is smooth and shows normal haustration. When there is total involvement of the colon the terminal ileum is usually involved also and this may help to differentiate the condition from ulcerative colitis. Other differential features are listed in Table 34.1.

The ulceration in the colon may appear similar to that seen in the small intestine. The ulceration may be longitudinal or transverse, a combination of the two forms giving rise to a *cobblestone* appearance. Deep *rose-thorn* ulcers may be seen at the margins of the colon; there may be irregularity of outline with asymmetrical involvement, and nodularity of the colon may be seen, particularly after evacuation. Fistulae are less common than in Crohn's disease of the ileum.

When the disease is confined to the colon it may not be possible to make a firm diagnosis on the first examination. The clinical course of the disease, subsequent involvement of the ileum, the development of fistulae or the finding of granuloma on rectal biopsy may confirm the diagnosis of Crohn's disease at a later date. Until a firm diagnosis is reached it is best to refer to 'colitis', type unknown, rather than to attach a possibly incorrect diagnostic label.

Differential diagnosis. In many instances of Crohn's disease the appearances are characteristic and the diagnosis not difficult. A number of conditions may display features seen in some cases of Crohn's disease.

Tuberculosis of the small bowel may simulate Crohn's disease completely. Stenotic lesions are common and may be multiple. The terminal ileum, caecum and ascending colon are often affected in continuity and the

Table 34.1 Comparison of Crohn's disease and ulcerative colitis

	Ulcerative colitis	Crohn's disease
Clinical features		
Rectal bleeding	Virtually always	50%
Abdominal pain	Uncommon	50%
Abdominal mass	Never	Common at some stage
Anal lesion	25%	75%
Colon involved	Distal colon always	Predominantly right-sided
Colonic Features		
Distribution of lesions	Rectum in 95% in continuity	Rectum in 30% Discontinuous; normal patches in diseased areas, asymmetrical
Ulceration	Shallow and granular	Deep, rose-thorn
Haustra	Lost early in disease	Incomplete loss
Small bowel	If involved, in continuity with caecum Ileo-caecal valve patulous Terminal ileum dilated	Often discontinuous Ileo-caecal valve narrow or normal Terminal ileum stenosed and thickened
Complication		
Fistula and sinuses	Never	Common
Toxic dilatation	Common	Rare
Perforation	Uncommon	Rare
Carcinoma of colon	High risk in total colitis	Rare
Associated conditions	Arthritis Sclerosing cholangitis	

caecum may become extremely contracted (Figs. 34.12 and 34.13). Internal fistulae and external sinuses frequently occur. Tuberculosis of the gut is not necessarily associated with involvement of the lung. The presence of calcified mesenteric lymph nodes cannot be used as a differentiating feature from Crohn's disease because calcified tuberculous mesenteric glands may be seen in both conditions.

Infection of the terminal ileum with *yersinia enterocolitica* which usually occurs in females aged 10–30 years, may cause colicky pain and tenderness in the right iliac fossa closely mimicking appendicitis or Crohn's

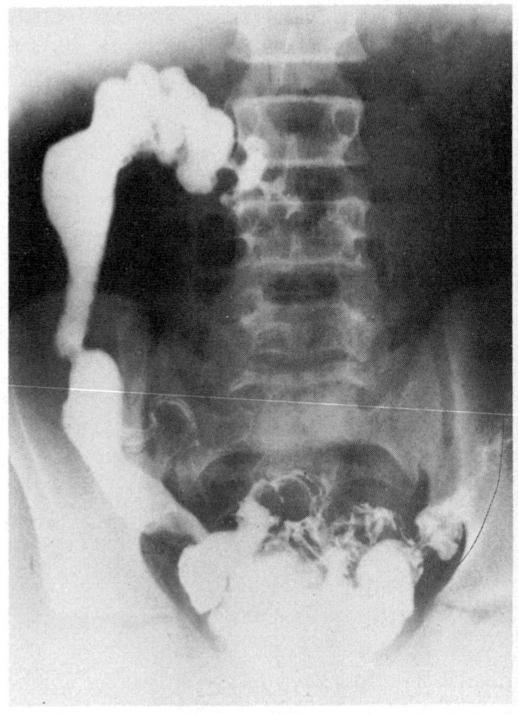

Fig. 34.12 Hyperplastic tuberculosis of the caecum in an adolescent aged 14. The caecum is very contracted and the terminal ileum moderately dilated.

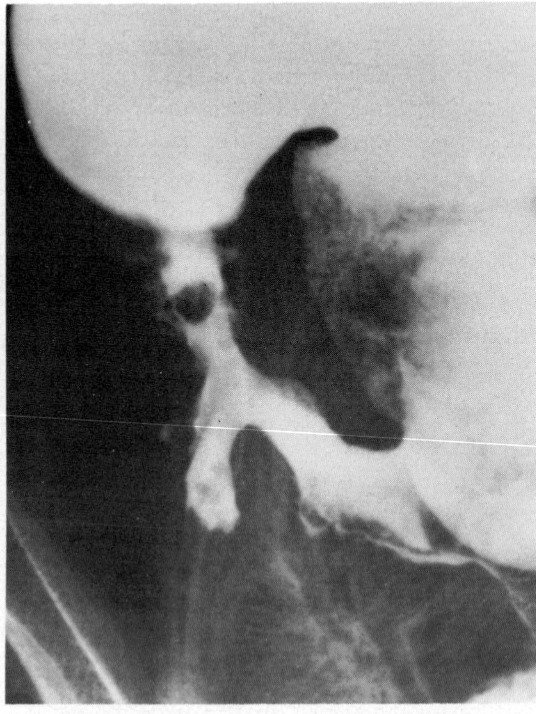

Fig. 34.13 Hyperplastic tuberculosis affecting the terminal ileum, caecum and ascending colon. The caecum and ascending colon are fibrosed and contracted and the ileo-caecal valve is patulous.

disease. There are exacerbations and remissions and the general course is more benign than Crohn's disease. Radiologically, small irregular filling defects may be shown in a thickened and tender terminal ileum. Deep ulceration does not occur and the colon is not demonstrably involved. The filling defects, due to inflammatory oedema, are larger and more irregular than those seen in nodular lymphoid hyperplasia (1–3 mm).

Lymphosarcoma may simulate non stenotic regional ileitis with ulceration, thickening and blunting of folds, and fistula formation. However, in lymphosarcoma the lumen tends to be eccentric, intraluminal nodules are common and stenotic areas are rare. *Hodgkin's disease* appears similar to lymphosarcoma but, being more fibrotic, stenotic lesions are more common and fistulae rarely occur.

Segmental *infarction* of the small bowel may show rapid changes from severe oedema, ulceration and spasm to a fibrotic stricture. Progression is rapid and the history may be helpful. Similar changes may be seen in *radiation ileitis*. *Carcinoid* tumours are occasionally multiple and may cause stenotic lesions in the ileum. *Actinomycosis* of the caecum is extremely rare and is diagnosed with certainty only by the detection of sulphur granules and microscopic demonstration of the ray fungus in the discharging sinus or on histological examination of a biopsy specimen from the tissues. Bone involvement is more frequent in actinomycosis than in any of the other granulomatous lesions.

VASCULAR LESIONS

Primary vascular lesions affecting the small bowel may cause acute or chronic ischaemia.

Acute ischaemia may result from arterial embolization or thrombosis of an atheromatous artery. It presents as a surgical emergency. Initially there may be a local ileus and oedema of the affected segment of gut. This may improve or progress to gangrene, rupture of the gut wall and generalized peritonitis. The plain films will show dilated fluid-filled loops of small bowel, possibly with air in their wall. Later there may be free gas in the peritoneal cavity. If the gut becomes infected with gas-forming organisms gas may be seen in the portal vein or in the intrahepatic branches, a sign of impending death.

In acute ischaemia barium examination is contra-indicated. In a few cases emergency angiography has demonstrated the cause, usually an embolus in a major vessel, and allowed restorative vascular surgery. Most patients with acute ischaemia of gut are dealt with as a surgical emergency, the aim being to preserve as much viable gut as possible and the delay for arteriographic examination is seldom tolerated.

Chronic ischaemia may result from atheromatous narrowing of arterial ostia, arteritis, fibromuscular hyperplasia or pressure on the coeliac axis artery by a band or the crus of the diaphragm. There is such a rich anastomosis between the coeliac axis and the superior and inferior mesenteric arteries that a gradual narrowing or occlusion of one main vessel may give rise to no symptoms and is often a chance finding at aortography. If two major vessels are affected mid gut ischaemia may result.

Unfortunately, the symptoms of chronic ischaemia, so-called intestinal angina, are non-specific, so that it is difficult to select the right patients for full angiographic examination. Pain after meals, steatorrhoea and other types of malabsorption and severe loss of weight may occur. An abdominal bruit may be heard. It is likely that many cases of ischaemia pass unrecognized.

Plain films may be normal or show dilatation of loops of small bowel. Barium examination may show thickened, rigid loops of intestine, some being dilated, with thickened oedematous folds. A featureless 'hosepipe' small bowel appearance has also been described. The appearances may very closely mimic coeliac disease or regional enteritis.

A mainstream aortogram to show the overall circulation and anastomoses is essential but it is the lateral view of the aortogram which gives the most information about the pathological anatomy and the exact site of the stenotic lesions. The gut is supplied by three main arteries with rich anastomotic connections of the coeliac axis, superior and inferior mesenteric arteries. It is necessary for at least two of these arteries to be significantly narrowed for symptoms to occur. The lateral view shows the site and extent of the stenosis; the anterior view the attempt at collateral circulation.

Reconstructive arterial surgery is hazardous and not uniformly successful but relief of symptoms may sometimes follow operation for pressure on the coeliac axis artery from a band or the crus of the diaphragm. The acceptance of the chronic mid-gut ischaemia is not universal and some authorities deny its existence (Morson, 1977).

Infarction of bowel due to mesenteric venous thrombosis may be even more difficult to recognize unless there are venous thromboses elsewhere in the body. A barium small bowel examination may show distorted inactive segments of bowel with 'fingerprint' deformities in the wall caused by mucosal and submucosal haemorrhages. Ulceration in the affected loops may also occur.

TUMOURS

Tumours of the small bowel are relatively rare, the majority are usually malignant (*adenocarcinomata*).

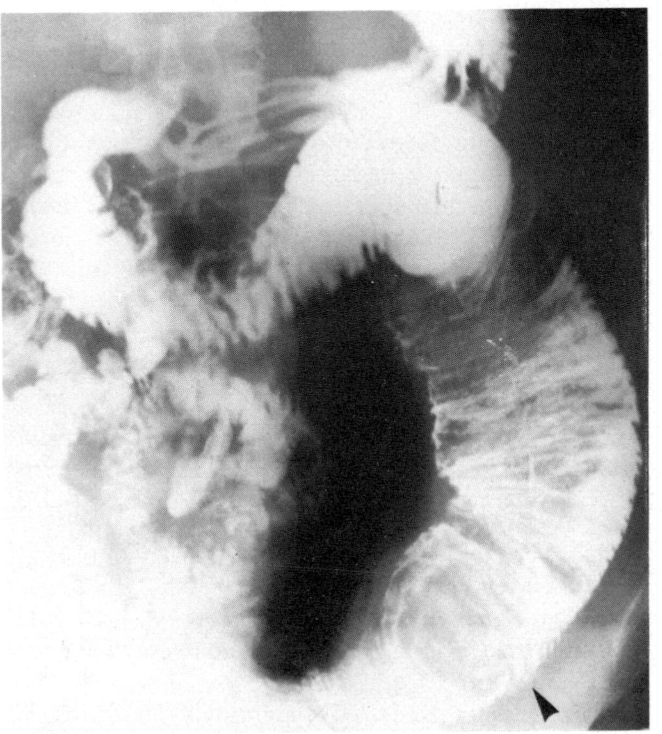

Fig. 34.14 Lymphosarcoma of jejunum. The jejunum is expanded by a partially intraluminal soft tissue tumour (*arrow*).

Benign *adenomata* and *lipomata* are usually only of clinical interest in that they frequently form the apex of an intussusception.

Malignant tumours are a less common cause of intussusception as they spread circumferentially around the wall and do not usually possess a pedicle. Owing to the fluid nature of the contents of the small bowel such growths do not produce obstructive symptoms until they are advanced. Polypoid carcinomata may, on rare occasions, give rise to intussusception and the associated obstruction may give rise to signs at an earlier date.

Sarcomata of the small bowel are usually *lymphosarcomata* and can sometimes be differentiated radiologically from carcinomata by the fact that, unlike carcinomata, they expand (Fig. 34.14) rather than constrict the bowel lumen (Fig. 34.15).

Carcinoid tumours radiologically manifest themselves as a filling defect mimicking a carcinoma and usually occur around the ileo-caecal region or in the appendix. Carcinoid tumours which produce endocrine secretions and the clinical syndrome associated with the production of serotinin are usually highly malignant and are frequently associated with liver metastases when these endocrine changes are present.

Metastatic (serosal) deposits of growth on the small

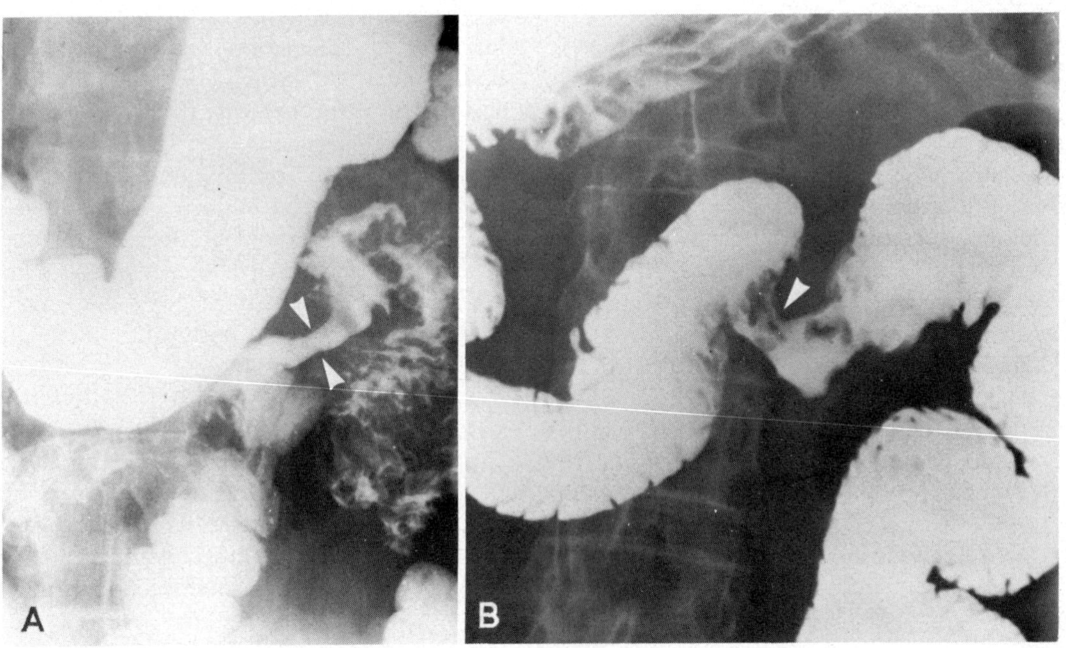

Fig. 34.15A Carcinoma of the first coil of jejunum demonstrating a constricting lesion lying just below the stomach in the left hypochondrium (*arrow*). B Further jejunal carcinoma causing stenosis of the lumen and destruction of the mucosa of a segment of proximal small bowel (*arrow*).

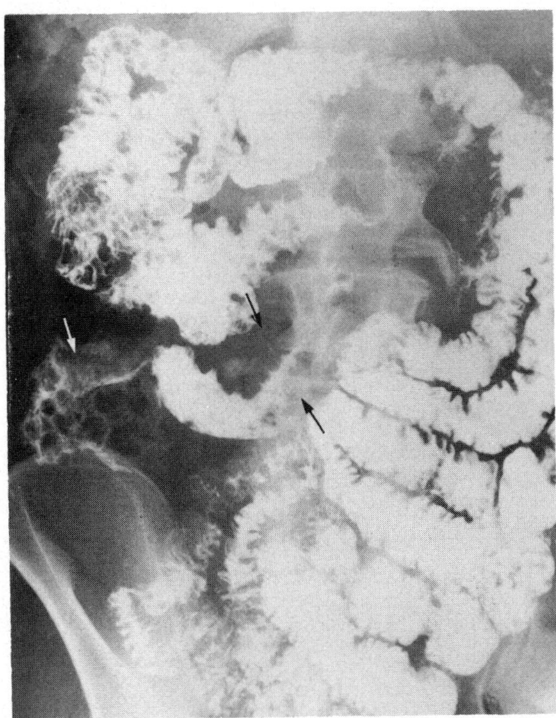

Fig. 34.16 Metastaic lymphosarcoma of the small bowel and caecum. Metastatic tumours, either sarcomatous or carcinomatous, arise on the serosal surface and produce bizarre deformities without mucosal ulceration. Changes in coils of small bowel and the caecum are indicated (*arrows*).

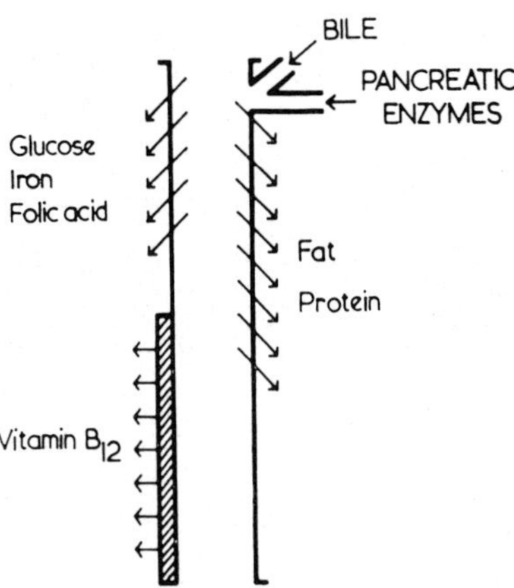

Fig. 34.17 Diagram of the sites at which different substances are absorbed in the small intestine.

bowel give the greatest difficulty in diagnosis as the defects they produce are shallow and are seldom associated with mucosal ulceration (Fig. 34.16). *Melanoma* and *carcinoma of the stomach* or *ovary* may all give such intestinal deposits, obstruction is marked only when there is associated extensive involvement of the peritoneum.

MALABSORPTION SYNDROMES

Absorption and malabsorption

An understanding of the physiology of digestion and absorption is essential if patients with malabsorption are to be investigated by radiological means to the best effect. After homogenization and lubrication in the mouth food is swallowed into the stomach, where further homogenization occurs and digestion begins. The chyme is then propelled through the pylorus into the small intestine where digestion and absorption are completed. The sites at which different substances are absorbed in the small intestine are illustrated in Fig. 34.17. Substances which require no digestion, such as glucose, inorganic iron and folic acid appear to be absorbed as soon as they reach the small intestine. Fat and protein, however, require preliminary emulsification and digestion by the bile and pancreatic enzymes and are therefore absorbed more slowly. These substances may be absorbed in the upper jejunum but it is probable that the motility of the upper intestine propels them more distally than glucose, before absorption is complete. The absorption of B_{12} is remarkable in that it is absorbed only from the distal ileum.

From this it will be seen that folic acid deficiency or a flat glucose tolerance test usually indicates a diffuse abnormality of the small intestine, the cause of which is often more accurately diagnosed by a biopsy than by radiology. Steatorrhoea, on the other hand, may be due to a failure of emulsification and digestion caused by a lack of bile or pancreatic enzymes, or to failure of absorption, caused by a widespread intestinal abnormality. Both radiology and biopsy are required in such cases. Pure B_{12} deficiency, if pernicious anaemia is excluded, is occasionally due to disease or resection of the distal ileum, but may be due to bacterial contamination of the small bowel, the bacteria competing with the host for the vitamin. Radiology has an essential part of play in this group of patients, since clinical symptoms of small bowel disease may be minimal, or absent, as in jejunal diverticulosis.

Gastrectomy may cause malabsorption in a number of ways. Severe deficiencies are not common after the Bilroth type of operation, since there is frequently a relatively large gastric remnant, some control of the rate of emptying of the stomach is retained and the continuity of the alimentary tract is not interrupted, so that normal mixing of chyme with bile and pancreatic enzymes occurs. After a Polya type of gastrectomy there are several potential reasons for severe malabsorption. There may be B_{12} deficiency due to lack of intrinsic factor, due to a small or atrophic gastric remnant. There is loss of the normal mixing and homogenization of food in the stomach, and this ill-prepared chyme may enter the small intestine at a rapid rate. Because of this and the discontinuity of the alimentary tract the chyme does not mix properly with bile and pancreatic enzymes so that digestion is impaired. A stagnant, afferent loop may cause malabsorption by pooling bile and pancreatic enzymes so that they do not mix with chyme and perhaps enter the jejunum at times when there is no food present, causing a gastritis and oesophagitis. Infection of this stagnant afferent loop may cause bacterial contamination of the alimentary tract. Any form of gastrectomy may unmask previously sub-clinical malabsorption. For example, adult coeliac disease or disaccharidase deficiency may become clinically important after gastrectomy although not recognized before operation.

Radiological investigation

The term 'malabsorption syndrome' is sometimes used as though it was a firm diagnosis (sometimes even synonymous with adult coeliac disease) instead of a general statement about a condition for which one or more of many causes could be responsible. It is no more precise as a diagnosis than 'shortness of breath' and requires the same detailed investigation in which radiology is important but must be correlated with all the other clinical data. Before a patient with malabsorption is examined radiologically it should be known what type of malabsorption or deficiency is suspected or proven, and what type of abdominal surgery, if any, has been performed. The examination can be planned accordingly and the findings are subsequently fitted into the whole clinical picture.

From the radiological point of view the malabsorption syndromes may be divided into two main groups (Table 34.2). The first group contains those conditions in which the radiological features are mainly those associated with steatorrhoea. In this group the radiological features are usually non-specific and a firm diagnosis depends on other methods, usually small bowel biopsy. Even in this group, however, radiology is frequently indicated in order to rule out some local anatomical cause for malabsorption (listed in Group 2). The second group contains conditions with specific radiological features. It is in this group, particularly when there is some anatomical lesion of the small bowel, that radiology may be of great value and is frequently the only method of arriving at a firm diagnosis.

Table 34.2 Malabsorption

GROUP 1 Radiological features mainly those of steatorrhoea

A. Diffuse lesions of the intestinal mucosa:
- Coeliac disease
- Idiopathic steatorrhoea (adult coeliac disease)
- Tropical sprue
- Infiltrations—Whipple's disease
  —amyloidosis

B. Defects of digestion:
- (*a*) Deficiency of bile
  - Obstructive jaundice
  - Biliary cirrhosis
- (*b*) Deficiency of pancreatic enzymes
  - Cystic fibrosis
  - Chronic pancreatitis
  - Pancreatectomy

C. Post-gastrectomy steatorrhoea

GROUP 2 Conditions with specific radiological features

A. Localized (often multiple) lesions of the small intestine:
- Regional ileitis
- Hodgkin's disease
- Lymphosarcoma
- Diffuse sclerosis (scleroderma)

B. Anatomical lesions of the small intestine:
- (*a*) Resection
  - Proximal resection
  - Distal resection
- (*b*) Bacterial contamination
  - Jejunal diverticulosis
  - Stagnant loop
  - Ileal stricture
  - Fistula
- (*c*) Mixed lesions (resection plus bacterial contamination)

C. Disaccharidase deficiency
- Hypolactasia
- Hyposucrasia

Group 1 (Radiological features mainly those of steatorrhoea)

(a) **Diffuse lesions of the intestinal mucosa.** In this group of conditions a firm diagnosis rests on intestinal biopsy but suspicion may be raised and a presumptive diagnosis made on the radiological appearances. Idiopathic steatorrhoea is an unfortunate term since it is not idiopathic but due to gluten sensitivity and steatorrhoea need not be present in a patient presenting with symptoms due to malabsorption of substances other than fat. Adult coeliac disease, or gluten-induced enteropathy, are better names for this condition in which there is partial or sub-total villous atrophy. The main radiological abnormalities are dilation of the jejunum and flocculation of the barium sulphate preparation.

Most modern barium sulphate preparations contain suspending agents designed to prevent flocculation or clumping together of the barium particles in the presence of mucus. Flocculation of undiluted barium sulphate suspension (Micropaque, Baritop) in the small intestine of an adult in the United Kingdom is abnormal, provided no gastric residue was present before the barium was administered and that food has not been taken after the barium. Steatorrhoea secondary to adult coeliac disease is the most likely cause and biopsy is needed for confirmation. However, many patients with steatorrhoea do not flocculate barium and there is no correlation between the amount of flocculation and the severity of the steatorrhoea or the degree of villous atrophy present. When flocculation occurs, radiographs show only the barium particles clumped together in the sump of individual coils of bowel. Coating of the mucosa does not occur and no details of the intestinal anatomy can be made out. A repeat examination with a 'non-flocculating' barium may be necessary to exclude localized lesions such as strictures. There is no completely non-flocculating barium preparation, but some resist flocculation more than others. A flocculation-resistant preparation such as

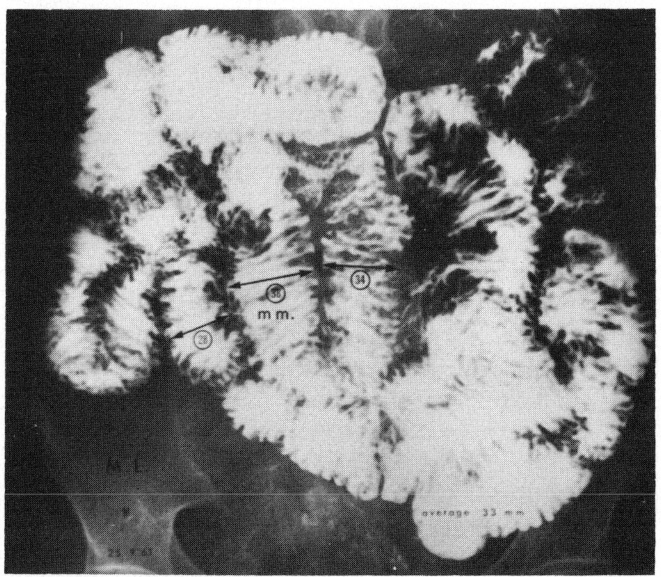

Fig. 34.18 Adult coelic disease. Moderate dilatation of the jejunum in a patient with diarrhoea due to steatorrhoea. Biopsy showed subtotal villus atrophy.

Micropaque is useful in that it is sufficiently resistant for flocculation to arouse suspicion of steatorrhoea and lead to biopsy.

Dilation of the jejunum results in the secondary folds being smoothed out, revealing the primary transverse folds, the valvulae conniventes. Normally individual folds of mucosa cannot be traced completely across the lumen of the jejunum, except transiently during the passage of a bolus. If several coils of bowel on one film show this smoothing out of the secondary folds the appearances are abnormal (Fig. 34.18).

In adult coeliac disease there is a correlation between the calibre of the small bowel and the clinical state of the patient (Fig. 34.20A). Those patients who are most severely ill show the most severe dilatation. All patients with hypokalaemia show moderate or severe dilatation but equal dilatation may be seen in those with normal serum potassium levels (Fig. 34.20B). Moreover, restoration of serum potassium to normal does not necessarily result in a reduction in the calibre of the small bowel. However, the calibre of the small bowel does mirror the clinical state quite closely, in that patients who respond to a gluten-free diet show a similar improvement in the radiological appearances of their small bowel (Fig. 34.19). On relapse the small bowel calibre increases. If a patient on a gluten-free diet shows a worsening radiological picture one should suspect that either the diet is not being adhered to, or that some complication has occurred such as the development of a reticulosis or a carcinoma of the gastro-intestinal tract.

At the other end of the spectrum of disease some

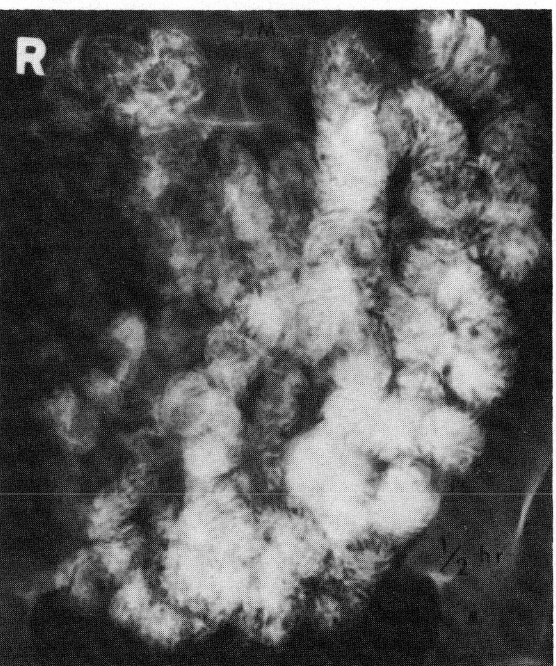

Fig. 34.19 Adult coeliac disease. Normal small bowel appearances in a patient with megaloblastic anaemia but no intestinal symptoms. Biopsy showed partial villous atrophy.

patients with villous atrophy have few or no intestinal symptoms and present with a mild, macrocytic megaloblastic anaemia. Such patients usually have either a completely normal small bowel appearance or show minimal dilatation. A normal radiological appearance in no way excludes partial or sub-total villous atrophy but such patients are not clinically ill (Fig. 34.19).

Radiological appearance of the small bowel in tropical sprue is identical to that of gluten-induced enteropathy. The degree of dilatation correlates roughly with the severity of the clinical illness and improvement follows successful treatment with a broad spectrum antibiotic (Fig. 34.21).

In intestinal lipodystrophy (Whipple's disease) there may be the non-specific changes found in patients with steatorrhoea from any cause—dilatation and sometimes flocculation. In addition there may be evidence of en-

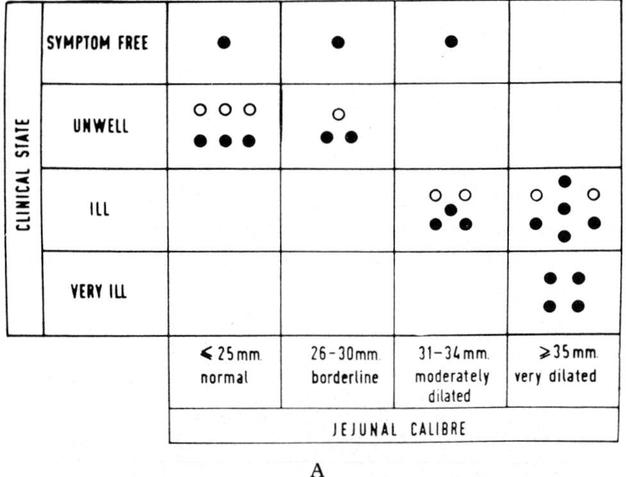

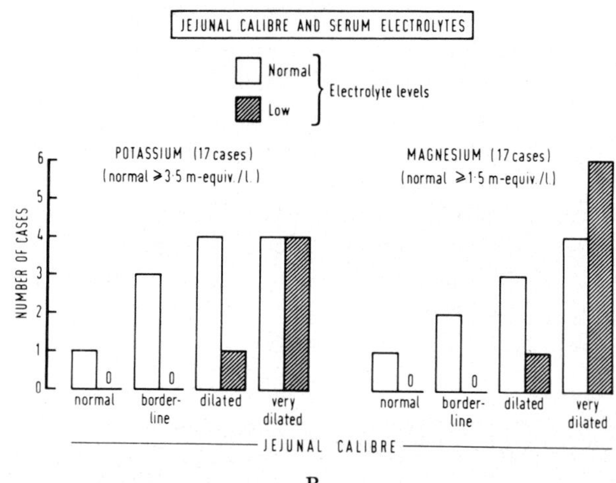

Fig. 34.20A Relationship between jejunal calibre and clinical state in 28 patients with adult coeliac disease. (Closed circles indicate subtotal villus atrophy. Open circles indicate partial villus atrophy.) B The realtionship between jejunal calibre and serum electrolytes in 23 patients with adult coeliac disease. All patients with hypokalaemia had dilated jejunal coils but equal dilatation also occurred in patients with normal electrolytes.

larged abdominal lymph nodes, bone changes, particularly in the spine and resembling rheumatoid arthritis as well as sclerosis of the sacro-iliac joints. The diagnosis, as in amyloid infiltration, depends on intestinal biopsy.

(b) **Defects of digestion.** In this group of conditions there may be malabsorption of fat, but the radiological changes associated with the steatorrhoeas are usually not as severe as when there is generalized abnormality of the intestinal mucosa. The underlying cause of the digestive defect may be demonstrated, for example, gallstones or pancreatic carcinoma may account for an obstructive jaundice, and pancreatic calcification may indicate the presence of chronic pancreatitis.

(c) **Post-gastrectomy steatorrhoea.** In most cases malabsorption following gastrectomy is a defect of digestion, due to poor mixing of food with bile and pancreatic enzymes, and radiology has little part to play. Stagnation in the afferent loop, either due to kinking or undue length, is a rare cause. This dilated afferent loop may be demonstrated by barium meal but frequently fails to fill as peristalsis tends to prevent filling. Filling may sometimes be obtained by inhibiting peristalsis by Probanthine (30 mg intravenously) and by placing the patient in the right lateral or prone position. Examination several hours after intravenous injection of Biligrafin may occasionally demonstrate a collection of opacified bile within a dilated stagnant afferent loop.

Sideropenic webs may occur between two and twenty years after gastrectomy and be associated with iron deficiency anaemia, dysphagia, glossitis and angular

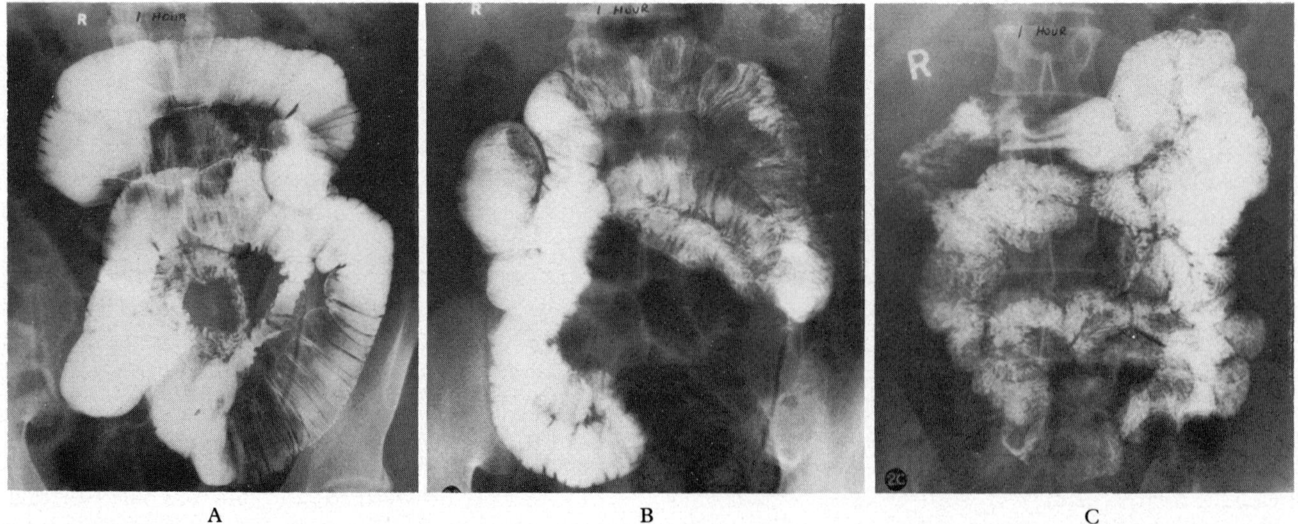

Fig. 34.21 Tropical sprue showing response to treatment with a broad spectrum antibiotic. A Patient severely ill with diarrhoea and megaloblastic anaemia. Moderate dilatation of the jejunum. B One month after treatment. Patient recovering and small bowel returning to normal. C Three months later. Patient has completely recovered and the small bowel appearances are normal.

stomatitis. Whereas the webs of the Plummer-Vinson syndrome are seen only in women, post-gastrectomy webs also occur in men.

Group 2 (Conditions with specific radiological features)

(a) **Localized (often multiple) lesions of the small intestine.** Although some form of malabsorption is common in Crohn's disease it is rarely if ever caused by destruction of absorbing surface alone. When malabsorption is severe there are usually multiple lesions throughout the small bowel causing stagnation in individual loops, and fistulae may be present. There is often the added problem of previous surgical resection and the possibility of stagnant loops following surgery. Loss of protein from the ulcerated lesions of regional ileitis further contribute to the patient's malnutrition. Demonstrations of the areas of small bowel affected by Crohn's disease, the extent of stagnation in different loops and the presence of fistulous connections between different loops of small bowel require very detailed radiological examination. Paired erect and supine films should be taken and the examination continued until all barium has left the small intestine, in order to assess the extent and demonstrate the site of stagnation.

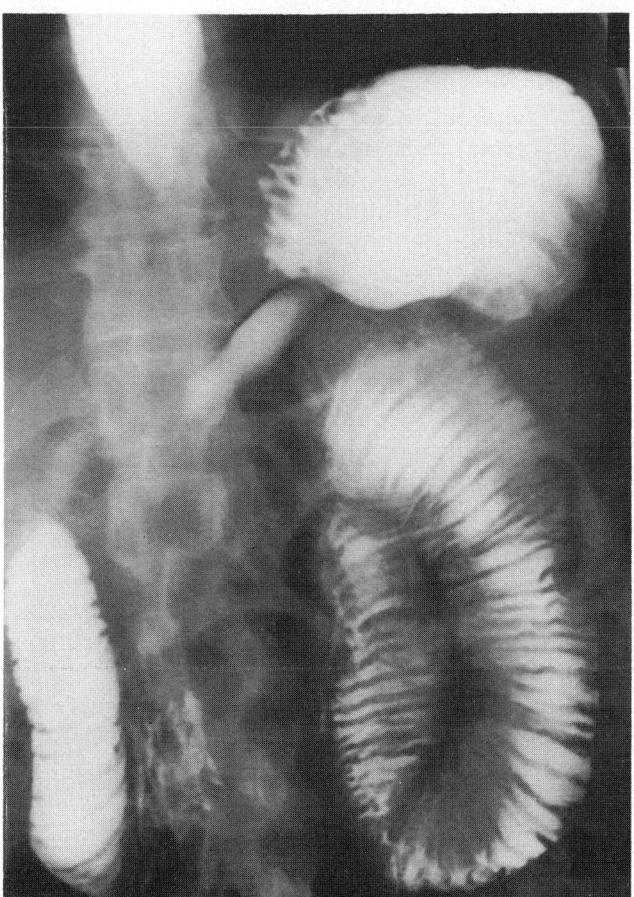

Fig. 34.22 Scleroderma affecting the oesophagus, duodenum and jejunum.

Hodgkin's disease of the small bowel is often associated with villous atrophy and may complicate longstanding gluten-induced enteropathy. Multiple ulcerated filling defects or rigid areas devoid of mucosa may be seen in the small bowel. These may cause partial but rarely complete obstruction. Enlarged lymph nodes in the mesentery may displace the gut and an enlarged spleen may be seen.

In diffuse sclerosis (*scleroderma*) the duodenum is often severely dilated together with other loops of proximal small bowel (Fig. 34.22). Although the loops may be very dilated the folds are not thickened and there is no evidence of ulceration. There are, in effect, multiple sites of functional obstruction because of lack of effective peristalsis. Severe stagnation in dilated loops may be demonstrated by continuing the examination until nearly all the barium has left the small bowel, up to 24 or 48 hours if necessary.

(b) **Anatomical lesions of the small bowel.**

A. Resection

Examination of the small intestine after resection is carried out for the following reasons.

(i) In order to assess the length and normality of the remaining small intestine. Massive resections are often carried out for infarction of bowel and surgical details of emergency operations are not always available. It is possible for up to one-quarter of the small intestine to be resected without it being recognizable radiologically.

(ii) In order to exclude a recurrence of the disease or the formation of a stricture or a blind loop at the site of anastomosis.

The radiological appearances will depend not only on the length of bowel resected, but also whether a proximal or distal resection has been carried out.

Peristalsis is more active in the jejunum than in the ileum so that chyme, and hence barium, moves through it relatively rapidly. After a massive resection of jejunum, usually following infarction, the overall transit time from stomach to caecum remains normal or is only slightly reduced, provided the slower moving ileum and ileocaecal valve is retained. Malabsorption is unlikely to occur since the ileum is capable of taking over most if not all of the functions of the jejunum. The follow-through examination is likely to appear normal except for some recognizable shortening of small bowel.

The ileum is resected far more often than the jejunum, usually for Crohn's disease; sometimes for tumour, adhesions or infarction. Since the active jejunum is retained the transit time from stomach to caecum is much reduced, especially if the ileo-caecal valve has been resected also. Malabsorption is more likely to occur and specific vitamin B_{12} deficiency develop if the distal ileum has been resected.

If less than a quarter of the jejunum has been resected and the ileo-caecal valve remains intact the radiological appearances may be entirely normal. With more massive jejunal resection the transit time is reduced and fluid levels may be seen in the colon and ascending colon. These fluid levels are commonly seen after massive distal resections and should not by themselves be accepted as evidence of obstruction (Fig. 34.23). Normally following distal resection there is no hypertrophy or dilatation of the remaining bowel unless only a few feet of jejunum remain. Dilatation of the small bowel following a distal resection is almost invariably due to a recurrence of the disease, adhesions, or stricture at the site of the anastomosis.

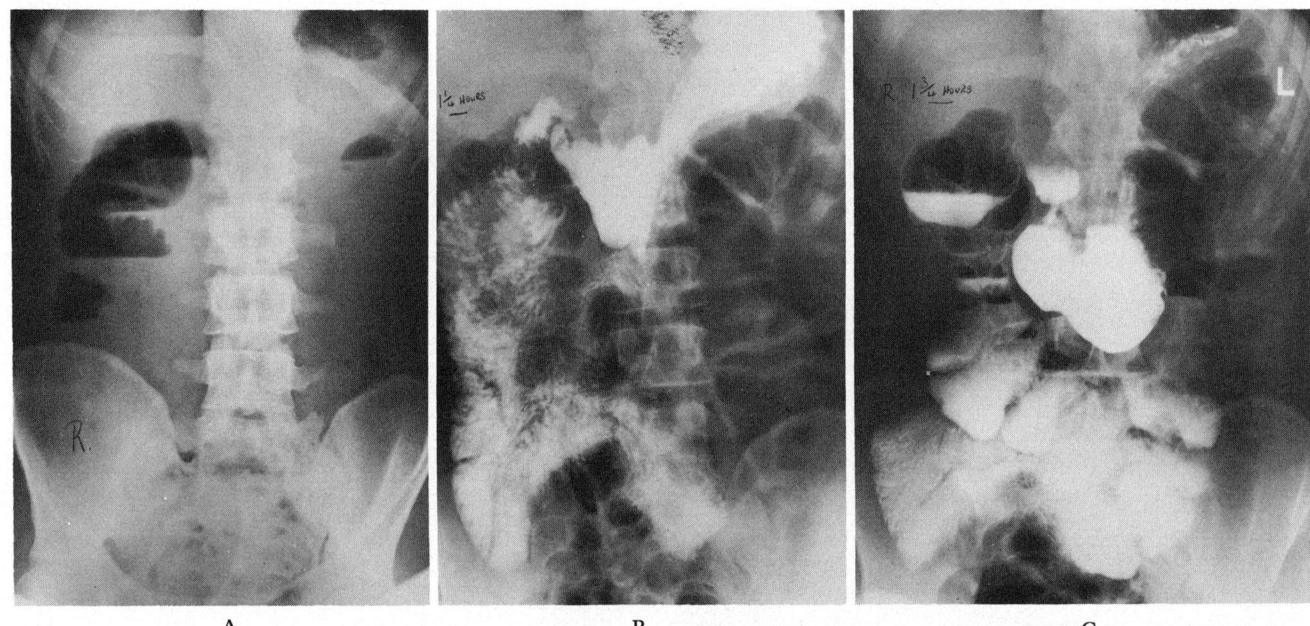

Fig. 34.23 Massive resection of distal small bowel without obstruction All except 4 ft of jejunum have been resected for volvulus. A Straight radiograph. Patient erect showing fluid levels. These do not indicate obstruction. B Barium follow-through examination. One and one-quarter hour film showing jejunum of normal calibre. C One and three-quarter hour film. The fluid barium in the colon demonstrates the site of the fluid levels in Figure 34.23A.

B. Bacterial contamination

Bacterial contamination in the small intestine of sufficient severity to cause malabsorption is usually due to the stagnation of intestinal contents, the extent of which can be estimated on the barium follow-through examination, provided the films are taken until most of the barium has passed into the colon. Films taken 24, 48, or even 72 hours after the ingestion of barium may be necessary. Much less commonly bacterial contamination may be due to a fistula.

Jejunal diverticulosis. Diverticulosis sufficiently severe to cause malabsorption can be recognized on the follow-through examination provided excessive flocculation of barium does not occur. Erect films with and without barium will show fluid levels within the diverticula and may simulate small bowel obstruction, except that no dilated bowel is seen on the supine film (Fig. 34.24). The diverticula themselves are commonly seen as round, oval or flask-shaped structures leading from the bowel lumen. Mucosa leading into the neck of individual diverticula may be shown and is the most certain method of diagnosis (Fig. 34.25). Occasionally accurate localization of the diverticula may be important, because if they are confined to one loop or a short segment of jejunum, resection with cure may be possible. In selected cases intubation of the lower jejunum or ileum may be useful by demonstrating the normality of the ileum before withdrawing the tube and showing segments of bowel affected by diverticulosis (ratio of jejunal to ileal diverticula, 29:1). However, since these patients are usually elderly and their anaemia can usually be controlled by antibiotics and replacement therapy, this localization is not needed in most cases.

Stagnant loops. A distinction should be made between blind and stagnant loops. A blind loop is closed at one end. Only a small proportion of blind loops are stagnant and not all stagnant loops are blind. If peristalsis tends to keep the loop empty (iso-peristaltic loop) there is no stagnation of contents and no malabsorption. The ascending colon following an end-to-end ileo-transverse anastomosis is an example of such a loop and causes no disability. If peristalsis in the loop tends to keep it full (retro-peristaltic loop) stasis of contents occurs and the loop may dilate to hold a large volume of stagnant intestinal contents. This type of blind loop occurs after

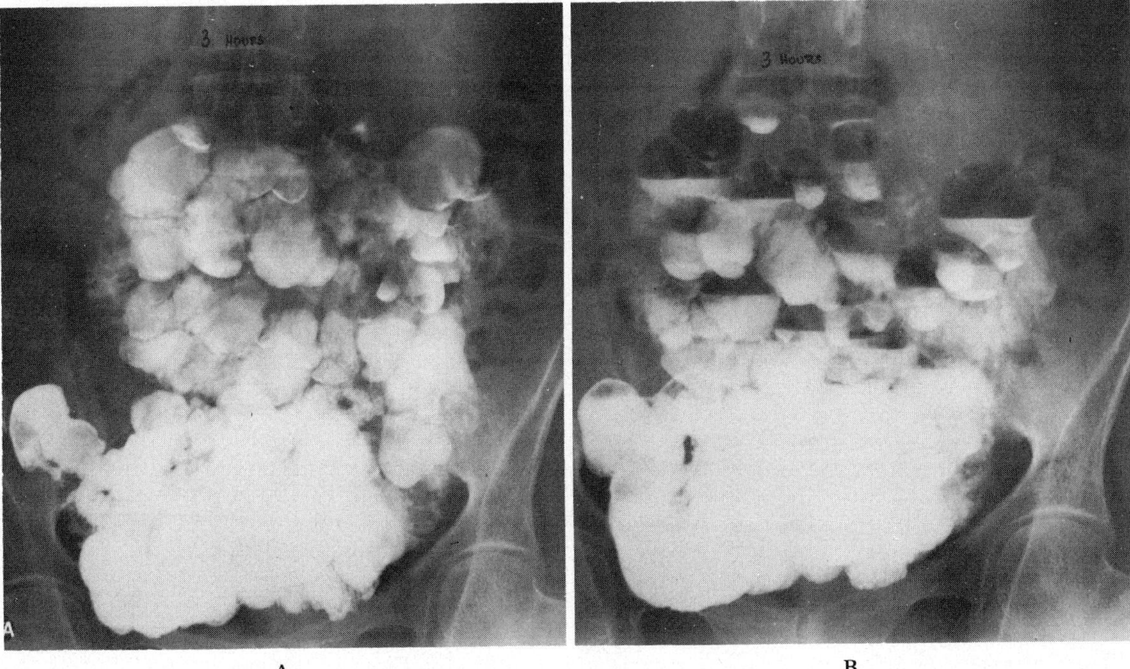

A B

Fig. 34.24 Jejunal diverticulosis. A Barium follow-through examination showing dilute barium in the diverticula resembling flocculation. B An erect film taken at the same time demonstrates the diverticula containing fluid levels.

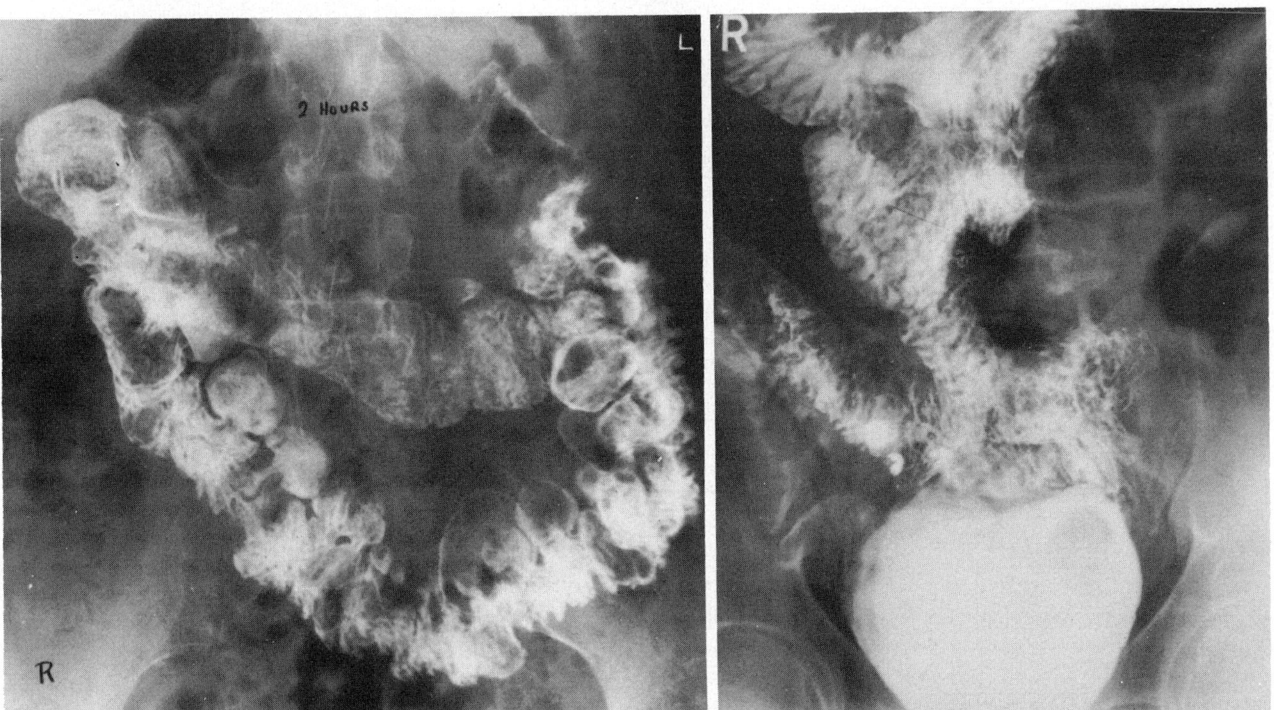

Fig. 34.25 Jejunal diverticulosis. Multiple diverticula are shown on the mesenteric border of a loop of jejunum. The mucosal folds entering the neck of the diverticula are well seen.

Fig. 34.26 Stagnant loop. Resection of distal ileum with side-to-side anastomosis following gunshot wound. A large stagnant loop of ileum has developed. A faecolith within this gave rise to ulceration and iron deficiency anaemia in addition to the megaloblastic anaemia caused by the bacterial contamination following stagnation.

a side-to-side entero-anastomosis, around an obstruction or after resection. Faecoliths may occur in these loops causing ulceration, haemorrhage and iron deficiency anaemia (Fig. 34.26). Fortunately only a small proportion of people with blind loops get malabsorption, the important factor being stagnation. Of course, many stagnant loops are not 'blind' but are incompletely obstructed loops in the mainstream of the ileum.

Stricture. Strictures of the jejunum usually present as an acute or sub-acute surgical emergency and rarely cause malabsorption. Ileal strictures, on the other hand, are often of sufficient chronicity to cause stagnation and malabsorption. Crohn's disease, tuberculosis and adhesions are the common causes. There may be surprisingly few intestinal symptoms even though there is gross dilatation of the ileum (Fig. 34.27). A follow-through examination shows progressive dilution of the barium sulphate suspension as it enters the dilated ileum. Thickened walls due to muscular hypertrophy may be seen in the less dilated proximal loops. The site of stricture can often be demonstrated by careful fluoroscopy, with separation of the loops by compression and local views. The size and length of the stricture should be noted, together with any evidence of ulceration, fistula formation or associated soft tissue mass. In severe and long-standing cases, however, the actual size of the obstruction may be difficult or impossible to demonstrate even after intubation of the ileum because of dilution and stagnation of barium. It may be possible to show the stricture by retrograde examination after barium enema.

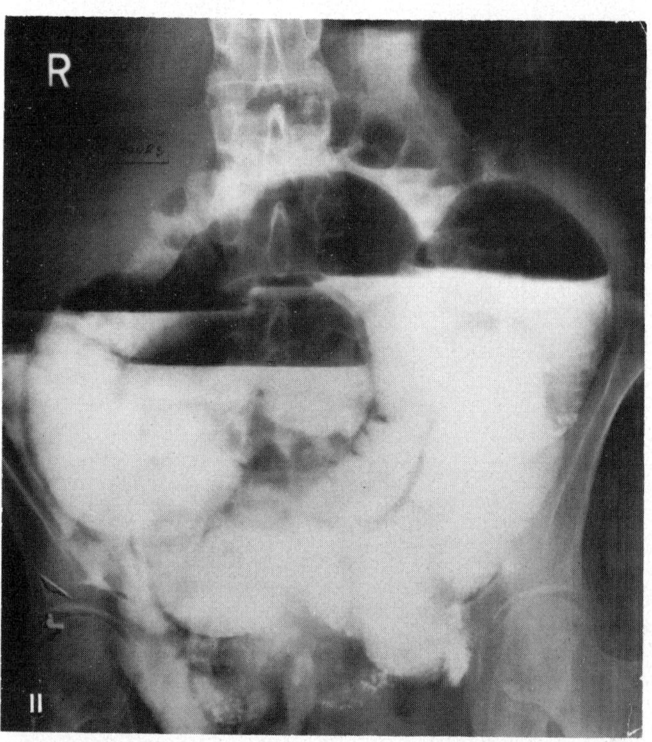

Fig. 34.27 Chronic ileum obstruction. The patient had a previous entero-enteric anastomosis for intestinal obstruction. Dilatation of this degree could not be due solely to a stagnant loop and must indicate main steam obstruction. Laparotomy revealed a carcinoid tumour of lower ileum.

Fistula. A large fistula may cause malabsorption by allowing contents of the gut to short circuit the absorbing mucosal area of the small intestine. On the other hand, even a small fistula between the colon and the proximal gut may cause malabsorption by bacterial contamination with colonic organisms. The pressure in the colon is usually higher than in the stomach or small intestine, so that in gastro-colic or ileo-colic fistulae the intestinal contents usually pass from the colon into the stomach or small bowel. Thus, these fistulae are more easily demonstrated by barium enema than by barium meal follow-through examination (Fig. 34.28). Unless the fistula is large it may be impossible to demonstrate it conclusively on a follow-through examination, whereas it is usually obvious on barium enema. Occasionally intubation of the small bowel may be the only conclusive method of demonstrating an entero-colic fistula.

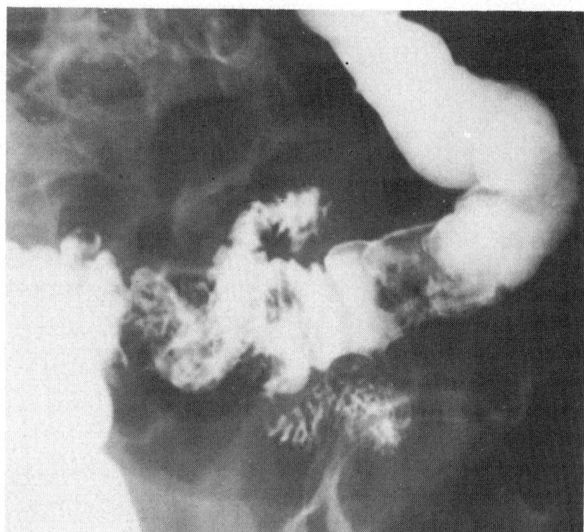

Fig. 34.28 Ileo-sigmoid fistula. A fistula formed spontaneously between the ileum and a diverticulum in the sigmoid. Barium follow-through examination was normal. Barium enema demonstrates the fistula.

Very rarely malabsorption following gastrectomy may be due to an error of surgical technique, when a gastro-ileal instead of a gastro-jejunal anastomosis has been performed, thus causing a short circuit of the jejunum.

C. Mixed lesions

Sometimes malabsorption is due to a combination of a number of factors. This is especially true of patients with Crohn's disease who have had surgical treatment. There may be loss of absorbing surface following resection as well as due to the primary disease. Bacterial contamination of intestinal contents may be due to the presence of fistulae as well as stagnant loops. Sinuses may be present.

Many forms of radiological investigation may be needed. The follow-through examination gives an idea of the sites of maximum stagnation within the gut. Barium enema may be needed to demonstrate the fistulae involving the colon. Sinography usually demonstrates the site or sites of leakage from the bowel. The radiological investigation of these patients leading to a full demonstration of the disorder anatomy can be very difficult and requires great patience. In no field is closer co-operation and understanding between radiologist and surgeon more important.

(c) **Disaccharidase deficiency.** The common disaccharides in our diet, *lactose, sucrose* and *maltose*, have to be split into monosaccharides by enzymes in the microvilli of the brush border of the small intestinal epithelial cell before they can be absorbed. Deficiency of one or other of these enzymes results in the large unsplit molecule remaining in the lumen of the small bowel where it causes an osmotic diarrhoea. Subsequently the unabsorbed sugar passes into the large bowel where it is fermented by intestinal bacteria. The commonest disaccharidase deficiency is *hypolactasia.* In some it appears to be genetically determined, being more common in some races (Greeks, Indians, Pakistanis) than others (white Caucasian). It is found in some cases of adult coeliac disease where there is atrophy of the villi as well as the microvilli, and it may occur temporarily after severe infective enteritis. *Hyposucrasia* is rare and *hypomaltasia* does not occur except as part of a multiple enzyme deficiency as seen in the kwashiorkor syndrome.

Adults with hypolactasia rarely present with a history of milk-induced diarrhoea, but often state they seldom drink milk. More frequently they have rather ill-defined complaints such as abdominal discomfort, distension, excess flatulence and occasional diarrhoea, which they do not relate to the ingestion of milk. Often they are subjected to many investigations, including barium studies of the whole intestine, without a firm diagnosis being made. Some of them are regarded as suffering from 'spastic colon'; others are considered to be neurotic. The assurance that there is a rational explanation for their symptoms is one of the chief benefits of diagnosing hypolactasia.

Hyposucrasia is rare but may cause severe symptoms since it is difficult to avoid cane sugar in modern diets. Two teaspoonfuls of sugar or two segments of chocolate may cause abdominal discomfort, distension and diarrhoea.

The diagnosis of disaccharidase deficiency is made by estimating the enzyme activity in the biopsy of jejunal mucosa. Supporting evidence may be obtained by a sugar tolerance test, but the results of these may be difficult to interpret and occasionally misleading. A reliable diagnosis can be obtained by observing the radiological appearance of the small bowel after the

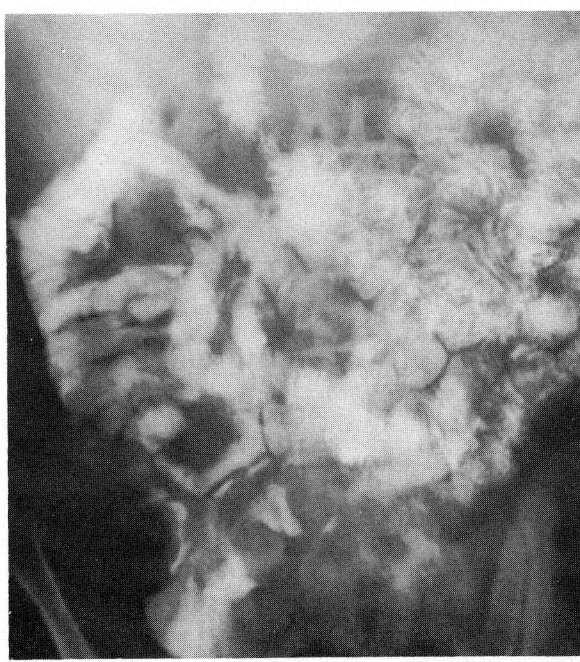

A

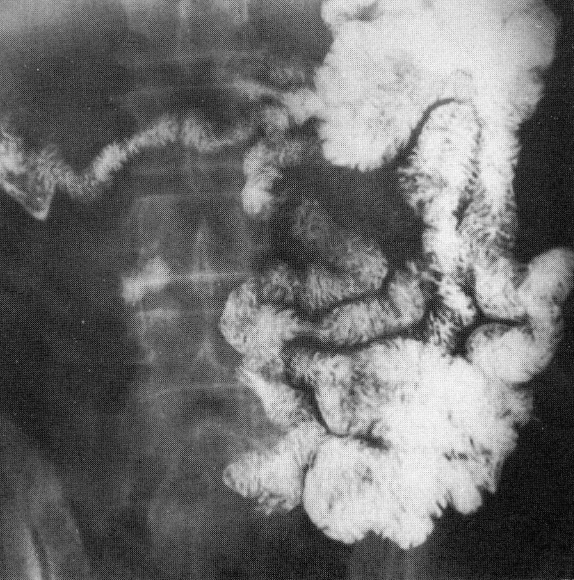

B

Fig. 34.29 Hypolactasia. A Radiograph taken 1 hour after lactose-barium mixture showing a large part of the small intestine filled with dilute contrast medium and some barium in the ascending colon (lactase level 0.0 units). B Same patient 1 hour after sucrose barium mixture showing the normal appearance of concentrated barium in the small bowel (sucrase level 7.3 units).

ingestion of a barium preparation to which a test sugar has been added. This simple radiological method is useful as a screening test in patients with vague abdominal symptoms and in carrying out population surveys.

Method. Twenty-five grams of the test sugar is added to 4–6 oz of barium sulphate preparation which should contain no disaccharide and no hydroscopic agent, such as sodium carboxymethyl cellulose or sorbitol. Micropaque is suitable in this respect. A formal barium meal examination of the oesophagus, stomach and duodenum can be carried out if desired. The patient then lies on his right side and a film is taken after 60 minutes with the patient supine. If the transit time is expected to be shorter than usual, as after gastrectomy or resection of the distal small bowel, the film should be taken at 30–45 minutes, before all the barium has passed into the colon.

In normal patients the presence of the test sugar will not be detectable and the normal appearance of concentrated barium sulphate suspension will be seen. If dissaccharidase deficiency is present there will be dilution of the barium sulphate suspension and a large part of the small intestine will be filled with dilute contrast medium. At the end of an hour some barium is usually in the colon (Figs. 34.29 and 34.30).

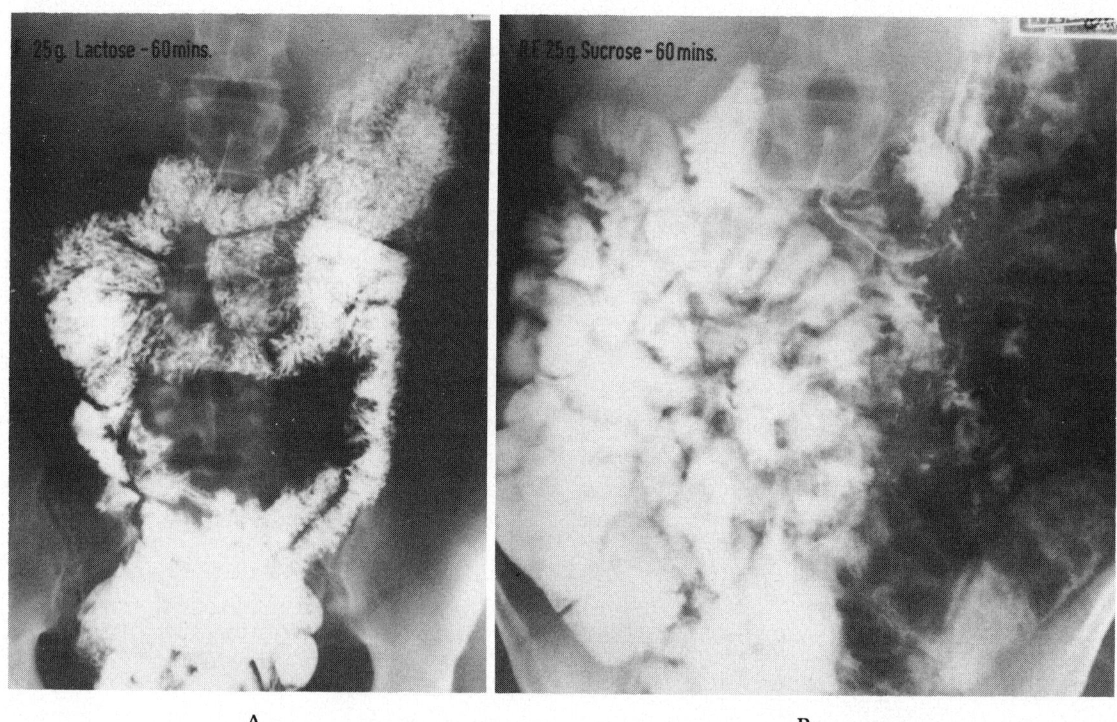

Fig. 34.30 Hyposucrasia. A Radiograph taken 1 hour after lactose-barium showing normal appearance of the small bowel (lactase 2.4 units). B One hour after sucrose barium showing dilute barium in the ileum and transverse colon (sucrase 0.0 units).

This combination of *dilution* of contrast combined with relatively *rapid transit* is easily recognized and is diagnostic. In some disorders, such as idiopathic steatorrhoea with severe intestinal symptoms, the intestine may be dilated and contrast medium may appear dilute but the transit in these patients is slow, the radiographic appearances sometimes resembling an ileus (Fig. 34.31). In addition, in idiopathic steatorrhoea the mucosal folds are often thickened, a feature not seen in disaccharidase deficiency demonstrated by this method. Again, in subacute obstruction of the ileum there may be dilatation of the intestine with dilution of contrast medium but the rate of transit of barium in these patients is reduced. On the other hand, rapid transit is sometimes seen in healthy people, the contrast medium reaching the colon in well under an hour. When this happens the small intestine is not dilated and the contrast medium not diluted either in the small or large intestine (Fig. 34.32).

In patients with an anatomical normal small intestine this test gives a clear-cut result, although if the disaccharidase level is borderline the radiological appearances may be difficult to interpret. Comparison with films taken after using Micropaque alone or with another test sugar usually lead to a definite diagnosis. If transit of barium is so rapid that it is all in the colon at 60 minutes the diagnosis can still be made because dilution of barium can be recognized in the colon just as readily as in the small intestine.

The addition of a disaccharide to Micropaque does not interfere with the examination of the small bowel

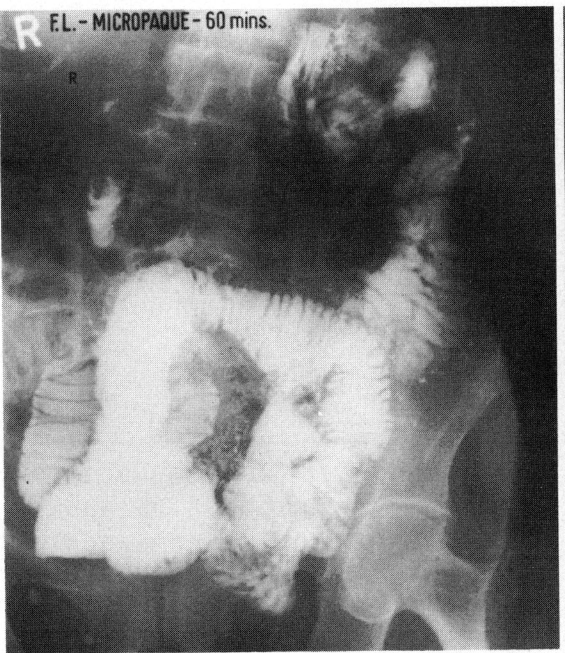

Fig. 34.31

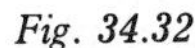

Fig. 34.32

Fig. 34.31 Dilution but no hurry. Coeliac disease showing dilatation of the jejunum and dilution of barium with slow transit.

Fig. 34.32 Hurry but no dilution. Normal patient in whom the barium has reached the colon in 15 minutes but in whom no dilution has occurred. The mucosal pattern is normal.

provided the patient has a normal disaccharidase level. If there is disaccharidase deficiency the dilution of barium and its rapid transit through the small bowel may prevent adequate demonstration of the anatomy of the small bowel. This is not always the case (Fig. 34.33) but the examination may have to be repeated using barium sulphate preparation alone.

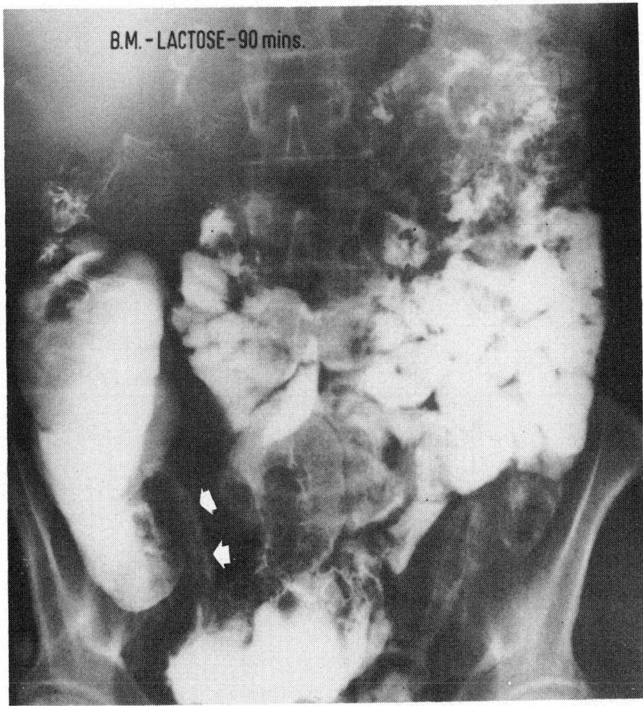

Fig. 34.33 Crohn's disease associated with hypolactasia. Dilution of contrast medium in the small bowel and colon has not prevented the demonstration of a narrowed segment of terminal ileum due to Crohn's disease (*arrows*). Radiograph taken 90 minutes after ingestion of lactose-barium.

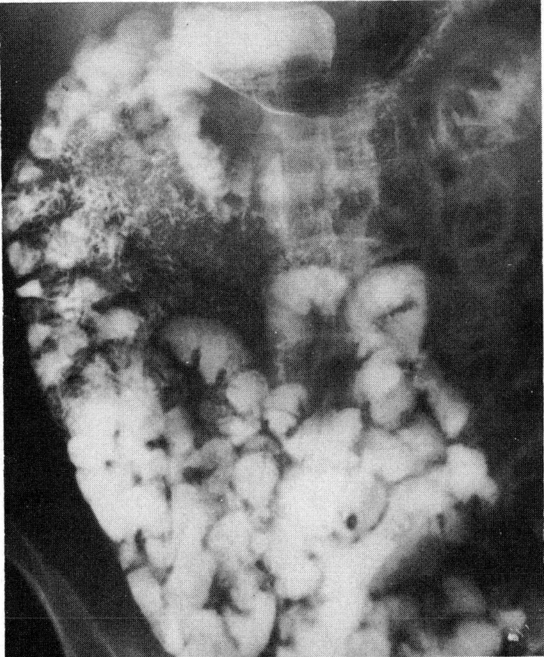

Fig. 34.34 Normal patient 1 hour after taking 120 ml of Micropaque and 16 g of magnesium sulphate. Dilution and hurry has occurred similar to that seen in patients with hypolactasia given 25 g of lactose in barium.

Hypolactasia occurs in some patients with subtotal villous atrophy due to gluten-induced enteropathy, presumably because of damage to the microvilli in the brush border of the small intestinal cell. When such a patient responds to a gluten-free diet the hypolactasia also improves.

The radiological appearances in patients with hypolactasia following a lactose barium sulphate meal are similar to those seen when a similar osmolar load of magnesium sulphate and barium sulphate are given to a normal subject (Fig. 34.34). These appearances are at least in part due to the osmotic effect of the unsplit disaccharide within the lumen of the small intestine. The dose of lactose used in the test (25 g) seldom causes unpleasant symptoms and is only half that usually given for a lactose tolerance test.

PROTEIN-LOSING DISORDERS OF THE GASTROINTESTINAL TRACT

Protein is continually entering the lumen of the gut in the form of shed mucosal cells, lymph and other secretions. In the normal most of it is reabsorbed. In a wide variety of conditions there may be excessive loss of protein so that the protein balance becomes negative. Isotope techniques, particularly the use of $_{131}$I-labelled polyvinylpyrrolidone, a synthetic polymer about the same molecular size as albumin, allows a quantitative assessment of the amount of protein leaking from the gastrointestinal tract to be made.

These patients usually present with oedema associated with a marked reduction in plasma protein for which no obvious cause can be found. Some have no intestinal symptoms while in others the protein loss complicates known organic disease of the gut. One classification is shown in Table 34.3.

Table 34.3 Diseases associated with protein-losing enteropathy

Lymphatic
Intestinal lymphangiectasia Whipple's disease (intestinal lipodystrophy) Mesenteric lymphatic obstruction —reticulosis —retroperitoneal fibrosis —non-specific granuloma Thoracic duct fistula, ligation or damage
Venous
Congestive heart failure Constrictive pericarditis Tricuspid disease Thrombosis —superior mesenteric vein —portal vein —inferior vena cava
Ulceration
Tumours, especially —carcinoma of the stomach —carcinoma of the colon —villous adenoma Regional enteritis Ulcerative colitis Radiation enteropathy
Unknown mechanism
Ménétrier's disease (giant hypertrophy of gastric mucosa) Gluten induced enteropathy, coeliac disease Tropical sprue Eosinophilic enteropathy Chronic intestinal ischaemia

Giant hypertrophy of the gastric rugae was first described by Ménétrier (1888). The most striking radiological feature is the presence of giant rugal folds in the stomach, particularly on the greater curvature. There is no evidence of rigidity or ulceration, although the lumen may be narrowed by the enlarged folds. Peristaltic activity may be slightly diminished. The maximal gastric acid output may be low or nil; the folds weep protein, not acid.

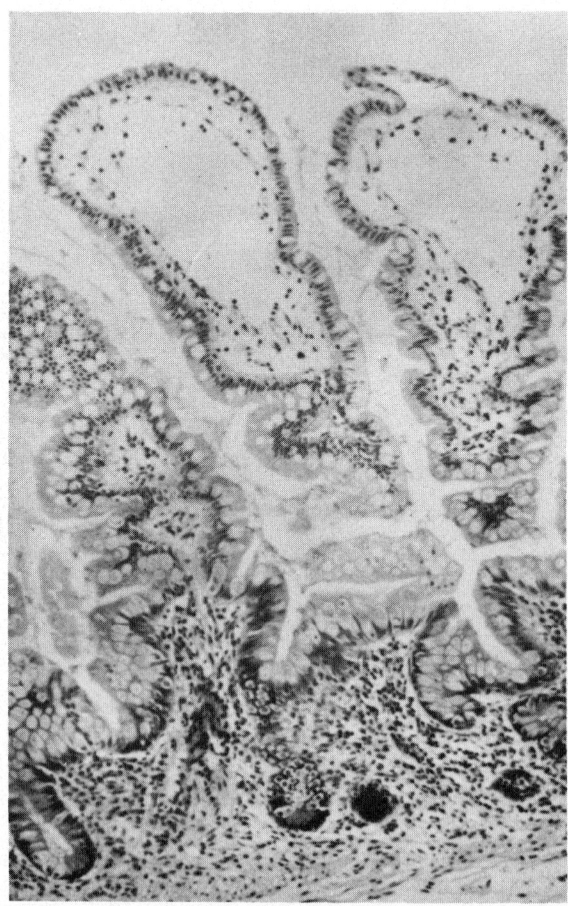

Fig. 34.35 Intestinal lymphangiectasia. Biopsy showing villi containing grossly dilated lymph spaces.

Intestinal lymphangiectasia chiefly affects children but may persist into adult life or at least first present then. There is commonly oedema of the lower limbs associated with hypoalbuminaemia but the condition may present with rickets due to failure of absorption of vitamin D. The patients do not always have steatorrhoea. The lymphatic vessels in the mesentery and frequently in the lower limbs are hypoplastic. Biopsy of jejunal mucosa shows dilated lymph spaces in oedematous villi (Fig. 34.35). The barium follow-through examination shows thickening of rugal folds in the small intestine due to widespread oedema of the intestinal wall (Fig. 34.36). The thickened folds give the edge of the jejunum a 'cog-wheel' appearance. Lymphangiography often shows hypoplastic lymphatics in the legs and occasionally contrast medium may be seen entering the lumen of the gut, possibly through ruptured lymph vessels, indicating the site of maximum protein loss. However, it is possible that lymphangiography may increase the protein loss by damaging the already inadequate lymphatic drainage of the gut and so should be used with circumspection.

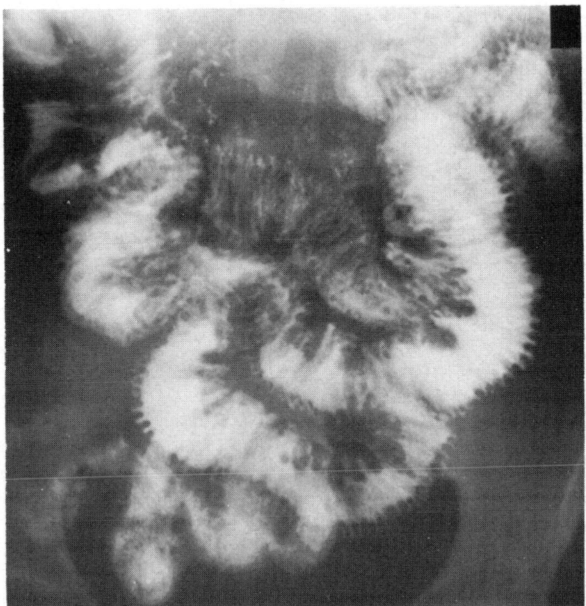

Fig. 34.36 Intestinal lymphangiectasia. Oedematous small bowel in a boy aged 14 who presented with hypoalbuminaemia and rickets due to vitamin D deficiency.

Villous adenoma of the colon, usually situated in the caecum, sigmoid colon or rectum, may give rise to severe hypo-albuminaemia or hypokalaemia. Because they weep protein these tumours do not coat easily with barium and are easily mistaken for faecal residue on barium enema examination. They are very soft and may be impalpable even at laparotomy. Protein loss into the gut may be a prominent clinical feature of some cases of gut carcinoma and lymphosarcoma, especially when the stomach is involved.

Table 34.4 Factors contributing to generalized oedema of the small bowel

Low plasma albumen (less than 2.0 g/100 ml)	as in	Nephrotic syndrome Cirrhosis of the liver Protein-losing gastro-enteropathy Villous adenoma
Lymphatic	(*a*)	Hypoplasia —intestinal lymphangiectasia
	(*b*)	Obstruction—reticulosis —tumour
	(*c*)	Obliteration—X-irradiation
Venous	(*a*)	Superior mesenteric vein thrombosis
	(*b*)	Portal hypertension
	(*c*)	Budd Chiari syndrome
	(*d*)	Constrictive pericarditis
	(*e*)	Tricuspid insufficiency

In *regional enteritis* there is frequently severe loss of protein as well as malabsorption. In addition, protein loss may be a feature of certain patients with *coeliac disease, mesenteric vascular occlusion* and *ulcerative colitis*.

It will be seen that widespread thickening of mucosal folds due to oedema of the small bowel may be seen in a variety of conditions. The mechanisms are similar to those which cause oedema elsewhere; raised venous pressure, lymphatic insufficiency, lowered plasma osmotic pressure and altered capillary permeability. Sometimes more than one mechanism may be present in the same patient, as when a patient with intestinal lymphangiectasia passes protein into the lumen of his gut so that the plasma albumen falls to a level at which oedema occurs in the gut and elsewhere in the body. Whenever the plasma albumen falls below 2.0 g per 100 ml oedema of the small bowel may occur, but it is usually not severe unless there is some complicating factor such as a raised portal pressure in a patient with cirrhosis of the liver. Thus whenever widespread oedema of the small bowel is demonstrated radiologically it is necessary to consider what mechanism or mechanisms may have operated to bring it about (Table 34.4).

EOSINOPHILIC GASTRO-ENTEROPATHY

In this uncommon condition there is a diffuse infiltration of eosinophils into one or more segments of the alimentary tract, usually the small bowel and gastric antrum. This is associated with oedema, thickening of the affected parts, sometimes with ascites. There is usually a blood eosinophilia. There may be a history of allergy but the causative agent is seldom discovered.

Patients present with recurrent attacks of abdominal pain, often colicky, with episodes of diarrhoea or vomiting or both. The condition responds to steroid therapy but may run a course of several years, relapsing when steroids are withdrawn.

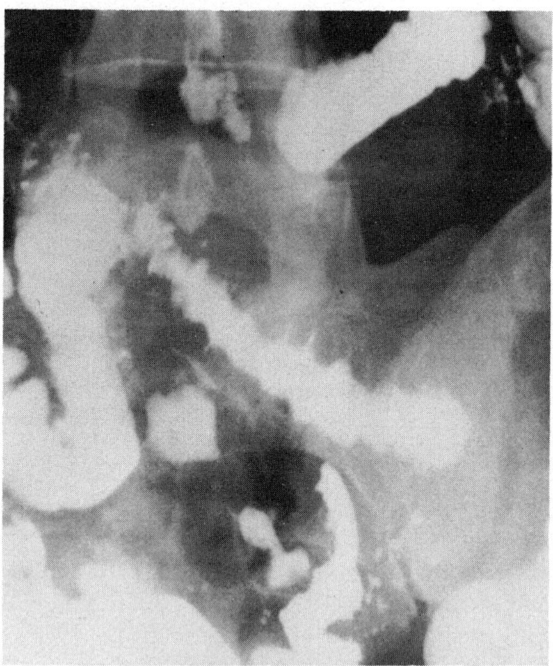

Fig. 34.37 Eosinophilic enteropathy showing a thickened irregular segment of jejunum with apparent ulceration similar to that seen in Crohn's disease. The appearances returned to normal with steroid therapy but relapsed when steroids were withdrawn.

Radiologically, the affected loops of bowel are thickened, with widened and blunted mucosal folds (Fig. 34.37). The lumen becomes narrowed, causing some degree of obstruction. These appearances closely mimic regional enteritis but fistulae do not occur and ulceration is not a prominent feature, though it has been seen in resected specimens.

MASTOCYTOSIS

Urticaria pigmentosa is an uncommon skin condition in which there is infiltration of the dermis with mast cells. In some cases the mast cell proliferation involves the reticulo-endothelial system and many organs may be affected. Mast cells produce histamine, heparin and hyaluronic acid which have the effect of producing local urticaria and stimulating fibrosis.

Involvement of the small intestine gives rise to nausea, vomiting and abdominal pain. There may be malabsorption associated with villous atrophy. The radiological changes are non-specific and include oedema of the mucosa, with thickening of the valvulae conniventes and the appearance of many mucosal nodules 2–5 mm in diameter throughout the jejunum. Sclerotic bone lesions simulating osteoblastic metastases may occur. The association of sclerotic bone lesions in a patient with diffuse small bowel abnormality raises the possibility of mastocytosis.

PANCREATIC CYSTIC FIBROSIS

Pancreatic cystic fibrosis may show radiological changes in the large and small bowel in patients over 5 years of age. These include:

1. Loss of normal duodenal folds.
2. Hyperplasia and redundancy of folds affecting both large and small bowel.
3. In the large bowel, filling of dilated crypts and marginal nodularity associated with adherent indurated faecal masses at the lateral wall of the colon.
4. About 10 per cent of patients develop hepatic fibrosis, portal hypertension and oesophageal varices.

RADIATION CHANGES

The use of high-voltage X-ray therapy has of necessity increased the risk of damage to the intestine. The mobility of the small intestine to some extent protects it from harmful effects of radiation, but the colon in its fixed position and its closer proximity to sites being treated, e.g. carcinoma of cervix and bladder, is more liable to radiation damage.

The changes induced in the small and large bowel are those of oedema and congestion of the wall, appearing radiologically as narrowing of the lumen thickening, straightening and rigidity of mucosal fold or even complete loss of mucosal fold pattern, associated with fixity and loss of peristalsis (Fig. 34.38). These features may be transient and may give rise to no clinical changes. These findings may result in the barium presenting as a rounded pool caused by the matting together of many coils of small bowel. More severe changes may be associated with mucosal ulceration and gastrointestinal haemorrhage.

Peritoneal reaction may give rise to adhesions and kinking between coils of small bowel which may lead to functional or mechanical obstructions.

Later, damage to the vessels of the bowel wall may give rise to the development of ischaemic fibrosis and strictures of the bowel which may be of considerable length.

ILEO-CAECAL VALVE AND APPENDIX

The terminal ileum, ileo-caecal valve and appendix are frequently the focus of radiological investigation owing to the relatively large number of diseases which may affect this area.

The terminal ileum is the commonest site in the small bowel to be affected by pathological processes and these have been considered above.

The ileo-caecal valve presents more as a problem in radiological differential diagnosis of lesions occurring around the caecum rather than of disease affecting the valve itself.

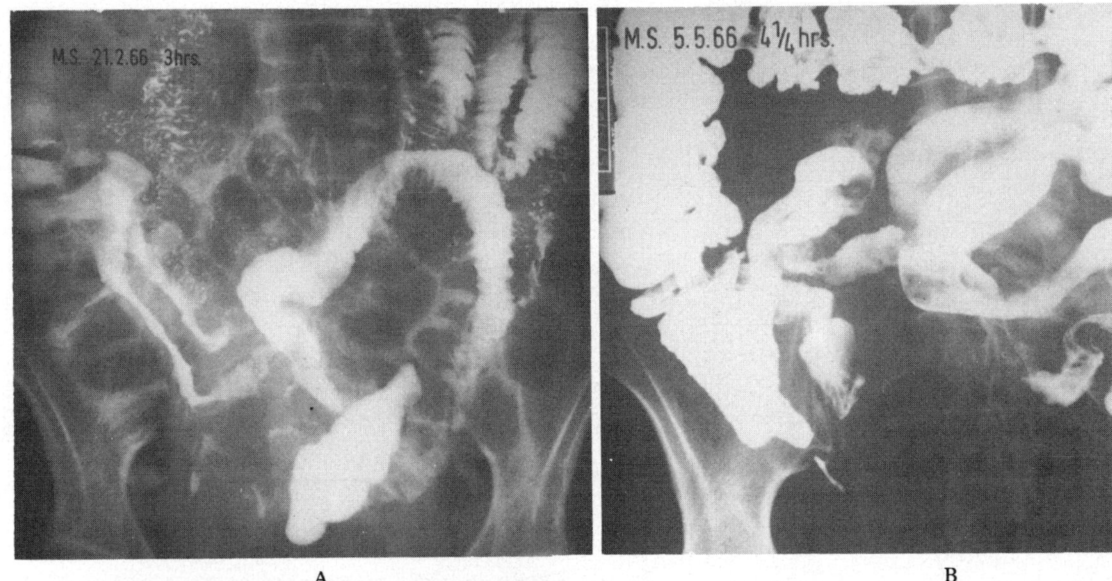

A B

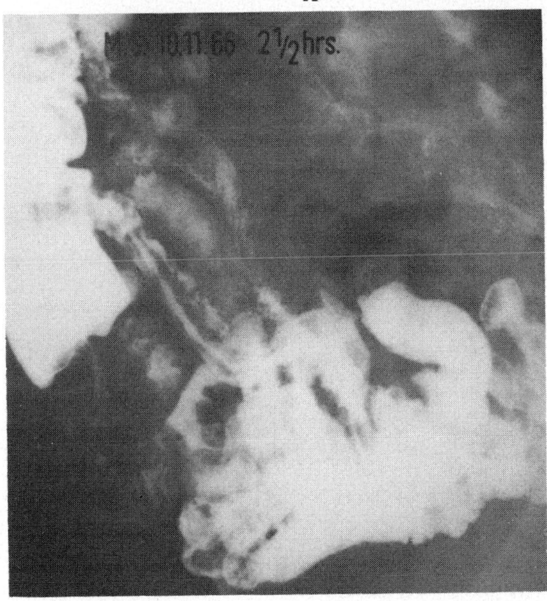

C

Fig. 34.38 Acute radiation ileitis following radiotherapy for carcinoma of the body of the uterus. Patient had severe diarrhoea, melaena, hypoproteinaemia and hypokalaemia. A There are narrowed coils of distal small bowel and also thickened loops with prominent folds more proximally. B Same case 10 weeks later with mucosal pattern destroyed and a featureless ileum. C Some 6 months later the ileum has almost returned to normal but several loops are matted together.

The ileo-caecal valve consists of an upper and well-developed lip covering a lower lip, both lips being continuous with mucosal frenulae which cross the posterior wall of the caecum in a horizontal direction.

The ileal opening appears as a transverse slit in the posterior wall of the caecum between these lips. The radiological appearances of the normal ileo-caecal valve depend on whether the valve is seen in profile on the medial wall of the caecum when it has been fancifully described as having a 'shark's mouth' appearance; or if it appears *en face* on the posterior wall when it appears as a round filling defect with a central stellate appearance due to mucosal folds (Fig. 34.39).

Enlargement of the lips of the ileo-caecal valve may follow fatty deposits in the caecal lips or, rarely, oedematous changes, and the condition has been described as hypertrophy of the ileo-caecal valve. This is a misnomer as no muscular hypertrophy is present and the condition is not associated with any obstruction of the terminal ileum.

The appearances have to be differentiated from 'appendicular stumps' and from polypoid lesions of the caecum. The identification of the mucosal folds in the ileo-caecal valve enables this differentiation to be made.

The appendix

The place of radiology in the investigation of acute appendicitis and appendix abscess is considered in Chapter 36.

Chronic appendicitis or recurrent appendicitis is a complex problem from the standpoint of radiological diagnosis as the actual clinical status of these two syndromes is not clearly defined.

It is doubtful to what extent radiological signs of chronic inflammation of the appendix are valid. The radiological signs on which chronic inflammation has been diagnosed are:

(a) Local tenderness over the barium filled appendix —this feature varies considerably with different reactions to palpation and is a difficult sign to evaluate.

(b) Fixity of the appendix as shown in a barium meal. Palpation under screen control confirms the fixity.

(c) Kinking of appendix—the appendix when filled with barium can be shown to be angulated. Barium

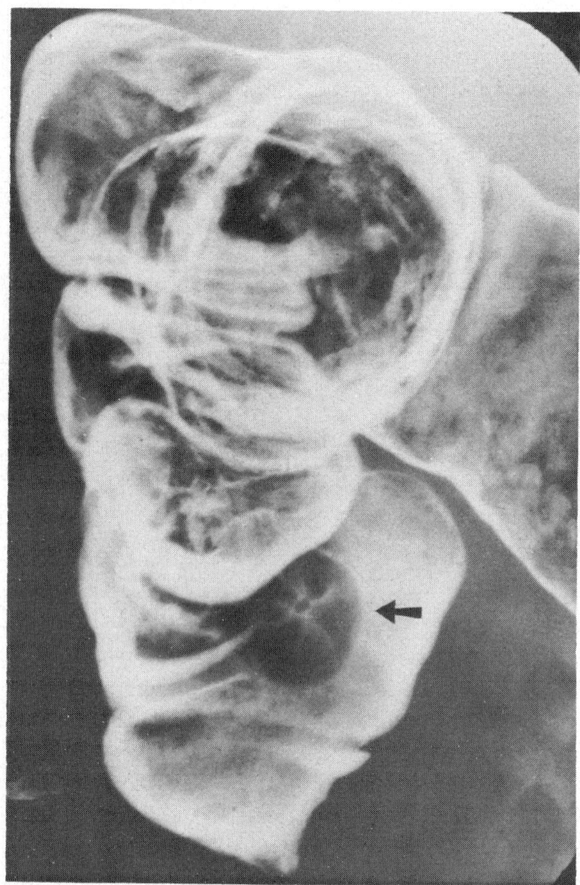

Fig. 34.39 Prominent ileo-caecal valve seen *en face* with stellate radiation of folds towards the valve. These appearances are frequently described as hypertrophy of the ileo-caecal valve but there is no thickening of the muscular wall and no obstruction is present.

remaining in the appendix after a barium meal frequently appears as segmented clumps of barium.

(d) Delay in emptying—delay in emptying of the barium from the appendix has been claimed as a radiological sign of chronic appendicitis. This sign is, however, so variable as to be worthless.

Mucocele of the appendix. Occasionally the appendix fills with mucus and forms a smooth round cyst-like structure, a mucocele. This may appear as a filling defect in the caecum pole. The outlines of the filling defect are smooth and rounded. On rare occasions it may show calcification in its wall.

In other instances the thickened omentum around an appendix which has been the seat of inflammation may produce a mass which indents the wall of the caecum when the caecum is distended by a barium enema.

Foreign bodies. Metallic foreign bodies lodged in the appendix and shotgun pellets in the appendix are not an infrequent finding in the game season.

Faecoliths in the appendix have to be differentiated from stones (enteroliths) in the alimentary canal, in diverticula, or in a Meckel's diverticulum. The site may be confirmed by a follow-through barium meal. An intraperitoneal appendolith may be the cause of a persistent discharging sinus following a ruptured appendix or appendix abscess. Calcified appendoliths are usually oval and laminated.

REFERENCES AND SUGGESTIONS FOR FURTHER READING

Bilbao, M. K., Frische, L. H. & Dotter, C. T. (1967) Hypotonic Duodenography. *Radiology*, **89,** 438–443.

Carlson, H. C. & Good, C. A. (1973) Neoplasms of the small bowel. Chapter 34 in Alimentary Tract Roentgenology, ed. Margulis, A. R. & Burhenne, H. J., 2nd edition. St. Louis: Mosby.

Crohn, B. B., Ginsburg, L. & Oppenheimer, G. D. (1932) Regional ileitis; a pathological and clinical entity. *Journal of American Medical Association*, **99,** 1323–1328.

Cummack, D. H. (1969) *Gastrointestinal X-ray Diagnosis.* Edinburgh: Livingstone.

Herlinger, H. (1978) A modified technique for the double contrast small bowel enema. *Gastrointestinal Radiology*, **3,** 201–207.

Herlinger, H., Glanville, J. N. & Kreel, L. (1977) An evaluation of the double contrast barium meal (DCBM) against endoscopy. *Clinical Radiology*, **28,** 307–314.

Kihara, T., Ohta, A., Ishihara, Y. & Morita, M. (1971) Hypotonic duodenography. *Clinical Radiology*, **22,** 251–256.

Kreel, L. (1975) Pharmacoradiology in barium examinations with special reference to glucagon. *British Journal of Radiology*, **48,** 691–703. the upper gastrointestinal tract. *Radiology*, **117,** 513–518.

Laufer, I. (1979) Double contrast gastrointestinal radiology with endoscopic correlation. London: Saunders.

Laws, J. W. & Neale, G. (1966) Radiological diagnosis of disacharidase deficiency. *Lancet*, **ii,** 139–143.

Laws, J. W., Booth, C. C., Shandon, H. & Stewart, J. S. (1963) Correlation of radiological and histological findings in idiopathic steatorrhoea. *British Medical Journal*, **1,** 1311–1314.

Laws, J. W. & Pitman, R. G. (1960) The radiological investigations of the malabsorption syndromes. *British Journal of Radiology*, **33,** 211–222.

Lennard-Jones, J. E., Lockhart-Mummery, H. E. & Morson, B. C. (1968) Clinical and pathological differentiation of Crohn's disease and procto-colitis. *Gastroenterology*, **54,** 1162–1170.

Lockhart-Mummery, H. E. & Morson, B. C. (1960) Crohn's disease (regional enteritis) of the large intestine and its distinction from ulcerative colitis. *Gut*, **1,** 87–105.

Marshak, R. H. (1975) Granulomatous disease of the intestinal tract (Crohn's disease). *Radiology*, **114,** 3–22.

Marshak, R. H. & Linder, A. E. (1972) Roentgen features of Crohn's disease. *Clinics in Gastroenterology*, **1,** No. 2, 411.

Marshak, R. H. & Lindner, A. E. (1976) Malabsorption syndrome: Sprue in *Radiology of the Small Intestine*, 2nd edition. Philadelphia: Saunders.

Marshak, R. H., Wolf, B. S., Cohen, N. & Janowitz, H. D. (1961) Protein-losing disorders of the gastrointestinal tract: Roentgen features. *Radiology*, 77/**6,** 893–905.

Miller, R. E. (1965) Complete reflux small bowel examination *Radiology*, **84,** 457–463.

Roswit, B. (1974) Complications of radiation therapy: the alimentary tract. *Seminars of Roentgenology*, **9,** 51–63.

Scott-Harden, W. G. (1960) Examination of the small bowel. In *Modern Trends in Diagnostic Radiology*, ed. McLaren, J. W. New York: Harper and Row.

Sellink, J. L. (1976) *Radiological Atlas of Common Diseases of the Small Bowel.* 1st edition. Massachusetts: Stenfert Kroese.

CHAPTER 35

THE COLON

RADIOLOGICAL INVESTIGATION

The value of plain films in the erect and supine position in the detection of lesions of the colon is described in Chapter 36. It must be emphasized that when such films are taken soon after an enema or bowel washout, fluid levels in the colon are not uncommon and may mimic pathological changes.

The barium enema examination is the routine method of examination of the colon. Adequate preliminary cleansing of the colon is vital to remove faecal material prior to the administration of the barium enema (Fig. 35.1). Careful cleansing of the colon by the administration of an aperient within the previous 24 hours and a low residue diet for 48 hours prior to the examination assists in clearing of the colon of faecal material. However, a high colonic lavage of two or more pints of tap water is usually also necessary to remove small particles of faecal material which may mimic polypi or other tumours.

A barium sulphate and water mixture (25 per cent weight/volume) is administered through a rectal catheter by gravity from a height of 4 feet. In elderly subjects or patients with difficulty in retention of the enema, a balloon rectal catheter may help. Filling of the colon is watched under fluoroscopic control and localized films of the colon taken during the filling phase. Lateral views of the pelvi-rectal region should always be taken early during the filling stage to avoid overlap of the sigmoid colon. Likewise areas where redundancy and overlap of colonic loops are liable to occur, e.g. the splenic and hepatic flexure, merit special oblique views to 'iron out' these overlapping loops.

The addition of $\frac{1}{2}$ per cent tannic acid or a colon activator (Veripaque, Clysodrast, etc.) greatly assisted the evacuation of the enema and usually gave a good demonstration of the mucosal pattern. The contraction of the colon, however, did not allow the finer details of the mucosal pattern to be seen. The possible hepatotoxic effects of tannic acid have in addition largely contributed to its falling into disuse. Colon activators should not be used in the preliminary washout in cases of active ulcerative colitis or when rectal bleeding has been present; indeed no preparation at all may be called for.

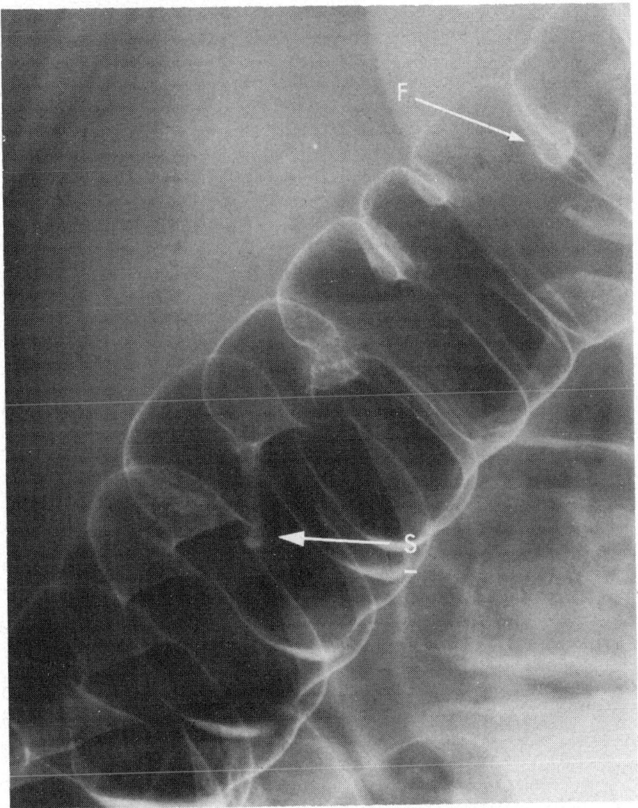

Fig. 35.1 Artefacts in double contrast enema. The folds of bowel wall (F) may simulate polypi, but oblique views usually unravel these appearances. 'S' is a stalactite appearance caused by a hanging drop of mucus coated with barium which resembles a polyp.

Double contrast examination. The use of a double contrast enema originally introduced for the diagnosis of polypi has now been widened to include a much more detailed study of the colonic mucosa. The adequacy of coating of the colonic mucosa depends on many factors, notably the amount of mucus present, as well as the type of barium mixture used.

Adequate double contrast enema can be obtained by

filling the colon with the selected barium sulphate preparation as far as the splenic flexure and then introducing air to drive the barium round to fill the right side of the colon.

By rolling the patient into the prone, supine and lateral decubitus positions and taking films with a fine focus tube, extremely fine mucosal detail can be seen. Two lateral decubitus films, oblique films of the hepatic and splenic flexures and oblique views of the sigmoid are routinely taken using a horizontal X-ray beam.

In cases where there is a spastic obstruction to the inflow of the barium enema the intravenous administration of an antispastic drug, e.g. Buscopan, may enable the spasm to be overcome. In other cases of diverticulitis or when a fistula is suspected a Gastrografin enema (100 ml of Gastrografin/100 ml of water) may allow the area of spasm to be traversed and the mucosal pattern to be visualized. This latter type of enema has been used in the treatment of meconium ileus in infants but should be used with caution because it is hygroscopic (see Ch. 33, p. 681).

Radiological anatomy

The hepatic and splenic flexures of the colon are relatively constant in position and displacements are usually evidence of enlargement of the adjoining solid viscera. At the hepatic flexure displacements are usually from liver or gall bladder enlargement; the splenic flexure is displaced by an enlarged spleen or a space-occupying lesion of the tail of pancreas or kidney. The origin of the transverse colon may overlap the hepatic flexure whilst a redundant loop of descending colon may overlap the splenic flexure. This overlapping is important as growths of these portions of the colon may be hidden behind the barium filled loops.

Likewise the pelvi-rectal junction is regularly obscured by the pelvic colon and lateral views and 'axial' views are needed to demonstrate changes in this site.

Certain areas of physiological narrowing, at times resembling 'sphincters', may occur during the filling of the colon by a barium enema. They are all transient and show normal mucosal pattern features which enable them to be differentiated from true strictures.

CONGENITAL LESIONS

Imperforate anus. This common deformity of the alimentary canal varies from a thin obstructing membrane (bulging with meconium) to a severe deformity where atresia of the rectum may be associated with other urogenital deformities and bony defects in the sacrum.

As the surgical management of imperforate anus is dependent on the extent of rectal atresia and associated anomalies, radiological demonstration of the exact anatomy of the defect is of utmost importance.

Low defects of the rectum where the gap between the anal dimple and rectal stump is relatively short are best dealt with by the perineal approach, whilst those cases with more severe degrees of rectal atresia should be treated via an abdominal approach, involving a preliminary defunctioning colostomy.

Radiological examination must not be carried out immediately after birth but should be delayed for 12 to 18 hours or so to allow sufficient swallowed air to reach and adequately fill the terminal rectal segment (Fig. 35.2A and B). The anal dimple is identified by a metallic marker and the infant held in the inverted position for a few minutes to allow the air to completely distend the rectal segment.

Films are then taken in the lateral and anteroposterior position with an anode film distance of 6 feet to minimize distortion. These are in addition to conventional supine and erect abdominal views.

The distance between the metal marker and the air-filled rectal segment is less than 1.5 cm in cases of low atresia (i.e. below the pelvic floor) whilst in high rectal atresia the distance is considerably greater. A line drawn between the terminal portion of the sacrum and the pubis in the lateral film is considered to indicate the level of the floor of the pelvis and as stated, lesions above this line must be regarded as requiring an abdominal surgical approach whilst lesions below are low and can be approached by the perineal route.

The presence of air in the bladder, uterus or Fallopian tubes indicates a vesico-colic or a vaginal fistula and indicates that the atresia is high and the presence of associated sacral deformities has the same significance (Fig. 35.3).

Plain film interpretation, however, must be made with great caution since the distal blind pouch may not always fill with gas or may be plugged with meconium. As pointed out above, the initial treatment of rectal agenesis involves the formation of a defunctioning loop colostomy. Subsequent contrast injection into the distal loop will then give precise information about the state of the distal bowel and the anatomy of any fistulous tracks to the genitourinary system or perineum.

Microcolon (atresia). Narrowing of a localized segment or of the whole of the colon may occur. Microcolon may be associated with other congenital abnormalities, for example duodenal atresia, and it must be remembered in such cases that the small colon may be the result of lack of distension by adequate quantities of meconium. These small colons may readily revert to a normal size when the obstruction is relieved.

Hirschsprung's disease (aganglionosis). Failure of development of the autonomic nerve (myenteric plexus) in the colon wall may occur in a localized segment,

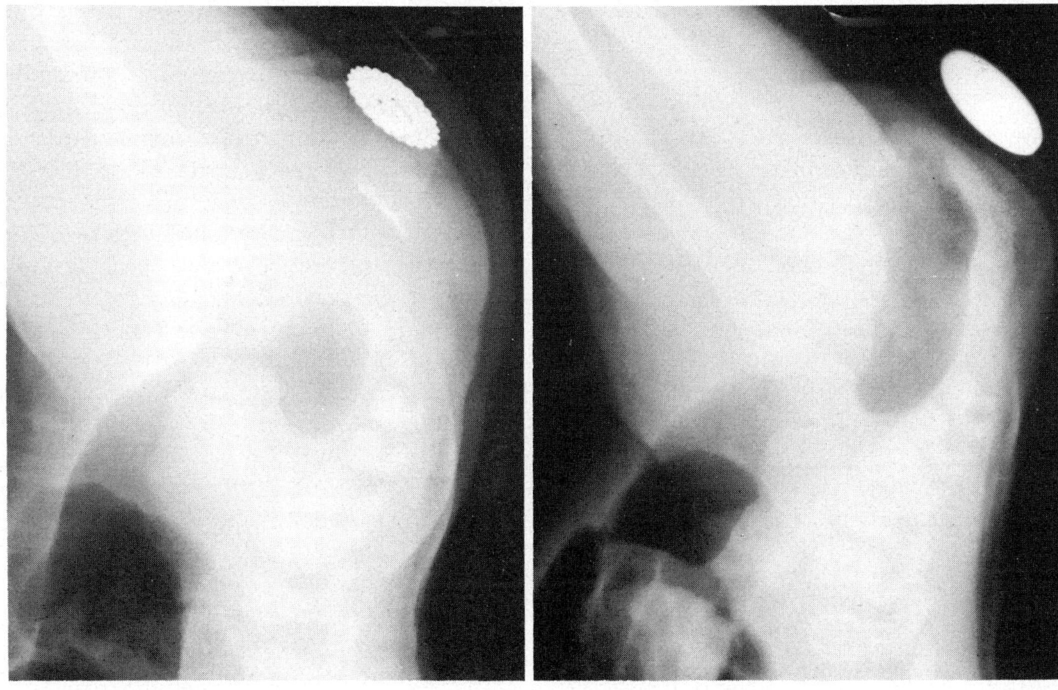

Fig. 35.2 Imperforate anus. A Film taken 3 hours after birth. B Same case after a further 6 hours giving time for the gas to reach the lower limits. (Reproduced by courtesy of *British Journal of Radiology*, **38,** 444–448, 1965.)

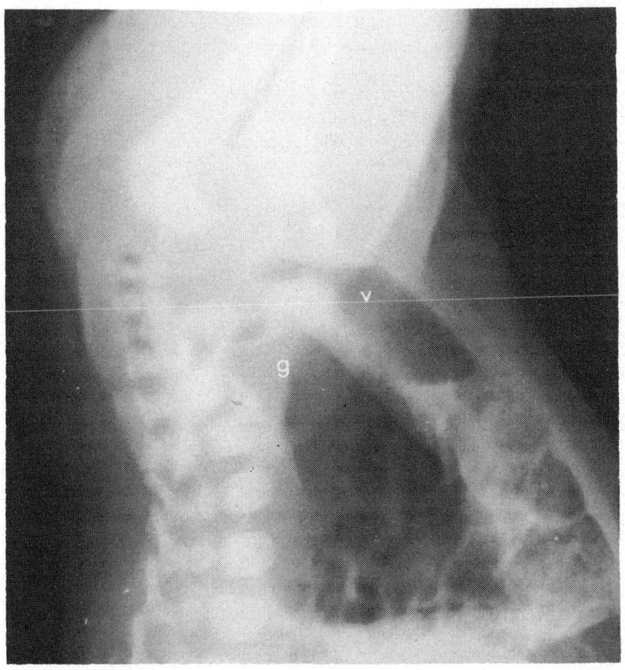

Fig. 35.3 High imperforate anus—the gas-filled terminal segment of colon (g) is situated at a considerable distance from the anus. The presence of gas in the genito-vesical organs (v) indicates that the colon has terminated above the pelvic floor level and surgical approach should be abdominal rather than perineal. (Reproduced by courtesy of *British Journal of Radiology*, **38**, 444–448, 1965.)

usually in the recto-sigmoid region, or rarely it may involve all or nearly all of the colon. In this rare latter condition the small bowel may be markedly distended and become larger than the colon.

Although the neurenteric defect is present at birth symptoms do not usually arise until the middle of the first decade of life when the constipation associated with overloaded and distended colon makes the clinical diagnosis usually obvious.

The plain films of the abdomen reveal a grossly distended pelvic colon with the characteristic mottled appearance caused by faeces admixed with gas. A contrast enema examination is necessary to exclude other forms of megacolon; some workers advocate barium but others prefer to use Gastrografin. Careful screening of the enema will reveal a narrowed segment of bowel which is the aganglionic segment. Great care must be taken in filling the rectum as the narrowed segment may be rapidly obscured by the distended colonic loops. The enema should be stopped as soon as the full length of the narrowed segment is demonstrated, as barium in the distended loop may give rise to faecal impaction. The use of Gastrografin obviates this possible complication.

In the neonate failure to expel normal meconium may be an indication of aganglionosis. Since there is little colonic distension at this early stage it may be impossible to demonstrate the transition zone between the aganglionic and normal colon. Ulceration may occur in the colon proximal to the functional obstruction.

Occasionally the aganglionic segment may be at a higher level in the bowel but the bowel filling should be persisted with until the transition between the narrow aganglionic colon and the proximal distended colon is demonstrated.

INFLAMMATORY LESIONS OF THE COLON

Changes in the mucosal pattern of the colon consisting of hyperaemia, cellular infiltration, increased mucus secretion and ulceration may be due to many causes. In some instances these changes may be limited to the mucosa itself in the early stages (e.g. ulcerative colitis), in others the process is more diffuse and involves the whole thickness of the bowel wall even at an early stage (granulomatous colitis).

The changes in the colon (colitis) may be grouped into:

(a) Colitis due to known organisms
(b) Ulcerative colitis
(c) Granulomatous colitis
(d) Ischaemic colitis

Colitis

Infection of the colon with specific organisms, e.g. *Shiga bacillus,* results in *bacillary dysentery* with inflammatory changes of the mucosa and an outpouring of fluid into the bowel lumen. Radiological examination is not an important factor in diagnosis but in the acute stage plain films may be requested to exclude other causes of acute abdomen. Plain films merely demonstrate a few gas-distended loops with a few small isolated fluid levels in the bowel.

Barium enema examination should not be performed in the acute stage but in the chronic stage it may be requested to distinguish from other forms of colitis. In *chronic bacillary dysentery,* loss of mucosal pattern, ulceration, fibrotic strictures and mucosal tags suggesting small polypi are seen.

Specific infections with saprophytic organisms, e.g. *monilia* or other *yeast infections,* may occur after antibiotic therapy. This so called *pseudo-membranous enterocolitis* may also occur in colonic obstruction or postoperatively. The radiological findings consist in alterations in the mucosal pattern with mucosal oedema, loss of normal haustration and a diffusely irregular and shaggy appearance of the outline of the bowel, resembling ulceration.

Infection with parasites, e.g. *entamoeba histolytica,* or *schistosomiasis,* may give rise to specific radiological appearances. *Chronic amoebic dysentery* usually presents with shrinking of the wall of the caecum and lack of distensibility of the caecum. These appearances are very similar to those seen in granulomatous colitis. Stricture formation especially on the left side of the colon may be a sequel of chronic amoebic colitis.

Amoeboma is a localized granulomatous lesion which produces one or more filling defects in the barium enema mimicking encephaloid carcinoma. In countries where amoebiasis is endemic multiple filling defects should always suggest the possibility of amoeboma. Rapid disappearance of the lesions with anti-amoebic therapy is the surest way of confirming the diagnosis.

Amoebic infection of the colon is frequently associated with a spread of the parasite of the liver giving rise to amoebic hepatitis or an amoebic abscess. Elevation of the right diaphragm associated with restriction of movement and a pleural reaction obscuring the right costophrenic angle are radiological signs indicating amoebic hepatitis. Isotope scans of the liver and ultrasound scans may be useful in hepatic abscess, indicating a localized nature of the lesion and that the defect is cystic and fluid-containing.

The appearances caused by schistosomiasis are described on page 758.

Cathartic colon

Prolonged ingestion of vegetable cathartics containing such irritants as podophyllin, jalap and colocynth in an attempt to correct chronic constipation is liable to produce radiologically demonstrable changes in the colon.

The radiological changes are first shown on the right side of the colon and consist in loss of haustral marking and the development of a smooth bowel wall. No rigidity or stiffening of the bowel wall occurs in the early stages but smooth tapering contractions of the colon walls do appear, mimicking strictures (pseudostrictures). However these can be shown to be inconstant.

The changes due to prolonged use of cathartics have to be differentiated from those of ulcerative colitis but the ragged mucosa, the true strictures and shrinkage of the colon wall seen in ulcerative colitis make differentiation possible.

With more advanced cases the whole of the colon may be involved and the appearances of atony and pseudostrictures are probably the result of gross neuromuscular dysfunction.

Metabolic changes consequent on the prolonged use of cathartics may occur and the commonest are hypokalaemia, hypopotassaemia, steatorrhoea and tetany. Permanent liver and renal demage may follow prolonged hypokalaemia consequent on prolonged and injudicious use of cathartics and at this stage the differentiation of induced from true metabolic disease may be extremely difficult.

Ulcerative colitis

The cause of ulcerative colitis is obscure though stress and autoimmune states have been suggested as possible causative factors.

Pathologically ulcerative colitis shows as oedematous inflammatory infiltration of the mucosa leading to mucosal ulceration and ultimately shortening and narrowing of the bowel. As viewed through a sigmoido-

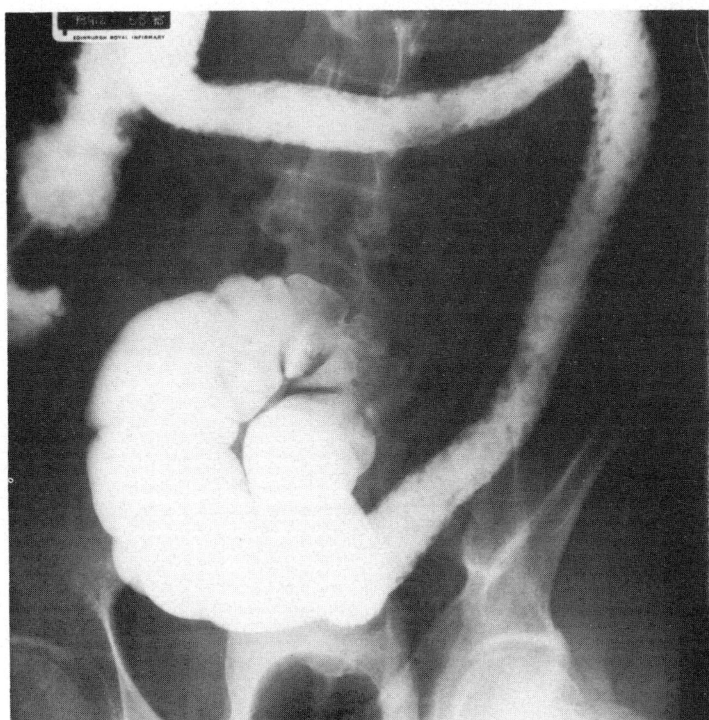

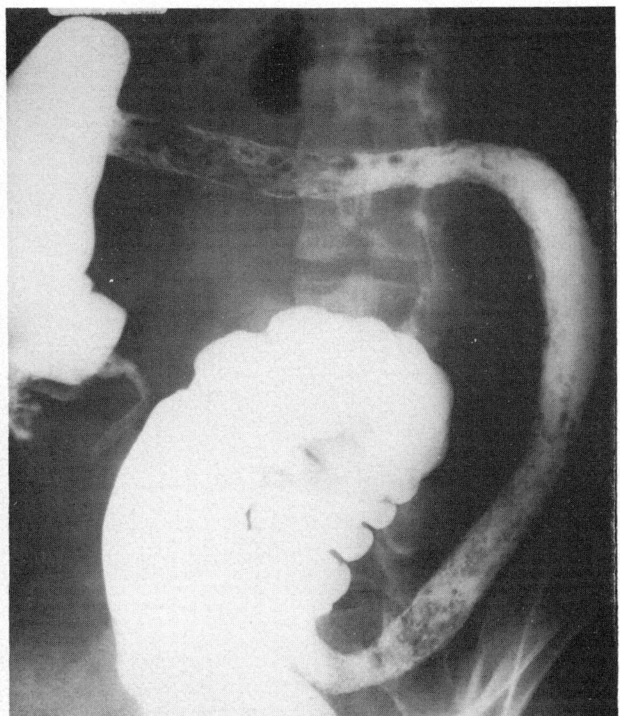

A B

Fig. 35.4 A Diffuse ulcerative colitis involving the descending and transverse colon and to a lesser extent the right side of the colon. Note the destroyed mucosal pattern and the narrowed lumen. B same case $2\frac{1}{2}$ years later. Some further narrowing of the colon has occurred. The descending colon has a 'pipestem' appearance and the mucosal pattern throughout the colon is shaggy.

scope, the mucosa in the early stages is seen to be red and swollen and bleeds readily to the touch. Later superficial ulcers and patches of mucus can be seen.

Double contrast studies of the colonic mucosa have shown an accurate correlation with the sigmoidoscopic findings and thus double contrast studies can be used to follow the course of the disease.

Ulcerative colitis predisposes to malignancy and the frequency of malignant change is related to the duration of the disease. In patients who have suffered from ulcerative colitis for more than 20 years the incidence of malignant change is 20 per cent. Carcinomatous change in ulcerative colitis arises diffusely in a flat mucosa. If the disease is treated by sub-total colectomy and ileo-rectal anastomosis, there is an ever-present risk of the development of malignant change in the rectal stump. Also with this procedure there may be problems because of active disease in the retained rectum, or subsequent relapse. These factors have tended to produce a surgical bias towards total protocolectomy and ileostomy, although each case requires an individual decision as to management.

Radiological appearances. In the single contrast enema the presence of mucosal disease is shown only at the margins of the barium-filled bowel, or on the after evacuation film. A much more precise delineation of the extent of the disease is afforded by the double contrast enema. Early changes show an alteration in the normal sharp mucosal line, which becomes blurred and slightly thickened; this change is accompanied by a fine granularity in the *en face* view. As the disease progresses, a coarse granular appearance is seen and the mucosal line, normally continuous, becomes clearly beaded. Frank ulceration is shown by projections of barium outside the mucosal line (Fig. 35.4) and as pools of contrast in the *en face* view. Larger ulcers tend to assume a collar-stud configuration and may coalesce (Fig. 35.5). Varying degrees of inflammatory polyposis may be seen. Whether mucosal involvement is mild or severe, disease tends to occur in continuity proximally from the rectum to involve a varying length of colon. As the disease progresses the colon may shorten and the lumen may narrow; haustral blunting and subsequent effacement occur (Fig. 35.6). These changes are due to a muscular abnormality rather than fibrosis which is not a feature of early ulcerative colitis but in the fully developed state produces the 'pipe stem' colon of late ulcerative colitis. It is seldom that the whole colon is in the same stage of evolution of disease and some of the older names of localized areas—regional colitis or ileocolitis—may represent areas of active disease in a colon that is more diffusely affected than appears from the barium enema examination.

Acute toxic dilatation of the colon occurs in a small proportion of patients with ulcerative colitis and it may be the presenting syndrome heralding the onset of the

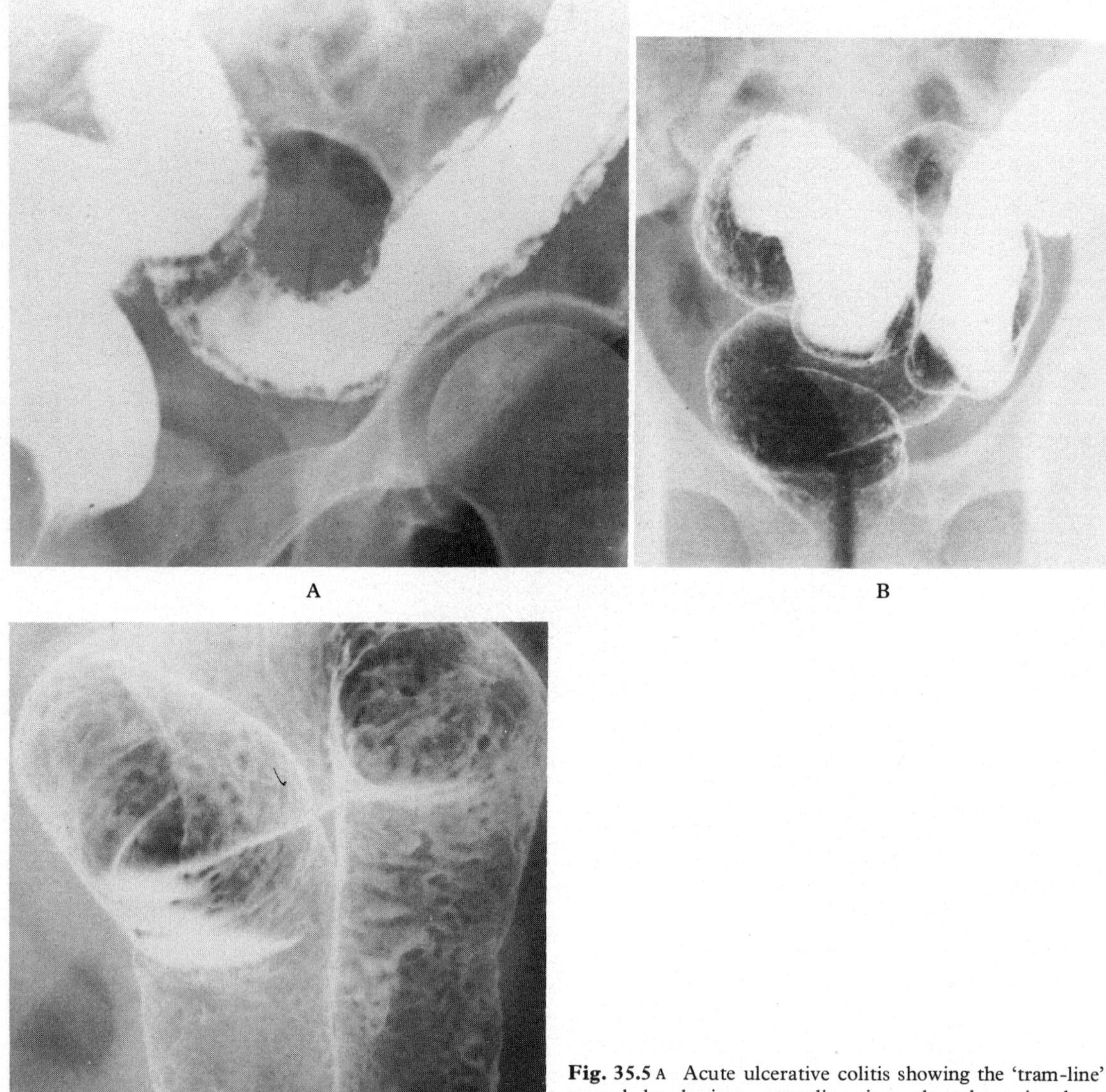

Fig. 35.5 A Acute ulcerative colitis showing the 'tram-line' appearance caused by barium extending into the ulcers in the sub-mucosa. B Coarse granularity in the rectum and deep ulcers in the distal sigmoid in ulcerative colitis. C Post-inflammatory polyposis in ulcerative colitis.

disease or it may develop in cases of established ulcerative colitis (Fig. 35.7). Toxic dilatation may also occur in Crohn's disease and occasionally in other conditions including ischaemia, dysentery and amoebiasis. The patient is acutely ill with a rapid pulse, low fever, diarrhoea and hypokalaemia.

The plain radiographs of the abdomen show a gas-filled dilated colon involving the whole or a segment of colon. The transverse colon is particularly affected and transverse measurements of more than 6.5 cm indicate that toxic dilation of the colon is present. The normal haustrations in the affected portion of colon may be blunted or effaced and the wall may show thickening with mucosal excrescences giving an irregular outline to the gas-filled colon—so-called mucosal islands. The affected portion of the colon is paralysed, causing a functional obstruction so that there is dilation and retention of fluid in the colon proximal to the area of toxic dilation.

Perforation of the affected oedematous segment or of the over-distended caecum is a very serious complication. Linear streaks of gas in the colon wall are indicative of potential necrosis and likely rupture of the bowel wall.

Carcinoma of the colon is a further complication which develops in long-standing ulcerative colitis and may occasionally be multifocal. Malignant change when it develops is usually a plaque-like or scirrhous carcinoma, the latter causing a stricture which must be differentiated from the more common benign stricture produced by hypertrophy of the muscularis mucosa (Fig. 35.8). This can be very difficult and colonoscopy with biopsy is now an important method of investigation in these patients. A full double contrast enema is necessary for

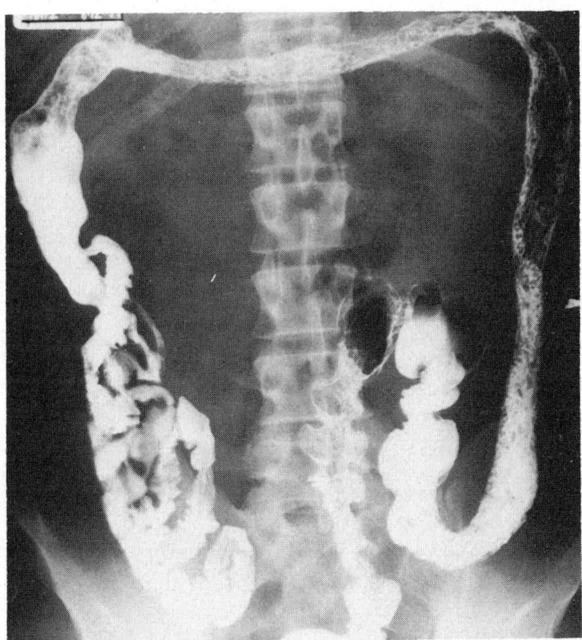

Fig. 35.6 Ulcerative colitis. Some air is present in the colon giving a double contrast appearance. Note the shortening of the right side of the colon and the generalized narrowing and loss of haustration present throughout the colon.

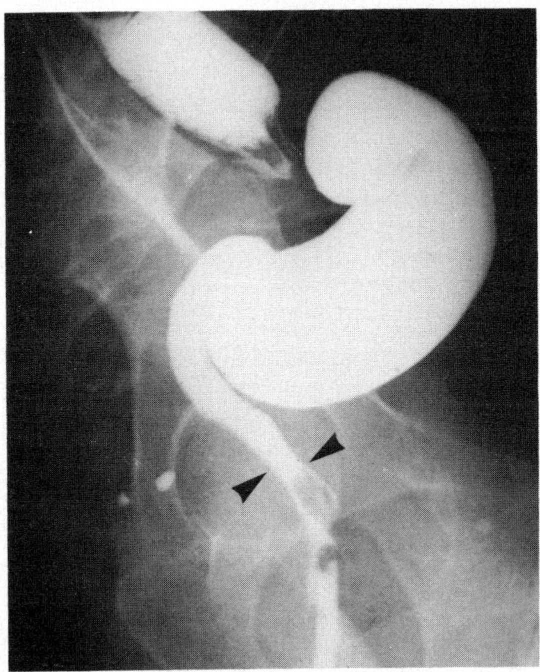

Fig. 35.8 Stricture of the rectum associated with ulcerative colitis. Lateral view shows narrowing of the rectum (*arrows*) with a loss of the mucosal pattern associated with a lack of distensibility.

the radiological investigation of patients in the high risk group.

Granulomatous colitis (Regional enteritis, see p. 718)
Granulomatous colitis (Crohn's disease) is a transmural inflammatory lesion of the colon which has to be differentiated from localized ulcerative colitis.

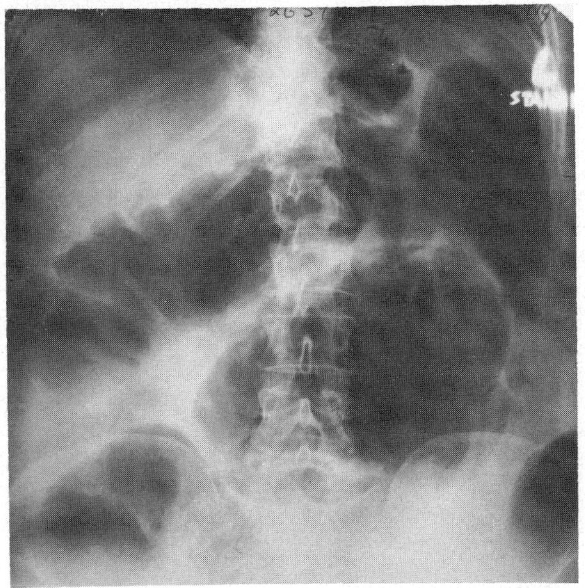

Fig. 35.7 Fulminating ulcerative colitis. Supine plain film of abdomen showing gas-distended colon with thickened walls. The erect film showed no fluid levels in the colon despite the marked distension.

Involvement of the caecum occurs to a varying degree with regional ileitis and the pathological process in the caecum is similar to that in the terminal ileum.

Localized lesions may, however, occur in other parts of the colon without any lesion in the terminal ileum.

Histologically there is an inflammatory change involving the whole thickness of the bowel wall; granulomatous lesions with giant cells without any necrosis and deep fissures and fistulae are seen.

Radiological appearances. In Crohn's disease the changes found differ in degree and distribution in comparison with ulcerative colitis although radiological differentiation is not always readily made. The disease process is characteristically discontinuous, both along the length of the bowel and circumferentially. Mucosal involvement tends to be patchy and the even granularity of ulcerative colitis is uncommon. One of the earliest roentgen features of Crohn's disease anywhere in the gut is the appearance of an *aphthoid ulcer*. These appear as small, central collections of barium surrounded by a radiolucent halo. These may produce a 'bull's eye' or 'target' lesion, often best seen in the colon where it may be surrounded by normal mucosa (Figs. 35.9A and B).

Although suggestive of Crohn's disease ophthoid ulcers are not specific but may be seen in Yersinia enterocolitis and amoebic colitis. In contrast, early cases may show discrete ulceration within an otherwise normal mucosa which is quite unlike the appearances of ulcerative colitis. Pathologically, ulceration tends to be deeper and

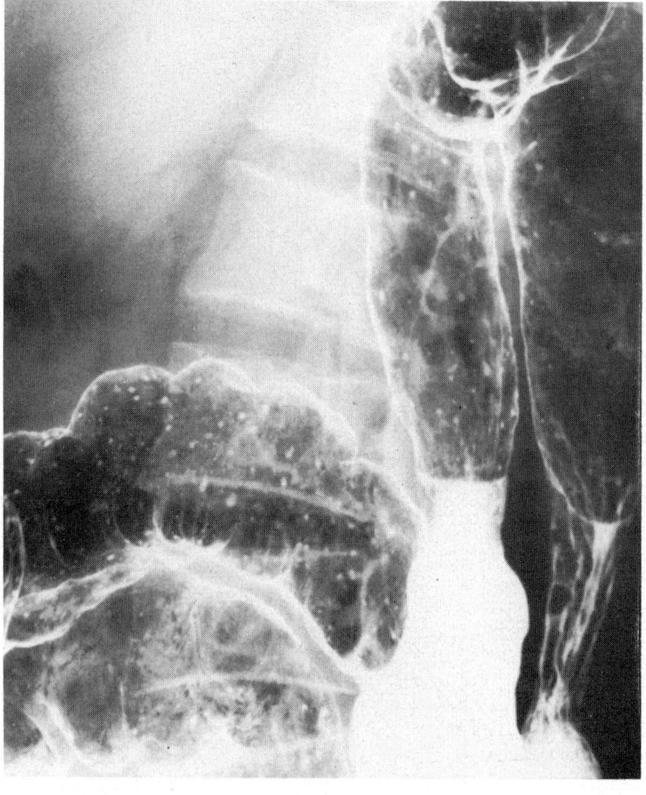

A

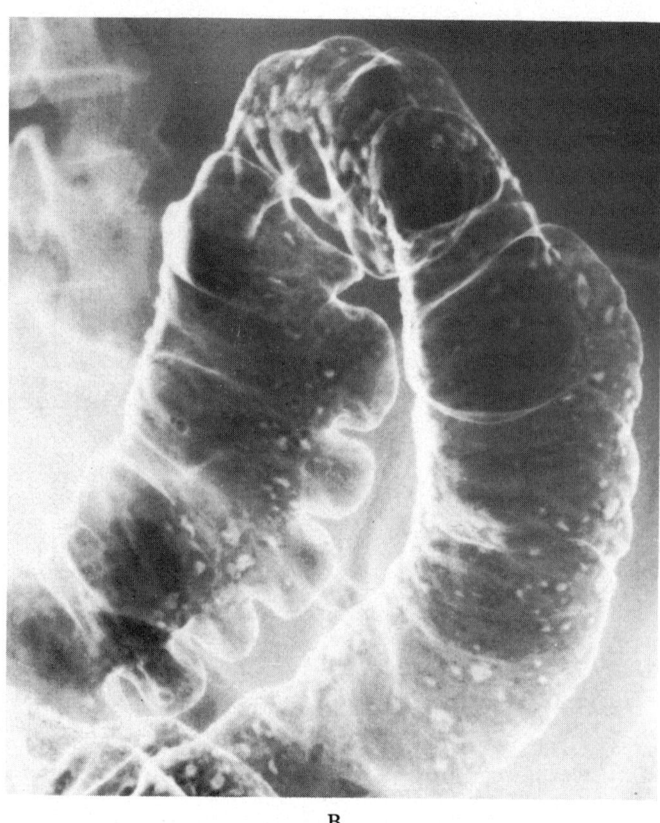

B

Fig. 35.9 Aphthoid ulcers in the colon in Crohn's disease. A The small, central collections of barium are surrounded by a radiolucent 'halo'. Note the asymmetrical haustra in ulceration of the walls of the colon. (Courtesy of Dr. K. C. Simpkins). B Aphthoid ulcers in the colon in Crohn's disease.

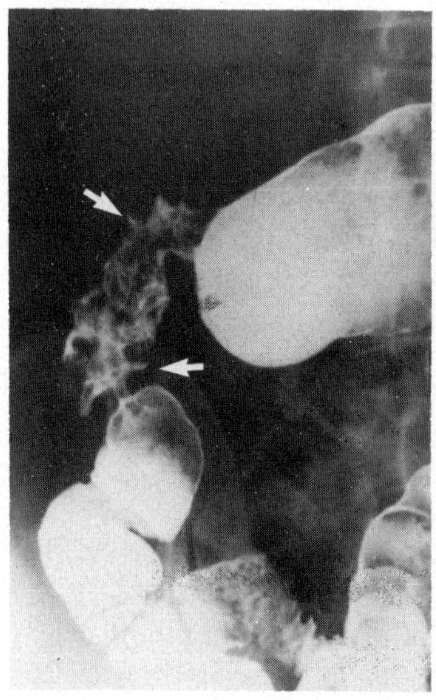

A

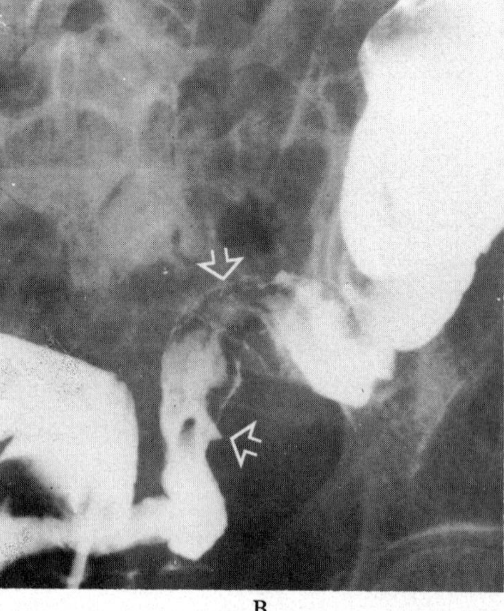

B

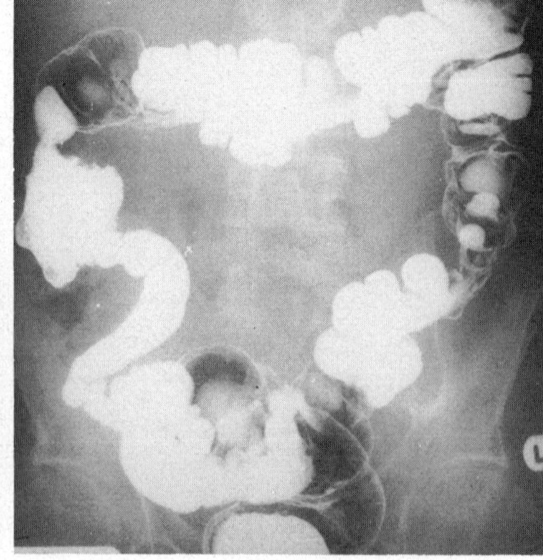

C

Fig. 35.10 Inflammatory granuloma (Crohn's) of right side of colon showing distortion of mucosal pattern, narrowing of bowel lumen and 'rose-thorn' spikes of barium (*arrows*) caused by filling of deep clefts into the bowel wall indicating the transmural nature of the disease. B Similar granulomatous lesion (Crohn's) involving the pelvic colon. The lesion shows a loss of mucosal pattern imperceptably blending with normal bowel and a single large 'spike' present in the bowel wall. C Crohn's colitis showing multiple strictures, ulceration and eccentric haustral loss.

is often linear in configuration; the combination of linear ulceration and mucosal oedema produces the so-called 'cobblestone' appearance of the mucosa. Together with deep ulcers, fissuring is a characteristic feature with fine thorn-like projections of barium extending outwards into the wall of the colon (Fig. 35.10). Haustral loss is often irregular and eccentric with folds effaced on one side of the lumen and preserved on the other. The rectum is frequently spared (in approximately 50 per cent of patients with Crohn's colitis), but in cases which do show rectal involvement deep ulcers and fissures are often seen. Skip lesions with intervening areas of normal mucosa are also characteristic and strictures are common. Internal or entero-cutaneous fistulae are also features of this disease. There may, of course, also be concomitant narrowing, cobblestoning or other mucosal abnormalities of the terminal ileum. Differentiation in particular must be made from ulcerative colitis; this presents no problem when classical features of Crohn's disease are present, such as a severe right-sided colitis with deep ulcers and fissuring, skip lesions and a normal distal bowel (see p. 722). Inevitably there is, however, an overlap in appearances in individual cases. Crohn's disease must also be distinguished from ileo-caecal tuberculosis—which is, however, now very uncommon in this country—and also from secondary carcinoma and ischaemia.

Differentiation from primary growths of the colon can be made by the destruction of mucosa present with neoplasm. However serosal deposits in the colon or involvement of the colon by growths from adjoining strictures, e.g. ovary, may cause difficulties in diagnosis as in such instances the mucosa may be intact in the area of involvement.

Ischaemic colitis

Interference with the arterial or venous supply of the colon may result in infarction of a segment of colon and, depending on the extent and rapidity of collateral circulation and revascularization, the affected segment of the colon may undergo necrosis with gangrene (acute) or may more slowly be affected with the development of a 'pseudotumour'. Less commonly revascularization may result in complete resolution of the lesion or in fibrosis with the development of stricture. With slow and insidious mesenteric arterial occlusion, as in atheromatous aortic thrombosis or abdominal aortic aneurysm, the excellent collateral circulation usually proves adequate to maintain the vitality of the bowel and produce no change (see Ch. 29). Vascular lesions of the colon may be classified as in Table 35.1.

Table 35.1 Ischaemic colitis (vascular obstruction)

	Pathological changes	Radiological appearances
Acute	Infarction with necrosis of right side of colon	Acute intestinal obstruction with fluid levels and gas distension of right half of colon
Subacute	Often venous infarction following peritoneal infection results in oedema and haemorrhages in the bowel wall.	May slowly resolve or form strictures
Reversible	Collateral circulation is almost adequate and thickening of the bowel walls and intramural haemorrhages occur	Barium enema shows narrowing of the bowel lumen and 'fingerprint' deformities. Pseudotumour appearances can be seen
Chronic	Collateral circulation usually adequate	Normal

Acute infarction. Obstruction of the main stem of the superior mesenteric artery is associated with infarction of the small bowel and the right half of the colon. Clinically this presents as an acute obstruction and radiologically the features are those of small fluid levels in the gas-distended right side of the colon. Fluid levels and gas distension of the affected small bowel are also present (Ch. 36). Barium examination is seldom undertaken at this stage as the clinical condition is too acute.

Subacute vascular lesions. If the vascular obstruction affects the vein rather than the artery the develop-

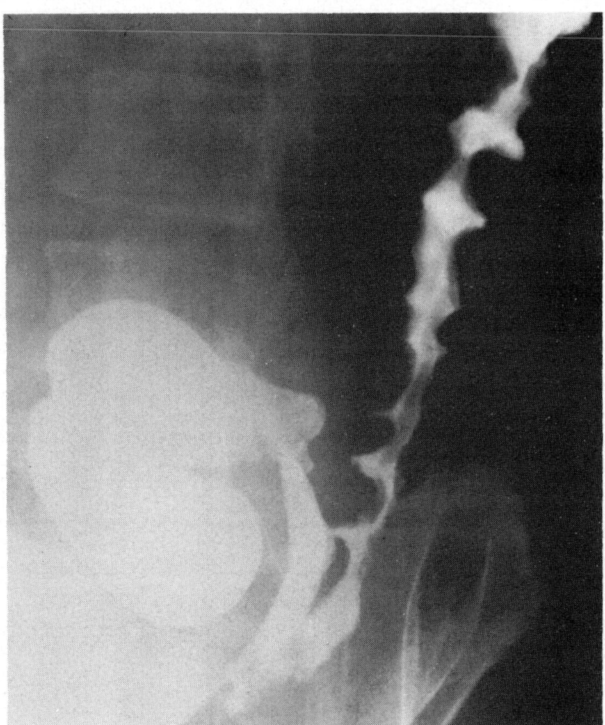

Fig. 35.11 Ischaemic lesion of the colon. Barium enema showing the classical 'fingerprint' deformities in the wall of the descending colon caused by areas of oedema and haemorrhage. These changes may regress completely with treatment or may result in fibrosis and stricture formation.

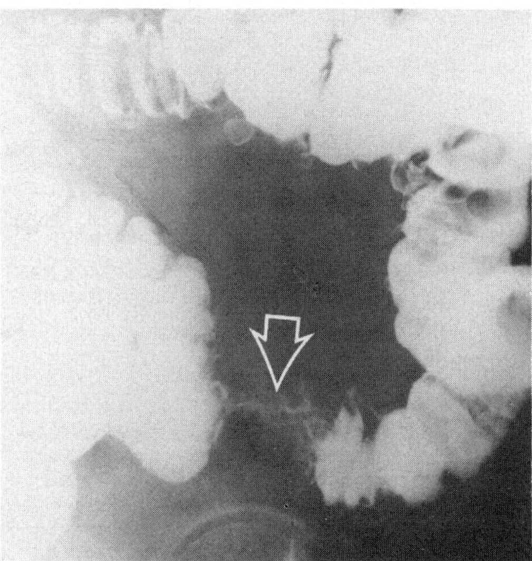

Fig. 35.12

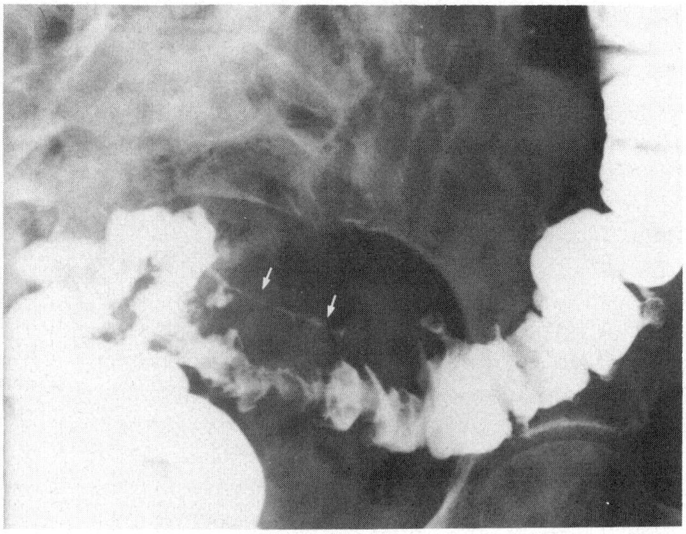

Fig. 35.13

Fig. 35.12 Diverticular disease. A segmental area of diverticular disease in the colon shows intact mucosa and spiky outlines (↓). Note that throughout the colon there are other diverticula present.

Fig. 35.13 Diverticular disease localized to the sigmoid colon showing a fistulous track (*arrows*) which indicates an inflammatory change.

ment of the bowel changes may be slower. Venous thrombosis may also be a sequel of intraperitoneal infection or strangulation of the bowel. The barium enema shows a localized lesion (pseudo-tumour) with thickening of the wall and large fingerprint deformities caused by areas of intramural haemorrhage or oedema (Fig. 35.11).

With venous thrombosis barium enema examination may show a deformity of the colon with a pseudo-tumour formation. Differentiation from granulomatous lesions may be difficult and even malignant tumours may be mimicked.

Reversible vascular lesions. As these lesions resolve spontaneously their pathology is largely conjectural, but by comparison it would appear that the lesion consists of oedema of the bowel wall associated with haemorrhage into the wall. The degree of vascular impairment, arterial or venous, is such that necrosis and gangrene of the bowel wall do not result and revascularization of the bowel through the establishment of collaterals occurs.

The radiological features are those of a pseudo-tumour as described above, but although complete resolution may occur in some cases, in others fibrosis with stricture formation may occur.

The arteriographic changes in reversible colonic ischaemia are as follows:

1. Increased blood supply to the diseased segment with dilated arteries.
2. An increased number of dilated vasa recta.
3. Early dense filling of the draining veins.

These features are, however, applicable to all inflammatory disease and are non-specific.

DIVERTICULAR DISEASE OF THE COLON

Colonic diverticula have long been regarded as representing mucosal herniations through the muscular wall of the colon along the sites of arterial branches of the colonic vessels, and consequent on weakening of the colonic wall by fatty infiltration at these points of arterial penetration. This concept has now been discarded.

The work of Morson (1963), Williams (1963) and others has drawn attention to the gross changes in the muscularis mucosa of the colon which occur in diverticular disease. The circular muscle of the colon is thickened and fasiculated and the diverticular protrusions occur between these hypertrophied muscle fibres. Funnel-shaped dimples of mucosa occur at sites not strengthened by muscular bands and it is from these that the diverticula arise (Fig. 35.12). Pressure measurements and motility studies have shown that considerable muscular dysfunction of the colon is present.

The ease of filling of a diverticulum by barium enema varies with the stage of muscular contraction of the colonic wall, and also with the amount and consistency of faecal material within the diverticulum.

The 'saw-tooth' pattern (serrated or accordion pattern) previously accepted as indicative of inflammatory change is now thought to be produced by thickened and coarsened circular muscle fibres. These are formed by merging and confluence of some widened muscle bundles in the circular muscle of the colon (Fig. 35.13).

The shortening and narrowing of the pelvic colon and descending colon found in this stage is also considered to be the result of thickening and shortening of the longitudinal muscular coat. Morson (1963) in a third of his cases found no evidence of inflammatory change in resected segments of colon for diverticulitis and considers that the appearances seen are due to changes in the quantity and arrangement of the colon musculature rather than to inflammatory conditions.

Fleischner, Ming and Henken (1964) believe that the underlying cause for the alteration in muscular appearances is muscular spasm consequent on the development of the spastic colon syndrome.

Radiological investigation. Although the diverticula can be seen in a barium meal follow-through examination a true appreciation and an understanding of the disease are best obtained from a barium enema examination. The radiological appearances are:

(a) *Diverticula.* These appear as flask-like outpouching from the bowel wall. The neck of the diverticulum is narrow and depending on the amount of faecal content it may appear as a flask-like, a crescentic, or a cut-off barium filled shadow.

(b) *Spasm.* The muscular hypertrophy described earlier results in local contraction which gives rise to a saw-tooth appearance or a spiky appearance of the affected area. Except in the acutely inflamed conditions, much of the spasm can be relieved by an anti-spasmodic such as Buscopan 20 mg i.v.

(c) *Shortening and stiffening.* The affected segment of the colon is usually shortened, thickened and tender on palpation.

Complications

Perforation. Perforation of a diverticulum is seldom associated with a pneumoperitoneum and general peritonitis as the leak is usually a more gradual process giving rise to a pericolic or paracolic abscess.

Pericolic abscess formation presents as an extrinsic filling defect associated with narrowing of the lumen of the bowel. The defect is usually eccentric (Fig. 35.14) and careful fluoroscopic examination shows that the mucosa, although more complex in character than normal, is not invaded or destroyed as would occur with a malignant tumour. Expansion of the colonic lumen is not diagnostic of a tumour as on rare occasions it may be seen with a pericolic abscess.

Perforation of the colon may be associated with the spread of gas into the retroperitoneal tissues, recognized by the 'soap bubble' appearance in the retroperitoneal tissues. Occasionally the abscess may track some distance from the colon, appearing at the inguinal ring and mimicking a psoas abscess.

Fistula. Fistula formation between the colon and the bladder is one of the commonest and most distressing complications of pelvic colon diverticular disease. The fistula itself is seldom demonstrated by barium enema as the symptoms produced by spread of infection to the urinary bladder demand treatment before the fistula is large enough to allow the passage of contrast medium. Less frequently an internal fistula may form between the colon and small bowel.

Malignant change. There is little evidence to show that diverticular disease predisposes to malignancy. Detection of malignant change is, however, more difficult and as the malignant tumours are usually strictures rather than encephaloid types of growth they tend to be obscured by the diverticular disease (Fig. 35.15).

Haemorrhage. Severe bleeding is not an infrequent complication of diverticular disease. The bleeding is usually brisk and of short duration unlike the steady ooze usually associated with carcinoma. Selective arteriography of the mesenteric arteries is an important investigation in the detection of the bleeding site, which is

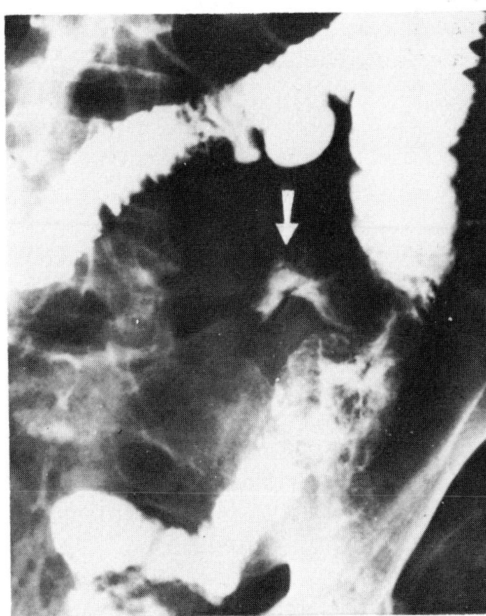

Fig. 35.14 Pericolic abscess associated with diverticulitis. Barium has extruded outside the lumen of the colon and a fistulous track is seen (↓).

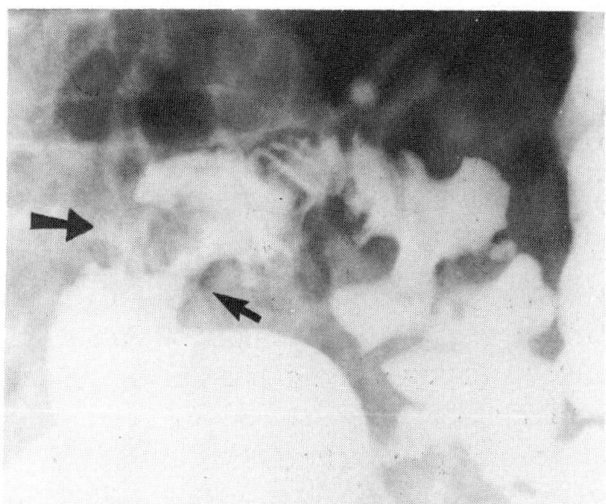

Fig. 35.15 Malignant change in an area associated with diverticulitis showing a circumferential lesion in the distal sigmoid with complete destruction of the mucosal pattern (*arrows*).

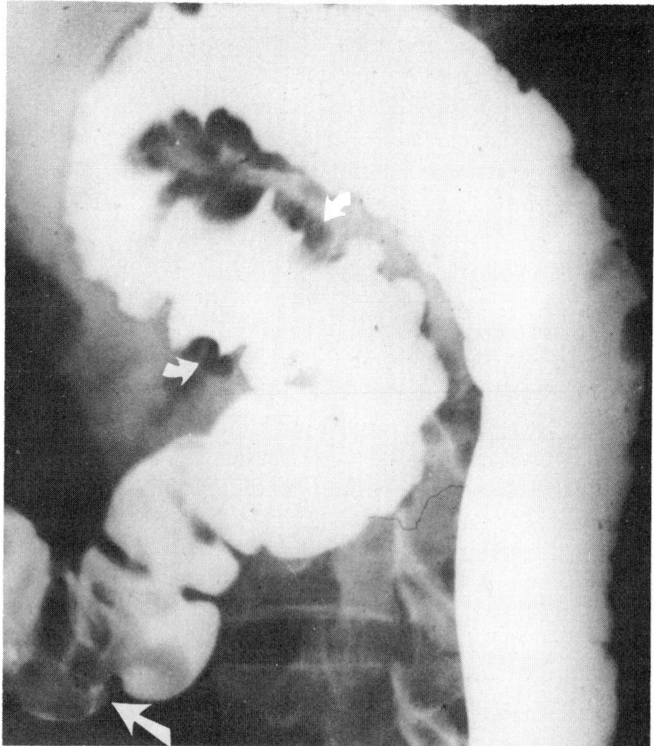

Fig. 35.16 Pneumatosis coli. In the filled barium enema the gas cysts (*arrows*) show as defects in the wall of the colon not dissimilar to polypi.

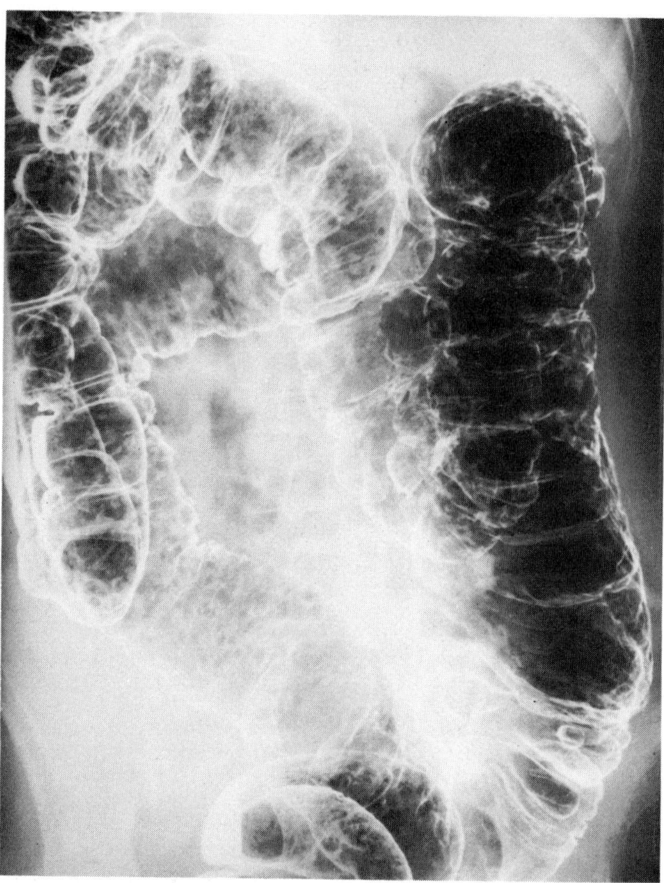

Fig. 35.17 Double contrast film of a patient with pneumatosis coli showing gross cystic changes present throughout the colonic wall.

often in the ascending colon. Characteristic arteriographic changes affect the vasa recti and consist of intimal thickening and focal thinning of the media. Severe degrees of eccentricity of intimal thickening towards the lumen of the diverticulum were seen exclusively in bleeding cases (Meyers, Alonso and Baer, 1976).

PNEUMATOSIS COLI

Small gas-filled cysts may occur in the wall of the colon and small bowel. The source of the gas-filled cysts has been attributed to the spread of air from the mediastinum. Pneumatosis coli is associated with chronic obstructive respiratory disease but pneumatosis of the small bowel is more frequently associated with duodenal or gastric ulceration.

Rupture of the cysts may be associated with a pneumoperitoneum but the cysts themselves may cause no clinical symptoms. Radiologically the gas-containing cysts can be seen as a collar-like chain or radiolucent filling defects following the line of the colon. Barium enema examination may show filling defects which may appear not unlike polypi (Figs. 35.16 and 35.17). Many of the cysts are subserosal and as such only show slight indentations of the barium-filled colon.

The gas-filled cysts may be either mainly subserous, submucosal or intramuscular. When the cysts are confined to the muscular wall they are generally small and may be difficult to see. In these circumstances the barium enema may give an irregularity of outline which suggests a granulomatous lesion.

TUMOURS OF THE COLON

POLYPOID LESIONS OF THE COLON

Histologically polyps occurring in the colon may be classified as:

(a) Adenomatous polyps
(b) Villous papilloma
(c) Juvenile polyps
(d) Peutz-Jegher's polyps
(e) Post-inflammatory polyps

The histological varieties of polyps cannot be differentiated on radiological grounds alone.

Adenomatous polyps may be single (Fig. 35.18) or multiple, sessile or pedunculated; they occur characteristically in large numbers in familial polyposis of the colon and Gardner's Syndrome.

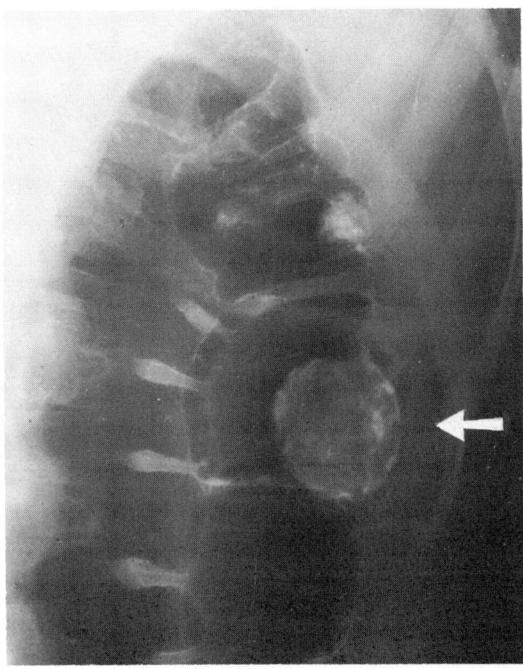

Fig. 35.18 Colonic polyp. Double contrast film showing a polyp arising from the wall of the descending colon and coated with barium. The smooth outline of the tumour can be seen.

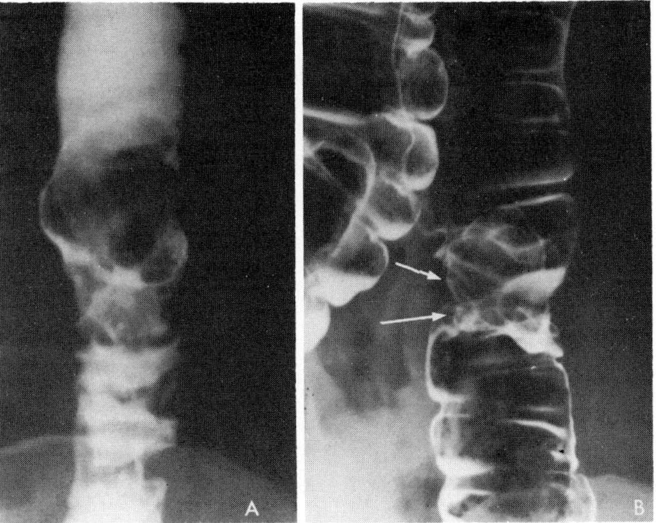

Fig. 35.19 Colonic polyp showing malignant change. A The filled colon reveals the polypoid appearance of the tumour. B The double contrast film shows a broad sessile base suggesting a malignant change.

Histologically they are composed of adenomatous glands and certain radiological features may help in differentiating benign and malignant polyps.

Familial polyposis of the colon is inherited as a Mendelian dominant; all cases develop malignant change if untreated. The double contrast barium enema shows multiple round filling defects characteristically involving the whole colon and always involving the rectum. The individual polyps vary in size from a pin-head to a large conglomerate mass. Polyps which have a broad sessile base must be regarded as especially prone to malignant change (Fig. 35.19). Likewise, a rapid increase in size of the tumour with thickening of the base may be indicative of malignant change before the development of overt carcinoma.

Gardner's syndrome consists of adenomatous polyposis of the colon, multiple osteomata of the skull and mandible, multiple epidermoid cysts and soft tissue tumours of the skin. The risk of malignant change is the same as in familial polyposis of the colon.

Table 35.2 Radiological differentiation of benign and malignant polyps

Benign	Malignant
Diameter less than 10 mm	Size increasing on serial examination
Pedunculated polyp with a long stalk	Sessile polyp with diameter of base greater than height
Smooth surface	Irregular surface
Colon contour unaffected by polyp	Indentation of colonic wall at base of polyp

Certain other lesions may be found with this syndrome including small bowel adenomas and carcinoma of the thyroid but the most important association is with carcinoma of the peri-ampullary region of the pancreas.

Villous papilloma may produce a polyp-like appearance and characteristically the tumour is composed of a frond-like soft mass; they occur most frequently in the lower bowel. They may be associated with a protein-losing or potassium-losing enteropathy.

Radiologically they appear as flat sessile masses with the interstices of the polyps filled with barium presenting a characteristic appearance of a tumour covered with frond-like stalks.

Juvenile polyps are particularly common in childhood and often present with symptoms of rectal bleeding. They do not predispose to malignant change and may undergo spontaneous regression. They have to be differentiated from adenomatous polyps and it was confusion with the latter that caused many patients suffering from juvenile polyposis to be subjected to unnecessary surgical measures. They appear on double contrast enemas as smooth, rounded masses usually with a well-defined pedicle. Histologically, these polyps are *hamartomas*.

Peutz-Jegher's syndrome consists of mucosal and circumoral pigmentation and gastrointestinal polyposis. In this condition the colon is involved in approximately 50 per cent of cases and the colonic polyps, when they occur, tend to be relatively few in number. The polyps in this syndrome are hamartomas, as in juvenile polyposis, and do not have the same predilection to malignant change, which does, however, occasionally occur usually as a carcinoma in the upper gastrointestinal tract.

Ovarian tumours are sometimes associated with this syndrome.

Post-inflammatory polyps. These polyps which occur in ulcerative colitis and other inflammatory diseases represent islands of surviving mucosa and granulation tissue in varying stages of inflammation and repair. As such they cannot be regarded as true polyps. Radiologically they may be few in number or multiple, segmental or widespread in distribution and may appear frond-like or resemble adenomatous polyps.

MALIGNANT TUMOURS

The vast majority of tumours of the colon are derived from the mucosa with the result that they are columnar cell tumours or adenocarcinoma depending on the degree of differentiation. Rarely the glands may be active and secretion of mucus may give rise to colloid-containing tumours.

Spread of the growth occurs along the bowel and circumferentially, ulceration of the tumour may occur with perforation, whilst in other instances a scirrhous reaction may produce stricture formation. The sites of growth in the colon appear to have some effect on the type of growth that occurs— encephaloid growths tending to occur in the right side of the colon or in the rectum, whilst scirrhous growths occur most frequently on the left side of the bowel.

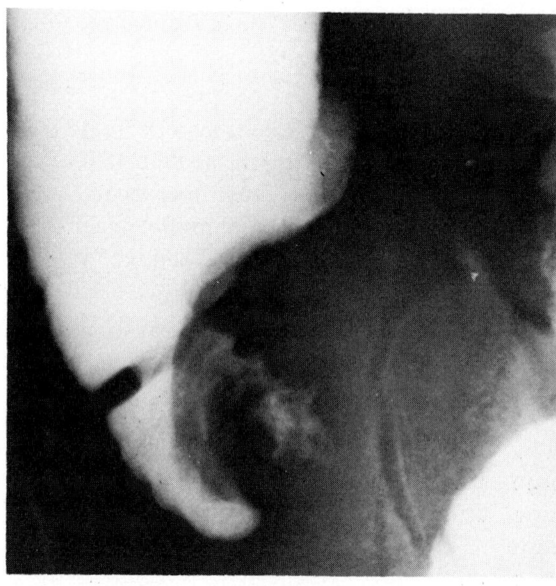

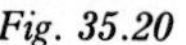

Fig. 35.20

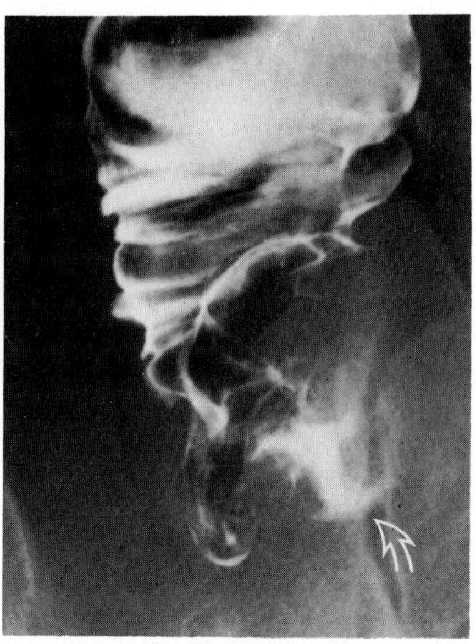

Fig. 35.21

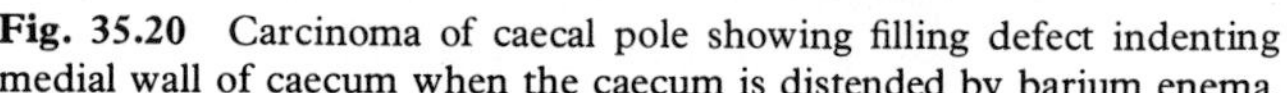

Fig. 35.20 Carcinoma of caecal pole showing filling defect indenting medial wall of caecum when the caecum is distended by barium enema.

Fig. 35.21 Carcinoma of caecum. Mucosal outline of caecum demonstrated after evacuation of barium demonstrating mucosal destruction (*arrow*) and the polypoid tumour. No barium has entered the terminal ileum.

Growths of the colon spread to the lymphatic glands at the root of the mesentery and via the superior mesenteric and portal veins to the liver.

The radiological appearances are those of:

(*a*) A filling defect projecting into the colonic lumen separated from normal mucosa by a sharp margin often having a shoulder-like deformity.

(*b*) Destruction of the mucosal pattern again with a sharp margin separating the growth from normal mucosa.

(*c*) A tumour mass projecting into the barium filled colon having the classical half shadows and irregular deformities (Figs. 35.20 and 35.21). In the double contrast enema the tumour mass coated with barium can be seen.

(*d*) Occasionally in the constricting type of lesion all that can be visualized is a narrowed stricture and often as the colon proximal to the lesion is distended (Figs. 35.22 and 35.23), the overlapping coils of bowel with retained faeces may make the demonstration of the features of the stricture difficult.

Retrograde intussusception of the bowel over the growth may occur if the distal bowel is distended to too great a degree during the performance of the enema. In other tumours, especially those developing from polypoid lesions, intussusception of the bowel may occur and the presenting features both clinical and radiological are those of intussusception (Fig. 35.24).

Metastatic spread to the liver is best investigated by ultrasound examination and by isotope scans. Pulmonary metastases from bowel tumours is uncommon.

Sarcomata of the large bowel are usually reticulum-celled and less commonly fibrosarcoma arising from benign lesions (e.g. leiomyoma). They are highly cellular with little fibrous stroma. They consequently tend to be

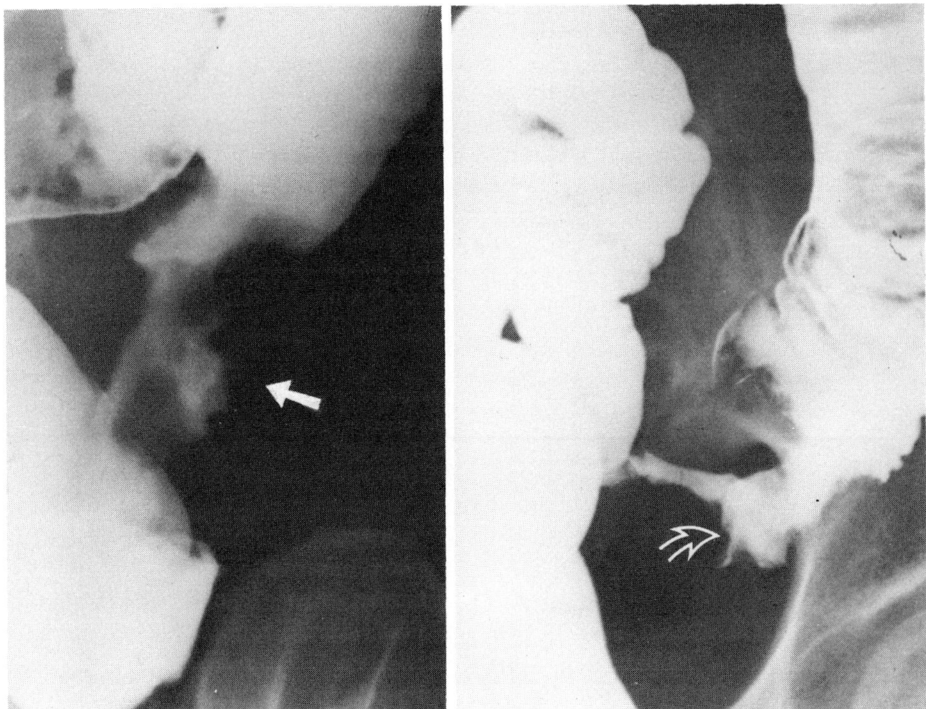

Fig. 35.22 *Fig. 35.23*

Fig. 35.22 Carcinoma of descending colon. The filling defect with sharp edges associated with some ulceration in the growth (*arrow*) is indicative of a carcinoma.

Fig. 35.23 Carcinoma of pelvic colon. An annular carcinoma surrounding the pelvic colon and narrowing the lumen is seen. There is distension of the colon proximal to the growth and the sharp margin (shoulder) between the tumour and the normal colon is seen (*arrow*).

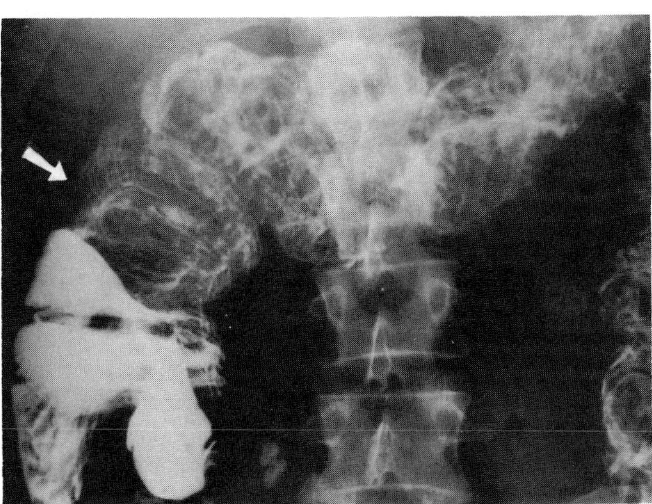

Fig. 35.24 Chronic intussusception of the right side of the colon associated with a polypoid carcinoma showing the classical 'watchspring' appearances produced by barium in the sheath between the intussusception and the intussuscipiens.

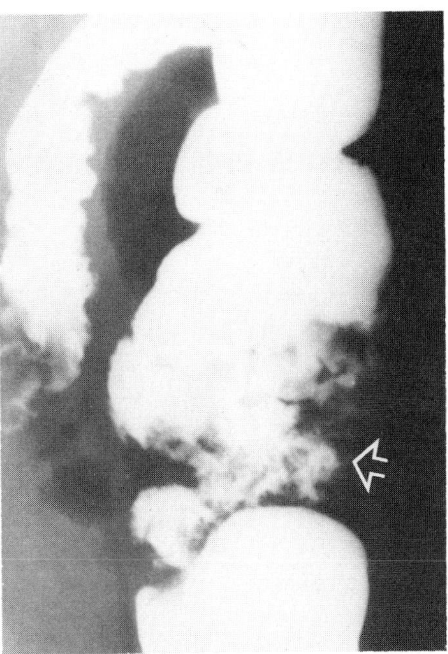

Fig. 35.25 Mucus-secreting villous adenopapilloma of the colon. The patchy appearance of the filling defect is fairly characteristic. Histology showed mucin secreting adenopapilloma. (*Courtesy of Dr. T. Philp.*)

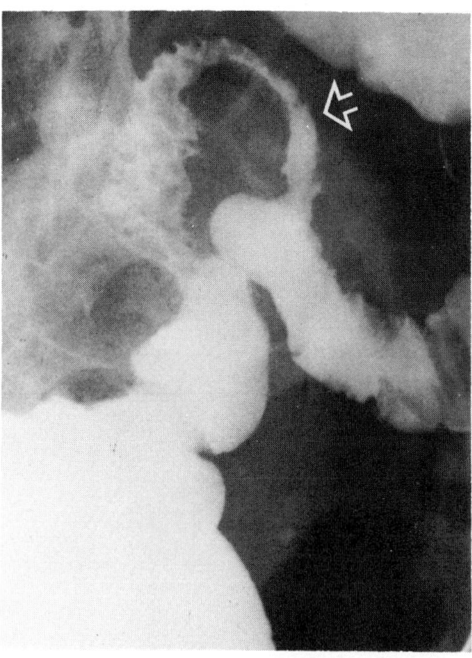

Fig. 35.26 Metastatic growth of the colon(←). Growths arising elsewhere may metastasize onto the serosal surface of the colon and give rise to filling defects in the colon. These filling defects as they arise from the serosal surface may show no mucosal destruction but they should be considered in any atypical filling defect in the colon.

large tumours which cavitate, giving rise to abscess formation, and produce expanding lesions of the bowel.

Mucus secreting tumours of the bowel may develop speckled calcification and this feature may be replicated when metastatic tumours occur in the liver (Fig. 35.25).

Differential diagnosis. Primary carcinoma of the colon has to be differentiated from the following conditions:

(*a*) Secondary malignancy affecting the bowel.
(*b*) Local spread from a primary tumour elsewhere, especially stomach and pancreas.
(*c*) Adhesions.
(*d*) Amoebiasis, Tuberculosis and Crohn's disease.
(*e*) Simple spasm, mimicking a stricture.

Malignant deposits in the bowel may be extensive and infiltration of the wall may cause relatively long areas of narrowing (Figs. 35.26 and 35.27). A similar appearance may be produced by a primary colonic tumour of the linitis plastica type.

Local spread from tumours arising elsewhere tends to produce a large, extracolonic component and adhesions may produce local narrowing and deformity but leave the mucosa intact.

Carcinoma may mimic amoebiasis and ileo-caecal tuberculosis, but other features of these diseases may aid in differentiation.

Crohn's disease may be distinguished from colonic growths by the following characteristics:

1. The edge of a granulomatous lesion blends imperceptibly with normal mucosa and the sharp cut-off of a shoulder is absent.
2. The length of bowel involved is often considerably greater than in carcinoma, and the lesions are often multiple.
3. The mucosal pattern although markedly distorted is not actually destroyed and often shows ulceration and fissuring.
4. There may be evidence of regional ileitis.

Simple spastic strictures should be distinguished by preservation of a normal mucosal pattern and absence of a filling defect.

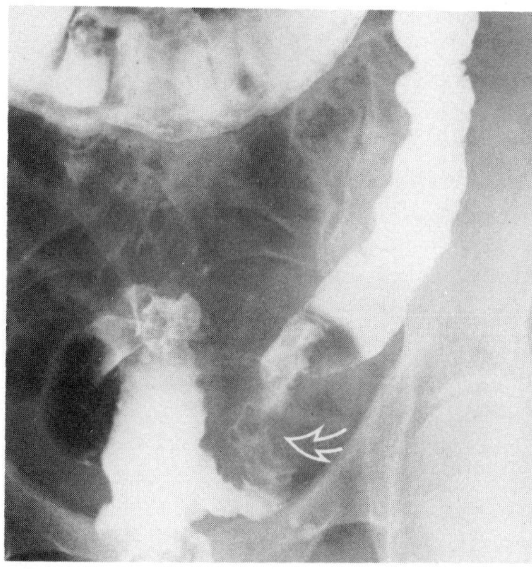

A

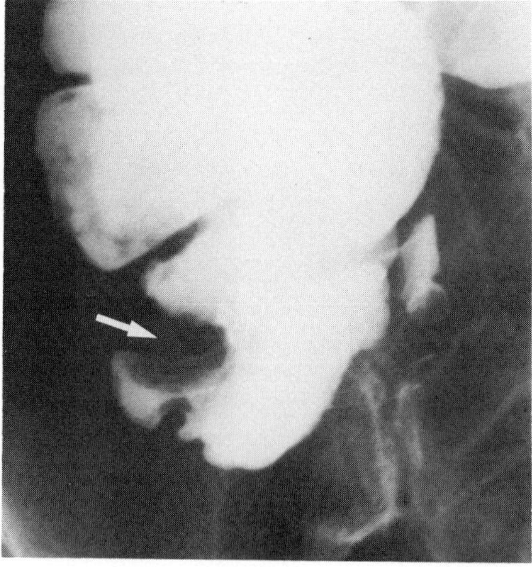

B

Fig. 35.27 Metastatic deposits on the colon wall mimicking primary colonic growths. A Shows a deposit on the pelvic colon but the mucosa is intact. B Shows a similar lesion on the lateral wall of the caecum. Both lesions were from a primary growth of the gall bladder.

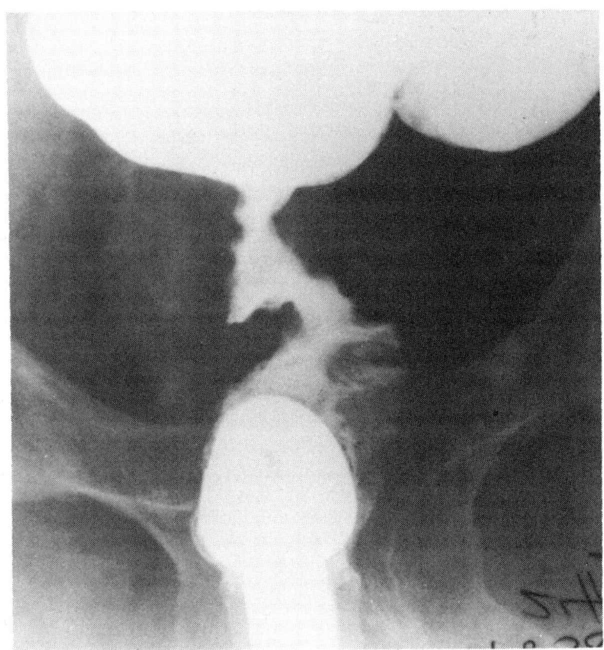

Fig. 35.28 Carcinoma of the rectum. The radiological features are similar to those of carcinoma in other parts of the colon. Carcinoma of the recto-sigmoid junction is more of a diagnostic problem than carcinoma of the rectum which should be diagnosed by local inspection. Lateral views of the pelvi-rectal junction during barium enema examination are mandatory to exclude lesions in this site.

POST-OPERATIVE COLON

Investigation of the colon after colostomy may present a difficult radiological problem as retention of the enema is difficult owing to the absence of sphincteric control at the colostomy site.

A catheter with a small balloon is inserted into the colostomy and gently filled with air to occlude the colostomy stoma. Overdistension of the balloon must be avoided and care must be taken to avoid perforation of the colon when the catheter is inserted.

The major problem in the performance of enema after colostomy is the detection of possible recurrence of the original growth for which colonic resection may have been originally undertaken. Recurrent growths may occur near the colostomy and produce extrinsic filling defects. Those defects have to be differentiated from adhesions due to kinking or surgical sewing. Filling defects in other parts of the colon have the same appearances as the defects caused by primary tumours, and destruction of the mucosal pattern and infiltration of the colonic wall by recurrent growth is much easier to detect at some distance away than when near the colostomy opening.

RADIATION CHANGES IN THE COLON

In the treatment of deep-seated intra-abdominal malignancy some radiation damage to the adjoining bowel is almost inevitable. The more intensive treatment of *cervical cancer* has resulted in a higher proportion of rectal injuries becoming apparent. It is thought that rectal injury from radiation occurs in 2.4 per cent of cases treated.

Some degree of reaction in the bowel must be accepted as an inevitable price for successful radiation therapy but more severe changes may result in necrosis and perforation with fistula formation showing a marked resemblance to acute diverticulitis.

Healing of these changes may be associated with fibrosis and stricture formation and these changes usually appear several years after treatment. Barium enema examination in such cases reveals a narrowed lumen of the bowel often associated with a smooth mucosal pattern and the appearances may be very similar to those of a long-standing ulcerative colitis. In the more acute phase there may be local spasm and overhang of the edges resembling a carcinoma.

Damage to other parts of the bowel such as the small intestine may occur if the loop of bowel is fixed by adhesions in the pelvis. It may also follow radiation therapy for testicular and ovarian neoplasms. These changes may be acute or, like those in the colon, may only be present years later as the result of fibrosis. They are probably the result of progressive endarteritis as a result of radiation damage to the vessels.

Radiologically the appearances are those of a stenotic lesion of the affected portion of bowel, or of ulcer formation in the rectum.

RECTUM AND ANUS

Most lesions of the anus and rectum can be directly inspected by proctoscopic examination and radiology is seldom required for the investigation of these structures (Fig. 35.28).

Cases of perirectal fibrosis and stricture, however, can only be assessed by radiology as direct inspection by proctoscopy may be impossible. Such cases usually follow trauma, frequently due to an incorrectly administered enema or to post-operative radiation, or, less frequently, to infective conditions such as lymphogranuloma inguinale.

The radiological features of perirectal fibrosis are those of general narrowing of the rectum with a loss of mucosal pattern. The appearances of perirectal fibrosis due to the different causes noted above are the same and usually give no clue as to the cause.

Although the rectum is most easily examined by proctoscopy, certain nodular contour defects may be noted on barium enema examination. They may be classified as follows:

Inflammatory lesions

1. Idiopathic ulcerative proctitis
2. Crohn's proctitis

} Both these may produce nodular masses with oedematous rectal mucosa and ulceration

3. Ulcerating granulomas of Schistosomiasis.
4. Amoebiasis usually gives rise to shallow ulcers.
5. Lymphogranuloma venereum may produce nodular rectal masses with ulceration before progression to rectal stricture.

Schistosomiasis, Lymphogranuloma, active Mycosis and Tuberculosis usually present as rectal stricture but in the pre-stricture phase they may give rise to nodular mucosal contour.

Malignant tumours

6. Villous adenoma, adenocarcinoma, lymphoma may all produce small nodular defects associated with a rectal mass.
7. Cloacogenic carcinomas occur as rare tumours.
8. Endometrial implants may give multiple small nodular lesions.

Colitis cystica profunda

Nodular plaque-like or polypoid lesions may be produced usually in the rectum or sigmoid colon. Histologically vast numbers of dilated mucous glands are seen surrounded by fibrous tissue. The condition may be mistaken for malignant invasion.

REFERENCES AND SUGGESTIONS FOR FURTHER READING

BARTRAM, C. J. (1977) Radiology in the current assessment of ulcerative colitis. *Gastrointestinal Radiology*, **1**, 383.

BARTRAM, C. J. & HALE, J. E. (1970) Radiological diagnosis of recurrent colonic carcinoma at the anastomosis. *Gut*, **11**, 778–781.

BARTRAM, C. J. & WALMSLEY, K. (1978) A radiological and pathological correlation of the mucosal changes in ulcerative colitis. *Clinical Radiology*, **29**, 323–328.

BROOKE, B. N. & COWE, D. (1973) Radiological pseudotumour in chronic ulcerative colitis. *British Medical Journal*, **1**, 293–294.

CALENOFF, L. (1970) Rare ileocaecal lesions. *American Journal of Roentgenology*, **110**, 343–351.

CREMIN, B. J. (1971) Radiological assessment of anorectal anomalies. *Clinical Radiology*, **22**, 239–250.

DODDS, W. J. (1976) Clinical and roentgen features of the intestinal polyposis syndromes. *Gastrointestinal Radiology*, **1**, 127.

EDLING, N. P. G. & EKLOF, O. (1963) The retrorectal soft tissue space in ulcerative colitis. A roentgen diagnostic study. *Radiology*, **80**, 949.

FERRUCCI, J. T. *et al.* (1976) Double tracking in the sigmoid colon. *Radiology*, **120(2)**, 307–312.

FLEISCHNER, F. G., MING, S. C. & HENKEN, E. M. (1964) Revised concepts on diverticular disease of the colon 1. Diverticulosis: emphasis on tissue derangement and its relation to the irritable colon syndrome. *Radiology*, **83**, 859–872.

FRASER, G. M. & FINDLAY, J. M. (1976) The double contrast enema in ulcerative and Crohn's colitis. *Clinical Radiology*, **27**, 103–112.

GOHEL, V. K., KRESSEL, H. Y. & LAUFER, I. (1978) Double contrast artifacts. *Gastrointestinal Radiology*, **3(2)**, 1939–46.

JOFFE, N. (1977) Localised giant pseudopolyposis secondary to ulcerative or granulomatous colitis. *Clinical Radiology*, **28**, 609–616.

LANE, N. & FERROGLIO, C. M. (1976) Observations on the adenoma as a precursor to ordinary large bowel carcinoma. *Gastrointestinal Radiology*, **1**, 111.

LAUFER, I., MULLENS, J. E. & HAMILTON, J. (1976) Correlation of endoscopy and double contrast radiography in the early stages of ulcerative and granulomatous colitis. *Radiology*, **118**, 1–5.

LENNARD-JONES, J. E., LOCKHART MUMMERY, H. E. & MORSON, B. C. (1968) Clinical and pathological differentiation of Crohn's disease and proctocolitis. *Gastroenterology*, **54**, 1162–1170.

LAWSON, J. P., MYERSON, P. J. & MYERSON, D. A. (1976) Colonic lymphangioma. *Gastrointestinal Radiology*, **1**, 85.

MCNAIR, M. & TRAPNELL, D. H. (1971) Calcification in lymph node metastases from adenocarcinoma of the colon. *British Journal of Radiology*, **44**, 468–471.

MEYERS. M. A., ALONSO, D. R. & BAER, J. W. (1976) Pathogenesis of massively bleeding colonic diverticulosis: new observations. *American Journal of Roentgenology*, **127**, 901–908.

MORSON, B. C. (1963) The muscle abnormality in diverticular disease of the sigmoid colon. *British Journal of Radiology*, **36**, 385–392.

MORSON, B. C. (1974) The polyps-cancer sequence in the large bowel. *Proceedings of the Royal Society of Medicine*, **67**, 451–457.

NORLAND, C. G. & KISNER, J. (1969) Ulcerative colitis. *Medicine*, **48**, 229.

O'CONNELL, D. J. & THOMPSON, A. J. (1978) Lymphoma of colon—the spectrum of radiolchanges. *Gastrointestinal Radiology*, **2(4)**, 377–387.

PARKS, T. G., CONNELL, A. M. & GOUGH, A. W. (1968) Volvulus of the sigmoid colon. *British Medical Journal*, **1**, 264–265.

Seminars in Roentgenology (1976) **2**, 1–137. Seven articles dealing with colonic lesions.

SIMPKINS, K. C. (1977) Aphthoid ulcers in Crohn's disease. *Clinical Radiology*, **28**, 601–608.

SIMPKINS, K. C. & STEVENSON, G. W. (1972) The modified Malmo double contrast barium enema in colitis. An assessment of its accuracy in reflecting sigmoidoscopic findings. *British Journal of Radiology*, **45**, 486–492.

TEPLICK, S. K. & STARK, P. *et al.* (1978) The retrorectal space. *Clinical Radiology*, **29**, 177.

THOMAS, B. M. (1979) The 'instant enema' in inflammatory disease of the colon. *Clinical Radiology*, **30**, 165–173.

WILLIAMS, I. (1963) Changing emphasis in diverticular disease of the colon. *British Journal of Radiology*, **36**, 393–406.

WILLIAMS, I. (1965) Innominate grooves in the surface of mucosa. *Radiology*, **84**, 877.

WYATT, A. P. (1972) Pneumatosis cystoides intestinalis. *Proceedings of the Royal Society of Medicine*, **65**, 780–782.

CHAPTER 36

THE ACUTE ABDOMEN

Radiography is of such great value in the diagnosis and management of the acute abdomen that it has become an integral part of the surgical management of that condition.

Plain radiography of the abdomen, a relatively simple procedure but one demanding meticulous technique, can provide invaluable information in trauma, infections, perforations, obstructions and other pathological states producing acute abdominal conditions.

Radiography of the acute abdomen should consist of at least three films. One film should be taken with the patient *supine*; using a vertical X-ray beam—and including the diaphragms and inguinal regions. A second should be taken with a horizontal X-ray beam to demonstrate fluid levels. For this the patient may be *upright* or, if too ill to sit up or stand, in a *lateral decubitus* position preferably right side up. This position has the added advantage in pancreatitis that gas and fluid may accumulate in the second part of the duodenum due to a local ileus. In addition, a chest film should be taken to help exclude pulmonary lesions such as pneumonia or pulmonary infarction which may mimic an acute abdomen. This film will show free gas below the domes of the diaphragm in cases of perforation.

If a rupture or dissection of the aorta is suspected, a conventional left lateral film will enable calcification in the aortic or aneurysmal wall to be more readily seen clear of the lumbar spine. The supine film may show the retroperitoneal extravasation of blood by the increased density of the psoas shadow and obliteration of the muscle markings.

TRAUMA

Closed abdominal trauma is becoming commoner because of the increasing number of motor vehicle accidents. The trauma may occur from impact injury (e.g. from the steering wheel) or may occur from damage from the seat belt. Both solid and hollow intra-abdominal viscera may be injured. Hollow viscus injuries are particularly liable to follow seat belt injuries.

The duodenum from its fixed position is most frequently injured and the injury may consist of rupture with intraperitoneal or retroperitoneal perforation, or an intramural haematoma. Traumatic perforation of the duodenum, if intraperitoneal, results in free gas which can be demonstrated beneath the diaphragm in the erect position. In the supine position the accumulation of gas

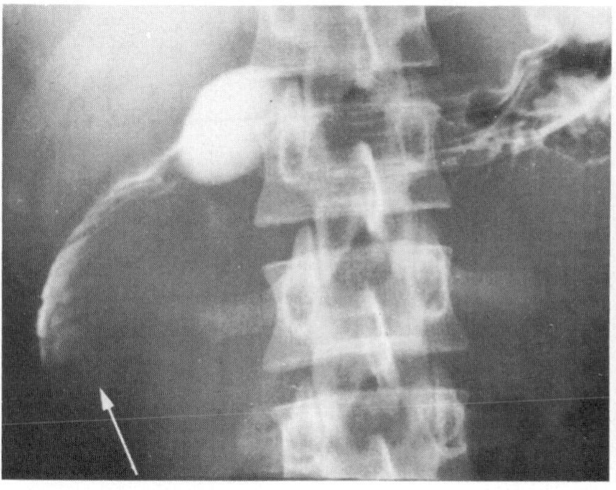

Fig. 36.1 Barium meal showing coiled spring appearance with an intramural haematoma. Arrow points to the obstruction in the duodenum and the stretched mucosal pattern.

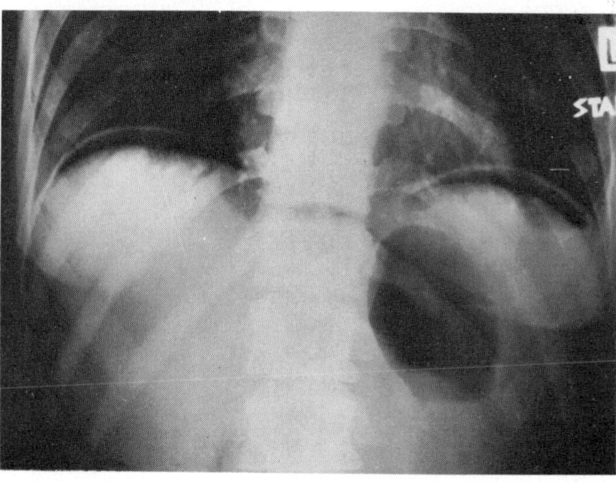

Fig. 36.2 Free gas beneath both diaphragms following a perforated peptic ulcer.

may be seen along the falciform ligament or collected anteriorly as a sharp circular area of increased radiolucency (the 'Dome Sign').

Intramural haematoma, if large, may result in complete obstruction of the duodenum (Fig. 36.1). In milder cases, the spread of blood between the thickened mucosal coils gives rise to a circular shadowing ('stacked coin' appearance) on contrast examination. It must be remembered that intramural haematoma may occur after relatively mild trauma in patients who are on anticoagulant therapy. Spontaneous resolution of the haematoma usually occurs in a few weeks.

Other injuries to the bowel may result in rupture of the small bowel or colon (from malpositioned seat belts) but in neither case is the demonstration of free gas a common sign. Contrast barium meal studies may show thickening of the wall or 'thumbprint' defects indicating intramural oedema or haemorrhage.

The colon is particularly liable to be injured at its fixed points, e.g. descending colon and sigmoid, and extensive damage to the colon and sigmoid mesentery may occur with relatively few radiological signs. Ischaemic changes in the colon mucosa may follow injury and barium enema examination will show the mucosal swelling, 'thumbprint' defects and nodularity. The condition usually resolves but may progress to perforation when localized retroperitoneal gas may be seen. A local stricture of the colon may occur as a late sequel.

Rupture of the diaphragm usually affects the left leaf and the presence of bowel (large or small) or a solid viscus, e.g. spleen, in the thoracic cage may give a ready diagnosis. More important is the rupture when the bowel herniates some time after the injury; this almost invariably results in strangulation of the herniated bowel.

Perisplenic, perirenal and extrahepatic haematoma occurring after surgery to the spleen, kidney and liver can be confirmed by ultrasound or C.A.T. Detailed assessment may require angiography of the affected organ.

PERFORATIONS

The most frequent cause of perforation of the gastro-intestinal tract is *peptic ulceration* of the duodenum or stomach, less frequently inflammatory disease such as *diverticulitis* and more rarely still *malignant growths*. Free gas in the peritoneal cavity is constantly present after *laparotomy* but usually disappears in 5 to 10 days unless some complicating factor such as peritonitis occurs. Rarer causes of free gas are *intestinal pneumatosis*, *necrotising enteritis* or *ischaemic disease* of the bowel with perforation. In these conditions there is usually evidence of intramural gas in the bowel wall.

Free gas can be demonstrated in the erect position beneath the diaphragm (Fig. 36.2) but smaller quantities can be recognized between the liver and lateral abdominal wall in the left lateral decubitus film. As little as 10 ml of free gas in the abdomen can be recognized by this method and approximately 75 per cent of perforated ulcers of more than 3 hours duration show free gas.

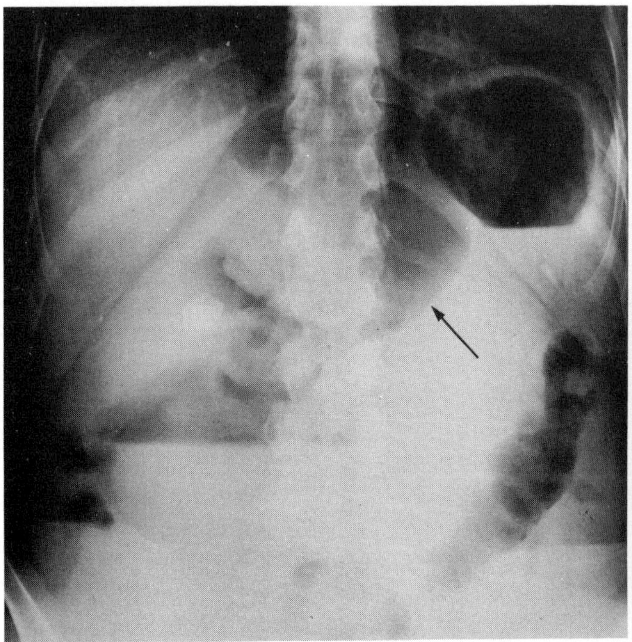

A

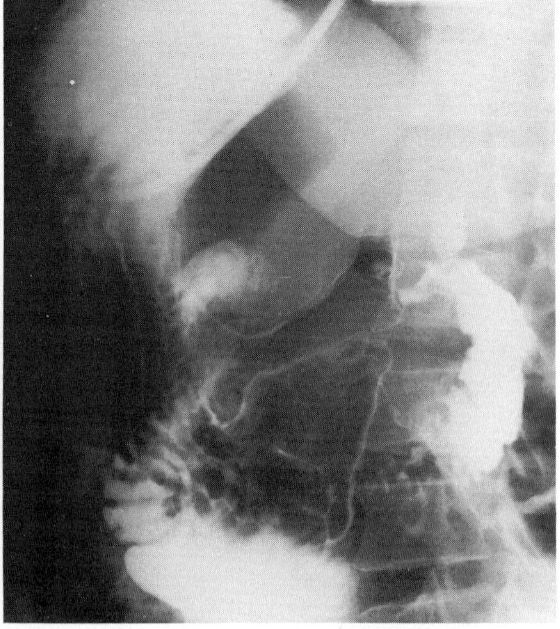

B

Fig. 36.3A Perforation into lesser sac. Erect film showing fluid levels in stomach and small bowel associated with a collection of gas in the midline (*arrow*). B Gastrografin examination revealing the gas lying behind the stomach, in the right lateral position.

Free gas in the lesser sac of the peritoneal cavity may be difficult to distinguish from the gas bubble normally present in the stomach (Fig. 36.3A and B). In the supine film the gas may be seen localized to the left hypochondrium.

Mention has already been made of the signs of free peritoneal gas in the supine film but gas on either side of the bowel wall, outlining the bowel wall, implies perforation associated with obstruction.

In those cases of perforation (approximately 20 per cent) where no radiological signs can be seen on the plain film, administration of water soluble contrast medium (Gastrografin or oral hypaque) may demonstrate the perforation. Fifty ml of water-soluble contrast medium diluted with 50 per cent water are swallowed or passed through a nasogastric tube and the patient is kept in the right lateral decubitus position for at least 15 minutes. Prone films at this time will usually demonstrate the leak of contrast medium into the peritoneal cavity (Fig. 36.4). Failure to demonstrate a perforation by this method is usually due to failure of the contrast medium to reach the perforation. This occurs when the patient has been kept in the supine position and the gastrografin remains in the fundus of the stomach. In some perforations due to the sealing of the perforation no escape of contrast medium occurs, in others the leak may be so small as to be unrecognizable. Delayed films (3 hours) may however show contrast medium in the bladder due to absorption of contrast medium from the peritoneum which is taken as indicating perforation of the bowel.

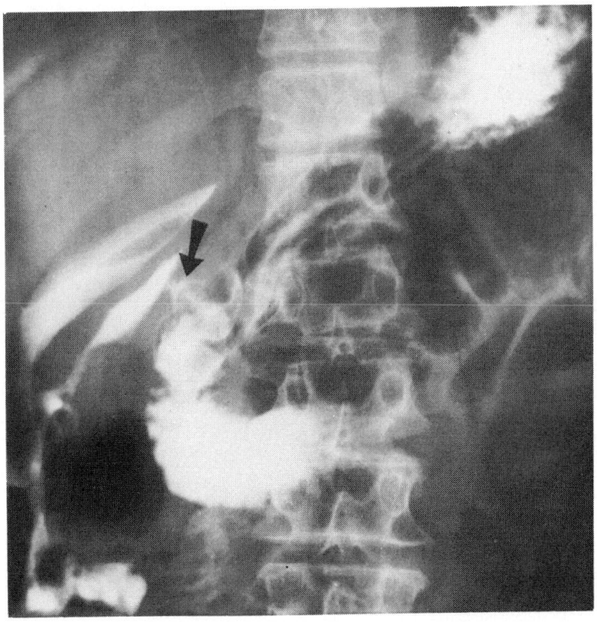

Fig. 36.4 Gastrografin demonstration of perforated ulcer (*arrow*). The site of perforation and the spread of contrast into the peritoneal space can be seen.

The use of water-soluble contrast medium in infants must be carefully controlled as this is a hypertonic solution and relatively small quantities may result in hypovolaemia in a young infant.

Rarely the presence of gas bubbles in the wall of the bowel (pneumatosis intestinalis) may indicate the source of the pneumoperitoneum. The appearance of linear streaks of gas, however, usually indicates the presence of intramural gas of a more sinister type and usually indicates necrosis of the bowel wall in necrotising enteritis or ischaemic lesions of the bowel.

Perforations due to inflammatory disease usually follow diverticulitis of the colon and in such cases the gas is usually paracolic or localised in the adjoining retroperitoneal tissues. Free peritoneal gas is an extremely unusual finding in perforated diverticulitis. Spread of gas associated with abscess formation after a perforated diverticulitis may present in unusual sites, for example in the groin or loin, and it is associated with an abscess tracking along tissue planes (Fig. 36.5).

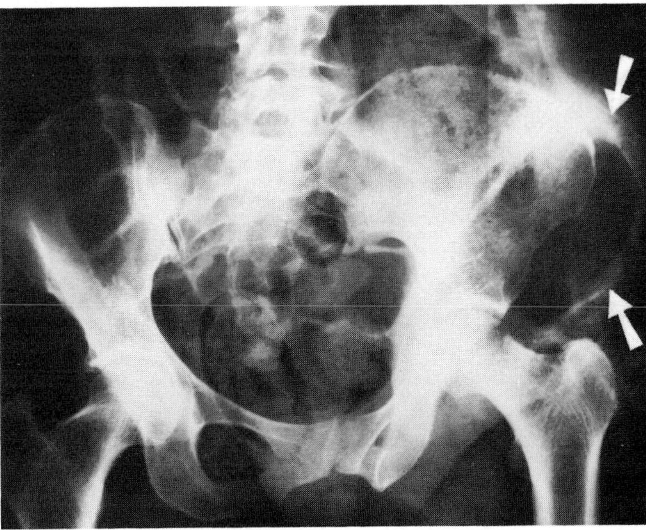

Fig. 36.5 Perforated diverticulitis with gas-filled abscess (*arrows*) extending into inguinal region.

Perforations of the bowel from specific inflammatory diseases such as typhoid or paratyphoid seldom present as radiological problems.

Perforation following malignant growths usually occurs in the elderly patient and generally follows carcinoma of the colon. The perforation may occur at the site of growth or proximally to the growth (usually the caecum) where the perforation may occur in an ischaemic or stercoral ulcer. The radiological signs of perforation in such instances are usually complicated by the signs of obstruction and the presence of gas in both sides of the bowel wall is a valuable diagnostic sign.

It is important to remember that in the elderly,

perforation of the colon may be associated with relatively few constitutional signs and the radiological signs may be all important in the early recognition of intestinal perforation.

In ulcerative colitis, especially when there is toxic dilatation, perforation of the colon may occur. Usually the dilated transverse colon is completely aperistaltic and causes a functional obstruction giving rise to gross dilatation of the caecum. Perforation usually occurs in the transverse colon or caecum. Occasionally gas may be seen in the necrotic wall of the gut before perforation occurs.

INFECTIONS

Acute appendicitis

The commonest infective condition which presents as an acute abdomen is acute appendicitis. Radiological examination of the abdomen is needed only where there is doubt about the diagnosis and renal or ureteric calculi need to be excluded.

There are no specific radiological signs associated with acute appendicitis but when the process is established and a degree of local peritonitis is present a distension of one or more coils of ileum indicating a local ileus may be seen. A laminated oval calcification in the right lower abdomen should raise the possibility of an appendicolith.

Cholecystitis

In acute cholecystitis plain film examination of the abdomen shows opaque gall stones in less than 10 per cent of cases. This is partly due to the relatively small number of stones which contain sufficient calcium to be seen on plain films and partly to the obscuring gas and faecal shadows in the hepatic flexure which are usually present.

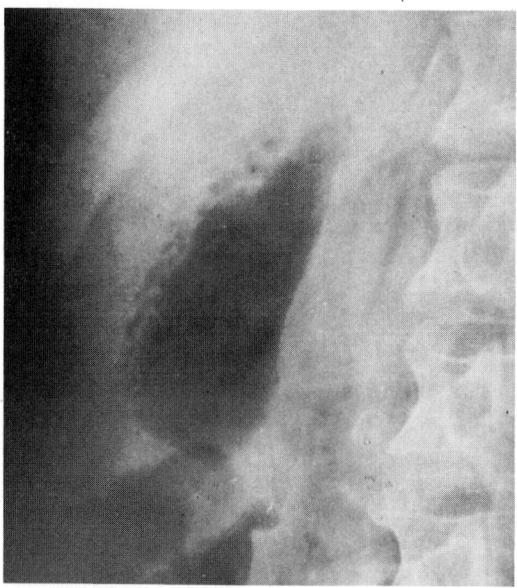

Fig. 36.6 Emphysematous cholecystitis. The gas-filled gall bladder and lace-like chain of gas bubbles around the gall bladder indicate gas in the wall of the gall bladder.

Distension of a coil of small bowel and hepatic flexure usually implies a degree of ileus of these structures associated with spread of inflammatory change outside the gall bladder or the formation of a localized abscess.

Rapid intravenous injection of 40 ml of hypaque or similar preparation and tomography of the right hypochondrium may allow the wall of the gall bladder to be seen especially when thickened and inflamed as in acute cholecystitis.

Rarely gas forming organisms may fill the gall bladder with gas and the outline of the gas filled gall bladder can be seen (Fig. 36.6).

In acute cholecystitis differentiation of the acutely obstructed from the non-obstructed gall bladder is important as the management of the former is essentially surgical, whilst the latter can be dealt with conservatively by medical measures. An intravenous cholangiogram may help by showing filling of the gall bladder unless the cystic duct is obstructed or there is extensive liver damage present. In the former the extrahepatic ducts will be seen to be normal and differentiation of both conditions is possible.

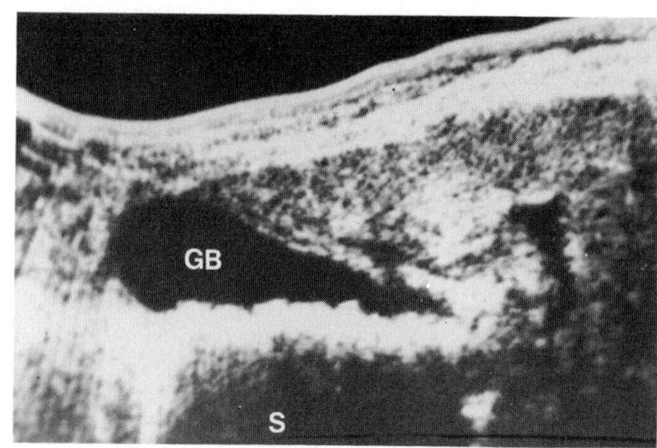

Fig. 36.7 Longitudinal ultrasound scan showing distended gall bladder (GB) as a transonic zone and the acoustic shadowing (S) noted by the absence of echoes behind the gall bladder caused by the layer of stones in the gall bladder.

If cholecystitis is associated with jaundice and an elevated serum bilirubin of 2 to 3 mg per 100 ml or more, the intravenous cholangiogram usually fails to visualize the extrahepatic ducts and the examination is worthless. Also, the administration of 30 ml of biligram to a jaundiced patient adds an unnecessary burden to a damaged liver and may result in acute liver necrosis. *Ultrasound* examination of the abdomen in suspected cases of acute cholecystitis has rendered intravenous

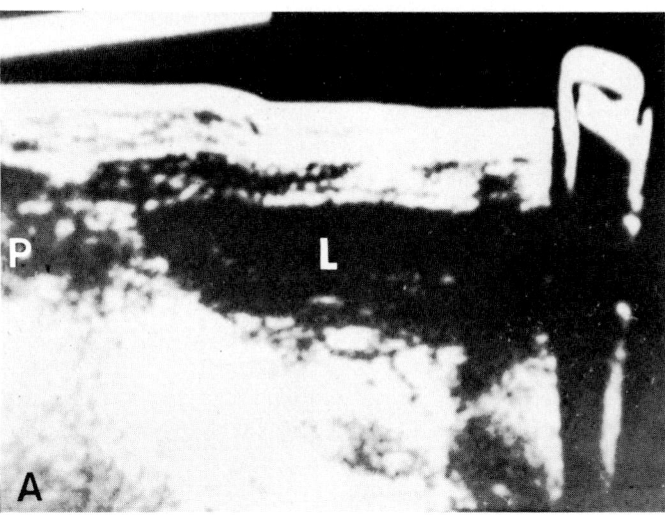

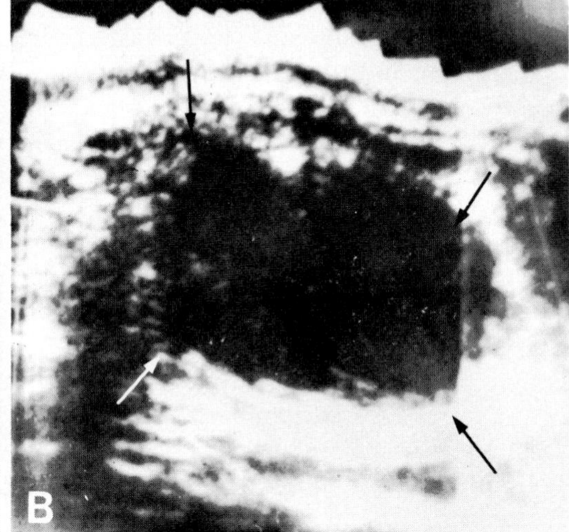

Fig. 36.8 Ultrasound of pancreatic cyst—longitudinal scan. L=liver. C=cyst. P=portal vein. S=solid component. (*Courtesy of Dr. G. B. Young.*)

cholangiography largely unnecessary as both the distended gall bladder and any stones that may be present are readily visible (Fig. 36.7).

Acute pancreatitis

Acute pancreatitis seldom results from acute bacterial invasion; reflux of bile along the pancreatic duct or ischaemic changes are more probable aetiological causes. The severity of the disease varies from the milder types associated with mumps, to the severe haemorrhagic type associated with marked shock and collapse. The diagnosis is usually established by urine amylase estimation.

The radiological signs of acute pancreatitis are:

(*a*) A 'gasless abdomen'. In the early stages of pancreatitis absence of the normal bowel gas from the abdomen may be seen.

(*b*) Inflammatory changes in the head of the pancreas may cause a local ileus in the duodenum. Thickening of the mucosal folds particularly along the medial wall of a gas distended duodenum is seen in films taken in the left lateral decubitus position.

(*c*) Inflammatory change in the body and tail of the pancreas may involve a coil of the upper jejunum and a single or several small fluid levels may develop in these coils.

(*d*) Absence of gas from the mid part of the transverse colon (Stewart's Sign) is unreliable as a sign of pancreatitis.

(*e*) The development of an abscess or pseudo-cyst in the lesser sac may occur later in the disease. This can be demonstrated by a fluid level in the sac (in abscess) but far more readily by ultrasound examination which shows a transonic mass in the lesser sac. The same technique can be used to watch the progress of the cyst and the swelling of the pancreas in the acute stage and as the disease progresses (Fig. 36.8) or resolves.

Contrast examination of the upper gastrointestinal tract allows the mucosal changes consisting of thickened folds and saw-tooth edges of the affected loops to be seen (Fig. 36.9). The C curve of the duodenum may also be expanded by the swollen head of pancreas. When the body and tail of the pancreas are involved similar changes may be seen in the duodenojejunal flexure.

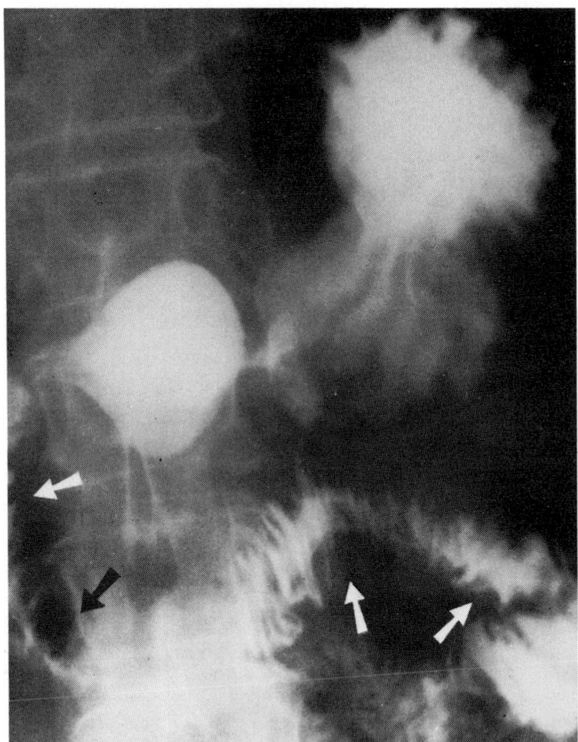

Fig. 36.9 Pancreatitis. Supine film after the administration of Gastrografin showing the distortion of the second part of the duodenum and of the duodeno-jejunal flexure by the inflammatory process in the pancreas involving these two portions of small bowel (*arrows*).

Calcification in the pancreas may be seen after attacks of recurrent pancreatitis and is a valuable sign in diagnosis. The calcification is often most clearly seen on the lateral view.

Pelvic inflammatory states. *Salpingitis* and *tubo-ovarian abscess* may present as an acute abdomen. Involvement of the ileum which normally lies in the pelvis gives rise to a local ileus which appears as a few slightly distended loops with a few small fluid levels present.

Involvement of the pelvic colon by a tubo-ovarian abscess may be recognized as an inflammatory granulomatous lesion during a barium enema examination.

Ultrasound examination may be helpful in cases of tubo-ovarian cysts or abscesses but frequently the presence of gas in the bowel detracts from the value of ultrasound examination.

Tubal pregnancy or *endometriosis* with spillage of blood into the pelvis may give rise to appearances not dissimilar to salpingitis from involvement of the ileum in the spilled, clotted blood. Ultrasound examination may prove extremely useful in both these conditions.

INTESTINAL OBSTRUCTION

Mechanical obstruction of the small or large bowel due to whatever cause gives rise to a recognizable pattern on the plain films. The accumulation of gas and fluid within the bowel lumen above the site of obstruction can be readily seen in that fluid levels occur when the patient is examined in the erect position. Fluid levels in the small bowel tend to be shorter than those occurring in the obstructed colon and are central in position as opposed to those in the colon which are usually longer and occur in the flanks.

The gas filled loops of bowel give characteristic appearances depending on the portion of the bowel involved. Thus the jejunum shows the circular lines of the valvulae conniventes whilst the lower ileum shows the smooth pattern of ileal mucosa. The colon on the other hand shows characteristic haustration. Consideration of these patterns and of the distribution of fluid levels will enable a reasonable approximation of the site of obstruction to be made.

However, difficulties may arise when the obstructing lesion is in the colon; the appearances will vary depending on whether or not the ileo-caecal valve is competent. When the valve is shut, the distension and fluid levels are confined, at least during the early stages, to the colon. The caecum may become grossly distended and may perforate. If the valve is incompetent, the colon may be slightly distended and the main fluid levels occur in the small bowel. The appearance is then similar to that seen in low small bowel obstruction.

The demonstration of fluid levels does not necessarily imply mechanical obstruction as such levels may be seen in metabolic or electrolyte disturbances which cause an accumulation of gas and fluid in the bowel. Uraemia and

Fig. 36.10 A 'False' fluid levels associated with a generalized infection—abortus fever. B 'False' fluid levels associated with metabolic disturbance.

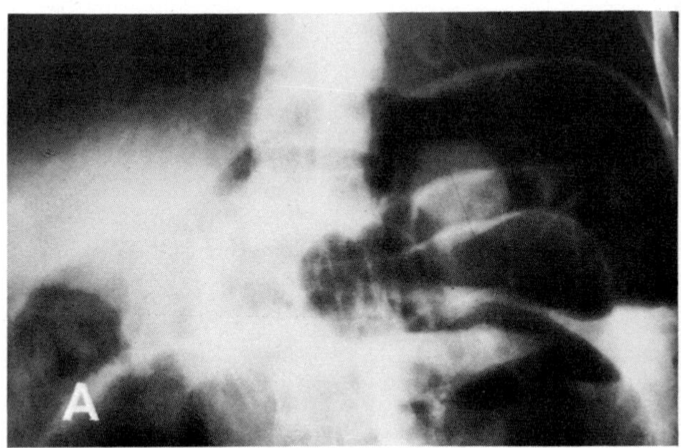

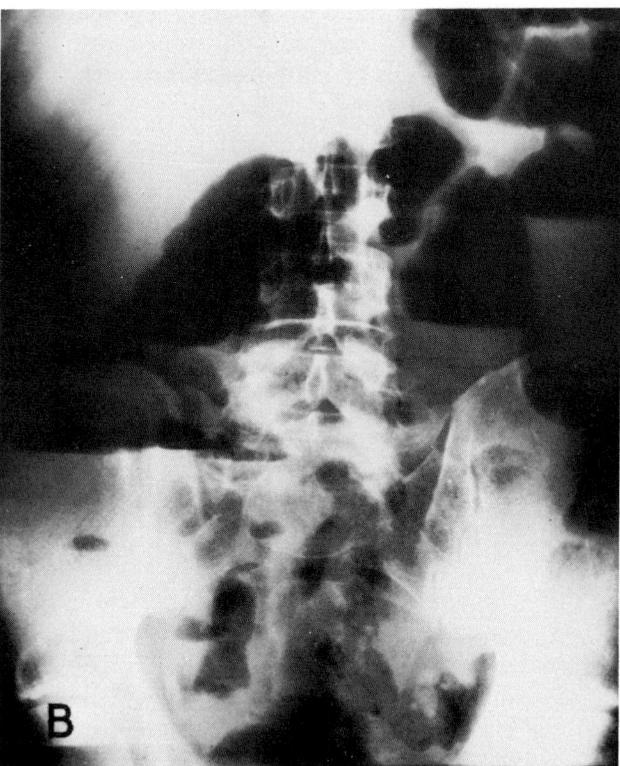

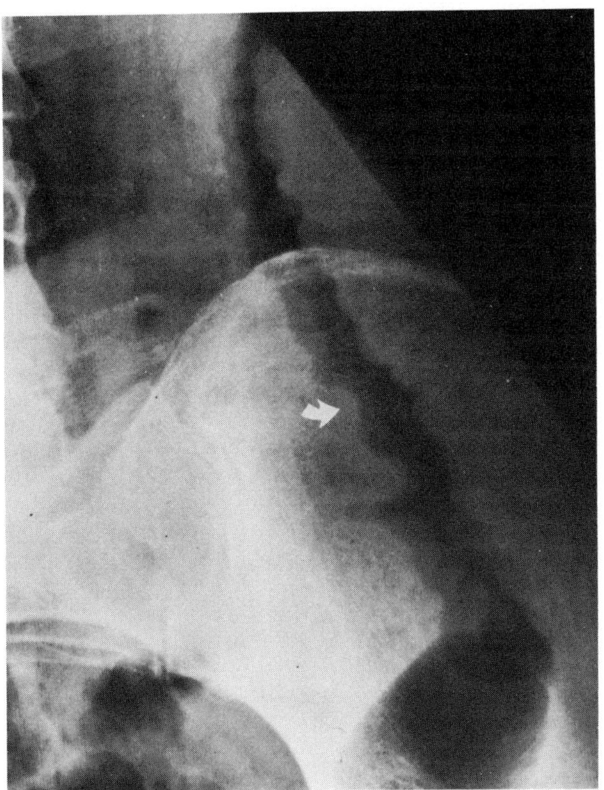

Fig. 36.21 Ischaemic changes in the colon. Plain film showing the 'thumbprinting' of the wall caused by oedema and submural haemorrhages (*arrow*).

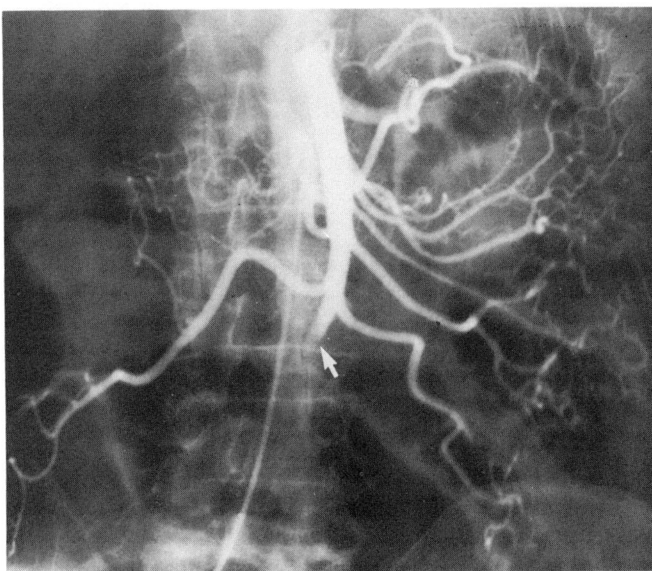

Fig. 36.22 Selective arteriogram of superior mesenteric artery in the case of mesenteric occlusion. The main stem artery is filled and the site of occlusion clearly marked by an arrow. The distended and thickened walls of gas-filled small bowel can be seen in the lower part of the illustration. (*Courtesy of Dr. T. A. S. Buist.*)

Leakage or dissection of the abdominal aneurysm is almost invariably associated with abdominal meteorism and this frequently obscures the soft tissue mass caused by the haematoma obscuring the muscle lines on the posterior abdominal wall.

As the atherosclerotic process frequently contains calcific plaques, the displacement of these plaques in their relationship to the soft tissue shadows frequently indicates an aneurysm or dissection. The lateral view is particularly helpful in demonstrating calcified plaques in the aneurysmal wall.

Positive confirmation of a leaking or dissecting aneurysm of the aorta can be obtained by retrograde femoral arteriography when the aneurysmal sac or the double lumen of the dissected aorta may be seen. Ultrasound examination is a non-invasive method of detecting and estimating the size of abdominal aneurysms but if surgical treatment is contemplated abdominal aortography is usually required. In more severe ruptures, however, surgical interference may be urgently required leaving no time for aortography to be carried out.

CONTRAST STUDIES

The administration of a contrast medium to outline a suspected organ in the acute abdomen can be undertaken in most cases if the clinical condition allows. Thus intravenous cholangiography to outline the gall bladder or pyelography for the demonstration of a suspected renal or ureteric stone can be used with care. Even if a ureteric stone is not immediately demonstrated, delayed films up to 24 hours will usually reveal the actual site of an obstructing calculus. The initial films usually shows a dense nephrographic effect and a delay in the appearance of the pyelogram is usually sufficiently suspicious for delayed films to be taken without clinical apprehension of overlooking some other pathology. Tomography after intravenous injection of contrast medium may visualize the thickened and oedematous wall of the gall bladder in acute cholecystitis. Ultrasound however is now the preferable investigation if this condition is suspected.

Water-soluble media (Gastrografin, Hypaque, etc.) can be safely administered by mouth for the demonstration of leaks and perforations from the upper gastrointestinal tract and may be particularly valuable in assessing the post-operative integrity of a bowel anastomosis.

The appreciation that many of the ischaemic lesions of the bowel are often subacute in nature has allowed the use of barium sulphate mixtures to outline the bowel loops and demonstrate the thickened and oedematous mucosa and intramural haemorrhages.

Probably the most controversial aspect of the investigation of the acute abdomen is the place of the contrast examination in **haematemesis** and **melaena**. The wider

Table 36.2

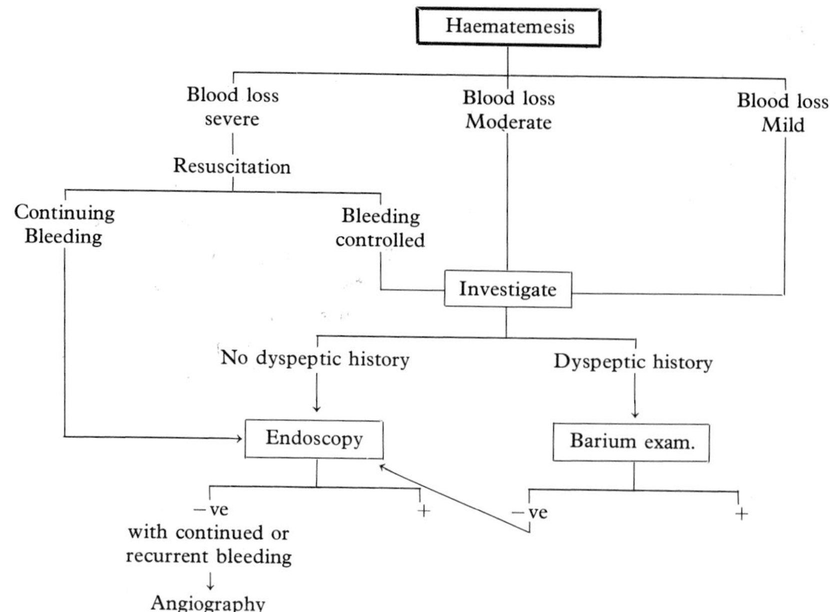

use of fibre optic endoscopes has resulted in an opinion being expressed that the barium meal or gastrografin meal has no place in the investigation of this condition. Whilst there can be no doubt that a lesion demonstrated at radiological examination is not necessarily the 'bleeder' as endoscopy has often demonstrated, it is equally valid that lesions have been overlooked by endoscopy and the success rate of the endoscopy diagnosis varies with the experience of the observer. Table 36.2 illustrates a suggested routine for investigation of haematemesis.

There is no doubt that radiological examination in

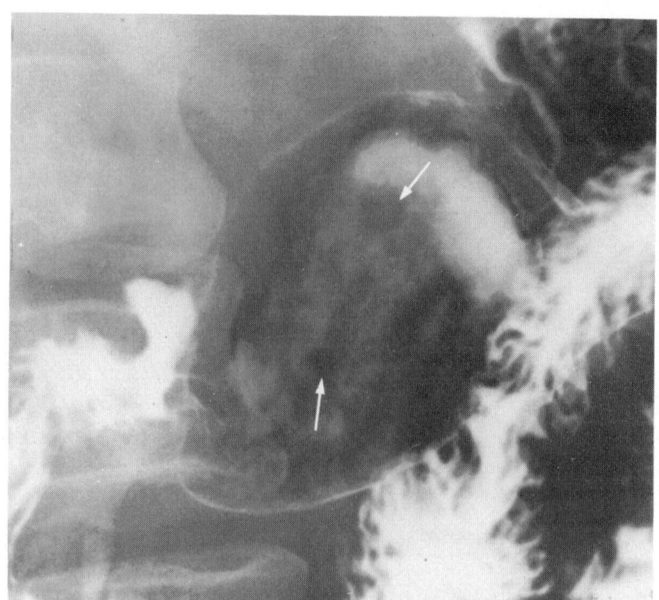

Fig. 36.23 Acute erosions. Double contrast view of pyloric antrum showing shallow erosions with areas of oedema around the crater (*arrows*).

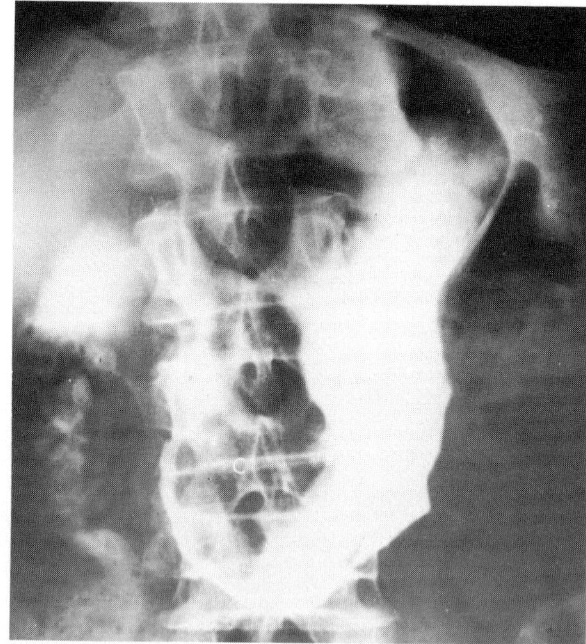

Fig. 36.24 Blood clot in stomach producing a filling defect. C = clot.

haematemesis will demonstrate the chronic type of gastric or duodenal ulcer having the classical radiological features. However, attention should also be devoted to the superficial mucosal erosion or ulcer which may equally produce brisk haemorrhages. Mucosal studies in such cases will reveal 'ring', 'arc' or other signs indicating superficial erosions (Fig. 36.23). Some authors have claimed that a barium smudge around the ulcer indicates actual bleeding; barium being removed from one edge of the ulcer by the steady ooze of blood.

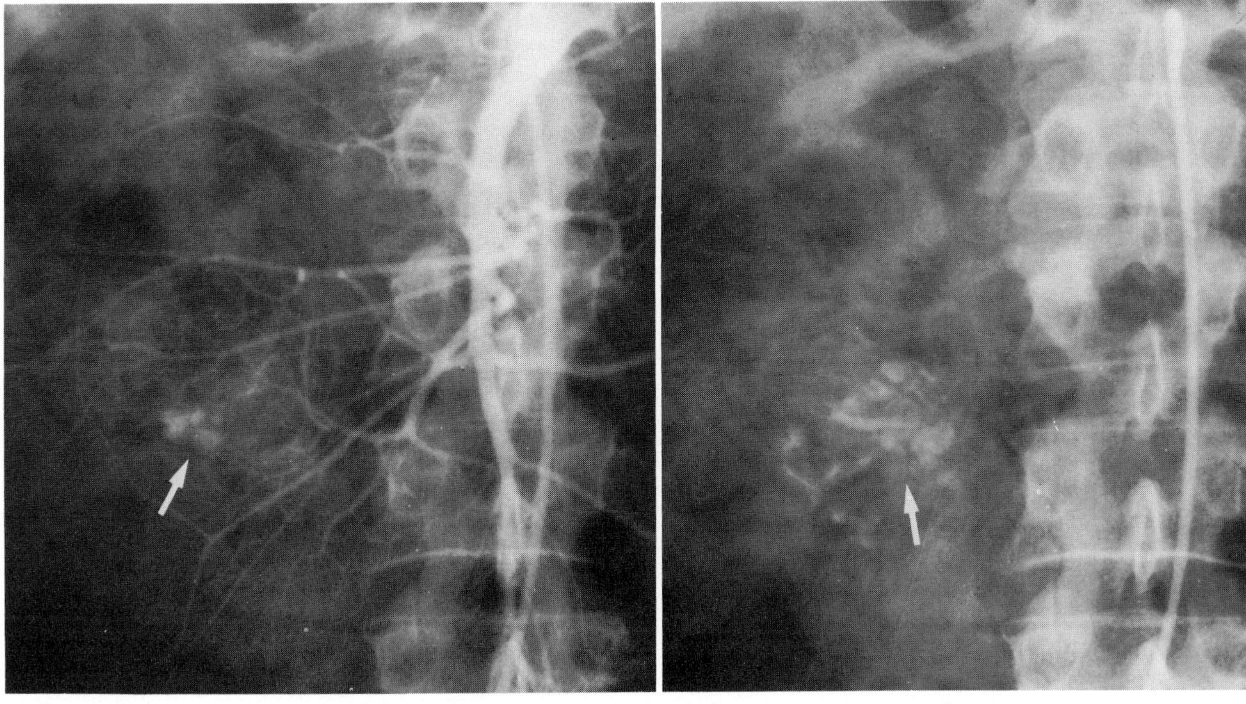

A B

Fig. 36.25A Angiodysplasia of caecum. Selective arteriography of the superior mesenteric artery. Arterial phase showing escape of contrast into the caecum in the case of unexplained recurrent intestinal bleeding.

B Later phase of Fig. 36.25A case. The staining of the caecum can be clearly seen. (*Courtesy of Dr. T. A. S. Buist.*)

Clot formation in the stomach may obscure the source of bleeding (Fig. 36.24) but this may be equally true when endoscopy is used.

In acute or subacute bleeding suspected to arise from the upper gastrointestinal tract **selective arteriography** of the vessels may show extravasation of contrast into the viscus (Fig. 36.25) and indicate the source of bleeding. For this investigation to be successful the patient must be bleeding briskly at the time of the examination (e.g. 2–4 ml per mm). The method may also be used to control bleeding from a peptic ulcer by the introduction of vasoconstrictor drugs through the catheter (see Ch. 29).

Patients with recurrent gastrointestinal bleeding in whom no source is found by routine barium, Gastrografin, or endoscopic examination may require selective mesenteric angiography in order to demonstrate a possible lesion in the small bowel or right side of the colon. A *tumour* may be revealed or there may be *angiodysplasia*. This condition usually affects the caecum or ascending colon and consists of a minute network of abnormal vessels in the mucosa. These vessels may be shown, together with early filling of draining veins and contrast in the lumen of the gut, if the patient is bleeding during the examination (Fig. 36.25). These lesions are usually too small and soft to be found at laparotomy so that resection is performed on the radiological evidence alone.

Selective arteriography also has considerable value in demonstrating the extent of liver, renal and splenic damage in cases of closed abdominal trauma. Rarely, hepatic angiography may demonstrate a cause for haemobilia.

POST-OPERATIVE ADBOMEN

The development of acute abdominal symptoms post-operatively provides one of the most complex diagnostic problems for the radiologist.

Normally free air is present in the abdominal cavity after laparotomy and is gradually absorbed over a period of 7 to 10 days. Persistence of gas beyond this period usually implies some complication such as peritoneal infection or post-operative fistula. The major abdominal complications are:

(*a*) Post-operative obstruction (ileus)
(*b*) Inflammatory changes

A degree of meteorism also invariably occurs after operation but the gas is mainly collected in the colon although some degree of small bowel distension may be present.

Fluid levels in the small bowel usually imply a degree of post-operative ileus and the appearances are similar to those of an incomplete small bowel mechanical obstruction.

Infective changes may be due to peritoneal soiling at operation or due to a post-operative leak from a surgical anastomosis. They may be diffused or localized and account for many cases of post-operative ileus. Localized infective changes are particularly liable to occur in the subphrenic spaces.

SUBPHRENIC ABSCESS

Radiological investigation plays an important part in the diagnosis of subphrenic abscess. In the early stages of infection of the subphrenic spaces before abscess formation has occurred, limitation of movement of the diaphragm (especially on forced inspiration) may be seen on fluoroscopy.

Later as abscess formation occurs and the diaphragm may form part of the abscess wall it becomes elevated and fixed. Pleural reaction over the diaphragm occurs, the costophrenic angle is obliterated and the lower part of the lower lobe obscured by fluid.

When gas occurs in the subphrenic abscess a fluid level is visible in the erect position and careful fluoroscopy will determine whether the anterior or posterior compartment of the subphrenic space is involved.

Fluid levels in subphrenic abscesses have to be differentiated from other causes of fluid level below the diaphragm. Interposition of the colon on the right side may cause some confusion with a subphrenic abscess, but the presence of colonic haustral markings enables interposition of the colon to be recognized.

Free air under the diaphragm from a perforated bowel has also to be differentiated from a subphrenic abscess and perforation into the lesser sac may cause difficulties in differential diagnosis in relation to left-sided subphrenic abscess.

Subphrenic abscess when associated with an effusion into the pleural cavity obscures the outline of the diaphragm and makes the differentiation of infrapulmonary effusions from subphrenic abscesses difficult. On the left side the position of the fundal gas bubble may be of help, or a barium swallow may show the position of the fundus of the stomach which is of inestimable value in differentiating the two conditions.

Ultrasound examination has greatly added to our ability to diagnose subphrenic abscesses and scans of the upper abdomen, particularly on the right side, will show the position of the liver, the diaphragm and the abscess cavity appearing as a transonic zone (see Ch. 67).

After drainage of a post-operative abscess or a fistula from an abdominal wound *sinograms* with a polythene catheter into the sinus and the introduction of water soluble contrast medium will determine the site of origin of the intestinal fistula. Fluoroscopic control of injection of contrast medium and films in the antero-posterior and lateral planes are necessary.

REFERENCES AND SUGGESTIONS FOR FURTHER READING

Bakhda, R. K. & McNair, M. M. (1977) Useful radiological signs in acute appendicitis in children. *Clinical Radiology*, **28,** 193–196.

Burrel, M., Toffler, R. & Lawrence, R. (1973) Blunt trauma of the abdomen. *Radiologic Clinics of North America*, **XI(3),** 561.

Cotton, P. B. (1973) Fibre optic endoscopy and the barium meal. Results and implications. *British Medical Journal*, **2,** 161–165.

Dahl-Frimahn, J. (1975) *Roentgen Examinations in Acute Abdominal Disease*. 3rd edition. Springfield: Thomas.

Deffeure, P. (1924) Appearance of intestinal gas in the newborn. *Annales de radiologie*, **17,** 335.

Frazer, G. M. & Frazer, I. D. (1974) Gastrografin in perforated duodenal ulcer and acute pancreatitis. *Clinical Radiology*, **25,** 397–402.

Goldman, H. & Antoniole, D. A. (1977) Barium studies in small bowel infarction, radiological pathology correlation. *Radiology*, **12(3),** 303.

Meyers, M. A., Alonso, D. R. & Baer, J. W. (1976) Pathogenesis of massively bleeding colonic diverticulosis. New observations. *American Journal of Roentgenology*, **127,** 901–908.

McCort, J. (1978) Intraperitoneal and retroperitoneal haemorrhage. *Radiology*, **391,** 14.

Osborn, D. J., Elickman, M. G., Gonja, V. & Ramsay, G. (1973) The role of angiography in abdominal non renal trauma. *Radiologic Clinics of North America*, **XI(3),** 579.

Santulli, T. V., Schullinger Jnr., Gingerware, W. C., Wigger, R. D. Jnr., Barlow, B., Black, W. A. & Berdon, W. E. (1976) Acute necrosing enteritis in infancy: a review of 64 cases. *Radiology*, **118,** 245.

Schuffler, M. D., Rohrman, C. A. & Templeton, F. (1976) Radiological manifestations of idiopathic intestinal pseudo-obstruction. *American Journal of Radiology*, **127,** 729–736.

Schwartz, S. (1973) Differential diagnosis of intestinal obstruction. *Radiology*, **109,** 753.

Young, W. S., Engelbrecht, H. E. & Stoker, A. (1978) Plain film analysis in sigmoid volvulus. *Clinical Radiology*, **29,** 553–560.

CHAPTER 37

THE BILIARY TRACT, PANCREAS, LIVER AND SPLEEN

A. BILIARY TRACT

PLAIN RADIOGRAPHY

It is essential that plain radiographs be taken before any examination of the biliary tract. Opacities in the right hypochondrium may be characteristically biliary or renal in appearance thus giving vital information at the beginning of the examination. In this respect it should be remembered that only 33 per cent of gallstones are radio-paque, whilst 90 per cent of renal stones are. A negative simple X-ray examination is therefore of little value in excluding gallstones.

The common faceted multiple gallstones are easily recognizable on the plain film as are the laminated round stones. The opacity of gallstones varies with the content of calcium salts, the uncommon calcium carbonate stones (Fig. 37.1A) being the densest and most homogeneous, while the calcified pigment stones are the faintest and most easily missed. The latter may be invisible when surrounded by contrast medium, a fact which emphasizes the diagnostic importance of the preliminary film. The pure cholesterol and pure pigment stones are, of course, invisible on plain radiographs. However, in the presence of contrast medium they will show as translucent defects within the medium. Rarely, translucent stones may contain gas in their centres which is visible on the plain X-ray (Fig. 37.2). This is the result of the presence of gas forming organisms in the stones.

Among patients with multiple stones in the gall-bladder, about 15–20 per cent will be found to have stones in the common duct at operation. From these figures it might be expected that 6 per cent of duct stones would show in the plain radiograph, but in practice the figure is much lower than this, probably 1–2 per cent. Why this should be is not understood. It follows that when the preliminary plain film of an oral cholecysto-gram shows multiple opaque gallstones in the gall-bladder region, there is much to be said for abandoning

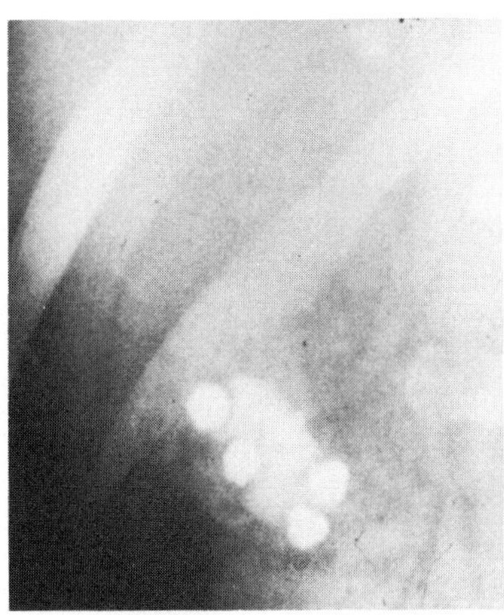
A

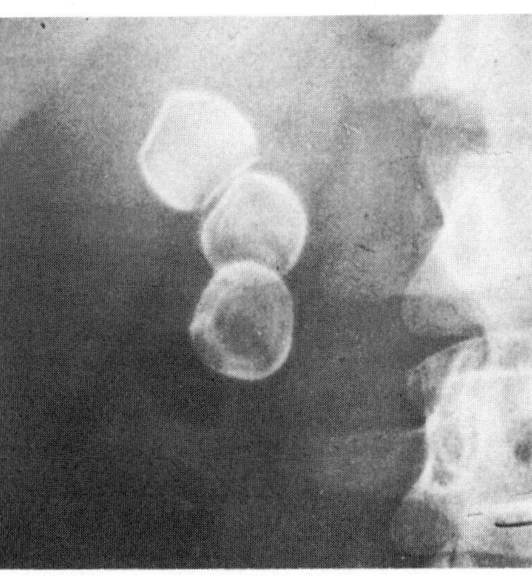
B

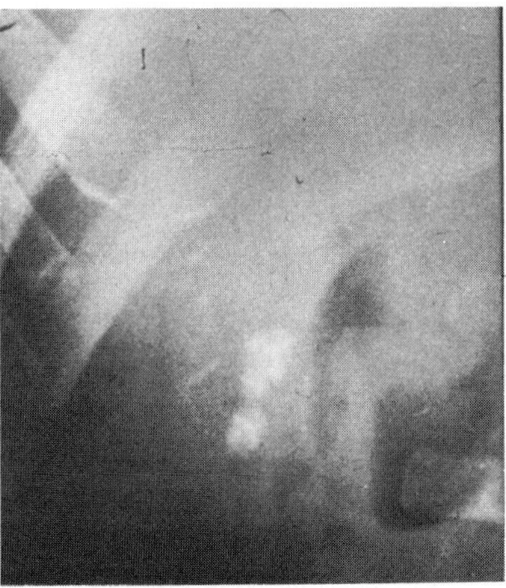
C

Fig. 37.1 A Calcium carbonate stones, 'biliary sand' ('limy bile'), as discrete mulberry-shaped stones, one of which is lying in Hartmann's pouch blocking the cystic duct (intravenous cholangiogram). B 'Mixed stones' showing lamination and facets. C Gallstones resembling calcified glands.

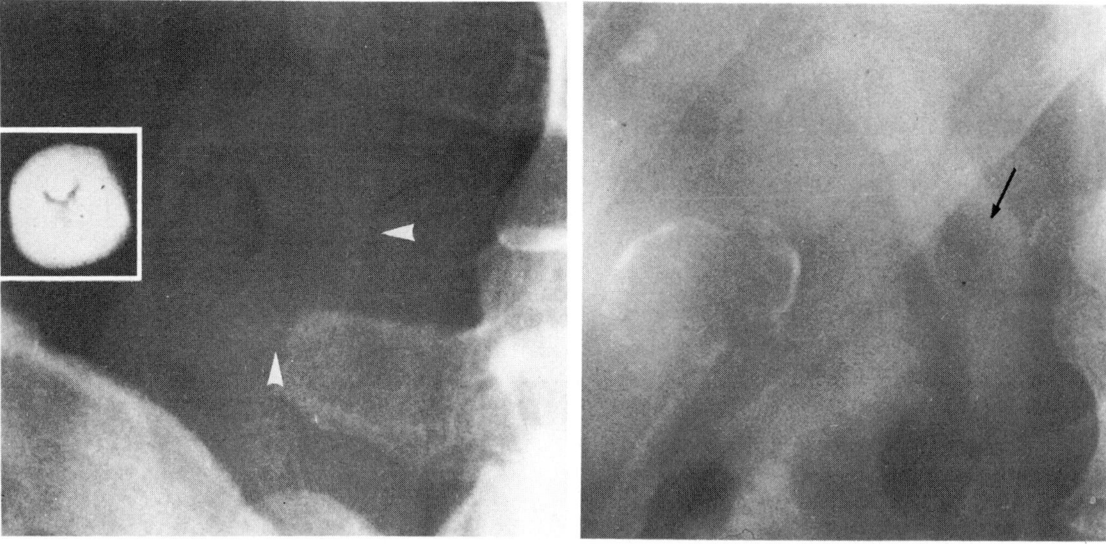

Fig. 37.2 *Fig. 37.3*

Fig. 37.2 'Mercedes Benz' stone; characteristic appearance on the plain radiograph (*arrows*) and after removal (*insert*).

Fig. 37.3 Calcified gallbladder; the common duct is dilated and contains a large stone (*arrow*).

the oral examination and proceeding to examine the common duct by intravenous cholangiography instead.

Occasionally, the appearances of gallstones may mimic renal stones or even calcified glands (Fig. 37.1C); less often, their appearances are frankly atypical. Fine calcific deposits can give rise to so called 'milk of bile' or 'biliary sludge'. This gives rise to radiopaque deposits in the gall bladder with a fluid level between the opaque and non-opaque bile in the erect position.

Very rarely, the wall of the gallbladder affected by chronic inflammatory disease may undergo calcification. Such cases of 'porcelain gallbladder' will show on the plain radiographs (Fig. 37.3). The cystic duct in such cases is usually blocked. Occasionally it is possible to see a faint shadow of the normal gallbladder in thin patients on the preliminary film; this is not to be interpreted as abnormal.

CONTRAST EXAMINATIONS

ORAL CHOLECYSTOGRAPHY

The development of radiology of the biliary tract has been punctuated at intervals by advances of prime importance. The first of these was the development of oral cholecystography. This closely followed Graham and Cole's (1924) initial opacification of the gallbladder using intravenous sodium tetrabrom-phenolphthalein.

Subsequent improvements in the radiopacity and tolerance of oral contrast media did not alter the basic nature of the test. For success this depends upon adequate absorption of the oral medium from the small intestine, excretion from the liver with the bile, patency of the cystic duct and finally adequate concentration by the gallbladder. This requires 10 to 12 hours for completion.

1. Adequate absorption of the medium from the gut

Failure can be attributed to non-absorption in cases of unsuspected achalasia of the cardia or pyloric stenosis, both of which effectively prevent the medium reaching the small gut. In addition, the absorption of oral media such as Telepaque may be impaired in the absence of bile salts and therefore the instruction to avoid fat before ingesting oral media is mistaken. All oral and intravenous media are transported in the blood bound to plasma albumen which reduces the chance of renal excretion. (Berk and Loeb, 1976).

2. Excretion from the liver with the bile

Technical failure can occur in cases of unsuspected cirrhosis of the liver or other causes of liver insufficiency. Obviously in cases of jaundice the chances of a successful examination are minimal.

Like Bilirubin, oral media are converted to and excreted as soluble glucuronides conjugated in the bile, while intravenous media (Biligrafin, Biligram) are excreted unchanged (Berk and Loeb, 1976).

3. Patency of the cystic duct

A blocked cystic duct is the commonest cause of repeated failure to obtain a shadow after oral cholecystography and always indicates a pathological gallbladder. The obstruction in the duct is commonly due to stones but occasionally to an inflammatory stricture.

4. Adequate concentration of medium in the gallbladder.

As the concentration of oral contrast media in the hepatic bile is usually too low to cast a shadow, no image of the gallbladder will show until its contents are concentrated. This requires both time and a normal gallbladder mucosa. By taking the oral contrast medium overnight, full opportunity is given to the gallbladder to fill, retain and concentrate its contents; especially important also in this respect is the entero-hepatic recirculation which all oral media normally undergo. This is in distinct contrast to intravenous media which are *not* reabsorbed from the gut.

Modern oral contrast media. The media in common use today are shown in Table 37.1, together with the manufacturing laboratory and the chemical composition. Modern media depend for their radio-opacity on 3 iodine atoms in the molecule and they contain between 60 per cent and 68 per cent iodine by weight. The dosage is usually 3 g taken at night 12 hours before radiography, although the amount can be increased in large patients.

Advances in oral technique have been the introduction of sodium ipodate (Biloptin) and calcium ipodate (Solu-Biloptin). These media, like intravenous compounds, are concentrated sufficiently by the liver to be demonstrable in the hepatic bile. As a result, by using the medium at night in the usual way but supplementing this with another dose by mouth 2 hours before the examination, the common duct can be visualized in a high proportion of cases before the gallbladder contracts and even if it does not fill.

The following advantages of this technique over others therefore became evident:

1. The incidence of non-opacifying gallbladders is lower, as visualization no longer depends on gallbladder concentrating power alone—a patent gallbladder with a damaged mucosa will now show.

2. Delineation of the hepatic bile flowing down the common duct indicates adequate absorption and excretion; a non-opacifying gallbladder in these circumstances must be due to cystic duct obstruction and is, therefore, unquestionably pathological. Confirmation by repeat oral or intravenous techniques is consequently rendered superfluous.

Table 37.1

Contrast medium (registered name)	Manufacturer	Chemical name	Formula
Telepaque	Bayer Products Ltd.	Iodopanoic Acid	Benzene ring with I, H_2N, H, I, I; CH_2-CH-COOH with CH_3
Biloptin	Schering, A.G., Berlin	Sodium Ipodate	Benzene ring with I, I, I; N.CH.N(CH_3)(CH_3); CH_2CH_2COO-Na(BILOPTIN)
Solu-Biloptin	Schering, A.G., Berlin	Calcium Ipodate	CH_2CH_2COO-$\frac{Ca}{2}$(SOLU-B)
Biligram	Schering, A.G., Berlin	Meglumine Ioglycamate	$C_{32}H_{46}I_6N_4O_{17}$

3. The calibre of the duct, if excessive, will indicate that it is partially obstructed; in addition, it produces a record of calibre for possible future use if symptoms recur post-operatively.

Toxicity. In general, toxic reactions from modern oral media are slight and consist of mild headache, occasional nausea, diarrhoea and sometimes dysuria. Iodism from organically bound iodine compounds is extremely unlikely. Undue sensitivity, however, does occasionally occur and is related to the chemical structure of the compound. Such allergic reactions may be accompanied by urticaria, oedema of the face, eyes and rarely the larynx. In doubtful cases a small test dose can be given at the time of the preliminary film, with appropriate instructions; if reaction occurs, a different chemical compound will usually be satisfactory. There is also a relation between the degree of protein binding in the blood and the toxicity of the contrast agents; for example, intravenous Biligrafin is the most highly bound and also the most toxic of the biliary media (Berk and Loeb, 1976).

Technique. The importance of the preliminary radiograph has already been stressed. Thorough preparation of the patient in order to dispense with bowel shadows is advisable. As the vast majority of gallbladder examinations are performed to confirm or exclude calculi, the radiographic technique is designed to make the diagnosis as infallible as possible. Coned films using a low K.V. technique are taken in the prone oblique position for the fundus; in the supine position for the neck and Hartmann's pouch; and in the erect or decubitus positions (or both) to distinguish loose stones which will sink or occasionally float, from fixed mural translucent filling defects and extraneous shadows. Similarly, films after the gallbladder has contracted may show small lesions more readily, or fill areas behind strictures, or show Rokitansky-Aschoff sinuses not previously visualized. Commonly the cystic duct may be seen and also the bile duct. The optimum time for taking these films is between half to 1 hour after a fatty meal. Commercial products such as Prosparol and Sorbital may be used with equally good results as may a simple chocolate bar and without the patient leaving the department. Serial films show that the process of gallbladder emptying occurs over a considerable period, up to 30 minutes or more. Such films often show the common duct throughout its length (Fig. 37.4).

Cholecystokinin cholecystography. The concept of biliary dyskinesia has been entertained for decades to explain those cases of clinical typical biliary pain associated with an apparently radiologically normal biliary tract. The concept is based upon the observation that the opacified gallbladder contracts poorly and simultaneously results in the reproduction of the patient's clinical symptoms.

To test this hypothesis, a slow intravenous injection of the soluble porcine cholecystokinin is given after oral cholecystography and subsequent radiographs in a constant position are taken at short intervals such as 1, 3, 5, 10 and 15 minutes. A positive result consists of (a) reproduction of the pain and symptoms of the patient together with (b) poor gallbladder contraction, the latter often assuming a round shape. Such findings indicate either partial cystic duct obstruction or gallbladder disease invisible radiologically.

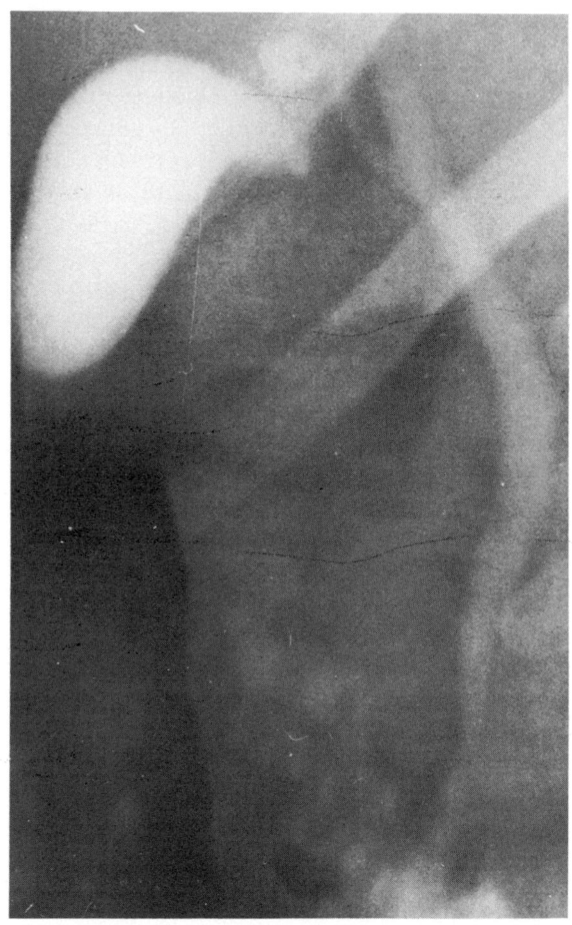

Fig. 37.4 Common duct outlined after gallbladder contraction—oral cholecystography.

It must be emphasized that to be of value this test must be strictly controlled; most studies indicate it has a place in the detection of non-calculous gallbladder or cystic duct disease in those patients with typical biliary symptoms and that cholecystectomy will benefit such patients, provided other lesions of the gastro-intestinal tract have been excluded (Goldberg, 1976).

There is therefore good evidence to show that a normal, routine cholecystogram does not necessarily exclude non-calculous gallbladder disease; careful clinical selection of cases combined with the use of specialised cholecystography techniques, as described above, can result in cure following cholecystectomy in about 80 per cent of cases (Gough, 1977).

Accuracy. The reliability of the examination with modern media is of a high order. If observer error is eliminated, mistakes in normally opacified gallbladders are usually due to cholesterosis and to moderate cholecystitis without stones. In a few instances mistakes can be attributed to failure to take preliminary films or films after contraction of the gallbladder. Such films may occasionally be the only ones to show small or faint lesions.

Non-opacifying gallbladders (no visible calculi). The chances of error are greater in these cases because of the possibility of technical defect; in spite of these possibilities, however, the vast majority of non-opacifying gallbladders are in fact pathological and contain calculi at surgery. Nevertheless Baker and Hodgson (1960) using Telepaque found 5 out of 229 non-opacifying gallbladders to be normal at surgery (2.2 per cent); Stenhouse (1956) had similar results (3.6 per cent).

2. INTRAVENOUS CHOLANGIOGRAPHY

The next advance of importance was the introduction of intravenous cholangiography and cholecystography (Biligrafin) in 1953. (A newer intravenous medium, Biligram, is referred to below.) For the first time opacified bile could be observed in transit down the common duct whether a gallbladder was present or not; this was and remains the most important role of i.v. cholangiography. In addition it offered an alternative technique of examination, particularly important in cases of non-opacifying gallbladders at oral cholecystograms. Studies with this medium confirmed that these non-opacifying gallbladders were pathological in the majority of cases due to cystic duct obstruction (usually by stone) but they were occasionally patent. Reports of normal intravenous examinations following upon failed oral cholecystograms appeared (Stenhouse, 1958) which confirmed and approximated to the normal surgical findings quoted above. Less common was the converse of this phenomenon, i.e. failure of a normal gallbladder to fill on the intravenous examination whereas it filled and concentrated normally on the oral cholecystogram. A similar parallel series using surgery as the control of normality showed 6 out of 46 non-filling gallbladders over a two hour period with intravenous iodipamide (Biligrafin) were normal (13 per cent) (Wise, Johnston and Salzman, 1957).

Technique. Owing to the fact that the methyl glucamine ioglycamate molecule is large and contains only 48 per cent iodine, the radio-opacity of the medium in the common duct is not great. Consequently films should be taken with a small cone, a low K.V. technique and with the patient slightly prone oblique to cast the duct clear of the spine.

It is obviously important to obtain a maximum concentration of the intravenous medium in the bile Experimental work has shown that this is best achieved by slow administration over 10–15 minutes either by syringe or by a drip technique in saline. This may increase the concentration by increasing the proportion bound to plasma albumen (so reducing the renal excretion) resulting in a 10 per cent improvement in the density of the image.

In addition, all intravenous cholangiographic media are cholagogues; by reducing the bile flow before the examination to a minimum, relatively low dose cholangiography (with consequently reduced toxicity) is feasible. Bile salts have a similar choleretic effect and the enterohepatic recirculation of these can be reduced to a minimum by fasting, so reducing the bile flow; consequently the examination should be performed in a fasting state (Berk and Loeb, 1976).

The medium appears in the duct 15–20 minutes after injection and begins to fall off in density after 1 hour. Better results are obtained if the patient is left on the table between exposures. Gallbladder filling commences early in many cases, but occasionally is delayed; most gallbladders will fill in 2 hours. A film at this time must be done if the gallbladder is present but has not filled by 1 hour.

In the examination of the common duct, tomography is useful when the presence of overlying gas or faeces makes interpretation difficult.

Indications for use. (a) Whenever a detailed examination of the common duct is required. This may be in primary examinations with a history suggestive of stones in the duct, as well as in post-cholecystectomy patients with recurrent biliary symptoms. In the former group, a combined examination with oral cholecystography will take less time. Recent investigation, however, has shown that the incidence of toxic reactions is slightly higher in the combined examination; consequently, some radiologists feel it is wiser to examine such cases initially by intravenous cholangiography. Alternatively, an interval of 24–48 hours after oral cholecystography can be allowed.

(b) In primary examinations which have failed to show an opacified gallbladder on oral cholecystography. Most of these will show an obstructed cystic duct, indicating the gallbladder is pathological; a few gallbladders will fill and may show stones or, rarely, appear normal. If the common duct does not opacify, the fault lies in the liver; in these circumstances, the medium is excreted by the kidneys.

(c) For rapid cholecystangiography.

COMPARISON OF TECHNIQUE (ORAL AND INTRAVENOUS)

It is the natural conclusion from the above considerations that, provided that the gallbladder opacifies, either technique (oral or intravenous) will give comparable results. The oral method does, however, have technical advantages.

1. It is simple, safe and quick, rendering it suitable for out-patient examinations in a busy X-ray department.

2. The entero-hepatic recirculation of all oral media ensures the maximum opportunity for gallbladder filling and concentration over 10–12 hours at night.

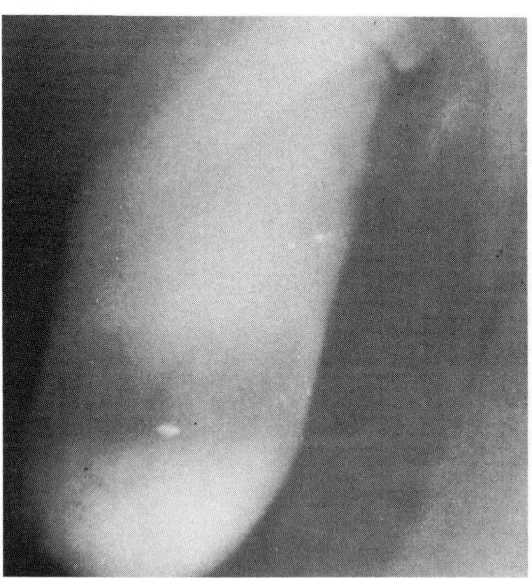

Fig. 37.5

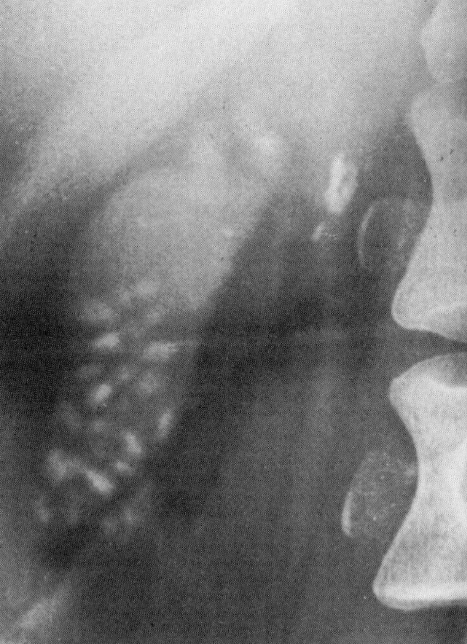

Fig. 37.6A

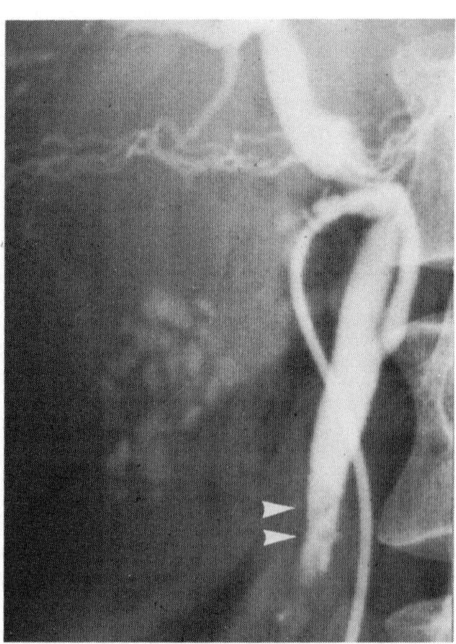

Fig. 37.6B

Fig. 37.5 Erect film (Biligram) showing translucent horizontal band due to poor mixing.

Fig. 37.6 A Intravenous examination showing gallstones and a normal common duct. The opacity overlying the common duct is in costal cartilage. B Four days later, the duct contains stones (*arrows*) (pre-exploratory operative cholangiogram). Note (i) medial insertion of the cystic duct, (ii) absence of flow into the duodenum.

Per contra, intravenous examinations are time consuming and, while they depict more of the biliary apparatus than oral cholecystograms giving a detailed common duct examination of all cases, the media are more toxic. A recent addition to this series—Biligram—is less toxic and has virtually displaced Biligrafin as the intravenous medium of choice. Apart from this, poor mixing with the bile may cause troublesome layering in erect films resembling floating stones (Fig. 37.5). Unlike oral media, no entero-hepatic recirculation occurs with these compounds and, while the medium is concentrated by the liver, no further concentration occurs in the gallbladder unless the examination is prolonged.

The above discussion about non-opacifying gallbladders indicates that in order to avoid errors due to false positive results, it may be necessary occasionally to do both oral and intravenous examinations irrespective of which is used initially. The explanation of a non-opacifying but otherwise normal gallbladder occurring by one or the other technique is not obvious. The experience with the intravenous cases suggests that possibly the gallbladder is already full at the time of the examination and cannot therefore accommodate the opacified bile flowing down the common duct. With the entero-hepatic recirculation of oral media, however, this explanation is unlikely; it may be that 2–4 per cent of normal gallbladders do not concentrate adequately and hence give a poor or absent shadow with Telepaque.

The choice of technique. The primary examination of the gallbladder is preferably performed with an oral medium. The entero-hepatic recirculation ensures the maximum opportunity for gallbladder filling. By using a second dose of Solu-Biloptin on the morning of the examination additional information regarding non-filling gallbladders and duct calibre is obtained. Only if neither gallbladder nor common duct are seen with this medium is Biligram indicated, and this is uncommon in the absence of jaundice; Biligram usually fails also in such cases.

The examination of the common duct in detail is best performed with i.v. Biligram. The advantages of a routine detailed duct examination in primary cases are offset by the additional time and inconvenience to the patient; in addition, it may give a false sense of security if there is an appreciable interval between the examination and the operation. During such an interval, stones may pass from the gallbladder into the common duct (Fig. 37.6).

THE PATHOLOGICAL GALLBLADDER

Gallstones

Most stones are of the mixed type and are composed of cholesterol, calcium and bile pigment, with traces of iron, phosphorus and carbonate, together with some protein. These stones are usually laminated giving a characteristic appearance on the plain radiograph. They are often also faceted when multiple, due to rubbing against each other (Fig. 37.1B).

Pure cholesterol stones contain 96 per cent or more of cholesterol, the remainder being composed of some pigment as well as protein. Typically large and single, they may also exist as multiple small round calculi which are not visible until surrounded by contrast medium and frequently float in erect films (Fig. 37.7); alternatively, they may only show when aggregated together by suitable positioning of the patient (Fig. 37.8) or after the gallbladder has contracted.

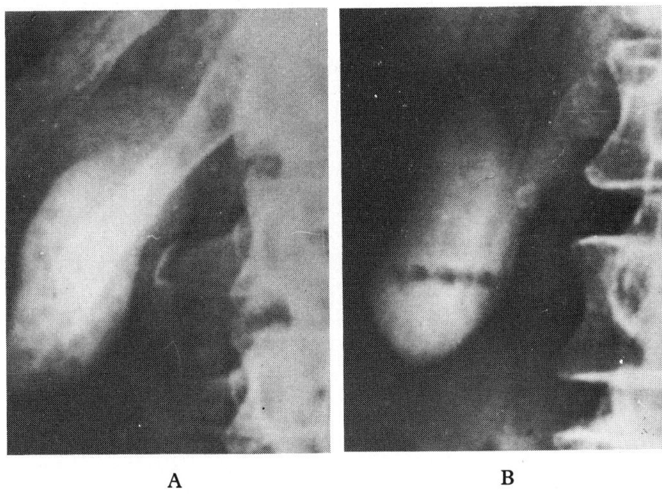

Fig. 37.7 Small cholesterol calculi which float in the erect posture (A) prone (B) erect.

Pigment stones are composed of calcium bilirubinate and are usually small and multiple. The cholesterol content of these stones is low, seldom exceeding 25 per cent, whereas the mixed stones may contain up to 70 per cent (Palayew, 1976).

Pure calcium carbonate stones are rare and exist in two forms—as fine granules (biliary sand) and as separate, discrete mulberry shaped calculi, which are the most radio-opaque gallstones encountered (Fig. 37.1A).

Incidence of gallstones. The frequency of cholelithiasis is increased in certain patient populations as well as in women. It is claimed that there is a higher incidence of cholesterol stones in post-vagotomy patients and that about a third of patients with Crohn's disease have gallstones of a similar constitution. Pigment stones are well

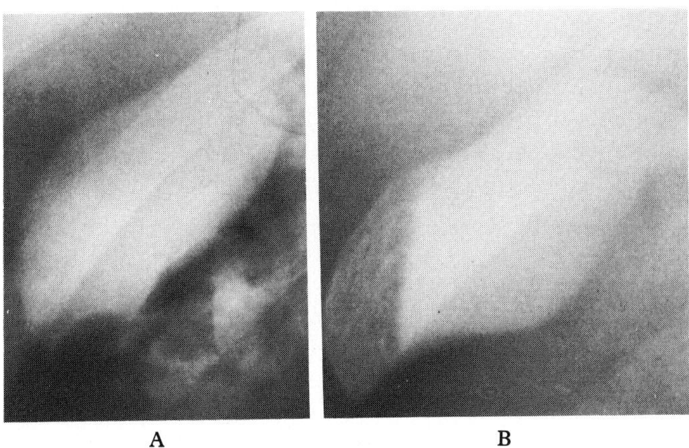

Fig. 37.8 Multiple small translucent calculi invisible in prone film (A) but easily seen in lateral decubitus film (B).

known to be increased in frequency in patients with haemolytic anaemia as the result of excessive red blood cell destruction.

Pigment stones are commonly associated with infection and contain 40–60 per cent Bilirubin, which is non-conjugated, due to the action of the enzyme B-Glucuronidase present in bile infected with *E.coli*. This organism releases the enzyme, forming free Bilirubin from the normally conjugated pigment in the bile and this combines with calcium to form calcium bilirubinate (Palayew, 1976).

The mechanism of the formation of calcium carbonate stones is not known.

The pathogenesis of cholesterol stone formation is considered below.

Stones are usually freely mobile within the cavity of the gallbladder as seen when the patient is radiographed in various positions. Exceptions occur when a stone is impacted in Hartmann's pouch (Fig. 37.1A) or confined by a stricture (Fig. 37.9). A stone impacted in the former position may obstruct the cystic duct: a stone in the

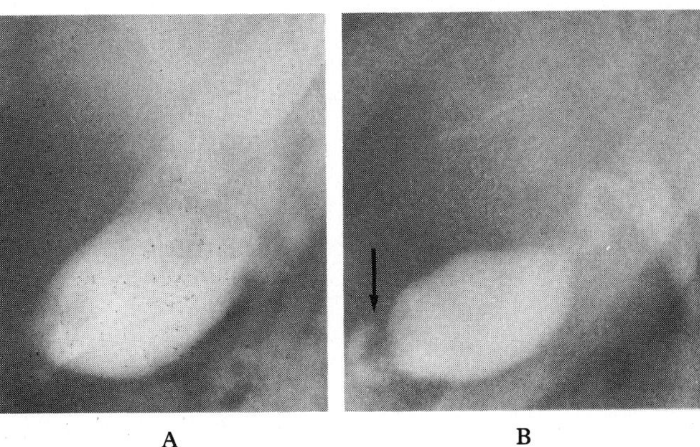

Fig. 37.9 A Prone film (oral cholecystography); the gallbladder appears normal. B After contraction, a stone confined by a stricture in the fundus is revealed(↓).

latter position may be missed if it is not opaque and if the stricture is sufficiently tight to prevent the contrast medium from reaching the stone. Most stones sink in the mixture of bile and contrast medium and the medium itself tends to sink as it has a higher specific gravity than the bile. Floating stones are usually composed of cholesterol and find a level in this uneven mixture (Fig. 37.7).

Finally small gallstones are occasionally seen to disappear. This is usually due to their passage into the common duct where they may or may not be retained. This can happen at any time (Fig. 37.6) and is not necessarily accompanied by symptoms. This is one of the main justifications for operative choledochography.

Cholesterosis ('strawberry gallbladder')

The common form of this condition is a diffuse deposition of cholesterol on the mucosa of the gallbladder

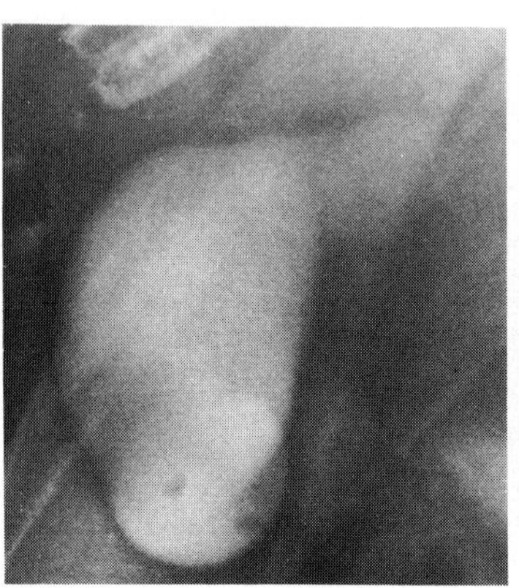

Fig. 37.10

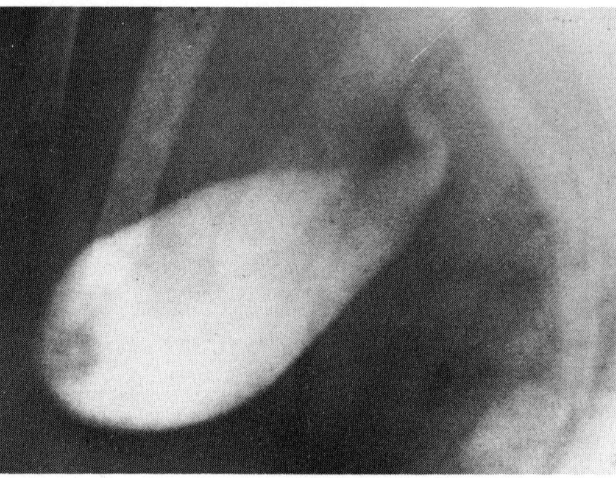

Fig. 37.11A

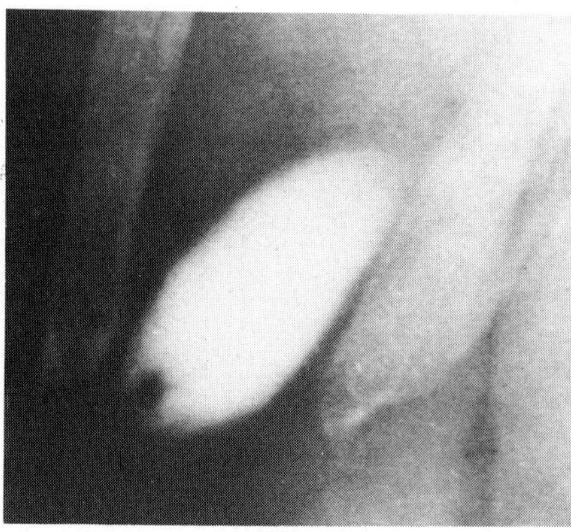

Fig. 37.11B

Fig. 37.10 Cholesterosis, showing fixed mural defects.

Fig. 37.11 Fundal nodule (adenomyomastosis) showing muscular contractions with gallbladder emptying. Note also the long cystic duct on the medial side.

and as such it cannot be diagnosed radiologically. The gallbladder shadow appears normal and concentrates and contracts normally.

When cholesterol deposits measure 2 mm or more they may be detectable, particularly on films after gallbladder contraction. Such cases mostly show a single fixed mural defect, although at surgery many more deposits may be visible. It may be impossible to distinguish such a filling defect from a polyp which is a potentially malignant lesion. Multiplicity of fixed mural defects, however, is absolutely characteristic of cholesterosis as multiple polyps are extremely rare. Unfortunately only about 10 per cent of those cases with positive radiological signs show the characteristic multiple defects (Fig. 37.10). Nevertheless the most likely diagnosis in the case of a single fixed mural filling defect is cholesterosis unless the lesion is large, when a new growth should be suspected. When stones are also present or when the concentration of the medium is poor. such lesions are commonly missed.

Cholecystitis glandularis proliferans (adenomyomatosis. Cholecystosis)

This condition is of unknown aetiology although it is suggested that it is associated with chronic biliary obstruction. Such obstruction may be located in the cystic duct, when the whole organ may exhibit this disease. In other cases, and these are more frequent, the gallbladder is only partially involved; in these only that part of the gallbladder proximal to a stricture will show changes. This limited involvement of the gallbladder wall is an important differential feature from chronic cholecystitis; another is the relatively infrequent association with stones.

The pathology is associated with localized muscle hypertrophy, formation of epithelial mucosal sinuses (Rokitansky-Aschoff sinuses) and round cell infiltration.

The radiological appearances reflect the macroscopic changes in the gallbladder wall. The three characteristic signs of the disease are:

1. *A fundal nodular filling defect*, sometimes umbilicated (Fig. 37.11). These nodules have often been dismissed as adenomata in the past. Such true tumours in the fundus are very rare.

2. *A stricture*. The stricture may be situated anywhere in the gallbladder and may be sharply localized or a more diffuse narrowing (Fig. 37.13). Its muscular origin is often manifest after gallbladder contraction when the stricture narrows still further. The fundal nodule may show similar changes in shape for similar reasons (Fig. 37.11). This feature of the strictures due to cholecystitis glandularis proliferans serves to distinguish them radiologically from congenital partial septa (Fig. 37.12) which are usually sharply localized to the fundal area ('Phrygian cap') but occasionally appear in the waist or neck of the viscus. Postural kinks may be similarly excluded.

3. *Epithelial sinuses* (*Rokitansky-Aschoff sinuses*). These may fill and become visible only after gallbladder con-

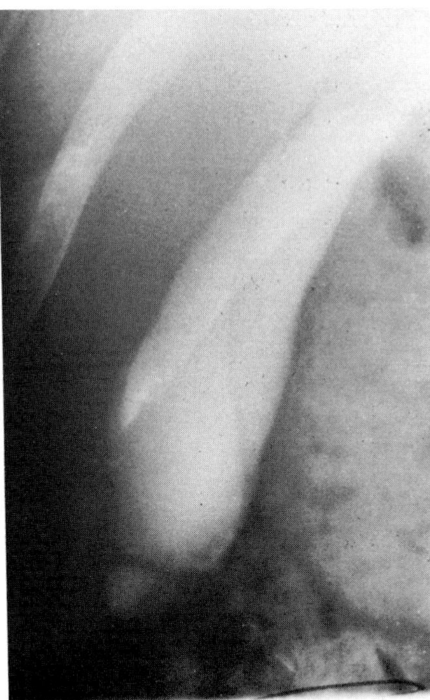

Fig. 37.12A

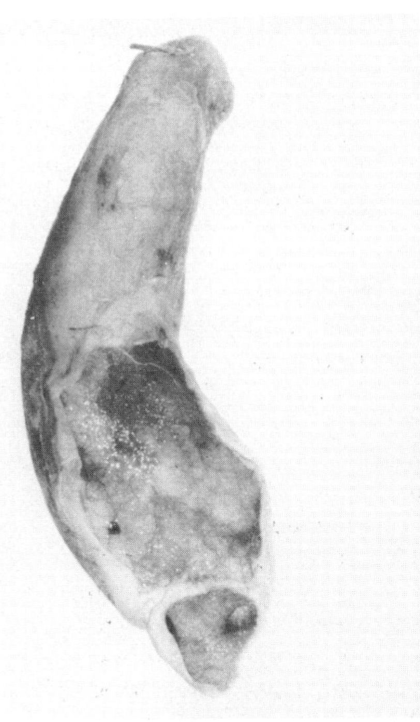

Fig. 37.12B

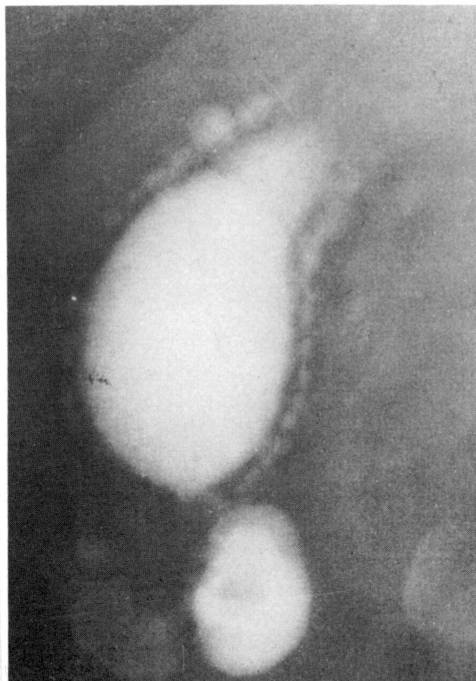

Fig. 37.13

Fig. 37.12 Partial septum across the fundus of an otherwise normal gallbladder; the septum contained normal mucosa and muscle. A Cholecystogram. B Specimen.

Fig. 37.13 Gross adenomyomatosis showing sinuses and a stricture, with a stone distal to it.

traction (Fig. 37.13). On the other hand, they may not be obvious radiologically nor are they essential to the diagnosis although they are always present pathologically.

While the natural history of this condition is not known, it is evident that it may remain static over long periods. There is no evidence that it predisposes to stone formation, but a stone forming behind a stricture in the affected segment may prevent filling of this segment and lead to an erroneous diagnosis (Fig. 37.9). There is also no evidence that the condition is pre-malignant but it may be responsible for symptoms of a biliary nature.

Acute cholecystitis

Radiology is seldom called upon to assist in this diagnosis, which is usually obvious clinically. In doubtful cases there is a place for emergency intravenous cholangiography. If the gallbladder opacifies, acute cholecystic can confidently be excluded, as the cystic duct is very likely to be obstructed in this condition. If this obstruction is due to temporary oedema and the case is treated conservatively, further assessment at a later date may show normal filling of the gallbladder. It is wise, therefore, always to re-examine the gallbladder before late elective surgery is performed. Re-examination is also advisable in all cases of biliary disease in which the interval between the radiological assessment and the operation is more than a few weeks.

Carcinoma of the gallbladder

In spite of modern methods of investigation, this diagnosis is rarely made radiologically. The growth is uncommon and is nearly always associated with gallstones. It is, therefore, commoner in females, but only a small proportion of women over 50 with gallstones are likely to develop carcinoma. The other possible predisposing cause already mentioned is the rare polyp. Usually the tumour is found as an unpleasant surprise at cholecystectomy for stones. Radiologically, a non-filling gallbladder on both oral and intravenous examinations is the rule—results which are indistinguishable from an obstructed cystic duct due to inflammation or stones. On the few occasions that filling occurs, any deformity present is indistinguishable from chronic cholecystitis accompanying gallstones.

CONGENITAL ABNORMALITIES OF THE GALLBLADDER

1. Absence of the gallbladder in the presence of an otherwise normal biliary tree is extremely rare. Most recorded cases occurred in infants in association with congenital absence of the extrahepatic bile ducts. Necropsy evidence in adults puts the incidence at between 0.03 and 0.07 per cent.

2. Double gallbladder occurs in about 1 case in 4000 in man. The usual type consists of a longitudinally septate viscus with a single cystic duct; very rarely, two

separate gallbladders each with a separate cystic duct occur. Rarer still, one of such a pair may be attached to the left lobe of the liver and drain into the left hepatic duct. A solitary gallbladder may occupy a similar position.

3. Partial transverse septa may be seen either in the neck or near the fundus, when they can give rise to the so-called Phrygian cap deformity (Fig. 37.12). They rarely interfere with the filling or emptying of the viscus, but they need to be differentiated from postural kinks and from the strictures of cholecystitis glandularis proliferans.

THE RADIOLOGY OF THE COMMON BILE DUCT

The methods available for the study of the common duct and the indications for each may be summarized as follows.

1. **Pre-operative (primary) cholangiography.** (a) *Oral cholangiography* is combined with oral cholecystography. The advantages of this technique have already been discussed; in brief, this method reduces the incidence of non-opacifying gallbladders, provides visible evidence of absorption and excretion of the contrast medium, gives valuable evidence of obstructed cystic duct and of obstructed common duct (Fig. 37.14), and provides a record of duct calibre.

(b) *Intravenous cholangiography* (Biligram) either alone or combined with oral cholecystography, in selected cases where detailed information about the common duct is desirable. Such cases might include primary examinations of patients with a previous history of obstructive jaundice.

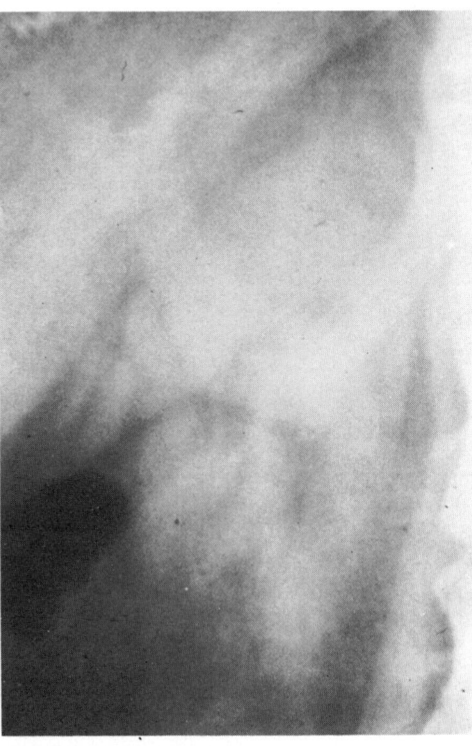

Fig. 37.14 Oral cholangiography showing obstructed cystic duct and stasis in a dilated (obstructed) common duct.

2. **Operative cholangiography.** This examination, performed in the operating theatre, has a twofold function:

(a) The purpose of the pre-exploratory operative cholangiogram is to determine whether or not the common duct contains calculi or shows obstructive features and so requires exploration. This examination is performed before cholecystectomy by injecting contrast medium via a catheter in the cystic duct and taking three serial films.

(b) The post-exploratory operative cholangiogram is performed through the T-tube after the common duct has been explored. The purpose is to ensure that no stones have been overlooked before the abdomen is closed.

3. **Post-operative cholangiography.** (a) T-tube cholangiography in the immediate post-operative period; before removing the tube (7–10 days post-operatively), performance of this examination ensures that the common duct is normal and free from obstruction.

(b) Intravenous cholangiography with Biligram in the late post-operative period. This is used particularly to exclude obstruction of the duct in patients who have had recurrent symptoms of possible biliary origin some tine after cholecystectomy.

4. **Four-day Telepaque test (see below).**

5. **Percutaneous transhepatic cholangiography (P.T.C.) (see below).**

6. **Endoscopy and retrograde choledocho-pancreatography (ERCP).**

7. **Duodenography (see under Pancreas).**

8. **Ultrasound.**

9. **Nuclear scanning.**

10. **Computer assisted tomography (CAT).**

Methods 4 to 10 are used in suspected obstructive jaundice; ERCP is used in any case in which both oral and intravenous methods have failed.

The purpose of the radiological examination directed specifically at the common bile duct is to confirm or exclude any existing obstruction of the duct. Such obstruction may be chronic or intermittent, mild or severe; it may be due to tumours or strictures, but the commonest cause is stone. In assessing the condition of the duct, attention must be focused on three main aspects, whatever the method of investigation. These aspects are:

1. The calibre of the duct.
2. The ease of flow of contrast medium into the duodenum.
3. The visualization of an obstructing agent.

Two further points must be remembered; firstly, not every duct which is partially obstructed will necessarily exhibit all three basic abnormalities; secondly, the assessment of any one aspect may be much easier in some examinations than in others. Thus the measurement of duct calibre seldom presents any obstacle, but the ease of flow into the duodenum may be difficult to assess on intravenous examinations, though simple by post-operative T-tube cholangiography. Likewise, calculi are easy to identify on T-tube cholangiograms but often difficult to visualize on intravenous examinations. It is obvious that of all forms of cholangiography, the T-tube examination technique gives the most accurate results.

THE CALIBRE AND ANATOMY OF THE COMMON DUCT

Duct calibre

It is well known that normal common bile ducts vary in size. Several series of studies have shown that the duct calibre as measured on films exposed at the usual film focus distance of 36 cm may range from 1–14 mm. Over 95 per cent of ducts have a calibre between 2 and 10 mm as measured on the radiographs. It is thus reasonable to suspect dilatation in any duct measuring 11–12 mm or more at its widest point.

It has also been shown convincingly that cholecystectomy has no effect on the calibre of the common duct and that ducts which have become dilated owing to partial obstruction do not return to normal dimensions after the obstruction has been removed.

It follows from these observations that the discovery of a dilated common bile duct must be interpreted quite differently in pre-operative (or operative) and in late post-operative examinations. In the former group, a dilated duct signifies an obstructed duct which requires surgical exploration even if the cause of the obstruction is not obvious (Fig. 37.14); in the latter examination, a dilated duct is of no significance in itself, unless pre-operative, operative or post-operative T-tube radiographic records are available for comparison. If this comparison shows that the duct has increased in size during the post-operative period, then this important discovery signifies that the duct is partially obstructed (Fig. 37.15B and C). Conversely, if it can be shown from such records that post-cholecystectomy symptoms are not associated with any increase in duct calibre, the duct is unlikely to be obstructed. The interpretation of intravenous cholangiograms in post-operative patients is therefore considerably aided by previous records of duct calibre, whether these exist as operative or post-operative T-tube cholangiograms or as pre-operative oral or intravenous cholangiograms. The routine use of Solu-Biloptin in all primary cholecystographic examinations in order to record duct calibre can prove of great value in those cases which develop recurrent symptoms post-operatively.

When no previous records are available, the problem is more difficult. On the one hand, a duct may be partially obstructed and dilated and yet fall within the

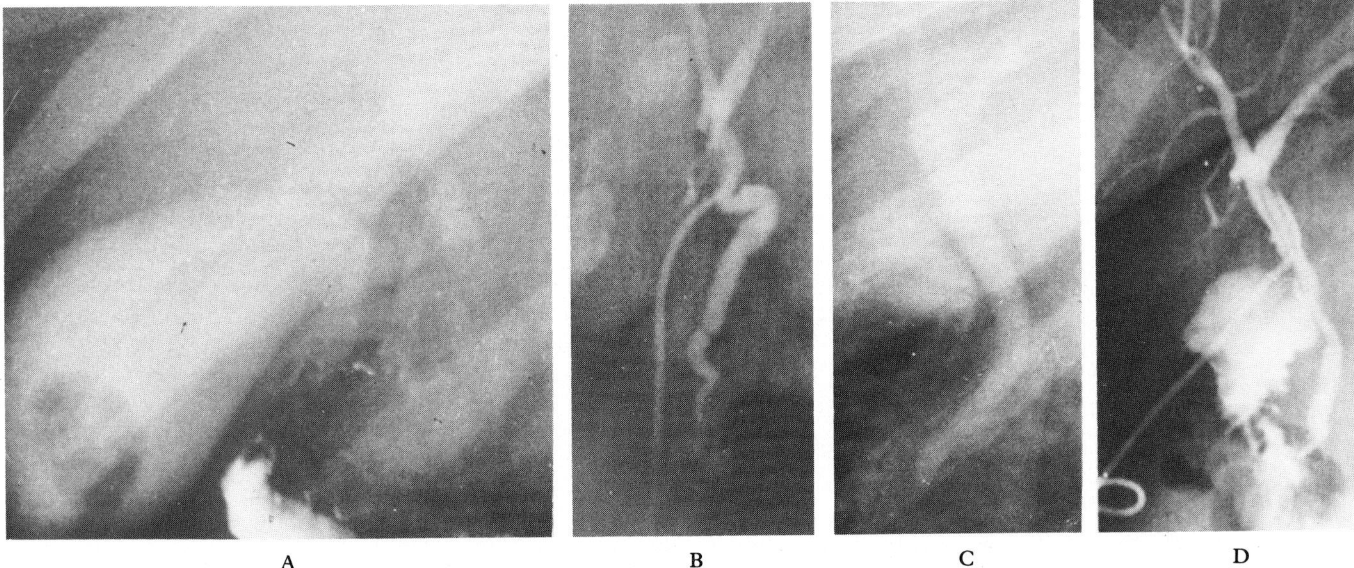

Fig. 37.15 A Oral cholecystogram showing a large solitaire stone and normal calibre duct. B Operative cholangiography shows an apparently normal duct also. C Intravenous cholangiography 6 months post-operatively shows slight increase in calibre and particularly stasis, with distended hepatic radicles. D Post-operative T-tube examination shows normal appearances following sphincterotomy. Diagnosis—ampullary stenosis.

normal variation of measurement; on the other, obviously dilated ducts may not be obstructed. Consequently, in the assessment of partial obstruction in post-operative intravenous cholangiograms, an isolated observation of calibre is of limited value. In this context also it has been shown recently by operative cholangiography in a series of 400 patients that two fifths of the patients with duct stones at surgery had ducts of normal calibre (i.e. less than 12 mm in diameter); in addition, one-third of ducts at this upper limit of normal calibre were shown to contain stones (Faris *et al.*, 1975).

The anatomy of the common duct. A few anatomical points need to be stressed. The duct contains no muscle in its walls except in the intra-mural portion as it pierces the duodenum obliquely and for 5 mm outside it (Fig. 37.16). This portion of the duct shows a narrow lumen and is observed radiologically most readily on operative and post-operative T-tube cholangiograms (Fig. 37.15D). Visualization may be obscured by over-filling the duodenum so it is important, both at operative and at T-tube examinations, to take an early film with only 2–3 ml of contrast injected into the duct. This intra-mural segment is seldom observed on intravenous examinations and often appears as a 'gap' between the duct and the duodenum; such appearances are not to be interpreted as abnormal.

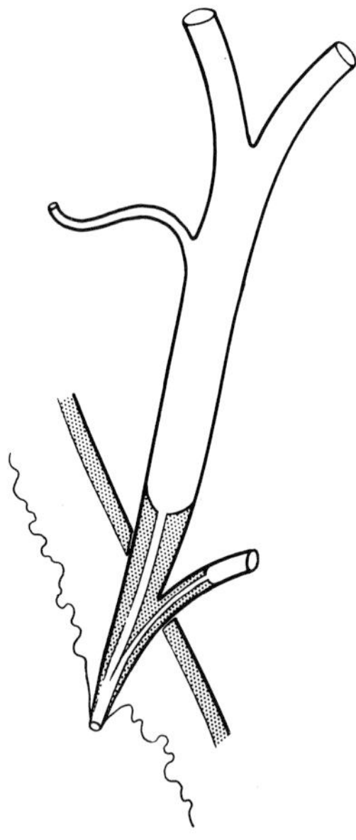

Fig. 37.16 Lower end of normal common duct to show terminal narrow segment and thickened wall. The shaded portions represent muscle.

There are several congenital variations affecting the cystic and common duct which are of importance surgically and radiologically. Instead of entering the common duct on its lateral border, the cystic duct may enter on its medial border; a common variation of this finding is a long cystic duct which runs down closely bound to the medial aspect of the common duct and enters it low down on its medial border (Fig. 37.11A). Again, the right and left hepatic ducts may join very low and the cystic duct enter the right hepatic duct (Fig. 37.17).

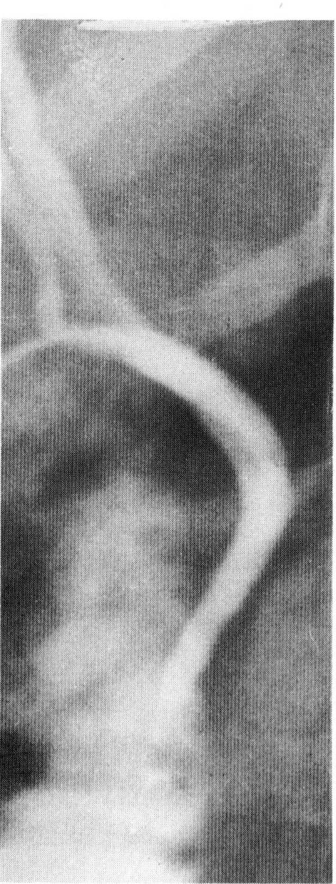

Fig. 37.17 Normal pre-exploratory operative cholangiogram showing low junction of the right and left hepatic ducts with the cystic duct entering the right hepatic duct.

The position of the ampulla of Vater may vary from just distal to the duodenum bulb to a location in the third part of the duodenum (Fig. 37.18). In about 75 per cent of cases the pancreatic duct joins the common duct in the intramural segment to form a small common chamber prior to entering the duodenum. Reflux up the pancreatic duct is not uncommon in operative and T-tube cholangiograms and does not appear to be related to the presence or absence of duct obstruction.

THE EASE OF CONTRAST MEDIUM FLOW INTO THE DUODENUM

Operative cholangiography. (*a*) *Pre-exploratory.* The meticulous attention to technical detail that this examination demands renders it unsuitable for a full description here. In practice, three films are taken after the introduction of 3 ml, 7–8 ml and 10–12 ml of 25–35 per cent of Hypaque or other equivalent contrast medium

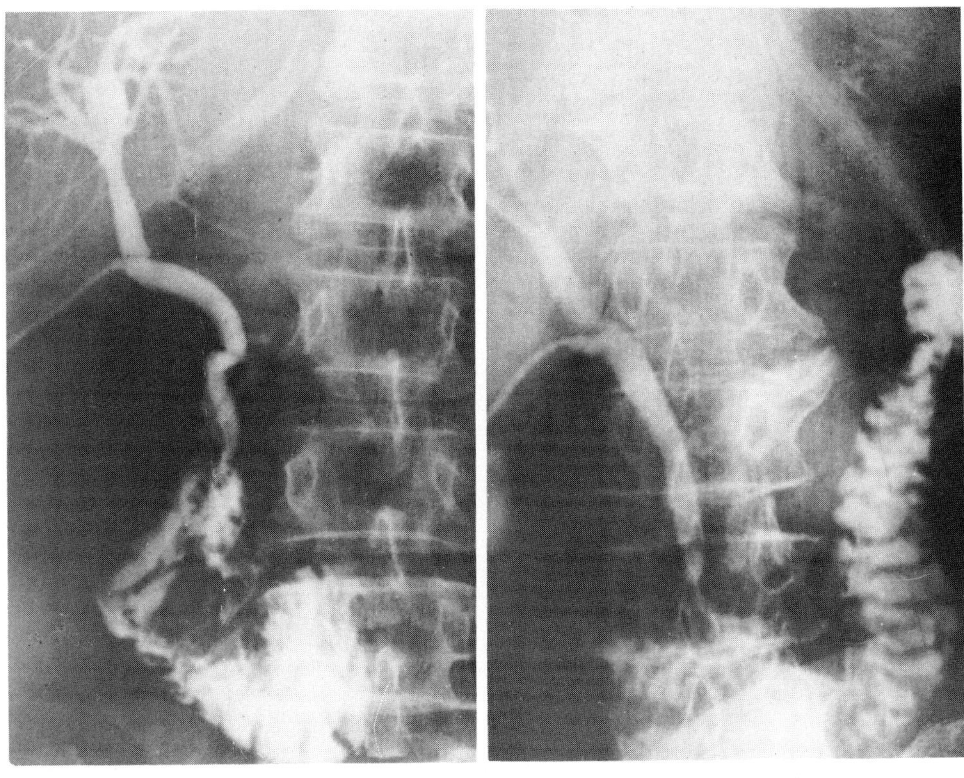

A B

Fig. 37.18 (A and B) Normal pre-exploratory operative cholangiograms in two patients showing the limits of variation in the position of the ampulla of Vater.

into the common duct. This is done on the operating table via a catheter in the cystic duct.

The assessment of flow is made by demonstrating that each film shows an increasing amount of contrast medium in the duodenum, including some flow in the first film after 3 ml injection. In addition, free flow is characterized by absence of excess retrograde filling of the intrahepatic ducts. It is noted also that the first film with its small amount of contrast medium will show the narrow terminal segment best before the opacified duodenum obscures it. Failure to demonstrate free flow in any pre-exploratory examination, irrespective of calibre and of filling defects, is an absolute indication for duct exploration. It must also be remembered, however, that in some cases a calculus may not interfere with free flow nor may there be a history of colic or jaundice.

(*b*) *Post-exploratory*. Basically the technique of this examination is the same as above, the amounts of contrast medium being increased to allow for the dead space of the T-tube.

One important problem in the post-exploratory examination stems from the oedema of the lower end of the duct following instrumentation during duct

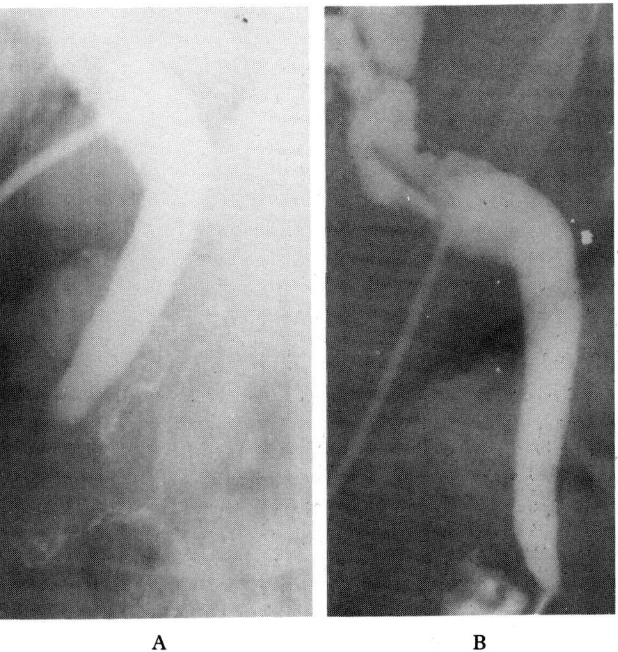

A B

Fig. 37.19 A Post-exploratory operative cholangiogram following removal of two stones. Note absence of flow following instrumentation. B. T-tube examination showing normal flow 10 days later.

exploration. This frequently interferes with free flow of bile, with the result that failure to observe the narrow segment and to demonstrate free flow are not of themselves proof of residual duct obstruction requiring further operative exploration (Fig. 37.19).

As an adjunct to post-exploratory operative cholangiography, operative choledochoscopy using the flexible fibre optic Olympus CHF–B2 series instrument has a place, particularly in those cases where there is real doubt whether residual stones remain after exploration.

This technique does not, however, compete with operative cholangiography as the method of choice in deciding whether the duct should be opened or not. As the instrument is 5.7 mm in diameter, its use is confined to ducts greater than this. It is particularly useful for removing stones in the hepatic ducts by its facility to allow the passage of small balloon catheters under direct vision (Ashley, 1976).

Post-operative T-tube cholangiography. The routine use of post-exploratory operative cholangiography in all cases of duct exploration has reduced almost to zero the incidence of residual stones found at the post-operative T-tube examinations. Owing to the difficulties with free flow at operation mentioned above, the post-operative examination must not be omitted. As stated previously, it is the most accurate of all forms of cholangiography.

Flow is assessed by the introduction of a small quantity of contrast medium under screen control: appropriate films are then taken (Fig. 37.15D). These show ease of entry of the medium into the duodenum, the narrow segment and any small filling defects. Films after further injection confirm the flow, outline the duct

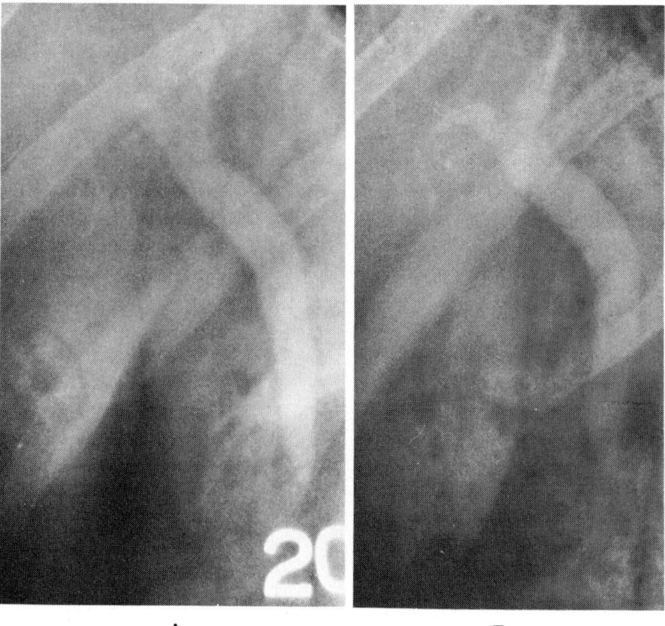

Fig. 37.20 A Obstructed dilated duct at 20 minutes (intravenous cholangiography) showing stasis. Solitary stone in the gallbladder. B Confirmation at 2 hours showing no diminution of duct density, together with the signs of obstruction. Ampullary stenosis.

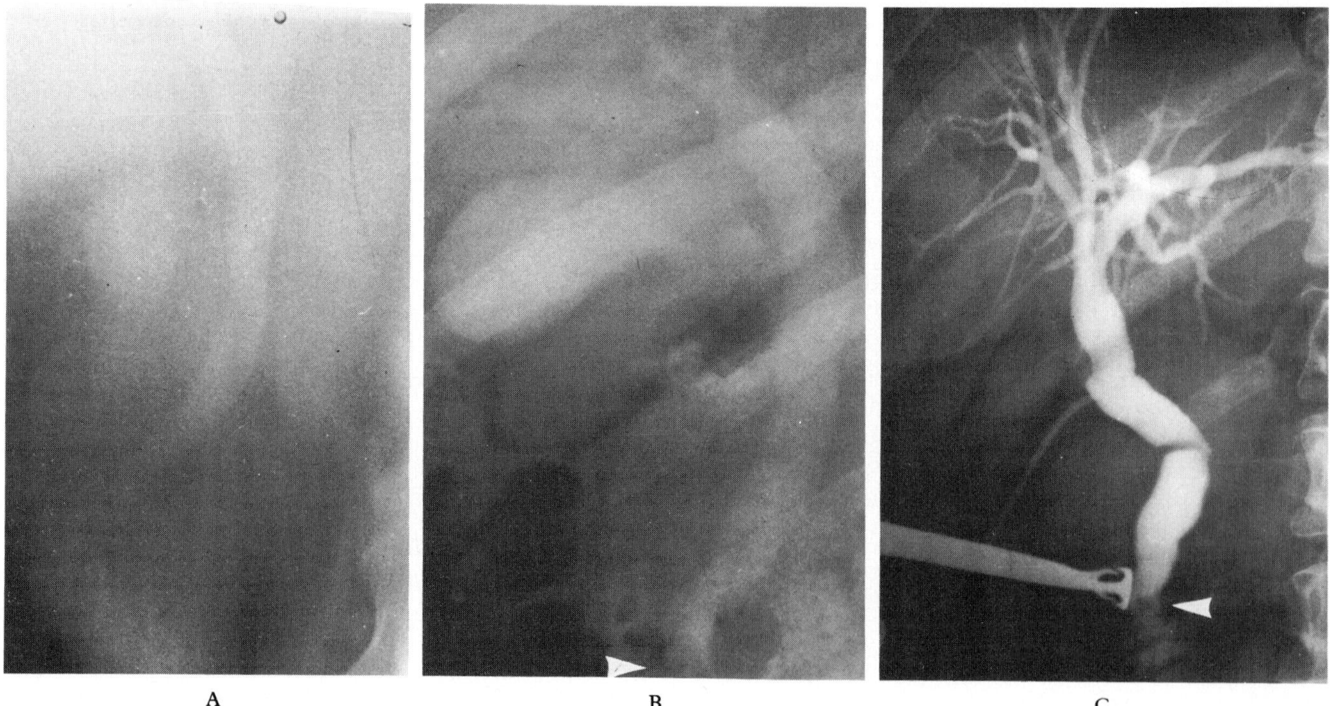

Fig. 37.21 A Intravenous cholangiogram (30 minutes tomograph). Apparently normal duct. B Two hour film, showing increase in duct distension, stasis and suspicion of stones at the ampulla (→). Shrunken gallbladder containing no stones. C Operative cholangiography confirmed the presence of duct stones (←). No stones found in gallbladder.

and its hepatic radicles and record its calibre. The use of a water-soluble contrast medium, such as Urografin 35 per cent, Conray 35 per cent or Hypaque 25 per cent and the exclusion of air bubbles are essential, as in operative cholangiography.

Post-operative intravenous cholangiography. In this examination the assessment of the ease of flow into the duodenum is much more subtle. Minor degrees of obstruction may be impossible to detect radiologically and the diagnosis is certainly not to be influenced by the presence or absence of visible contrast medium in the duodenum.

The diagnosis of partial obstruction is reached if *stasis* can be demonstrated. This feature is most reliable in post-cholecystectomy patients or in those pre-operative cases in which the cystic duct is obstructed ('pathological cholecystectomy'). It is made manifest by:

1. An overfull common bile duct remaining distended to its maximum capacity irrespective of calibre.
2. Corresponding distention and overfilling of the hepatic radicles rendering these unusually visible (Fig. 37.15c).
3. Failure of diminution of the density of the duct on a film taken 2 hours after injection (Fig. 37.20). Normally visualization of the duct decreases markedly in density at this time.

Stasis means existing obstruction and any increase in calibre is corroborative evidence of this (Fig. 37.15B and C). Conversely and obviously, absence of stasis and no increase in calibre indicates no obstruction. If the duct increases in size post-operatively but there is no detectable stasis, this suggests either the obstruction has been overcome (e.g. passage of a calculus previously retained) or that it is intermittent in character (ball-valve calculus Fig. 37.21).

THE VISUALIZATION OF AN OBSTRUCTING AGENT

The appearances of calculi in the duct are well known and common to all forms of cholangiography. They are most easily detected in T-tube cholangiograms where even the smallest may be visible, often accompanied by secondary signs of obstruction.

Stones may also be shown in the hepatic radicles (Fig. 37.22). These are sometimes responsible for recurrent stone formation in the common duct in cases which have been otherwise normal on post-operative T-tube examinations. Their position may indicate that they are quite inaccessible to the surgeon but their presence will affect the prognosis.

It is important to remember that the presence of a stone in the common bile duct does not necessarily result in obvious stasis or dilated duct. As a result, it is unsafe to rely upon normal calibre and the absence of stasis without a thorough search for filling defects (Fig. 37.23). In intravenous work small calculi may be difficult to detect and the routine use of tomography with good technique is all important.

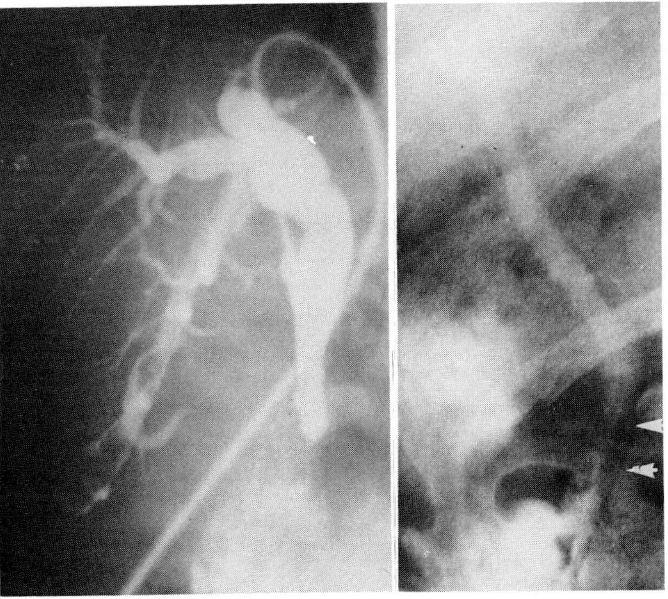

Fig. 37.22 *Fig. 37.23*

Fig. 37.22 T-tube cholangiogram showing stones in the lower branches of the right hepatic duct.

Fig. 37.23 Stones visible in the common duct (*arrows*). Note absence of obstructive signs, i.e. no dilatation, no stasis.

Differential diagnosis of duct obstruction

The importance of the stasis concept is best illustrated by those post-operative cases in whom no previous records of duct calibre are available and no calculi can be seen (Fig. 37.24). In this respect two separate series of cases 14 years apart by different authors have arrived at similar conclusions, *viz*: that the presence of stones in the duct proved subsequently at surgery was visible in only 60 per cent of cases on previous intravenous cholangiography; in one series, duct stones were seen in 86 per cent at subsequent operative cholangiography (Wise, 1962; Faris *et al.*, 1975).

The importance, therefore, of the indirect signs of duct obstruction cannot be emphasised too strongly in all forms of cholangiography; only in the T-tube examinations does stone visualization approach 100 per cent.

In post-operative intravenous cholangiography, therefore, the differentiation of obstruction due to stone which is not visible from that due to ampullary stenosis or chronic pancreatitis may not be possible radiologically, especially in the absence of pre-operative or other radiographs of duct calibre or operative surgical findings. In these cases the only diagnosis possible is 'obstructed duct, cause not evident'.

On the other hand, when such records are available they may reveal that a previously normal common duct not containing stone associated with a patent distensible gallbladder has dilated and shown stasis following the cholecystectomy. In some of these cases the cholecystectomy will have revealed evidence of chronic pancreatitis; a few of these may have shown corroborative radiological pancreatic calcification and/or compression on the pancreatic portion of the duct (Fig. 37.25). Other cases on re-exploration (Fig. 37.15c) will disclose ampullary stenosis.

It would seem that in these cases the patent distensible gallbladder has been acting as a pressure safety valve in the pre-operative period. If the cystic duct becomes obstructed ('pathological cholecystectomy') then any common duct signs of obstruction due to chronic pancreatitis or to ampullary stenosis would already be established. As examples, Wise (1962) described a series of 22 patients with primary chronic pancreatitis; of these 16 had normal common ducts associated with patent gallbladders. Of the remaining 6, 2 showed signs of duct stasis with a patent gallbladder while 3 showed duct stasis with obstructed cystic duct. The remaining case had stones in the duct. Similarly, in 12 patients with ampullary stenosis, the only 2 normal ducts were cases associated with patent gallbladders.

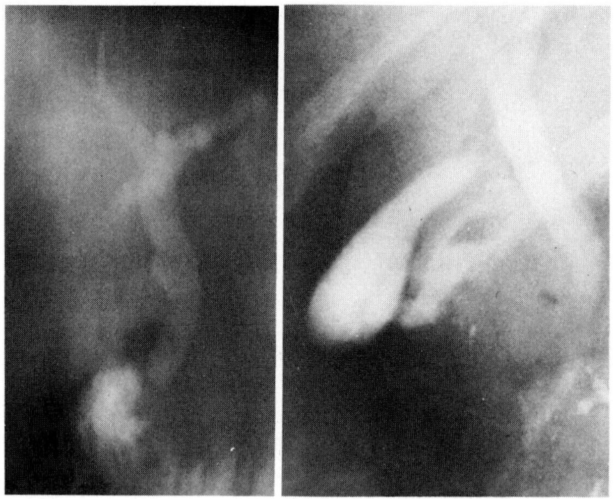

Fig. 37.24 *Fig. 37.25*

Fig. 37.24 Obstructed duct showing stasis, dilatation but no visible calculi. Note that visibility of contrast medium in the duodenum is not relevant. Ampullary stenosis at surgery.

Fig. 37.25 Chronic pancreatitis showing calcification, compressing the pancreatic portion of the duct and causing obstructive signs.

It would appear, therefore, that in post-cholecystectomy cases showing signs of duct stasis and obstruction, a differential diagnosis from stone is possible, provided:

1. A patent distensible gallbladder was present pre-operatively.
2. The common duct and biliary tree were unequivocally free of stone at operation and yet signs of obstruction and stasis have developed post-operatively.
3. No stone is visible.

For this differentiation to be valid, only the strictest criteria of a duct system free from stone at operation are acceptable, e.g. a first class operative choledochogram (if the duct was not explored), or a negative exploration followed by a good post-operative T-tube examination, absence of stone in the hepatic tree etc.

This 'safety valve' phenomenon may therefore mask the true state of affairs pre-operatively. Even at operation and post-operatively, nothing abnormal may be suspected until a return of symptoms results in re-examination and discovery of an obstructed duct. In the known absence of pancreatitis, the alternative diagnosis of ampullary stenosis is likely.

JAUNDICE

When the obstruction is severe enough to cause clinical jaundice, the oral and intravenous methods of examination usually fail, although they may be worth trying if the serum bilirubin is below 2 mg per cent and if the jaundice is waning.

Clinical problems frequently arise in the differentiation of hepatocellular ('medical') from extrahepatic obstructive ('surgical') jaundice. The latter needs surgery while the former must be protected from it. It is evident that a critical discriminating factor in this differentiation is the cholangiogram and the techniques available to obtain it in these patients. There is now little or no place for the 'wait and see' approach to cases of jaundice of obscure origin unless there is a strong clinical bias towards intrahepatic cholestasis.

Other problems may be concerned with the possible presence of liver metastases. Both isotopic liver scans and grey scale ultrasonography can diagnose liver masses (Taylor, 1976) and the latter can often delineate dilated obstructed ducts in extrahepatic obstructive jaundice; being non-invasive, perhaps this should be the first examination in jaundice of obscure origin. Computer tomography is not likely to be generally available for these purposes for some time (Stern *et al.*, 1975).

Four-day Telepaque test. If a non-opaque stone is suspected, as in some cases of obstructive jaundice, it may sometimes be rendered opaque to X-rays by giving the patient 3 g of Telepaque daily for 4 days. If the surface of the stone contains bile pigment it will combine with the medium and may become visible on X-ray. Negative results in this test, as occur with pure cholesterol stones, are consequently of no value, but suitable stones may be rendered opaque in this way, both in the gallbladder and in the common bile duct.

Percutaneous transhepatic cholangiography (PTC). The modern approach is to use a fine Chiba ('skinny') needle of flexible steel (outside diameter 0·71 mm, internal diameter 0·42 mm). This is introduced under basal and local anaesthesia through the skin in the 8th or 9th intercostal space anteriorly in the axilla. It is thrust rapidly and horizontally into the liver in the direction of 12th dorsal vertebra. During slow withdrawal under fluoroscopic control, a continuous trickle of contrast medium such as Conray 280 is injected until a biliary radicle is seen to be tapped. If this is obviously dilated, further contrast medium alternating with aspiration of bile is introduced to outline the system without raising the biliary pressure. A tilting table is required to obtain radiographs in the erect position and so outline the obstruction more clearly. Finally, aspiration prior to the removal of the needle is performed to decompress the system (Jain *et al.*, 1977).

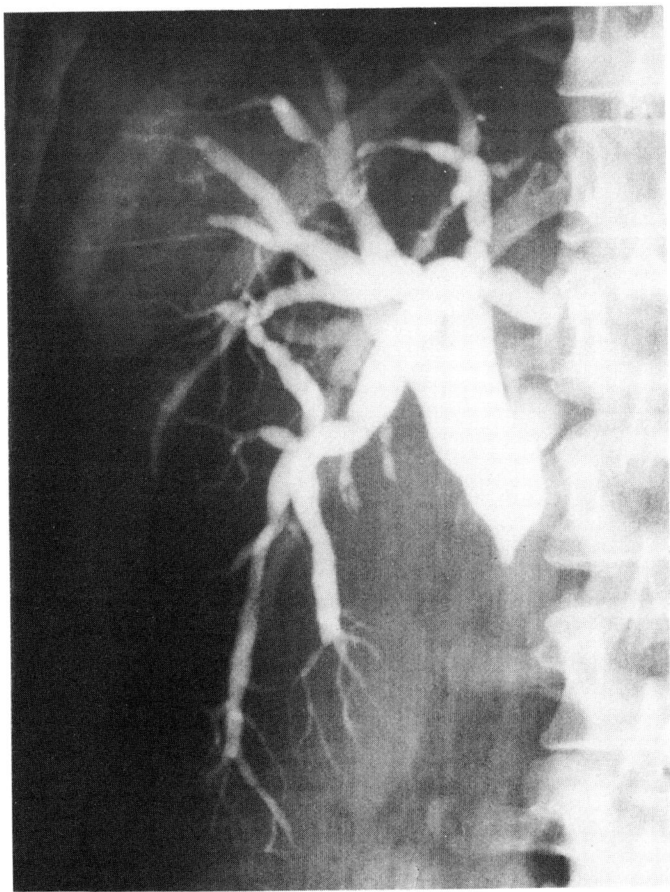

Fig. 37.26 Percutaneous transhepatic cholangiogram showing extrinsic compression of the duct by carcinoma of the head of the pancreas.

It is perfectly possible to puncture a normal biliary system with this technique, but the success rate is lower (60–80 per cent, as against 80–100 per cent in dilated systems). Up to five punctures in slightly different directions is commonly practised, if no radicle is tapped.

Complications. Cholangitis in obstructed cases may occur in about 6 per cent and there is also a risk of biliary peritonitis following leakage after withdrawal of the needle. The examination is therefore preferably performed as a pre-operative investigation under antibiotic cover. These complications occur only after successful puncture of obstructed systems; with a Chiba needle using the technique described, the incidence of leakage is very low (3 per cent—Elias *et al.*, 1976).

Advantages. The cost is low, the personnel do not require great skill and the accuracy is high in diagnosing extrahepatic obstructive jaundice (Fig. 37.26). More recently the technique has been used therapeutically in the jaundice of inoperable cholangiocarcinoma (Fig. 37.36). A P.T.C. catheter sheathed needle is introduced and a guide wire used after a duct has been punctured. This is manipulated through the malignant stricture and used to site an endoprosthesis (a 10 cm Teflon tube with side holes). Excellent palliative results can be achieved and additional prolongation of a comfortable existence ensured for one to two years, since these tumours grow quite slowly.

Endoscopy and retrograde cholangiopancreatography (ERCP). As an alternative examination to transhepatic cholangiography, the development of fibro-endoscopes, such as the Olympus J.F.B., has a definite place in the investigation of jaundice of obscure origin.

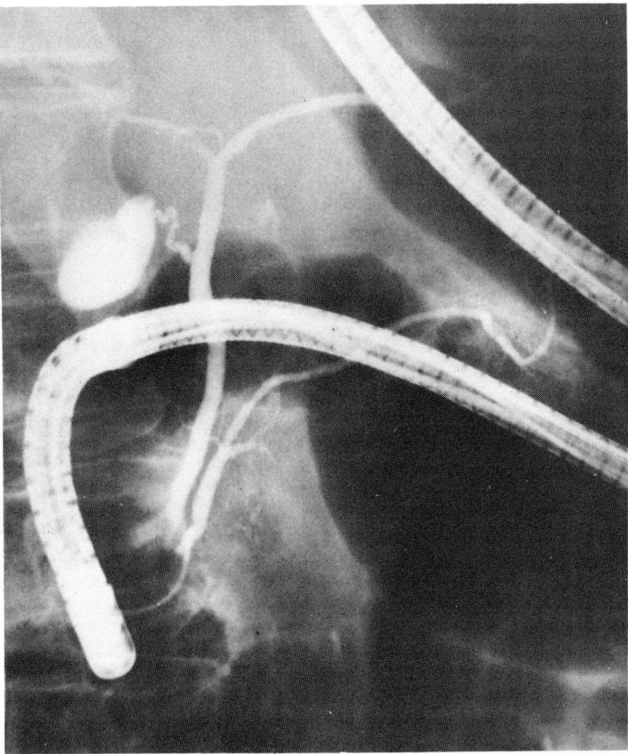

Fig. 37.27 Normal ERCP of biliary and pancreatic duct systems.

ERCP is a difficult technique requiring an experienced endoscopist, an enthusiastic radiologist and at least one technical assistant. Under local and sedative anaesthesia the instrument is passed through the stomach into the duodenum where, with its lateral viewing lens, manually controlled flexible tip and facilities for the passage of a 1.6 mm Teflon catheter, the papilla of Vater is cannulated under image intensifier control. Aqueous contrast is gently introduced to outline the common bile duct from below. In the best and the most experienced hands the success rate is about 90 per cent and the examination may take up to one hour to perform (Fig. 37.27).

Indications. ERCP should be used in three possible situations: (i) persistent or recurrent jaundice of obscure origin; (ii) hepatic disease (e.g. biliary cirrhosis) in which orthodox intravenous cholangiography has failed; (iii) known or suspected pancreatic disease (see below).

Contra-indications. The examination should not be used following a recent attack of pancreatitis or in the presence of Australian antigenaemia; the latter entails a risk of spread of infection to subsequent patients as the instrument is difficult to sterilize effectively.

Morbidity. Complications are uncommon; the serum amylase rises between 5 and 15 hours after the examination in about 30 per cent of cases and may be associated with some abdominal discomfort. It usually settles to normal values in 2 to 5 days. Occasional cases of Gram negative septicaemia have been described following this examination, but they usually respond to antibiotic treatment. ERCP is therefore preferably performed on in-patients under local anaesthesia.

Advantages. ERCP can be used early in the disease without waiting for the jaundice to wax or wane and can provide unequivocable evidence of both intra- and extra-hepatic cholestasis. While it would seem, therefore, that it should be the next cholangiographic investigation in obscure jaundice, it is only likely to be available in major centres for some time to come. The instrument is expensive and the technique requires significant commitment of resources and trained endoscopic workers.

Comparison of PTC and ERCP. These two examinations are complementary in some cases. A randomized trial of these two techniques showed that PTC was most effective in extra-hepatic obstructive jaundice with dilated hepatic radicles, while ERCP was more valuable when the ducts were normal (Elias *et al.*, 1976). In addition, ERCP has visual and biopsy advantages in the stomach, duodenum and at the level of the papilla, as well as advantages in the assessment of both the biliary and pancreatic duct systems at one examination; furthermore, there are also therapeutic possibilities in those cases with retained duct stones after surgery (see below). Finally, ERCP enables samples of both pancreatic and biliary secretions to be obtained for analysis (Cotton and Heap, 1975).

THE PASSAGE OF STONES

The stones found in the common duct originate in the gallbladder in the vast majority of cases. Such stones may either pass into the duodenum (Fig. 37.28) or alternatively remain in the duct. Movement of stones can occur at any time and may take place between the radiological examination and operation (Fig. 37.6). Lack of symptoms is no proof that stones have not entered the common duct. It is for these reasons that pre-exploratory operative cholangiography, which assesses the state of the duct at the time of operation, is preferable to pre-operative oral or intravenous examinations which may give a false sense of security.

The factors controlling the passage of stones are not known. There is no doubt that stones left behind at operation may occasionally be passed, particularly if a sphincterotomy has been performed (Fig. 37.28). More commonly, however, a second operation is required for their removal. The value to both the patient and surgeon of making the diagnosis by post-exploratory operative cholangiography at the time of the primary operation is obvious.

An occasional case of stone in the common duct without stones in the gallbladder may be encountered. In our series this occurred in about 2 per cent of all cases of gallstones coming to surgery (Fig. 37.21B).

Non-surgical removal of retained duct stones. In spite of the use of operative cholangiography stones are still occasionally left behind after surgery. An alternative technique has been developed for their removal which requires fluoroscopic assistance. Patients who are relatively poor surgical risks are particularly suitable for consideration in this respect and fall into two groups:

A. Patients with a T-tube in situ (immediate post-cholecystectomy cases—Fig. 37.29A).

B. Post-cholecystectomy patients without a T-tube (late post operative) with or without obstructive jaundice (Fig. 37.23).

Group A. (1) If the stone is not large (less than 8 mm in diameter) successful passage may occur with irrigation of the duct for several days at the rate of 30cc/hour, using either simple saline or attempting simultaneous dissolution with sodium cholate or heparin.

(2) ERCP papillotomy (see below), followed by infusion as in (1).

(3) ERCP with removal of stones by use of a Dormia basket or balloon catheter if (2) has failed after about a week.

(4) Removal of residual stones by Dormia basket via the T-tube track.

On discovery of retained stones post-operatively, the patient is discharged from hospital for 5 weeks to allow formation of a fibrous wall round the T-tube; on returning, the T-tube cholangiogram is repeated in case the stones have passed spontaneously. If they have not,

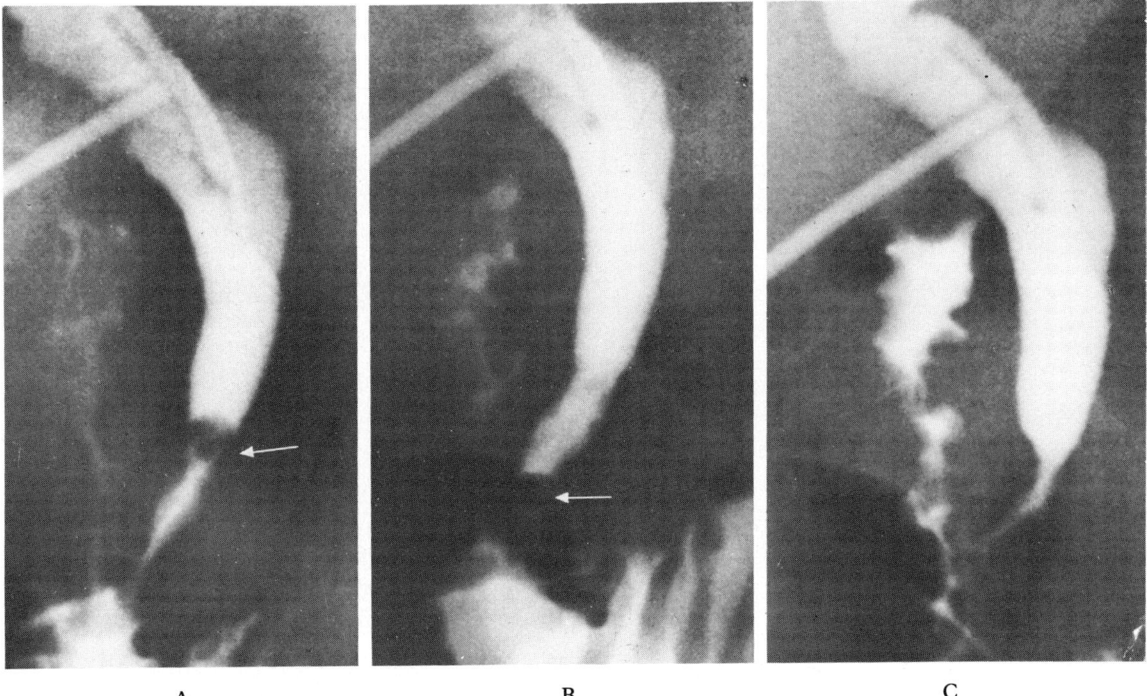

Fig. 37.28 Post-operative T-tube cholangiogram showing a stone being passed during the examination (A and B *arrows*) A sphincterotomy had been performed.

the T-tube is removed either over a Seldinger wire previously introduced or, alternatively, a steerable catheter is guided into the track and introduced beyond the visible stones under fluoroscopic control; through this a Dormia basket is threaded, positioned beyond a stone and then opened to snare it and so remove it via the T-tube track. Provided that the latter is at least 14F in size, a skilled operator can expect 95 per cent success

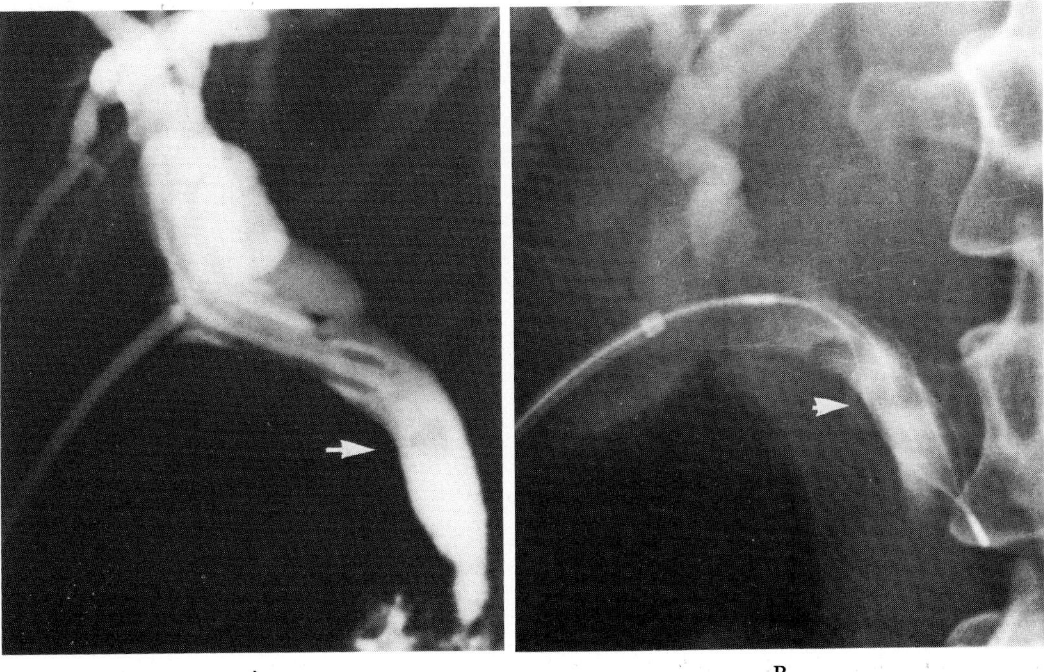

Fig. 37.29 A Retained stone on T-tube examination 5 weeks after cholecystectomy (→). B Snaring a stone in Dormia basket via the T-tube track (→).

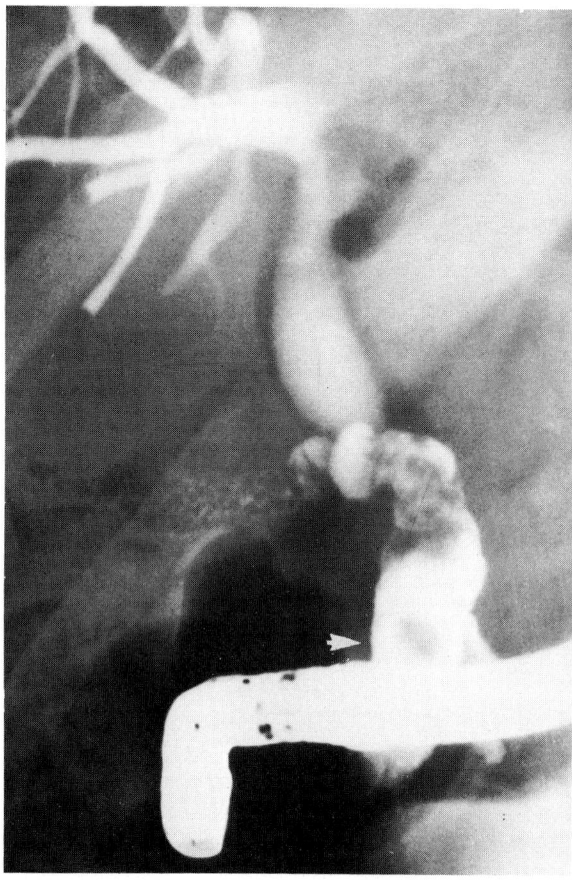
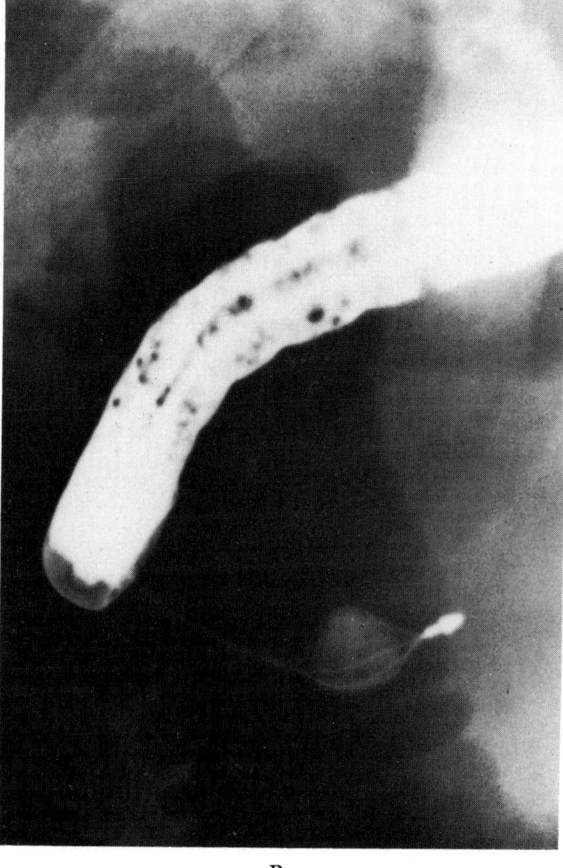

A B

Fig. 37.30 A ERCP showing stone (*arrow*) remaining in lower end of duct following unsuccessful attempt at removal via the T-tube track. Papillotomy performed. B Successful removal with Dormia basket one week after papillotomy.

with no mortality and only about 5 per cent morbidity (pancreatitis, infection, bile extravasation—Burhenne 1976) (Fig. 37.29).

Another modern variation of technique is the extraction of residual duct stones through the T-tube tract using direct vision by means of a choledochoscope. This has the advantage of saving both time and irradiation as it has both balloon and basket facilities. A wide T-tube tract however is essential.

Group B. In these cases the diagnosis of extra-hepatic obstruction by stone is confirmed by ERCP prior to attempted removal. This entails performing papillotomy under Diazepam sedation through the roof of the papilla, using a diathermy wire via an insulated duodenoscope. Re-examination a week later by ERCP will determine both the size of the papillotomy and whether (as is usual) the stones have passed spontaneously; if not, they are extracted using a Dormia basket or balloon catheter through the instrument under fluoroscopic control (Fig. 37.30). With stones of 1 cm diameter or less, a skilled endoscopist can expect success in over 80 per cent of cases. (Cotton *et al.*, 1976; Safrany, 1977). Complications (haemorrhage, perforation, pancreatitis) are uncommon (2 deaths in a series of 130 cases—Rosch, 1975).

A similar approach can be used in cases of papillary stenosis; the abnormal kinetics associated with this are helpful in confirming the diagnosis prior to diathermy by showing a dilated duct which is apparently free of stones and yet shows poor flow. In general the sphincter becomes incompetent following papillotomy in about 60 per cent of cases (Safrany, 1977).

As an alternative technique, a fine catheter can be left in the duct following papillotomy, bringing the endoscope out over it; this can be used for subsequent cholangiography to see if the stones have passed.

GAS IN THE BILIARY TRACT

A plain film of the upper abdomen may show the gall-bladder and/or the bile ducts outlined by gas. The possible causes are:

1. Operative. Gas in the biliary tree may be seen following operations such as cholecystojejunostomy performed for inoperable carcinoma of the pancreas in

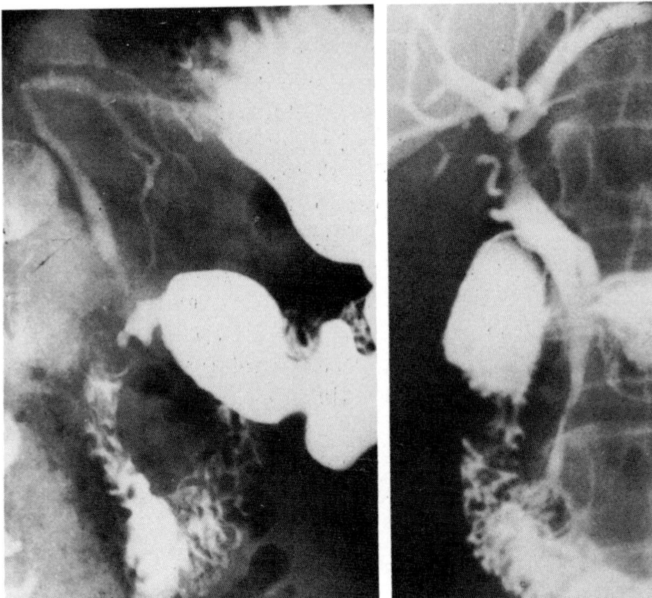

Fig. 37.31 *Fig. 37.32*

Fig. 37.31 Barium entering the common duct from a penetrating duodenal ulcer.

Fig. 37.32 Barium entering the common duct via the ampulla of Vater following extensive sphincterotomy.

order to relieve jaundice. The implantation of the common duct into the small bowel during operations such as partial pancreatectomy and duodenectomy will also result in gas in the biliary tract, as will ERCP papillotomy (60 per cent).

2. Spontaneous biliary fistulae. These cases are due to large stones in the gallbladder ulcerating through into the neighbouring alimentary tract, to which the chronically inflamed gallbladder has become adherent. Commonly, the hollow viscus involved is the duodenum, but occasionally the colon is implicated. Other cases may be due to chronic duodenal ulcer penetrating the common duct. In these cases the diagnosis can be confirmed by an opaque meal or enema (Fig. 37.31).

If gas is seen in the biliary tree on radiographs taken for intestinal obstruction, the possibility of gallstone ileus due to impaction of a large stone in the small gut must be remembered; if the stone is opaque, a definite diagnosis can be made.

3. Regurgitation through the ampulla of Vater. This is an uncommon cause of gas in the bile duct but may occur after operations on the sphincter of Oddi (sphincterotomy, Fig. 37.32). A careful barium meal examination will differentiate this condition from the spontaneous biliary fistulae into the duodenum described above. Incompetence of the sphincter may also follow the passage of stones, but this is rarely seen.

4. Emphysematous cholecystitis. Infection with gas-forming organisms is a rare condition usually associated with diabetes. The gas may be intramural as well as intraluminal; erect pictures will show a fluid level in the gallbladder. Owing to inflammatory obstruction of the cystic duct, the gas does not enter the bile duct; this is a differential diagnostic point from the other causes of gas in the gallbladder (Fig. 37.33).

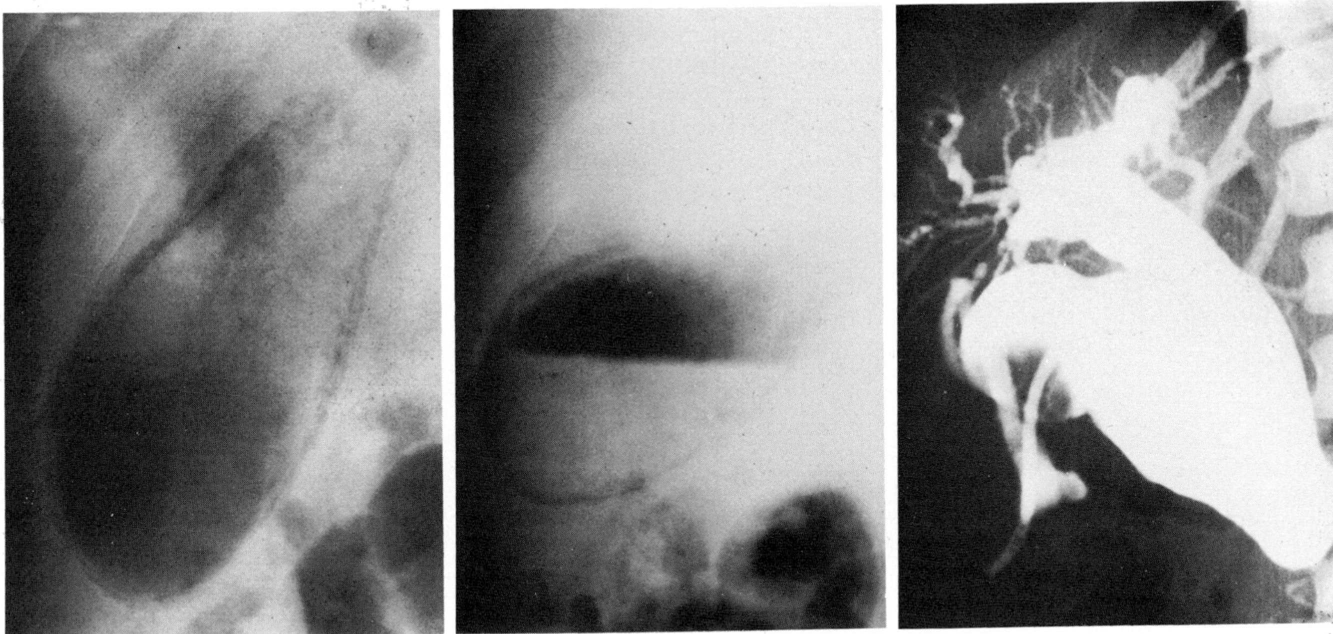

Fig. 37.33A *Fig. 37.33B* *Fig. 37.34*

Fig. 37.33 Emphysematous cholecystitis showing (A) gas in the lumen and wall of the gallbladder (B) a gas fluid level in the erect posture.

Fig. 37.34 Choledochal cyst (operative cholangiogram).

CONGENITAL ABNORMALITIES OF THE BILE DUCTS

Some of the common congenital variations of the normal duct system which may be discovered at operative or intravenous cholangiography have been described above.

Biliary atresia. The degree and extent of biliary atresia varies from case to case and determines the possibility of successful operative intervention. These patients present with deepening jaundice noted soon after birth and the radiological investigation is therefore almost entirely confined to the operating theatre. Cholangiograms performed at operation via a patent gallbladder will give information useful to the surgeon.

Choledochal cyst. This condition is characterized by a cystic dilation of the common duct. It usually affects the supraduodenal portion and may also involve the hepatic and cystic ducts. It is four times commoner in females than in males. Most cases present in the first two decades of life with pain, intermittent jaundice and a palpable mass.

Radiologically, the cyst shows as a soft tissue mass separate from the kidney. It may displace the stomach and duodenum, and also the hepatic flexure (Fig. 37.34). Contrast medium examinations are often unsuccessful, but repeated doses of oral media may show the gallbladder and also on occasions the choledochal cyst, especially if the jaundice is not severe. In more severe cases ultrasonography, computerised tomography and radioisotope scanning may be helpful.

Choledochocoele (Fig. 37.35). This is a rare anomaly consisting of either a ureterocoele-like dilatation of the lower end of the common bile duct, or alternatively, as a lateral diverticulum of the same region. It may cause episodic pain, jaundice and vomiting and present as a negative filling defect at the ampulla on the medial wall of the duodenum during barium studies and be confused with the other causes of this appearance (Fig. 37.46). It does not fill with barium and yet is usually lined with duodenal and not common duct mucosa (Hatfield, Scholtz and Wise, 1976).

TUMOURS OF THE BILE DUCTS

(*i*) *Benign.* These are rare and occur in the ampullary region, a papilloma or adenoma being the commonest. They may cause obstructive jaundice and are usually mistaken for calculi on cholangiography.

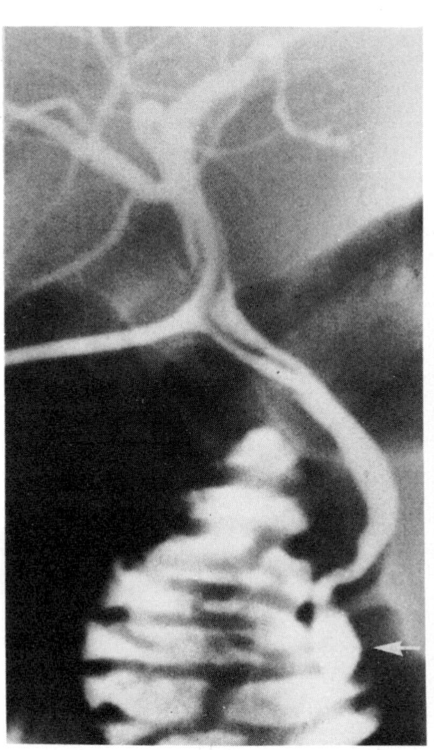

Fig. 37.35

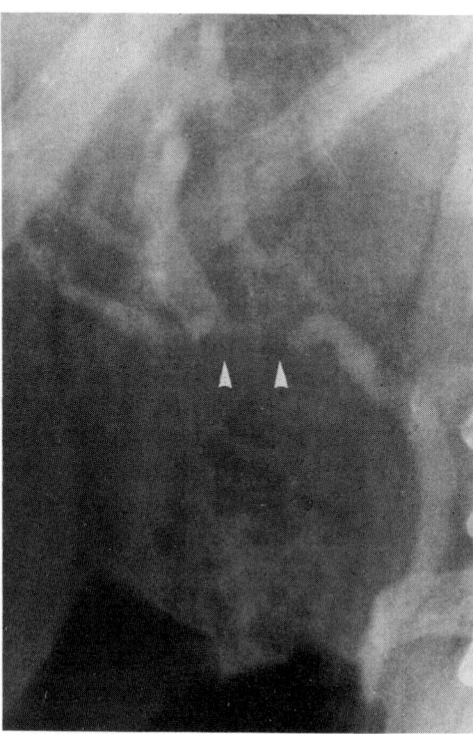

Fig. 37.36

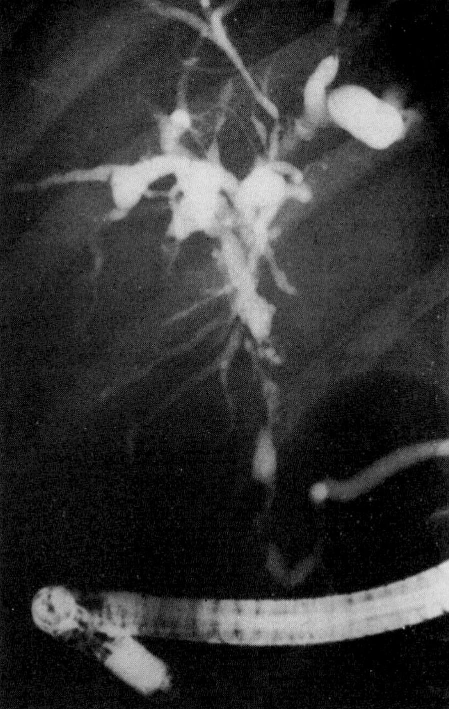

Fig. 37.37

Fig. 37.35 Choledochocoele (←). Accidental finding on postoperative T-tube examination.

Fig. 37.36 Carcinoma of the right hepatic duct (*arrows*) causing a stricture (intravenous cholangiogram).

Fig. 37.37 Sclerosing cholangitis (ERCP) showing multiple strictures in the hepatic and common ducts.

(*ii*) *Malignant.* The commonest tumour is an adenocarcinoma but it is still a rarity. The patient is usually obstructively jaundiced and the diagnosis is therefore dependent on one of the cholangiographic techniques already described, mainly PTC with ERCP. Operative cholangiography will also confirm. (Fig. 37.36).

INFECTIONS

Sclerosing cholangitis. This is a rare disease of unknown origin associated with ulcerative colitis in about 30 per cent of cases. The main appearances are those of multiple strictures of the intrahepatic ducts with beading and dilatations. The extra-hepatic and common ducts also show similar changes and there is often secondary cirrhosis of the liver; consequently, intravenous cholangiography is rarely successful and the best method of demonstrating the condition is by ERCP (Fig. 37.37). The disease is associated with fever, jaundice, hepatomegaly and splenomegaly and has a high mortality.

Parasites. Patients infected with *Ascaris lumbricoides* may present with symptoms of cholangitis or cholecystitis and are found to have a migrating worm in the common bile duct and/or gallbladder (Fig. 37.38). The diagnosis may be suspected on oral or intravenous cholangiography.

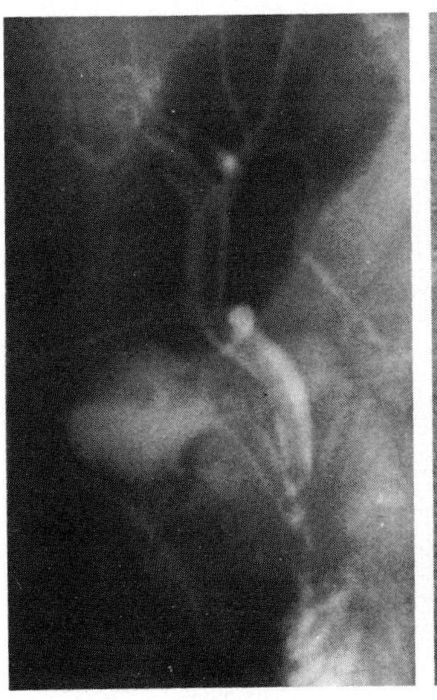

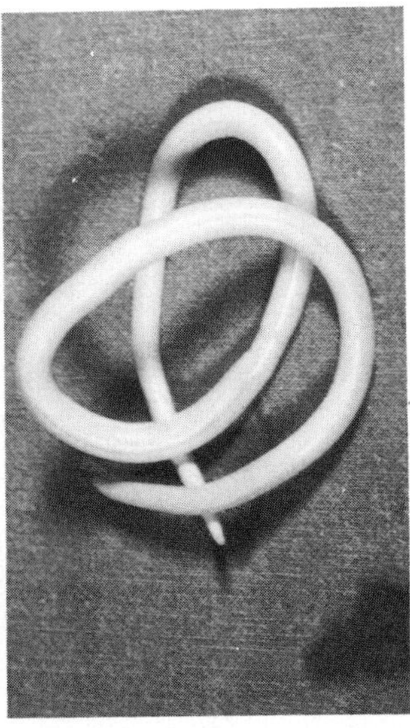

A B

Fig. 37.38 A Ascaris worm in the biliary ducts. B Specimen after surgical removal.

Clinorchis sinensis. This is a liver fluke, which may also occasionally occupy the bile ducts and can be seen as curved crescentic defects on cholangiography.

B. THE PANCREAS

Radiological demonstration of the pancreas has been difficult until recent years. Simple X-rays and barium studies will only demonstrate large masses displacing other organs, or the occasional calcification seen in chronic pancreatitis. However, in recent years new and improved techniques of imaging have changed the situation and a whole battery of new tests is now available. These include:

1. Hypotonic duodenography
2. ERCP (endoscopic retrograde choledochopancreatography)
3. Angiography
4. Isotope scanning
5. Ultrasound
6. CAT (computerised axial tomography)

The methods used will depend on the clinical problem and to some extent on the apparatus and expertise available at individual centres. Generally speaking, however, the simpler non-invasive techniques such as ultrasound and simple X-rays should be used in the first place. CAT can provide vital diagnostic information with most pancreatic masses and cysts and, if available, should be used where ultrasound produces doubtful or equivocal results. Isotope scanning has proved rather disappointing because of the high rate of false positives and false negative results (see Chapter 66). It should be regarded as a complementary technique to confirm or give evidence against equivocal results by other methods. The more invasive techniques of angiography and ERCP should be reserved for cases which cannot be confidently diagnosed by non-invasive techniques. However, they may be essential in certain cases, e.g. the localization of small islet cell tumours by angiography.

In this section we are concerned largely with the simpler radiological methods and ERCP; fuller details about ultrasound, isotope scanning and CAT will be found in the chapters devoted to these subjects in Part VIII and angiography is discussed in Chapter 29.

Swellings in the head of the pancreas may affect the pyloric antrum, duodenal bulb or duodenal circle; the common bile duct may be obstructed (Fig. 37.39). The use of hypotonic duodenography, with or without the double contrast technique, has undoubtedly added to the accuracy of diagnosis of lesions affecting the duodenal circle. While it is more time consuming, it is

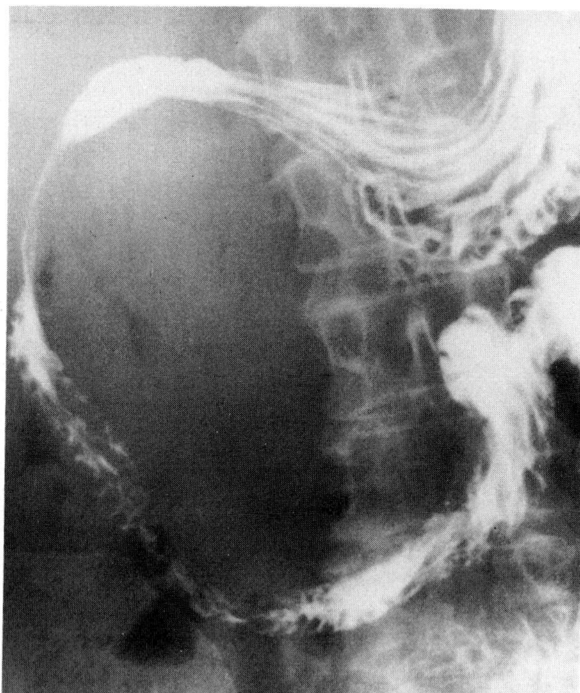

Fig. 37.39

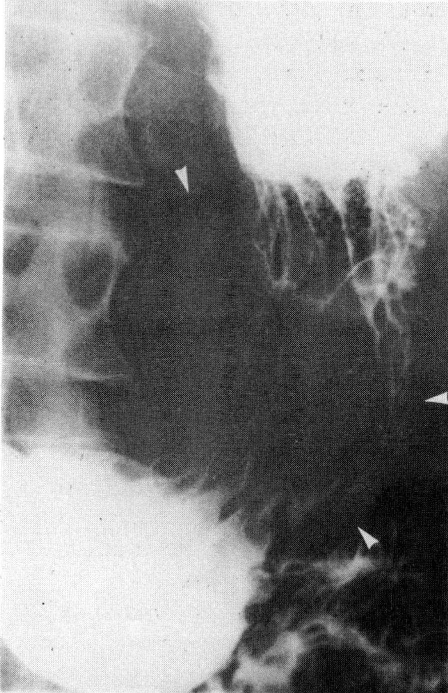

Fig. 37.40

Fig. 37.39 Large carcinoma of the head of the pancreas displacing and compressing the pyloric antrum and duodenal circle.

Fig. 37.40 Soft tissue mass in the tail of the pancreas, indenting the body of the stomach (*arrows*). This proved to be an adenocarcinoma at surgery.

particularly indicated in most patients in whom the activity of the pylorus and duodenum renders it impossible to obtain good distention pictures by the conventional methods. In enlargement of the body and tail of the pancreas, the stomach will be displaced and the duodeno-jejunal flexure may be depressed (Fig. 37.40). Such displacements, however, can be closely mimicked by large swellings of the left kidney or adrenal gland, by enlargement of the spleen or by an abscess or cyst in the lesser sac.

Congenital abnormalities—annular pancreas

In this condition, the descending loop (second part) of the duodenum is narrowed or occluded by the pressure of an annular band of normal pancreatic tissue. The condition is uncommon and usually presents in infancy with signs of pyloric obstruction. As with infantile pyloric stenosis, male cases predominate, but in duodenal obstruction the vomit contains bile. Some cases present in adults (Fig. 37.41).

Plain radiography will show a gas-distended stomach and duodenal bulb, with little or no gas in the rest of the bowel. In infants, differentiation from congenital duodenal stenosis may be difficult or impossible even with the use of an opaque meal. About half the cases show other anomalies such as malrotation of the gut, oesophageal atresia, congenital heart disease or Down's syndrome.

Acute pancreatitis

While the majority of patients show elevation of the serum amylase, about 5 per cent do not and radiology and even laparotomy may be necessary to establish the diagnosis.

Plain radiography is useful to exclude a perforation or an obstruction. It may also assist by showing retroperitoneal oedema with obliteration of the psoas shadows, general ileus of the gut and occasionally gallstones, the latter being associated with about half the cases in this country (Trapnell, 1974). In sub-acute cases (or even acute cases) a barium or gastrografin study will show obvious swelling of the pancreatic head displacing the duodenal circle (Fig. 37.42); gastrografin can also be used with safety in the differentiation from perforated peptic ulcer (Fraser and Fraser, 1974), especially in those cases in which no air is seen beneath the diaphragm on erect plain films.

Ultrasound is of great value in the detection of subsequent pseudocyst development, and particularly in differentiating this diagnosis from pancreatic abscess or carcinoma which is often not possible radiologically (Fig. 37.40;—Duncan *et al.*, 1976). Pseudocysts appear to occur more frequently in those cases associated with alcoholism than those with biliary disease. The majority of acute cases, however, have an idiopathic background. There is an appreciable mortality, particularly in the

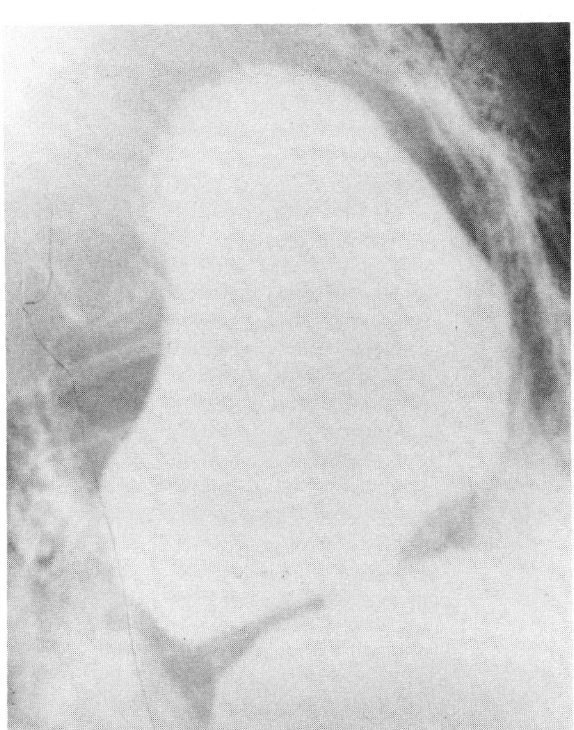

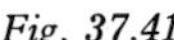

Fig. 37.41

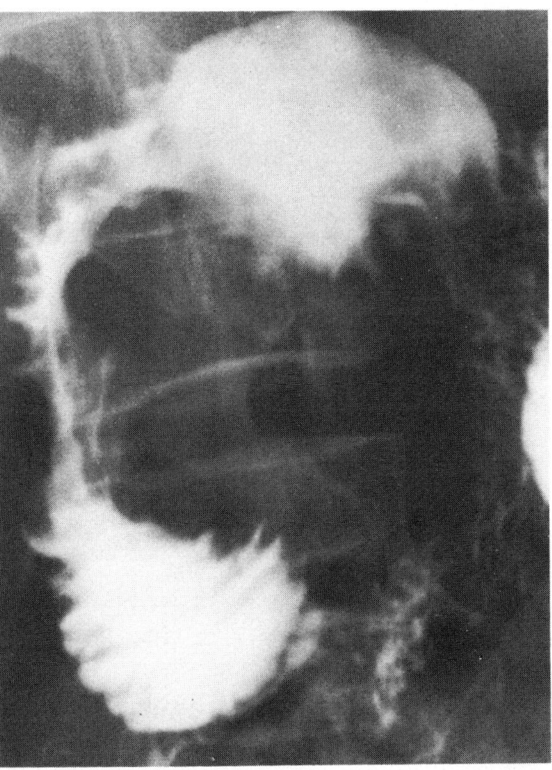

Fig. 37.42

Fig. 37.41 Post-bulbar duodenal obstruction by annular pancreas presenting in an adult.

Fig. 37.42 Swelling of the head of the pancreas due to sub-acute pancreatitis.

elderly and in alcoholic cases. Alcoholism plays a large part in the U.S.A. and is showing an increasing importance as an aetiological agent in the U.K. (Trapnell, 1974).

Chronic pancreatitis

In most cases, no positive radiological signs can be detected either with plain films or on barium studies. Calcification occurs late and infrequently in chronic pancreatitis (Fig. 37.43) and is therefore of limited clinical value. Pancreatic isotope scanning with 75 Se-Seleno-methionine proved disappointing because of the significant incidence of false negative results (21 per cent—Baron, 1975).

Similarly, arteriography, which is a difficult technique requiring much experience, cannot exclude chronic pancreatitis or even carcinoma if its findings are normal; moreover, even in abnormal cases the differentiation of these two conditions can be difficult and this applies also to isotope scanning (Agnew *et al.*, 1976).

ERCP in pancreatitis. By careful manipulation of the catheter, the expert can selectively fill the pancreatic duct. ERCP is a powerful tool in the investigation of obscure abdominal pain, even in the absence of jaundice, as it allows a complete survey of stomach, duodenum, papilla, biliary and pancreatic systems (Fig. 37.27). In experienced hands a successful pancreatogram can be obtained in 90 per cent of cases. Depending on the stage and severity of any case of chronic pancreatitis, ERCP may show duct stenosis and/or obstruction (Fig. 37.44B, C). It may even be normal in mild cases, leaving the diagnosis in doubt, yet pure pancreatic juice can be obtained for analysis and in any case such findings will guide the clinician away from surgery.

When this examination shows an obstructed main duct, differentiation from a carcinoma may be difficult on radiological grounds alone; in such cases cytology may

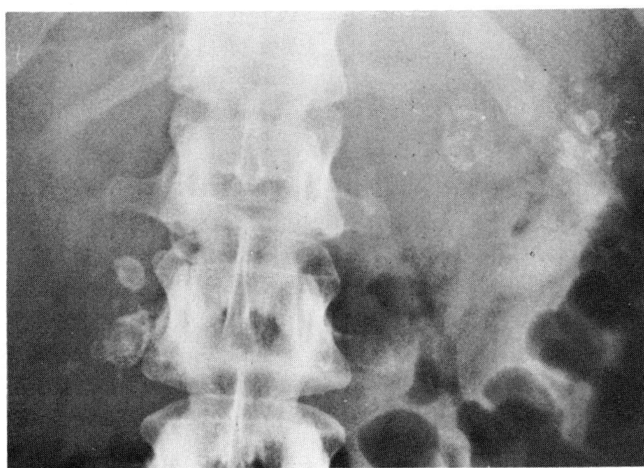

Fig. 37.43 Chronic pancreatitis showing typical calcification across the upper abdomen.

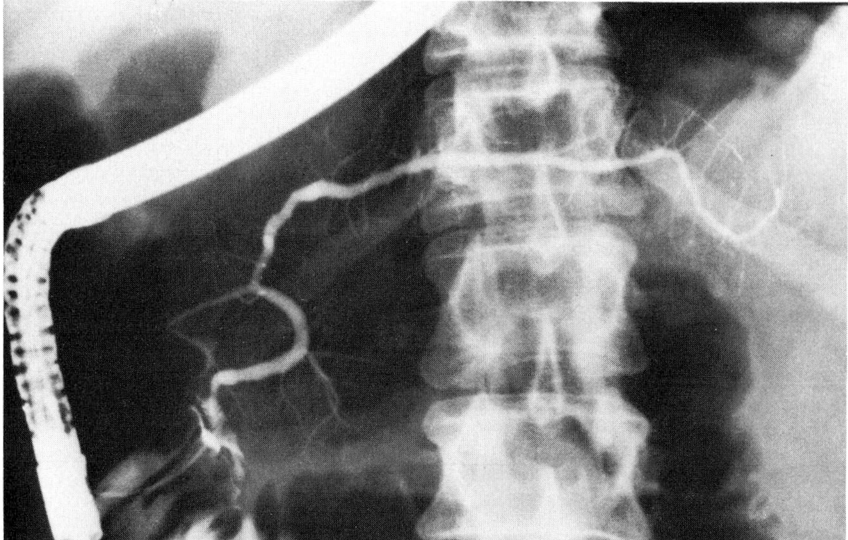

A

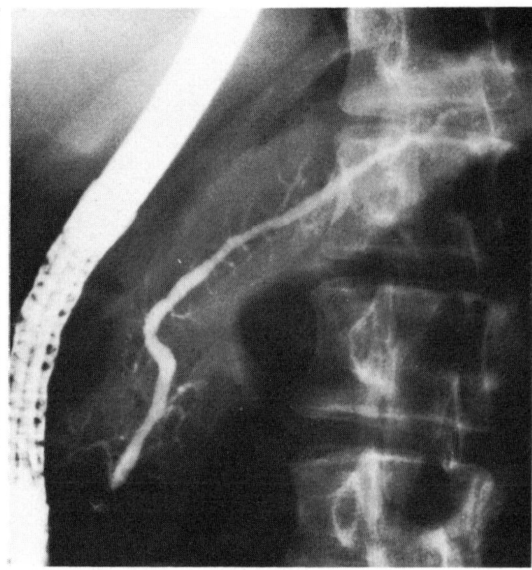

B

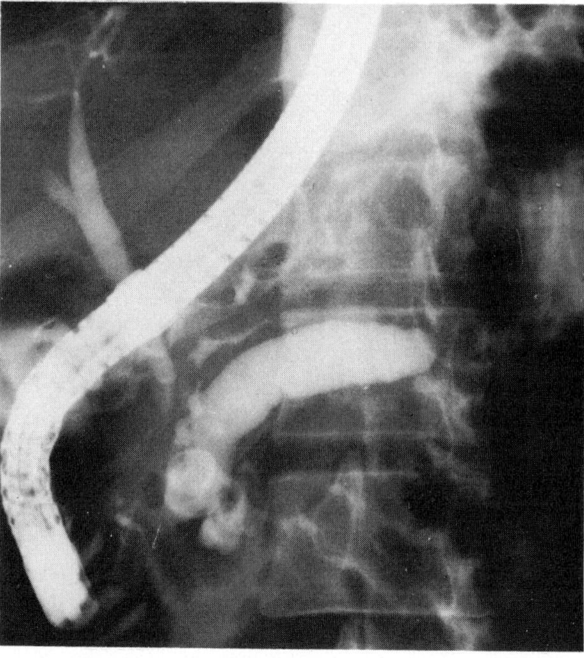

C

Fig. 37.44 A Normal pancreaticogram. B Chronic pancreatitis showing irregularity and stunting of the branches of the duct and shrinkage of the gland. C Gross chronic pancreatitis with marked dilatation of the main duct, very few patent branches and obstruction of the duct near the tail. The common bile duct is normal.

be helpful. Pseudocysts rarely fill with contrast medium and consequently ERCP is of little value in their diagnosis, unlike grey scale ultrasound and computed tomography which have definite places in the diagnosis of pancreatic masses generally (Burger and Blauenstein, 1974; Kreel, 1977).

Complications. As in operative pancreatography, acute pancreatitis may develop following this examination in about 1 to 2 per cent of cases and, as stated above, 30 per cent will show changes in the serum amylase.

Congenital pancreatic duct variation. Variations occur as the result of the fact that the pancreas develops from two distinct parts—a ventral portion forming the head of the organ which springs from the lower end of the biliary duct with its own draining duct of Wirsung and a dorsal portion which develops quite separately arising from and opening into the duodenum. The latter is by far the larger part and consequently most of the duct of the pancreas originates from this section which fuses with the ventral portion. The ducts also fuse, the proximal portion of the dorsal pancreas (duct of Santorini) losing its opening and becoming a tributary and the junction quite often being sharply angulated (Fig. 37.44A).

In some cases the opening of the duct of Santorini into the duodenum may persist and the ducts may fail to fuse. Two pancreatic papillae are then present, the former proximal to the latter; consequently ERCP may outline the head only and a search must then be instituted for the second opening to complete the examination. Other variations consist of (i) two openings in spite of successful fusion of the ducts (ii) a blind end to the duct of Santorini proximally and finally (iii) complete obliteration of this proximal portion.

Pancreatic cysts. The retention cyst is the result of obstruction following pancreatitis and may reach a large size. False cysts may also occur in the lesser sac from pancreatitis or trauma. These cysts are usually palpable and may grow rapidly. Rarely hydatid cyst may occur.

Radiologically, a large cyst may cast a soft tissue shadow on the plain film. The cyst may also displace portions of the upper or lower intestinal tract according to its position in the pancreas but without signs of invasion (Fig. 37.40). Apart from renal masses, differentiation from other retroperitoneal swellings may not be possible.

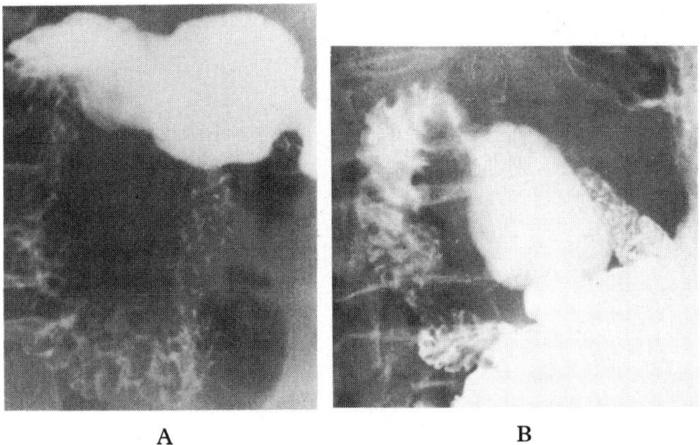

A B

Fig. 37.45 Narrowing of the post-bulbar portion of the duodenum (A) by an encircling new growth of the pancreas (B) by an otherwise silent carcinoma of the right kidney.

Even renal tumours, however, may affect the duodenal circle on the right side (Fig. 37.45B) or the duodenal jejunal flexure on the left and pyelography must be performed in doubtful cases.

TUMOURS OF THE PANCREAS

1. Carcinoma of the ampulla of Vater

Owing to their situation, these tumours may be detected radiologically in a high percentage of cases, provided a meticulous technique is employed. The object is to obtain good filling of the duodenal circle in the right anterior oblique position and this is best done in the horizontal posture.

Spot films may show (1) an extrinsic filling defect constantly present at the site of the ampulla, (2) barium entering the ampulla, (3) actual duodenal invasion in advanced cases. Several examples are illustrated in Fig. 37.46. Such cases will have obstructive jaundice and will need to be differentiated from carcinoma of the pancreatic head and, more closely, from a mass of stones in the lower end of the dilated common bile duct bulging into the lumen of the duodenum; rarely, residual oedema of the ampulla following the passage of a stone may simulate a tumour (Fig. 37.47). In such cases ERCP with its biopsy facility is usually decisive.

2. Carcinoma of the pancreas

This tumour commonly presents in the head of the gland and obstructs the pancreatic portion of the common duct. The findings on transhepatic choledochography (PTC) is a tapering, smooth extrinsic pressure defect occurring in a dilated duct (Fig. 37.26).

The positive results with duodenography, even in the best hands, probably do not exceed 66 per cent. For success it is essential that films in full duodenal distention are obtained; to this end hypotonic duodenography using Probanthine and double contrast study may be required, particularly if the activity of the pylorus and duodenum prevents satisfactory distention.

The tumour will encroach upon the duodenal wall showing a pressure defect on the medial aspect of the mucosa. Eccentrically situated tumours of the head will press upon the pyloric antrum or occasionally invade the duodenum itself. A similar picture can occasionally be produced by the oedematous swelling of the head

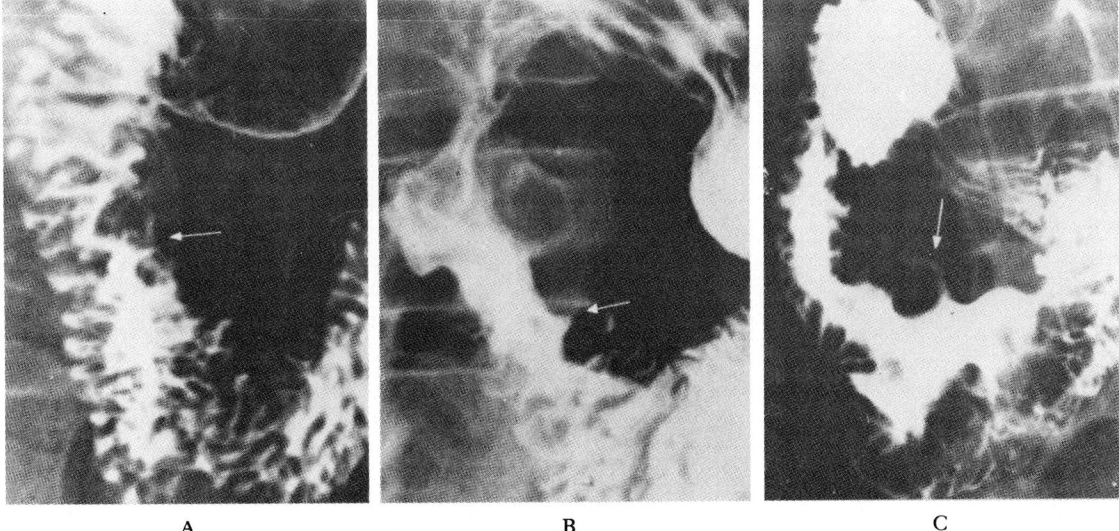

A B C

Fig. 37.46 Three cases of ampullary carcinoma. Note the position of one tumour (C) in the horizontal portion of the duodenum (see Fig. 37.18).

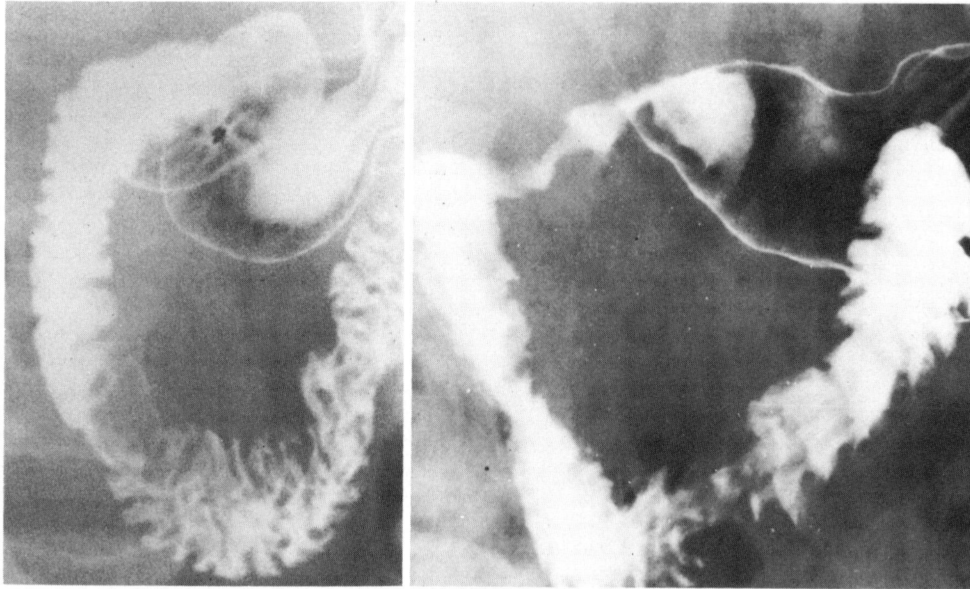

Fig. 37.47 *Fig. 37.48*

Fig. 37.47 Oedema of the ampulla following natural passage of a stone which had caused obstructive jaundice. A mural leiomyoma would show a similar smooth appearance.

Fig. 37.48 Penetrating chronic duodenal ulcer causing oedematous swelling of the pancreatic head and obstructive jaundice.

resulting from a penetrating duodenal ulcer (Fig. 37.48). Other differential diagnoses include duodenal involvement by tumours of the gallbladder and silent tumours of the lower pole of the right kidney.

In the absence of clinical jaundice a suspected mass of the pancreatic head may narrow and/or displace the intra-pancreatic portion of the common bile duct. Differentiation from chronic pancreatitis may be difficult (Fig. 37.25) as it may also be with ERCP (see under Chronic Pancreatitis). Grey scale ultrasound and/or computer tomography may be necessary to arrive at a definitive diagnosis.

Conclusion. The differing imaging techniques available for pancreatic diagnosis depend as much on the skill and diligence of the investigator for success as on the technique employed, whether this be isotope scanning, ultra-sonography, C.T., duodenography, arteriography or ERCP. The choice of examination must depend on the availability of apparatus and expertise as well as the relevance of the clinical problem.

C. THE LIVER

Plain radiography. The liver casts an appreciable shadow by virtue of its bulk. The boundaries of the right lobe merge with the right hemi-diaphragm above, and the right lateral edge and the lower border sloping upward and medially are usually obvious enough. The left lobe, however, cannot be seen so easily because of its more central position and smaller size.

Generalized enlargement of the liver may be due to a number of causes, and these may be:

(*a*) Vascular—right heart failure.
(*b*) Biliary—obstructive jaundice.
(*c*) Hypertrophic cirrhosis.
(*d*) Infective—amoebiasis, portal pyaemia, hydatid disease.
(*e*) Neoplastic—secondary deposits or, less commonly, primary hepatoma.

The radiological assessment of liver size is relatively inaccurate compared with clinical methods. The relation of the costal margin to the lower edge of the liver is seldom obvious as the costal cartilages do not commonly calcify and, when they do, they may obscure the liver edge. Similarly, the left lobe is easier to feel when enlarged than to see on a film. By the time positive signs appear on the radiograph, clinical methods assess the

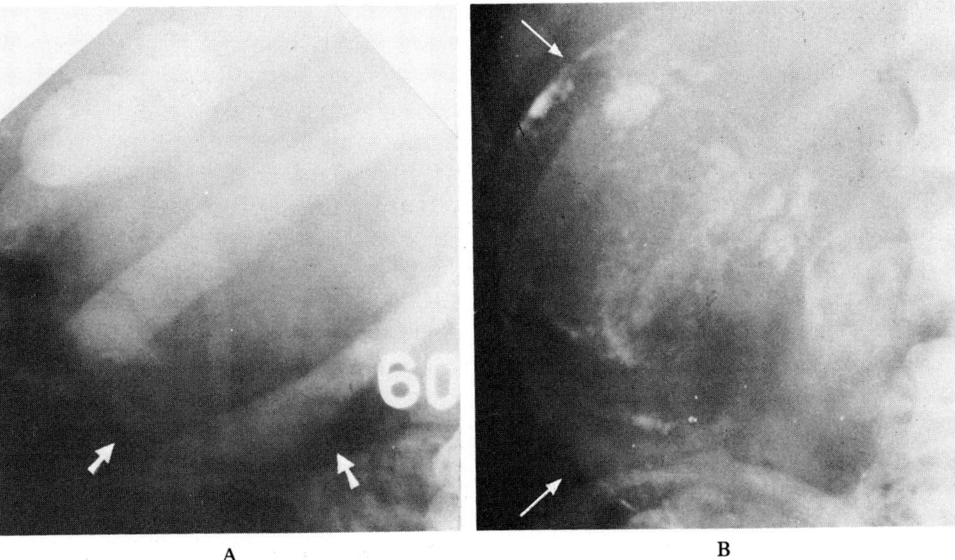

Fig. 37.49 Hydatid cysts of the liver (*arrows*) A stretching the common duct and displacing the gallbladder upwards, B showing cystic calcification.

degree of enlargement as considerable. These radiological signs are:

(*a*) *Right lobe*
(i) Elevated right diaphragm.
(ii) Depressed hepatic flexure.
(iii) Depressed right kidney.
(iv) Low liver edge.
(*b*) *Left lobe*
(i) Displaced gastric fundus in a downward and lateral direction.
(ii) Elongation of the intra-abdominal oesophagus.
(iii) Extrinsic pressure on the lesser curve of the stomach.

Localized masses in the liver due to lesions such as hydatid cyst, primary hepatoma or large solitary amoebic abscess may be evident if they present near one of the visible linear borders. Inflammatory masses under the right diaphragm (e.g. subphrenic abscess) will cause not only elevation localized to a part of the diaphragm and impede movement of that part, but also a pleural effusion.

Calcification may be seen in solitary masses and occasionally also in multiple hepatic lesions. An hydatid cyst of the liver may present as a localized bulge (Fig. 37.49A) but will not calcify unless it dies (Fig. 37.49B); the calcification may be typically spherical but is often not characteristic of a cyst. Secondary deposits in the liver are impossible to diagnose on plain radiography; occasionally, however, colloid carcinoma of the colon will give rise to deposits showing very faint granular calcification in multiple areas. Old healed tuberculous lesions will often calcify and are commonly multiple.

Portal venography in cases of portal hypertension is dealt with elsewhere (see Ch. 30).

Hepatic arteriography is discussed in Chapter 29. Highly vascular lesions such as rare arterio-venous angiomas and vascular tumours can be well shown, but

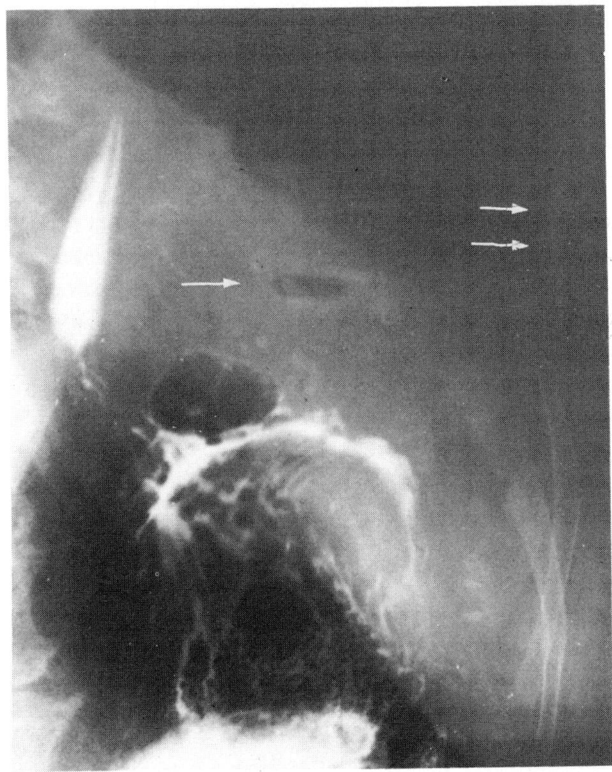

Fig. 37.50 Left subphrenic abscess showing gas in the abscess (→) downward displacement of the gastric fundus and a pleural effusion (⇉).

in general the simpler and non-traumatic technique of **isotope scanning** is the investigation of choice in patients with suspected liver tumours or masses (see Ch. 66).

Ultrasound is often decisive in outlining the presence of a liver mass and diagnosing its nature i.e. whether cystic or solid (see Ch. 67).

Computed tomography, when available, is also invaluable in this respect (see Ch. 65).

Subphrenic abscess. This can occur on either side and is commoner on the right, where it occurs occasionally as a complication of perforated ulcer, gallbladder disease or appendicitis. Characteristically, such patients run a swinging temperature about a week after surgery and show a rising white cell count.

The abscess on the right side occurs between the liver and the diaphragm, and on the left between the gastric fundus, spleen and diaphragm.

Radiological features. In early cases, fluoroscopy will give the most information. The affected diaphragm will show diminished excursion and may be raised and immobile; the contour is seldom affected. At this stage there is probably only interstitial cellulitis without actual abscess formation and so no displacement of the gastric fundus may be seen in left-sided cases.

When an abscess forms, it will manifest its presence most readily on the left side by displacing the gastric fundus (Fig. 37.50); on the right, this feature is not visible; occasionally, however, the organism responsible is gas-forming, such as *B. welchii* (Fig. 37.50). It is thus easier to locate the position of subphrenic abscesses on the left side than on the right; in either case, pleural effusions occur as a result of irritation of the parietal pleura by the inflammatory process (Fig. 37.50).

It is important to remember that after any laparotomy, gas may persist in the peritoneal cavity for 7–10 days and consequently erect films may show subdiaphragmatic gas in cases falsely suspected of harbouring an abscess. The differential diagnosis will lie with the diaphragmatic position and movement and it is imperative therefore that all cases are screened, in addition to having erect and supine films of the diaphragm. In doubtful cases, serial examinations may show increase in the gas and fluid under one diaphragm and this is diagnostic of abscess.

The differential diagnosis from pulmonary post-operative collapse with effusion or pulmonary infarct may present difficulties. Both may show a raised and relatively immobile diaphragm with effusion. The former occurs in the immediate post-operative period which is early for subphrenic abscess: the onset of the latter is sudden about a week post-operatively and may be accompanied by haemoptysis. Paradoxical diaphragmatic movement on sniffing on the affected side is common with subphrenic abscess but may occur also with other conditions affecting the diaphragm.

D. THE SPLEEN

Plain radiography. The outline of the spleen is usually visible on radiographs of good quality. The normal spleen lies under the left leaf of the diaphragm and forms part of the stomach bed. By virtue of its smaller size and close relation to the stomach, diaphragm and splenic flexure, a reasonably accurate assessment of its size can be made; on occasions, it is possible to suggest splenic enlargement before clinical signs become obvious.

The causes of enlarged spleen are numerous and include:

(*a*) Blood disorders: leukaemia, pernicious anaemia, haemolytic anaemia, myelosclerosis.

(*b*) Disorders of the reticulo-endothelial system: Gaucher's disease, Hans-Schuller-Christian disease, Niemann-Pick disease, Hodgkin's disease.

(*c*) Infective causes: malaria, kala-azar, hydatid disease.

(*d*) Hepatic cirrhosis: portal hypertension, Banti's disease.

(*e*) Trauma: rupture and haematoma.

As might be expected, the splenic flexure is commonly depressed (Fig. 37.51), the stomach displaced forwards and medially and the left diaphragm raised. The left kidney may or may nor be depressed; such displacement usually accompanies only massive enlargements of the spleen.

There is usually no obvious way of differentiating the causes of splenic enlargement radiologically.

The exceptions are:

(i) Myelosclerosis—the film will show the typical changes in the bones.

(ii) Trauma—there may be an associated fracture in a lower rib and the history of trauma. There may also be loss of the clear outline of the enlarged spleen.

Calcification in the spleen. The splenic artery or vein may be calcified in the aged and is easily recognizable as such. Calcified splenic artery aneurysms are also readily identified. Phleboliths in the spleen are also easily recognized by their close resemblance to those commonly seen in the pelvis.

Multiple calcified nodules are commonly tuberculous.

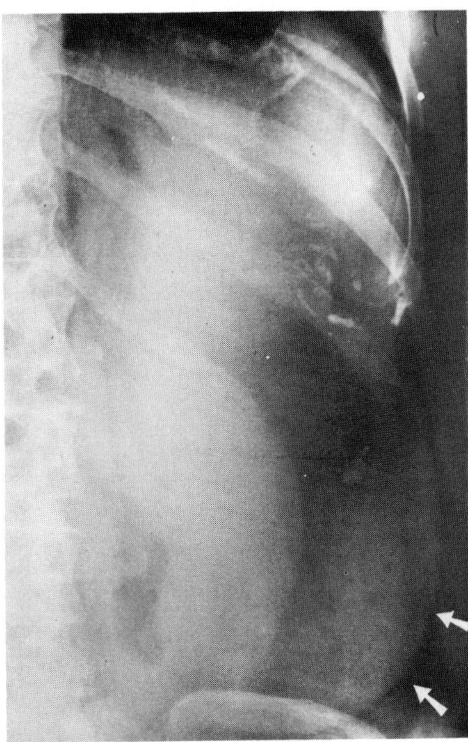

Fig. 37.51 Enlarged spleen (*arrows*) causing elevation of the left diaphragm and depression of the splenic flexure.

Rarely splenic hytadid cysts or splenic infarcts may calcify.

Contrast examinations. Splenic arteriography will outline the spleen but is seldom necessary.

If imaging of the spleen is required, this can now be done easily and without trauma by radioisotopes or by CAT.

REFERENCES AND SUGGESTIONS FOR FURTHER READING

AGNEW, J. E., MAZE, M. & MITCHELL, C. J. (1976) Review article—Pancreatic scanning. *British Journal of Radiology*, **49,** 979–995.

ASHBY, B. S. (1976) Operative choledochoscopy: technique and indications. *Proceedings of the Royal Society of Medicine*, **69,** 331–333.

BAKER, H. L. & HODGSON, J. R. (1960) Further studies on accuracy of oral cholecystography. *Radiology*, **74,** 239–245.

BARON, J. H. (1975) Pancreatic function tests. In *Topics in Gastroenterology—3*, pp. 129–152, ed. Truelove, S. C. & Goodman, J. Oxford: Blackwell.

BERK, R. N. & LOEB, P. M. (1976) Pharmacology and physiology of the biliary radiographic contrast materials. *Seminars in Roentgenology*, **11,** 147–156.

BOUCHIER, I. A. D. (1976) Diseases of the alimentary system—gallstones. *British Medical Journal*, **2,** 870–872.

BURGE, J. & BLAUENSTEIN, U. W. (1974) Current aspects of ultrasonic scanning of the pancreas. *American Journal of Roentgenology*, **122,** 406–412.

BURHENNE, H. J. (1976) Non-operative extraction of stones from bile ducts. *Seminars in Roentgenology*, **XI,** 213–217.

COTTON, P. B. & HEAP, T. R. (1975) The analysis of pancreatic juice. *British Journal of Hospital Medicine*, **14,** 659–666.

COTTON, P. B., CHAPMAN, M., WHITESIDE, C. G. & LE QUESNE, L. P. (1976) Duodenoscopic papillotomy and gallstone removal. *British Journal of Surgery*, **63,** 709–714.

DUNCAN, J. G., IMRIE, C. W. & BLUMGART, L. H. (1976) Ultrasound in the management of acute pancreatitis. *British Journal of Radiology*, **49,** 858–862.

ELIAS, E., HAMLYN, A. N., JAIN, S., LONG, R. G., SUMMERFIELD, J. A., DICK, R. SHERLOCK, S. (1976) Randomized trial of percutaneous transhepatic cholangiography with the Chiba needle versus endoscopic retrograde cholangiography for bile duct visualisation in jaundice. *Gastroenterology*, **71,** 439–443.

FARIS, I., THOMSON, J. P. S., GRUNDY, D. J. & LE QUESNE, L. P. (1975) Operative cholangiography: a re-appraisal based on a review of 400 cholangiograms. *British Journal of Surgery*, **62,** 966–972.

FRASER, G. M. & FRASER, I. D. (1974) Gastrografin in perforated duodenal ulcer and pancreatitis. *Clinical Radiology*, **25,** 397–402.

GOLDBERG, H. I. (1976) Cholecystokinin cholecystography. *Seminars in Roentgenology*, **XI,** 175–179.

GOUGH, M. H. (1977) The cholecystogram is normal . . . but . . . *British Medical Journal*, **1,** 960–962.

HATFIELD, P. M., SCHOLTZ, F. J. & WISE, R. E. (1976) Congenital diseases of the gallbladder and bile ducts. *Seminars in Roentgenology*, **XI,** 235–243.

JAIN, S., LONG, R. G., SCOTT, J., DICK, R. & SHERLOCK, S. (1977) Percutaneous transhepatic cholangiography using the 'Chiba' needle —80 cases. *British Journal of Radiology*, **50,** 175–180.

KREEL, L. (1977) Computerised tomography using the EMI general purpose scanner. *British Journal of Radiology*, **50,** 2–14.

PALAYEW, M. J. (1976) Chronic cholecystitis and cholelithiasis. *Seminars in Roentgenology*, **XI,** 249–257.

ROSCH, J. (1975) Workshop: operative endoscopy. *Endoscopy*, **7,** 156–157.

SAFRANY, L. (1977) Duodenoscopic sphincterotomy and gallstone removal. *Gastroenterology*, **72,** 338–343.

STENHOUSE, D. (1956) On the relative merits of the oral and intravenous methods of cholecystography. *British Journal of Radiology*, **29,** 498–503.

STENHOUSE, D. (1958) Biligrafin and the non-visualized gallbladder. *Journal of the Faculty of Radiology*, **9,** 223–225.

STERN, R. B., KNILL-JONES, R. P. & WILLIAMS, R. (1975) The use of a computer programme for the diagnosis of jaundice in a District Hospital and a specialized liver unit. *British Medical Journal*, **2,** 659–662.

TAYLOR, K. J. W. (1976) Grey scale ultrasound B-scanning for the assessment of the liver and kidney. *British Journal of Clinical Equipment*, **1,** 113–121.

TRAPNELL, J. E. (1974) Acute pancreatitis. *British Journal of Hospital Medicine*, **12,** 193–203.

WISE, R. (1962) *Intravenous Cholangiography*. Springfield, Illinois: Thomas.

WISE, R. E., JOHNSTON, D. O. & SALZMAN, F. A. (1957) Intravenous cholecystographic diagnosis of partial obstruction of the common bile duct. *Radiology*, **68,** 507–525.

CHAPTER 38

THE ADRENAL GLANDS

The adrenal glands are, for their size, among the most important structures in the body. The function was quite unknown until 1855 when Addison first described the syndrome resulting from their destruction. In 1856 Brown-Séquard showed that their removal led to death in animals.

The adrenal glands lie just above the kidneys and are composed of a *cortex* and a *medulla*. The medulla has a totally different embryonic origin to the cortex, and arises with the sympathetic nervous system. Both cortex and medulla secrete hormones.

Since 1927 there have been many advances in evaluating the biochemistry of the adrenal hormones and several have been synthesized.

Three main groups of hormones are secreted by the adrenal **cortex**. These are all chemically related and have a similar basic chemical structure. They are:

(1) *The glucocorticoids*. The secretion of these is controlled by the pituitary gland through its adrenocorticotrophic hormone (ACTH). The most important glucocorticoid is hydrocortisone (Cortisol) and this is normally secreted at the rate of about 20 mg per day. The glucocorticoids have many actions, such as stimulation of protein breakdown, antagonism to the action of insulin, and the inhibition of tissue response in injury.

(2) *Mineralocorticoids*. Aldosterone is the most important of these. Its secretion is mainly controlled by the renin-angiotensin system and by the level of plasma potassium. Aldosterone stimulates the reabsorption of sodium in the distal renal tubules of the kidney in exchange for potassium.

(3) *The androgens*. Though they are produced in relatively large amounts, the adrenal androgens are very weak compared with testosterone.

The **medulla** also secretes hormones, mainly adrenalin and noradrenalin.

ANATOMY

The right adrenal gland is triangular and is closely related to the upper pole of the right kidney. The left adrenal is crescent shaped and is related to the upper and medial part of the left kidney. The average size of the adrenals varies from 3 to 5 cm in length by 2 to 3 cm in width and their average thickness is only about 5 mm. The average weight is 3 to 5 g of which 90 per cent is contributed by the cortex.

The blood supply is of considerable importance in radiology and it is therefore important to know the vascular anatomy. Anatomists describe three main arteries of supply (Fig. 38.1):

(*a*) An inferior adrenal artery arising from the renal artery.
(*b*) A middle adrenal artery arising from the aorta.
(*c*) A superior adrenal arising from the inferior phrenic artery.

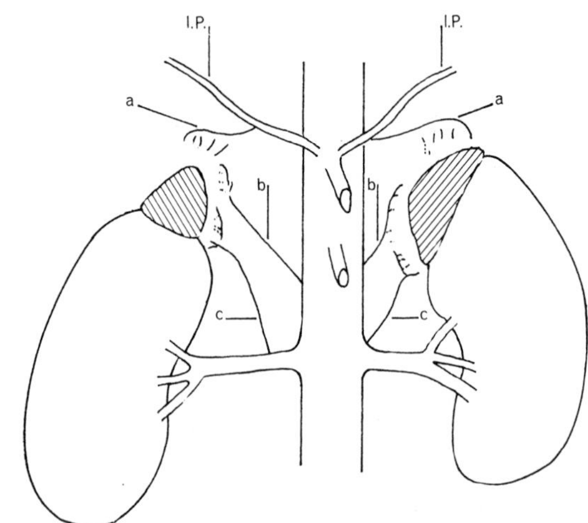

Fig. 38.1 Arterial supply of the adrenals. I.P. = Inferior Phrenic Artery. a = Superior Adrenal Artery. b = Middle Adrenal Artery. c = Inferior Adrenal Artery.

However, this anatomy is subject to considerable variation. Thus the inferior phrenic artery can arise direct from the aorta or from the coeliac axis, or from other vessels. There may also be arteries of supply from other adjacent large arteries. The major arteries of supply break up into numerous smaller branches before entering the gland, which thus has multiple small vessels of supply.

The venous drainage of the adrenals (Fig. 38.2) is also of considerable importance since adrenal phlebography is an established radiological technique. There is usually a fairly large adrenal vein on the *left* which passes downwards medial to the upper part of the kidney to join the main renal vein, and lies just lateral to the left vertebral border. This vein may also have connections with the inferior phrenic vein and veins from the kidney.

On the *right* side, the anatomy is quite different since the adrenal vein has only a very short trunk which passes straight from the right adrenal into the postero-lateral aspect of the inferior vena cava at a level just above the upper pole of the right kidney. Occasionally it may pass to an accessory hepatic vein before entering the inferior vena cava.

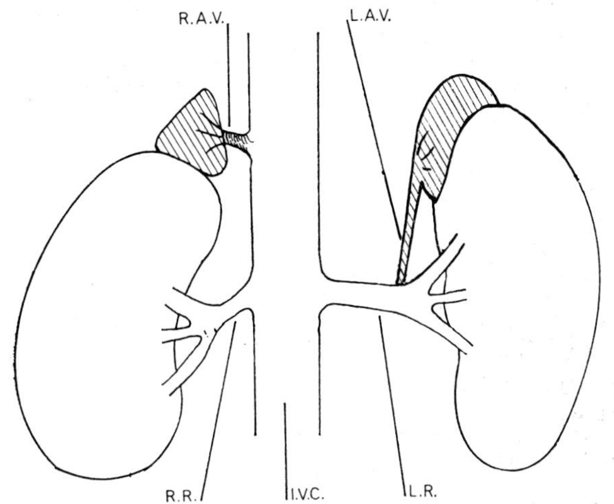

Fig. 38.2 Venous drainage of the adrenal gland. R.A.V. = Right Adrenal Vein. L.A.V. = Left Adrenal Vein. L.R. = Left Renal Vein. I.V.C. = Inferior Vena Cava.

PATHOLOGY

Disorders of the adrenal gland may be due to *infections*, either acute, as in meningococcal or other fulminating septicaemia, or chronic, as in tuberculosis or histoplasmosis. Adrenal *haemorrhage* (adrenal apoplexy) is usually associated with overwhelming septicaemia, and characterized by acute adrenal insufficiency. This may also occur without infection, as in neonatal birth trauma. It can also occur in pregnancy and in severe hypertension, or following adrenal vein thrombosis or severe convulsions in epilepsy. Most of the above conditions are of little radiological interest with the exception of the chronic infections, which may give rise to adrenal calcification and Addison's syndrome. The latter, however, is nowadays more commonly associated with *auto-immune disease.*

Of greater radiological interest are *tumours* of the adrenal gland and *bilateral hyperplasia.* These may be associated with a variety of clinical syndromes including:

(1) Addison's disease
(2) Cushing's syndrome
(3) Conn's syndrome (hyperaldosteronism)
(4) The adrenogenital syndrome
(5) Adrenalism and noradrenalism (pheochromocytoma)
(6) Abdominal tumour
(7) Metastases to bone or liver in childhood
(8) Wolman's disease.

Most patients with suspected adrenal disorder present with one or other of the syndromes or clinical manifestations just described.

Radiological investigation is aimed mainly at those cases thought to be suffering from adrenal tumours in the hope of demonstrating and localizing the lesion.

RADIOLOGICAL INVESTIGATION

The methods available include:

(1) Simple X-ray and tomography
(2) I.V.P. and high dose I.V.P. with tomography
(3) Retroperitoneal air insufflation
(4) Arteriography
(5) Phlebography
(6) Vena caval and adrenal vein blood sampling
(7) Isotope scanning
(8) Ultrasound
(9) C.A.T.

Apart from simple X-ray and tomography the techniques listed above are used largely for the assessment of suspected adrenal tumours.

Simple X-ray. In a suspected adrenal lesion plain radiology of the abdomen with or without tomography may help in two ways.

First, a **mass** in the adrenal area may be obvious and may be seen to be displacing the kidney. This is particularly evident with large tumours but can occasionally be seen even with relatively small lesions provided there is a fair amount of perinephric fat present to help contrast. In general, however, masses smaller than 5 cm in diameter are not likely to be visualized. There are several important aspects of differential diagnosis, thus all the following structures have been known to stimulate a mass in the adrenal area and must be borne in mind:

(*a*) Renal cysts or tumours
(*b*) Spleen and accessory spleen
(*c*) Pancreatic cyst or tumour
(*d*) Liver mass
(*e*) Para-aortic glands
(*f*) Retroperitoneal tumour
(*g*) Stomach mass.

Of considerable importance are the normal fluid-filled gastric fundus in the supine position, which can simulate a mass over the left kidney, and also the fluid-filled antrum or duodenal bulb, which can simulate a mass over the right kidney. As long as these possibilities are borne in mind there is usually little difficulty in differential diagnosis, though occasionally erect films or even barium contrast will have to be used to exclude fluid in the stomach simulating a mass.

The second abnormality which may be seen on plain X-ray is **calcification** in the adrenal area. This may be seen both in tumours and in non-tumourous conditions (Table 38.1).

So called *'idiopathic' calcification* may be found as a chance finding on routine abdominal examination of patients with no relevant symptoms of adrenal disease. It is possible that such calcification may be the result of old haemorrhage or infection in infancy or childhood which has healed with no effect on function (Fig. 38.3).

Table 38.1 Adrenal calcification.

1. Idiopathic–(Normal patient)
2. Addison's Disease
3. Neoplasm
   - (*a*) *Medullary*
     - Neuroblastoma
     - Ganglioneuroma
     - Phaeochromocytoma
   - (*b*) *Cortical*
     - Adenoma
     - Carcinoma
4. Inflammatory. Tuberculosis
   Histoplasmosis
5. Cystic Disease
6. Old Haemorrhage
7. Wolman's Disease

When tuberculosis was common in Britain, involvement of the adrenals was said to be the commonest cause of *Addison's disease* and to be frequently followed by adrenal calcification. However, tuberculosis is now rare in our indigenous population and most of the cases seen today are due to 'atrophy'. This is thought by many to be an auto-immune disease since it may occur in association with such conditions as Hashimoto's thyroiditis and with pernicious anaemia.

Circulating antibodies to the adreno-cortical tissue has been shown in the serum of such patients.

Addison's disease is not caused by primary tumours but it can be due to secondary carcinomatosis. The adrenals are frequently involved, for instance in bronchial carcinoma. Addison's disease may also occur with non-tumourous mass lesions such as amyloidosis. The clinical features are largely due to the resulting deficiency of glucocorticoids and mineralocorticoids. The former leads to anorexia, nausea, vomiting and later to pyrexia, hypotension and hyperglycaemia. The latter causes sodium depletion with dehydration and hypotension. Abnormal brown pigmentation of the skin, involving in particular parts exposed to the sun and pressure areas occurs. In addition, there are deposits of pigment in the mouth and conjunctival mucous membrane.

Wolman's disease is a lipoidosis which was formerly confused with Neiman Pick disease. It is associated with hepatomegaly, splenomegaly and a characteristic calcification of the adrenal glands which are enlarged. It was first defined in 1961 and many well documented cases have since been reported. Most of the affected infants died in the first six months of life. Abdominal X-ray in these infants show large adrenals with diffuse stippled calcification which is virtually diagnostic.

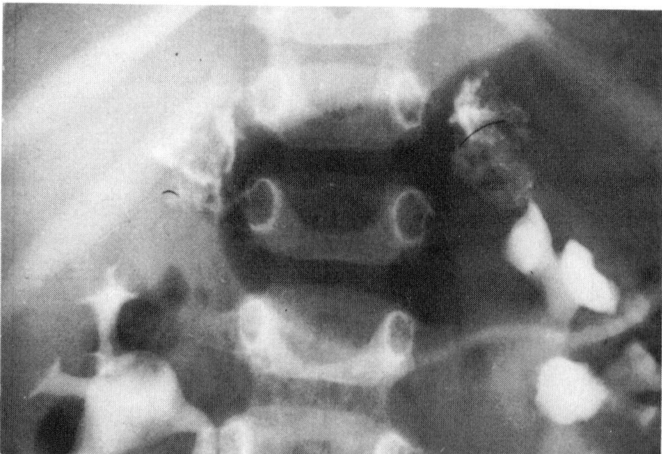

Fig. 38.3 Calcified adrenals in a child. These were a chance finding, the I.V.P. being performed for urinary infection.

Benign cysts of the adrenal, possibly of haemorrhagic origin, and in patients with no symptoms of adrenal pathology, may show *arc-like marginal calcification*. Similar calcification has been described in patients with phaeochromocytoma but is very rare.

Irregular calcification has been described in most adrenal tumours but is very uncommon except in malignant tumours. It is said to occur in about one third of *carcinomas* usually as faint irregular calcification. It also occurs in *neuroblastomas* in about one third of cases. The calcification is usually stippled and non-homogeneous (Fig. 38.5). In this respect, it is interesting that liver metastases from neuroblastoma may also calcify.

Ganglioneuromas which may be regarded as a mature type of neurogenic tumour also calcify frequently, the calcification being similar to that in neuroblastomas (see Fig. 38.6). The majority of ganglioneuromas are extra-adrenal in origin, arising from sympathetic ganglia along the sympathetic chain.

Intravenous urography. In the investigation of

suspected adrenal tumours intravenous urography is often very helpful by differentiating between a mass in the upper pole of the kidney and one in the adrenal. In this respect high dose urography with tomography will frequently define the kidney quite clearly and show whether it is normal. Occasionally it will accentuate a mass in the adrenal and show it more clearly. Downward displacement of an intact kidney by a large suprarenal mass is usually well shown.

Retroperitoneal air insufflation. In the past this method was fairly widely practised for the demonstration of adrenal masses. It was largely replaced by angiographic techniques. There are several methods of performing retroperitoneal air insufflation.

One simple method is to premedicate the patient and then, under local anaesthesia, insert an 18 S.W.G. needle. The point of puncture is midway between the coccyx and the anus. After preliminary sterilization of the skin, the needle passes upwards and backwards through the anococcygeal raphe into the hollow of the sacrum. Some 400 to 500 cc of gas are injected slowly with the patient first lying on one side and then on the other. The procedure is done cautiously with intermittent checking by withdrawing the piston to ensure that the tip of the needle is not in a vein.

Air embolus has been reported as a complication of this procedure with a significant number of fatalities. Because of this, many workers prefer to use CO_2 rather than air. Once the gas has been injected into the presacral retroperitoneal tissues it tracks upwards and passes around the kidneys and the adrenals. These can then be well shown by plain films and tomography. While large tumours are well shown there can be considerable difficulty in determining whether a small tumour is present or not. A retrospective study showed a high incidence of false positives and false negatives from this investigation.

Arteriography. Where simple X-ray and pyelography have failed to show a tumour or have given equivocal results arteriography can be a most useful procedure. Simple flush aortography may show tumours such as large carcinomas, neuroblastomas, or phaeochromocytomas. However, smaller tumours may require selective techniques for their demonstration and even these may be unsuccessful. Phaeochromocytomas are sometimes poorly vascularized and may also need selective techniques for adequate visualization.

Phlebography. Selective adrenal vein phlebography can be performed on both sides and proved a most reliable method for demonstrating small tumours such as occur in primary hyperaldosteronism. The adrenal veins can be catheterized percutaneously from the femoral vein. The right adrenal vein is the more difficult to catheterize, but using specially designed catheters a high success rate can be achieved on both sides. Care must be taken not to overfill the glands by using excessive doses of contrast media or excessive injection pressures. We use hand injections only. On the left side 5–8 ml of a water-soluble contrast medium such as Urografin 60 are used, and on the right side 2 ml are usually adequate. In both cases the volume necessary can be judged by small test doses observed with an image intensifier.

Serious complications such as adrenal infarction have been recorded from using excessive doses.

Inferior vena cavography. This procedure may occasionally prove useful when the vein is displaced by an ectopic tumour (see Fig. 38.18).

Hormone assay. Catheterization of the vena cava can be performed for blood sampling at different sites and levels in suspected phaeochromocytomas. This is usually done when other techniques have failed to localize a suspected tumour. Samples are usually taken from the renal veins, and high and low in the inferior vena cava. Since these tumours can be intrathoracic or in the pelvis samples may also be taken from the superior vena cava and the iliac veins. The technique of blood sampling and hormone assay is also used in suspected Conn's tumours. Samples are taken from the adrenal veins or as near to their mouths as possible. Some consider that adrenal vein aldosterone is diagnostic in cases of Conn's tumour even without phlebography, the value being abnormally high on the tumour side and normal on the other. In cases of bilateral hyperplasia the aldosterone level is elevated on both sides.

Isotope scanning. Conn *et al.* 1972 first reported the successful demonstration of Conn's tumours by radioisotope scanning. Unfortunately the isotope first used gave a rather high radiation dose but later radio pharmaceuticals have been produced which give more acceptable doses. Where the technique is available it is a useful non-invasive method of investigating Conn's tumours. However, there are pitfalls and we have seen a tumour diagnosed in a patient with a normal gland and a non-functioning gland on the opposite side. Isotope scanning can also be used to demonstrate the adenoma of Cushing's disease but so far the method has proved of little use in commoner adrenal tumours, such as phaeochromocytoma.

CAT scanning. Adrenal tumours can be readily shown by CAT body scanning, and normal adrenals can also be visualized. It is already suggested that the technique will even show small adenomas such as are seen in Conn's syndrome and the results of further experience in this field are awaited with interest (see Ch. 65).

Ultrasound (see Ch. 66). Large tumours should be readily diagnosable by ultrasound but it is unlikely that the method will prove of much use with the smaller lesions, or with ectopic tumours, unless large. However, in expert hands some surprisingly accurate results have been claimed for this technique (Bernardino *et al.*, 1978). To date, this work awaits more widespread confirmation.

Choice of investigation. It is clear from the above discussion that there are now a large battery of tests available using radiology or imaging to show adrenal tumours. On general principles the least invasive techniques will be used first. Simple X-rays or tomography with high dose I.V.P. are relatively cheap and easily available. Of the newer imaging techniques ultrasound is the cheapest and most widely available. However, it is unlikely to be helpful with very small or ectopic lesions. Isotope scanning is useful with small tumours such as Conn's but is time consuming and of little use with other tumours; C.T. scanning is the most promising of all the non-invasive new imaging techniques but it is expensive and not widely available except in highly developed countries. It seems likely therefore that the invasive techniques of angiography and phlebography will still be necessary in many areas. However, where the modern imaging techniques are freely available, invasive methods should be reserved for the difficult or problem cases, e.g. the ectopic phaeochromocytoma which other methods have failed to show, or the possible small Conn's tumour where imaging methods are negative or equivocal.

NEUROBLASTOMA

Chracteristically these tumours occur in children and present either with an abdominal mass or with manifestations of secondary deposit. Over half of them arise in the adrenals, but they can arise from sympathetic tissue anywhere in the body.

Radiological investigation by plain X-rays can be very helpful. They may show an abdominal mass visible by virtue of its size, or by downward displacement of the kidney, or by the presence of calcification. The latter has been noted to occur in about one third of cases. An I.V.P. may be helpful in confirming the kidney displacement.

Sometimes it is very difficult to differentiate between a renal mass such as Wilm's tumour and a suprarenal mass on simple X-ray and even on I.V.P. Calcification, if present, is an important point in favour of neuroblastoma since it is rare in Wilm's tumour. In these cases, angiography may be very helpful and will usually settle the differential point (Fig. 38.4). Both Wilm's tumour and neuroblastoma can be quite vascular but are sometimes very poorly vascularized. However, a Wilm's tumour is more likely to show a florid pathological circulation than a neuroblastoma. The latter usually displaces the kidney downwards and produces extrinsic distortion of its outline, but the renal substance, as shown in the nephrogram, is seen to be intact.

While radiology and particularly angiography will usually settle the problem of differential diagnosis, one should nevertheless be prepared for the occasional surprise, since many mass lesions can occur in this region. Hydronephrosis and pyonephrosis must be considered particularly when involving the upper part of a duplex kidney. Rarer lesions include retroperitoneal sarcoma, liver tumour, and enteric duplication cyst.

Although occasional rarities such as these must be

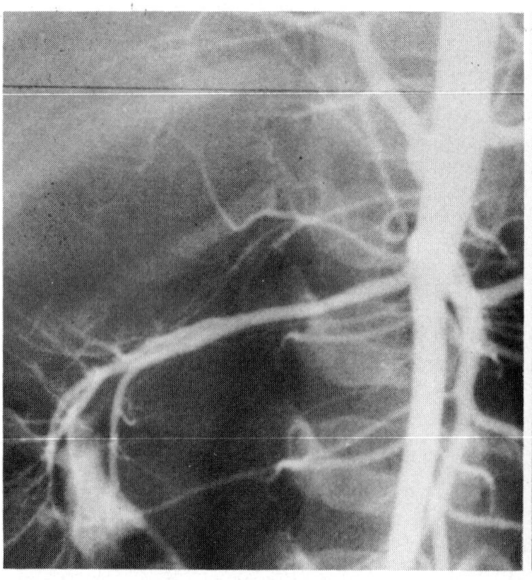

A

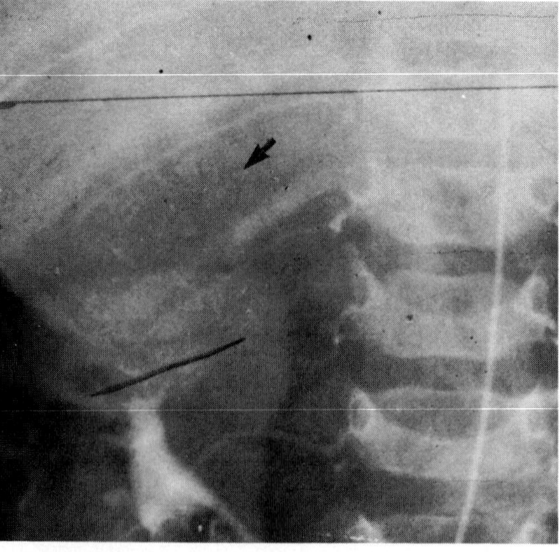

B

Fig. 38.4 (A and B) Renal arteriogram in a child with neuroblastoma. The nephrogram shows clearly that the mass lies above the kidney. There is a limited pathological circulation supplied by a hypertrophied middle adrenal artery. (*Courtesy of Dr. F. Starer.*)

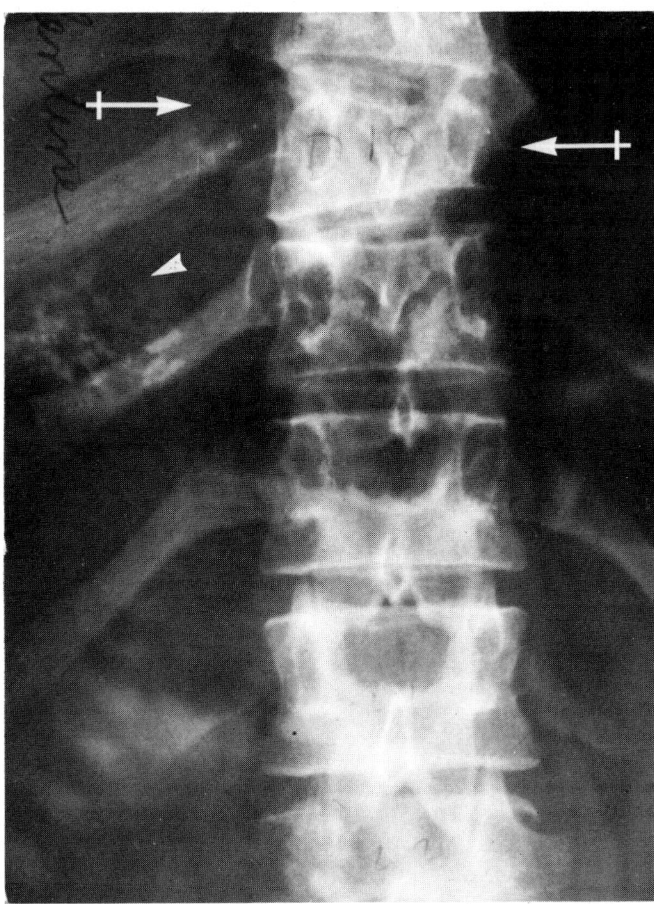

Fig. 38.5 Calcification in a neuroblastoma presenting in pregnancy (↙). There is a secondary deposit in the 10th dorsal vertebra extending into the transverse process of the 10th right rib (→←). (*Courtesy of Dr. J. Haggar.*)

borne in mind, it is nevertheless true that the usual differential diagnosis of an apparent mass above the kidney in a child is between neuroblastoma and Wilm's tumour.

It should not be forgotten that neuroblastoma can occasionally present in adults. Figure 38.5 is the X-ray film of a young woman who developed crippling back pain in the later stages of pregnancy. As a result of this, and despite the pregnancy, a simple X-ray was taken. This revealed a vertebra eroded by a metastasis but also showed the calcified neuroblastoma from which it had arisen.

GANGLIONEUROMA

This is a mature form of neurogenic tumour. Apart from arising in the adrenal, these tumours can, like neuroblastoma, arise from the parasympathetic system elsewhere along the spine, particularly in the thorax.

Like neuroblastomas they are commoner in children but although 60 per cent occur before the age of 20 a good proportion present in adults.

Ganglioneuromas occurring in children may also show calcification which can help in suggesting a diagnosis of neurogenic tumour (Fig. 38.6).

Occasionally, as in this case, ganglioneuromata invade the spinal canal. In these cases there is not only an extraspinal mass but also an intraspinal component causing neurological symptoms either from cord compression or from involvement of the cauda equina. These rare cases are usually mistaken for dumb-bell neurofibromata.

If the lesion presents in a child and calcification is present in the paraspinal mass the diagnosis of ganglioneuroma should always be considered. It is interesting that some of the recorded cases were first reported histologically as neuroblastomas but a second and later biopsy showed ganglioneuroma. It is now well recognized that neuroblastomas can sometimes mature into the more benign and well differentiated tumour.

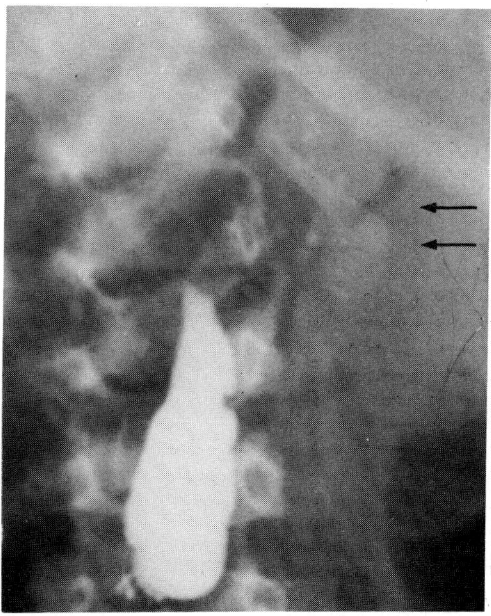

Fig. 38.6 Calcification in a dumb-bell ganglioneuroma (arrows). The child presented with evidence of a spinal tumour and showed an almost complete block at myelography.

CUSHING'S SYNDROME

Most cases we now see are iatrogenic due to treatment with cortisone. There are many interesting radiological features of patients presenting with Cushing's syndrome. Thus there is an unusual central type of osteoporosis which may be associated with pathological fractures that can go unrecognized. These are particularly common in the ribs and in the pelvis.

The radiologist is frequently asked to X-ray the skull in patients presenting with Cushing's syndrome, but this is rarely necessary since pituitary tumours in this condition are usually microscopic and do not produce enlargement of the sella. There are occasional exceptions to this rule. In particular, patients who have been treated by adrenalectomy may develop large adenomas which enlarge the sella (Nelson's syndrome).

As regards the adrenal lesion it is unusual to demonstrate a tumour in Cushing's syndrome, though both adenomas and carcinomas in the adrenal gland can present in this way. In the majority of cases (over 80 per cent) there is merely bilateral hyperplasia of the glands. The decision as to whether the patient has a tumour and not bilateral hyperplasia is usually made on biochemical evidence.

The radiological investigation commences with a simple X-ray in the hope of demonstrating a mass. At this stage it is appropriate to remember some of the diagnostic snares already noted. Thus on the right side the gastric fundus, and on the left side the antrum of the stomach, can simulate a rounded mass above the kidney. If there is any clinical doubt it may be necessary to put contrast into the stomach or to rotate the patient to confirm that the apparent lesion is an artefact.

A high degree of success in the diagnosis of cortical adenomas in Cushing's syndrome has been claimed for the relatively simple technique of high dose I.V.P. with tomography. It is said that this technique will demonstrate tumours larger than 1 inch in diameter. However, as most cases do not have tumours this is not very helpful. Furthermore, such cases as have tumours demonstrated may show equally well with simple tomography.

Cases of Cushing's syndrome associated with bilateral hyperplasia can be very difficult to assess by radiology. In the past, retroperitoneal air insufflation was widely used both to demonstrate adenomas and to show bilateral hyperplasia.

As already emphasized, however, the interpretation of such air insufflation pictures presented considerable difficulties and the accuracy of diagnosis with small lesions was poor. Of the invasive methods now in use adrenal phlebography seems to be the method of choice and is usually preferred to arteriography for demonstrating adenomas. If available, however, ultrasound or CAT should be tried before invasive methods are used.

CONN'S SYNDROME

Primary hyperaldosteronism, or Conn's syndrome, is characterized by hypokalemia, weakness and hypertension. It is known that in most cases the cause is a small adenoma of the adrenal. The demonstration of such a small lesion by radiological methods was, until recent years, not possible. Certainly, plain X-ray or even arteriography could hardly hope to show lesions 1 cm or less in size. Historically it was the development of adrenal phlebography which first made it possible to demonstrate these small adenomas in Conn's syndrome (Sutton, 1968). The characteristic feature is usually an arc-like vein in the circumference of the tumour, which is relatively avascular (Fig. 38.7).

Larger Conn's tumours are occasionally seen and Figure 38.9 shows such a case.

Calcification has not been recorded in Conn's tumours but was present in one of our cases. It was thought that this was due to haemorrhagic cysts in the tumour. Larger Conn's tumours like this may even be shown by selective adrenal arteriography (Fig. 38.9).

If bilateral adrenal vein catheterization has failed to

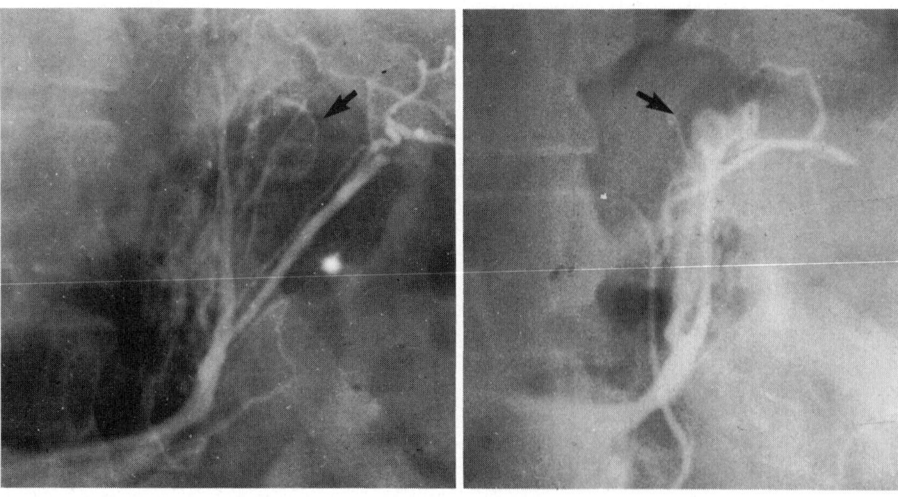

A B

Fig. 38.7A Left adrenal phlebogram showing small Conn's tumour (↙).
B Right adrenal phlebogram showing small Conn's tumour (↘).

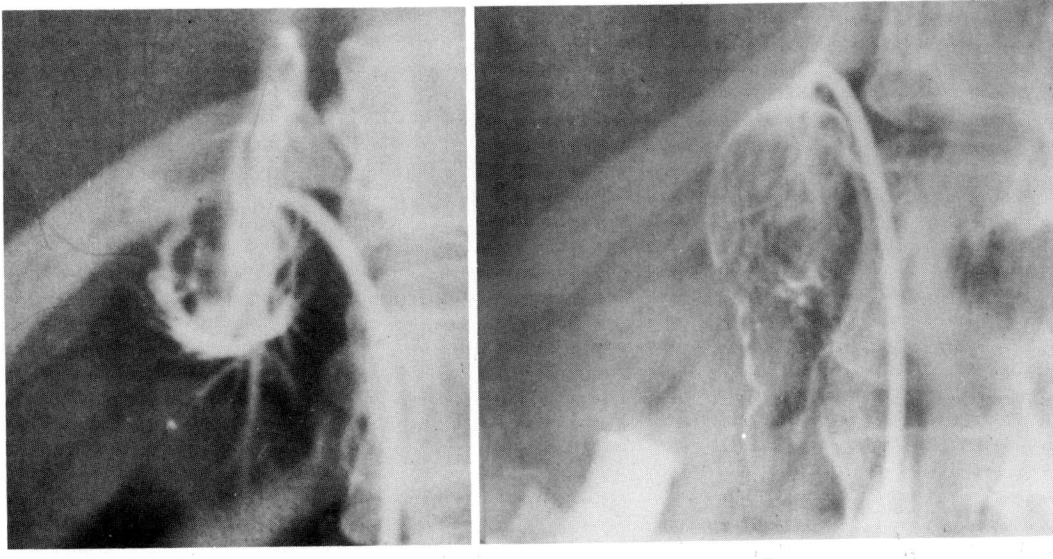

Fig. 38.8 (A and B) Right adrenal phlebograms showing Conn's tumours. Two different patients.

demonstrate a small Conn's tumour and the diagnosis is clinically and biochemically certain then bilateral hyperplasia is likely to be the cause.

Bilateral adrenal vein sampling for aldosterone estimation in the venous blood can be carried out at the time of adrenal vein catheterization.

Figure 38.10 is from a patient who also presented with Conn's syndrome and underwent adrenal phlebography. This was clearly a very large tumour and the connections with other retroperitoneal veins raised the possibility of malignancy. Operative removal confirmed that this was an adrenal carcinoma.

As noted above C.T. and isotope scanning offer less invasive methods of diagnosing the small Conn's adenoma.

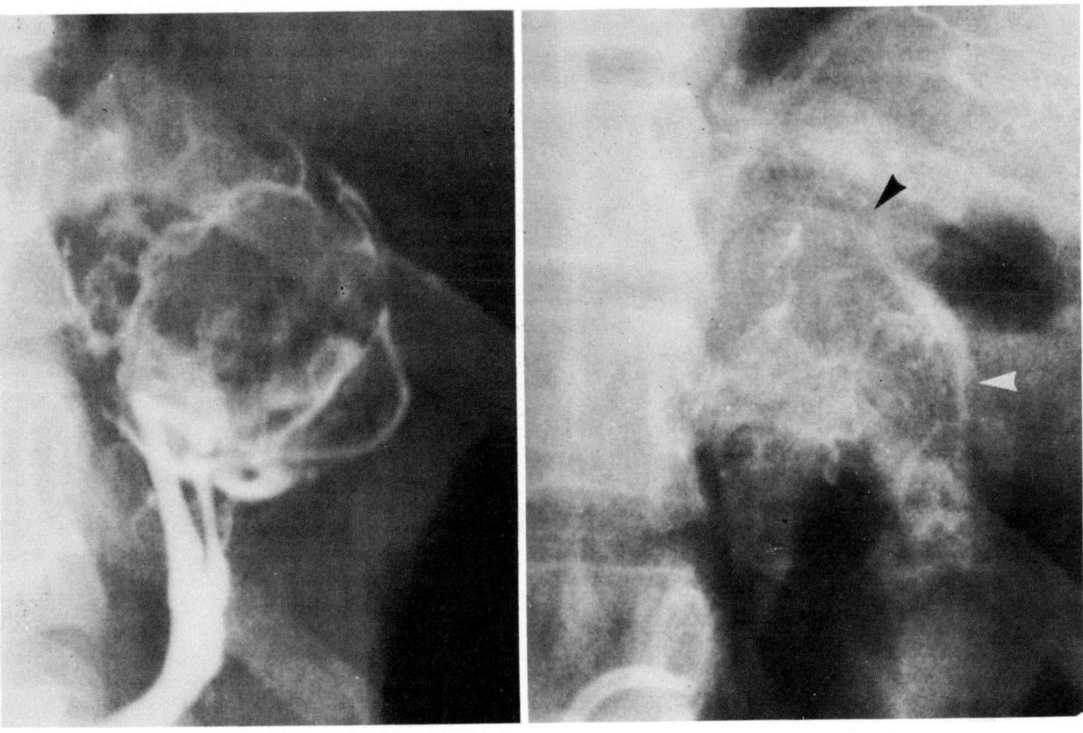

Fig. 38.9A Left adrenal phlebogram showing large Conn's tumour. B Selective inferior phrenic arteriogram showing the same tumour (arrows) as in Figure 38.9A.

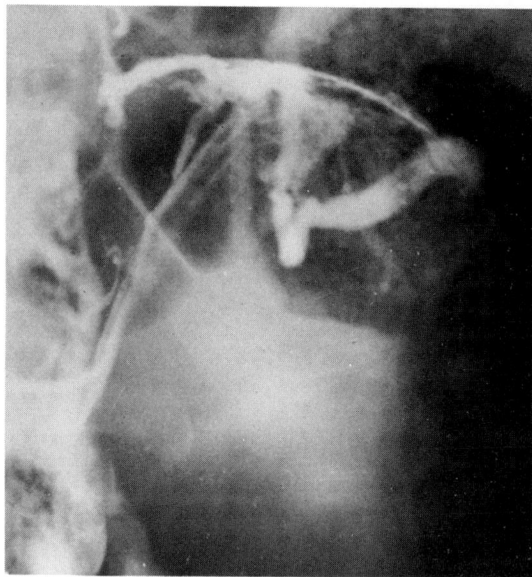

Fig. 38.10 Left adrenal phlebogram. This shows a large adrenal mass which has drainage veins communicating with other retroperitoneal veins. The patient presented with Conn's syndrome due to an adrenal carcinoma.

ADRENAL CARCINOMA

This is sometimes described as being particularly associated with the *adreno-genital syndrome.* In practice it may present in any of several different ways, and has been encountered with:

(1) Cushing's syndrome
(2) Conn's syndrome
(3) The adreno-genital syndrome
(4) An abdominal mass only.

One third of adrenal carcinomas may show calcification which is usually patchy and irregular. Thus simple X-ray can be helpful in suggesting the diagnosis where there are no endocrine changes. Many of these adrenal carcinomas can become very large before discovery. The average size of the mass in one series was about 6 inches in diameter, and the mass is often obvious at simple X-ray.

Apart from the plain X-ray changes just mentioned, one would expect the I.V.P. to show downward displacement of the kidney. Ultrasound or CAT should also readily show such large masses. Invasive methods will be reserved for equivocal cases or problem cases where the localization of the mass remains unclear. The adrenal phlebogram may show irregular vessels communicating with veins around the tumour (Fig. 38.10). Arteriography may show hypertrophied adrenal arteries supplying pathological vessels and tumour cuffing around vessels of supply. Clearly these changes would best be shown by selective adrenal arteriography though they may be visible at flush aortography (Fig. 38.11).

THE ADRENO-GENITAL SYNDROME

When this occurs in infants it is usually due to so called 'congenital bilateral hyperplasia'. In older children and

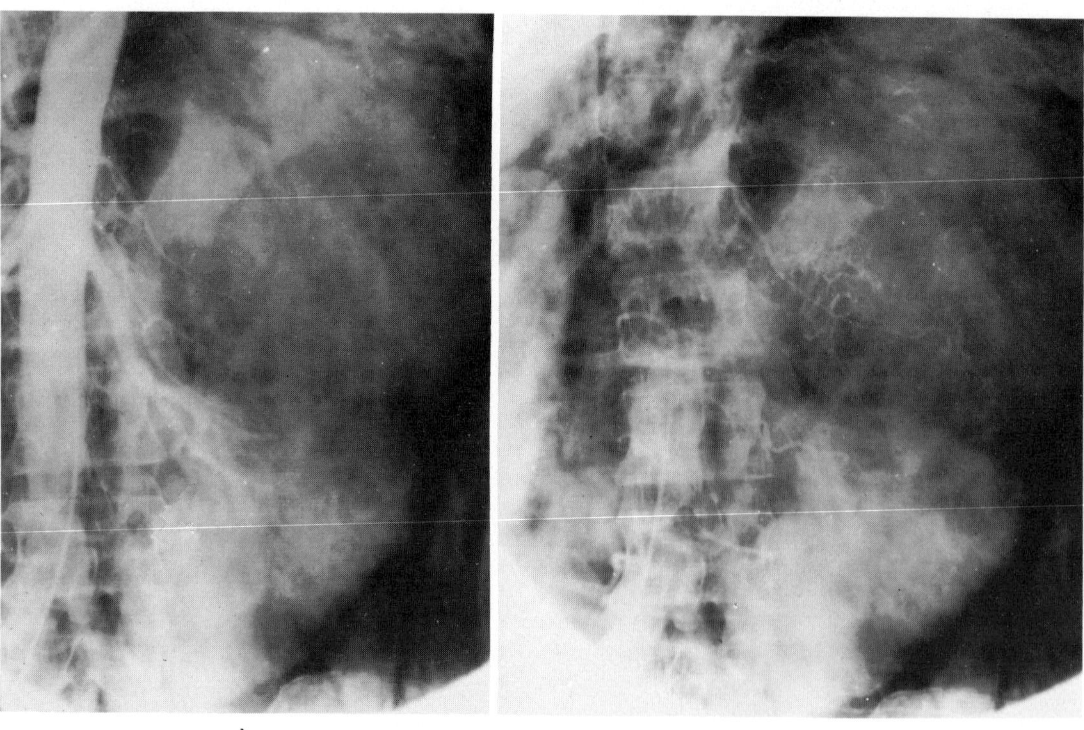

A B

Fig. 38.11 (A and B) Adrenal carcinoma shown by flush aortogram. There is a pathological circulation supplied by hypertrophied adrenal arteries. The nephrogram of the kidney is displaced downwards.

adults it is usually due to a tumour. This is more commonly a carcinoma, but it can be an adenoma. If the tumour is large, as most carcinomas are, simple methods of X-ray with tomography will usually localize the lesion. If not, ultrasound or CAT may be tried. Invasive methods should only rarely be required.

PHAEOCHROMOCYTOMA

This is the most frequent type of adrenal tumour to be seen in clinical practice. The value of plain X-rays in this condition has already been discussed. Calcification in our experience is very rare (one in 40 cases) but if curvilinear it may suggest the possibility of a phaeochromocytoma. Such curvi-linear calcification is, however, more frequent in simple haemorrhagic cysts.

The very large tumours are fairly easy to demonstrate by simple X-ray with tomography, or by I.V.P. with tomography, or by air insufflation. We have already noted, however, that the interpretation of air studies can be difficult and has many pitfalls, particularly with smaller tumours. When air insufflation was more widely practised we found that lateral tomograms were very helpful in these cases. This is because phaeochromocytomas can be abnormal in situation and they may be anterior to the kidney or in other ectopic positions in more than 10 per cent of cases.

In the 1950s angiography was tentatively used for the diagnosis of phaeochromocytomas, but the method gained a rather sinister reputation following three reports of fatalities. These appeared to have resulted from hypertensive crises. As a result, the method became for a time contra-indicated. However, during the 1960s it began to be used again, particularly with catheter techniques. It was pointed out that if a patient should develop a crisis, hypotensive drugs could readily be administered, if necessary through the catheter. Angiography thus became the most accurate and extensively used method of localizing phaeochromocytomas in the decade from 1965 to 1975. In the last few years *ultrasound* has been widely practised in the investigation of abdominal masses. It will no doubt readily confirm the site of normally or even abnormally sited tumours if these are large. However, it is unlikely to be of much help with the smaller and ectopic tumours. CAT should also show many phaeochromocytomas, but again there may be difficulty with ectopic or multiple tumours. These new non-invasive techniques will undoubtedly reduce the need for angiography.

As regards the technique of angiography, most people

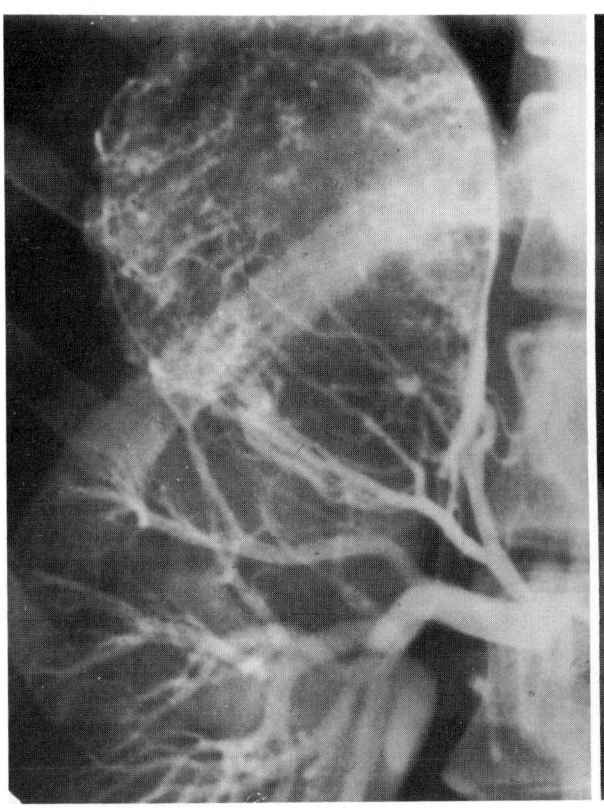

A

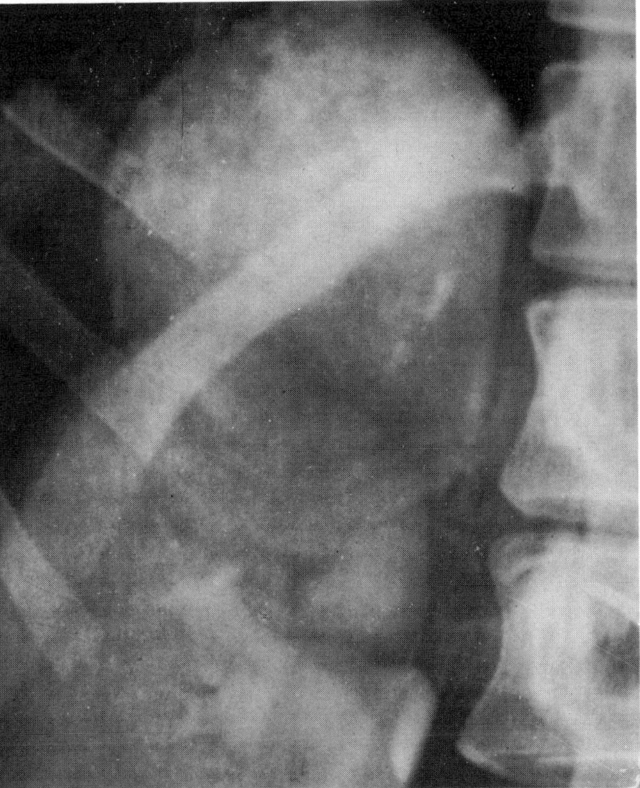

B

Fig. 38.12 (A and B) Large vascular phaeochromocytoma shown by selective right renal angiography with the catheter tip in the hypertrophied right inferior adrenal artery.

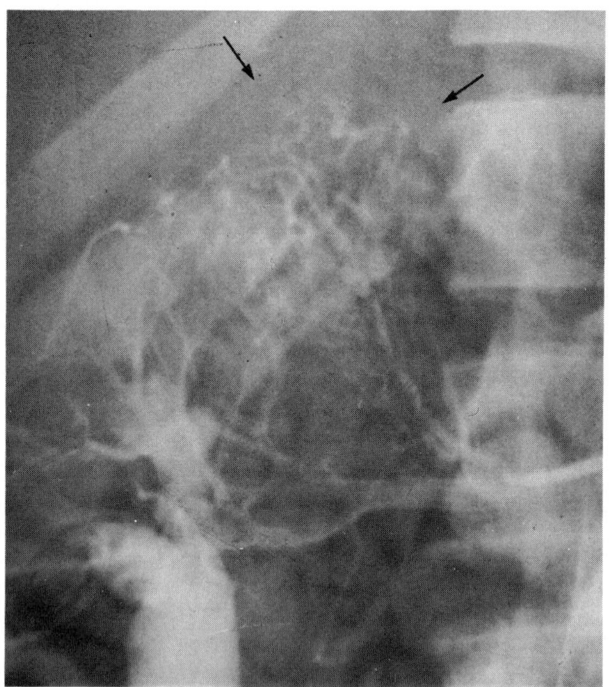

Fig. 38.13 Smaller phaeochromocytoma shown by the same technique as in Figure 38.12.

in the past have used direct injection of the aorta (flush aortography).

Selective adrenal arteriography has also been safely used. It will be remembered that there are said to be three main arteries supplying the adrenal. The most common arrangement is an inferior adrenal artery arising from the renal, a middle adrenal artery arising direct from the aorta, and a superior adrenal artery arising from the inferior phrenic artery. However, this anatomy is subject to great variation, and the inferior phrenic artery itself can arise either from the aorta or from the coeliac axis or other vessels. It can thus be a most difficult and tedious examination to attempt selective injection of all the adrenal arteries. We found by experience that a simpler and quicker method of approach in most cases was to perform selective renal angiography with the catheter tip near the origin of the renal artery. Even if the inferior adrenal artery is tiny it will still show quite well by this method, particularly on the right side. If it is enlarged (as with tumours) it can often be entered selectively.

Since the adrenal arteries anastomose fairly freely, injection of the renal artery and thus of the inferior adrenal will usually show tumours well, if they are normally sited and supplied. In our hands this has proved a most useful and rewarding technique.

Figures 38.12, 38.13 and 38.14 illustrate cases which showed readily by this technique. Figure 38.14 illustrates a case which underwent flush aortography which was regarded as negative. The tumour was poorly vascularized but it showed readily at selective renal angiography. A vascular phaeochromocytoma is supplied by hypertrophied adrenal arteries. These give rise to a fine reticular network followed by a homogenous stain throughout the tumour (Figs. 38.12 and 38.14).

Sometimes the arteries follow the periphery of the

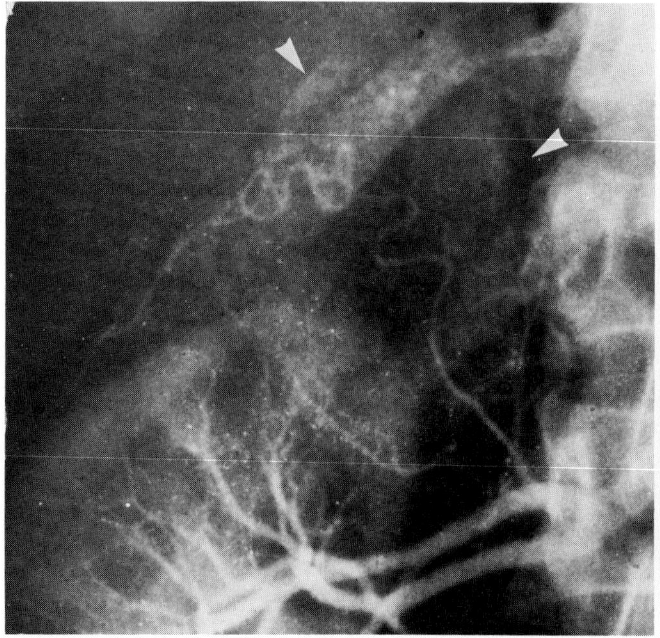

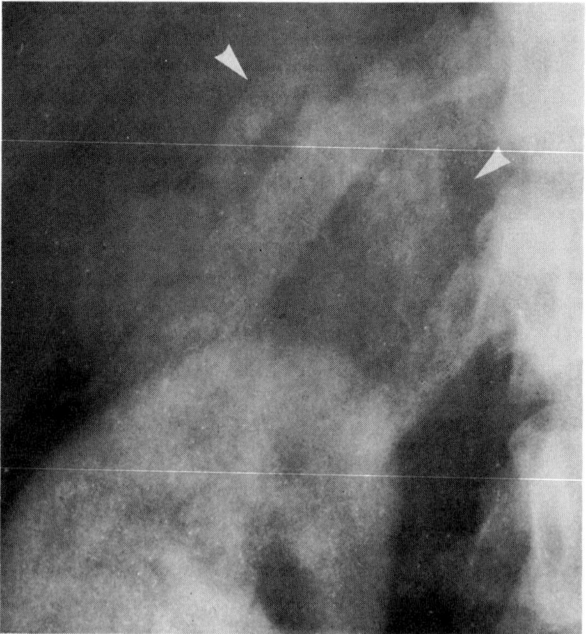

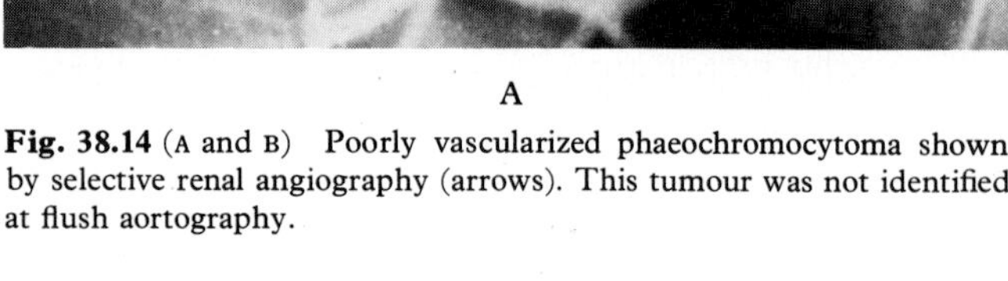

A B

Fig. 38.14 (A and B) Poorly vascularized phaeochromocytoma shown by selective renal angiography (arrows). This tumour was not identified at flush aortography.

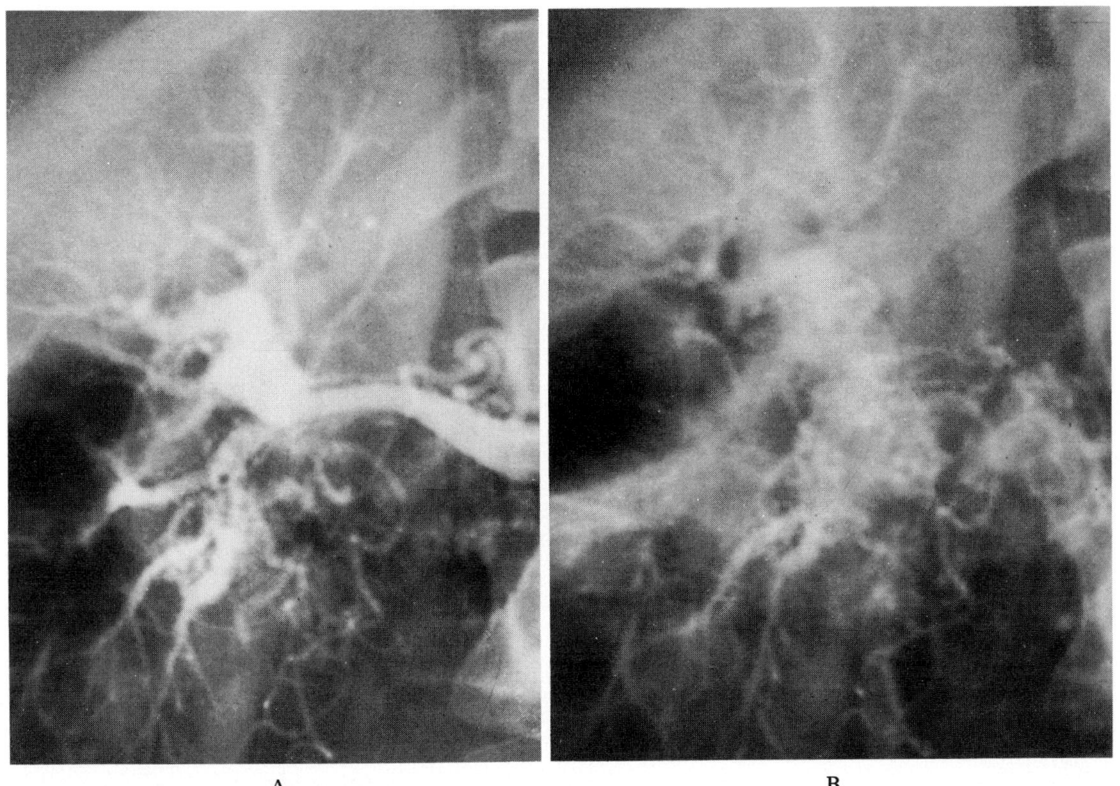

A B

Fig. 38.15 (A and B) Vascular phaeochromocytoma below right renal artery which is stretched over the tumour.

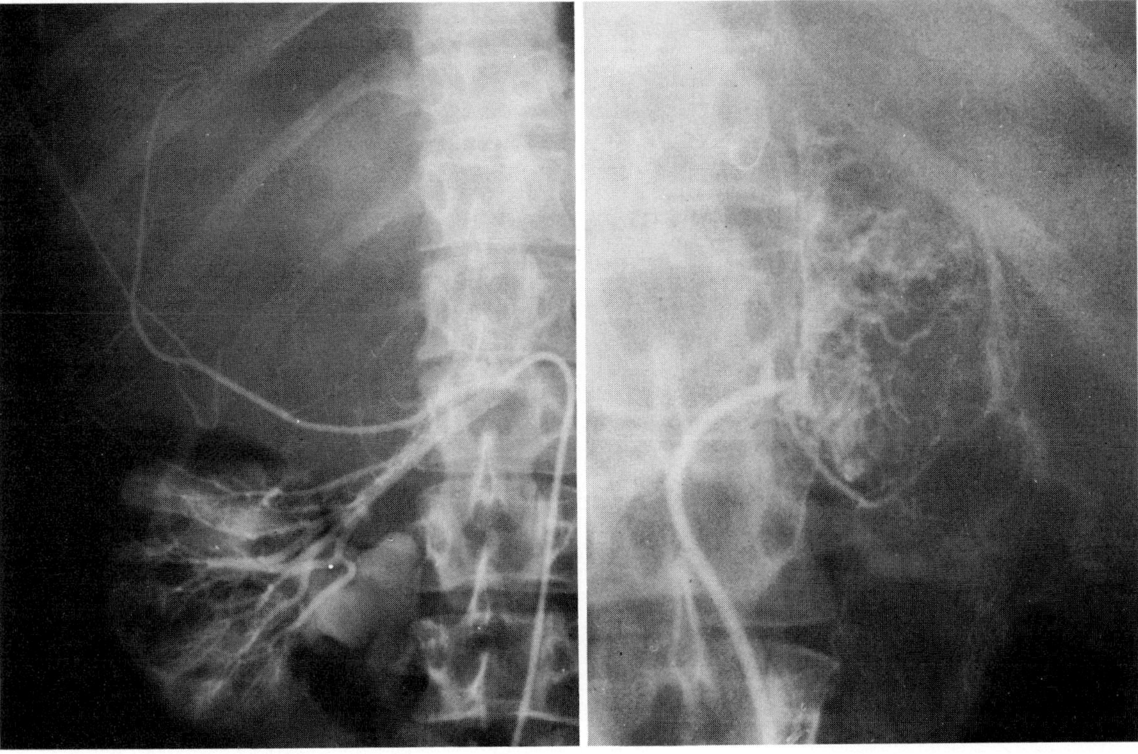

A B

Fig. 38.16A Huge non-vascular phaeochromocytoma above right kidney which is displaced downwards. The tumour was cystic. B Small vascular phaeochromocytoma in left adrenal of same patient.

tumour maintaining a similar calibre throughout (Figs. 38.12 and 38.16A). Rarely, wide capsular veins are seen encircling the mass. Other tumours appear to show a tangle of tortuous vessels (Figs. 38.15 and 38.17).

Whilst the increasing use of angiography resulted in improved diagnosis and localization of phaeochromocytomas it is not the complete answer and several problems still remain. Angiographic techniques, even of the best quality, will still fail to diagnose and localize a proportion of phaeochromocytomas. The problems are of four kinds:

(1) The non-vascular or poorly vascularized tumour.
(2) Multiple phaeochromocytoma.

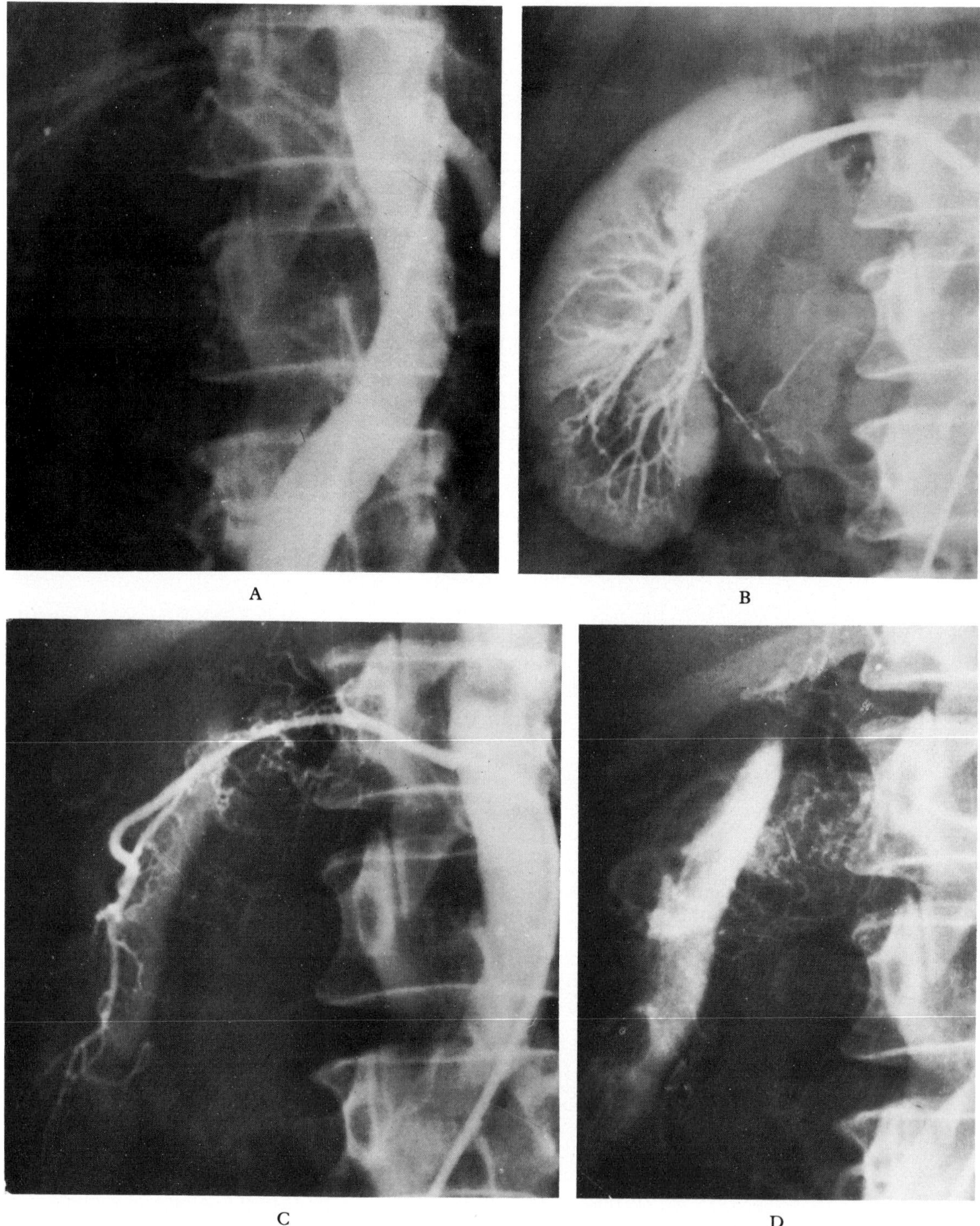

Fig. 38.17A Flush aortogram. B Selective arteriogram of main right renal artery. (C and D) Selective arteriogram of accessory right renal artery. The tumour is mainly supplied by the accessory artery. A pathological circulation is evident which was not seen on flush aortography.

(3) The ectopic phaeochromocytoma.
(4) Association with renal artery stenosis.

1. **The poorly vascularized phaeochromocytoma.** While many phaeochromocytomas are quite vascular and show readily at angiography, a significant proportion are very poorly vascularized (Figs. 38.14 and 38.16A). If such a tumour is large it may be diagnosed by the mass causing displacement of the adjacent kidney or other structures. If it is small a good quality selective arteriogram may identify the lesion, as in cases illustrated. However, good selective angiograms may not always be possible, particularly with the very small tumours or with ectopic tumours whose exact arteries of supply are not easily identified. In these cases adrenal phlebography may occasionally succeed in demonstrating a lesion in the region of the left adrenal, as in two of our own cases. In other cases selective injection of the ectopic artery of supply may succeed (Fig. 38.19).

2. **Multiple phaeochromocytomas.** According to the literature these are not uncommon and the situation is claimed to be present in up to 10 per cent of cases. Thus it is advisable to perform flush aortography as well as selective renal angiography as a routine. Selective angiography should then be attempted of any suspicious or equivocal area. Figure 38.16A shows a giant right phaeochromocytoma which was easily palpable and obvious on simple X-ray. The tumour was very poorly vascularized for its size, but a concomitant small left-sided tumour would not have been suspected without a prior flush aortogram. The suspicion was confirmed by selective injection of the enlarged left middle adrenal artery noted at the midstream aortogram.

3. **Ectopic phaeochromocytoma.** About 10 per cent of phaeochromocytomas are ectopic in situation. The majority of these show local ectopia in the region of the kidney and we have seen such tumours behind the inferior vena cava or between the inferior vena cava and aorta (Fig. 38.18), and at the hilum of the kidney (Fig. 38.15). In two separate cases we have shown phaeochromocytomas lying below the left kidney and supplied only by the inferior mesenteric artery (Fig. 38.19). Other tumours may be found in more remarkable positions, well away from the kidney, and even outside the abdomen. Cases have been described with phaeochromocytomas in the bladder wall and such cases have been diagnosed by angiography. These patients are said to show a characteristic syndrome of attacks of palpitation, sweating or

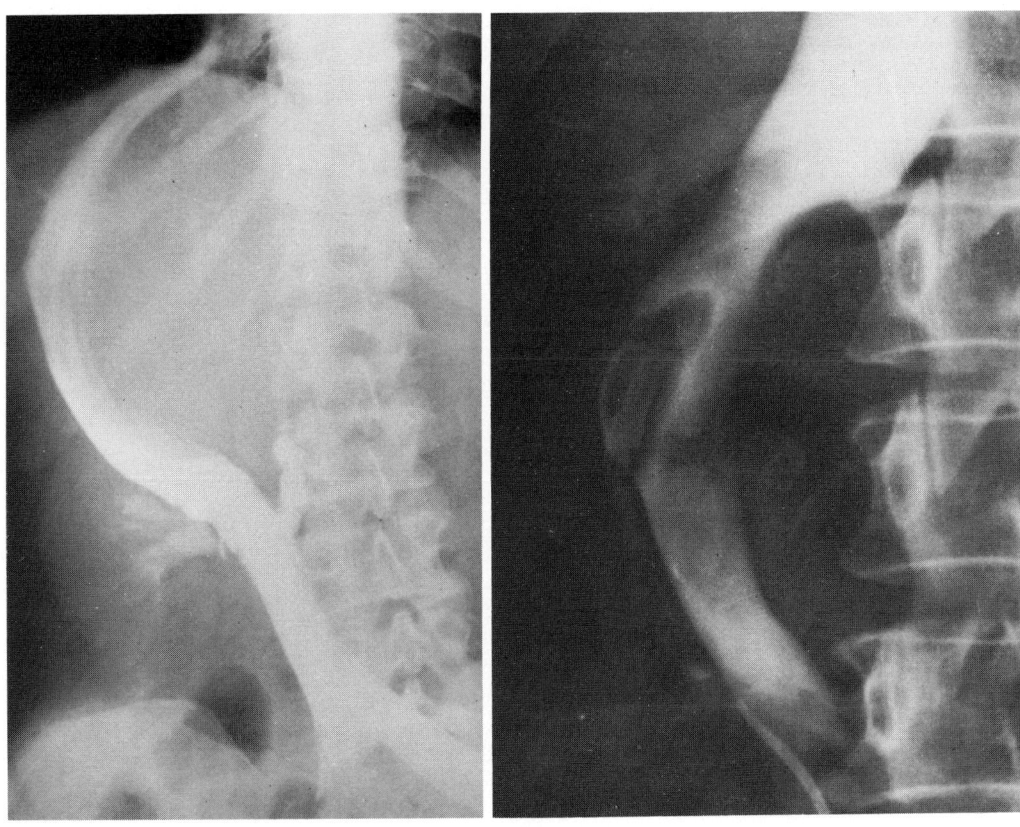

Fig. 38.18 (A and B) Inferior vena cavography in two different patients, each with phaeochromocytomas lying medial to the inferior vena cava.

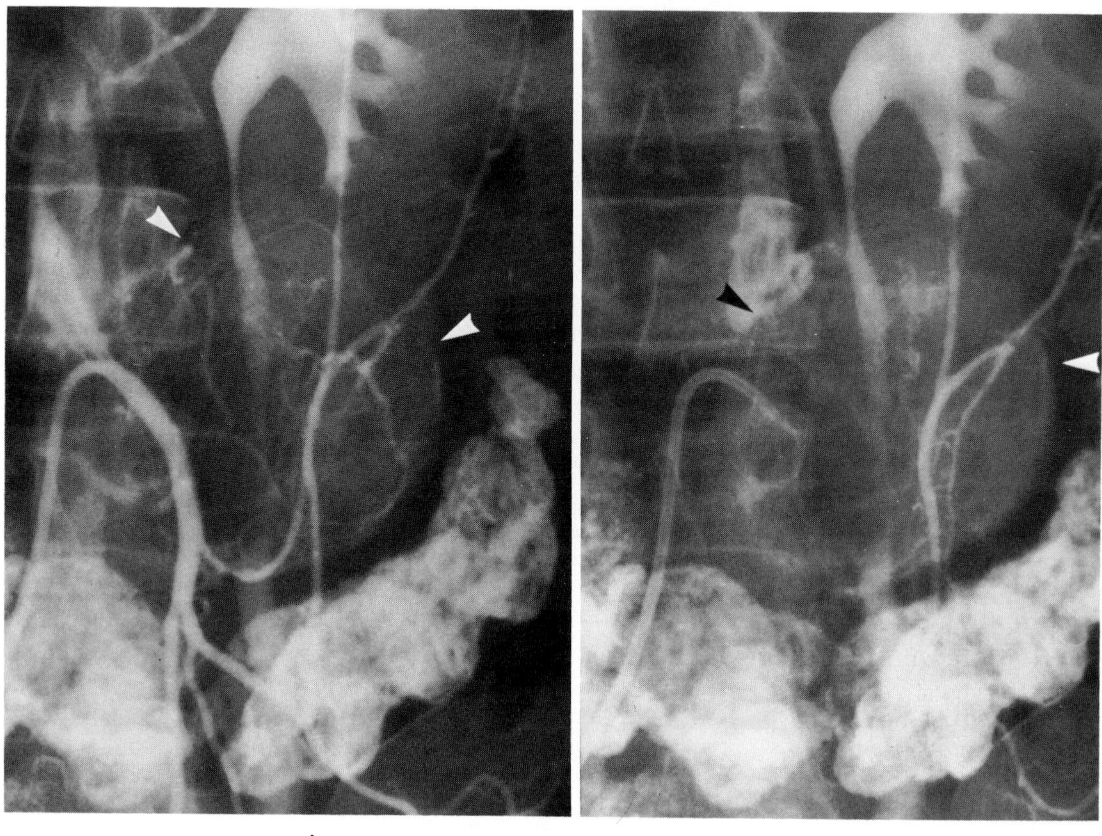

Fig. 38.19 (A and B) Phaeochromocytoma lying below the left kidney and only shown by selective inferior mesenteric arteriography. It had no other arteries of supply.

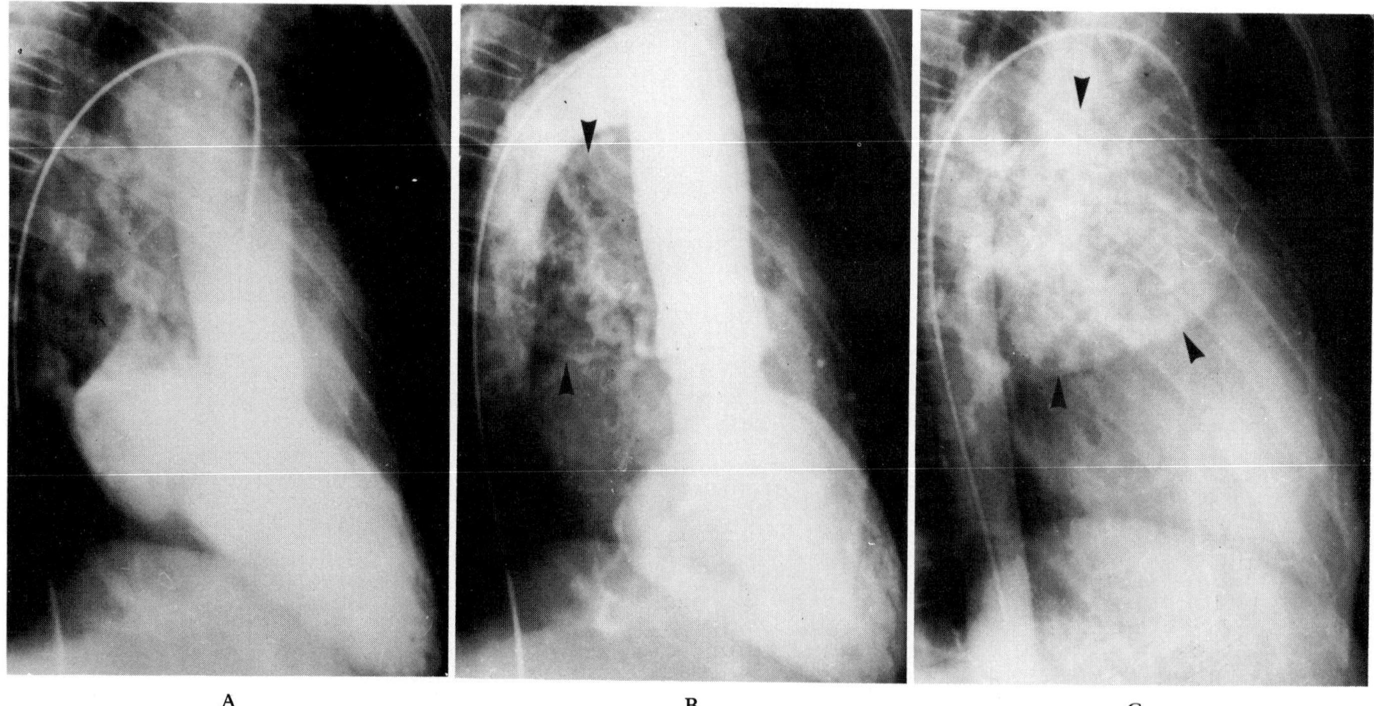

Fig. 38.20 Left ventricular angiocardiogram. A There is evidence of marked mitral incompetence. B and C Pathological vessels are shown arising from the aorta to supply a large vascular mass above the left auricle.

even fainting brought on by micturition. Other ectopic phaeochromocytomas have been demonstrated in the paravertebral gutter in the thorax, and in the neck, and these presumably arise from sympathetic tissue. The most remarkable ectopic tumour in our experience was found to lie above the left auricle of the heart to which it was closely attached. This particular patient underwent every known investigation including simple X-ray, retroperitoneal air insufflation, abdominal aortography, selective adrenal angiography, and adrenal phlebography. Even a laparotomy was negative, and it was not until a subsequent admission, when she presented with increasing cardiac symptoms, that the tumour was diagnosed by left heart angiocardiography (Fig. 38.20). This case serves to emphasize that while a phaeochromocytoma can be among the simplest of tumours to diagnose and localize, it can also be among the most difficult.

Even large tumours which at first sight seem normal in situation can be shown to be locally ectopic if adequately investigated (Fig. 38.18).

4. **Renal artery stenosis in phaeochromocytoma.** The problem of the occasional association of renal artery stenosis or obstruction with phaeochromocytoma has already been touched on (Figs. 38.15 and 38.17). There are a number of such cases described in the literature. In most of these the renal artery was either stretched or compressed by a tumour in the renal hilum, as in the cases described above. In many of these reported cases the artery or kidney had to be sacrificed at operation.

It is important that in these cases the possibility of a phaeochromocytoma should be considered since they can present clinically as apparent cases of vascular hypertension. This implies the routine performance of biochemical tests to exclude phaeochromocytoma even in patients with persistent hypertension and apparent unilateral renal ischaemia.

REFERENCES AND SUGGESTIONS FOR FURTHER READING

Bernardino, M. E., Goldstein, H. M. & Green, B. (1978) Grey scale ultrasonography of adrenal neoplasms. *American Journal of Roentgenology*, **130,** 741–4.

Cremin, B. J. & Kaschula, R. O. C. (1972) Arteriography in Wilms tumour. *British Journal of Radiology*, **45,** 415–22

Farah, J. (1971) New pre-formed catheter for right adrenal phlebography. *Radiology*, **101,** 274.

Hanafee, W. N. (1972) *Selective Angiography*. Baltimore, Maryland: Williams & Wilkins.

Hartmann, C. W., Witton, D. M. & Weeks, R. E. (1966) The role of nephrotomography in diagnosis of adrenal tumours. *Radiology*, **86,** 1030–1034.

Kahn, P. C. & Nickros, L. V. (1967) Selective angiography of the adrenal glands. *American Journal of Roentgenology*, **101,** 739–749.

Korobkin, M., White, E. A., Kressel, H. Y., Moss, A. A. & Montagne, J. P. (1979) Computed tomography in the diagnosis of adrenal disease. *American Journal of Roentgenology*, **132,** 231–238.

Kyaw, M. M. (1972) Simple pre-shaped catheter for bilateral adrenal vein catheterisation. *Radiology*, **105,** 201.

McLachlan, M. S. F. & Beales, J. S. M. (1971) Retroperitoneal pneumography in the investigation of adrenal disease. *Clinical Radiology*, **22,** 188–197.

Queloz, J. M., Capitanio, M. A. & Kirkpatrick, I. A. (1972) Wolman's disease. Roentgen observations in three siblings. *Radiology*, **104,** 357–359.

Rossi, P., Young, I. S. & Panke, W. F. (1968) Techniques useful for hazards of arteriography in phaeochromocytoma. *Journal of the American Medical Association*, **205,** 547–571.

Salz, N. J., Luttwak, E. M., Schwarz, A. & Goldberg, G. M. (1956) Danger of aortography in the localisation of phaeochromocytoma. *Annals of Surgery*, **144,** 118–21.

Starer, F. (1970) The radiology of suprarenal masses. *British Journal of Hospital Medicine*, **4,** 207–212.

Straube, K. R. & Hodges, C. V. (1966) Phaeochromocytoma and renal artery stenosis. *American Journal of Roentgenology*, **98,** 222–234.

Sutton, D. (1968) Diagnosis of Conn's and other adrenal tumours by left adrenal phlebography. *Lancet*, **1,** 453–455.

Sutton, D. (1975) The radiological diagnosis of adrenal tumours. *British Journal of Radiology*, **48,** 237–258.

Wolman, M., Sterk, V. V. & Gatt, S. (1961) Primary familial xanthomatosis with adrenal calcification. *Journal of Paediatrics*, **28,** 742–757.

Yun Ryo, U., Johnston, A. S., Kim Ilsup & Pinskey, S. M. (1978) Adrenal scanning uptake with ^{131}I 6β Iodomethyl/Nor Cholesterol. *Radiology*, **128,** 157–161.

PART 5

THE UROGENITAL TRACTS

CHAPTER 39

THE URINARY TRACT: METHODS OF EXAMINATION

INTRAVENOUS UROGRAPHY

The greatly improved results obtained by intravenous urography in recent years are partly due to refinements in the technique of the examination and partly to the introduction of the tri-iodinated salts of diatrizoate, iothalamate and metrizoate. There is little difference between the modern triodinated contrast media as regards mode of excretion, toxicity and frequency of side effects but there is evidence that for a given intravenous dosage of iodine the contrast media containing the sodium salts achieve slightly higher concentration of iodine in the urine.

In patients with normal renal function some 98 per cent of the injected diatrizoate and iothalamate salts is excreted by the kidneys within 24 hours. The remaining 2 per cent is excreted by the liver and the small intestine. Increased extrarenal excretion, leading to opacification of the biliary tree, the small and the large intestine, may occur when high dosages are used in patients with impairment of renal function. It may also occur in the presence of unilateral and bilateral ureteric obstruction without an apparent impairment of function tests (Fig. 39.1). With large doses of the metrizoate salt (Triosil) extrarenal excretion is not uncommonly seen even in the complete absence of evidence of renal disease. It seems likely that the increased protein binding ability of this salt is responsible for the increased extrarenal excretion.

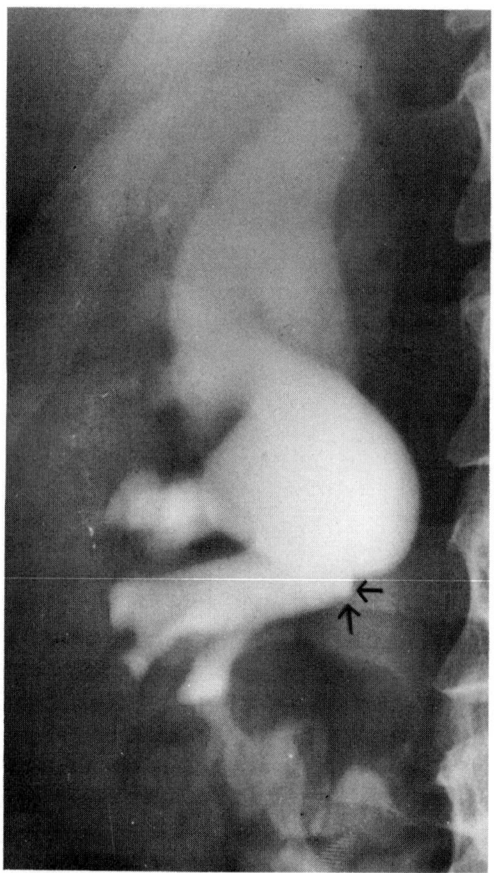

Fig. 39.1 Gallbladder opacification with high dose urography in the presence of renal pelvic obstruction (arrows).

Urinary excretion occurs by glomerular filtration. The concentration of contrast medium in the glomerular filtrate is the same as the concentration in the plasma, and thus is dependent on the injected dose and the body weight. There is still doubt as to whether there is any excretion by the renal tubular cells. Certainly in the presence of normal glomerular function tubular excretion is unlikely to exceed 2 per cent of the total urinary excretion. Reabsorption of sodium and water from the filtrate in the proximal renal tubule results in a marked increase in the concentration of the contrast medium within the proximal tubule, which is independent of the state of hydration. Further reabsorption of water in the distal tubule is controlled by the circulating level of anti-diureteric hormone, the level of ADH being increased by fluid deprivation. Very large doses of contrast medium produce an osmotic diuretic effect competing with the normal tubular concentrating mechanism and thus leading to a lower concentration within the tubule.

The nephrogram is mainly due to the accumulation of contrast medium within the proximal tubule and is thus the result of glomerular filtration. Its density is maximal at the end of a rapid intravenous injection corresponding to the maximum plasma concentration and its density will be directly proportional to the dose of contrast medium. The nephrographic density is unaffected by water deprivation but will be affected by radiographic factors, overlying soft tissue thickness, the renal substance thickness and the number and volume of the functioning nephrons.

The radiographic density of the collecting systems is also influenced by radiographic factors and soft tissue thickness but is mainly determined by the total amount of contrast medium in the calyces and renal pelvis, i.e. on the product of the concentration and volume of the contrast medium. Dehydration leading to an increase in the level of circulating ADH results in increased water absorption in the distal tubule and thus gives a denser shadow in the collecting system.

CONVENTIONAL DOSAGE UROGRAPHY

A strict routine cannot be laid down for intravenous urography. Each examination must be carefully supervised by a radiologist at every stage and modified according to the results obtained.

A period of preliminary preparation is desirable. Intestinal gas shadows are most troublesome in patients confined to bed and whenever possible the examination should be performed on outpatients. The bowels should be cleared by aperients taken on the two nights prior to the examination and only a light dry breakfast should be allowed on the morning of the examination.

The use of high dosages of contrast medium makes it possible to obtain adequate results without preliminary dehydration but dehydration does increase the concentration of iodine in the distal renal tubules and pelvicalycine systems. For the conventional examination in adults the intake of all fluids should be restricted to 1 pint (560 ml) over the preceding 24 hours and no fluid is permitted during the 12 hours immediately preceding the examination. This strict regime should not be enforced in infancy and childhood. In infancy the examination is best carried out immediately before the next feed is due and in childhood a period of 12 hours dehydration is adequate. Dehydration must be avoided in the presence of proteinuria from multiple myeloma and also when renal function is impaired.

Plain films of the kidneys, ureters and bladder must be taken and viewed before the intravenous injection of contrast medium. Twenty ml of Conray 420 (8 g of iodine) or an equal iodine dosage with some other contrast medium will produce a satisfactory urogram in a normal well-dehydrated patient. Greatly improved results are obtained with the use of higher dosages and it is recommended that 40 ml of Conray 420 or similar contrast medium (16 g iodine) be administered for the routine examination of the average adult of 70 kg. In the obese patient the dosage should be increased to 60 or 80 ml (25–32 g iodine). Neonates, infants and small children may be given 1 ml per lb of body weight of Conray 280 (2·2 ml per kg) up to a maximum of 20 ml. In recent years much larger doses of contrast medium have become routine at many centres but it is possible that the routine use of very large doses may be responsible for an apparent increase in the mortality of this examination.

The pelvis of young patients is protected with a lead sheet and the first film 'coned down' to the kidneys should be taken 3 minutes after the injection; ureteral compression is then applied. A second 'coned' film of the kidneys is taken 15 minutes after the injection and, provided that the pelvicalycine systems have been well demonstrated, compression is released, the protection removed and a full-length film taken of the kidneys and ureters. If the kidneys have not been well demonstrated ureteral compression is maintained, further films are taken at 10 minute intervals and further injections of contrast medium given if necessary until the upper urinary tract is adequately demonstrated. After release of compression an A.P. film is taken of the full bladder, supplemented when necessary by oblique views, and is followed by an after micturition film.

Modifications and additional views

Inspiratory, expiratory and oblique views may be required to demonstrate the relationship of opacities and filling defects to the kidneys, ureters and bladder.

Tomographic cuts may be required to demonstrate accurately the renal outlines and to overcome obscuring intestinal shadows particularly in infancy and childhood. Thick cuts (1 to 2 cm) produced by a short tube swing are usually all that is required.

Prone films are of great value in the investigation of the pelvi-ureteric junction and of ureteric obstruction. These should be taken when the renal pelvis or calyces have been well filled, after which the patient may be sat up for a few minutes before being turned into a prone position. In this position heavy contrast-laden urine lying in the dorsally situated calyces and renal pelvis will gravitate down to the site of the obstruction.

Rapid sequence urography should be a routine procedure in hypertensive patients. Films of the kidneys are taken at 2, 4 and 6 minutes following the injection of contrast medium; it is thus possible to compare the rate of excretion of contrast medium from each kidney.

A *water load* of 500 ml given by mouth is of value in exaggerating the increased density of the excreted contrast medium in unilateral renal ischaemia. A 'water load' may also be of value in the investigation of suspected cases of pelvi-ureteric junction obstruction—the increased diuresis producing distension of the renal pelvis. This technique for demonstrating pelvi-ureteric junction obstruction can be further improved if the water load is followed by the intravenous injection of a diuretic such as frusemide.

Delayed films taken at hourly intervals up to 24 hours may be necessary to demonstrate the actual site of ureteral obstruction.

An *immediate after micturition* film of the kidneys and ureters may demonstrate ureteral dilatation in the presence of vesico-ureteral reflux, the patient being asked to micturate whilst lying on the table. The absence of ureteral dilatation does not exclude reflux.

Ureteral compression cannot be tolerated in the presence of renal colic and is inadvisable in the investigation of renal trauma; effective compression is also impossible in the presence of large abdominal masses and a distended bladder. It is unnecessary once the diagnosis of ureteral obstruction is established.

HIGH DOSE UROGRAPHY

High dose urography is indicated in the investigation of renal failure and ureteric obstruction. It is also indicated for nephrotomography and for emergency urography when it is not possible to introduce a preliminary period of dehydration. It is occasionally of value in opacifying the bladder for cysto-urethrography when urethral catheterization cannot be carried out.

High dose urography in renal failure. Intravenous urography has been considered to be a dangerous and unrewarding procedure in patients with renal failure but it is now clear that very large doses of contrast medium may be safely administered to patients with renal failure without severe oliguria. The use of large doses of contrast medium in conjunction with tomography will almost always produce a nephrogram and allow an estimation of renal size. The pelvicalycine systems may be only faintly demonstrated, but the results are usually adequate to demonstrate the presence or absence of extrarenal obstruction. Retrograde urography with its attendant hazards can be almost completely eliminated in the investigation of these patients.

Dialysis prior to the examination improves the urographic results; lowering of the blood urea level leads to a diminished osmotic diuretic effect and an increased tubular concentration of contrast medium. The failing kidney is incapable of concentrating urine, so the surviving nephrons must carry an increased volume of water and dehydration therefore produces a negative fluid balance which is almost certainly a greater danger than the injection of contrast medium. It must be emphasized that patients must always be well hydrated before injecting large doses of contrast medium. One ml of Conray 280 (or equivalent contrast medium) per lb of body weight (2·2 ml per kg) is given intravenously by injection. There is no advantage in using the drip infusion method where the contrast medium is diluted with 5 per cent dextrose. The infusion of large volumes of fluid is in fact contraindicated in the presence of cardiac failure and in these patients it is also preferable to avoid the sodium salts.

In the normal patient the density of the nephrogram is proportional to the plasma concentration of contrast medium and it is at a maximum at the end of the injection. In the presence of hypotension or renal ischaemia the appearance of the nephrogram will be delayed. With extra- and intrarenal obstruction the nephrogram persists and increases in density over several hours. A similar state of affairs is seen in any condition in which glomerular filtration continues in association with tubular stasis. These include acute extrarenal obstruction, renal vein thrombosis, tubular block in acute pyelonephritis, acute medullary necrosis, acute tubular necrosis, multiple myeloma and Tamm Horsfall proteinuria. The nephrogram is usually of uniform and homogeneous density though segmental defects may be seen with peripheral infarcts Polycystic disease produces multiple rounded defects and a patchy irregular nephrogram may be seen in acute pyelonephritis and acute renal venous thrombosis. Glomerular disease, on the other hand, produces an immediate faint persistent nephrogram.

The plasma concentration of contrast medium falls slowly in renal failure allowing adequate time for tomography. A number of tomographic cuts should be taken at the end of the injection at levels 1 cm apart (usually 7, 8 and 9 cm from the table top for the average adult). Subsequent cuts are made at the optimum level at 10 minute intervals for 30 minutes. If no contrast is seen in the collecting systems delayed films at hourly intervals for the first few hours may demonstrate dilated calyces and 12- and 24-hour films will be of value in localizing the site of ureteric obstruction.

The liver and the small intestine normally excrete only 2 per cent of the injected contrast medium but when renal function is impaired a much higher percentage is excreted extrarenally. Visualization of the gallbladder, the bile ducts and the intestine is frequently seen on delayed films in these circumstances (Fig. 39.1). It should be noted, however, that when high doses of metrizoate salts are used delayed films may show evidence of extrarenal excretion in the complete absence of evidence of renal disease.

High dose urography has also been used in the investigation of oliguric and anuric renal failure and also in the presence of combined renal and hepatic failure. In this latter group of patients one of the extrarenal excretion pathways is blocked and very high contrast medium levels persist in the plasma. In the small number of patients so far reported in these two groups there has been no further impairment in the renal or hepatic function. It is too early to assess the safety of this investigation in these patients and the examination should only be done when facilities for dialysis are readily available.

If both kidneys are reduced in size with smooth outlines renal failure is almost certainly due to end stage chronic renal disease—glomerulonephritis, nephrosclerosis, bilateral renal arterial disease, etc. A reduction in size with coarse scarring of the renal surface indicates a diagnosis of chronic pyelonephritis or multiple infarcts.

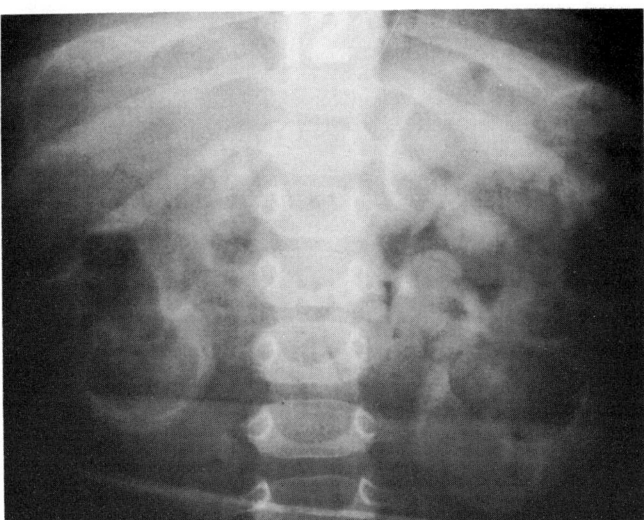

Fig. 39.2 'Crescents' in obstructive uropathy.

These two conditions will be distinguished by the absence of calyceal deformity in patients with infarction.

Enlargement of the kidneys may indicate infiltration of the kidney by lymphoma or amyloid; bilateral acute pyelonephritis; acute tubular or cortical necrosis; polycystic disease; or obstruction.

Polycystic disease will in the majority of cases be associated with lobulation of the outline, calyceal deformity and cystic defects in the nephrogram.

The main objective of this examination is to rule out an obstructive nephropathy as the cause of renal failure. In extrarenal obstruction the kidney is usually markedly enlarged and a dilated renal pelvis may be visible as a large soft tissue mass. Even in the presence of complete ureteral obstruction tubular reabsorption of sodium and water continues, the resultant reduction in the pressure and volume of tubular fluid enables glomerular filtration to proceed. The nephrogram is thus delayed and slowly increases in density, the concentrated opacified fluid in the tubules may be seen as 'crescents' around the radiolucent dilated calyces, or as a narrow rim of surviving renal tissue outlining the kidney (Fig. 39.2). As the dilated collecting system opacifies the nephrogram slowly fades, and films taken up to 24 or even 48 hours after injection may demonstrate the site of obstruction.

NEPHROTOMOGRAPHY

Nephrotomography has been used for many years particularly in the United States for the demonstration of renal masses. Preliminary tomographic cuts of the renal area should be obtained to determine the level which best demonstrates the kidney. When all is set for tomography at this preselected level a high dose of contrast medium (e.g. $\frac{2}{3}$ ml Conray 420 per lb of body weight) is rapidly injected intravenously. The simultaneous injection of half the total dose into each arm ensures rapid introduction of the medium. The tomographic cut is made at the end of the injection. With vascular tumours a pathological circulation may be seen and the blotchy nephrogram contrasts with the well-demarcated defect produced by a renal cyst or intrarenal haematoma. Nephrotomography is a useful method for demonstrating the multiple nephrographic defects of polycystic disease and it may also be used to demonstrate the size of the adrenal glands. Selective renal angiography with angiotomography (a tomographic cut at the end of a renal arterial injection) is, however, much superior for the differentiation of renal cyst from renal tumour. When dealing with renal masses nephrotomography should be reserved for those patients in whom angiography has proved to be difficult or is considered to be hazardous, i.e. the elderly and patients with arterial disease.

ADVERSE REACTIONS

The majority of reactions occur quite unpredictably and severe reactions may occur even when there has been a previous uneventful examination but the incidence of reactions is considerably higher in patients with a history of allergy or sensitivity of one type or another. Patients suffering from asthma or angioneurotic oedema are particularly prone to quite severe reactions and about one-third of patients with a history of a previous reaction will react to subsequent injections.

Major reactions may occur after minute doses but there is evidence to suggest that there is an increased incidence of reactions when high doses are administered, particularly in infancy, old age and in the presence of renal failure. Animal experiments also indicate that there is increased toxicity with high dosage. In infancy the hyperosmolar effect of high doses may produce pulmonary and cerebral oedema and, in renal failure, anuria and increase in serum creatinine may follow high dosage urography even in the well hydrated patient.

The rate of injection of urographic contrast media does not seem to have any effect on the incidence of reactions but if there appears to be an increased risk of a reaction it is prudent to inject 1 ml of contrast and wait a few minutes before proceeding with a slow injection of the full dose.

The occurrence of renal failure following intravenous urography in *multiple myeloma* is an unusual event but several cases have been described in patients with Bence Jones protein-uria. Renal failure in these cases is due to the deposition of protein casts in the tubules leading to blockage and subsequent atrophy of nephrons. It is possible that this cast formation is due to dehydration and not the direct result of contrast medium. Intravenous urography should only be carried out on patients with Bence Jones proteinuria when there are definite indications that it is likely to produce useful information; preliminary dehydration of these patients must be avoided.

In terms of toxicity there is little difference between the available contrast media, all contrast media and particularly the methylglucamine salts can act as histamine-releasing agents.

Many of the symptoms and signs of contrast media reactions are similar to those produced by allergy but it now seems unlikely that they can be entirely explained on an allergic basis and it is more likely that several factors are involved. Histamine release, hypertonicity, enzyme inhibition have all been incriminated and it is possible that anxiety may play a part.

Figures for the mortality rate of intravenous urography vary widely from 1 in 40 000 to 1 in 117 000. In a recent United Kingdom survey the mortality rate was given as 1 in 40 000, the incidence of severe non-fatal reactions was 1 in 14 000 and intermediate reactions 1 in 2000 examinations. Minor reactions occur in about 10 per cent of examinations. The introduction of new, apparently less toxic, contrast media and more effective methods of resuscitation appear to have had little effect either on the incidence of reactions or on the mortality rate. This surprising finding is probably due to the recent more extensive use of high dosage urography in infancy, old age and in the very ill patient.

Minor reactions take the form of arm pain, nausea, vomiting, a sensation of heat, sweating, headache, abdominal pain and rigors. These are usually mild and transitory and require no treatment apart from reassurance but minor reactions may precede a more severe reaction. Arm pain due to venous spasm is commoner with high concentrations of sodium salts and it should be distinguished from the severe localised pain produced by perivenous injection which may be followed by a phlebothrombosis. Unexplained rigors may be delayed up to six hours following the injection of contrast medium.

Immediate and severe reactions

Skin rashes of various types may occur and include diffuse erythema, urticaria, periorbital oedema, and angioneurotic oedema.

Iodine effects. A very small amount of free iodine is present in all contrast media, this may lead to interference with radioactive iodine tests of thyroid function. Salivary gland enlargement, often delayed for several days, after the examination is a rare manifestation of iodism.

Bronchospasm and glottic oedema. These are most commonly seen in asthmatics and if severe may result in cyanosis and respiratory and cardiac arrest.

Convulsions and tetany. Convulsions are usually secondary to hypotension but in infancy may also be due to cerebral oedema produced by high dosage. Tetany may result from overbreathing in anxious patients but may also be produced by lowering of the serum calcium.

Hypotension. Syncope may result from obstruction to venous return by abdominal compression, it is relieved by releasing compression and tilting the patient's head downwards. Hypotension also occurs in the absence of abdominal compression, the patient is pale, cold, clammy with bradycardia and if there is a profound fall in blood pressure, consciousness may be lost with a consequent risk of airways obstruction.

Arrhythmias and cardiac disorders. Cardiac arrest, arrhythmias and electrocardiographic changes are commoner in older patients with heart disease. They may be due to a direct toxic effect of the medium on the myocardium possibly aggravated, when large doses are used, by a high sodium load.

Pulmonary oedema may occur in infancy and as a complication of pre-existing heart disease in the older age groups. It is a result of hypervolaemia produced by the osmotic effect of the contrast medium and the infusion of large volumes of fluid.

Prevention and treatment

Even when full precautions are taken adverse reactions will occasionally occur and although the administration of hydrocortisone may decrease the incidence of minor reactions, it appears to have little effect on the incidence of severe reactions.

Test doses have proved unreliable although they have often been given in the past to satisfy a possible medico-legal need and deaths have followed a negative response to a test dose. It is much more important to take a proper history and to see that the staff is properly trained and equipped to deal with a reaction.

In patients with no history of sensitivity to food, drugs or contrast medium and when there is no history of asthma, urticaria, hayfever, etc., the full dose of contrast medium may be given without any preliminary precautions.

In cases with a history of allergic illness or of sensitivity to food or drugs (other than severe reaction to contrast medium) the injection of the medium should be preceded by an intravenous injection of hydrocortisone 100 mg. This should be injected through an indwelling needle or catheter and a venous line should be preserved throughout the examination. After an interval of 30 minutes 1 ml of the contrast should be injected and if there is no reaction the full dose may be given after a delay of a few minutes. Antihistamines appear to have no effect on the development of severe reactions, they may produce undesirable side effects and their *routine* prophylactic use should be abandoned, although they still retain a place in the treatment of allergic reactions with urticaria and angioneurotic oedema and may be useful prophylactically in patients with an 'allergic' history. A number of commonly used contrast media and antihistamines are incompatible and when mixed produce a precipitate. Intravenous antihistamines must not therefore be given in the same syringe as the contrast medium and should preferably be given at a separate site.

When there is a history of previous reaction it is important to assess the nature of the previous reaction and to reconsider the necessity for the examination. The examination should not be repeated unless it is absolutely necessary. If the examination is considered to be essential one should use a contrast medium different from the one to which the patient previously reacted. If the facilities are available the patient should be referred for immunological tests to determine whether there is evidence of sensitivity to the chosen contrast medium. Hydrocortisone 150 mg should be given 30 minutes before the injection of contrast medium through an indwelling venous catheter.

If a severe reaction occurs abdominal compression must be released, the patient's head should be tilted downwards and assistance immediately summoned. *Allergic reactions* should be treated by intravenous chlorpheniramine maleate (Piriton) 10–20 mg followed if the symptoms or signs worsen by hydrocortisone 100 mg slowly intravenously. In all severe reactions intravenous steroids should be administered immediately, larger doses may be effective when smaller doses have failed; an initial dose of 300 mg of hydrocortisone intravenously may be required followed by further doses of 200 to 300 mg every two hours. *Bronchospasm* may be relieved by 0·5 ml of adrenaline 1 in 1000 intramuscularly into the deltoid or by a single slow intravenous injection of aminophylline 250 to 500 mg in 500 ml of saline but corticosteroids must not be withheld. Oxygen is required whether or not cyanosis is detected and an adequate airway must be maintained. If laryngeal oedema does not respond a surgeon should be summoned to carry out a tracheostomy but the radiologist must be prepared to relieve the respiratory obstruction by laryngostomy. *Bradycardia* may be relieved by atropine 1 to 2 mg intravenously and severe hypotension should be treated with intravenous methedrine 3 mg, repeated if necessary. Intravenous diazepam, 10 to 15 mg for an adult, may be used to control convulsions, but it may produce a fall of blood pressure and respiratory depression.

Respiratory and cardiac arrest require immediate steps to ensure an adequate airway, artificial respiration and external cardiac massage whilst assistance is being summoned. Prolonged shock may be due to hypovolaemia which will require correction by plasma expanders.

RETROGRADE UROGRAPHY

The need for retrograde urography, with its risks of infection, septicaemia, ureteric obstruction due to oedema of the ureteric orifice, renal papillary necrosis and extravasation (Fig. 39.3), can be almost completely eliminated if intravenous urography is properly carried out and full use made of delayed films and high dosage. When retrograde catheterization is required merely to determine whether or not an opacity is produced by a ureteric stone, an A.P. and an oblique view is all that is required, In these cases it is usually unnecessary to inject contrast medium. If injection of contrast medium is necessary a dilute contrast medium is less likely to obscure small filling defects. Diodone $17\frac{1}{2}$ per cent, Conray 280 diluted with an equal volume of water, and similar dilution of other commonly used contrast media are all suitable.

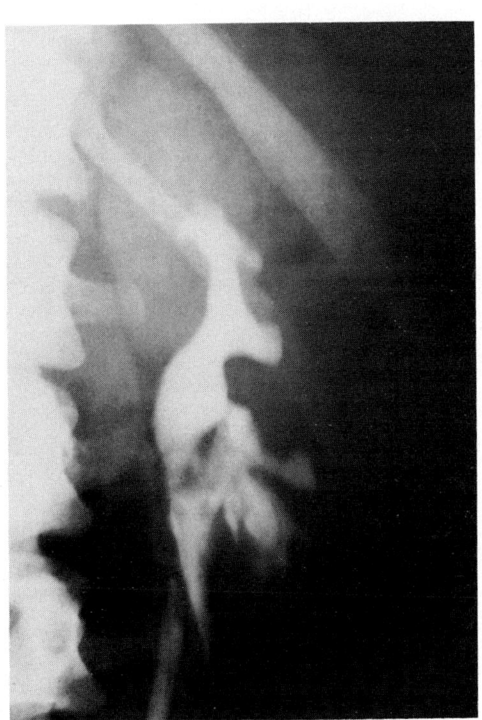

Fig. 39.3 Extravasation during retrograde urography.

More concentrated solutions may be necessary in the very obese or if the contrast medium is diluted by urine in a greatly dilated renal pelvis. The contrast medium should be injected under fluoroscopic control. Films may then be taken in the best position for demonstrating the suspected lesions.

EXTRAVASATION OF CONTRAST MEDIUM

Pyelotubular 'extravasation' due to filling of the collecting tubules is a common normal finding in retrograde urography and also, particularly when ureteral compression is used, in excretion urography. It produces a tuft-shaped or brush-like opacity within the renal pyramid consisting of very fine linear opacities radiating from the minor calyces into the renal medulla and in extreme cases to the cortex (Fig. 39.4A and B). It should not be confused with the larger, more irregular, dilated tubules seen in the *medullary sponge kidney* nor with an early tuberculous erosion.

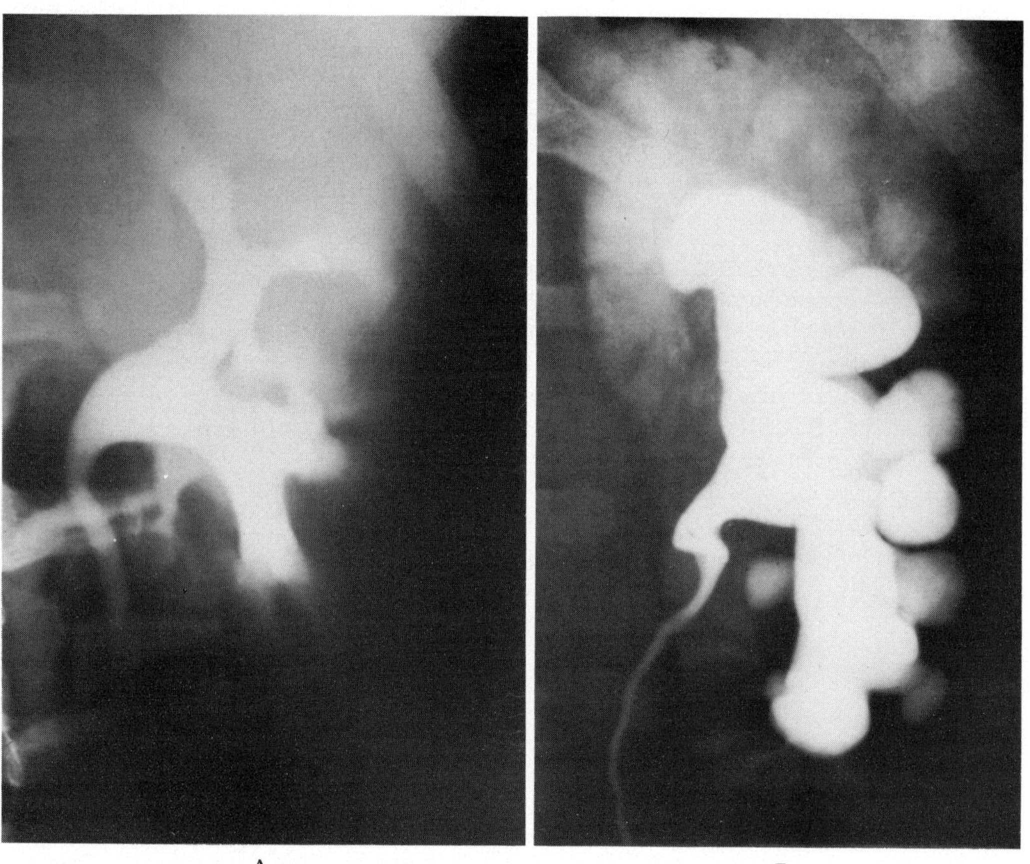

Fig. 39.4 A. Normal compression I.V.U. with tubular extravasation. B. Retrograde urogram, obstructive atrophy with pyelotubular 'backflow' or intrarenal reflux.

Pyelosinous extravasation of contrast medium may be produced by overdistension during retrograde urography and less commonly during intravenous urography. Spontaneous extravasation during intravenous examination usually indicates the presence of ureteral obstruction and is not uncommonly seen when urography is carried out in the investigation of renal colic. It is occasionally seen in the complete absence of any other demonstrable lesion. The extravasation is probably the result of rupture of the calyceal fornix and it produces irregular or horn shaped opacities extending from the minor calyces (Fig. 39.5).

The other types of extravasation are usually more extreme forms of pyelosinous extravasation.

In peripelvic extravasation the contrast medium extends around the renal pelvis and ureter (Fig. 39.6). It is possible that this is one of the mechanisms responsible for the formation of acute perinephric abscess and it has been suggested that chronic retroperitoneal inflammatory changes resulting in pelvic or ureteral obstruction may be produced in this manner.

Pyelolymphatic extravasation occurs following pyelosinous extravasation but may rarely be seen in patients with chyluria as a result of lymphatic obstruction and rupture of a dilated lymph vessel. It produces fine linear opacities extending from the hilum of the kidney to the para-aortic region (Fig. 39.5).

So-called **'Pyelovenous' extravasation** with the production of arcuate opacities in the renal substance is almost certainly due to *peri*vascular extension of pyelosinous extravasation and does not represent contrast medium within the lumen of the veins.

'Pyelointerstitial' extravasation following pyelosinous extravasation produces irregular collections of contrast medium within the renal substance and may rarely extend to the renal capsule and perinephric tissues with the formation of a *perirenal pseudocyst*.

Percutaneous nephrostomy is a useful temporary procedure to provide drainage and maintain function of an obstructed kidney.

The examination is preceded by high dose intravenous urography and tomography to delineate the position and size of the obstructed kidney, premedication is not usually required. With the patient prone and under Image Intensifier control a catheter-over-needle assembly is inserted under local anaesthesia through the loin into the obstructed kidney. On entry into the pelvicalyceal system urine is aspirated and replaced by a slightly smaller quantity of contrast medium. The aspiration of urine and injection of contrast medium may be repeated to promote full mixing of the contrast medium and urine and so delineate the site of obstruction. When the patient's condition permits low ureteric obstruction may be best demonstrated by tilting the patient into the erect position, the catheter may then be left *in situ* to decompress the pelvicalycine system.

If a temporary nephrostomy is to be maintained the simple catheter should be replaced by some form of self-retaining catheter such as a balloon or pigtail catheter.

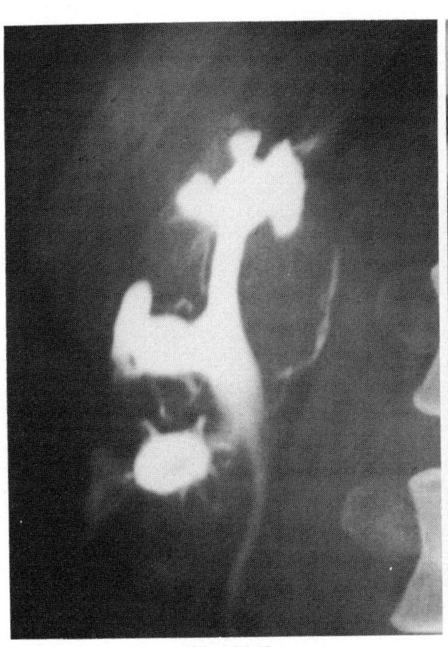

Fig. 39.5

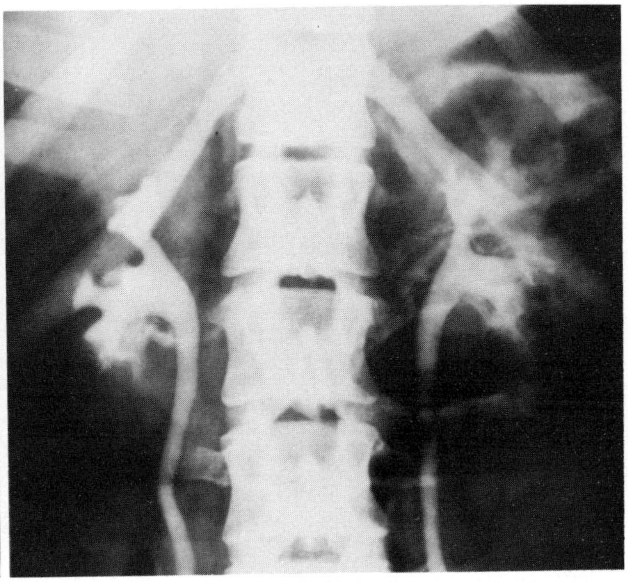

Fig. 39.6

Fig. 39.5 Pyelosinous and lymphatic extravasation.

Fig. 39.6 Peripelvic extravasation during I.V.U.

PERCUTANEOUS UROGRAPHY AND NEPHROSTOMY

Percutaneous urography is a useful adjunct to the investigation of selected cases of obstruction to the upper urinary tract. Intravenous urography with tomography will in most cases establish the diagnosis of obstruction and will also often demonstrate the site and nature of the obstructing lesion. Retrograde ureteric catheterization may then be needed to confirm the diagnosis and to establish drainage of the obstructed renal tract. Percutaneous urography and nephrostomy is indicated in those few cases in whom retrograde ureteric catheterization is impossible, for instance—patients with an ileal loop, patients whose condition precludes general anaesthesia and patients in whom there may be a danger of producing a pyonephrosis with retrograde catheterization.

RENAL MASS PUNCTURE

Percutaneous needle biopsy of renal masses following angiography, nephrotomography, ultrasound examination or C.T. scanning has become increasingly popular. When combined with cytological examination of the aspirate it provides a definite diagnosis and, in the case of simple cysts, a method of treatment which avoids the morbidity of surgical removal. The likelihood of disseminating malignant disease by this examination is very remote and the incidence of significant complications is less than 1·5 per cent. Reported complications include haemorrhage, pneumothorax, arteriovenous fistula, traumatic urinoma and infection.

The examination is conducted with the patient prone, a long needle or a catheter-over-needle is introduced into the renal mass under local anaesthesia with fluoroscopic or sonographic guidance and localization. Entrance into a cyst is indicated by a sudden 'give' similar to that experienced when performing a lumbar puncture and clear straw coloured fluid escapes. The cyst may then be emptied and its contents sent for cytological examination. An alternative method is to aspirate some 20 to 30 ml of fluid and introduce a slightly smaller quantity of water-soluble contrast medium. Films are then taken to ensure that the cyst corresponds with the whole of the space-occupying lesion and that there are no filling defects within it. A further elaboration is to produce a double contrast examination by introducing contrast medium and air. The use of an oily contrast medium (Myodil) is said to reduce the incidence of cyst recurrence. If the cyst contains a filling defect or the aspirated fluid contains blood or altered blood surgical exploration is indicated, even in the absence of positive cytology. In countries where hydatid disease is common cyst puncture should not be undertaken unless hydatid disease has been excluded. If the renal mass proves to be an avascular tumour the characteristic 'give' is not felt on puncture, no fluid escapes but blood or blood-stained fluid is obtained on aspiration. This fluid should be preserved for cytological examination and a few millilitres of contrast medium should be injected to confirm that the puncture has been done at the site of the mass.

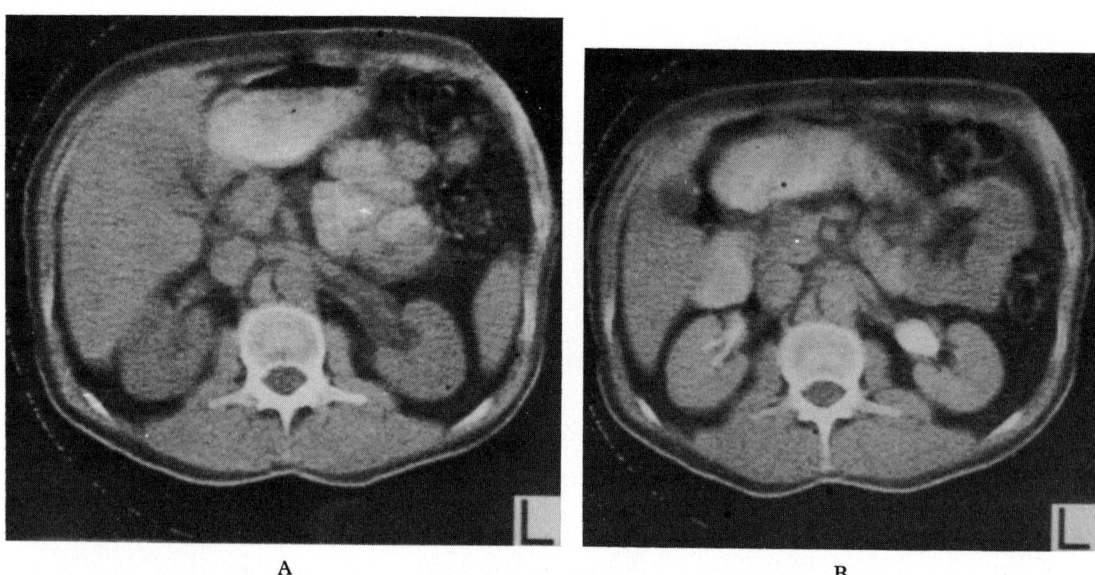

Fig. 39.7 C.T. through kidneys (A) before I.V. contrast, (B) after I.V. contrast Gastrografin in the stomach and small intestine.

COMPUTERIZED TOMOGRAPHY (see Ch. 65)

The kidneys surrounded by fat in the retroperitoneal space are particularly suitable for demonstration by computerized tomography. Scans of the kidney with a slice thickness of 13 mm are usually taken at 15 mm intervals along the long axis lengths of the kidneys but in the investigation of small renal masses it may be necessary to obtain overlapping slices at narrower intervals if narrower collimators are available. Selected slices may then be repeated, when indicated, after enhancement by intravenous urographic contrast medium given either as a bolus injection or as a continuous infusion.

Retroperitoneal structures are clearly demonstrated, the renal outlines can be clearly defined, the cross-sectional size of the kidney and the thickness of its parenchyma can be accurately measured (Fig. 39.7A and B). The renal parenchyma is of homogeneous density (30 to 50 Hounsfield units) and it is not possible to differentiate between cortex and medulla. The calyces and renal pelvis, approximate to water density (0 Hounsfield units) and are visible without the aid of contrast medium enhancement.

The place of computerized tomography in the investigation of *renal masses* is not yet fully determined. It will demonstrate masses projecting from the anterior or posterior surface of the kidney even when the urogram is normal and it can differentiate with a high degree of accuracy between benign renal cyst and tumour. Benign cysts are round or lobulated (unless compressed by adjacent structures) with well defined margins, thin smooth walls and low attenuation approaching that of water (0 Hounsfield units), they do not enhance following contrast medium injection. Tumours are irregular with ill-defined margins and attenuation approximating to that of renal parenchyma but as a result of necrosis may contain areas of low attenuation (0 to 20 Hounsfield units). Very low attenuation is seen in angiomyolipoma. Contrast enhancement occurs even when tumours appear to be avascular on angiography. In the investigation of a renal mass the main advantages of C.T. scanning seem to be:

1. Ability to demonstrate extrarenal extension through the renal capsule into the perirenal tissues.
2. It can demonstrate anterior and posterior subcapsular masses when the urogram is normal.
3. Ability to demonstrate metastatic deposits in lymph glands, liver and lungs.
4. In cystic disease ability to demonstrate the presence of associated cystic disease of the liver and pancreas.
5. It has better resolution than ultrasound and is less dependent on the skill of the operator.

Computerized tomography is of value in the investigation of *renal failure*. The renal size can be accurately measured and hydronephrosis and hydroureter demonstrated either with or without contrast enhancement. It also provides an alternative method to fluoroscopic or ultrasonic guidance for *percutaneous antegrade urography*.

Except when there is gross weight loss the *perinephric spaces* are well demonstrated. Computerized tomography is therefore of particular value in elucidating the cause of *renal or ureteral displacement* and in the investigation of *renal trauma*. Subcapsular and perirenal haematomata are readily visualized and serial scans in these cases will demonstrate changing absorption coefficients indicating liquefaction and dissolution of the blood clot.

The diagnosis and intraluminal extent of *bladder cancer* is established by urography, cystoscopy and biopsy. There are many available radiographic methods (cystography, lymphography, angiography, ultrasonography, intra and perivesical gas insufflation) for assessing the extraluminal extent of the disease but all are inaccurate. Early results indicate that computerized tomography is not only valuable for assessing disease but can also accurately demonstrate intramural and extravesical extension.

MICTURATING CYSTOGRAPHY

Micturating cysto-urethrography is indicated for the following purposes:

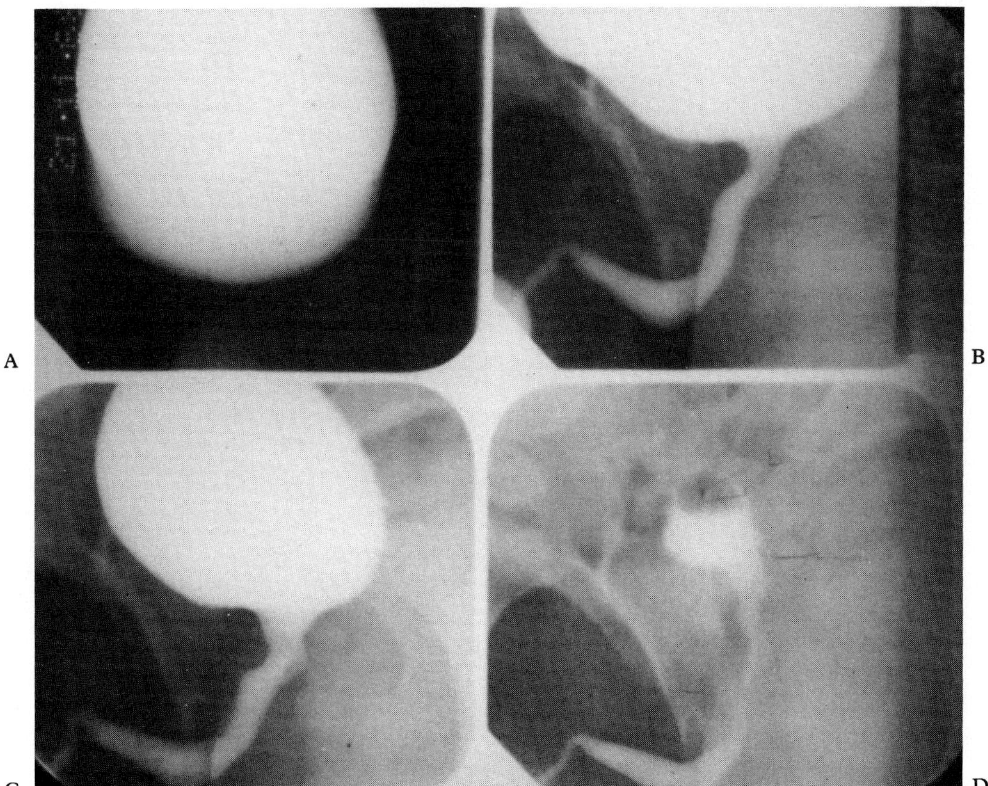

Fig. 39.8 Normal male micturating cystogram.

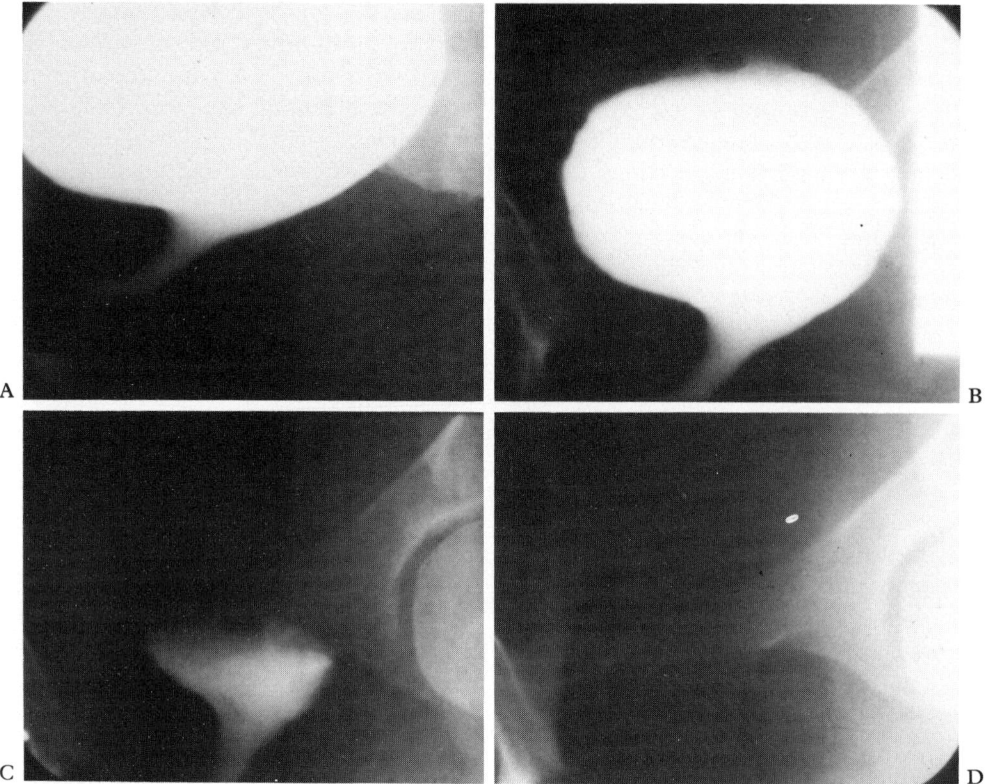

Fig. 39.9 Normal female micturating cystogram.

1. Demonstration of the ability of the bladder to contract.
2. Demonstration of the peripheral control of micturition.
3. Assessment of vesical diverticula.
4. Investigation of anatomical abnormalities of the bladder neck and urethra.
5. Recognition of vesico-ureteric reflux.
6. Investigation of recurrent urinary tract infection.

The examination is contraindicated in the presence of acute infections of the bladder and urethra.

The patient is asked to empty the bladder and the male urethra is anaesthetized with a 1 per cent Lignocaine gel before introducing a urethral catheter. Any residual urine is measured and the bladder filled to full capacity with contrast medium, either Diodone in strengths between 15 and 50 per cent according to the patient's size or Sterile Barium Sulphate 15 to 20 per cent. The latter

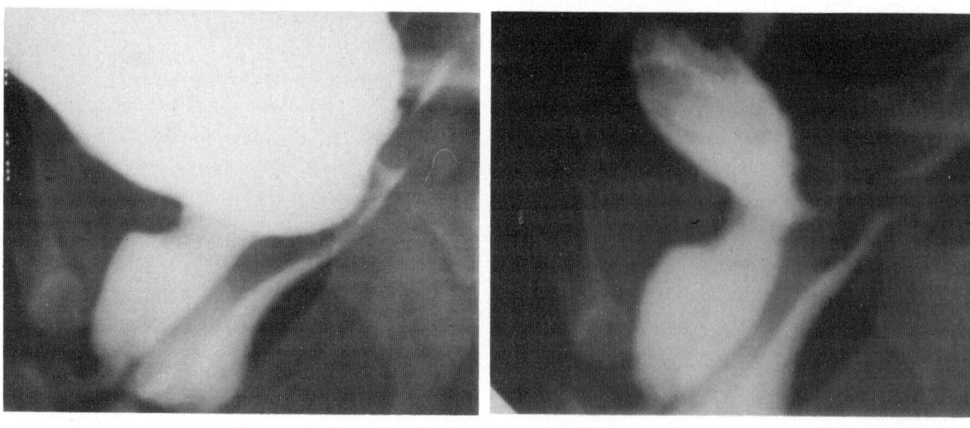

Fig. 39.10 Vaginal reflux.

should be avoided in the presence of diverticula, of a residue greater than 30 ml, and when vesico-ureteric reflux is suspected. A film of the filled bladder is taken in the oblique position and further views may be required at this stage for the demonstration of vesical diverticula. The whole examination is conducted under fluoroscopic control. At least three and preferably four serial film exposures of the entire process of micturition are then obtained. It is essential to rotate the patient into a lateral or oblique position to adequately demonstrate the bladder neck and posterior urethra (Figs. 39.8 and 39.9). The region of the lower ureters must be included on the films so that transient reflux is not missed. Alternatively the examination may be recorded on cine film. Vaginal reflux is a common normal finding in the female (Fig. 39.10).

Infection from the urethral catheterization is the chief hazard. A scrupulous aseptic technique is essential and sulphonamides should be given for four days after the examination.

If urethral catheterization is not possible the bladder may be filled by percutaneous suprapubic catheterization or by high dosage urography but, as already mentioned, it may not be possible to recognize the presence of reflux with certainty if the intravenous route is used.

THE SIMPLE CYSTOGRAM

This examination is rarely indicated, and it is unreliable as a means of diagnosis of bladder tumour. Vesical diverticula are well demonstrated but as these are often secondary to bladder neck or urethral obstruction a micturating cystogram is essential.

THE STRESS CYSTOGRAM

The investigation of stress incontinence demands the demonstration of the position of the bladder base, the size of the cysto-urethral angle and the state of the bladder neck. A sterile 50 per cent suspension of barium sulphate in water is an excellent contrast medium provided that the contra-indications already discussed are observed. In order not to disturb the anatomical relationship of the urethra to the bladder base it is essential that an old soft rubber catheter is used. The bladder is filled with contrast medium, the catheter is opacified with a viscous contrast medium ('Umbradil') and kept in position by strapping to the inner thigh. An erect resting lateral 'Bucky' film is then taken with the tube centred 2 inches above the greater trochanter and this is followed by another film centred in the same place with the patient straining. It is essential to include the tip of the sacrum and the pubic symphysis on both films. A routine micturating cysto-urethrogram should then be carried out and a record obtained of the control of micturition by instructing the patient to interrupt the stream.

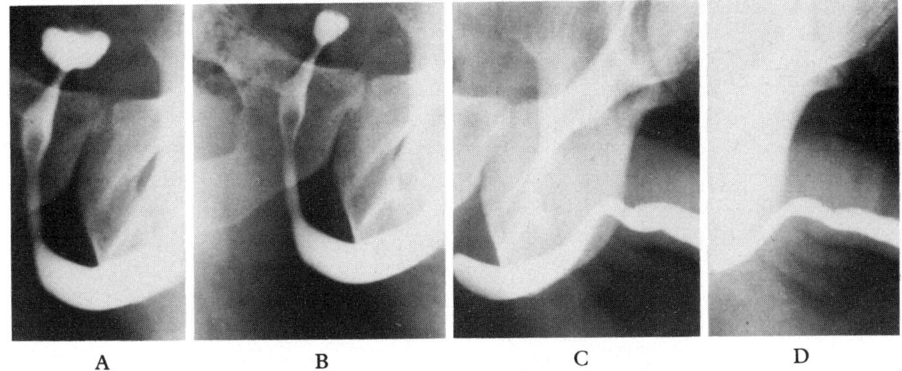

Fig. 39.11 Normal male retrograde urethrogram. The spindle-shaped filling defect in the posterior urethra is produced by the normal verumontanum.

DOUBLE CONTRAST CYSTOGRAPHY

Double contrast cystography gives more information than simple cystography in the investigation of bladder tumours but even more information is normally obtained by cystoscopy.

RETROGRADE URETHROGRAPHY IN THE MALE

The indications are as follows:

1. Demonstration of urethral injuries.
2. Investigation of urethral stricture.
3. Demonstration of false passages.
4. Investigation of peri-urethral abscesses, fistulae, prostatic abscesses and cavities.
5. Investigation of prostatic enlargement.

The examination is contraindicated in the presence of acute urethritis and balanitis, a strict aseptic technique is essential and the examination should be followed by a four-day course of sulphonamides. In the absence of an impassable stricture the micturating cystogram is a better method of investigating urethral strictures and fistulae.

The patient is told to empty his bladder and the viscous contrast medium (Umbradil U) is introduced by means of a Knutsson penile clamp under fluoroscopic control. Several 'spot' films of the urethra are obtained in varying degrees of rotation so that short strictures are not missed (Fig. 39.11) and a lateral-oblique and P.A. view taken of the posterior urethra and bladder neck.

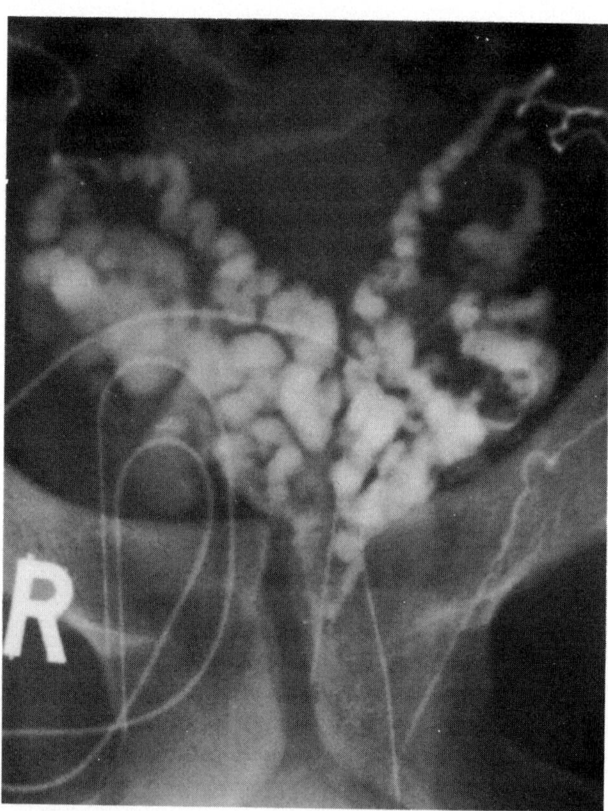

Fig. 39.12 Normal vesiculogram. Fine polythene catheters have been introduced into the vasa deferentia.

VESICULOGRAPHY

Vesiculography is mainly used to demonstrate patency of the genital tract in the infertile male. In the past it has also been used in the investigation of inflammatory disease of the seminal vesicle, epididymis and the prostate and also for the staging of prostatic carcinoma. About 2 ml of contrast medium (Conray 280 or similar) is injected into the exposed vas deferens under fluoroscopic control (Fig. 39.12). An alternative, but more difficult and less reliable, method is to cannulate the orifices of the ejaculatory ducts via a urethroscope.

ANGIOGRAPHY

Renal angiography is of great value in the investigation of renal lesions and in hypertension. It is discussed in detail in Chapter 29.

REFERENCES AND SUGGESTIONS FOR FURTHER READING

Ansell, G. (1970) Adverse reactions to contrast agents. *Investigative Radiology* **5**, 374–384.

Ansell, G. (1976) *Complications in Diagnostic Radiology*. London: Blackwell Scientific Publishers.

Brown, C. B., Glanney, J. J., Fry, I. K. & Cattell, W. R. (1970) High dose urography in oliguric renal failure. *Lancet*, **ii**, 952.

Fry, I. K. & Cattell, W. R. (1971) High dose urography. *British Journal of Radiology*, **44**, 198–202.

Grainger, R. G. (1972) Renal toxicity of radiological contrast medium. *British Medical Bulletin*, **28**, 191.

Sagel, S. S., Stanley, R. J. & Levitt, R. G. (1977) Computed tomography of the kidney. *Radiology*, **124**, 359–370.

Saxton, H. M. (1969) Review article. Urography. *British Journal of Radiology*, **42**, 372–377.

Saxton, H. M. & Strickland, B. (eds) (1972) *Practical Procedures in Diagnostic Radiology*. London: H. K. Lewis.

van Waes, Paul, F. G. M. (1972) High dose urography in oliguric and anuric patients. *Excerpta Medica*, Amsterdam.

Witten, D. M., Myers, G. H. & Utz, D. C. (1977) Seminal vesiculography. *Clinical Urography*, vol. **1**, 76–88. (W. B. Saunders Company, Philadelphia, London, Toronto).

Whole body computed tomography (1977) *Radiologic Clinics of North America*, **15**, No. 3, 401–441.

CHAPTER 40

CONGENITAL LESIONS

THE KIDNEY AND URETER

Renal dysplasia

The term dysplasia indicates some abnormality of development which results in the presence of abnormal tissue within the kidney—cartilage, muscle, primitive nephrons and cysts. The affected kidney may be grossly disorganized, as in the multicystic kidney, or may be macroscopically normal. In its most minor form it is probably of little clinical significance although it is possible that the abnormal tissue may act as a nidus for bacterial infection. Vesico-ureteric reflux or obstruction in early life may be predisposing factors.

The most common radiological appearance is that of a small kidney usually some 4 to 5 cm in length with a coarsely scarred surface and dilated calyces (Fig. 40.1).

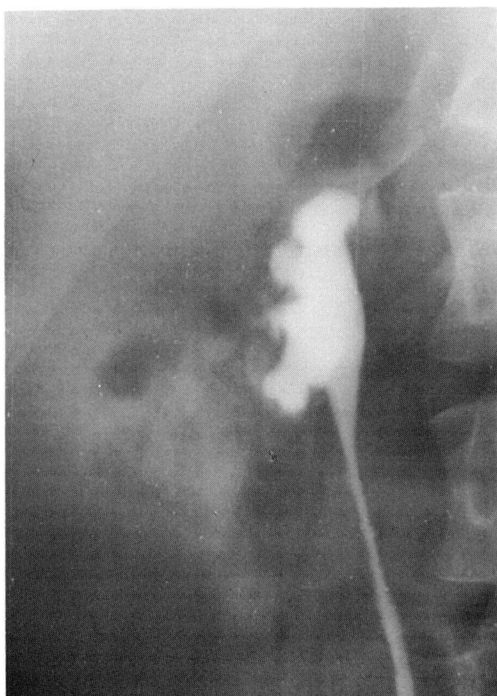

Fig. 40.1 Dysplastic kidney.

Aortography demonstrates a small thread-like renal artery.

In both their mode of presentation and in their radiological appearances these cases are indistinguishable from chronic pyelonephritis but it must be remembered that the great majority of small scarred kidneys with calyceal deformity are a manifestation of chronic pyelonephritis.

Multicystic kidney

This is an extreme form of renal dysplasia in which the entire kidney is composed of numerous cysts varying in size from a few millimetres to two or more centimetres in diameter, resembling a bunch of grapes. The condition is not familial, it is usually unilateral, bilateral disease being incompatible with prolonged extra-uterine existence. The cysts lined with cuboidal epithelium contain clear or straw-coloured fluid and are embedded in a stroma of undifferentiated mesenchymal tissue; primitive cartilaginous and lymphoid tissue may also be present but there is no identifiable renal tissue. The ureter draining the affected kidney is either completely absent or atretic, the renal artery is absent or very small and thread-like.

There is an increased incidence of congenital abnormalities in the contralateral kidney (most commonly pelvi-ureteric junction obstruction) and also in other systems (oesophageal atresia, tracheo-oesophageal fistula, imperforate anus, ventricular septal defect, patent ductus arteriosus, hydrocephalus and meningomyelocoele).

Unilateral multicystic kidney is the commonest cause of an abdominal mass presenting in infancy, it is otherwise asymptomatic and it rarely presents in adult life. Plain films of the abdomen will demonstrate a large mass extending from the loin, displacing loops of bowel medially and anteriorly. Calcification in the walls of the cysts may occur in cases presenting later in life resulting in multiple ring like densities which are said to be characteristic of the disease. There is no excretion of contrast from the affected kidney and there is no nephrogram. The contralateral kidney if healthy shows compensatory hypertrophy. The draining ureter is absent or atretic, ending blindly, and retrograde urography of the atretic ureter may demonstrate the presence of multiple ureteral saccules.

The main diagnostic difficulty is in differentiating the condition from Wilm's tumour and congenital hydronephrosis. In congenital hydronephrosis high dosage and delayed films will usually demonstrate some evidence of renal function. The 'crescent sign' produced by the compressed nephrogram is characteristic of hydronephrosis but may only be seen on tomography. Retrograde or antegrade urography will establish the diagnosis.

Wilms' Tumour, when extensive, may completely destroy the kidney and at this late stage there may be no evidence of renal function but such cases are rare and absence of demonstrable excretion in Wilms' Tumour is usually due to obstruction by tumour or blood clot. The visualization of a nephrogram or calyces, however deformed, completely excludes multicystic kidney.

Renal agenesis

The complete failure of development of both kidneys is incompatible with prolonged extra-uterine life. It is usually associated with a characteristic facies, oligohydramnios and abnormalities of the lower urinary tract.

Unilateral agenesis is an uncommon congenital anomaly, presumably due to failure of development of the ureteric bud from the Wolffian duct. It is often associated with other abnormalities of the urogenital tract. The single kidney is hypertrophied with a thick renal substance and a normal pelvicalycine system but may be in an abnormal position and may show anomalies of rotation. In all cases of apparent agenesis the lower abdomen and pelvis should be carefully scrutinized in order that a small ectopic kidney is not overlooked. Aortography will confirm the absence of the kidney and renal artery, and cystoscopy will, in the majority, reveal a single ureteric orifice with absence of the homolateral half of the trigone. This cystoscopic appearance is pathognomic of unilateral renal agenesis but a normally developed trigone is present in about one-third of the cases. When a complete trigone is present the ureteric orifice is either blind or absent.

Renal agenesis is commonly associated with anomalies of the genital tract or urethra and the homolateral adrenal gland may be absent.

Renal hypoplasia

True congenital hypoplasia may occur in the ectopic kidney. A small kidney in the normal position, with a normal renal outline, a reduced number of calyces but an otherwise normal collecting system may be the result of congenital hypoplasia. The kidney on the opposite side will be hypertrophied and angiography will demonstrate that the small kidney is supplied by a small but otherwise normal renal artery.

The urographic appearances may be indistinguishable from those seen with *unilateral renal ischaemia* and it is possible that similar angiographic appearances could be produced by recanalization of an occluded renal artery. Shrinkage produced by *chronic pyelonephritis* can be excluded by the presence of a diffuse uniform narrowing of the renal substance and by the absence of calyceal deformity and scarring of the renal outline.

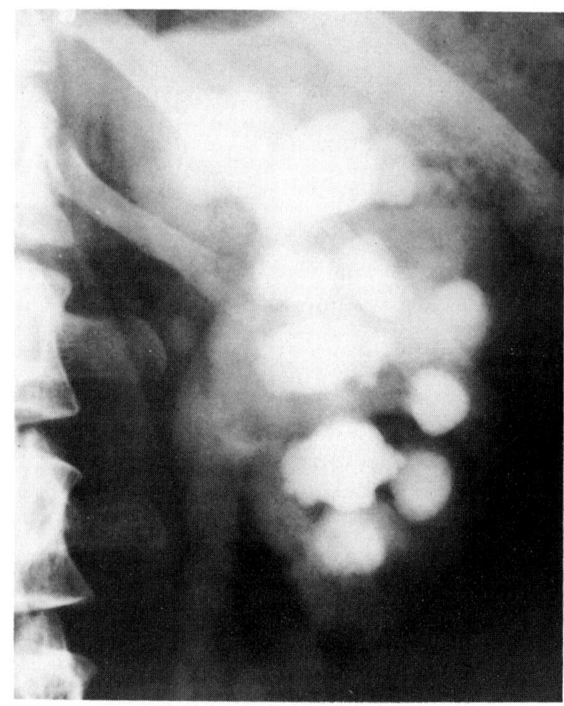

Fig. 40.2 Postobstructive atrophy.

A kidney which has been subject to *obstruction* in the past may also show considerable atrophy and become greatly reduced in size. Postobstructive atrophy produces a diffuse narrowing of the renal substance with a smooth renal outline, but unlike the ischaemic or hypoplastic kidney there is also a uniform dilatation of the minor calyces (Fig. 40.2).

Renal ectopia, malrotation and fusion

The foetal kidney develops in the pelvis by fusion of the ureteric bud arising from the Wolffian duct with the primitive nephrogenic tissue. In this position the renal pelvis lies anterior to the renal tissue, but as the kidney ascends to its normal position in the upper abdomen it rotates so that the pelvis comes to lie on its medial surface. During its ascent it also acquires a permanent blood supply from the upper abdominal aorta.

A failure of the normal ascent is a common congenital anomaly, the kidney remaining within the pelvis or in the

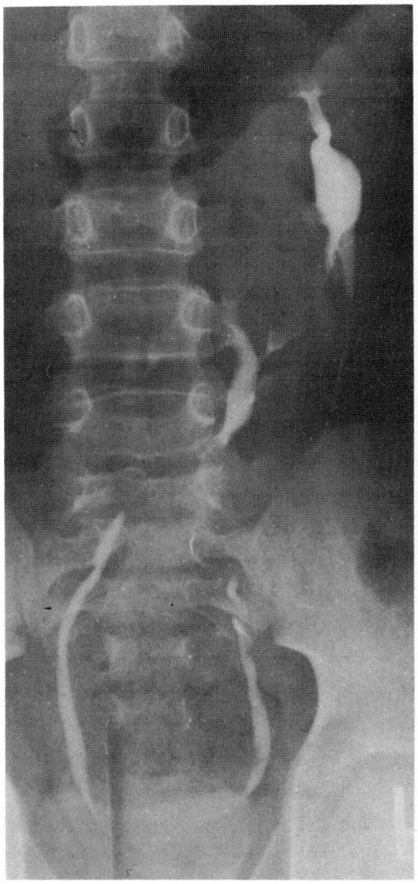

Fig. 40.3 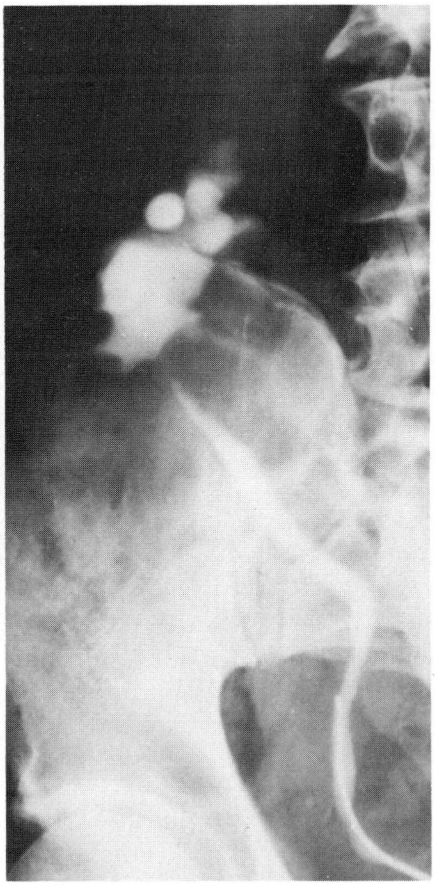 *Fig. 40.4A* 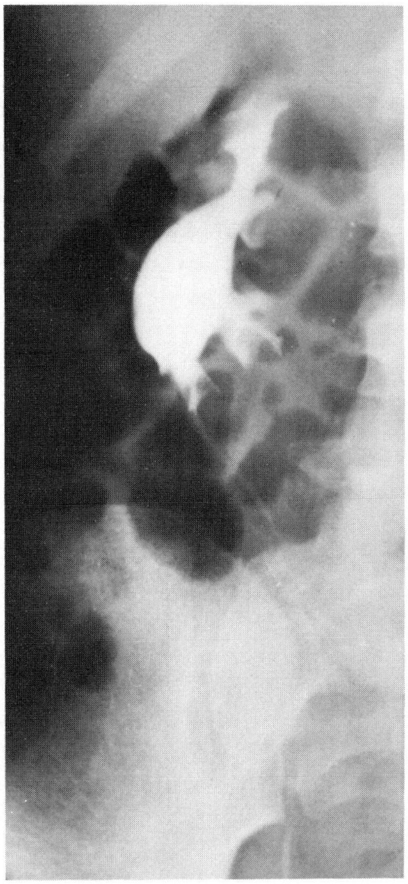 *Fig. 40.4B*

Fig. 40.3 Crossed ectopia producing unilateral fused kidney.

Fig. 40.4A and B Incomplete rotation.

lower abdomen and deriving its blood supply either from the iliac vessels or the lower abdominal aorta. A failure of ascent may be distinguished from ptosis by the absence of any redundancy in the length of the ureter, and by the frequently associated malrotation.

Crossed ectopia occurs when the kidney migrates to the opposite side, the ureteric orifice retaining its normal position in the bladder. The crossed ectopic kidney is low in position, usually malrotated and fused with the lower pole of the normal kidney producing the *unilateral fused kidney* (Fig. 40.3).

Incomplete or abnormal rotation is often associated with ectopia but may also occur in the normally positioned kidney. The commonest variety is that in which the renal pelvis retains its foetal relationship to the kidney tissue and the calyces are seen to lie posteriorly to, and on either side of, the pelvis (Fig. 40.4A). Reverse rotation in which the renal pelvis lies laterally is less common but is frequently seen in the fused kidney (Fig. 40.4B).

The commonest variety of renal fusion is the *horse-shoe kidney* in which the kidneys are united, in the great majority of cases at their lower poles, by a bridge of

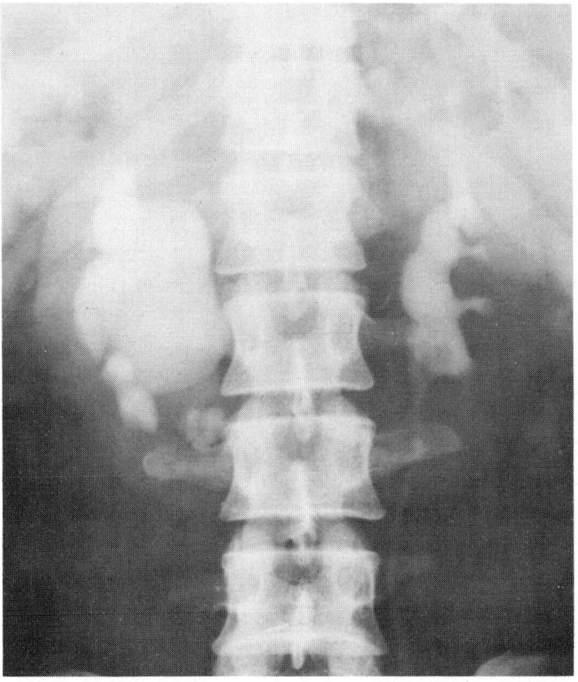

Fig. 40.5 Horseshoe kidney with bridge of renal tissue crossing the spine and obstruction of the right renal pelvis.

renal tissue crossing in front of the aorta, spine and inferior vena cava. The kidneys are low in position, lie close to the spine with their long axes parallel to the spine and the uniting bridge of renal tissue is frequently visible as a soft-tissue mass crossing the spine (Fig. 40.5). There is often an associated malrotation, the renal pelvis lying anteriorly with the calyces posteriorly, laterally or medially. A characteristic feature is the medially directed lower calyces passing into the bridge of renal tissue. Fusion of the upper poles is a much rarer anomaly.

The abnormal relationship of the renal pelvis to the renal vessels and tissue may lead to obstruction with infection, hydronephrosis and stone formation.

Intrathoracic kidney

An intrathoracic kidney may rarely be truly congenital in origin and result from migration of the primitive kidney above the level of the diaphragm before this structure is completely formed at three months gestation. More commonly, an intrathoracic kidney results from herniation through a congenital or acquired diaphragmatic defect.

Renal duplication

Completely separate supernumary kidneys are very rare but up to five kidneys in one individual have been described.

Duplication of the renal pelvis and ureter, the result of abnormal division of the ureteric bud, is a common anomaly.

Complete duplication involves the renal pelvis and whole length of the ureter so that each division of the pelvis is drained by its own ureter opening separately into the bladder. The ureters cross in the abdomen or pelvis so that the ureter draining the upper renal segment always opens below and medial to the ureteric orifice for the lower renal segment.

Incomplete duplication may be confined to the renal pelvis or also involve the ureter, but the ureteric divisions unite at a variable level in the abdomen or pelvis to open at a single ureteric orifice.

In all varieties of duplication the kidney is enlarged and when duplication is unilateral the affected kidney, if healthy, is larger than its fellow on the opposite side. An indentation on the renal outline may be seen corresponding to separate renal segments but complete separation of the renal substance with the formation of a supernumerary kidney is rare.

Uncomplicated cases are of little clinical significance but the presence of duplication must be recognized because of the associated renal enlargement (Fig. 40.6). Urinary infection is said to be commoner in the presence of duplication and minor congenital anomalies such as malrotation and ectopia are frequently associated. The

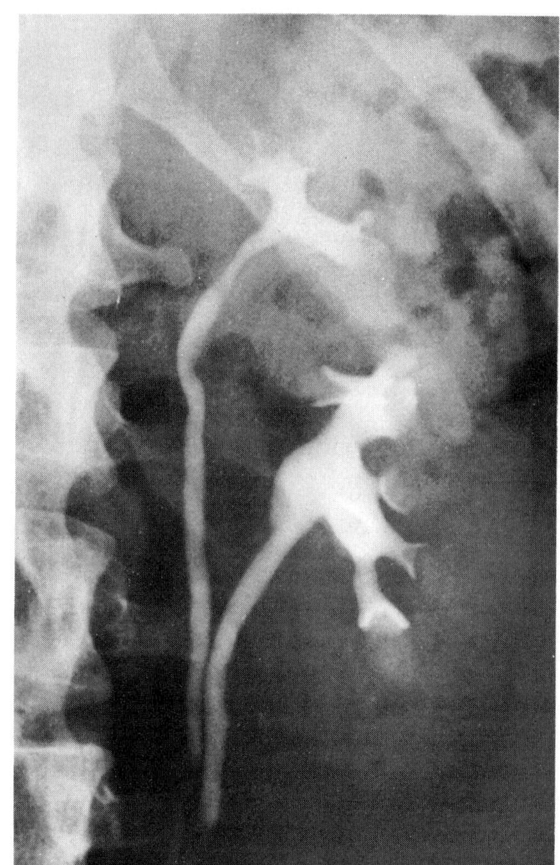

Fig. 40.6 Duplication of the renal pelvis and ureter.

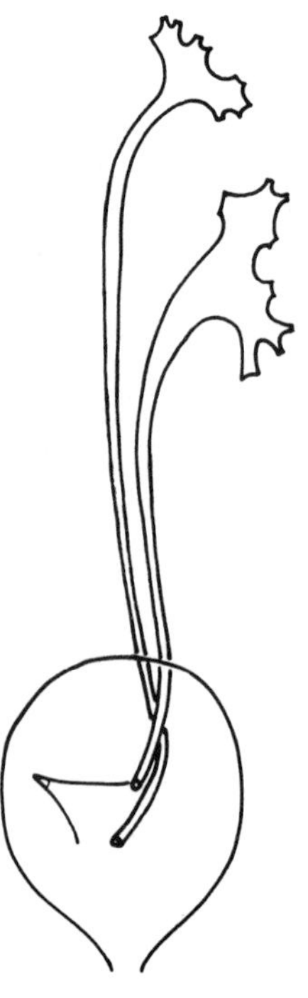

Fig. 40.7 Diagram of renal and ureteric duplication.

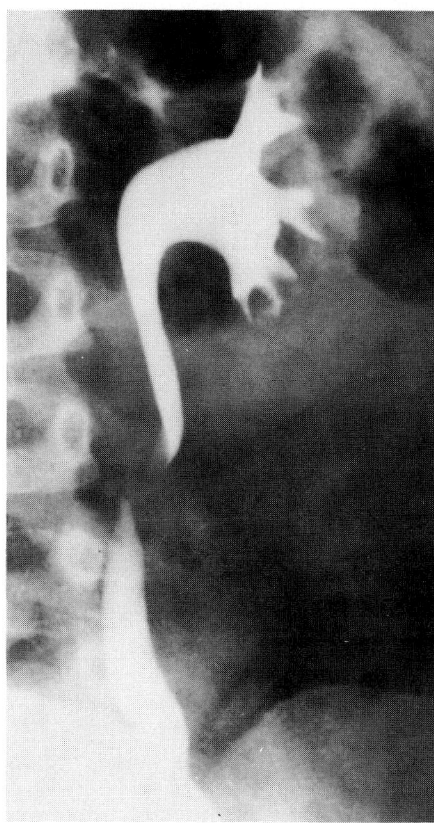

Fig. 40.8 Cystogram demonstrating reflux into the lower moiety of a duplication kidney.

ureter draining the lower renal segment has a shorter intramural course (Fig. 40.7) and is more prone to reflux in the presence of cystitis or lower tract obstruction (Fig. 40.8). Certain pathological conditions such as ureterocoele or ectopic ureteral orifice may also occur and may lead to serious diagnostic error if non-opacification of one renal pelvis remains unrecognized.

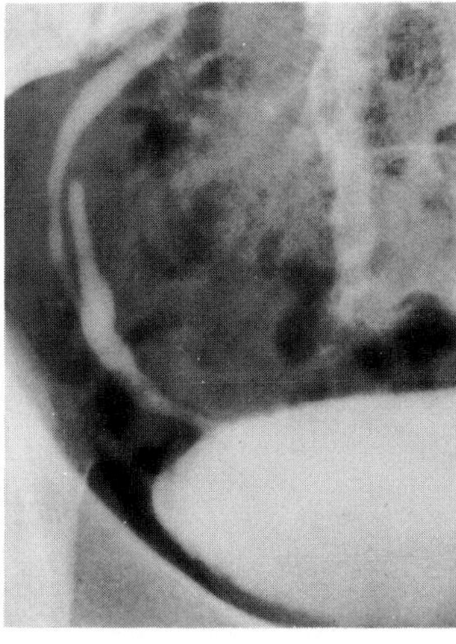

A

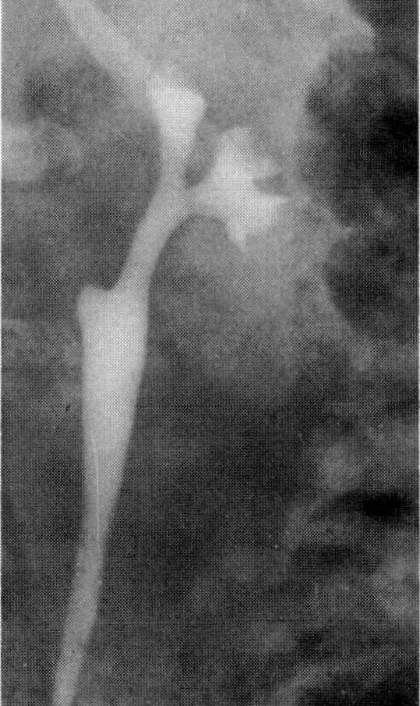

B

Fig. 40.9 A and B Ureteral diverticula.

Ureteral diverticula probably produced by abortive attempts to duplicate are rare; they are usually single but may be multiple (Fig. 40.9). They usually present with urinary infection or stone formation.

The megaureter

The term megaureter should be reserved for cases of unilateral or bilateral congenital dilation of the ureter when there is no evidence of organic obstruction or vesico-ureteric reflux. In some of these patients the bladder capacity is markedly increased (Megaureter-megacystis syndrome). Ureters which are dilated as a consequence of obstruction, infection or pregnancy should be referred to as hydroureters. The dilatation of the megaureter may affect the whole length of the ureter or may be confined to the pelvic segment of the ureter. Even when the abdominal and pelvic ureter is dilated there is often a short narrow supravesical segment and the intravesical segment appears to constitute a functional obstruction. However there is no organic obstruction and a ureteric catheter can be introduced without difficulty. Cineradiography demonstrates very active contractions together with reverse contractions starting at the lower end of the ureter. The cause of this condition is not known but it has been suggested that the functional obstruction at the ureterovesical junction is the result of an abnormal arrangement of the circular fibres of the ureteric musculature.

Congenital stenosis of the lower end of the ureter produces an organic obstruction at the ureterovesical junction which does not allow the passage of a catheter.

Retrocaval ureter

This is a rare anomaly in which the middle third of the right ureter curves medially behind the inferior vena cava and then forwards and laterally over its anterior surface to regain its normal paravertebral position (Fig. 40.10). The anomalous course may lead to obstruction of the upper ureter.

Ureterocoele

A ureterocoele is a congenital cystic dilatation of the lower end of the ureter; it is usually classified as simple when the orifice is within the bladder, and ectopic, when the ureteral orifice lies outside the lumen of the bladder. The simple form is frequently symptomless, but ureteral obstruction, with or without stone formation, commonly occurs.

The simple ureterocoele usually produces a characteristic appearance on the urogram. When filled with contrast medium the dilated lower end produces a circular or elliptical area of increased density within the bladder which is surrounded by a radiolucent halo produced by the ureterocoele wall. This, together with the lower end of

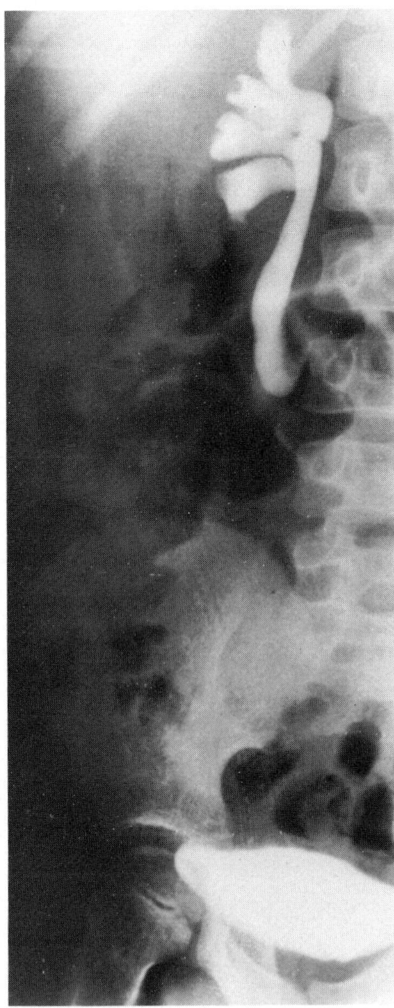

Fig. 40.10 Retrocaval ureter.

the ureter produces the classical 'cobra head' appearance (Fig. 40.12). When the ureterocoele is not filled with contrast medium it forms a round or elliptical filling defect (Fig. 40.11). When large the ureterocoele may almost completely fill the bladder and obstruct the ureters on both sides. In the absence of obstruction the upper urinary tract may be normal but obstruction frequently occurs with consequent dilatation of the ureter and renal pelvis. Stones are not uncommonly found within the dilated ureter.

Cysto-urethrography with dense contrast medium may completely obscure the simple ureterocoele and in the presence of a high intravesical pressure the ureterocoele may collapse or evaginate to form a diverticulum. The simple ureterocoele does not commonly reflux.

The 'cobra head' appearance may rarely be produced by transient dilatation and thickening of the ureteric wall following retrograde catheterization or impaction of a stone at the ureteric orifice. A similar appearance may also be produced by a bladder tumour arising close to and partially obstructing the ureteric orifice.

The ectopic ureter

Ectopia of the ureteric orifice occurs most frequently in females and the majority are associated with duplication of the whole length of the ureter. Whenever there is ureteral duplication the orifice of the ureter draining the upper renal moiety is always situated below and medial to the orifice of the ureter draining the lower moiety (Fig. 40.7). Intravesical orifices, even when situated in some position other than the normal at the lateral angles of the trigone, should not be regarded as ectopic; the term

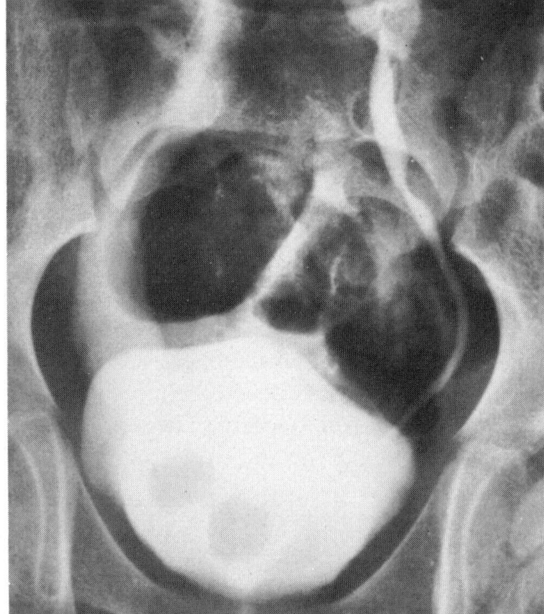

Fig. 40.11 Simple ureterocoele with stone formation producing 'cobra head' appearance.

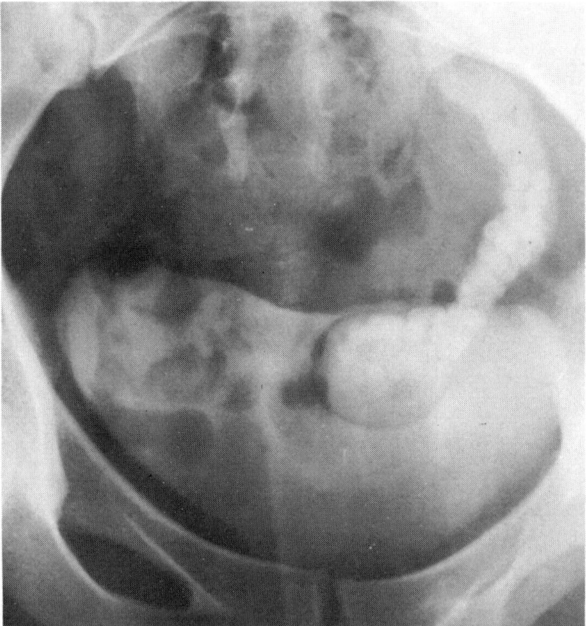

Fig. 40.12 Simple ureterocoele producing ureteral obstruction and filling defect in the bladder.

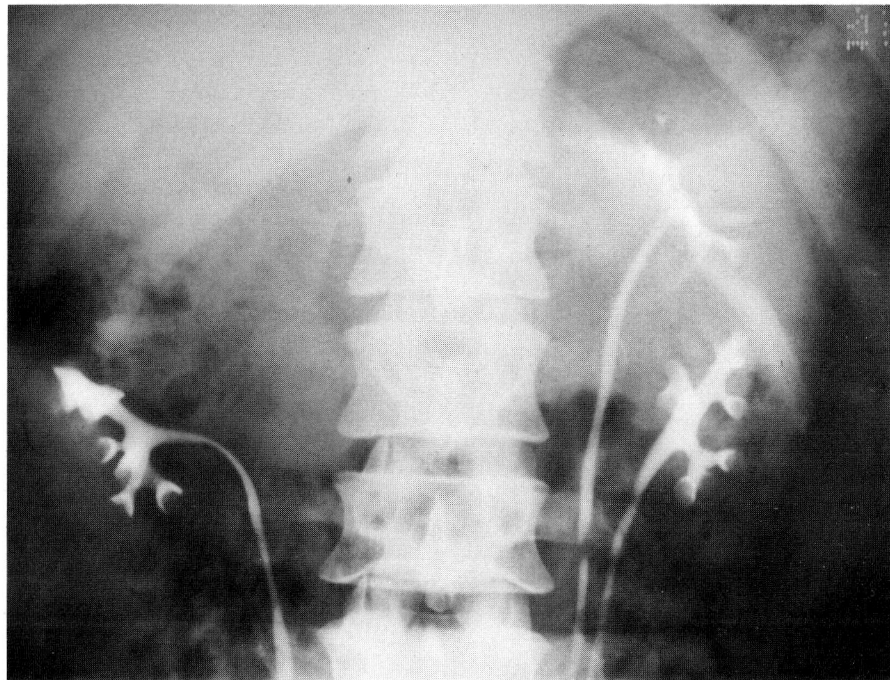

Fig. 40.13 I.V.U. obstructed ectopic ureterocoele producing 'drooping flower' appearance.

should be reserved for those cases in whom the orifice lies outside the bladder lumen. When ureteral duplication is present and only one orifice is ectopic, it is always the one draining the upper pole of the kidney.

In the male the ectopic orifice most commonly opens into the posterior urethra but it may also open into the seminal vesicle, the epididymis, the vas deferens, the ejaculatory ducts and at the bladder neck. In the female it

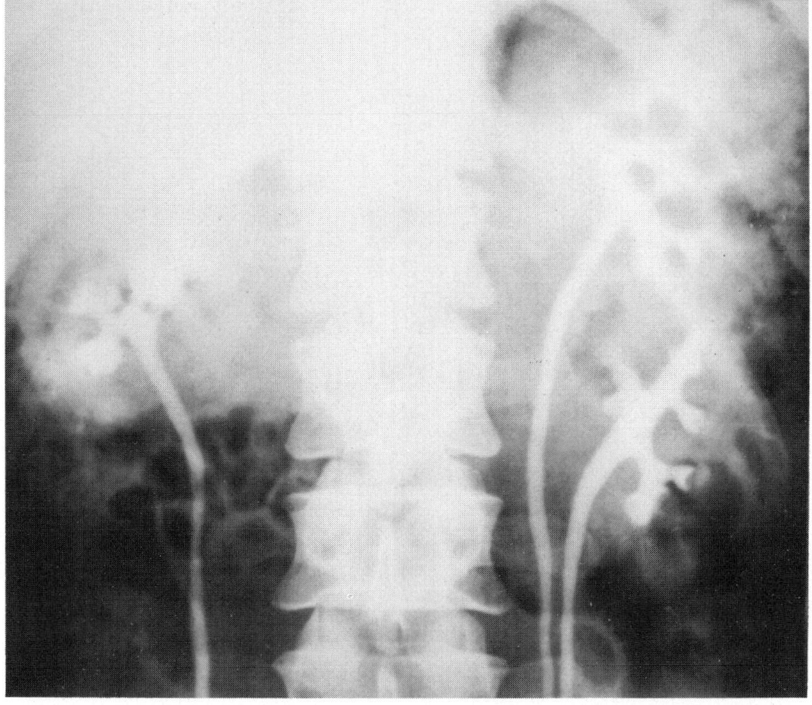

Fig. 40.14

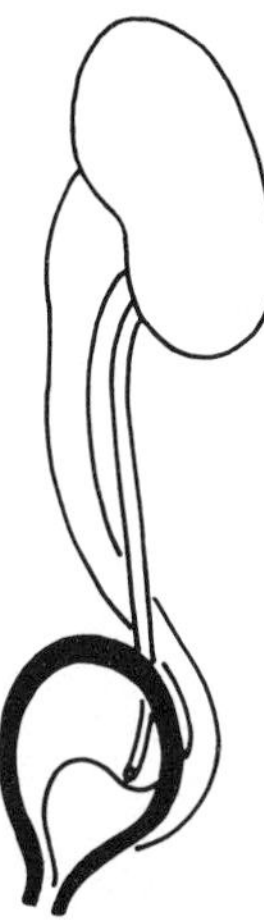

Fig. 40.15

Fig. 40.14 Obstructed ectopic ureter on the right side with an atrophic upper renal moiety.

Fig. 40.15 Diagram illustrating ectopic ureterocoele at the bladder neck.

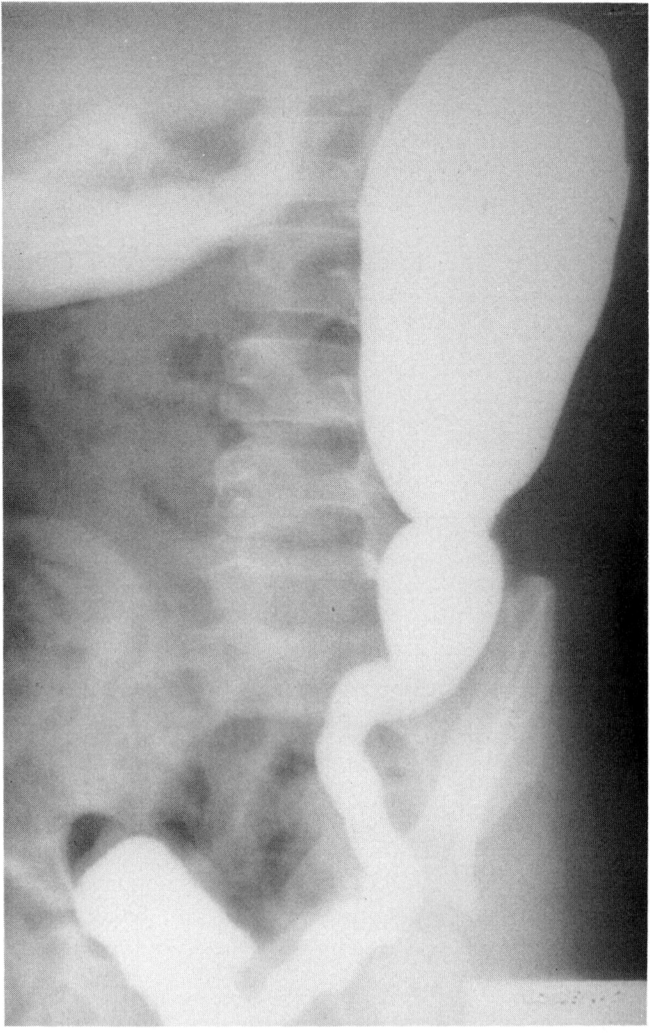

Fig. 40.16 Micturating cystogram demonstrating refluxing ectopic ureterocoele.

is most commonly situated in the vestibule but may also open into the urethra, the vagina, the cervix, the uterus, Fallopian tubes or the bladder neck.

Ectopic ureters are likely to become obstructed and when situated at the bladder neck or in the urethra may allow vesico-ureteral reflux to occur on voiding. Patients usually present in childhood with symptoms of urinary infection. When the orifice is beyond the bladder neck incontinence of urine will occur, provided the obstructed renal moiety excretes.

The urographic appearances are usually distinctive:

1. The renal shadow is enlarged, the increased size being produced by the dilated upper renal segment so that there is an increased renal substance thickness between the lower calyceal group and the top of the renal outline. Delayed films may demonstrate that this is occupied by the dilated upper renal pelvis and calyces.

2. The lower segment of the kidney is displaced downwards and laterally to produce the 'drooping flower' appearance (Fig. 40.13). Rarely the obstructed upper moiety of the kidney is atrophic and non-functioning. There is then no displacement and on the urogram the kidney on the affected side appears to be reduced in size with a deficiency in the number of its calyces as compared with the normal side (Fig. 40.14).

3. The ureter draining the lower renal segment may be deformed by the dilated ectopic ureter.

4. The bladder base may be elevated and deformed by the dilated ureter.

Ureterocoeles of the ectopic ureter are usually larger than the simple ureterocoele and unlike simple ureterocoeles frequently reflux (Fig. 40.16). They may elevate the

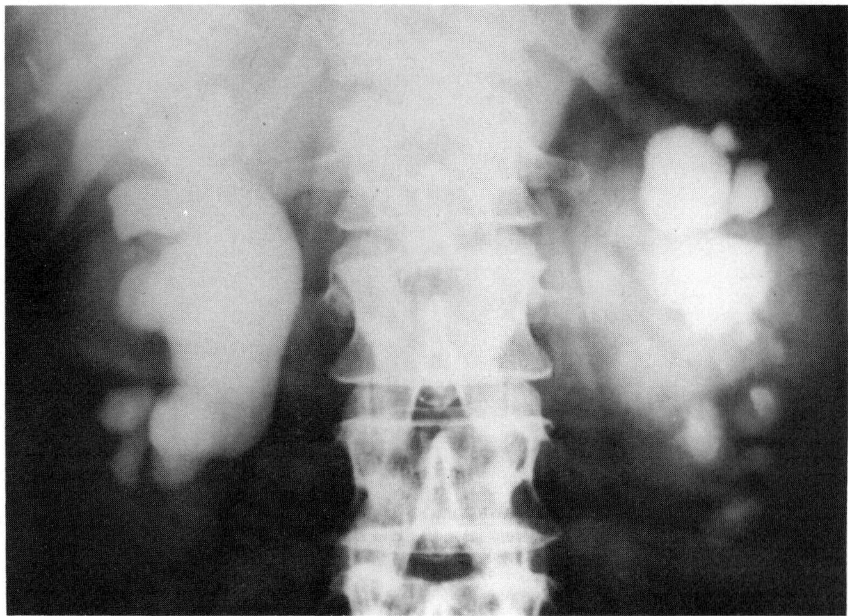

Fig. 40.17

Fig. 40.17 Bilateral congenital hydronephrosis.

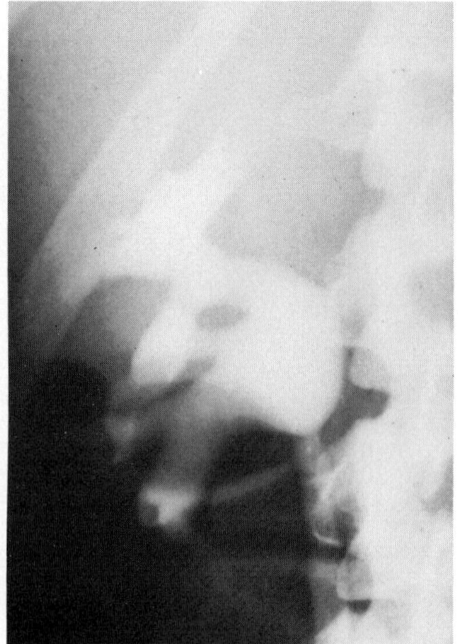

Fig. 40.18

Fig. 40.18 Minor degree of pelvi-ureteric obstruction with a high ureteric insertion producing a 'wine glass' appearance.

bladder base and appear as a huge intravesical mass obstructing the ipsilateral and contralateral ureters and also the bladder outflow tract (Fig. 40.15). The size of the mass varies with intravesical pressure, with high pressures during voiding it may be completely obliterated and even everted and appear as a bladder diverticulum. Prolapse of the ureterocoele into the urethra will produce urethral obstruction.

Lateral and downward displacement of the kidney may be produced by masses arising from the upper pole of the kidney or extrarenal masses arising in the suprarenal area. The intravesical filling defect may be mistaken for gas in the rectum, bladder tumour, or non-opaque calculus, and the deformity of the bladder base produced by the ectopic ureterocoele may simulate the lobulated filling defect of a rhabdomyosarcoma.

CONGENITAL HYDRONEPHROSIS

Hydronephrosis due to a functional obstruction at the pelvi-ureteric junction is a common anomaly occurring at all ages in childhood, and occasionally it may not manifest itself until adult life. The disease is not infrequently bilateral but it is usually more advanced on one side than the other. It usually presents with loin pain, urinary infection, an abdominal mass, or with stone formation. Congenital bands, adhesions, neuromuscular inco-ordination and aberrant vessels have all been suggested as the cause of the obstruction. It is almost certain that the apparent obstruction produced by renal arterial branches is the result of and not the cause of the pelvic distension. An organic stricture cannot be demonstrated and it seems likely that the functional obstruction is due to a failure of transmission of the renal pelvic contractions

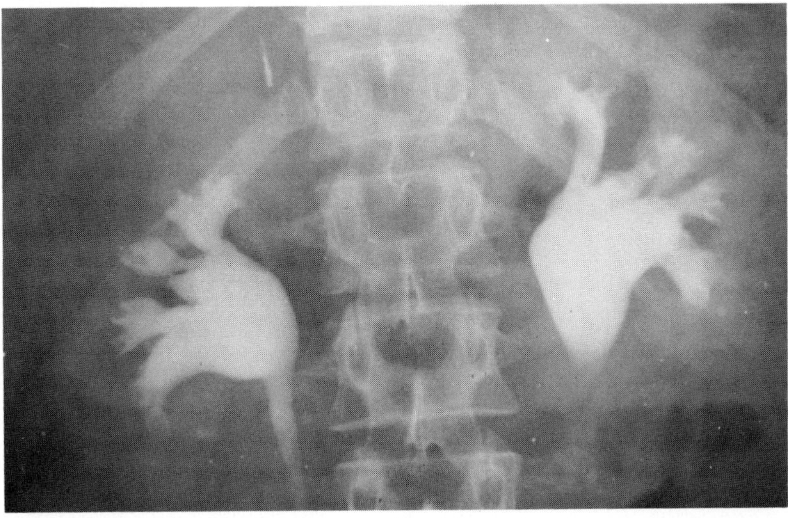

A

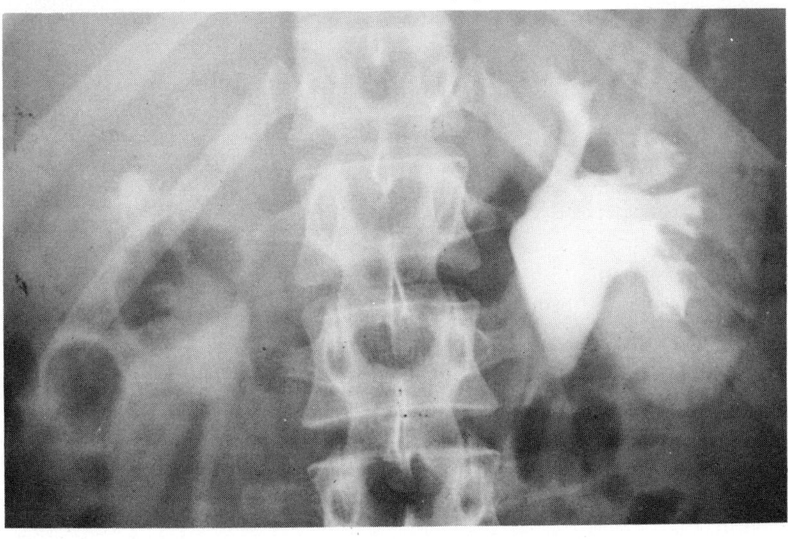

B

Fig. 40.19 Congenital pelvi-ureteric obstruction—(A) 15-minute film of I.V.U. following dehydration; (B) following hydration and I.V. Frusemide.

to the ureter. A characteristic feature is a large dilated extrarenal pelvis. Calyceal dilatation frequently appears late, but with advancing disease, the calyces dilate and there is progressive narrowing of the renal substance.

As in cases of hydronephrosis due to ureteric obstruction from other causes, the radiological appearances vary with the duration and the degree of obstruction.

In the most advanced cases with loss of glomerular function, there is a large soft tissue mass replacing the normal renal outline with no opacification of the collecting system on intravenous urography. Retrograde urography demonstrates a normal-sized ureter entering a very large renal pelvis and grossly dilated calyces surrounded by a narrow renal substance. The kidney on the opposite side is hypertrophied. Computerized tomography and ultrasonography is of particular value in these advanced cases.

In lesser degrees of obstruction when there are still functioning nephrons, tubular reabsorption of fluid leads to a lowering of intratubular pressure and allows glomerular filtration to continue (Fig. 40.17). It is in these cases that high dose urography has led to a dramatic decrease in the need for retrograde urography. The nephrogram demonstrates a thin rim of renal substance outlining the kidney and, on later films, crescent shaped opacities produced by dilated stretched tubules surround the markedly enlarged calyces which still contain non-opacified radiolucent urine (Fig. 39.2). Delayed films will show slow filling of the calyces and the renal pelvis and eventually, with the aid of prone films, the site of obstruction at the pelvi-ureteric junction.

In mild forms there may be little or no loss of renal substance and little or no dilatation of the calyces. The extrarenal pelvis shows little dilatation but has a convex lower margin producing a 'wine glass' appearance (Fig. 40.18). The ureter is not dilated and frequently has a high insertion into the renal pelvis—a feature that may only be demonstrated with the aid of lateral-oblique films. In other cases the ureter enters the renal pelvis in the normal position and a narrow segment of variable length is present at the pelvi-ureteric junction. The demonstration of a normal-sized or narrowed upper ureter localizing the site of obstruction to the pelvi-ureteric junction is of the utmost importance. It may only be accomplished by the use of delayed films and films taken in the prone position when sufficient contrast medium has accumulated in the dilated collecting systems.

The mildest forms, particularly when the patient is dehydrated, may show only minimal deviation from the normal appearances, with slight renal pelvic deformity, no calyceal dilatation and a normal ureter or high ureteric obstruction. In these doubtful cases the patient should be given a 'water load' and a further injection of contrast medium. Films taken at 10 minute intervals show little or no change in the normal, but in the presence of obstruction the renal pelvis distends. The effect of a water load can be increased by an intravenous injection of a diuretic, such as Frusemide.

A water load and intravenous Frusemide is of particular value in the investigation of patients with intermittent symptoms. Between the attacks the urogram may be normal but a diuresis will produce the characteristic dilatation of the renal pelvis with delayed emptying (Fig. 40.19).

Appearances similar to those seen in pelvic ureteric junction obstruction may be seen in patients with reflux extending up to the kidney. Cysto-urethrography is therefore indicated whenever there is doubt and particularly when there is ureteral dilatation.

THE BLADDER AND URETHRA

Duplication of the bladder and urethra

Duplication of the bladder is a rare congenital anomaly in which a vertical septum divides the bladder into right and left portions; it may be associated with urethral duplication. In the *'hour glass' deformity* (Fig. 40.20) a muscular ring incompletely divides the bladder into upper and lower chambers. The appearances in the resting state are similar to those produced by a urachal diverticulum. In the 'hour glass' bladder, however, both chambers contract normally during voiding whereas a diverticulum will distend as the bladder contracts. Urethral duplication may occur without vesical duplication; it may be complete, may take the form of a blind canal separate from the urethral lumen, or may form a urethral diverticulum.

Extrophy of the bladder, epispadias and hypospadias

Extrophy of the bladder produces wide separation of the symphysis pubis commonly associated with rotational deformities of the pelvic bones around the sacroiliac joints (Fig. 40.21). Epispadias also produces separation of the symphysis pubis together with funnelling and widening of the bladder neck and posterior urethra.

Severe degrees of hypospadias with a perineal opening and splitting of the scrotum are sometimes difficult to differentiate from intersex cases particularly if, as not uncommonly occurs, the testes are undescended. Injection of contrast medium into the perineal opening will, however, demonstrate a male type of urethra with

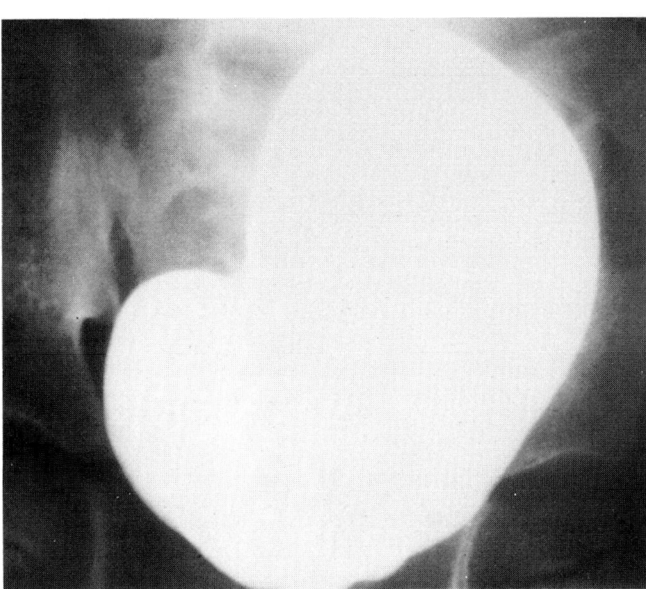

Fig. 40.20 'Hour glass' bladder.

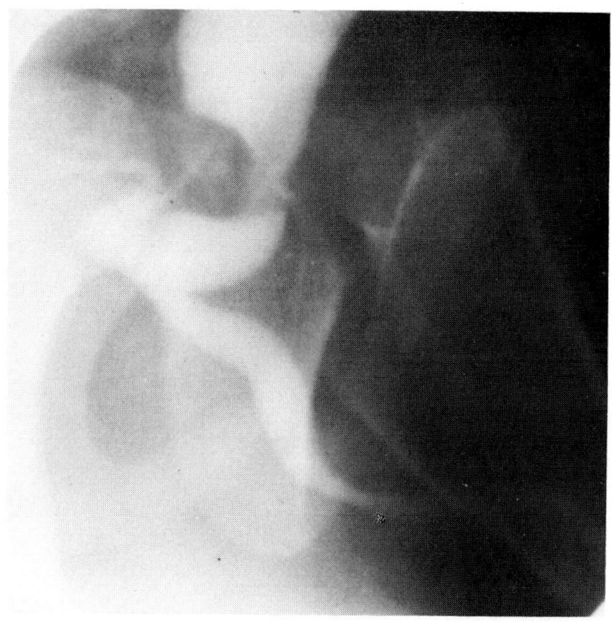

Fig. 40.22 Anal atresia with acute urethral angulation and an urethro-rectal fistula.

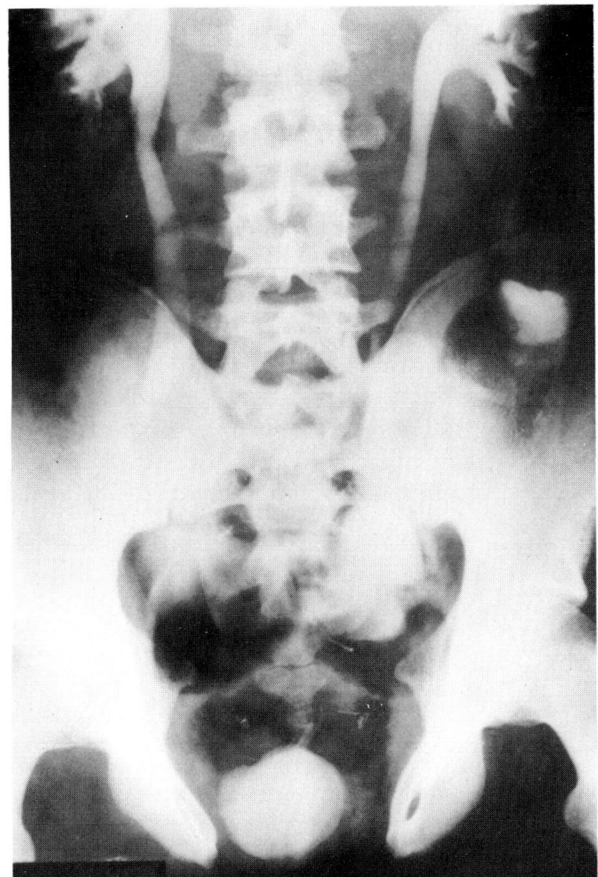

Fig. 40.21 Extrophy of the bladder; a urinary diversion procedure has been performed.

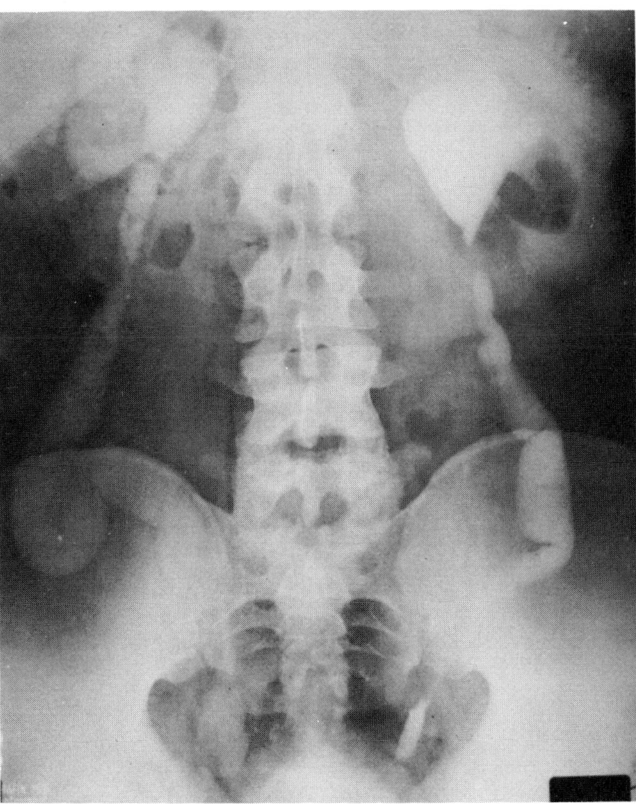

Fig. 40.23 I.V.U. in prune belly syndrome.

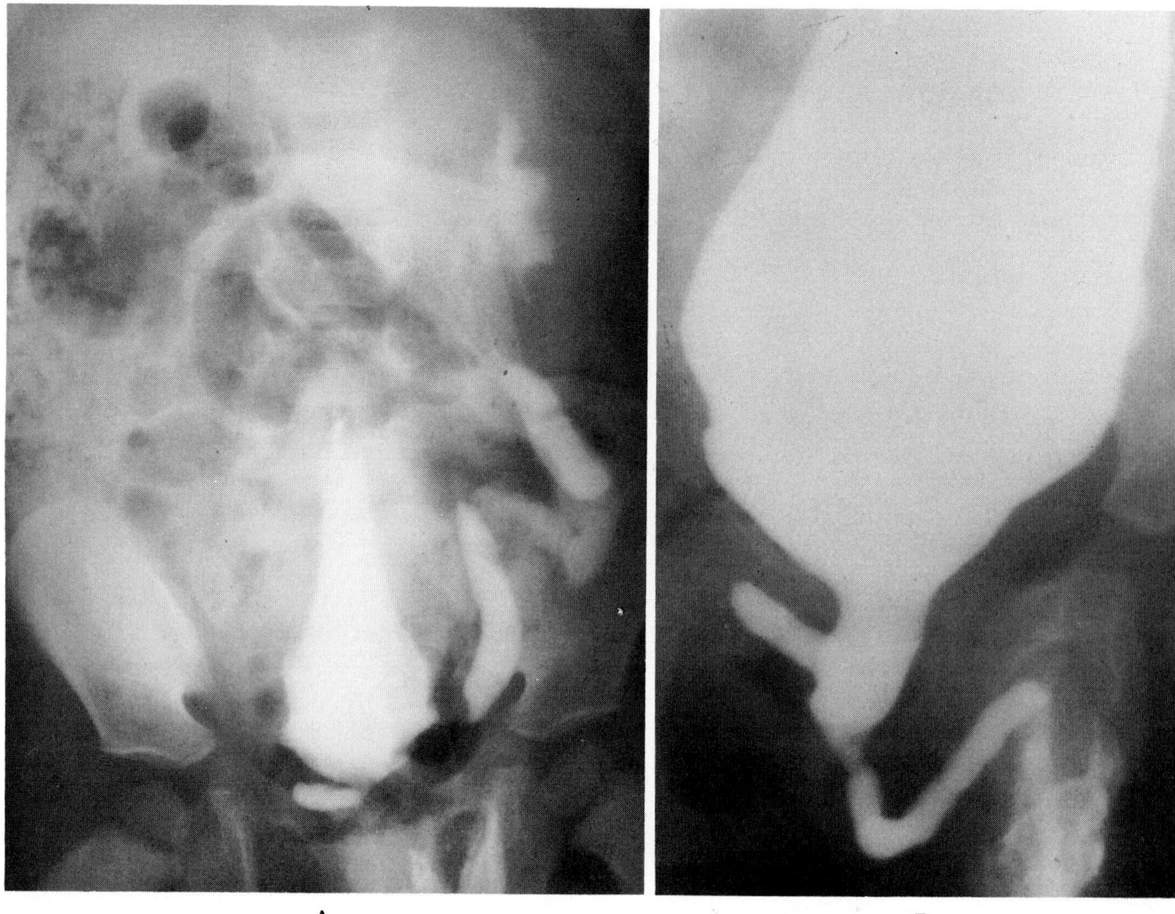

A B

Fig. 40.24 Micturating cystogram. Prune belly syndrome with characteristic deformity of the bladder, reflux into a dilated ureter, dilatation of the posterior urethra and a large prostatic utricle.

a verumontanum. In some cases there is a large utricle similar to that seen in the triad syndrome—this must not be assumed to be a vagina.

Anal atresia

The majority of cases of anal atresia have fistulae connecting the rectum with the bladder, urethra, vagina or the perineum (Fig. 40.22). In the absence of a fistula a fibrous cord running between the urethra and rectum causes acute angulation of the posterior urethra.

Urachal anomalies

Incomplete obliteration of the urachus produces an apical vesical diverticulum, a blind external umbilical sinus, or a urachal cyst which does not communicate with the bladder or the anterior abdominal wall. Persistence of the urachus leads to the presence of a fistula between the apex of the bladder and the umbilicus.

Prune belly syndrome (triad syndrome, agenesis of the anterior abdominal wall)

The prune belly syndrome is a rare congenital anomaly occurring almost exclusively in males and with a high mortality. The complete syndrome is characterized by dilatation of the upper urinary tract, lateral deviation of the dilated ureters, a large bladder with urachal anomalies, vesico-ureteral reflux, dilatation of the prostatic utricle, undescended testicles and patchy agenesis of the anterior abdominal wall (Figs 40.23 and 40.24). All of these manifestations are not necessarily present. The primary

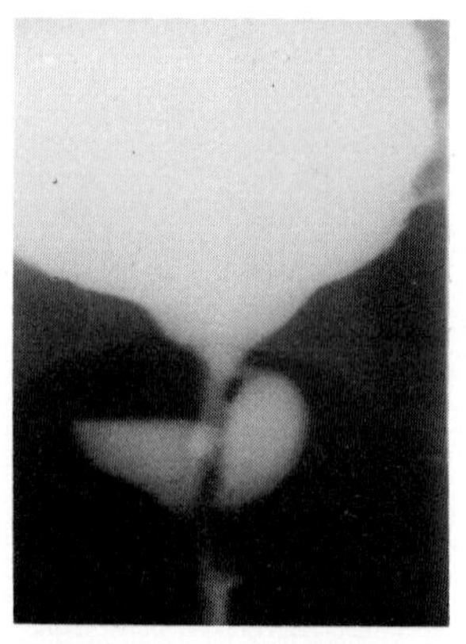

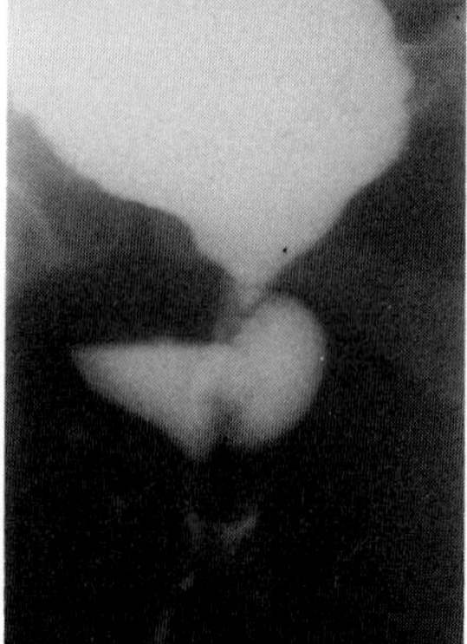

Fig. 40.25 Paired urethral diverticula.

anomaly is probably due to failure of development of the musculature of the urinary tract and abdominal wall. A high proportion of cases show evidence of urethral obstruction.

Urethral diverticula

Congenital diverticula may occur both in males and females, but the majority of those seen in the male are the result of peri-urethral abscess or trauma.

The diverticula may present in several ways. Stasis may lead to urinary infection, compression of the adjacent urethral lumen may produce obstruction and leakage of their contents may lead to incontinence of urine. Stone formation may rarely occur (Fig. 40.25).

Congenital lesions of the bladder, neck and urethra producing obstruction are discussed in Chapter 46.

REFERENCES AND SUGGESTIONS FOR FURTHER READING

ABRAHAMSON, J. (1961) Double bladder and related anomalies: clinical and embryological aspects. *British Journal of Urology*, **33,** 195–214.

BERDON, W. E., BAKER, D. H., SANTULLI, T. V. & AMOURY, R. (1968) The radiologic evaluation of imperforate anus. *Radiology*, **90,** 466.

CREMIN, B. J. (1974) Intersex states in young children: the importance of radiology in making a correct diagnosis. *Clinical Radiology*, **25,** 63–73.

FRIEDLAND, G. W. & DE VRIES, P. (1975) Renal ectopia and fusion: embryologic basis. *Urology*, **5,** 698–706.

HARTMAN, G. W. & HODSON, C. J. (1969) The duplex kidney and related anomalies. *Clinical Radiology*, **20,** 387–400.

KYAW, M. M. (1974) The radiological diagnosis of congenital multicystic kidney. *Clinical Radiology*, **25,** 45–62.

MALEK, R. S., KELALIS, P. P., BURKE, E. C. & STICKLER, G. B. (1972) Simple and ectopic ureterocoele. *Surgery, Gynecology and Obstetrics*, **134,** 611–616.

STEPHENS, F. D. (1963) *Congenital Malformations of the Rectum, Anus and Genito-Urinary Tracts.* Edinburgh: E. & S. Livingstone.

WILLIAMS, D. I. (Ed.) (1968) *Paediatric Urology.* London:Butterworth.

CHAPTER 41

TUMOURS OF THE KIDNEY AND URETER; CYSTIC DISEASE OF THE KIDNEY

RENAL CYSTS AND TUMOURS

Simple renal cysts and renal tumours produce similar urographic appearances and will therefore be considered together.

The **simple renal cyst** containing clear straw-coloured fluid may be single or multiple, unilateral or bilateral and may vary in size from a few millimetres to 25 cm or more in diameter. In the majority of cases of apparently solitary cyst careful autopsy examination has revealed the presence of more than one cyst and they are not infrequently associated with other disease in the kidneys. Unsuspected renal cysts are frequently discovered during computerized tomography or ultrasound even when the urogram is normal. The aetiology of simple cysts remains in dispute. They may arise from embryonic rests or as retention cysts due to tubular obstruction. Multiple cysts occur in *tuberous sclerosis*, they are usually small but may be several centimetres in diameter.

Haemorrhagic cysts are much less common. They may be due to haemorrhage into simple serous cysts or be produced by infarction; they may result from encapsulated haematoma or from cystic degeneration of a tumour, and 25 per cent of haemorrhagic cysts will be found to contain strands of malignant tissue in their walls.

Simple serous and haemorrhagic cysts are rare in children and usually present in middle life. The majority are clinically silent, but symptoms may be produced by compression of adjacent structures, by haemorrhage into the cyst and rarely by infection of the cyst.

Multilocular cysts (Fig. 41.1A and B) are rare hamartomas consisting of non-communicating loculi lined by epithelium and separated by septa consisting of fibrous tissue, muscle and rudimentary nephrons.

Tumours of the kidney comprise a complex group with, until recent years, a confused nomenclature produced by the extremely variable histology.

Benign renal tumours are usually small, varying in size from less than one to several millimetres in diameter and they are rarely of such a size as to manifest clinically. The majority are found at autopsy and are frequently multiple. The commonest benign tumour is the *adenoma*, followed by mesenchymal tumours such as *myoma*, *lipoma*, *haemangioma*, mixed *mesenchymal tumours* and *fibroma*.

Nearly all the clinically important tumours are **malignant**, and *adenocarcinoma* (*Grawitz tumour*, *hypernephroma*) is by far the commonest accounting for over 80 per cent of all malignant tumours. It is followed in frequency by the *epithelial tumours of the renal pelvis*, *nephroblastoma* (*Wilm's tumour*) and *sarcoma*. Adenocarcinoma is rare before the fourth decade. Nephroblastoma is practically the only renal tumour of the first decade of life and tumours of the renal pelvis and sarcomata tend to occur earlier than the adenocarcinoma.

Secondary metastatic renal tumours are not uncommon and are usually multiple. The kidney may also be infiltrated by neoplastic tissue in the *leukaemias* and *lymphomata*. Retroperitoneal tumours displace and distort the kidney but direct extension with penetration of the capsule is rare.

The malignant tumours frequently spread by direct extension into the renal veins, thus gaining access to the blood stream and early spread to the lungs is characteristic. The para-aortic lymph glands are involved early in the diseases and metastatic deposits are commonly found in the bones, liver, adrenal glands, the opposite kidney, the brain and the skin.

Classically the renal tumour presents with loin pain, haematuria and a palpable mass, but these signs may be entirely absent and the tumour silent until far advanced. Not uncommonly it may present with fever as the sole symptom, or a secondary deposit in the lung, brain or in a bone may be the only clinical manifestation. Renal

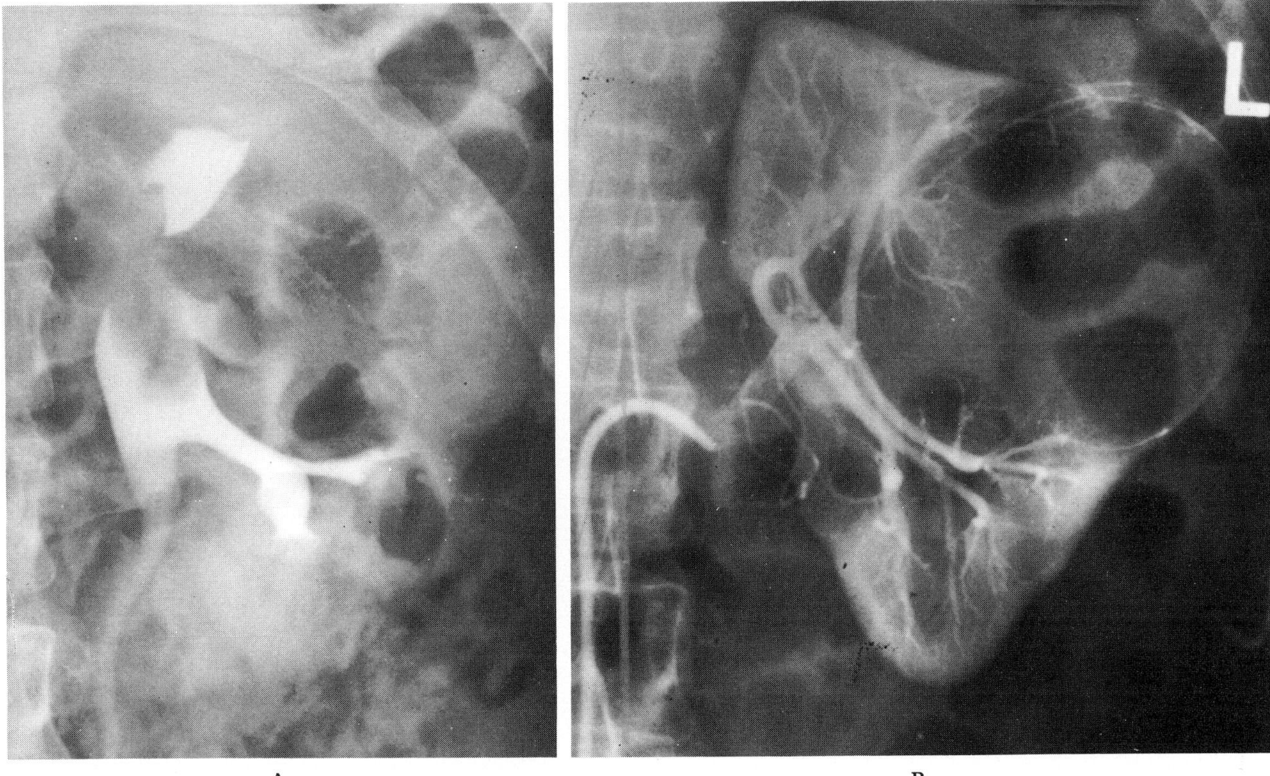

Fig. 41.1 Multilocular renal cyst. (A) I.V.U. (B) Renal angiogram—superficial resemblance to cyst, but note vessels within the lesion.

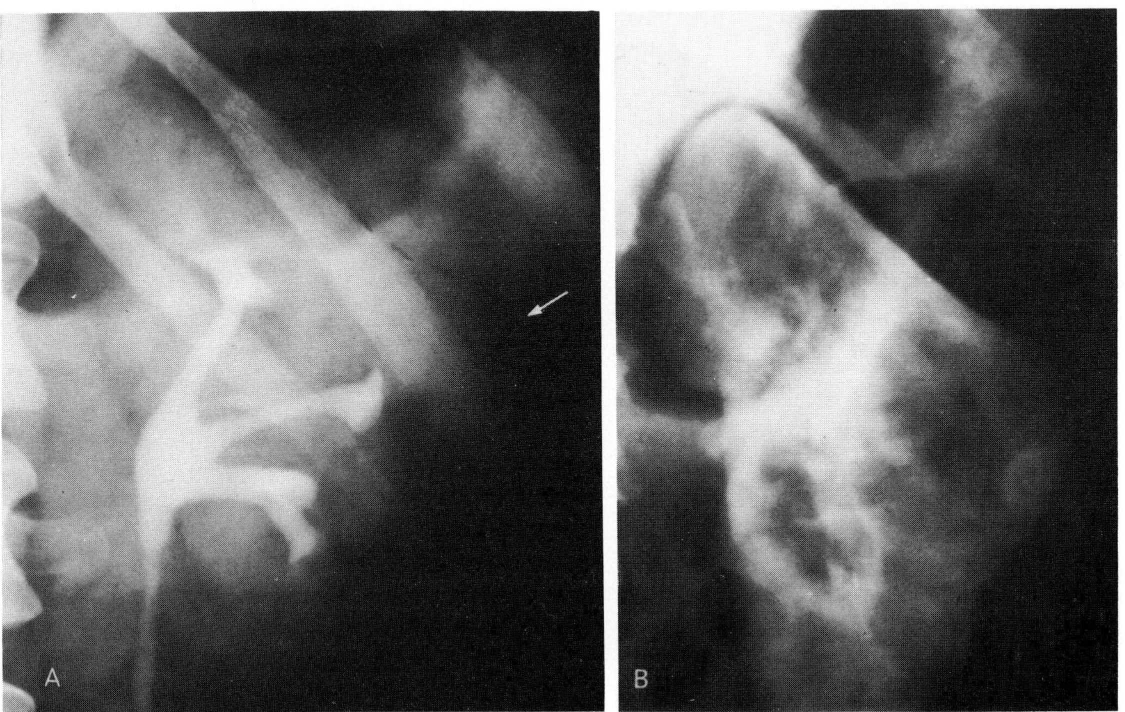

Fig. 41.2 (A) I.V.U. Normal lateral bulge on left renal outline. (B) Selective renal angiogram. Nephrogram phase.

tumours may also present with polycythaemia (due to the production of erythropoietin by the tumour), hypertension, hypercalcaemia and anaemia.

Radiological appearances

Mass lesions in the upper pole of the kidney may displace the kidney downwards, and tumours or cysts arising from the medial surface of the upper pole will displace the upper pole laterally so that the long axis of the kidney lies parallel to the spine.

The normal renal outline forms a smooth regular curve, a soft-tissue mass protruding from the renal surface always raises the probability of the presence of a renal cyst or tumour. A normal variant on the left side—the presence of a bulge on its lateral surface—may simulate an expanding lesion and it may be quite impossible without the aid of angiography to differentiate this normal appearance from that produced by a tumour. Usually, in the normal, the adjacent calyx is elongated into the bulge whereas if an expanding lesion is present the calyx will be displaced medially and distorted (Fig. 41.2). Cysts and tumours lying in the substance of the kidney may produce a diffuse enlargement of the kidney without a recognizable soft-tissue mass, and extension of the tumour into the renal vein or vena cava may also produce venous congestion and diffuse renal enlargement. The renal outline is preserved unless the tumour breaks

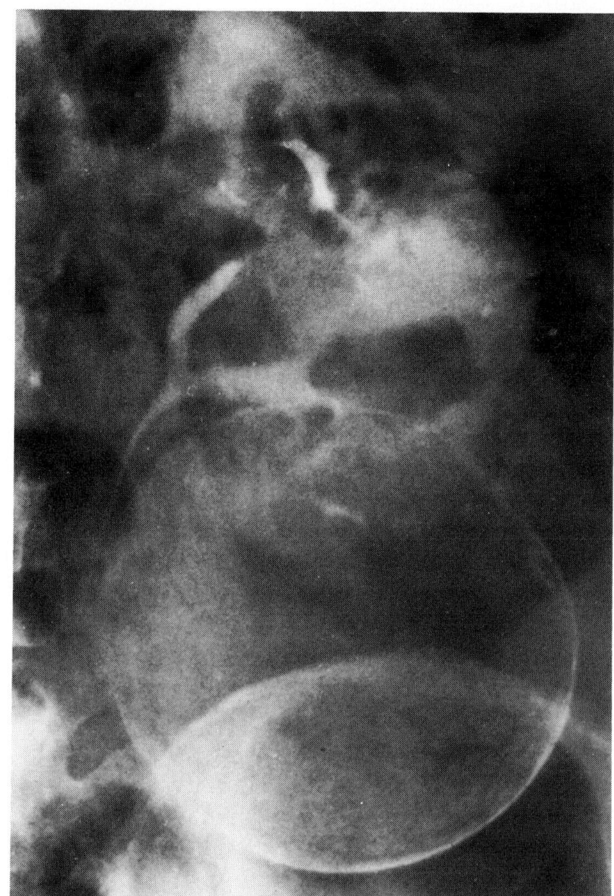

Fig. 41.3 Calcification in simple serous cyst.

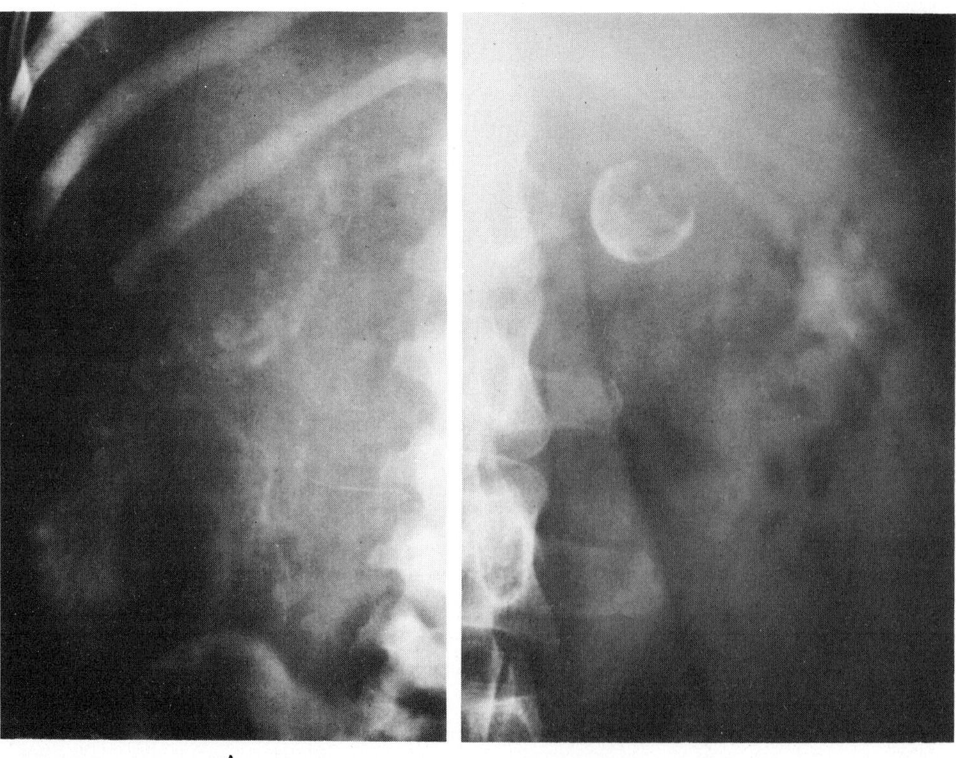

A B

Fig. 41.4 Calcification in renal tumours. (A) Diffuse irregular calcification in a nephroblastoma. (B) Ring-like calcification in an adenocarcinoma.

through the renal capsule to invade the perirenal areolar tissue.

Calcification occurs in 6 per cent of renal carcinoma and 3 per cent of renal cysts. Cystic calcification (Fig. 41.3) is much commoner in haemorrhagic than in simple serous cysts and usually takes the form of curvilinear peripheral streaks or a ring shadow. Tumour calcification may take the form of irregular areas scattered throughout the tumour (Fig. 41.4A), but a ring of calcification also occurs in tumours and it must be emphasized that the presence of a calcified ring within the kidney is more likely to be due to an area of cyst formation in a carcinoma than to a simple serous cyst (Fig. 41.4B).

Nephrotomography in both cysts and tumour demonstrates a defect in the renal parenchyma. In the case of a simple cyst the defect is sharply defined and regular and if the cyst protrudes from the renal surface a thin wall (about 1 mm to 2 mm) may be visible; an infected simple cyst may have a thick irregular wall. Where a cyst protrudes from the renal surface the adjacent renal tissue may be elevated around its margins in the form of well defined triangles (Fig. 41.8B). The nephrographic defect produced by a tumour is usually irregular with a thick wall, and mottled densities may be visible within it. (Fig. 41.5.)

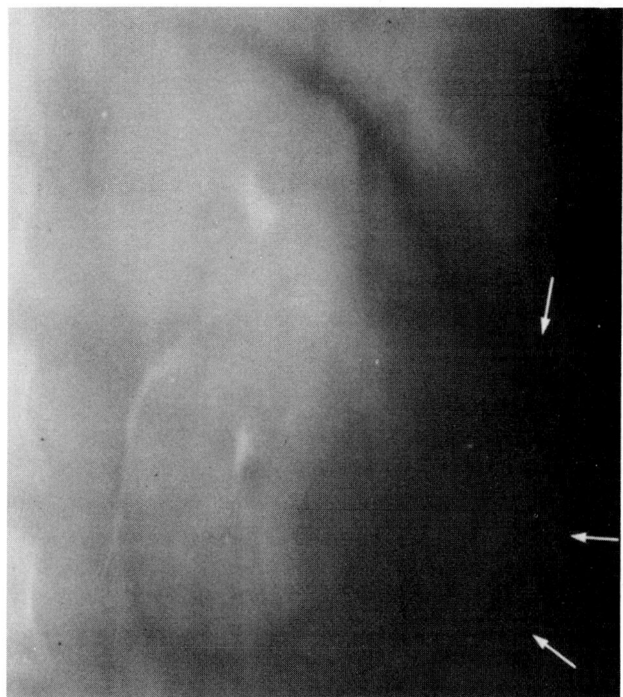

Fig. 41.5 Renal carcinoma with a 'thick wall'.

The distortion of the pelvicalycine system produced by renal tumours and cysts is dependent on the position and size of the lesion. Small tumours may not deform the pelvicalycine system and may only be revealed by angiography. Peripheral lesions may merely distort a single adjacent minor calyx. The calyx may be stretched and elongated or when lying on the surface of a tumour may be widened and apparently 'clubbed'. More centrally

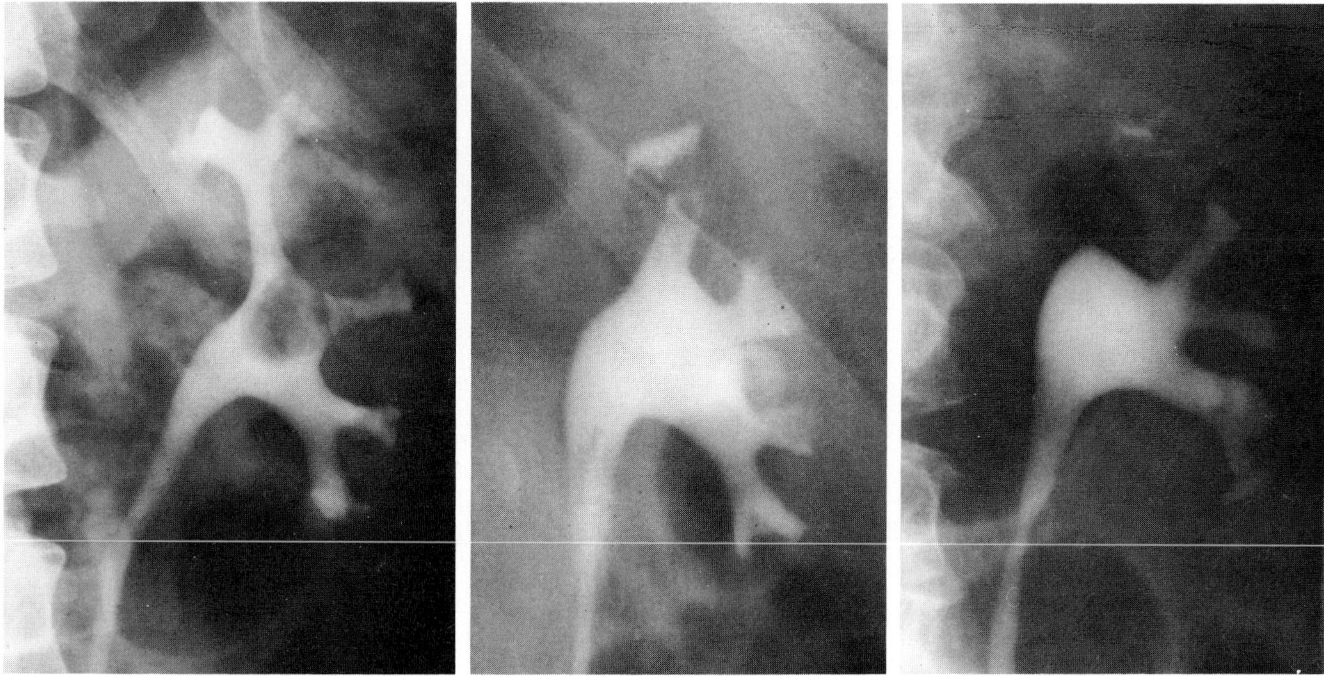

Fig. 41.6 *Fig. 41.7A* *Fig. 41.7B*

Fig. 41.6 Extension of adenocarcinoma into the renal pelvis.

Fig. 41.7(A) and (B) Adenocarcinoma extending into a calyx producing in (A) a filling defect and in (B) amputation of a calyx.

placed lesions will displace, elongate and separate adjacent major calyces, and if the calyceal lumen is obstructed the minor calyces will become dilated. Distortion and displacement of the renal pelvis and upper ureter may be produced by tumours or cysts in the hilum of the kidney. Compression and distortion of the ureter or pelvis may lead to hydronephrosis with a filling defect in the pelvis. Extension of a growth into the renal pelvis may produce a filling defect indistinguishable from a primary epithelial tumour or blood clot (Fig. 41.6). Extension into a calyx produces a filling defect or complete 'amputation' of the calyx (Fig. 41.7A and B).

Large tumours may cause partial or complete destruction of renal tissue—a few remaining calyces may be demonstrated or there may be a large 'non-functioning' kidney. Extension of the tumour through the renal capsule may lead to invasion of the upper ureter with the development of a hydronephrosis.

Occlusion of the renal vein or inferior vena cava by tumour tissue or thrombus will lead to diffuse renal enlargement with narrow elongated calyces.

Angiography is of great value in the differentiation of renal cyst from malignant tumour (see Chapter 29). A cyst is always avascular, renal arterial branches are displaced and elongated but are otherwise normal. (Fig. 41.8A and B). A partial selective angiogram when the apical segmental artery is not filled produces a well marked defect in the nephrogram which could be mistaken for a cyst (Fig. 41.9). When the cyst is more centrally placed, normal vessels lying on its anterior and posterior surface may conceal the avascular area, but this can be revealed by nephrotomography. A malignant tumour is only rarely avascular, but irregular avascular areas may be produced by necrotic tumour tissue. Irregular beaded pathological vessels will be present and irregular pools of contrast medium may be seen within the tumour. Arterio-venous anastomoses occur and anastomoses may be seen with capsular and extra renal vessels. Nephrotomography may show that the tumour is of equal or greater density than the surrounding renal substances and necrotic tissue will produce blotchy ill-defined radiolucent areas.

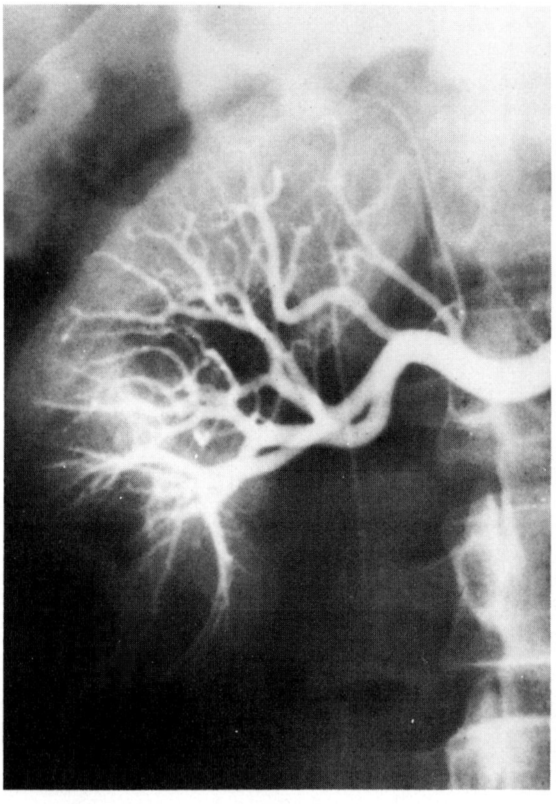
A

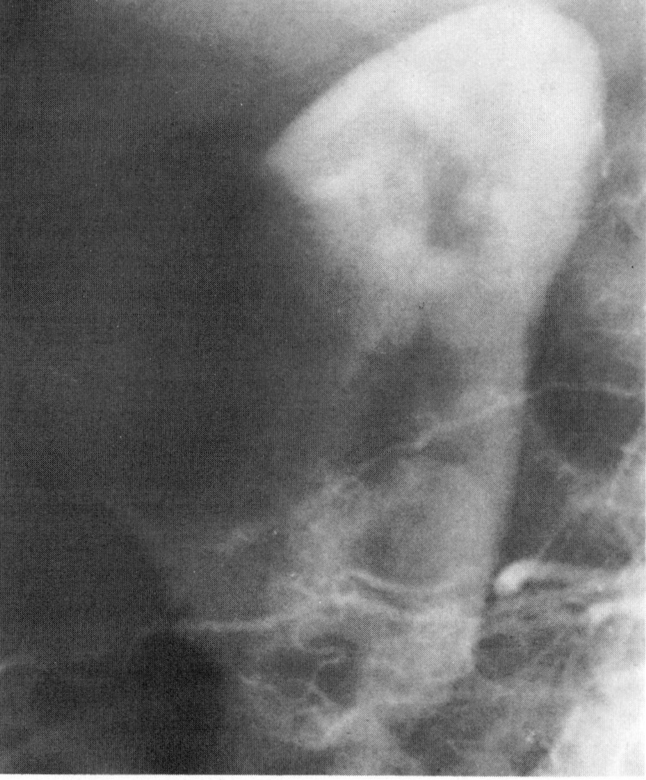
B

Fig. 41.8 Simple renal cyst. Selective renal angiograms. (A) Cyst in lower pole stretching renal arterial branches. (B) Nephrogram with well-demarcated radiolucency.

When angiography indicates the presence of a cyst, the cyst may be aspirated by percutaneous puncture and its contents partially replaced with contrast medium and air before complete evacuation (Fig. 41.10A and B). The majority of simple cysts contain straw-coloured fluid; the fluid may rarely be haemorrhagic or, in the presence of infection, turbid. The presence of haemorrhagic fluid and a thick irregular wall makes malignancy likely and the

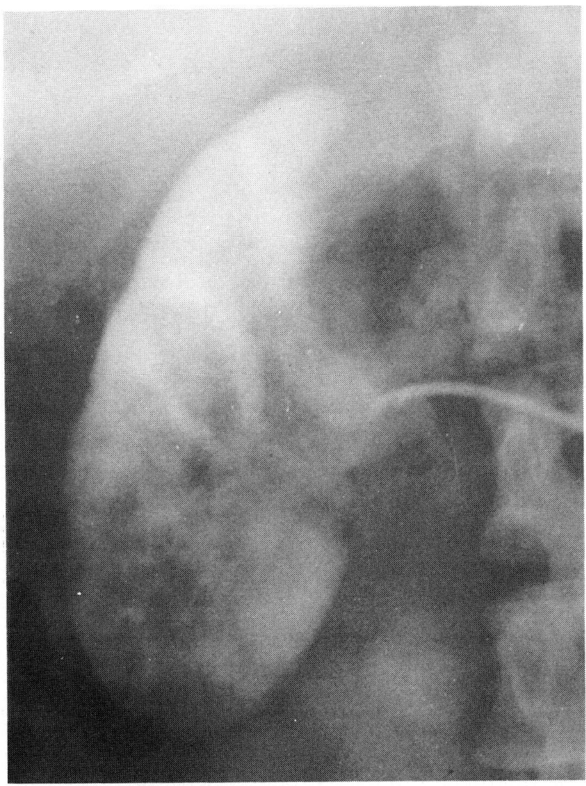

Fig. 41.9 Partial renal angiogram. Catheter advanced beyond origin of artery to upper medial pole.

diagnosis can be further supported by cytological examination of the aspirated fluid.

It is rarely possible to differentiate with certainty between cyst and tumour on the basis of the urographic changes alone. When the urogram is equivocal or suggests a fluid-filled mass an ultrasound examination should be the next step. If on ultrasound examination the mass is echo free it should be aspirated (Fig. 41.10) and the aspirated fluid examined for the presence of malignant cells. If internal echoes are present angiography should be carried out prior to surgical exploration or aspiration.

In those instances where the urogram indicates the presence of a solid tumour, angiography is probably the most useful second examination. If angiography confirms the presence of a tumour surgical exploration is indicated. When angiography produces equivocal results it would be reasonable to proceed with an ultrasound examination prior to surgery or needle aspiration.

Needle biopsy of solid lesions is probably associated with a slightly increased risk of complicating haemorrhage but when angiography is contra-indicated because of advanced age or presence of arterial disease, needle biopsy provides an excellent method of making a definitive diagnosis. The risk of tumour seeding along the needle track is remote.

Computerized tomography will demonstrate masses projecting from the anterior or posterior surface of the

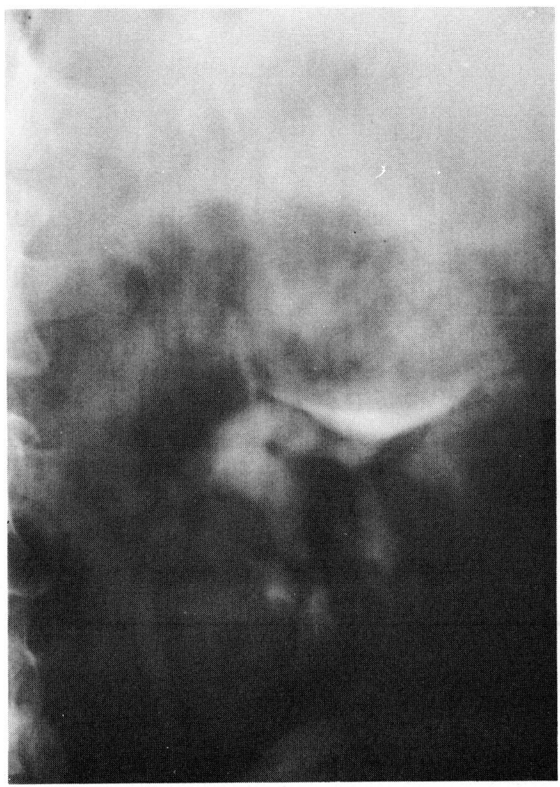

A

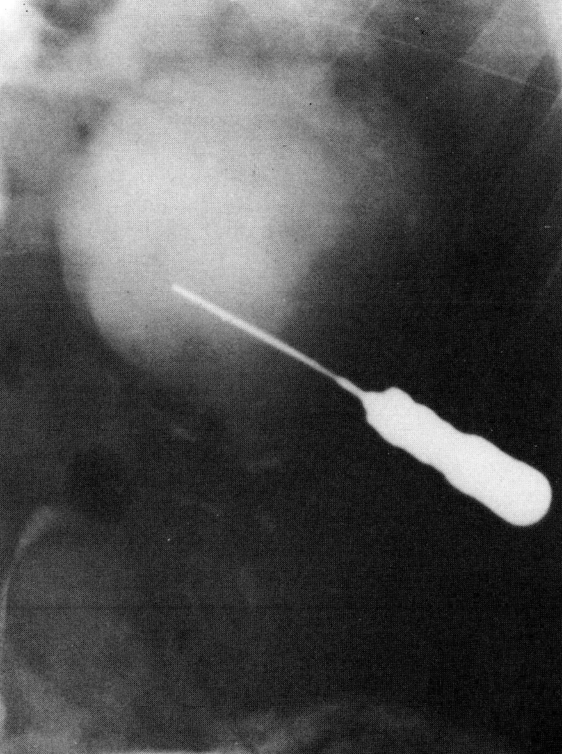

B

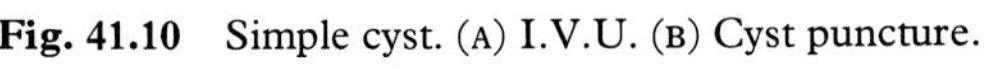

Fig. 41.10 Simple cyst. (A) I.V.U. (B) Cyst puncture.

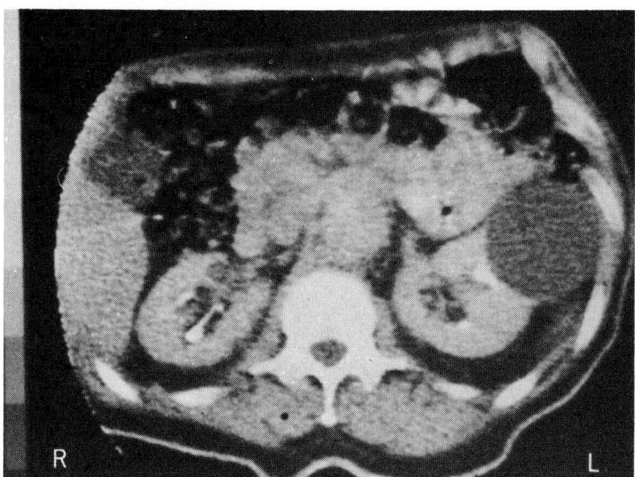

Fig. 41.11 C.T. Scan. Large simple cyst on the left side, small simple cyst on the right side. Normal I.V.U.

kidney even when the urogram is normal (Fig. 41.11) and it can differentiate with a high degree of accuracy between benign renal cyst and tumour (see Ch. 65).

Multiple renal masses

Multiple renal masses are usually cystic; benign tumours can be multiple but they are usually small and rarely diagnosed. Multiple cysts, multiple benign and malignant tumours may occur in Lindau-von Hippel disease. Malignant tumours (adenocarcinoma and nephroblastoma) are rarely bilateral but a carcinoma may occur in association with cystic disease. It can also occasionally metastasize to the contralateral kidney.

Metastatic disease of the kidney is a common autopsy finding particularly in patients dying of lung cancer but renal metastases rarely present clinically. Metastases are usually relatively avascular on angiography but pathological vessels may be present and renal arterial branches may show tumour encasement.

Infiltration of the kidney in the lymphomata, leukaemia and multiple myeloma usually produces diffuse renal enlargement with a normal outline and elongated attenuated calyces but single or multiple masses may also be seen.

Hamartoma (angiomyolipoma)

These benign, encapsulated, mixed mesenchymal tumours are most commonly seen in patients with tuberous sclerosis but also occur in the absence of other evidence of tuberous sclerosis. They are usually asymptomatic but haemorrhage into or necrosis of the tumour may produce abdominal pain, fever, raised sedimentation rate, etc.

When the tumour contains a high proportion of fat its true nature may be suspected on the intravenous urogram or nephrotomogram by the presence of radiolucent areas within the mass. C.T. will also show the presence of low attenuation areas. The tumour is extremely vascular with a characteristic angiographic appearance, which if not recognized will lead to a mistaken diagnosis of a highly malignant tumour (Fig. 41.12). It is supplied by wide tortuous vessels arising from the renal arteries and the capsular branches of the renal and lumbar arteries. Aneurysmal dilatation of the abnormal vessels is present and large vascular lakes with early venous filling may also be seen.

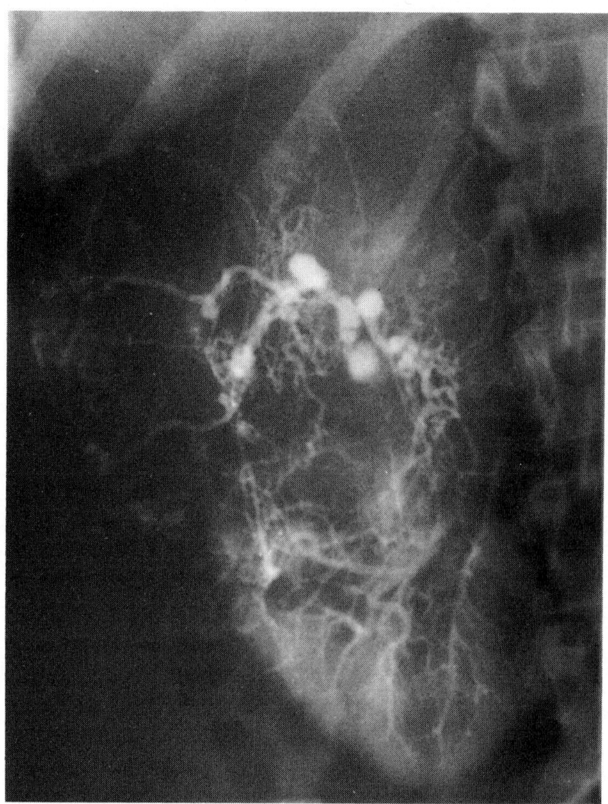

Fig. 41.12 Angiomyolipoma.

Pseudotumour of the kidney

Many pathological lesions of the kidney may mimic a renal tumour; *renal abscess* often gives rise to difficulty particularly as the angiographic changes—abnormal vessels with large capsular vessels and a thick irregular wall—may be mistaken for a malignant circulation. *Hypertrophy of normal renal tissue* adjacent to the scars of chronic pyelonephritis or renal infarcts produces a localized thickening of the renal substance with a bulge on the renal surface but the true nature of these lesions is usually evident on urography. *Fibrolipomatosis* of the renal hilum may occasionally cause elongation of the calyces and simulate a central or hilar renal mass (page 895, Fig. 44.19). An apparent renal enlargement with elongation of the calyces may also occur when the kidney

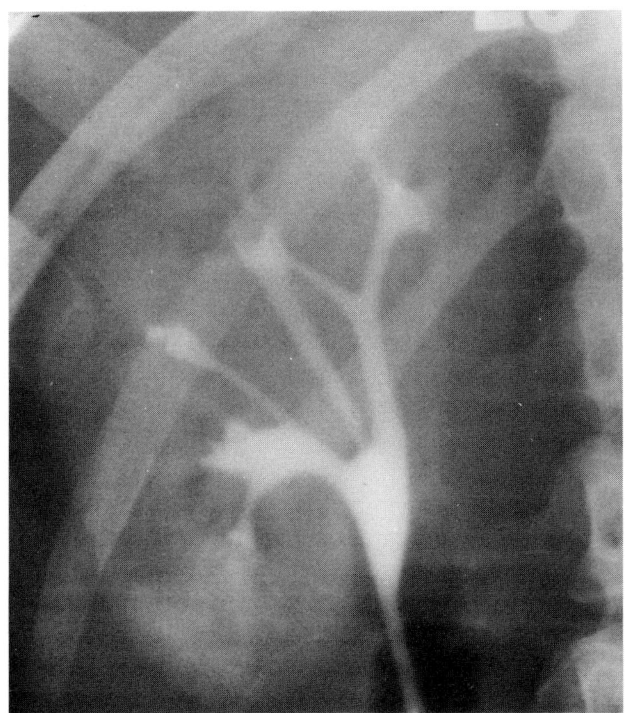

Fig. 41.13 Renal compression simulating a renal mass.

is compressed by an enlarged spleen or by a pararenal mass (Fig. 41.13).

In the normal kidney persistence of foetal lobulation may simulate a tumour and the frequent occurrence of a bulge on the normal left kidney has already been mentioned. Urographic appearances suggesting the presence of a tumour are occasionally produced by an *invagination of normal cortical tissue* towards the renal sinus. The added cortical thickness presents as a localized mass displacing adjacent calyces. This appearance is most commonly seen in the middle segment of a kidney in which some degree of duplication is present. In others when there is no urographic evidence of duplication the cortical infolding probably represents an abortive attempt at duplication. The condition can usually be recognized on nephrotomography, the infolded tissue producing a dense 'blush'. Angiography demonstrates displacement of interlobar arteries with normal arcuate arteries entering the mass and a dense 'blush' on the nephrogram simultaneous with the cortical nephrogram (Fig. 41.14A and B). There are no pathological vessels. Isotope scans in these cases show areas of increased activity whilst tumours and cysts give areas of decreased activity.

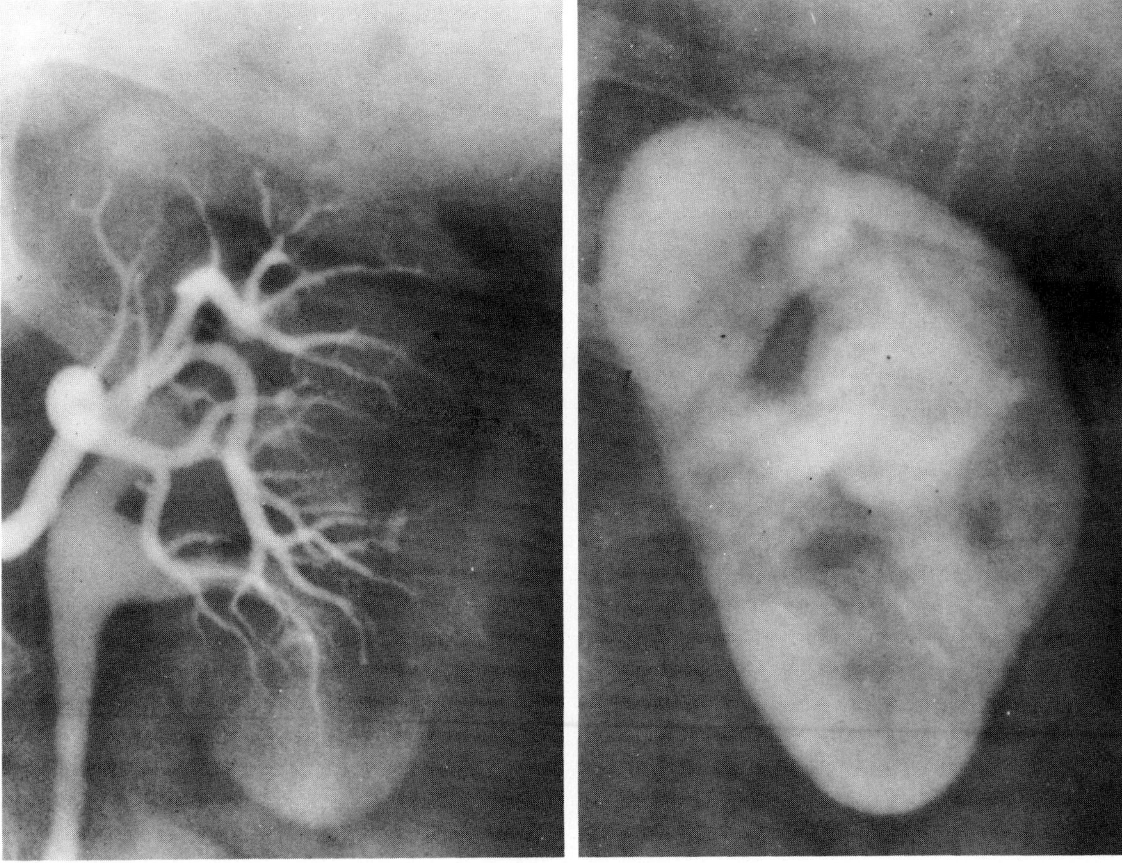

Fig. 41.14 'Pseudotumour'. Angiogram demonstrating spreading of the interlobar arteries and nephrographic blush.

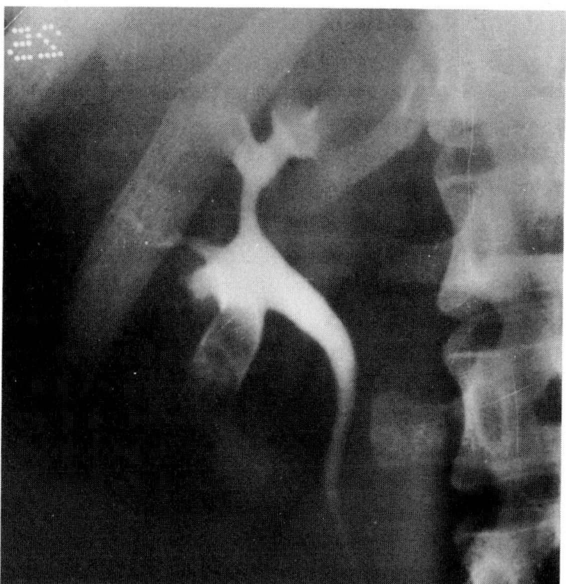

Fig. 41.15 Congenital hypertrophy of a renal papilla.

Congenital hypertrophy of a renal papilla with normal histology is a rare condition which may simulate a renal tumour. It produces a filling defect continuous with the papilla and protruding into a calyx (Fig. 41.15). Angiography does not demonstrate any abnormality and only nephrectomy will distinguish it with certainty from an epithelial tumour of the calyx.

TUMOURS OF THE RENAL PELVIS AND URETER

Benign tumours of the renal pelvis and ureter of non-epithelial origin, such as *haemangioma*, *fibroma*, *fibrolipoma* and *myoma* are rare and it is not possible to differentiate these on clinical or radiological grounds from malignant epithelial tumours.

Squamous metaplasia of the transitional epithelium, a possible precancerous condition, occurs rarely in association with chronic irritation from stone. The desquamated stratified squamous epithelium—a *cholesteatoma*—may form a filling defect indistinguishable from a true tumour. There is an increased incidence of urothelial tumour in association with analgesic abuse.

The epithelial tumours, more common in men than in women, should for practical purposes be regarded as **malignant** although it is probable that papillomata can be benign. Two main types are recognized, the transitional cell and the squamous cell carcinoma. The *transitional cell tumour* is usually papilliferous, it may be single but is often multiple, secondary lesions or seeds being found in the ureter below the primary and in the ipsilateral half of the bladder. Bilateral tumours are rare. The *squamous cell tumour* usually takes the form of an ulcerated plaque or stricture, it is usually single and in more than half of the cases is associated with stones.

Clinically the patients present with loin pain due to obstruction of the upper urinary tract and haematuria.

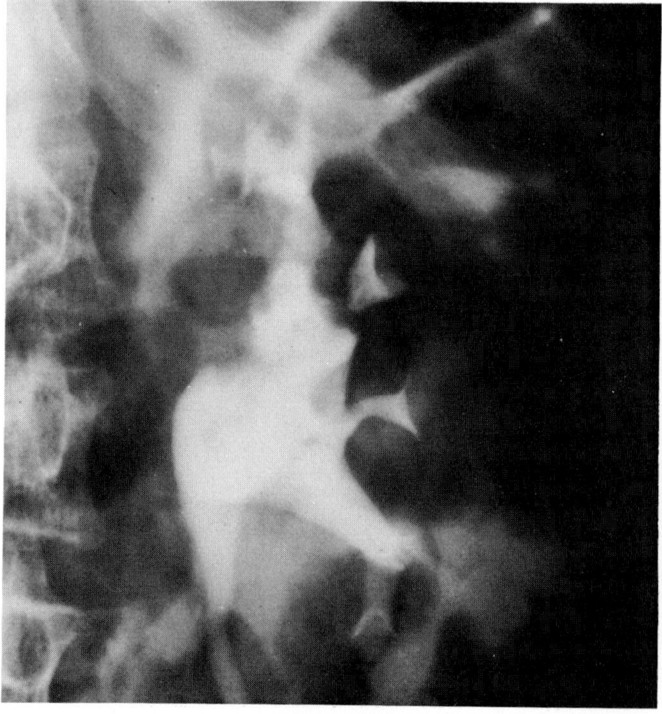

Fig. 41.16

Fig. 41.16 Carcinoma of renal pelvis producing irregular filling defect.

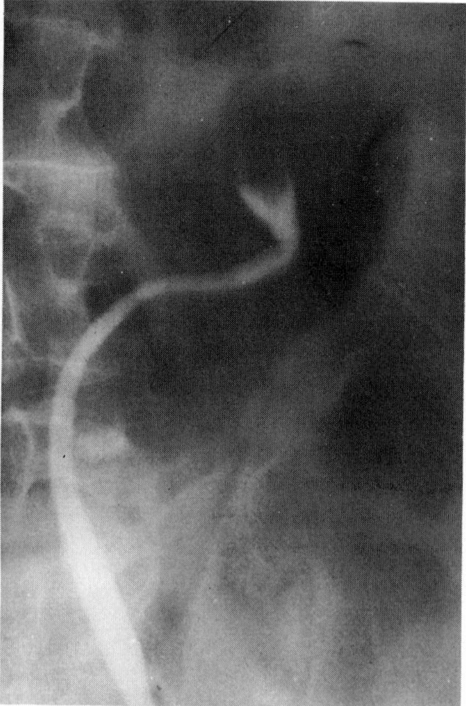

Fig. 41.17

Fig. 41.17 Ureteral tumour producing filling defect and 'wine glass' appearance.

Papillary tumours usually produce obstruction with dilation of the urinary tract above the tumour. Complete utereral or pelvic obstruction may lead to a large non-functioning kidney, and hydronephrosis or hydro-ureter in a man over the age of 40 should give rise to the suspicion that it may be due to a carcinoma. If the tumour is small and within a calyx, it gives rise to a localized dilatation or a complete amputation of the calyx.

The cardinal sign of a pelvic or ureteral papillary tumour is the presence of a filling defect often with a lobulated surface which may rarely be encrusted with calcium (Fig. 41.16). At the site of a papillary tumour the ureter dilates to accommodate the tumour and the dilation of the ureter may extend below the site of obstruction.

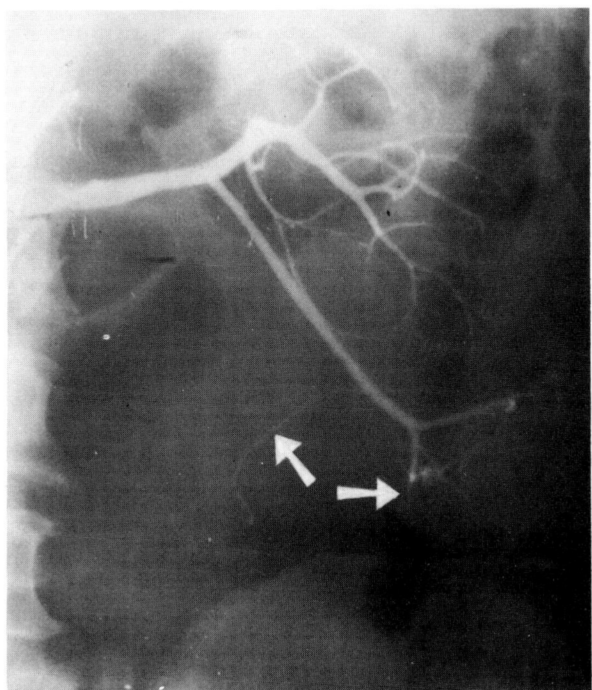

Fig. 41.18 Selective renal angiogram. Hydronephrosis due to carcinoma of the renal pelvis. Pathological vessels are present in the lower part of the dilated calycine system. A 'seed' in the upper ureter resulted in gross dilatation of the renal pelvis.

Retrograde urography may then produce a 'wine-glass' appearance due to protrusion of the tumour into the dilated ureteral lumen (Fig. 41.17) and the ureteral catheter may coil in the dilated ureter around the tumour mass.

In all cases of papillary tumours the whole renal tract must be carefully examined both radiologically and cystoscopically to exclude the presence of multiple tumours.

Squamous cell carcinoma of the ureter usually manifests itself as a stricture and there is no demonstrable filling defect. In the renal pelvis it may also present with obstruction and usually infiltrates widely into the peri-renal tissues before there is any sizeable intrapelvic mass.

Renal pelvic carcinomata are relatively avascular and a normal selective renal angiogram does not exclude the presence of a tumour. Invasion of the renal parenchyma may produce irregular filling defects in the nephrogram phase. Renal arterial branches may show evidence of tumour encasement and pathological vessels supplied by large uterero-pelvic vessels may be visible, particularly if the overlying renal vessels are separated by a dilated renal pelvis (Fig. 41.18). The tumour vessels are usually few in number and high-quality films are required for their demonstration. The renal vein is commonly occluded. The upper ureter is supplied by the uretero-pelvic branches of the renal arteries, and tumours in this area may also be demonstrated by selective renal angiography. The middle third of the ureter is supplied by the ovarian or spermatic artery and branches from the common iliac so that contrast medium should be injected into the lumbar aorta, the distal third supplied by the vesicovaginal or prostatovesical arteries can be demonstrated by common iliac artery injection.

Differential diagnosis

Blood clot in the renal pelvis may produce filling defects identical with those produced by an epithelial tumour.

Vascular impressions produced by an *angiomatous malformation* of the renal artery may mimic a renal pelvic or ureteral tumour. A similar appearance may be produced by *collateral vessels* in renal arterial or venous stenosis or occlusion.

Filling defects may also be produced by *non-opaque stones, sequestrated papillae, tuberculous granulation tissue, schistosomiasis, and, very rarely, fungal balls.*

CYSTIC DISEASE OF THE KIDNEY

Classification (Elkin, 1975)

1. Renal dysplasia
   a. Multicystic kidney
   b. Focal and segmental dysplasia
   c. Multiple cysts associated with lower urinary tract obstruction
   d. Hereditary and familial cystic dysplasia
2. Polycystic disease
   a. Polycystic disease of the young
      (i) Polycystic disease of the newborn
      (ii) Polycystic disease of childhood
   b. Adult type polycystic disease
3. Cortical cysts
   a. Trisomy syndromes
   b. Tuberous sclerosis
   c. Simple cyst (solitary or multiple; unilateral or bilateral)
   d. Multilocular cyst

4. Medullary cysts
   a. Medullary sponge kidney
   b. Medullary cystic disease (uraemic)
   c. Medullary necrosis
   d. Pyelogenic cyst
5. Miscellaneous intrarenal cysts
   a. Inflammatory (tuberculosis, calculus disease, echinococcus disease)
   b. Neoplastic (cystic degeneration of neoplasm)
   c. Traumatic (intrarenal hematoma)
6. Extraparenchymal cyst
   a. Parapelvic cyst
   b. Perinephric cyst

POLYCYSTIC DISEASE OF THE KIDNEYS

Polycystic disease of the young and adult polycystic disease have morphological similarities but they are almost certainly different entities.

Polycystic disease of the young. Polycystic disease of the young is a rare disease, inherited as an autosomal recessive, in which there is cylindrical and saccular dilatation of the tubules in the renal cortex and medulla with cystic changes and periportal fibrosis in the liver. The severity of the disease, its age of presentation and clinical features depend upon a very variable pattern of organ involvement. In those presenting early in life the renal changes dominate whilst later in childhood the periportal fibrosis is the dominant pathological change and there is a wide spectrum between the two extremes.

Infantile polycystic disease usually presents in the first few days of life with renal failure and the greatly enlarged kidneys may embarrass respiration. The renal parenchyma is almost entirely replaced by minute cysts representing dilated tubules and glomeruli, the cut surface of cortex and medulla having a sponge like appearance. The liver is enlarged. The outlines of the greatly enlarged kidneys are smooth, the lobulation so characteristic of the adult disease is not seen and the nephrogram has a mottled appearance. The impairment of renal function usually prevents demonstration of the calyces but when seen they are normal and dilated collecting tubules may be seen in the renal papillae. The majority of affected children die within a few days.

Childhood form. These usually present at about the age of 3 to 5 years or later, the cystic change in the kidneys which is most prominent in the medulla tends to be less evident and the hepatic fibrosis greater. These children usually present with symptoms and signs of portal hypertension, the renal disease is mild but it may progress to renal failure.

The kidneys are enlarged but not massive as in the infantile form, the outlines are smooth and the nephrogram may be mottled. In the mildest forms the only urographic change may be the *renal tubular ectasia* producing an appearance similar to that seen in adult sponge kidney.

Adult polycystic disease. The adult disease does not usually present until after the third decade, common presenting symptoms being loin pain, haematuria and renal colic, an abdominal mass, hypertension or renal failure. It is a familial disease transmitted through several generations. The renal parenchyma is almost entirely replaced by numerous cysts containing straw-coloured fluid and lined with flattened or cuboidal epithelium. Varying amounts of normal renal tissue is interspersed between the cysts, and with progression of the disease a gradual compression and destruction of nephrons occurs until death ensues from renal failure. The disease may be more advanced on one side than the other but is almost invariably bilateral. There are few authentic unilateral cases and it is probable that cases in whom the disease appears to be unilateral are examples of *unilateral multicystic kidney*.

The fundamental defect appears to be a failure of union of the tissues derived from the metanephros (glomerulus, convoluted tubule and loop of Henle), and the collecting tubules arising from the ureteric bud of the Wolffian duct. Others believe that the condition may be the result of separation of branches of the ureteric bud from the parent lumen with the formation of retention cysts. There may be associated cystic changes in the liver, pancreas and spleen.

Radiological appearances

Renal enlargement is invariably present and the kidneys may reach enormous proportions. Protrusion of the cysts from the kidney surfaces produces lobulation of the renal outlines and cysts protruding from the medial surface of the upper pole of the kidney will displace the upper pole of the kidney laterally so that its long axis comes to lie parallel to the spine. The lower pole of the kidney lying further from the midline is not usually displaced laterally by cysts on its medial surface.

When renal function is impaired, intravenous urography will fail to demonstrate the pelvicalycine system unless large doses of contrast medium are used. The degree of distortion of the pelvicalycine system varies with the size, number and position of the cysts. In the earliest cases the only abnormality may be the increase in size of the kidneys. Advanced disease will produce elongation and deformity of all major and minor calyces resulting in the characteristic 'spider leg' appearance. In less obvious cases the deformity may be restricted to one or two calyces in each kidney.

Minor calyces may be stretched by adjacent cysts, thus forming elongated crescents which are not 'clubbed' but retain their normal sharp angles. If a minor calyx is stretched over the surface of a cyst it may, when viewed in one plane, appear to be dilated and 'clubbed', mimick-

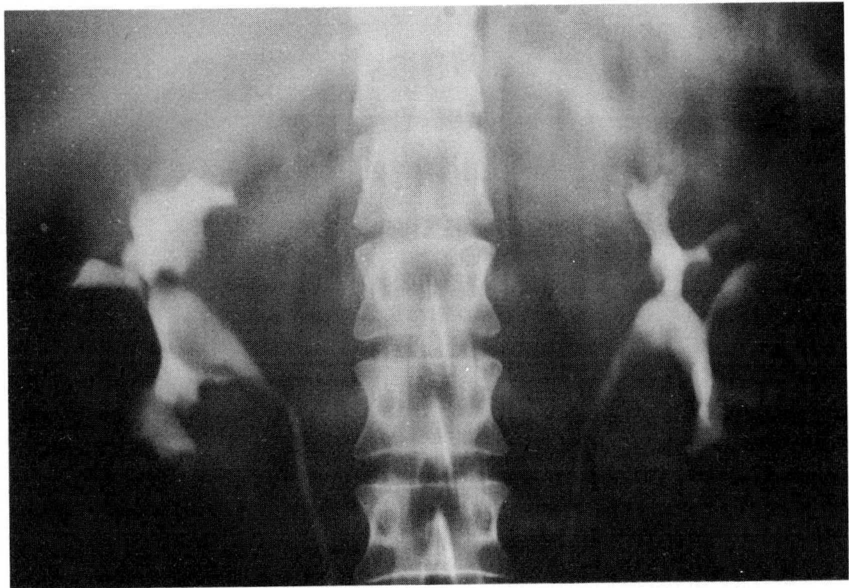

Fig. 41.19 Polycystic disease.

ing the appearance produced by obstruction to a major calyx.

Major calyces are displaced, elongated and narrowed by adjacent cysts, but when stretched over the surface of a cyst may appear to be widened (Fig. 41.19).

Protrusion of a cyst into the renal pelvis will produce deformity of the pelvis with a filling defect or half shadowing, and cysts protruding from the medial surface of the lower pole may displace the upper ureter and renal pelvis upwards and medially.

Occasionally a cyst may rupture into a calyx and the cyst cavity will fill with contrast medium.

Angiography and *nephrotomography* are only indicated in the less obvious cases when renal enlargement may be the only abnormality detected on urography. In these cases cysts approaching 2 cm in diameter produce characteristic multiple, well-defined, round defects in the nephrogram phase (Fig. 41.20), and larger cysts produce curvilinear displacement of renal arterial branches. There is an increased incidence of intracranial aneurysms in

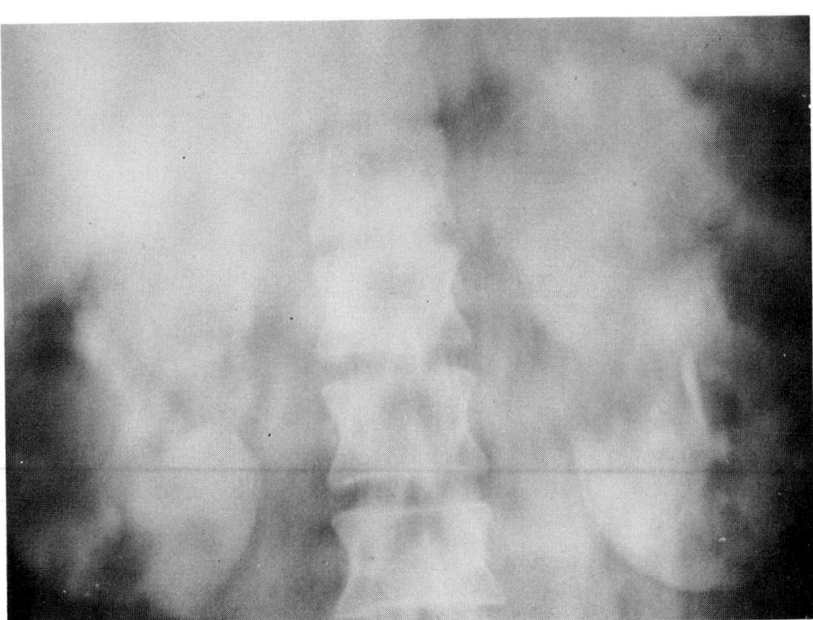

Fig. 41.20 Polycystic disease—renal enlargement with multiple rounded defects in the nephrogram.

patients with polycystic disease and cysts may be present in other organs, particularly in the liver and pancreas.

MEDULLARY SPONGE KIDNEY

Medullary sponge kidney is a congenital disease in which the renal medulla is replaced by numerous small cysts producing a sponge-like appearance. It is more common than would appear from the small number of cases reported, and is being increasingly frequently recognized.

The disease may affect the whole or the greater part of one or both kidneys, it may be confined to one segment or rarely one papilla of one kidney. The affected portions of the kidney are enlarged with enlargement of the adjacent calyx or calyces. The renal medulla is pale and cystic. The cysts which may contain areas of embryonic epithelium are most numerous at the papillary tips. They vary in size, usually 1 to 3 mm in diameter, but they may be microscopic and rarely they form large cavities. The majority of the cysts communicate with the tubules and the tubules themselves may be dilated and tortuous. *Calculi*, the result of retention and precipitation, are present within the cysts in 80 per cent of the cases. In the absence of complications the renal cortex and pelvis are normal.

Other malformations may be present in the urinary tract and cystic disease may also be present in the liver, pancreas and spleen.

The uncomplicated disease is clinically silent, but secondary infection or the passage of stones will produce symptoms. Renal function is unimpaired unless repeated attacks of infection or obstruction by stones produces renal damage.

Radiological appearances

When both kidneys are diffusely affected the kidneys will be enlarged with, in the absence of complications, smooth renal surfaces. If only one area of the kidney is affected, the increase in the renal substance thickness will be confined to the affected segment or papilla. An increase of the renal substance thickness may also be found in areas where no cysts can be demonstrated, presumably due to the presence of microscopic or non-communicating cysts.

Calculi varying in number from one to several hundred are visible in the majority of cases; they are usually small, very dense and are confined to the renal medulla. Calculi frequently occur in groups, producing a characteristic appearance like a bunch of grapes (Fig. 41.21). In other cases they may be diffusely distributed throughout the kidney.

The majority of the cysts fill with contrast medium on intravenous urography, but they may not fill with retrograde urography. The intravenous examination demonstrates that the calculi lie within the medullary cysts which

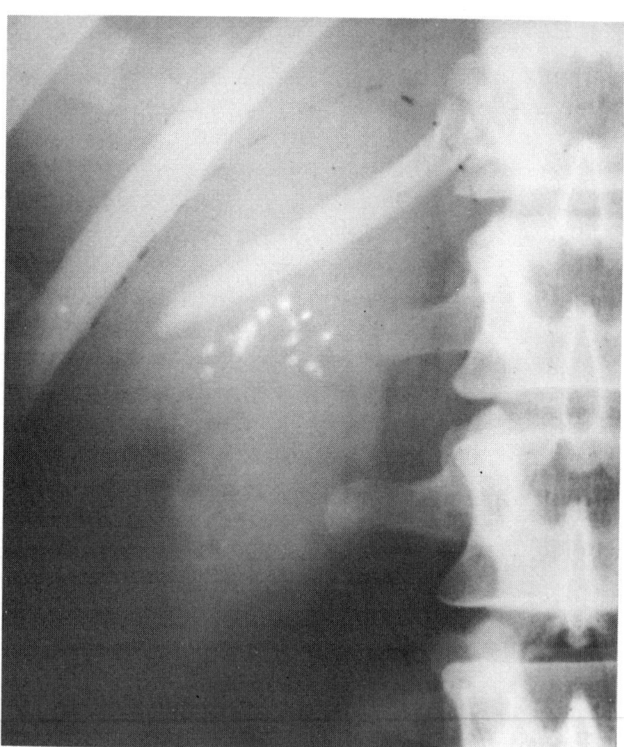

Fig. 41.21 Calculi in medullary sponge kidney.

are usually round and smooth, varying in size from the microscopic to one centimetre in diameter. The cysts may be irregular in shape, and linear, slightly irregular channels, produced by dilated tubules may be seen radiating into the medulla from the papillary tip. Contrast medium persists within the cysts after release of ureteric compression.

The minor calyx draining the affected segment will be enlarged, forming a wide arc, and protrusion of subepithelial cysts into its lumen may produce a finely blistered appearance (Fig. 41.22A and B).

Recurrent urinary infection may produce chronic pyelonephritic scarring, and back-pressure changes may result from obstruction due to the passage of stones.

The angiographic appearances are normal and angiography is of no value in this disease.

Differential diagnosis. The *normal renal tubular shadow* producing fine linear opacities radiating from the papilla should not produce difficulty, there being no papillary enlargement or cyst formation.

Calyceal diverticula or cysts are usually single, but may be multiple. They are usually 2 to 6 mm in diameter, smooth and round, lying between the papillae and connected to the infundibulum of a calyx by means of a narrow channel. They may contain calculi.

The appearances of early *tuberculous* erosion of a papilla may simulate the dilated tubules of the sponge kidney and a small well-defined healed tuberculous cavity may cause difficulty. Calcified and cavitated areas in renal

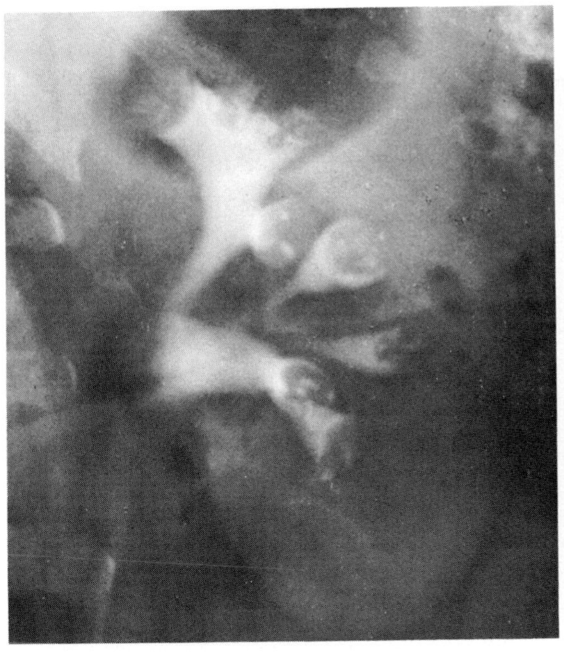

A

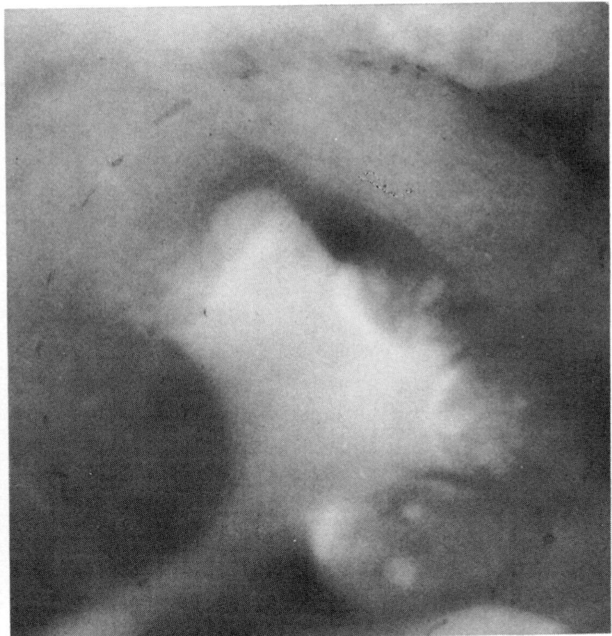

B

Fig. 41.22(A) I.V.U. Medullary sponge kidney demonstrating diffuse cyst formation and papillary enlargement. (B) Magnified view of affected calyces.

tuberculosis are usually larger and more irregular than those seen in the sponge kidney, and tuberculosis does not produce expansion of the pyramid and its calyx.

Renal papillary necrosis with cavitation and calcification rarely simulates this disease.

Nephrocalcinosis due to other causes does not produce the urographic changes of the sponge kidney.

Medullary cystic disease

This rare familial disease, presenting in childhood with renal failure or salt losing nephropathy, is distinct from medullary sponge kidney. The renal medulla is replaced by numerous cysts varying in size from pin points up to a few centimetres in diameter and there is a variable degree of interstitial fibrosis in both the cortex and the medulla. Unlike medullary sponge kidney the cysts are most numerous close to the corticomedullary junction. The kidneys may be large or small, calyceal deformity produced by the cysts may be evident in the early stages of the disease but usually high dose urography merely demonstrates the alteration in renal size and the nephrographic defects produced by the cysts.

DERMOID CYSTS

Dermoid cysts of the kidneys are rare. They frequently calcify and cannot be distinguished from calcified simple serous or haemorrhagic cysts.

EXTRA-PARENCHYMAL CYSTS

Most cysts which lie in the renal hilum are simple serous cysts. True **parapelvic cysts** lie in the hilum of the kidney outside the renal substance and are believed to be the result of lymphatic obstruction. There is usually a visible soft tissue mass, the renal pelvis is distorted by the mass and obstruction of the pelvis may produce a hydronephrosis.

Paranephric cysts (urinoma) form collections of clear fluid within the renal capsule surrounding the kidney. They are believed to be the result of extravasation of urine secondary to urinary obstruction or trauma. The urogram demonstrates enlargement of the renal outline, but it rarely opacifies during intravenous urography. The cyst may obstruct the renal pelvis.

REFERENCES AND SUGGESTIONS FOR FURTHER READING

BECKER, J. A., KINKHABIOLA, M., POLLACK, H. & BOSNIAK, M. (1973) Angiomyolipoma of the kidney. *Acta radiologica*, **14**, 561–568.

BOSNIAK, M. A. & AMBOS, M. A. (1975) Polycystic kidney disease. *Seminars in Roentgenology*, vol. 10, No. 4, p. 133–143.

CHOUKO, A. M. WEISS, S. M., STEIN, J. H. & FERRIS, T. F. (1974) Renal involvement in tuberous sclerosis. *American Journal of Medicine*, **56**, 124–131.

DANIEL, W. W., HARTMAN, G. W., WITTEN, D. M., FARROW, G. M. & KELALIS, P. P. (1972) Calcified renal masses. *Radiology*, **103**, 503–508.

ELKIN, M. & BERNSTEIN, J. (1969). Cystic diseases of the kidney. Radiological and pathological considerations. *Clinical Radiology*, **20**, 65–82.

ELKIN, M. (1975). Renal cystic disease—an overview. *Seminars in Roentgenology*, vol. **10**, No. 4, p. 99–102.

KING, M. C., FREEDENBERG, R. M. & TENA, L. B. (1968). Normal renal parenchyma simulating tumour. *Radiology*, **91**, 217–222.

Lucke, B. & Schlumberger, H. G. (1957) Tumours of the kidney, renal pelvis and ureter. *Atlas of Tumour Pathology*, Section 8, Fascicle 30, pp. 5–208. Washington, D.C.: Armed Forces Institute of Pathology.

Martinez-Maldonado, M. & Ramirez de Arellano, G. A. (1966) Renal involvement in malignant lymphomas. *Journal of Urology*, **95**, 485–488.

Richmond, J., Shermann, R. S., Diamond, H. D. & Craver, L. F. (1962) Renal lesions associated with malignant lymphomas. *American Journal of Medicine*, **32**, 184.

Stevenson, J. J. & Sherwood, T. (1971) Conservative management of renal masses. *British Journal of Urology*, **43**, 646–647.

CHAPTER 42

RENAL CALCULI; NEPHROCALCINOSIS

URINARY CALCULI

Stones in the urinary tract are most commonly seen in middle age and are uncommon in children unless there is some underlying structural or metabolic defect. The increased prevalence of stones in tropical countries is probably the result of dehydration with precipitation of crystalline debris, but dietary factors may also be involved. In many cases no cause can be found for the development of stones, but some underlying anatomical or metabolic disorder should always be suspected particularly in the presence of bilateral or repeated stone formation.

Congenital or acquired **structural abnormalities leading to stasis** predispose to stone formation. Thus pelvi-ureteric junction obstruction, horse-shoe kidneys, vesical diverticula and lower urinary tract obstruction are not infrequently complicated by calculi. Calculi may also be seen in medullary sponge kidney and calyceal cysts; in renal papillary necrosis the necrotic tissue may form a nidus for stone formation.

Metabolic disorders producing hypercalcaemia or hypercalcuria, particularly *hyperparathyroidism* and *idiopathic hypercalcuria* may be responsible for stone formation even in the absence of skeletal change. *Cystine* calculi only occur in patients with cystinuria, a familial disease in which there is a failure of the normal tubular absorption of amino-acids. *Uric acid* calculi occur as a familial disease in people of Eastern Mediterranean origin and also in diseases such as gout and polycythaemia in which there is disordered purine metabolism. *Xanthine* stones may occur when there is a failure of the normal oxidation of purines. *Primary hyperoxaluria* is a very rare disease presenting in childhood with repeated stone formation and nephrocalcinosis.

Secondary hyperoxaluria, the result of a disturbance of bile acid metabolism, is responsible for the increased incidence of oxalate stones in patients with inflammatory bowel disease. There is also an increased incidence of uric acid stones in these patients.

The great majority of stones are radio-opaque and consist of a fibrous matrix of muco-protein covered by crystals of calcium oxalate, calcium phosphate, calcium carbonate, ammonium magnesium phosphate and urates. Cystine stones are radio-opaque but less so than the above and frequently produce a characteristic 'milky' opacity. Pure uric acid and xanthine stones are radiolucent. Rarely radiolucent stones composed almost entirely of matrix are found in poorly functioning infected urinary tracts.

Calcium oxalate calculi are frequently laminated and have a nodular mulberry appearance or may form a 'jack stone' with a central nucleus and projecting thorn-

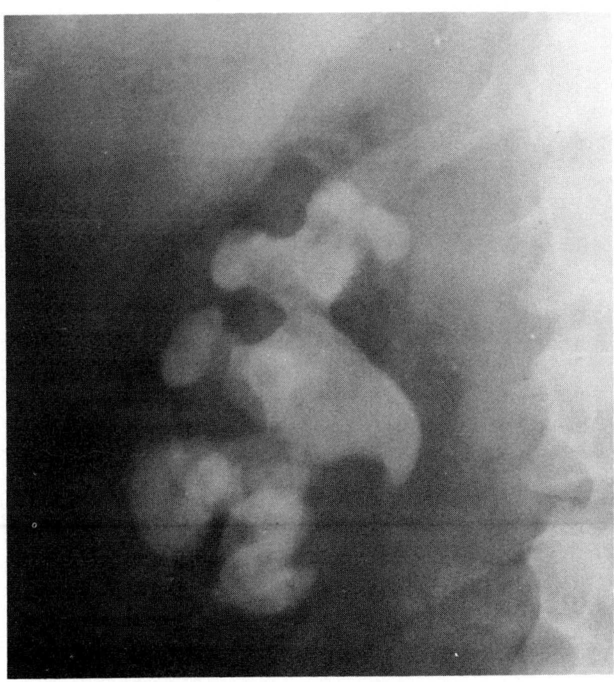

Fig. 42.1 Phosphate stone forming complete cast of the renal pelvis and calyces (staghorn calculus).

like processes. *Phosphate* calculi grow rapidly, often attain a great size and may form a cast of the renal pelvis and calyces (Fig. 42.1). '*Milk of calcium*' stones containing calcium carbonate may be seen within calyceal diverticula. They are usually asymptomatic and in the supine film produce a rounded opacity. Erect or lateral decubitus films demonstrate that the milky opacity gravitates to the bottom of the cyst. Ureteral stones are usually small and elongated in the line of the ureter, but may be very large when they occur in a dilated ureter. Bladder stones, when not lying within diverticula and when not displaced by an intravesical mass such as an enlarged prostate, usually lie in the midline.

Opaque calculi must be distinguished from other opacities in the region of the kidneys, ureters and bladder. *Calcified costal cartilages, gall stones, mesenteric glands,* the *tips of transverse processes, calcified iliac vessels, phleboliths and fibroids* may cause difficulty. Many of these have a characteristic appearance which makes recognition easy, but an extra-urinary origin can often only be proved by demonstrating that the opacities do not maintain a constant relationship to the kidney, ureter or bladder when films are taken in inspiration and expiration or in oblique views. It must be remembered that a stone lying in a duplicated ureter may appear to lie outside the urinary tract unless both ureters are demonstrated. Stones lying free within a dilated kidney or ureter may change in position relative to the renal outline or an ureteric catheter, but it will not be possible to 'throw out' the opacities when the urinary tract is opacified. A stone lodged in the infundibulum of a calyx may produce a localized calyceal dilatation and simulate a partially calcified tuberculous abscess. During an attack of colic a film of the abdomen may demonstrate contraction of the flank with obliteration of the psoas outline on the same side as the stone and a lumbar scoliosis with its convexity directed to the opposite side.

Intravenous urography supplemented when necessary by retrograde ureteric catheterization is essential in the investigation of calculi. Whenever possible, the intravenous examination should be carried out in the acute stage of renal colic. In these circumstances ureteric compression cannot usually be tolerated and is unnecessary; preliminary dehydration is also unnecessary provided that sufficient contrast medium is injected.

If obstruction is present, the affected kidney will be increased in size. There will also be delay in excretion, increased density and persistence of the nephrogram, with or without pyelo-tubular 'backflow', and dilation of the urinary tract down to the site of obstruction (Fig. 42.2A and B). Perirenal extravasation of contrast medium may result from acute calculus obstruction. The presence of obstruction will be established on the early films by the increase in the size of the kidney and the delay in excretion, but it may prove necessary to prolong the examination for up to 24 hours to establish the site and

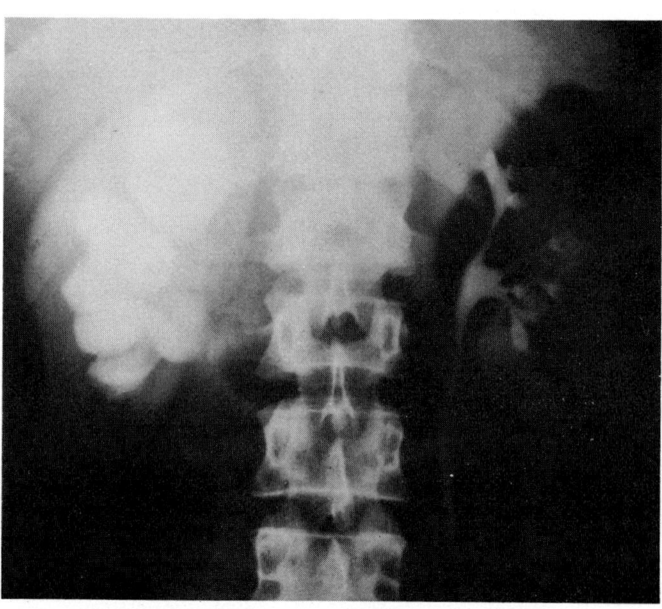
A

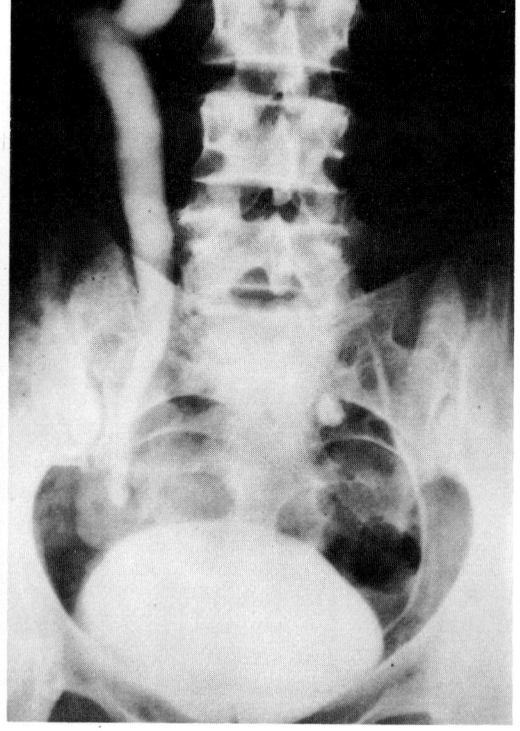
B

Fig. 42.2 I.V.U. during attack of right-sided colic due to a right ureteric calculus. (A) Early film of kidneys. (B) Later film of ureters.

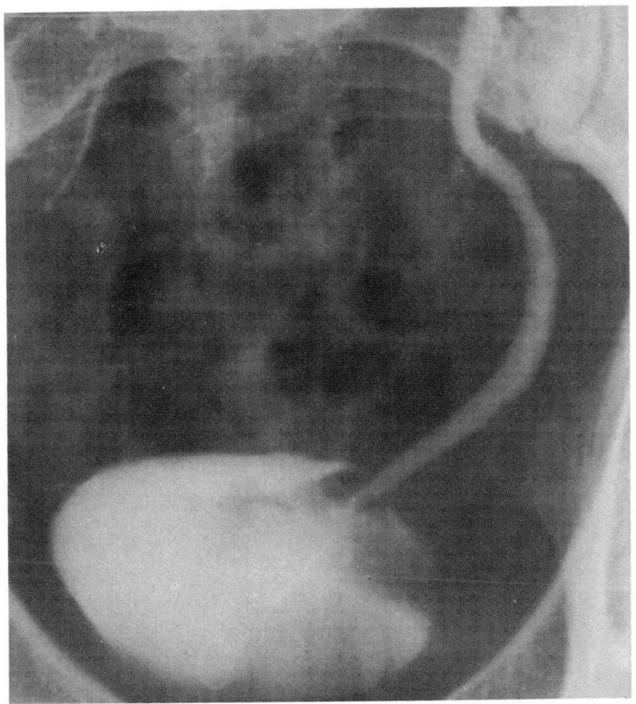

Fig. 42.3 Oedema around the ureteric orifice produced by a ureteric stone impacted at the orifice.

nature of the obstruction. The passage of a stone through the ureteric orifice or its impaction in the lower ureter produces oedema around the orifice. The resultant filling defect in the bladder may be quite extensive and may mimic the appearance of a carcinoma (Fig. 42.3). Identical changes may also follow ureteric catheterization.

Non-opaque stones if small may be quite impossible to demonstrate; larger radiolucent stones must be distinguished from other causes of a filling defect—tumour, blood clot, sequestrated papilla, fungal ball.

Ureteric obstruction, even when short-lived, may lead to permanent atrophy of the renal parenchyma, this *post-obstructive atrophy* produces a diffuse uniform narrowing of the renal substance thickness with flattening of the papillae and dilatation of the calyces.

NEPHROCALCINOSIS

The term nephrocalcinosis should only be used to describe a radiological appearance in which there is a deposition of calcium within the renal substance in the form of small rounded opacities or less frequently spicules (Fig. 42.4). Microscopic calcification and localized dystrophic calcification which may occur in renal tumour, cyst, tuberculosis, abscess or infarction should not be included.

Nephrocalcinosis may be (*A*) the result of hypercalcaemia or hypercalcuria or (*B*) due to the presence of biochemical or structural changes which favour the deposition of calcium.

A. Nephrocalcinosis due to hypercalcaemia and/or hypercalcuria

1. Hyperparathyroidism.
2. Renal tubular acidosis.
3. Idiopathic hypercalcuria.
4. Sarcoidosis.
5. Multiple myeloma and carcinomatosis.
6. Cushing's syndrome.
7. Steroid therapy.
8. Milk alkali syndrome.
9. Hypervitaminosis D.
10. Malignant disease (with or without bone secondaries).
11. Idiopathic infantile calcaemia.

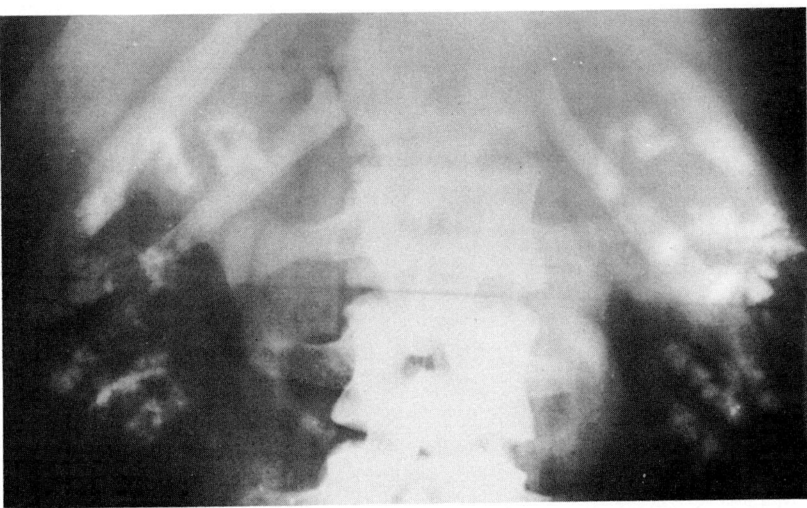

Fig. 42.4 Nephrocalcinosis.

B. **Nephrocalcinosis due to the presence of structural or biochemical changes favouring the deposition of calcium**

1. Medullary sponge kidney.
2. Renal medullary necrosis.
3. Excessive intake of alkalis.
4. Renal cortical necrosis.
5. Chronic glomerular nephritis.
6. Hyperoxaluria.

In a number of cases no cause can be found.

Diagnosis

In the majority of cases the aetiological diagnosis depends on biochemical investigation, but radiological investigation may often be helpful.

Nephrocalcinosis due to hypercalcaemia or hypercalcuria may be associated with osteoporosis in hyperparathyroidism, sarcoidosis, myeloma and carcinomatosis, Cushing's syndrome and hypervitaminosis D. Osteomalacia may be present in renal tubular acidosis and idiopathic hypercalcuria. The complete absence of skeletal changes, however, does not necessarily indicate that the nephrocalcinosis is not due to hypercalcaemia or hypercalcuria. The presence of osteolytic deposits would incriminate multiple myeloma or carcinomatosis and lung changes, sarcoidosis.

The detection of small areas of calcification demands carefully 'coned' films and low kilo-voltage. Tomography and oblique views are useful in establishing that the calcification is within the renal substance.

A decrease in renal size occurs as a result of renal damage and is more likely to occur with hypercalcaemia. An increase of renal size may indicate the presence of medullary sponge kidney and this may be confirmed by the distribution of the calcified deposits, which will be confined to the medulla, and also by the characteristic change in the calyces and pyramids. Renal granulomata are common in sarcoidosis and these may occasionally produce bilateral symmetrical enlargement of the kidneys.

Staghorn calculi are usually seen with hypercalcuria in renal tubular acidosis and idiopathic hypercalcuria. Dense confluent calcification in the renal medulla is characteristic of renal tubular acidosis.

Primary hyperoxaluria. Nephrocalcinosis is seen in the late stages of this rare condition in which there is a high excretion of oxalic acid with the deposition of calcium oxalate crystals in the tubules and the formation of calcium oxalate stones.

Chronic glomerulonephritis. Nephrocalcinosis producing a characteristic cortical calcification is a very rare occurrence in chronic glomerulonephritis.

Renal cortical necrosis. Cortical necrosis is a rare cause of renal failure usually occurring as a result of haemorrhage in late pregnancy. The kidneys are reduced in size and cortical calcification may occur, the appearances being similar to those seen in chronic glomerulonephritis. The calcification is best demonstrated by tomography and may take the form of double parallel 'tram' lines. Calcification may also be seen in the thrombosed ureteral veins.

CHAPTER 43

URINARY INFECTION

CYSTITIS

Bacterial cystitis, usually due to *E. coli* infection, is most commonly seen in young girls and adult women. In men it is usually a complication of incomplete bladder emptying. Clinically it presents with frequency, urgency, dysuria and suprapubic discomfort.

The inflammed bladder has a reduced capacity and is rounded or 'systolic' in shape. Irregularity of the bladder outline may be produced by mucosal oedema (Fig. 43.1) and the thickened mucosal folds are often well seen on the post-voiding film. Transient vesico-ureteric reflux occurs during acute infections as a result of oedema of the bladder wall. Chronic inflammatory changes with fibrosis leads to gross bladder contracture and permanent reflux.

Cyclophosphamide cystitis. A haemorrhagic cystitis occurs as a complication of cyclophosphamide therapy. It can produce severe haemorrhage, the bladder lumen being filled with large blood clots.

Cystitis emphysematosa. Gas within the bladder wall and within the urinary tract is usually due to *E. coli* infection in diabetics.

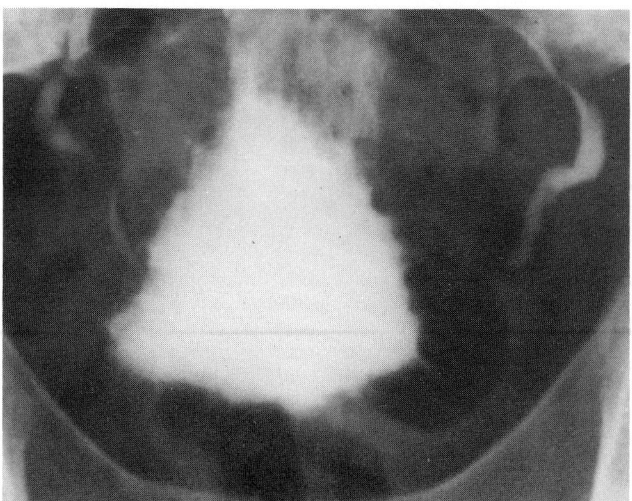

Fig. 43.1 Acute cystitis. Mucosal oedema producing irregularity of the bladder outline.

Irradiation and chemical cystitis. The bladder is relatively insensitive to irradiation but gross bladder contracture and vesico-ureteric reflux may occur as a result of irradiation and exposure to irritant chemical solutions.

Cystitis of unknown cause

1. Eosinophilic cystitis in which there is eosinophilic infiltration of the bladder wall.
2. Malacoplakia—histiocytic infiltration of the bladder and ureteral walls may produce an appearance simulating carcinoma.
3. Cystitis glandularis—hyperplasia of the urothelium may also simulate a carcinoma.
4. Cystitis cystica—see Pyeloureteritis cystica.

ACUTE PYELONEPHRITIS

Acute pyelonephritis is usually the result of infection by organisms normally present in the bowel which gain access to the bladder via the urethra. Vesico-ureteric reflux may then lead to transmission of the infection to the kidneys. The infection often complicates pre-existing lesions of the urinary tract leading to obstruction or reflux. Less commonly the infection is the result of haematogenous spread from a distant focus.

In the first year of life the disease is equally distributed between the sexes but later in childhood and also in adult life it is much more commonly seen in women, especially during pregnancy.

In the majority of cases in the absence of underlying renal disease the urogram is normal but during the acute stage of the disease there may be an increase in renal size with delayed excretion, impairment of concentration and, as a result of renal oedema, attenuation and elongation of the calyces. A dense persistent nephrogram with little or no pyelogram, presumably the result of tubular blockage by pus, has also been described. The infection rarely proceeds to abscess formation (Fig. 43.2A and B). Following the acute stage the kidneys return to normal in the great majority of cases. A small percentage of cases proceed to chronic pyelonephric scarring, the first sign of

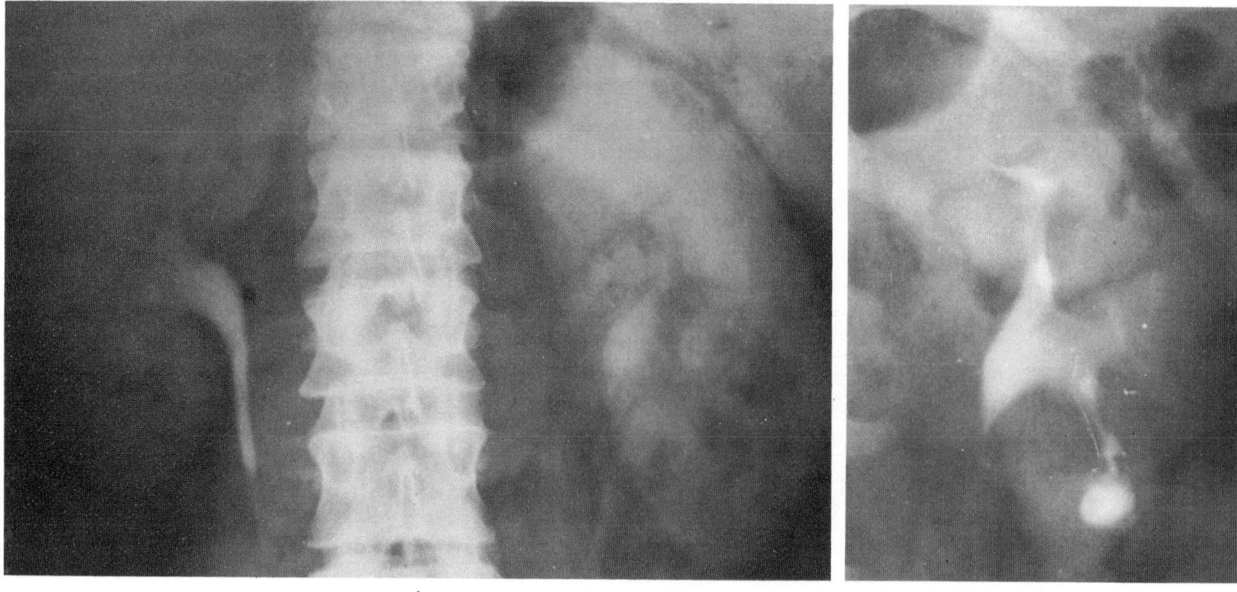

Fig. 43.2 Acute pyelonephritis. (A) Initial I.V.U. demonstrating left renal enlargement, persistent nephrogram and delayed opacification of the collecting system. (B) Two months later, abscess cavity in the lower pole of the left kidney.

permanent renal damage being a reduction in renal size.

Rarely, usually in diabetics, infection with *E. coli* may produce radiolucent gas shadows outlining the lumen of the urinary tract and gas may also be visible in the renal substance and retroperitoneal tissues. Clostridial infection of the urinary tract is very rarely seen and is then usually secondary to a septicaemia. Gas may also be seen in the urinary tract following instrumentation, as a result of penetrating wounds and fistulous communications with the gut—perforated duodenal ulcer, diverticular disease.

RENAL AND PERIRENAL ABSCESS

Renal abscesses are uncommon, the majority are the result of ascending infection with Gram-negative organisms from the bladder and are preceded by acute pyelonephritis. Haematogenous spread of staphylococcal and streptococcal infection is much less common but it does occur as a complication of septicaemia particularly in diabetics and 'main line' drug addicts.

An acute renal abscess produces the radiological changes of acute pyelonephritis together with evidence of a mass displacing the collecting system and possibly deforming the renal outline. Communication with a calyx will produce an irregular cavity similar to that seen in tuberculosis (Fig. 43.2B).

Perinephric abscesses usually result from extension of a renal abscess but may also occur as a result of direct extension of duodenal ulceration, pancreatic and colonic disease. Involvement of the perirenal space leads to fixity of the kidney (demonstrated by inspiratory and expiratory films), loss of definition of the psoas outline and a lumbar scoliosis concave to the affected side. There may be a localized ileus and a sympathetic pleural effusion with an elevated hemidiaphragm. Rarely, gas shadows may be seen in the perirenal tissues.

Renal angiography demonstrates a slow arterial flow in a diffusely enlarged kidney and a defect in the nephrogram. Abnormal vessels similar to those seen in malignant disease may also be demonstrated. Perinephric extension leads to enlargement and displacement of capsular vessels and feeding branches may arise from the lumbar arteries.

XANTHOGRANULOMATOUS PYELONEPHRITIS

This is an unusual form of renal infection in which renal tissue damaged by chronic infection is replaced by large lipid containing histiocytes. The chronic inflammatory process may extend into the perinephric space. It is more commonly seen in diabetics and in the great majority of cases arises as a complication of pyonephrosis due to renal pelvic or ureteral obstruction.

The commonest radiographic finding is a large 'non-functioning kidney' with a hydronephrosis. Less frequently there is diffuse swelling of the renal tissue and extension into the perinephric tissue may lead to localized or generalized loss of definition of the renal outline. The rare localized form produces a renal mass which may calcify, the urographic and angiographic appearances being indistinguishable from a renal carcinoma.

FUNGAL INFECTIONS

Infection of the urinary tract with *Candida albicans* is a rare condition which is usually secondary to systemic or ascending infection, the kidney is very rarely the only organ to be involved. It usually occurs in debilitated patients or following prolonged antibiotic, steroid or immunosuppressive drug treatment and is also seen in diabetics and drug addicts.

In the acute form the radiographic appearances are similar to those described in acute bacterial pyelonephritis, multiple parenchymal abscesses may occur and the disease if unchecked leads to rapid destruction of the kidney. Fungal balls producing filling defects within the renal pelvis, ureter or the bladder produce an appearance similar to non-opaque calculi, epithelial tumour, blood clot and sequestrated papillae.

Actinomyocosis very rarely involves the urinary tract and is usually secondary to the extension of intrathoracic disease across the diaphragm or direct spread from the gastro-intestinal tract. In the kidney it may produce an appearance similar to that produced by an ordinary renal carbuncle, infiltration of the retroperiotoneal tissues may produce unilateral or bilateral ureteric displacement and obstruction.

CHRONIC PYELONEPHRITIS

Chronic pyelonephritis is now the commonest cause of death from renal failure and hypertension in the British Isles and is almost invariably the result of infection and reflux during childhood. The disease may be symptom free until the onset of renal failure or severe hypertension. In some cases albuminuria may be discovered in a symptom-free patient during routine medical examina-

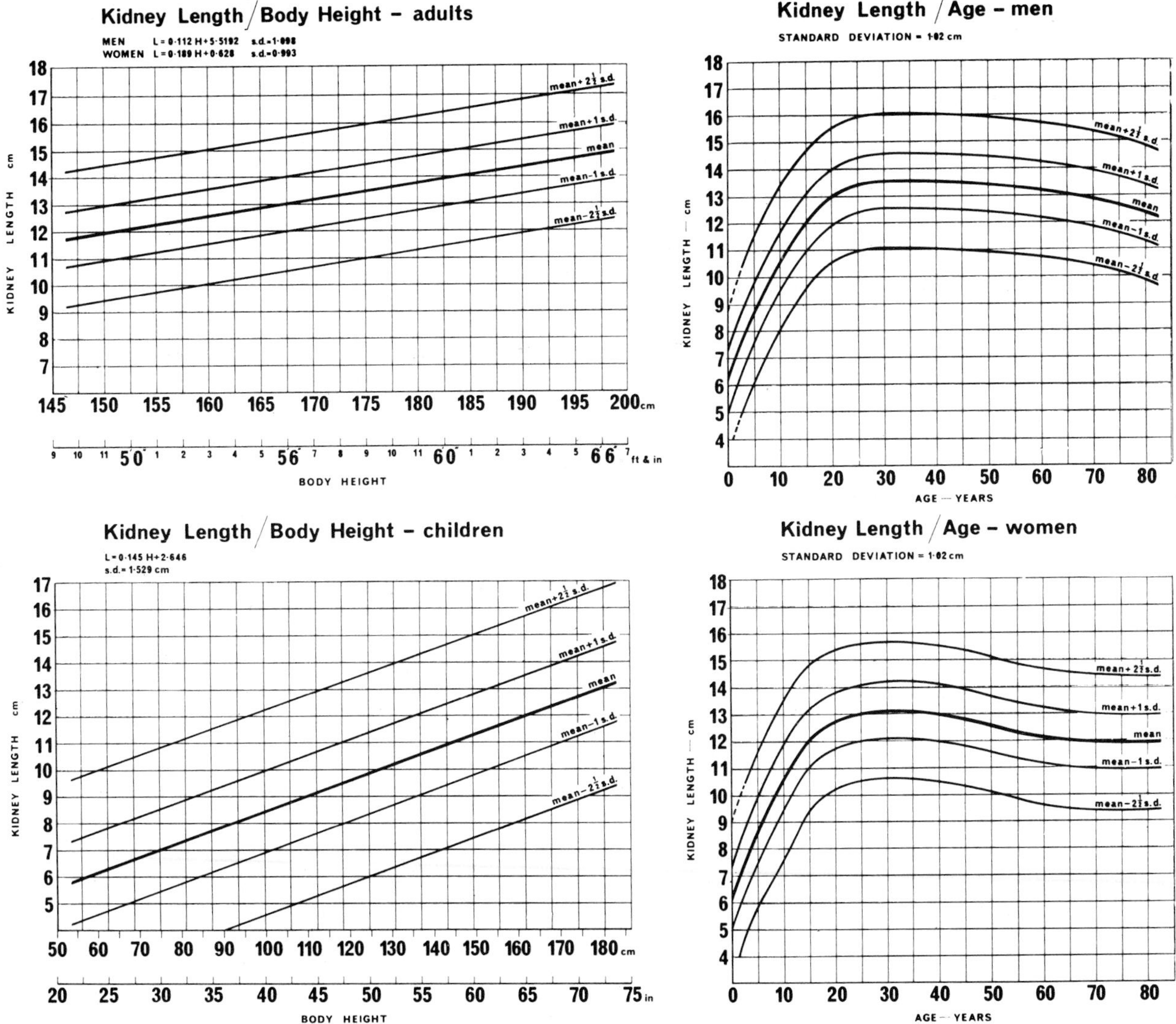

Fig. 43.3 Kidney size. Normal long axis length in children and adults as measured on films of the abdomen with an anode–film distance of 36 inches. (By courtesy of Dr C. J. Hodson.)

tion and others may present with recurrent urinary infection. It is the end result or chronic stage of bacterial infection of the renal substance.

The kidney is reduced in size, it shows coarse focal scarring with adjoining areas of normal hypertrophied renal tissue. The disease may be unilateral or bilateral and usually presents in childhood and early adult life, it is rarely seen over the age of 40 unless it complicates obstruction or reflux produced by operations on the lower ureter.

The radiological changes produced are:

1. Reduction in kidney size with irregularity of the renal surface.
2. Narrowing of the renal substance thickness.
3. Calyceal deformity.
4. Evidence of renal failure.

The renal outlines are usually visible on good-quality films taken during intravenous urography supplemented when necessary by tomography or high-dosage urography. In the absence of developmental anomalies such as reduplication and mal-rotation, or of displacement by adjacent organs, the kidneys are normally symmetrical in size. Even minor degrees of duplication such as a bifid renal pelvis will produce considerable asymmetry, the affected kidney, if healthy, being larger than its fellow on the opposite side. The long axis length of the kidney should be routinely recorded (Fig. 43.3) and in adults, any variation between the two sides greater than 1·5 cm should, in the absence of morphological differences, be regarded as being highly suggestive of renal disease. In children an asymmetry greater than 10 per cent of the long axis length should be regarded as significant. In unilateral disease the asymmetry is exaggerated by compensatory hypertrophy of the healthy kidney but even with bilateral disease asymmetry is usually present. A progressive reduction in renal size will be demonstrated if serial films are available over a period of several years.

Coarse scarring of the renal substance produces irregularity of the renal outline which is rendered more obvious by hypertrophy of adjacent healthy tissue within the diseased kidney. The initial scarring most commonly occurs at the renal poles. When confined to the upper pole it may be difficult to detect but with the loss of renal substance thickness the calyx of the affected pole will be seen to lie closer to the vertebrae body than the corresponding calyx on the healthy side (Fig. 43.4). In the presence of ureteral duplication both reflux and scarring is usually confined to the lower renal moiety (Fig. 43.5).

In the normal urogram a line drawn through the tips of the outer renal papillae describes a gentle curve with a constant relationship to the surface outline. The thickness of the renal substance is represented by the distance between this line and the renal surface and is normally found to be greatest at the upper and lower poles of the kidney (Fig. 43.6). Pyelonephritic scarring causes loss of

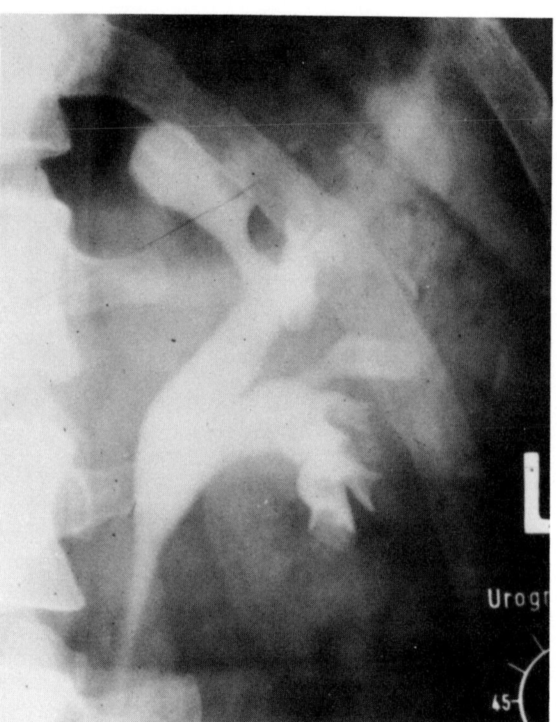

Fig. 43.4 Chronic pyelonephritic scarring confined to the upper pole.

the normal interpapillary line, one or more calyces will protrude beyond the line towards the renal surface with consequent narrowing of the renal substance thickness and there is an associated indentation of the renal outline. The affected calyces are dilated and distorted and in the presence of gross disease the whole calycine system

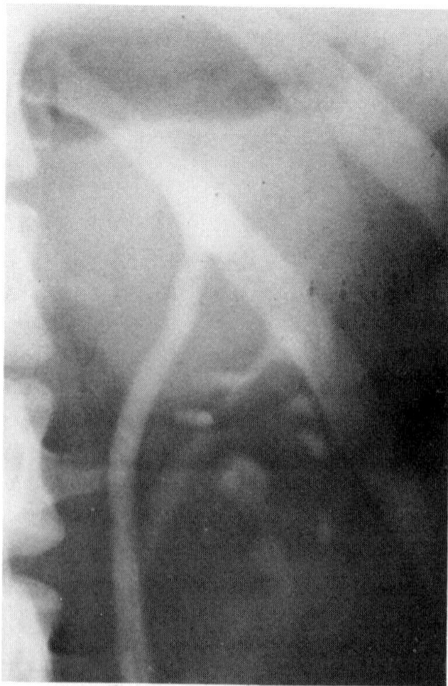

Fig. 43.5 Chronic pyelonephritic scarring confined to the lower pole of a duplicated kidney.

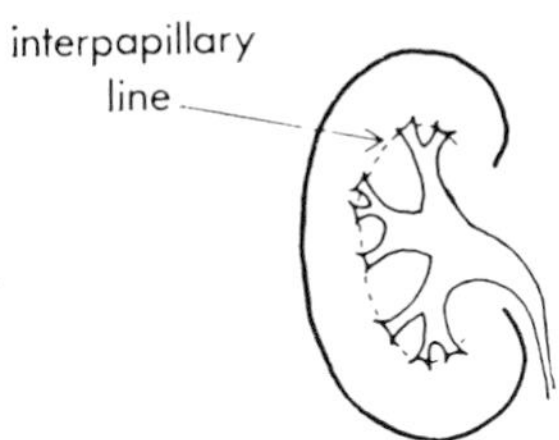

Fig. 43.6 Interpapillary line.

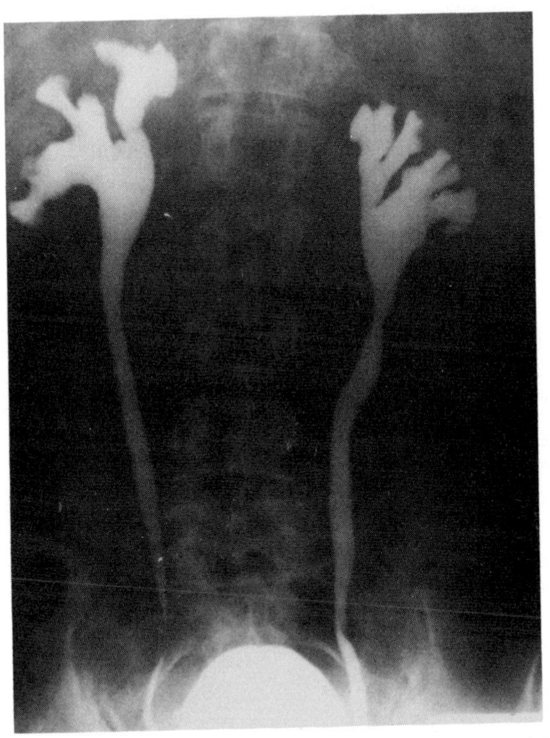

Fig. 43.8 Micturating cystogram. Bilateral chronic pyelonephritis with bilateral reflux.

is so distorted that it becomes quite impossible to make out the normal pattern (Fig. 43.7).

Owing to the hypertrophy of islands of surviving renal tissue, and possibly ischaemia, the concentration of contrast medium may be well maintained and the pelvicalycine systems well demonstrated even with extensive disease.

An overgrowth of fatty tissue in the renal sinus and perirenal tissues frequently accompanies marked shrinkage of the kidney.

Almost all the children and about half the adult patients with 'primary' chronic pyelonephritis show vesico-ureteric reflux (Fig. 43.8). Only rarely is this due to lower urinary tract obstruction, but any possible obstructing lesion must be excluded by micturating cysto-urethrography.

Differential diagnosis. *Foetal lobulation* produces smooth indentations of the renal outline between normal calyces. *Segmental infarction* may produce surface irregularity very similar to that produced by chronic pyelonephritis but the calyces are normal.

Back pressure atrophy unlike chronic pyelonephritis is not a focal disease, it produces a diffuse uniform narrowing of the renal substance with uniform 'clubbing' of the calyces. Unless complicated by chronic pyelonephritis there is no scarring of the outline and there is no interruption of the normal regular curvature of the interpapillary line.

Renal medullary necrosis does not produce coarse scarring of the renal outline unless it is complicated by chronic pyelonephritis but irregularity of the outline may occur as a result of hypertrophy of healthy renal tissue. Papillary sequestration, calcification and the characteristic 'horns' are not seen in chronic pyelonephritis.

Renal tuberculosis—calcification, abscess formation and cicatrization does not occur in chronic pyelonephritis.

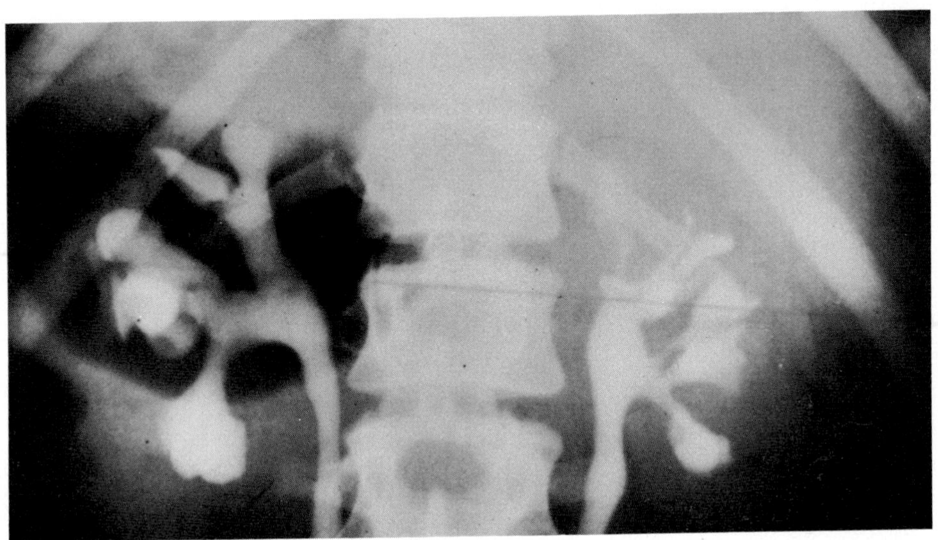

Fig. 43.7 Bilateral chronic pyelonephritis.

VESICO-URETERIC REFLUX

When urine enters the bladder from the ureters it normally stays there until it is passed via the urethra during the next act of micturition. The efficacy of the normal uretero-vesical junction in preventing reflux has long been known but it is only in recent years that the close association of reflux, urinary infection and renal disease has been recognized.

The competence of the normal uretero-vesical junction is dependent on three factors—the obliquity of the intramural course of the ureter, the surrounding bladder musculature and a mucosal flap valve produced by the intravesical, submucosal ureter. Certain pathological states may interfere with this valvular mechanism and allow reflux to occur. These include:

1. Congenital anomalies—Triad Syndrome, vesical diverticula, duplication of the ureter, ectopia of the ureter.
2. Cystitis—acute and chronic and following irradiation of the pelvis.
3. Carcinoma of the bladder.
4. Neurological lesions, congenital or acquired.
5. Surgical operations on the lower ureter.
6. Lower urinary tract obstruction.
7. Megaureter-Megacystis syndrome (page 843).
8. Primary reflux.

Diverticula of the bladder are not uncommonly due to a congenital deficiency in the bladder musculature and when they involve the ureteric orifice they may lead to vesico-ureteric reflux. Small para-ureteric diverticula (Fig. 43.9) produced by a localized herniation of the vesical mucosa through a congenital defect in the vesical musculature are not uncommonly seen in children with reflux.

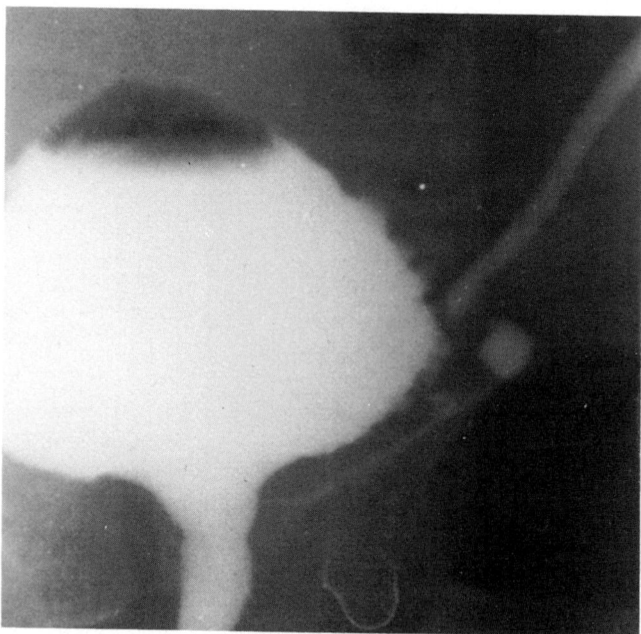

Fig. 43.9 Para-ureteric saccule and reflux.

Duplication. When there is complete duplication the ureter from the lower moiety of the kidney opens into the bladder above and lateral to the orifice of the ureter draining the upper moiety (page 844). This ureter, therefore, has a shorter and less oblique course through the bladder musculature and a less effective valvular mechanism. When reflux complicates this anomaly it is usually the ureter draining the lower moiety that is affected and any associated pyelonephritic scarring may be confined to the lower moiety.

Ectopia. When the ectopic ureter opens into the urethra, and provided that there is no stenosis of its orifice, reflux will occur into the ectopic ureter during micturition (page 846). This is a convenient method of localizing the site of entry of the ectopic ureter.

Cystitis. It is well recognized that cystitis may lead to reflux; oedema, rigidity and fibrosis interfering with the normal valvular mechanism. Chronic cystitis may produce irreversible changes and the reflux is permanent. Acute infection commonly leads to transient reflux in both children and adults.

Carcinoma of the bladder. The mechanism of reflux production in these cases is similar to the inflammatory lesions—infiltration by neoplastic cells around the ureteric orifice leads to rigidity and incompetence.

Neurological lesions. Vesico-ureteric reflux is most commonly seen when there is gross thickening of the bladder wall with sacculation and there may be evidence of obstruction at the level of the bladder neck or in the posterior urethra.

Surgical operations on the lower ureter. Reflux may result from reimplantation of the ureter, the slitting of an ureterocele or the removal of a calculus impacted at the ureteric orifice.

Lower urinary tract obstruction. Reflux is not invariably seen even in the presence of gross degrees of obstruction. When reflux does occur with lower tract obstruction it produces a rapid deterioration in the state of the upper urinary tract. It is possible that reflux is not merely due to raised intravesical pressure but occurs when a para-ureteric saccule involves the ureteric orifice or when infection supervenes.

Primary reflux and infection

Infection of the urinary tract is a common condition in childhood and one which if often overlooked. Many children with a significant bacteriuria are free from symptoms and symptoms referrable to the urinary tract are uncommon under the age of 2 years. The presenting symptoms in early childhood are usually non-specific—failure to thrive, feeding difficulties, fever and vomiting. It is not until the age of 5 years and over that the conventional symptoms of urinary infection are found—frequency, dysuria, loin pain and haematuria. Frequently the condition follows a benign course but in a significant proportion urinary infection is indicative of serious anomalies of the urinary tract which, in the presence of continuing infection, may lead to progressive renal damage, hypertension and chronic ill health.

In the majority of infected children the bladder is invaded by organisms originating in the bowel and ascending the urethra. Multiplication of organisms within the bladder is normally prevented by the natural defence mechanisms of the bladder, the most important being regular, complete emptying of the bladder. Interference with normal emptying induces stasis and formation of residual urine. In a small proportion this may be a result of obstruction, e.g. urethral valves or a functional obstruction due to a neurological defect. The return of refluxed urine to the bladder or retention of urine within a diverticulum are other mechanisms of residue formation. Stones may obstruct or irritate the bladder and predispose to infection. Finally local or general impairment of immunity will encourage multiplication of organisms within the bladder. The most severe renal damage follows infection of the obstructed urinary tract.

Vesico-ureteric reflux plays a crucial part in the production of renal damage, it allows organisms in the bladder to reach the kidney and the demonstration of reflux from the calyces into the collecting tubules—*intra-renal reflux*—suggests that organisms infecting the urine can be carried into the renal substance in this way. Anatomical differences in the circular openings of the collecting tubules in the upper and lower renal poles as compared with the more easily occluded slit-like orifices in the mid-zone papillae permit intrarenal reflux to occur more readily at the poles.

If the transient reflux of acute infections is excluded from consideration, by delaying the cystogram until infection has been controlled for a period of two weeks, one-third of children with a history of urinary infection will be found to have reflux. It is only rarely that one can detect an obvious cause for the reflux whereas in the later years of life reflux is commonly secondary to some other abnormality in the lower urinary tract. This *primary reflux* of childhood is presumably the result of some congenital anomaly at the ureterovesical junction. Some believe that it is the result of lateral recession of the ureteric orifice and consequent shortening of the intravesical ureter whilst others attribute the incompetence to a congenital deficiency or shortening of the submucosal ureteric segment with or without aplasia of its muscular coat.

It is convenient to classify reflux into four grades of severity.

Grade I. Reflux confined to the lower pelvic portion of a normal sized ureter.

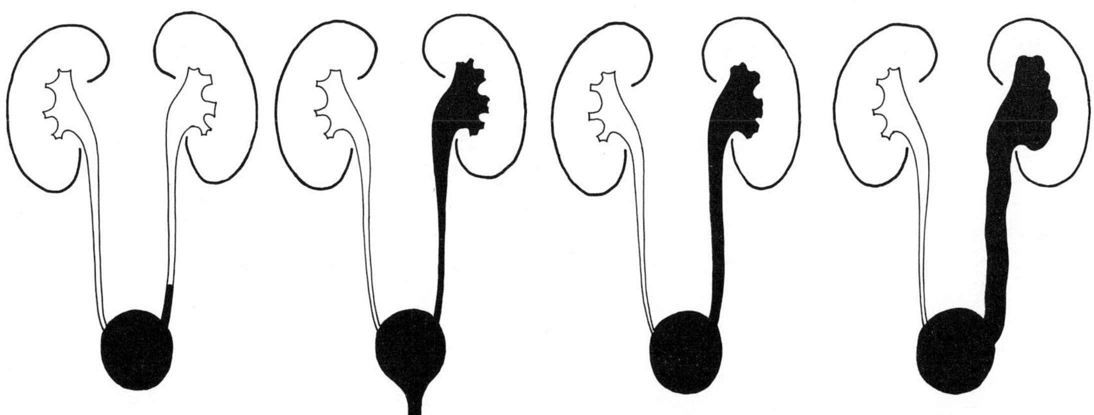

Fig. 43.10 Grades of reflux.

Grade II. Reflux extending up to the kidney on micturition only, no ureteral dilatation.

Grade III. Reflux extending up to the kidney in the resting state and also during voiding. No ureteral dilatation.

Grade IV. Reflux up to the kidney with dilatation of the upper tract (Fig. 43.10).

Follow-up studies indicate that primary reflux has a natural tendency to improve at any time during childhood, thus 80 per cent of ureters with grade I reflux will stop refluxing in the first few years but only 20 per cent of grade IV reflux will cease refluxing. Primary reflux in childhood is thus a condition with a natural tendency to improve. It is very commonly associated with chronic pyelonephritic scarring of the refluxing kidney but provided that infection is controlled refluxing kidneys will continue to grow normally and the development of fresh renal scars is very rare in the presence of sterile primary reflux. Surgical correction should therefore be confined to those patients in whom there is gross reflux and in whom long-term chemotherapy fails to control infection.

The association of renal disease with reflux is now well established. The most striking finding is the association of reflux with chronic pyelonephritic scarring of the kidneys. Pyelonephritic scarring is present in 50 per cent of patients with reflux and 70 per cent of all patients with chronic pyelonephritis have reflux. In childhood almost all children with pyelonephritic scarring have reflux and it seems likely that the great majority of cases of adult chronic pyelonephritis is due to infection and primary reflux during childhood and it has been suggested that the term chronic pyelonephritis should be replaced by *reflux nephropathy*. A less common radiological change in the affected kidney is one of diffuse narrowing of the renal substance with dilatation of the calyces—an appearance identical to that seen in postobstructive atrophy (Fig. 43.11). Occasionally the upper tract may show changes similar to those seen in congenital pelvi-ureteric obstruction but with reflux the ureter below the pelvi-ureteric junction is usually dilated.

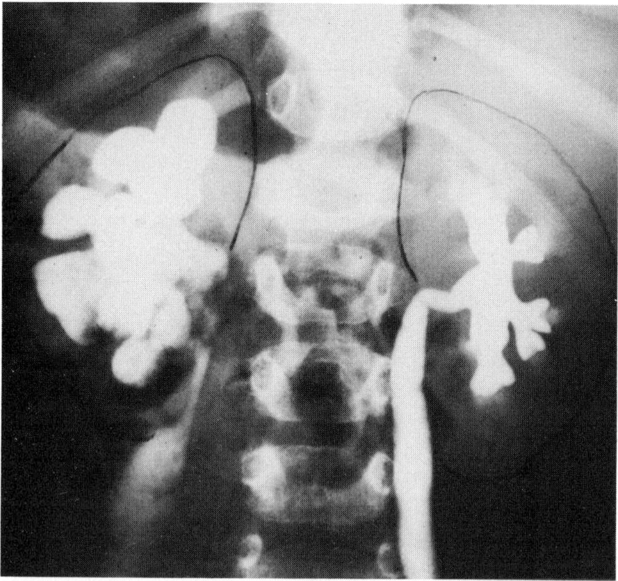

Fig. 43.11 I.V.U. Bilateral reflux with ureteral dilatation and renal changes similar to those seen in obstructive atrophy.

When the kidneys are normal other changes on the urogram which lead one to suspect the presence of reflux are—a vesical residue and ureteral dilatation. The residue of reflux is a false residue and does not necessarily indicate the presence of obstruction. In the absence of obstruction or a neurogenic lesion the bladder empties completely into the urethra and into the refluxing ureter. After micturition the detrusor relaxes, the ureteral residue drains downwards into the bladder producing a false vesical residue and a second act of micturition is then possible. Double and even triple micturition leads to a progressive reduction in the false residue and may usefully be employed with chemotherapy to rid the urinary tract of infection. Ureteral dilatation may be confined to the lower ureter or may involve its whole length; it may only be recognized if there is adequate ureteral compression or if an immediate postmicturition film is taken. Ureteral dilatation may be completely absent even in the presence of marked reflux.

RENAL TUBERCULOSIS

Renal tuberculosis is almost invariably secondary to tuberculous disease elsewhere, usually in the lungs or bones. Tubercle bacilli reach the kidney via the blood stream and are arrested in a glomerulus with the development of tubercles in the renal cortex. The tubercles are nearly always bilateral and the majority heal. The tuberculous foci may enlarge and coalesce and extension of the bacilli via the tubules leads to the formation of medullary lesions and papillary involvement. Ulceration into the renal pelvis produces urinary symptoms and may be followed by extension along the ureter to the bladder, prostate, seminal vesicles, vas deferens and epididymis.

In the early stages when the disease is confined to the renal cortex or medulla, radiological examination will be normal, and a normal urogram does not exclude renal tuberculosis.

Plain films of the abdomen may demonstrate changes in the renal outline and the presence of calcification. Changes in the renal outline are produced by the presence of tuberculous abscesses, fibrosis, ureteral obstruction and

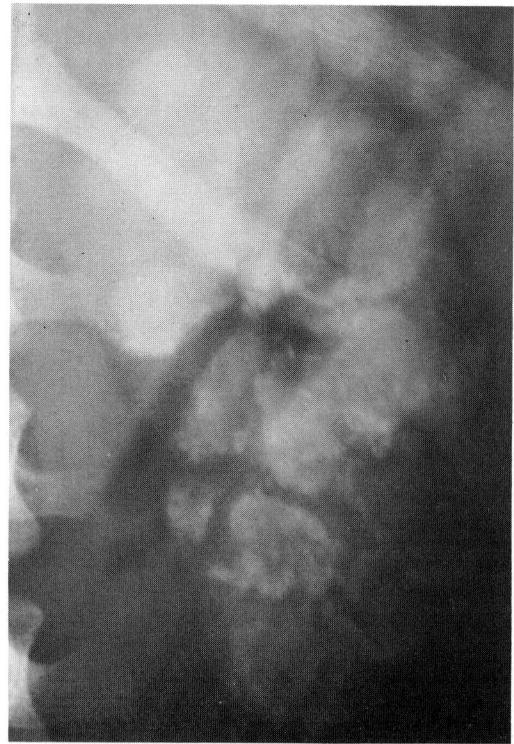

Fig. 43.12 Calcified tuberculous kidney.

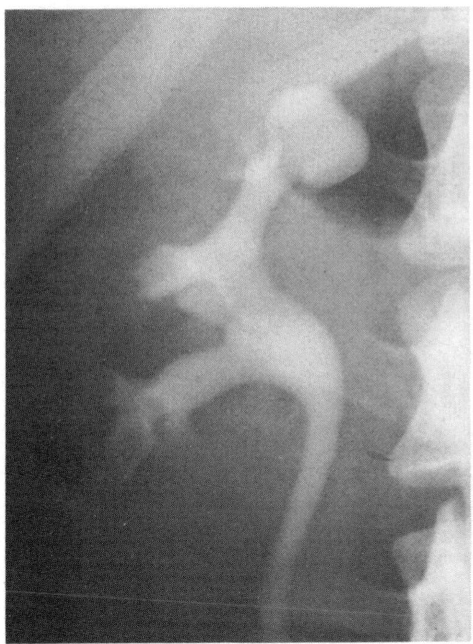

A

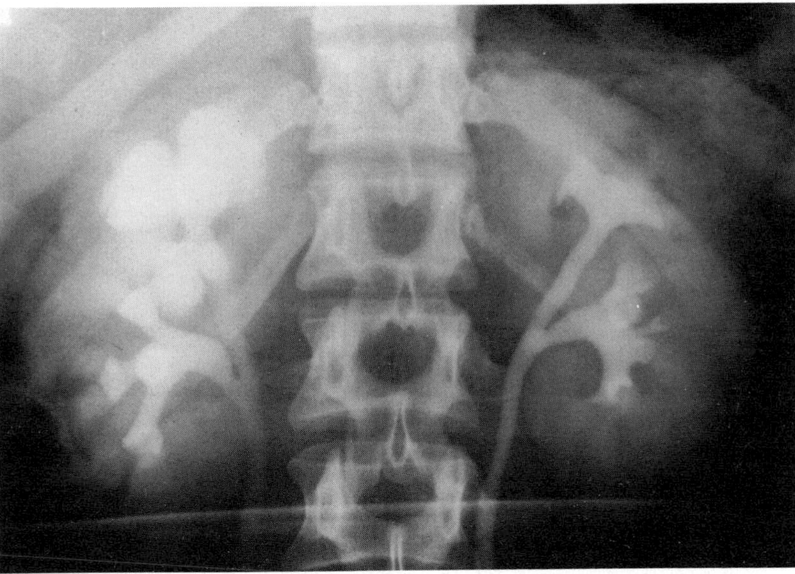

B

Fig. 43.13 (A) and (B) Tuberculous cavitation.

atrophy. An abscess may produce a bulge on the renal outline indistinguishable from that produced by a renal tumour or cyst. Fibrosis produces coarse scarring of the renal outline with a reduction in renal size as in chronic pyelonephritis or renal arteriolar infarction. Ureteric obstruction may produce a diffuse increase in the size of the whole kidney.

Calcification is commonly present, it varies in extent from a few minute areas to a complete cast of the kidney (Fig. 43.12). It usually produces irregular ill-defined areas lying within the renal substance but may mimic a calcified renal tumour or cyst. When the caseous material contains little calcium if forms a faint 'soft' opacity which has been likened to a cumulus cloud. Calcification in prostatic cavities is common, but it is often impossible to differentiate this from prostatic calculi. The seminal vesicles and vasa deferentia may also calcify, but it should be noted that such calcification may also occur in the absence of tuberculous infection, particularly in the elderly and in diabetics. Ureteral calcification is less common and calcification of the bladder wall is very rare in tuberculous disease.

The earliest change in the collecting system is a loss of definition of a minor calyx producing an indistinct feathery outline, its early stages being very similar to the normal tubular shadow. With progression of the disease a rounded cavity with irregular walls communicates with a deformed calyx (Fig. 43.13A and B). Destruction of renal substance with fibrosis may produce appearances identical to those seen in non-tuberculous chronic pyelonephritis with dilatation and deformity of the calyces, scarring of the renal surface and hypertrophy of the remaining normal renal tissue.

Calyceal stricture will cause narrowing of the calyx with dilatation proximal to the stricture and eventually a complete cut-off of the affected calyx (Fig. 43.14). A localized tuberculoma will produce displacement of the calyces identical to that produced by a renal tumour or cyst. With extensive disease gross deformity may occur with dilatation and cicatrical deformity of the calyces and a part or the whole of a kidney may be entirely destroyed.

Dilatation of the renal pelvis also occurs in the absence of ureteral stricture or reflux and filling defects within its lumen may be produced by caseous debris and granulation tissue.

Ureteral involvement produces irregular areas of dilatation and narrowing with a turtuous rigid appearance

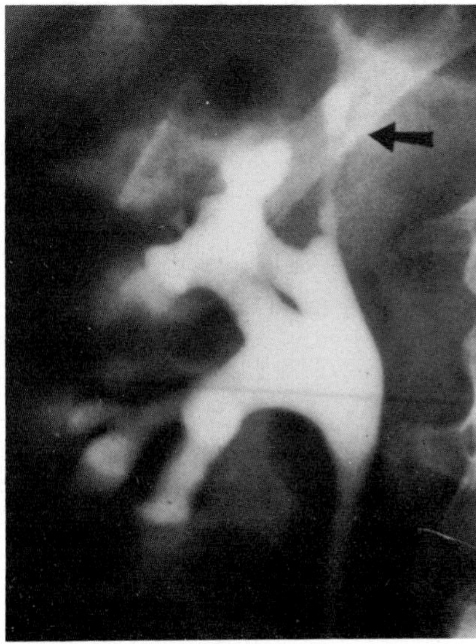

Fig. 43.14 Cicatrization upper pole calyx.

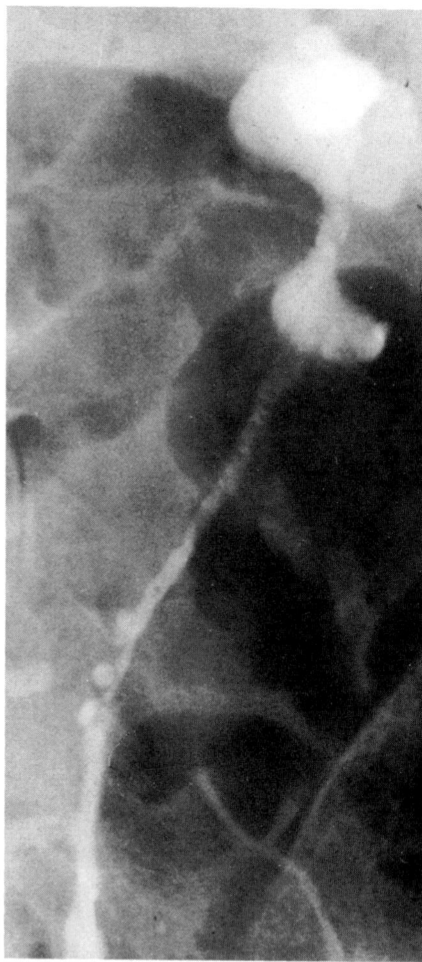

Fig. 43.15 Renal tuberculosis with ureteral involvement.

(Fig. 43.15). Shortening of the ureter by fibrosis obliterates its normal curvature so that it enters the bladder perpendicularly and its wide open 'golf hole' mouth may be clearly visible. Ureteral stricture will produce a hydronephrosis and hydro-ureter and, when complete obstruction ensues, a non-functioning kidney. Tuberculous intrapelvic abscess in the female may lead to displacement and obstruction of the ureters and bladder.

Tuberculous cystis leads to a reduction of the normal bladder capacity with a 'systolic' appearance (Fig. 43.16). Oedema of the bladder mucosa may produce a 'cobble-stone' appearance or filling defects very similar to those produced by a growth may be seen, particularly around the ureteric orifice. Advanced disease leads to gross irregular contracture of the bladder and free reflux into dilated ureters will be demonstrated on cystography. Tuberculous prostatic abscesses are best demonstrated by retrograde urethrography.

Angiography is of greatest value in cases with calyceal obstruction and no other sign of destruction of renal tissue and also as a preliminary to partial nephrectomy.

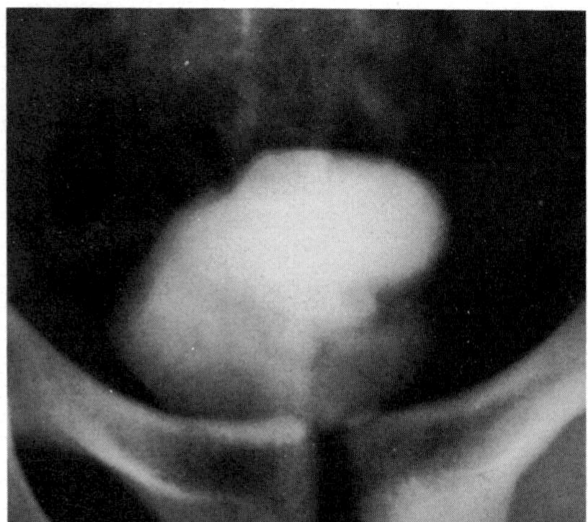

Fig. 43.16 Tuberculous cystitis with marked reduction of bladder capacity.

Tuberculous foci produce avascular areas, vessels may be displaced around an abscess cavity and scarring of the renal outline will be clearly demonstrated during the nephrogram phase.

URINARY SCHISTOSOMIASIS

Schistosomiasis is endemic in East and South Africa, Egypt, Arabia and in parts of the Eastern Mediterranean. It is produced by infestation by the worm *Schistosoma haematobium*.

The adult worm inhabits the submucosa of the bladder,

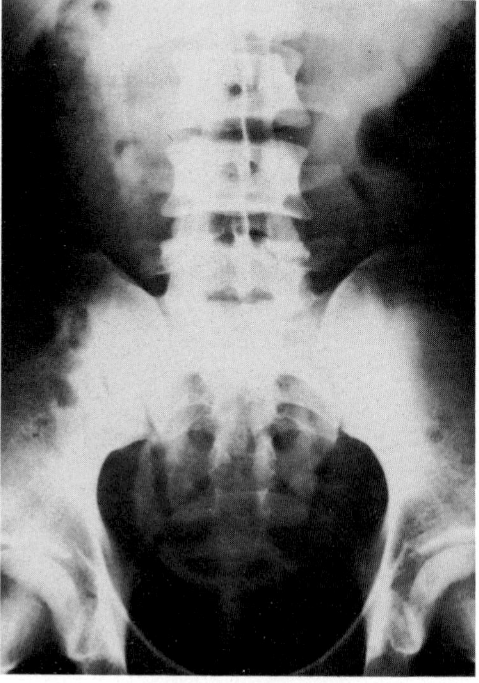

Fig. 43.17 Schistosomiasis. Curvilinear calcification of the bladder and calcification of the whole length of the right ureter.

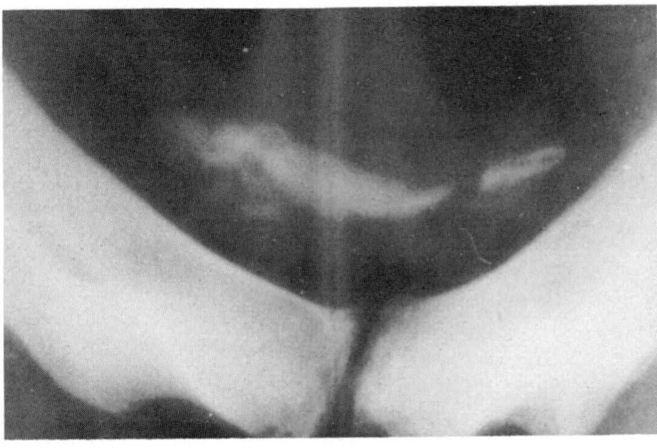

A

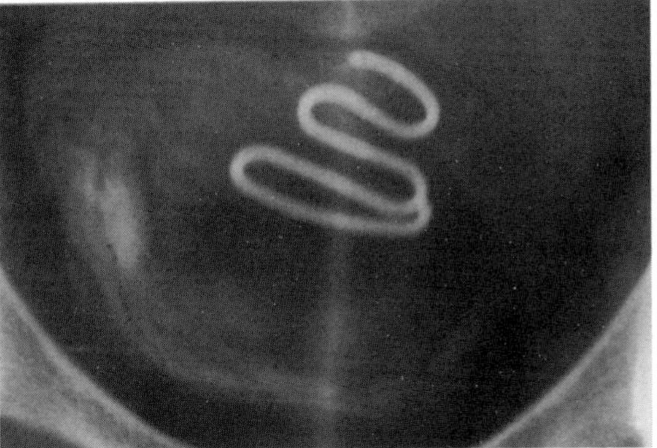

B

Fig. 43.18 (A) and (B) Bladder calcification in schistosomiasis. An I.U.C.D. is present in B.

where the ova are deposited by the female. The ova escape in the urine and on gaining fresh water develop into larvae which enter the intermediate host, a fresh-water snail. A free-swimming form, the cercaria, develops in the snail and when excreted into water penetrates the intact skin of man, the definitive host. In man the cercaria migrate via the pulmonary and portal circulation to reach the bladder. Ova are deposited in the submucosa of the bladder but may also to a lesser extent be found in the muscular and subserous layers and in the ureters. The ova calcify and excrete a toxin producing necrosis of tissue, granulomatous tubercles and eventually extensive fibrosis. The granulomatous tubercles may take the form of pedunculated tumours, and bladder neck fibrosis may rarely occur.

Calcification is the most important single diagnostic finding in schistosomiasis. It is very commonly seen in the bladder, less frequently in the lower ureters, and in advanced disease it may involve the whole length of the ureters (Fig. 43.17). The appearance of the calcified bladder varies with its degree of distension. When full it produces a thin linear opacity outlining the bladder margin, but when empty it takes the form of crowded linear opacities or even a calcified plaque (Fig. 43.18A and B).

The earliest change in the bladder on urography is a swelling of its mucosa, producing a cobblestone pattern (Fig. 43.19). With more advanced disease papillomatous granulomata may form filling defects within its lumen (Fig. 43.20), but it should be remembered that carcinoma is a not uncommon complication.

Ureteral dilatation and tortuosity occur even in the absence of obstruction. In its earliest stage dilatation is confined to the lower third, which has an irregular margin, and tubercles may produce small round filling defects within its lumen. In more advanced cases the dilatation may involve the whole length of the ureter and the renal pelvis, but when the whole upper urinary tract is dilated, it is usually the result of obstruction or reflux.

Ureteral strictures are most frequently seen at the lower end of the ureter, in its intravesical or pelvic portion;

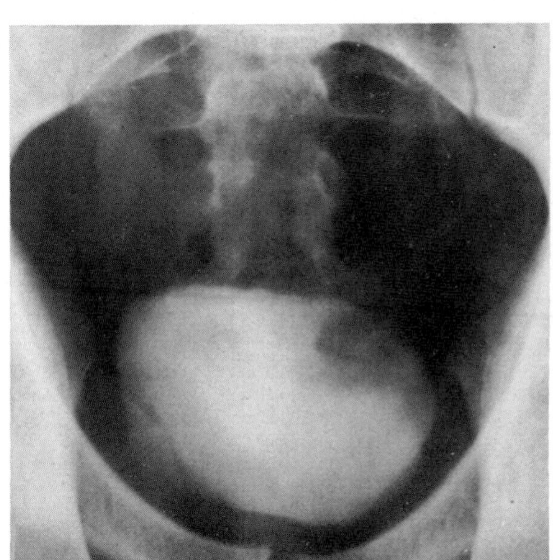

Fig. 43.19 Schistosomiasis. Granuloma at left ureteric orifice.

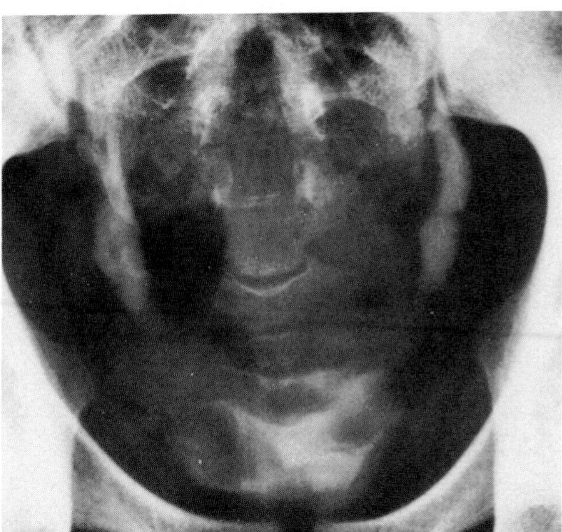

Fig. 43.20 Schistosomiasis. Numerous granulomata with dilatation of the lower ureters.

much less commonly they may occur at the level of the third and fourth lumbar vertebrae. Ureteral calculi are commonly present and are usually situated in a dilated ureter above a stricture.

The micturating cystogram is normal in the early stages and, as the ova are predominantly in the submucosa, even the heavily calcified bladder may have a normal capacity and contract normally. With advanced disease the bladder capacity may be greatly reduced and its wall thickened and irregular. In some cases extensive involvement leads to a large atonic bladder which fails to empty completely Reflux, due to inflammatory changes at the ureteric orifices, is a common occurrence, but it is not necessarily associated with ureteral dilatation.

Bladder neck obstruction due to fibrosis around the bladder neck and urethra is a rare manifestation.

HYDATID DISEASE

Renal hydatid disease usually starts in the cortex of the kidney. The cysts gradually enlarge and in a high proportion of cases they eventually rupture into a calyx.

When daughter cysts are not visible, the radiological appearances are indistinguishable from simple serous and haemorrhagic cysts. Calcification may or may not occur.

If the cyst wall calcifies, calcified daughter cysts may be visible within the parent cyst. Open cysts communicating with the calyces fill on intravenous and retrograde urography. Daughter cysts may then produce filling defects resembling a bunch of grapes within the parent cyst, an appearance which is diagnostic of hydatid disease. Occasionally the collecting system communicates with a space formed in the walls of the cyst and not with the cyst cavity. In these cases the presence of contrast medium in the cyst wall produces an ill-defined opacity around the cyst.

Severe anaphylactic reactions may occur from spillage of cyst contents following spontaneous or traumatic rupture of a cyst wall. Diagnostic needle biopsy must therefore be avoided when hydatid disease is suspected.

REFERENCES AND SUGGESTIONS FOR FURTHER READING

Clark, R. E., Minagi, H. & Palubinskas, A. J. (1971) Renal candidiasis. *Radiology*, **101**, 567–572.

Edwards, D., Normand, I. C. S., Prescod, N. & Smellie, J. M. (1977) Disappearance of vesicoureteric reflux during longterm prophylaxis of urinary tract infection. *British Medical Journal*, **ii**, 285–288.

Gingell, J. C., Roylance, J., Davies, E. R. & Pearcy, J. B. (1973) Xanthogranulomatous pyelonephritis. *British Journal of Radiology*, **46**, 99–109.

Hodson, C. J. & Edwards, D. (1960) Chronic pyelonephritis and visico-ureteric reflux. *Clinical Radiology*, **11**, 219–231.

Honey & Gelfan (1960) *The Urological Aspects of Bilharzia in Rhodesia*. Edinburgh & London: E. & S. Livingstone Ltd.

Hunt, V. C. & Mayo, C. W. (1932) Actinomycosis of the kidney. *Annals of Surgery*, **93**, 501–505.

Kirkland, K. (1966) Urological aspects of hydatid disease. *British Journal of Urology*, **38**, 241–254.

Ransley, P. G. & Risdon, R. A. (1974) Renal papillae and intrarenal reflux. *Lancet*, **ii**, 1114.

Rolleston, G. L., Maling, T. M. J. & Hodson, C. J. (1974) Intrarenal reflux and the scarred kidney. *Archives of Disease in Childhood*, **49**, 531–539.

Roylance, J., Penry, B., Davies, E. R. & Roberts, M. (1970) Radiology in the management of urinary tract tuberculosis. *British Journal of Urology*, **42**, 679–687.

CHAPTER 44

RENAL VASCULAR DISEASE: MISCELLANEOUS LESIONS

HYPERTENSION AND RENAL ARTERY STENOSIS

Hypertension is a very common disease from which patients tend to die prematurely. According to the Registrar General's report 11,000 people died of the disease in the United Kingdom in 1968. The most common cause of death in these patients is heart disease —coronary artery disease, congestive heart failure and left ventricular failure. The next most common cause of death is cerebrovascular disease—thrombosis, infarction or haemorrhage. Uraemia, usually the result of the malignant phase, caused by fibrinoid arteriolar necrosis or the progression of some primary renal disease is a less common cause of death.

Essential hypertension refers to the majority of patients with a high blood pressure reading who, after a complete evaluation, exhibit no evidence of a known cause. Secondary hypertension refers to a small proportion of patients in whom there is some discoverable cause for the elevated blood pressure (Table 44.1).

Table 44.1 Hypertension

1. Essential or primary hypertension
2. Secondary hypertension
    - Disease of the kidneys and urinary tract
        - Glomerulonephritis
        - Chronic pyelonephritis
        - Renal arterial disease
        - Polycystic kidneys
        - Renal stone and other obstructing lesions
        - Interstitial nephritis due to analgesics, gout, hypercalcaemia
        - Diabetes
        - Connective tissue disease, i.e. polyarteritis nodosa acuta, disseminated lupus, systemic sclerosis
        - Tumour
        - Radiation nephritis
        - Amyloid
        - Page kidney
    - Coarctation
    - Phaeochromocytoma
    - Cushings syndrome
    - Primary aldosteronism
    - Pre-eclamptic toxaemia of pregnancy
    - Post toxaemic hypertension
    - Miscellaneous conditions affecting the nervous system

The majority of patients with secondary hypertension are suffering from diseases of the kidneys, an adrenal tumour or coarctation; other conditions are much less common.

It is extremely difficult to assess the prevalence of renal hypertension amongst the hypertensive population, it is likely that its true incidence does not exceed 1 to 2 per cent of hypertensives. More than 30 per cent of hypertensive patients will be found to have renal artery stenosis on arteriography or on postmortem study but there is no relationship between the presence or degree of renal artery stenosis and the level of the diastolic blood pressure.

Intravenous urography is widely used as a screening procedure for the presence of renal vascular disease in hypertensives but the return from urographic screening of the hypertensive population is very low and it should be reserved for patients who fall into one or more of the following groups:

1. Hypertension in young people (under 40)—especially if there is no family history. Presence of a family history does not exclude a treatable cause.
2. Older patients with severe elevation of blood pressure (diastolic over 130 mmHg).
3. Rapidly advancing hypertension at any age.
4. Malignant phase of hypertension appearing in the elderly.
5. Clinical evidence of renal disease—
    - Loin pain, renal surgery or injury
    - Urinary infection
    - Previous renal disease e.g. proteinuria, polyuria, polydipsia
    - Bruit (not heard in 50 per cent patients with RAS).
6. Patients who do not respond to drug therapy.

Renal ischaemia may be produced by a number of conditions:

1. Aortic disease—artheroma, aneurysm, thrombosis, aortitis involving the renal artery ostia.
2. Renal arterial diseases. The commonest lesions are:
    - (a) Atheroma—this is the commonest lesion and usually involves the orifice or proximal third of the main artery; it may be bilateral.

(b) Fibromuscular hyperplasia—this usually affects the middle and distal third of the artery; it is more often seen in the younger age groups, and women are more commonly affected than men; it produces alternating areas of constriction and dilatation of the lumen.

Less common are:

(c) Thrombosis or embolism.
(d) Compression by tumour, retroperitoneal bands and fibrosis.
(e) Aneurysm.
(f) Angioma.
(g) Neurofibromatosis.

than or equal in size to its fellow on the opposite side. The majority of patients with bilateral renal artery stenosis also show asymmetry in renal size. When the stenosis affects the main renal artery there is a uniform reduction in size with uniform narrowing of the renal substance thickness. If a segmental artery is occluded or narrowed the reduction in renal substance thickness is confined to that segment. Multiple infarcts of small renal arterial branches produce scarring of the renal outline similar to that produced by chronic pyelonephritis but in ischaemia there is no associated calyceal deformity.

(b) *Delay in excretion.* A sudden complete occlusion of the renal artery leads to complete failure of excretion of

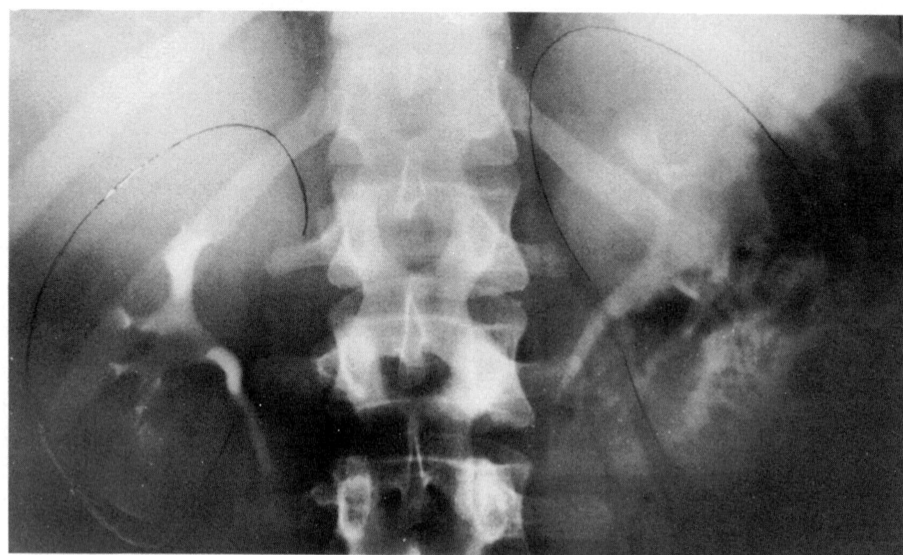

Fig. 44.1 Right renal artery stenosis with increased concentration and diminution in size of the kidney and its collecting system.

The urographic changes produced by significant stenosis of the renal artery are:

(a) Decrease in renal size.
(b) Delay in excretion.
(c) Increased concentration of contrast medium.
(d) Reduction in size of the collecting system.
(e) Ureteral notching.

(a) *A decrease in renal size* is the most reliable index of renal ischaemia, it may merely be due to reduction in the fluid volume of the kidney as a consequence of a reduced blood flow or may indicate the presence of ischaemic atrophy of the renal tissue. The long axis measurement of the normal kidney bears a close relationship to the patient's size and the kidneys are normally symmetrical. An asymmetry in the renal length of more than 10 to 15 mm is uncommon in the normal patient in the absence of morphological differences (page 874). It must be remembered that a duplicated ischaemic kidney may be larger

contrast; a small non-functioning kidney with a normal retrograde urogram being characteristic of a complete occlusion of acute onset. Renal arterial stenosis severe enough to produce elevation of the blood pressure is usually associated with a significant decrease in glomerular filtration rate and a consequent delay in the appearances of the nephrogram and in opacification of the calyces. This delayed excretion can be recognized by taking films 2, 4 and 6 minutes following the intravenous injection and before the application of compression.

(c) and (d) *Increased concentration of contrast medium and reduction in size of the collecting system.* Renal ischaemia results in an increased tubular reabsorption of sodium, chloride and water, this physiological change being the basis for differential tests of renal function in renal arterial disease. The concentration of the tubular fluid is increased, its volume is reduced resulting in an increased density of the calyces (Fig. 44.1). This is often a

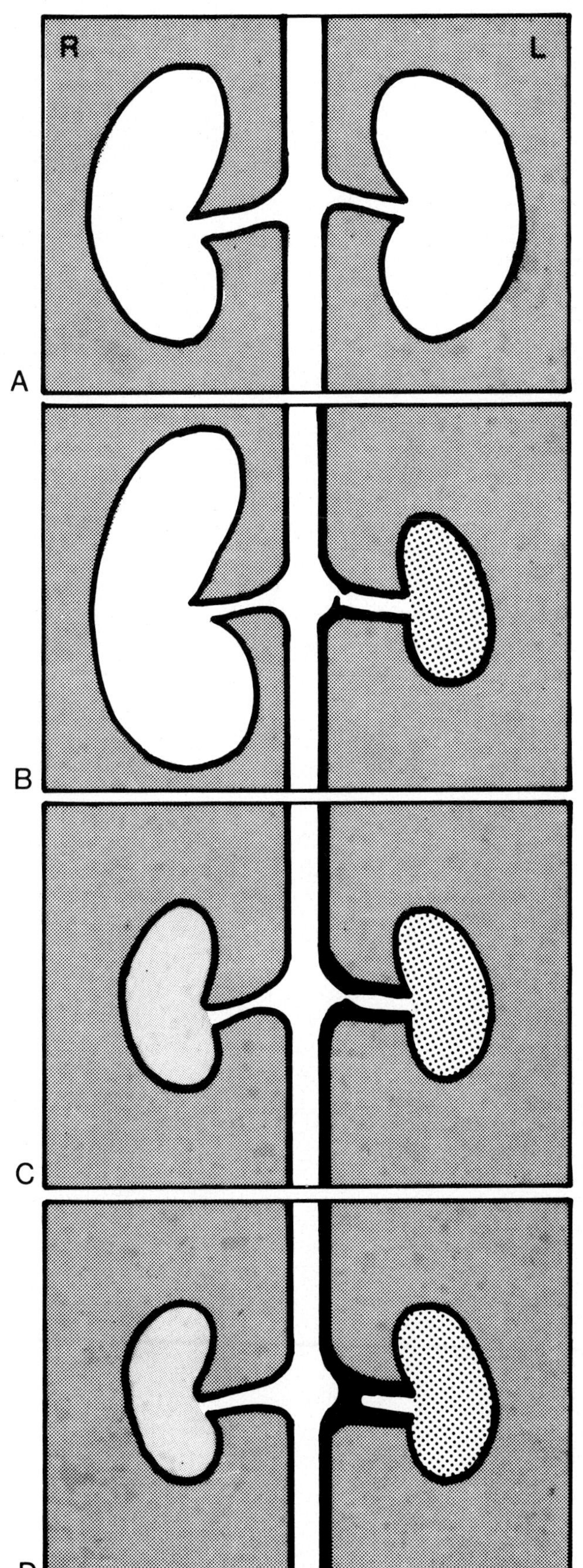

difficult sign to evaluate, the density being affected by the thickness and nature of overlying soft tissues.

It is also important to distinguish between concentration and density, a large collecting system being deeper will appear denser than a small system with equal concentration. In ischaemia the quantity of urine produced is reduced and this together with atrophy leads to a small dense collecting system. The disparity in concentration between the two sides may be augmented by inducing diuresis with simple hydration or with intravenous urea—the so called 'urea washout'. When severe structural changes occur in the kidney in response to ischaemia the concentration of the contrast medium will be impaired.

(e) *Ureteral notching*. Ureteral indentation may be produced by the development of a collateral circulation through the ureteral arteries from the lumbar branches of the aorta. They are usually seen in the upper ureter and are similar to those seen with venous occlusion. Similar vascular impressions may be produced by angiomatous malformations of the renal artery.

Effective medical treatment is now available for hypertension of renal vascular origin and surgical treatment is only indicated in a relatively small group of patients.

Acute complete occlusion of the renal artery produces an immediate decrease in renal size. The radiological appearances are those of a small non-functioning kidney with, on retrograde urography, a normal collecting system.

Renal angiography is not free from morbidity and should be reserved for patients with renovascular hypertension who are being considered for surgical treatment. The patient with a normal urogram has a less than 2 per cent chance of having surgically correctable renal vascular disease but angiography is probably indicated in hypertensive patients under the age of 30 even if the intravenous urogram is normal. Over the age of 40 angiography should be reserved for those patients who have rapidly accelerating hypertension or in whom medical control has been unsuccessful. When unilateral renal arterial stenosis causes hypertension the opposite healthy kidney is exposed to the effects of hypertension whilst the ipsilateral kidney is to a varying extent protected by the arterial stenosis (Fig. 44.2). It follows that some patients with renal failure and hypertension might be found in whom advanced hypertensive nephrosclerosis is confined to one kidney. Poor function or non-function of the other kidney being due to thrombosis of the renal artery consequent to stenosis. The kidney with the occluded artery may remain viable because of a collateral circulation and may

Fig. 44.2 Hypertension and renal failure: (A) normal kidneys with normal renal function; (B) left renal artery stenosis, hypertrophy of the right kidney, normal renal function; (C) secondary arterial disease in the right kidney, renal failure; (D) left renal artery thrombosis, rapidly accelerating renal failure.

have life-sustaining function following arterial reconstruction. Deterioration of renal function, an indication of bilateral disease, is thus not a contra-indication and indeed a rapid deterioration of renal function is a good indication for renal angiography.

ANEURYSM OF THE ABDOMINAL AORTA

The renal arterial orifices may be narrowed or occluded when involved in an aortic aneurysm. Renal ischaemia may also occur when the renal artery itself is compressed by an aneurysmal mass. An aneurysm or retroperitoneal haematoma may displace the kidneys and ureters laterally. Rarely the ureters may be involved in a fibrous retroperitoneal reaction around the aneurysm with consequent unilateral or bilateral medial ureteric deviation and obstruction—appearances similar to those seen in periureteric fibrosis.

SMALL ARTERY DISEASE

The kidneys are most commonly affected by arteriosclerosis secondary to essential hypertension, less commonly the kidneys may be involved in polyarteritis, systemic lupus, Wegner's granuloma and other systemic diseases.

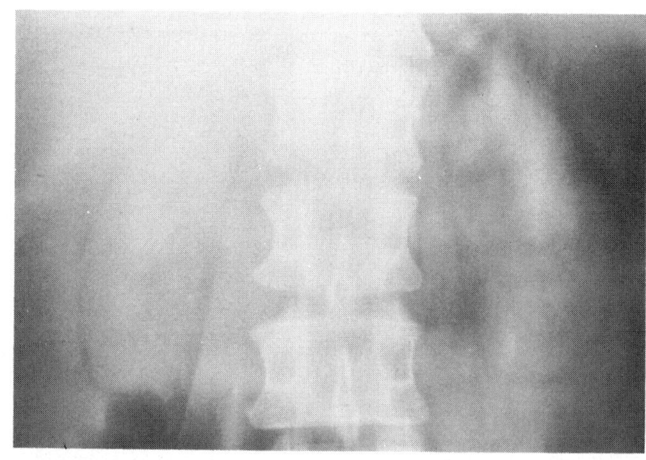

Fig. 44.3 Chronic glomerulonephritis.

In all these conditions there is bilateral reduction in renal size usually without a significant asymmetry in the long axis lengths of the kidneys. The renal outlines are usually smooth but minor irregularities may be produced by peripheral infarcts. In arteriosclerotic disease calcification may be visible in the renal arteries and their branches. Atrophy of renal tissue may be accompanied by an accumulation of fat in the renal sinus and perirenal space (renal fibrolipomatosis—page 895). Renal function may be grossly impaired and the reduction in the glomerular

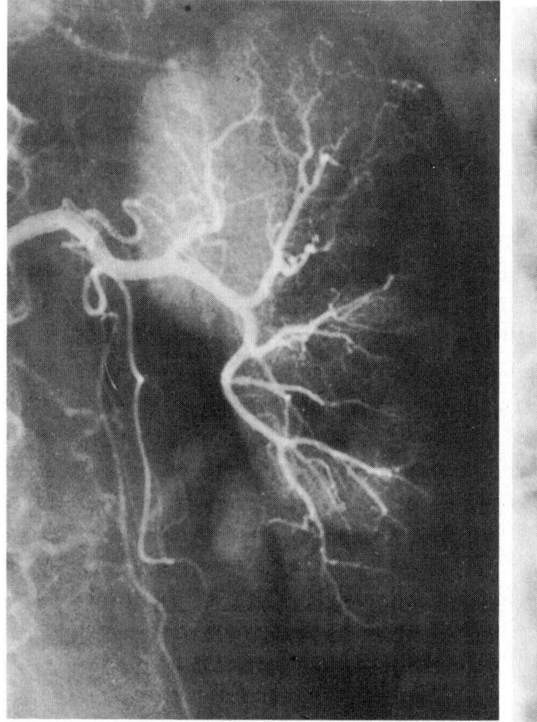

A

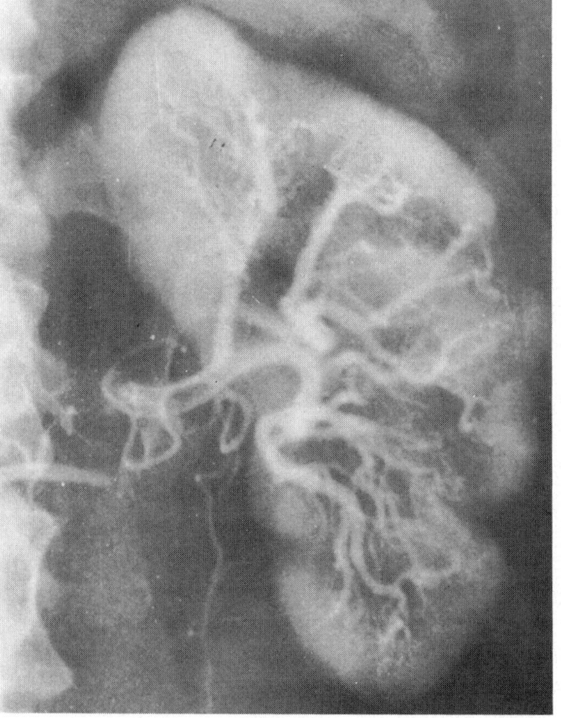

B

Fig. 44.4 (A) Selective renal angiogram. Polyarteritis with microaneurysms. (B) Arteriosclerosis with coarse 'oak tree' arterial pattern and peripheral infarcts.

filtration rate leads to delay in appearance and persistence of a faint nephrogram. The thickness of the renal substance is reduced, the normal collecting systems are usually poorly opacified. The appearances are very similar to those seen in chronic glomerular nephritis (Fig. 44.3). Angiography, which is rarely indicated, demonstrates a coarse irregular branching of the renal arterioles, and, in polyarteritis, multiple small renal arterial aneurysms (Fig. 44.4A). Wedge-shaped defects in the nephogram may be produced by renal infarcts (Fig. 44.4B).

Multiple small renal infarcts are not uncommonly seen as a result of embolism of the small arterioles in patients

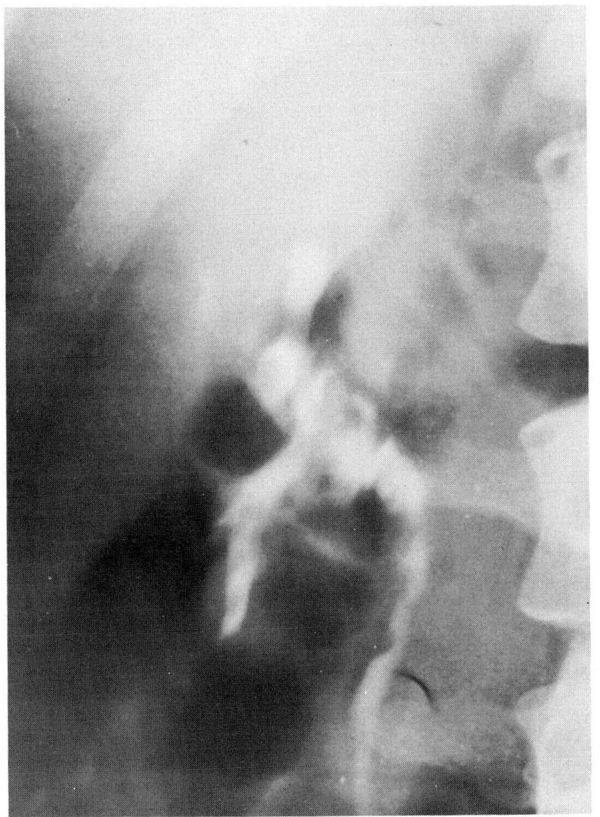

Fig. 44.5 Angiomatous malformation producing vascular impressions on the renal pelvis and upper ureter.

with mitral valve disease, auricular fibrillation, and also in myocardial infarction. The angiographic appearances of these cases must be distinguished from those produced by the partial selective angiogram as a result of non-opacification of the ventral or dorsal branches of the renal artery.

Radiation nephritis. Radiation nephritis occurs when one or both kidneys are subjected to high doses of therapeutic radiation. The basic lesion is ischaemia produced by radiation induced small artery disease confined to those portions of the kidney included within the field of irradiation. When both kidneys are affected the clinical picture is similar to that of chronic glomerulonephritis with uraemia, proteinuria, urinary casts and hypertension. Renal failure does not occur if only one kidney or part of the kidney is irradiated.

The radiological appearances are those of renal ischaemia—reduction in renal size with a smooth renal outline and a normal collecting system. In unilateral disease the contralateral kidney is hypertrophied. When only a portion of the kidney is subjected to irradiation the shrinkage of renal tissue is confined to the irradiated area.

Aneurysms and angiomatous malformations of the renal arteries are uncommon. They are usually congenital in origin but aneurysms are also seen distal to a stenosis in atheroma and fibromuscular hyperplasia. Microaneurysms are a characteristic feature of polyarteritis. An aneurysm of a renal arterial branch may produce an extrinsic filling defect in the renal pelvis which may closely simulate a renal tumour particularly when there is curvilinear calcification in its walls. Angiomatous malformations produce multiple small filling defects in the renal pelvis similar to those produced by a collateral arterial or venous circulation (Fig. 44.5).

Arteriovenous communications are seen in congenital cirsoid aneurysm but also occur in an alarmingly high proportion of patients subjected to renal biopsy. The majority of the postbiopsy fistulae appear to heal spontaneously.

RENAL MEDULLARY NECROSIS

Acute renal medullary necrosis produced by ischaemic infarction of the renal pyramids was, until recent years, only recognized as a terminal event in diabetics and in the obstructive uropathies. In the last few years acute medullary necrosis has also been recognized in infancy as a complication of severe illness producing dehydration, shock or anoxia (gastro-enteritis, asphyxia, congenital heart disease, etc.) and also as a complication of obstructive uropathy. In infancy, there is a short oliguric phase followed by polyuria with excessive sodium loss and mild elevation of the blood urea.

In the acute stage the characteristic radiological appearances are those of renal enlargement with an increasingly dense and persistent nephrogram. In oliguric patients there is little or no calyceal opacification but when polyuria occurs the calyceal pattern is seen to be normal. It seems likely that these radiological appearances are due to the fact that glomerular filtration continues but the contrast-laden tubular filtrate leaks through the damaged tubular walls into the interstitial tissue thus producing a rapid increase in the kidney density. A similar appearance is seen in acute tubular necrosis. In surviving patients follow-up urography has demonstrated the typical changes seen in the chronic form of the disease.

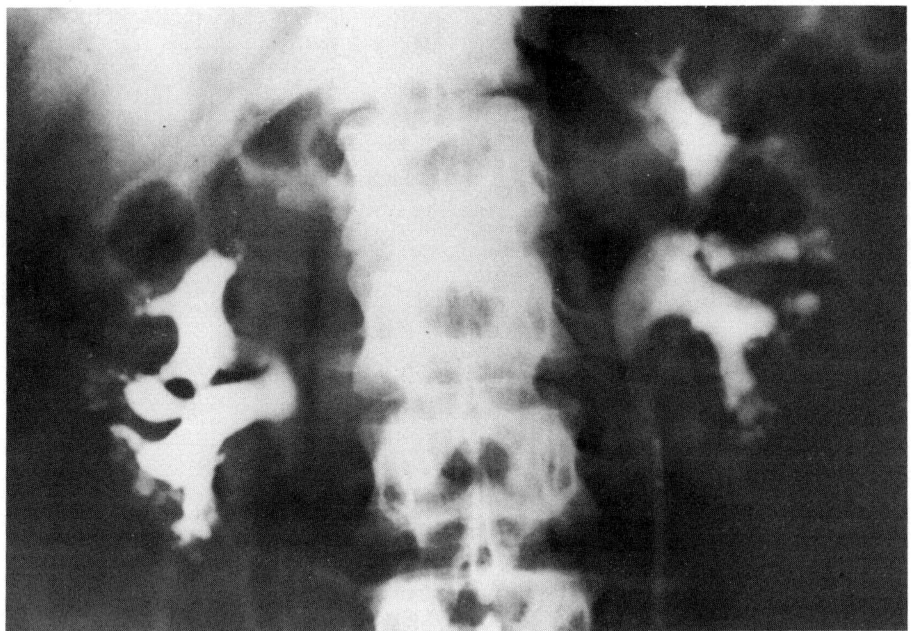

Fig. 44.6 Central form of renal papillary necrosis.

Chronic medullary necrosis. The chronic form of the disease is also the result of ischaemic necrosis of the pyramids. The blood supply to the renal pyramid is particularly vulnerable to diabetic arterial disease, infection and back pressure. The blood supply may also be impaired by arteriosclerosis, polyarteritis and thrombosis or embolism of renal arterial branches. The recent increase in the incidence of renal medullary or papillary necrosis appears to be associated with a high intake of analgesics containing phenacetin, codeine and aspirin. The duration of analgesic abuse, often understated by the patient, is usually greater than 8 years but the mode of action of these

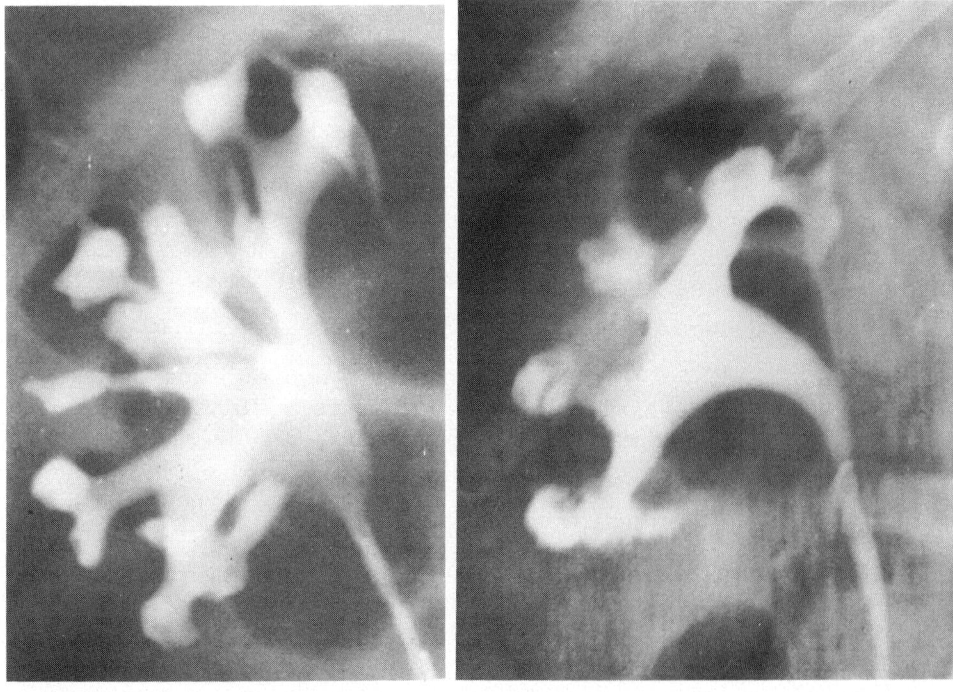

Fig. 44.7 (A) 'Horn' shadows in renal medullary necrosis. (B) Renal papillary necrosis with cavitation, ring shadows around separated papillae and horn-shaped protrusions in the lower pole.

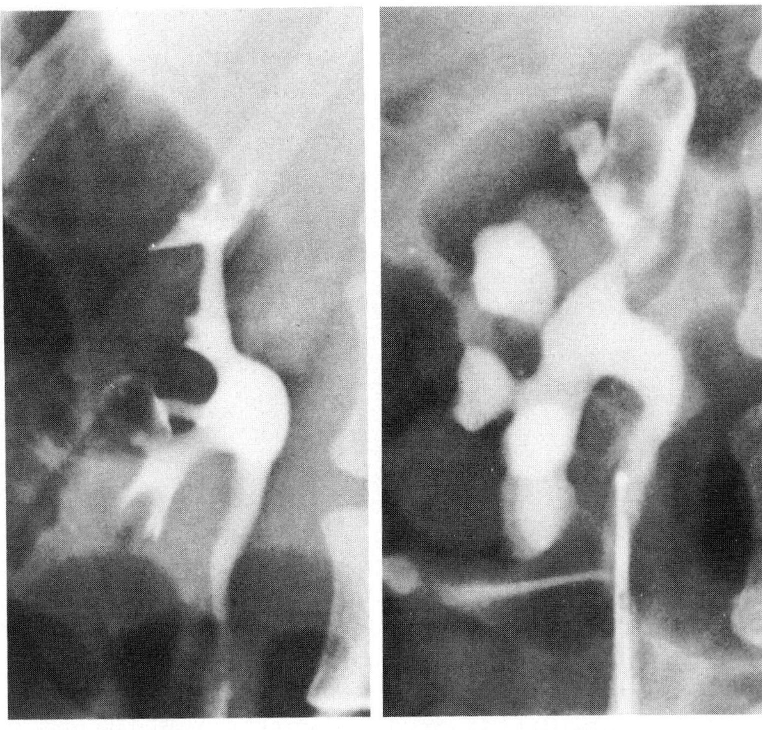

Fig. 44.8 *Fig. 44.9*

Fig. 44.8 'Sling' shadow around a necrotic papilla in the middle segment.

Fig. 44.9 Renal papillary necrosis with sequestration of a renal papilla.

drugs on the renal papilla is not understood. The condition has also been observed in patients with sickle-cell trait (SA) as well as in sickle-cell disease (SS).

The necrosis of the pyramid never extends to the cortex, it is often confined to the papilla and is sometimes centrally located in the papilla. The disease commonly affects more than one papilla, it is usually bilateral and necrosis of a papilla may be followed by sequestration of the papilla which may subsequently be passed in the urine. The resultant cavity may heal by epithelialization and it is possible that the diffuse pyramidal loss seen in long-standing obstructive uropathies is the result of healed papillary necrosis.

The sub-acute and chronic forms of the disease pursue a course varying from a few months to many years. Clinically the disease presents with urinary tract infection, renal pain and haematuria. Colic may occur with passage of pyramidal remnants in the urine and progression of the disease leads to renal failure with death from hypertension or uraemia.

The kidney size is reduced; this reduction in renal size may develop rapidly and become recognizable by serial examination over a period of a few months. The coarse focal scarring of chronic pyelonephritis is not commonly seen but hypertrophy of unaffected renal parenchyma may produce an irregular renal outline. Urography does not demonstrate any abnormality in the calyceal pattern until separation of the papilla occurs. In the central form small cavities may appear in the substance of the pyramid and calculi may form within them (Fig. 44.6). In the more common variety where the pyramidal tip is affected the earliest change is a loss of definition of the calyceal outline, very similar to the early lesion in tuberculous disease; this may be followed by characteristic irregular horn-shape projections into the renal medulla (Fig. 44.7A and B). With complete separation contrast medium may pass between the affected papilla and the base of the pyramid thus forming a 'ring' or 'sling' of contrast around the radiolucent papilla (Fig. 44.8). Complete separation of the papilla produces cavitation—at first with ill-defined outlines but later, if healing occurs, a well-defined, smooth-walled cavity may be present. The sequestrated papilla may then be seen as a filling defect in the calyx or renal pelvis (Fig. 44.9).

Loss of renal papillae, the end result of medullary necrosis, produces clubbed calyces with smooth rounded extremities an appearance which when it affects the whole kidney is indistinguishable from post-obstructive atrophy. Occasionally the necrotic papillae remain in position (*necrosis in situ*) and may subsequently calcify and even ossify (Fig. 44.10). Urography in these cases demonstrates small kidneys, the papillae are preserved

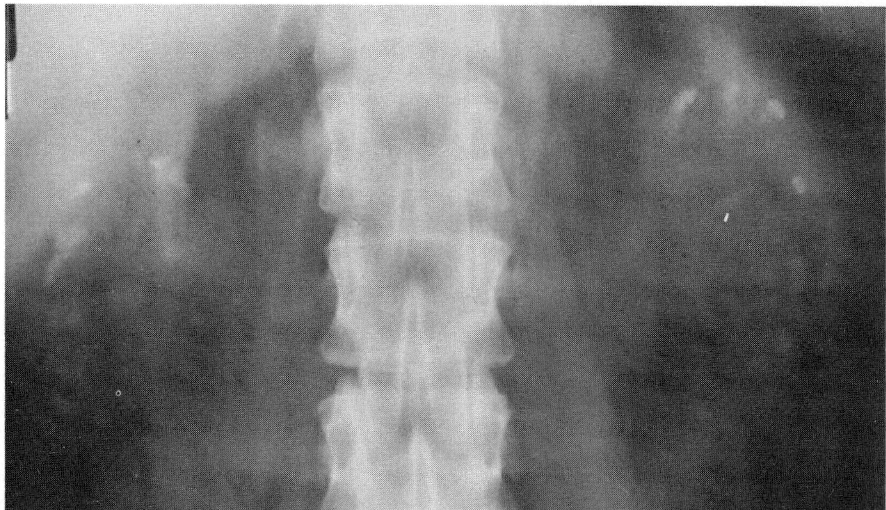

Fig. 44.10 Renal medullary necrosis *in situ*.

and may appear to be disproportionately large relative to the kidney size (Fig. 44.11).

Calcification may occur around the margins of the necrotic papilla producing a very characteristic appearance, the papilla forming a radiolucent centre to a stone, either attached to the pyramidal base or lying free in the renal pelvis (Fig. 44.12). Escape of the papilla into the ureter produces an appearance very similar to that produced by other varieties of ureteric calculi (Fig. 44.13).

Differential diagnosis. *Chronic pyelonephritis* is likely to cause most difficulty. In both diseases the kidney is reduced in size; scarring of the renal outline is not a feature of medullary necrosis unless there is superadded infection but an irregular outline may occur as a result of localized areas of hypertrophy. Calyceal deformity is common to both but papillary sequestration and calcification does not occur in chronic pyelonephritis. Horn-like protrusions into the pyramid are characteristic of medullary necrosis.

Renal tuberculosis may also produce changes similar to medullary necrosis. The early erosion of the papilla may be identical in both diseases and it may not be possible to distinguish between them on radiological evidence alone. Cavitation in tuberculous disease is not confined to the pyramid and strictures do not occur in medullary necrosis. Calcification in medullary necrosis produces a characteristic appearance quite distinct from that seen in tuberculous disease.

The medullary cysts in the *sponge kidney* bear some resemblance to the central type of medullary necrosis but they are usually much more numerous, smaller and lie within pyramids which are normal or increased in size.

Calyceal cysts or diverticula occur in otherwise normal kidneys, the cavities usually lie between the papilla and

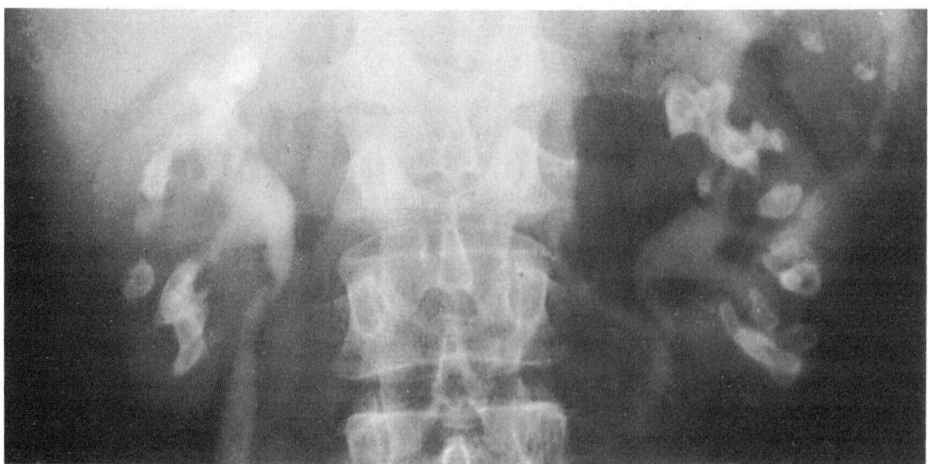

Fig. 44.11 Medullary necrosis *in situ* with bilateral reduction in renal size.

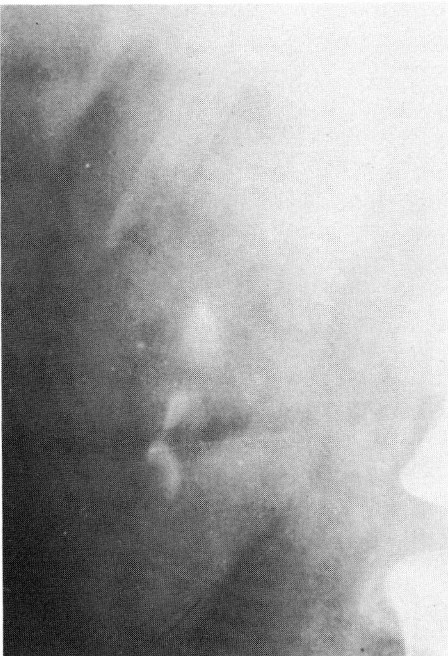

Fig. 44.12 Calcification in necrotic papillae.

communicate by a narrow channel with the infundibulum of the minor calyx (Fig. 44.14).

Other varieties of *renal* or *ureteric stones* can be distinguished by the absence of a central radiolucent papilla and absence of papillary destruction.

The acute form of the disease with symmetrical enlargement of the kidneys and impaired excretion of contrast medium produces appearances similar to those which may be seen in *acute pyelonephritis*, *acute tubular necrosis* and the *acute nephritides*. *Renal vein occlusion*, *amyloid disease*, *lymphoma* and *myeloma* may also produce similar appearances.

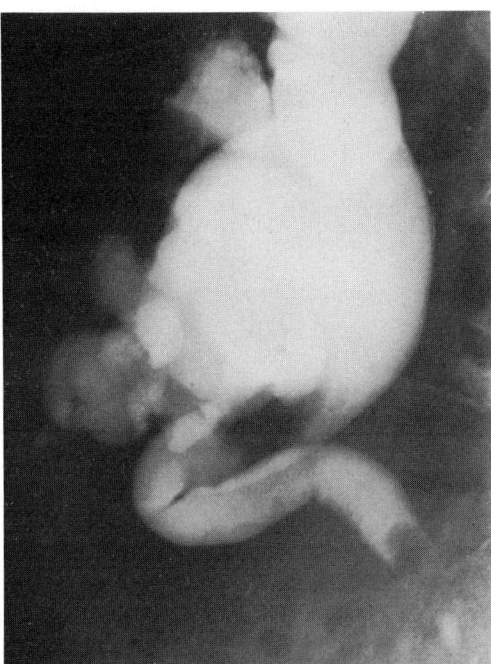

Fig. 44.13 Detached partially calcified papilla producing ureteric obstruction.

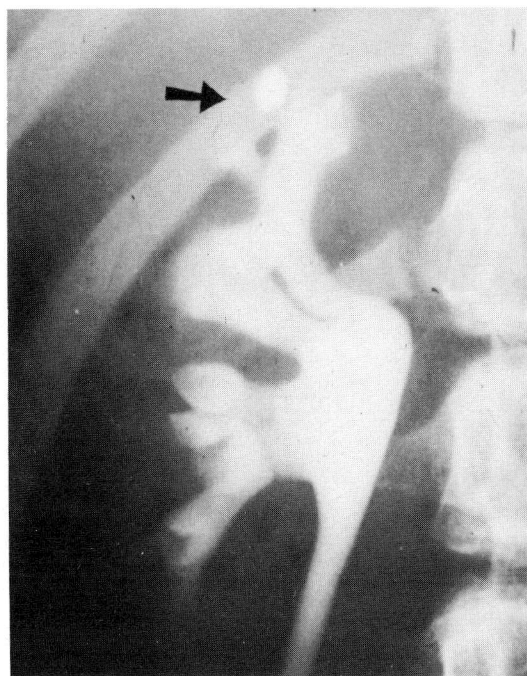

Fig. 44.14 Calyceal cyst.

When *renal failure* occurs in the chronic form with *necrosis in situ* the kidneys are symmetrically reduced in size and in the absence of calcification, the appearances are indistinguishable from *chronic nephritis* and *bilateral renal ischaemia*.

The intraluminal filling defects produced by *urothelial tumours* may mimic sequestrated papillae and it should be noted that an increased incidence of these tumours has been described in association with a high analgesic intake.

RENAL VEIN THROMBOSIS

Renal vein thrombosis is most commonly seen in infants as a complication of some other illness producing severe dehydration. The primary disease is rare in adults, it may occasionally be a result of trauma but in adults renal vein thrombosis is usually secondary to invasion of the vein by renal tumour or retroperitoneal malignant disease. It may also occur when renal blood flow is reduced as a consequence of renal disease, e.g. glomerulonephritis, amyloid disease and pyelonephritis. Thrombosis of the renal vein is occasionally the result of ascending thrombophlebitis from the pelvic or leg veins. The nephrotic syndrome has been associated with both unilateral and bilateral renal vein occlusion but patients with nephrotic syndrome have a thrombotic tendency and the evidence now suggests that renal vein thrombosis is an effect rather than a cause of the nephrotic syndrome.

Acute complete occlusion presents with severe loin pain, fever, leucocytosis, haematuria and usually but not invariably proteinuria. Thrombo-embolic complications, particularly pulmonary emboli are common. The kidney is congested, cyanosed and haemorrhagic infarction may be followed by renal rupture. When occlusion occurs more gradually congestion is less marked and symptoms and signs may be absent.

vasation of contrast medium into the interstitial tissue of the kidney. Alternatively it may be due to tubular obstruction as a result of oedema or may be a consequence of diminished arterial perfusion with resulting increased tubular reabsorption of water.

The presence of venous collaterals along the ureter produces notching of the ureteral lumen similar to that produced by arterial collaterals in renal arterial occlusion. Renal angiography gives more information than venography and is free from the possible hazard of pulmonary embolism following dislodgment of a thrombus. The

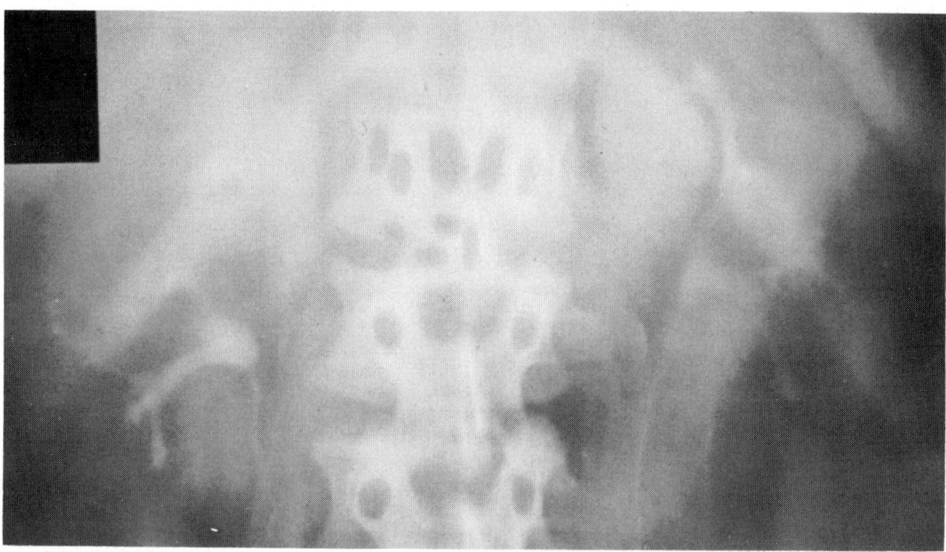

Fig. 44.15 Nephrotic syndrome with bilateral renal venous thrombosis.

In acute complete occlusion intravenous urography demonstrates a large non-functioning kidney and the retrograde examination reveals elongation of the major calyces with swelling of the renal substance. Angiography during this stage shows stretching and separation of the renal arterial branches with a diminished arterial flow rate and a poor, persistent nephrogram. There is no opacification of the renal vein. In the later stages the kidney becomes small and atrophic.

When occlusion occurs gradually a collateral circulation develops via the subcapsular veins to the adrenal, lumbar, ureteral and gonadal veins. Renal function is not impaired, proteinuria may be present but there may be no clinical signs or symptoms. In these cases the intravenous urogram demonstrates a large kidney with a poor, persistent nephrogram, a thick renal substance and elongation and splaying of the calyces (Fig. 44.15). An appearance which is similar to that seen when the kidney is infiltrated by abnormal tissue, e.g. amyloid, lymphoma.

A dense nephrogram developing over many hours without opacification of the calyces has also been reported in these cases. The mechanism producing this appearance is uncertain; it may be due to tubular damage with extra-

angiogram will confirm the presence of venous collaterals, the renal vein does not opacify and it may reveal the presence of primary disease in the kidney. If renal venography is considered to be necessary thrombosis of the inferior vena cava must be excluded before proceeding to selective renal vein catheterization.

It has recently been demonstrated that the non-invasive technique of CAT can diagnose a renal vein thrombosis.

RENAL TRAUMA

Injuries to the kidney usually follow blows or falls upon the loin. Penetrating wounds, renal biopsy, crushing accidents and falls upon the buttocks or feet may also produce renal rupture. Kidneys with pre-existing disease show an increased susceptibility to injury and rupture of a large hydronephrosis may occur as a result of a trivial injury. The ureter may be involved in penetrating wounds but ureteral injury most commonly occurs as a result of pelvic surgery or retrograde catheterization. Being well protected the ureter is rarely affected by blunt trauma but ureteral rupture is said to occur with extreme hyperextension of the lumbar spine.

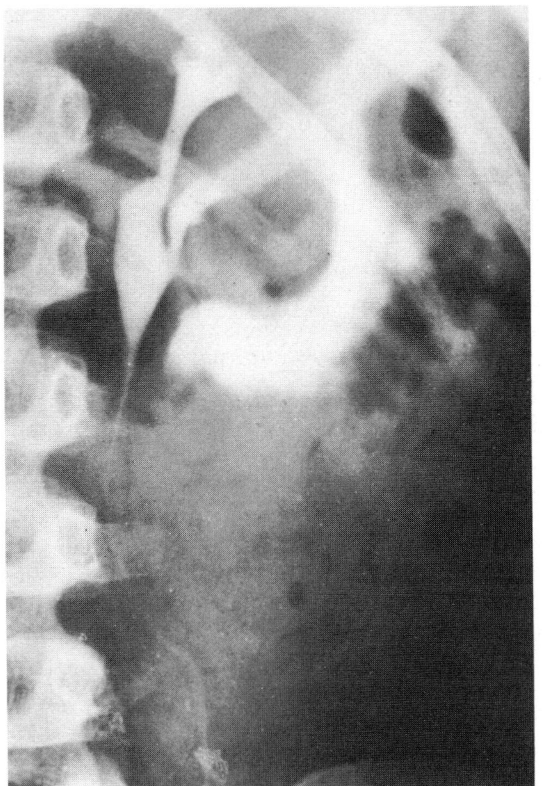

Fig. 44.16 Rupture of kidney with intra- and extrarenal extravasation. The perirenal haematoma produces medial displacement of the upper ureter.

Patients usually present with loin pain, haematuria and variable degrees of shock. Treatment is usually conservative but surgical treatment may be indicated in the presence of signs of continuing haemorrhage and irreversible shock. The chief value of radiology is the demonstration of a healthy functioning kidney on the uninjured side.

Plain films of the abdomen are frequently of poor quality due to the presence of meteorism, the distended coils of intestine obscuring the retroperitoneal structures. Fractures of the lower ribs and the transverse processes of the lumbar vertebrae are frequently seen and contraction of the psoas muscle may produce a scoliosis concave to the side of the lesion. The diaphragm on the affected side may be elevated and there may be a secondary pleural effusion.

Most information is obtained by high dose urography with tomography during the nephrogram phase, ureteric compression is to be avoided during the acute stage. An intrarenal haematoma produces a localized defect in the nephrogram with calyceal displacement. Subcapsular haematoma produces enlargement of the renal outline, compression of the renal parenchyma and displacement of the renal capsule which may be visible on nephrotomography as a fine line displaced away from the compressed nephrogram. Laceration of the renal capsule produces a perinephric haematoma with a soft tissue mass, loss of the renal outline and obliteration of the normal fascial planes. Compression of the renal pelvis may result in a hydronephrosis. When the laceration also involves the collecting system extravasation of contrast medium into the renal substance or the perirenal tissues occurs (Fig. 44.16), this is usually transient but may persist particularly in penetrating wounds with the formation of a *urinoma* which may require surgical drainage. Retrograde urography is rarely indicated but may be of value when there is no demonstrable excretion of contrast medium. This finding may be the result of obstruction by a blood clot, severe damage to the renal substance or it may result from injury to the vascular pedicle.

Computerized tomography is of particular value in the investigation of renal trauma. Subcapsular and perirenal haematomata are readily visualized (Fig. 44.17A and B)

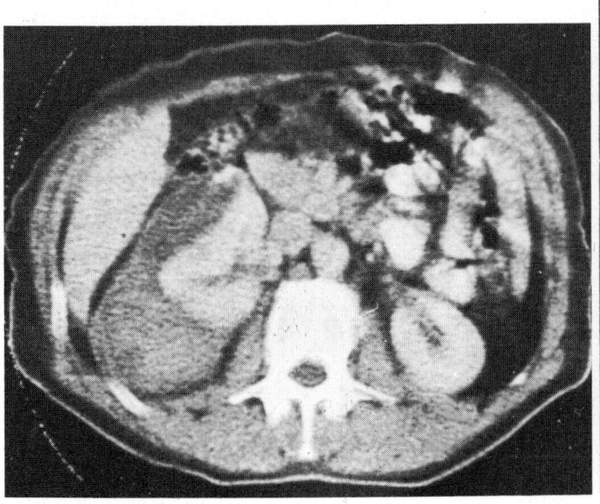

A

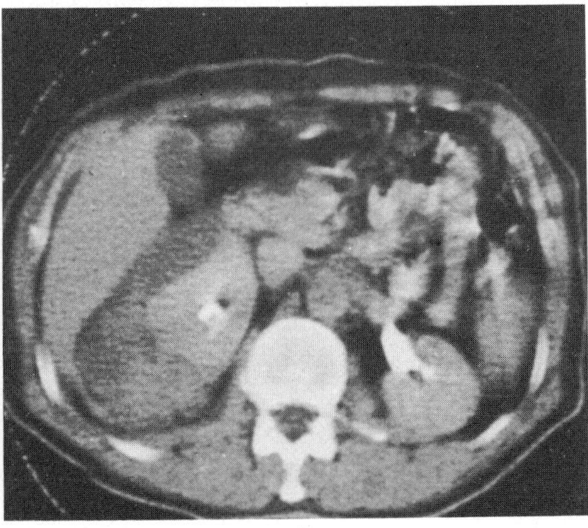

B

Fig. 44.17 C.T. scan: right perirenal haematoma. (A) Before contrast; (B) After I.V. contrast. L. + 58. W. 200.

and serial scans in these cases will demonstrate changing absorption coefficients indicating liquefaction and dissolution of the blood clot.

The information obtained by renal angiography gives a precise demonstration of the nature and extent of renal injury but it does not usually influence the clinical management of the patient and in the acute stage it is very rarely indicated. An intrarenal haematoma will cause displacement of the intrarenal branches with a defect in the nephrogram phase. A subcapsular haematoma will cause stretching of the capsular vessels around the haematoma and a rupture of the renal parenchyma will be visible as a break in the renal substance during the nephrogram phase. This nephrographic defect may be concealed if anterior posterior views are not supplemented when necessary by oblique views or tomography. Injury to the renal arterial supply may cause ischaemia of the whole kidney or a segment of the kidney and in these cases the main renal artery or one of its branches will be occluded or narrowed.

The great majority of patients recover completely, late complications are rare; arteriovenous fistulae usually occur as a result of penetrating wounds (including renal biopsy) and these usually disappear spontaneously. A transient increase in blood pressure may occur in the acute phase, persistent hypertension may rarely occur as a result of renal artery stenosis or occlusion and also as a result of compression of the kidney by organization of a perirenal haematoma (*Page kidney*).

RETROPERITONEAL FIBROSIS

Retroperitoneal fibrosis is a disease of unknown aetiology with features resembling an auto-immune reaction in which there is a proliferation of fibrous tissue in the retroperitoneal space. Several cases have been reported following the use of methysergide and other ergot derivatives in the treatment of migraine. The histological appearances range from a subacute cellular tissue to mature fibrous tissue. In the majority of cases there is a diffuse fibrosis usually starting at the brim of the pelvis and spreading upwards to the kidneys. The fibrosis may extend downwards into the pelvis and upwards through the crura of the diaphragm to involve the mediastinum. A localized form, in which a plaque of fibrous tissue surrounds the ureter, is much rarer. The process may involve any structure in the retroperitoneal space, particularly the inferior vena cava and the iliac veins. Involvement of the aorta, renal and iliac arteries, the common bile duct, the gut and the mediastinum (including the coronary arteries) has been reported.

Patients usually present with a long history of ab-

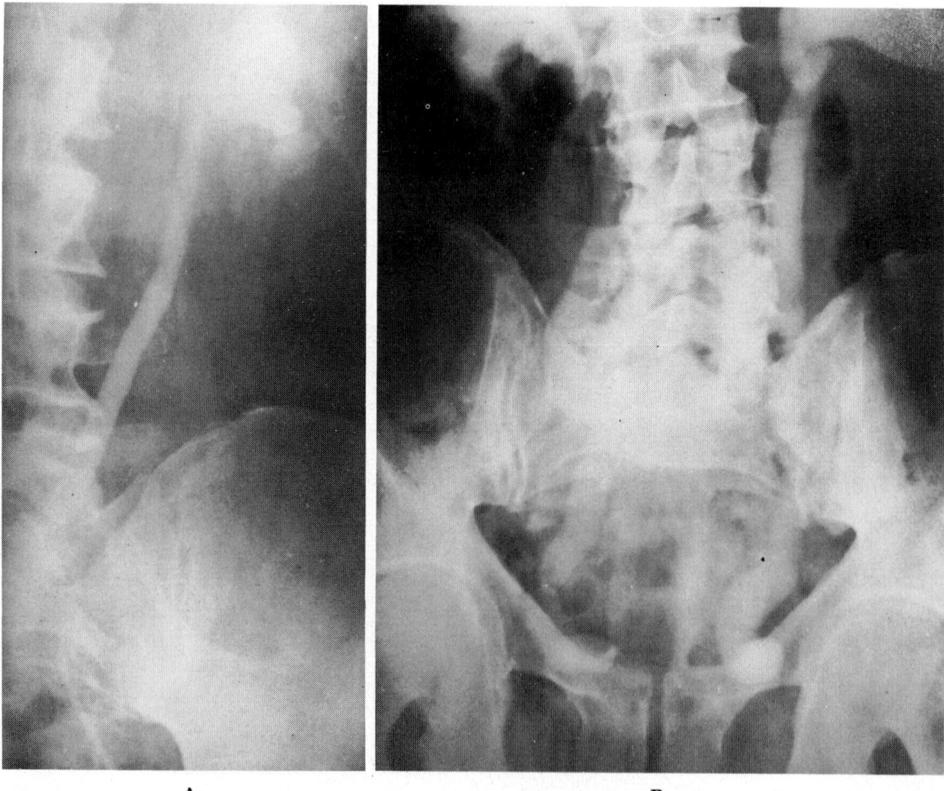

Fig. 44.18 (A) Retrograde urogram. Retroperitoneal fibrosis producing medial deviation and obstruction of the ureter at the level of S1. (B) I.V.U. retroperitoneal fibrosis producing obstruction low in the pelvis.

dominal or renal pain and urinary infection. There may be evidence of an inflammatory process in the form of malaise and fever. Eventually progressive ureteral obstruction leads to uraemia.

Radiological examination demonstrates ureteral deviation and obstruction (Fig. 44.18A and B). The most frequent site of ureteral obstruction is usually in its middle third, but obstruction of the upper or lower third is nearly as common. There is a variable degree of distension of the upper tract above the obstruction which tapers smoothly down to the narrowed segment. Contracture of the fibrous tissue leads to medial displacement of the ureter. A characteristic feature of the disease is that a retrograde catheter can be passed easily through the obstructed segment. Both ureters are usually involved, but the disease may be more advanced on one side than the other.

Venography may demonstrate obstruction or distortion of the inferior vena cava and iliac veins.

The ureteral distortion and obstruction is not pathognomic, the same appearances can be produced by retroperitoneal malignant growths and lymphomata. Involvement of the ureters in a chronic retroperitoneal inflammatory reaction as may occur in actinomycosis, Crohn's disease, diverticular disease and ischiorectal abscess may also result in ureteral obstruction and medial deviation. Abdominal aortic aneurysm usually produces lateral ureteral deviation but in a few cases medial deviation and obstruction may occur.

It must also be remembered that normal ureters may deviate medially at the level of the fourth and fifth lumbar vertebral. This medial displacement is particularly common in muscular subjects and in patients of West African origin.

CHRONIC GRANULOMATOUS DISEASE

This is a familial immunological disease of childhood in which polymorphonuclear leucocytes fail to kill off bacteria. Clinically it presents with protracted recurrent infection with a granulomatous tissue response involving many organs. The bladder may be contracted and deformed and involvement of the ureters in a retroperitoneal granulomatous reaction produces appearances similar to those seen in peri-ureteric fibrosis in the adult.

RENAL FIBROLIPOMATOSIS

A proliferation of fat within the renal sinus frequently occurs in response to atrophy of the renal substance and there may also be an increased deposition of fat around the renal capsule. Tomography, nephrotomography and computerized tomography demonstrates the radiolucent fat within the renal sinus extending along the calyces towards the periphery of the kidney. The major calyces are elongated and narrowed and the minor calyces may be impressed from the sinus side (Fig. 44.19). Its only clinical

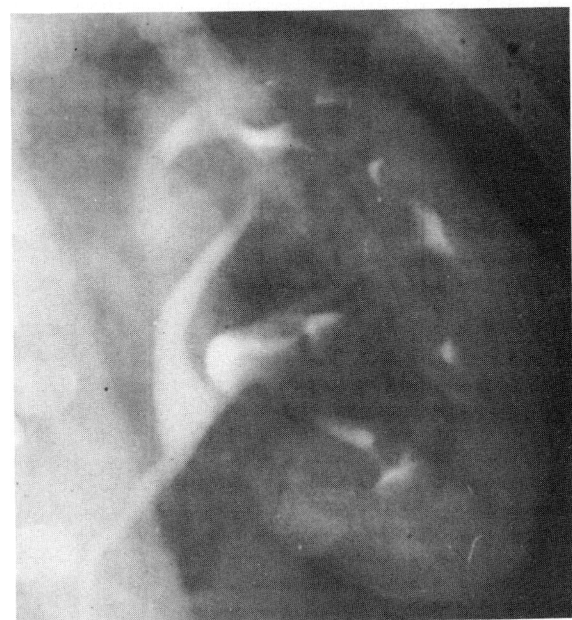

Fig. 44.19 Renal fibrolipomatosis.

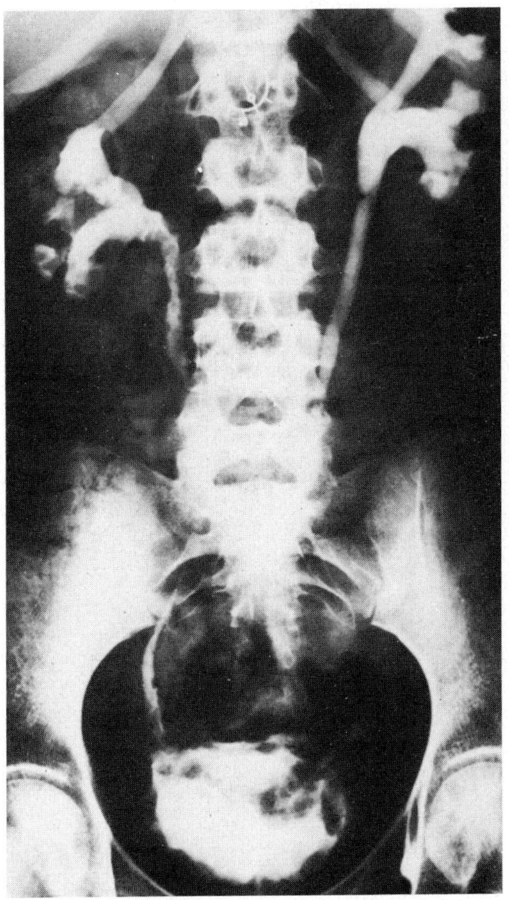

Fig. 44.20 I.V.U. pyelo-ureteritis cystica affecting the renal pelvis, ureter and bladder.

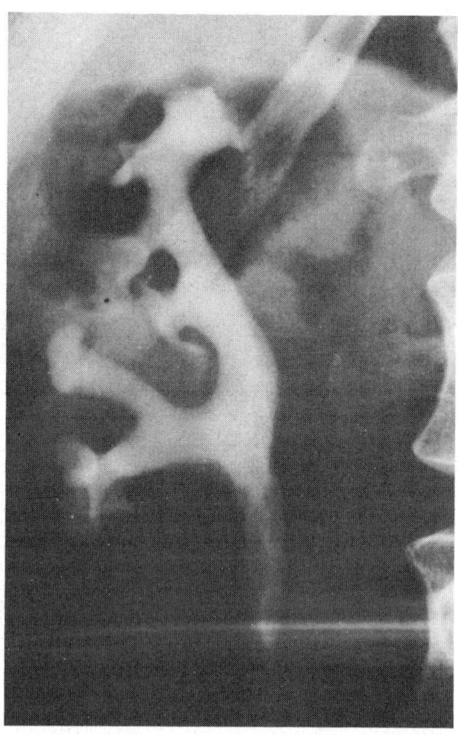

Fig. 44.21 Submucosal haemorrhage occuring during anticoagulant therapy.

significance is that the calyceal deformity is similar to that produced by a parapelvic cyst or tumour but the appearances on computerized tomography are characteristic.

PYELO-URETERITIS CYSTICA

This condition is characterized by the presence of small translucent greyish-pink cysts containing viscous fluid in the submucosa of the renal pelvis and ureter and occasionally in the bladder. Its aetiology is unknown, it is possible that it is the result of an inflammatory process and it is usually seen in patients with recurrent urinary infection.

The cysts produce multiple, small, round filling defects in the renal pelvis and ureter and, when seen in profile, scalloping of the pelvic and ureteral walls (Fig. 44.20).

The appearances are similar to those produced by air bubbles on retrograde urography, but air bubbles change position with changes of posture. The differential diagnosis also includes vascular impressions following renal arterial or venous occlusion or stenosis, epithelial tumour and intraluminal or submucosal haemorrhage. Both *intraluminal* and *submucosal haemorrhage* are a common complication of anticoagulant therapy (Fig. 44.21).

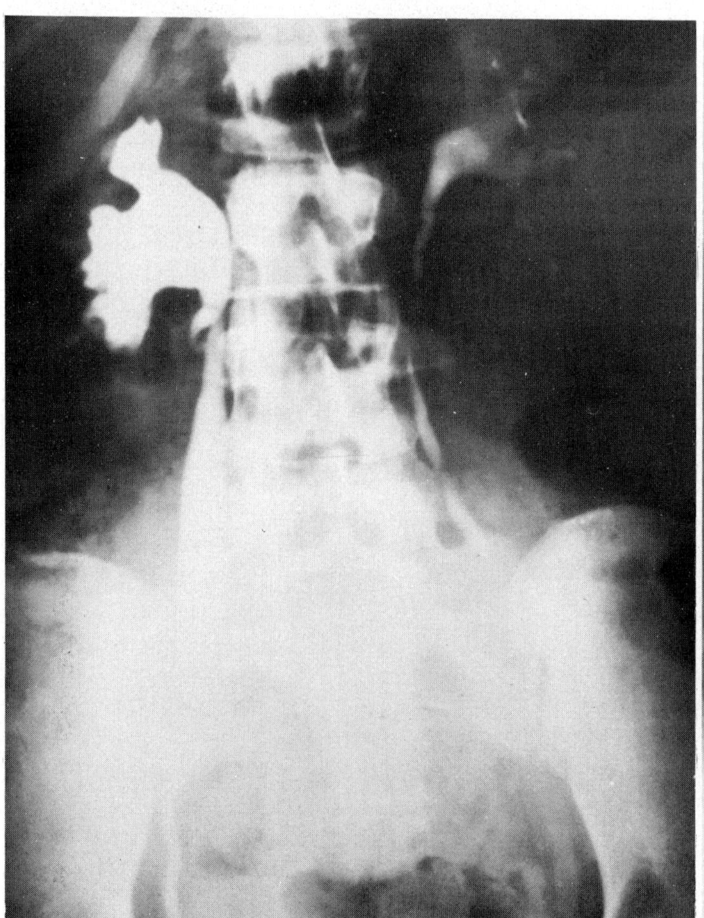

A

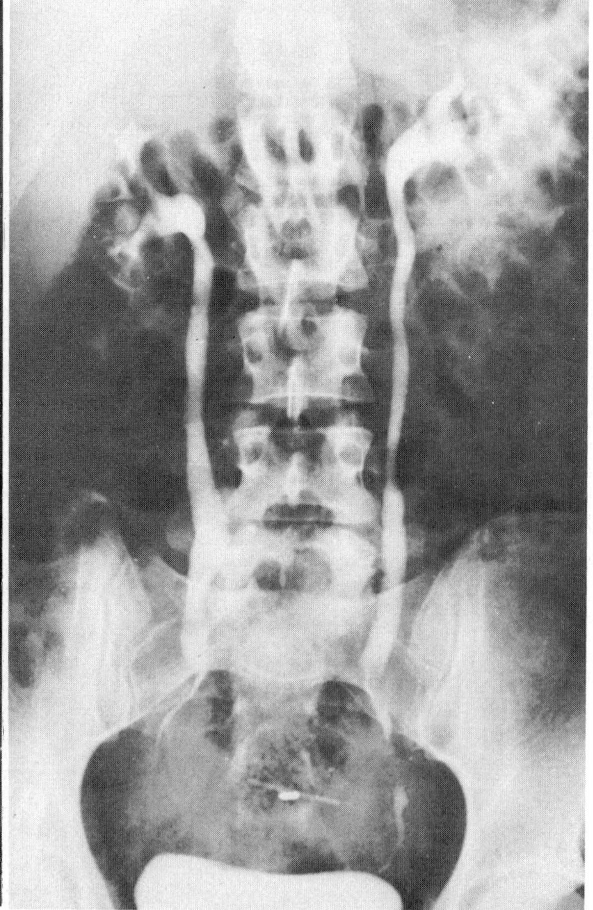

B

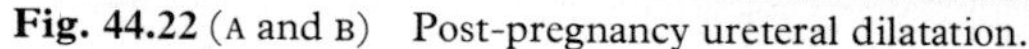

Fig. 44.22 (A and B) Post-pregnancy ureteral dilatation.

HYDRO-URETER OF PREGNANCY

Asymptomatic bacteriuria occurs quite commonly in early pregnancy and some 1 to 2 per cent of pregnant women develop symptomatic pyelonephritis which may be associated with vesico-ureteric reflux but radiographic examination of the urinary tract is contra-indicated during pregnancy unless there are very pressing clinical indications.

Dilatation of the renal pelves and ureters occurs to a greater or lesser extent during every pregnancy. These changes are usually transitory and a return to the normal state usually occurs within 14 weeks of delivery. Occasionally, particularly in multipara, the normal state may not be completely regained. The cause of these changes is not understood—hormonal factors, a changed muscle tone and obstruction by a gravid uterus are all possible mechanisms. The changes are usually bilateral but are often more marked on the right side and may be confined to this side (Fig. 44.22A and B). The calyceal outlines are blunted, the renal pelvis is dilated and the ureter dilated and tortuous. The ureteral dilatation rarely involves its lower pelvic portion.

The occurrence of these physiological changes makes accurate post-partum radiological evaluation extremely difficult and radiological investigation should whenever possible be postponed until 16 weeks after delivery.

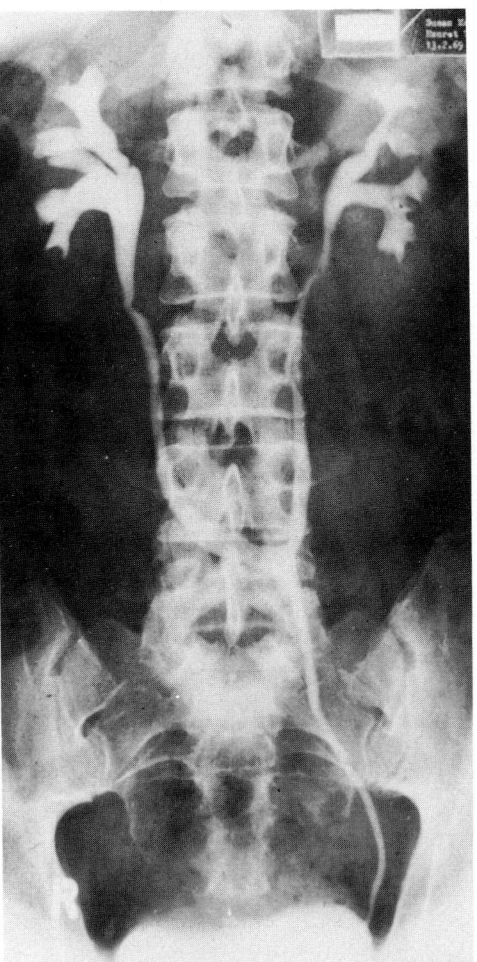

Fig. 44.23 Transuretero-ureterostomy.

URINARY DIVERSION

Nephrostomy is the most commonly used form of temporary urinary diversion. It may be performed percutaneously as an emergency procedure to preserve renal function until the patient's condition permits more definitive treatment (page 833).

The simplest form of urinary diversion at ureteral level is *cutaneous ureterostomy* but there are many technical difficulties in performing this operation and post-operative complications, particularly obstruction of the terminal portion of the ureter, are not uncommon. Retrograde injection of water-soluble contrast medium through the cutaneous stoma will demonstrate the site of obstruction and is indicated when impaired renal function prevents adequate demonstration by intravenous Urography.

Uretero-ureterostomy, the anastomosis of one ureter to the other, is usually indicated when a lower ureter is destroyed (Fig. 44.23). Post-operative urography may demonstrate dilatation of both upper tracts due to oedema at the anastomotic site, fibrosis at this site may lead to varying degrees of permanent dilatation of one or both upper ureters.

Uretero-ileal, uretero-colic anastomosis, the implantation of the ureters into the bowel may be used, when other methods fail, in the relief of incontinence, pain and distressing frequency. It may also be used in the treatment of malignant disease of the bladder and neurogenic lesions interfering with bladder emptying. The chief complications are electrolyte imbalance, infection from regurgitation of the gut contents into the ureters, ureteral obstruction at the site of anastomosis and renal stone formation. Infection and obstruction may lead to bilateral ureteral dilatation with hydronephrosis and impairment of renal function (Fig. 44.24).

RENAL TRANSPLANTATION

As in other immunologically suppressed patients there is an increased incidence of malignant disease in recipients and tumours have been reported in virtually every organ of the body. The common complications of renal transplantation are rejection, acute tubular necrosis and surgical complications occurring as a result of extravasation, obstruction of the ureter or the kidney, and narrowing or occlusion of the renal vessels.

Extravasation of urine may occur from the bladder or

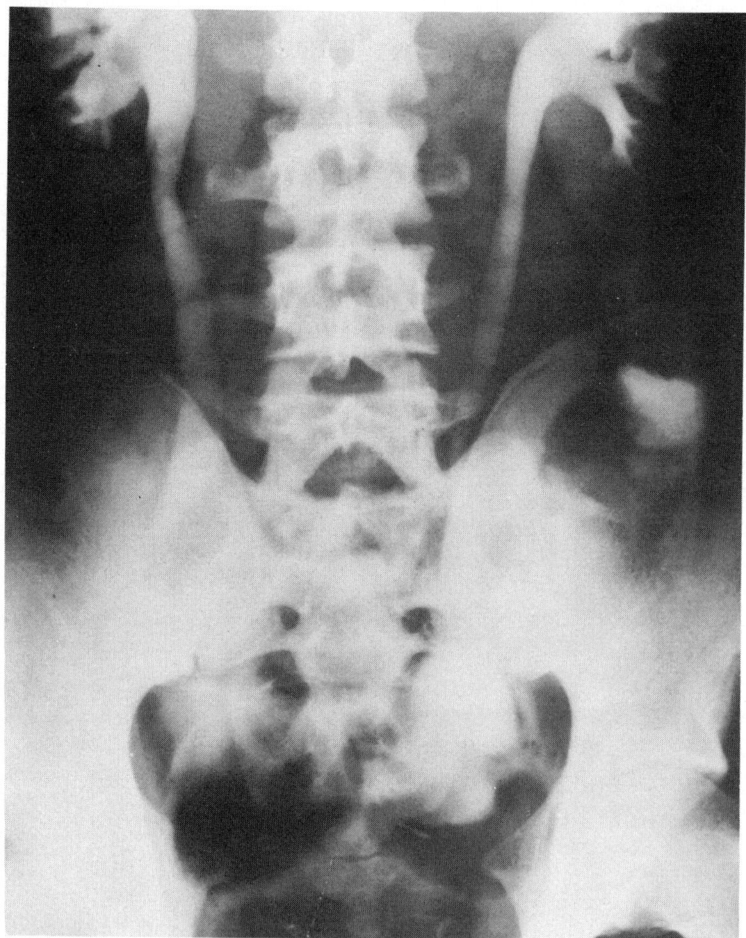

Fig. 44.24 I.V.U. ureterocolic anastomosis.

ureter at the site of implantation or from the donor kidney into the retroperitoneal tissues with the formation of a *urinoma*. Extravasation of lymph producing a *lymphocoele* is a late complication resulting from leakage of lymph from the interrupted lymph vessels of the recipient or from the surface of the donor kidney. A lymphocoele is rarely seen without previous episodes of rejection, it may compress the ureter or the kidney. *Ureteral obstruction* due to fibrosis at the site of anastomosis may be delayed for several years, it is less common with newer techniques of reimplantation. *Arterial stenosis* at the site of vascular anastomosis may lead to renal failure and exacerbation of hypertension; in some instances stenosis and thrombosis of the renal artery is a sequence of intravascular thrombosis occurring during a rejection episode. The renal vein may be compressed by a loculated collection of lymph or urine. *Vesico-ureteric reflux* occurs in about one-quarter of cases. *Rejection episodes* are common and may be preceded or followed by acute tubular necrosis—the result of renal medullary ischaemia.

Radio-isotope studies are of value in demonstrating the integrity of the vascular supply and will also demonstrate the presence of obstruction or extravasation of urine. A urinoma or lymphocoele will be demonstrated both by ultrasound and computerized tomography but the site of leakage or obstruction is best demonstrated by urography. Both rejection and acute tubular necrosis produce a diffusely enlarged kidney with elongated calyces. Urographic estimation of the renal size in these patients is unreliable because of the obliquity and anterior position of the kidney and urography is of no value in differentiating between rejection and acute tubular necrosis. Angiography is only indicated when there is clinical suspicion of renal arterial stenosis or renal venous thrombosis. The renal vessels may be concealed by the iliac arteries and oblique views may be needed. Angiography during rejection will demonstrate obliteration and narrowing of the intrarenal vessels with a mottled nephrogram and failure of opacification of the renal vein. In acute tubular necrosis the vessels are elongated and narrowed, there is a delayed but uniform nephrogram and late opacification of the renal vein.

REFERENCES AND SUGGESTIONS FOR FURTHER READING

BECKER, J. A. & KUTCHER, R. (1978) Urologic complications of renal transplantation. *Seminars in Roentgenology*, vol. XIII, no. 4, pp. 341–351.

BECKER, J. A. & KUTCHER, R. (1978) The renal transplant: rejection and acute tubular necrosis. *Seminars in Roentgenology*, vol. XIII, no. 4, pp. 352–362.

BROWN, J. J., OWEN, K., PEART, W. S., ROBERTSON, J. I. S. & SUTTON, D. (1960) Renal artery stenosis. *British Medical Journal*, **ii**, 327.

CHRISPIN, A. R. (1972) Medullary necrosis in infancy. *British Medical Bulletin*, **28**, 233–236.

DAWBORN, J. K., FAIRLEY, K. F., KINCAID SMITH, P. & KING, W. E. (1966) Renal papillary necrosis. *Quarterly Journal of Medecine*, **35**, 69–83.

EKELUND, J. & LINDHOLM, T. (1971) Artero-venous fistulae following percutaneous renal biopsy. *Acta radiologica*, **11**, 38.

HARE, W. S. C. & POYNTER, J. D. (1974) The radiology of renal papillary necrosis as seen in analgesic nephropathy. *Clinical Radiology*, **25**, 423–443.

LINDWELL, N. (1960) Renal papillary necrosis. *Acta radiologica*, Suppl. 192.

POUTASSE, E. F. & DUSTAN, H. P. (1957) Renal artery stenosis. *Journal of the American Medical Association*, **165**, 1521.

SUTCLIFFE, J. (1970) Chronic granulomatous disease. *Annals of Radiology*, **13**, 305–310.

SUTTON, D., BRUNTON, F. J. & STARER, F. (1961) Renal artery stenosis. *Clinical Radiology*, **12**, 80–90.

WEGNER, G. P., GRUMMY, A. B. & FLAKERTY, T. T. (1969) Renal vein thrombosis. *Journal of the American Medical Association*, **209**, 1661–1667.

CHAPTER 45

THE BLADDER AND PROSTATE

BLADDER TUMOURS

The bladder is the commonest site of neoplastic disease in the urinary tract. The majority of the tumours are of epithelial origin and these should all be regarded as malignant.

Epithelial tumours may take the form of papillary or non-papillary tumours. The *papilloma*, consisting of numerous, delicate, fern-like papillary processes covered with uro-epithelium, is frequently multiple, it may be secondary to tumours of the ureter and renal pelvis and is of low-grade malignancy. The *papillary carcinoma* resembles the papilloma, but its base is broader and its villi clubbed. Non-papillary epithelial tumours, *transitional cell carcinoma* and epidermoid carcinoma form flat plaque-like growths which infiltrate widely. Adenocarcinoma is a very rare mucus-secreting tumour which may calcify and is believed to arise from urachal remnants.

Bladder tumours may be produced by specific chemical agents in patients exposed to aniline derivatives and those employed in the rubber and cable industry: Leukoplakia of the bladder, a probable precancerous condition, may occur as a complication of chronic infection and lithiasis. There is an increased incidence of carcinoma in patients infected with *Schistosomiasis haematobium*, and also in association with analgesic abuse.

Tumours of non-epithelial origin (adenoma, neurogenic tumours, and angioma) are rare. Phaeochromocytoma rarely arise in the bladder, characteristically they present with haematuria and episodic attacks of 'phaeochromocytoma syndrome' precipitated by micturition. Sarcoma and tumours of muscular origin form a special group which will be considered separately.

Secondary tumours, apart from 'seeding' of renal pelvic and ureteral tumours, are rare and are usually malignant melanoma deposits lymphomatous in origin.

It is not possible to distinguish radiologically between benign and malignant tumours, and the diagnosis of bladder tumours is usually established by cystoscopy.

The main value of radiology is to demonstrate the presence of ureteric involvement, infiltration of the bladder wall and the presence of extravesical spread. Infiltration around the ureteric orifices may interfere with the valvular mechanism and produce reflux or may obstruct the ureter.

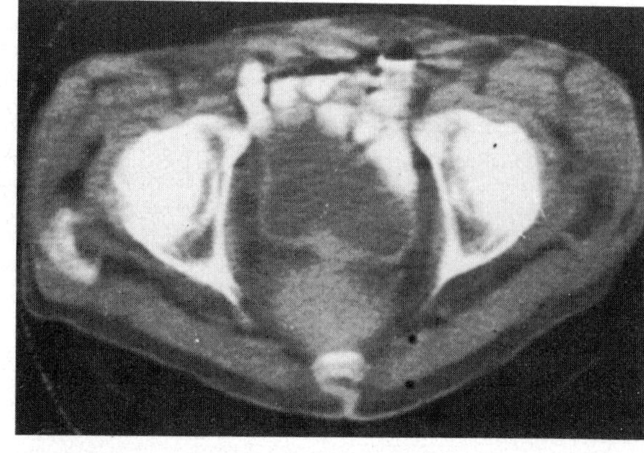

A

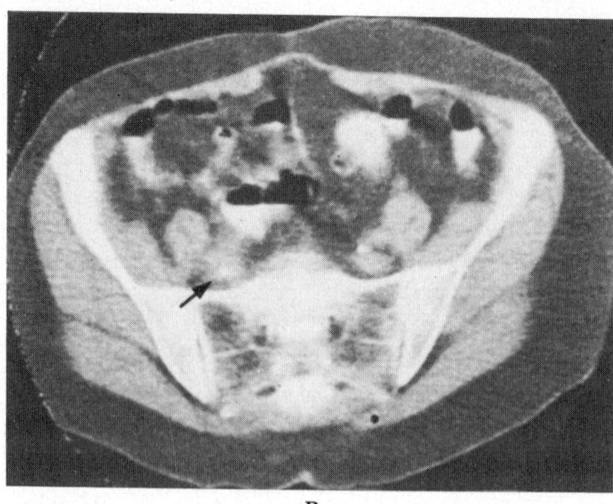

B

Fig. 45.1 C.T. scan. (A) Carcinoma of the bladder producing a localized thickening of the posterior bladder wall. (B) Peri-ureteric extension on the right side (the ureters are opacified following I.V. contrast medium). L. + 15. W. 200.

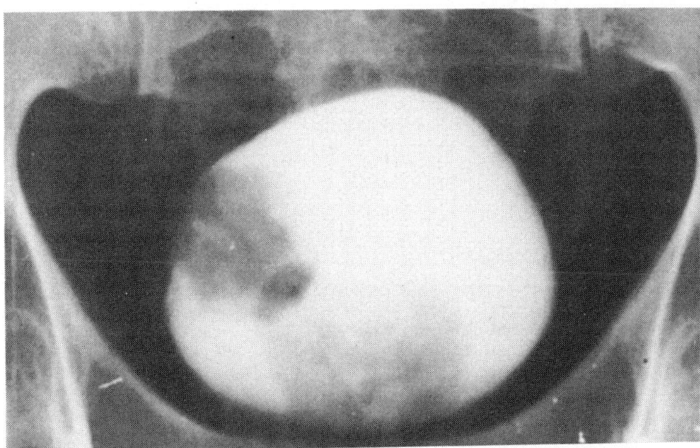

Fig. 45.2 Papillary tumour producing filling defect within the bladder.

Papillary tumours produce well-defined, frequently lobulated, filling defects in the bladder lumen and when large may almost completely fill the bladder (Fig. 45.2). Non-papillary tumours produce plaque-like irregular defects with ill-defined margins and occasionally encrustation of urinary salts on the surface of the growth may be visible on the plain film (Fig. 45.3). Occasionally bladder tumours may produce appearances very similar to those seen with ureterocoele. Localized mucosal oedema following ureteric instrumentation or the passage of a stone may also simulate a carcinoma.

The bladder may sometimes be outlined by the translucent perivesical fatty layer, this is inconstant but if the fatty layer is visible a localized loss of the radiolucent layer indicates extravesical spread and when the bladder lumen is opacified infiltration of its wall produces a localized or diffuse thickening. Extensive invasion of the pelvis may displace the bladder and retroperitoneal extension may lead to medial deviation and obstruction of the ureters. Early results of computerized tomography indicate that it is capable of demonstrating not only intravesical growth but also the intramural and extravesical extent of the disease (Fig. 45.1 A and B). Perivesical insufflation of carbon dioxide combined with opacification of the bladder lumen will also demonstrate increased bladder wall thickness but is rarely of value in the clinical management of a patient. Angiography is also rarely used, it is performed by bilateral femoral artery catheterisation, the catheter tips being placed at the orifices of the internal iliac arteries. Contrast medium is injected after distending the bladder with carbon dioxide. Tumours as small as 1 cm in size can be demonstrated by this method and the presence of pathological vessels in the bladder wall or in the perivesical tissues indicates the presence of an infiltrating growth, the demonstration of a blood supply from the obturator or internal pudenal artery invariably means involvement of the pelvic wall.

Lymphography via the usual pedal root does not demonstrate the obturator and internal iliac nodes which are the lymph glands first involved.

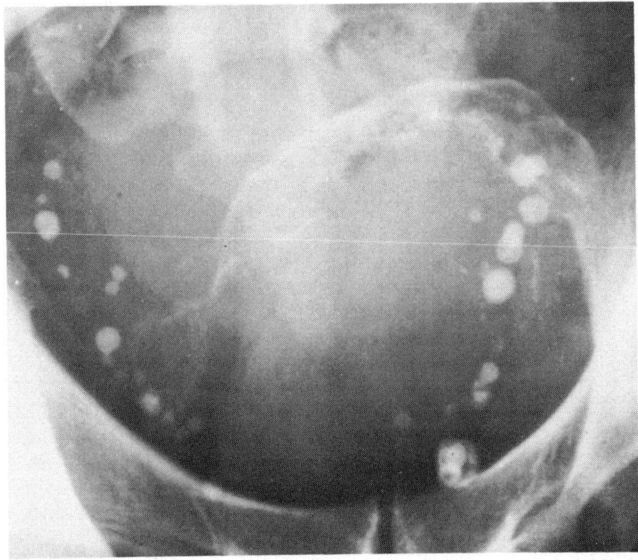

Fig. 45.3 Deposit of urinary salts on the surface of a large bladder tumour.

Sarcoma of the bladder

The sarcomata are mixed tumours of the bladder and prostate containing muscle elements and myxomatous tissue. They not infrequently present in childhood and may form a very large mass.

The bladder may be displaced out of the pelvis and there is often a characteristic elevation of the lower ureters. Multiple, smooth, round filling defects may be visible within the bladder, usually in its lower half, and the urethra may be elongated and stretched over the surface of the growth; filling defects may also be visible within the urethral lumen. Ureteric dilatation may occur as a result of involvement of the lower ureters or as a result of lower urinary tract obstruction.

VESICAL DIVERTICULA

True congenital diverticula do occur, possibly derived from supernumerary ureteric buds or in the case of apical diverticula from urachal remnants, and a small congenital saccule is occasionally seen alongside the orifice of the refluxing ureter. These congenital diverticula are not uncommon, but in the presence of a vesical diverticulum lower urinary tract obstruction should be assumed to be present until it has been excluded by cysto-urethrography.

Residual urine and stasis within the diverticula may lead to infection and stone formation and the diverticulum when large may deform or even obstruct the lower ureter. Reflux may occur if the ureteric orifice lies within the diverticulum. Diverticula may be single or multiple and

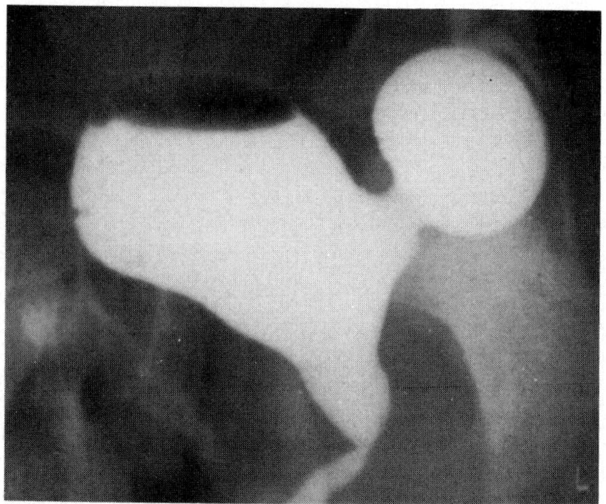

Fig. 45.4 Vesical diverticulum. No evidence of lower tract obstruction.

may be small or become very large, exceeding the size of the bladder.

The simple cystogram is an unreliable and incomplete method of investigation. Whenever possible, a micturating cystogram should be carried out so that the whole of the lower urinary tract is demonstrated (Fig. 45.4). Diverticula may not be visible or only one seen, on the simple cystogram when multiple diverticula are demonstrated on films taken during micturition. It is also fallacious to estimate the size of diverticula from the simple cystogram, the diverticula may be quite small on the resting film but become greatly distended during micturition. On completion of micturition and as the bladder relaxes, the contents of the diverticula empty back into the bladder, producing a large, and often misleading, vesical residue. As with a refluxing ureter these patients may then be able to carry out a double or triple micturition.

The small lateral pouches seen arising from the contracting female bladder are a normal finding and of no significance (Fig. 45.5). They should not be confused with true diverticula.

Vesical reduplication and the hour-glass bladder may mimic diverticula, but these contract normally and empty during micturition, unlike diverticula which usually increase in size as the bladder contracts.

Transitory herniation of the partially filled bladder through the inguinal ring is occasionally seen in normal infants. These anterior and lateral protrusions may simulate diverticula but they disappear with bladder distension and contraction.

THE NEUROGENIC BLADDER

A wide variety of lesions of the spinal cord and peripheral nerves may affect the normal control of micturition. Amongst those most commonly encountered are traumatic lesions of the cord, disseminated sclerosis, tabes dorsalis, congenital myelodysplasias, diabetes and those resulting from extensive pelvic operations such as abdominoperineal resection.

The radiological appearances of the lower urinary tract show a wide variation, and attempts to correlate these appearances with the site of the neurological lesion have not been entirely successful but it is generally recognized that most small spastic bladders are due to upper motor

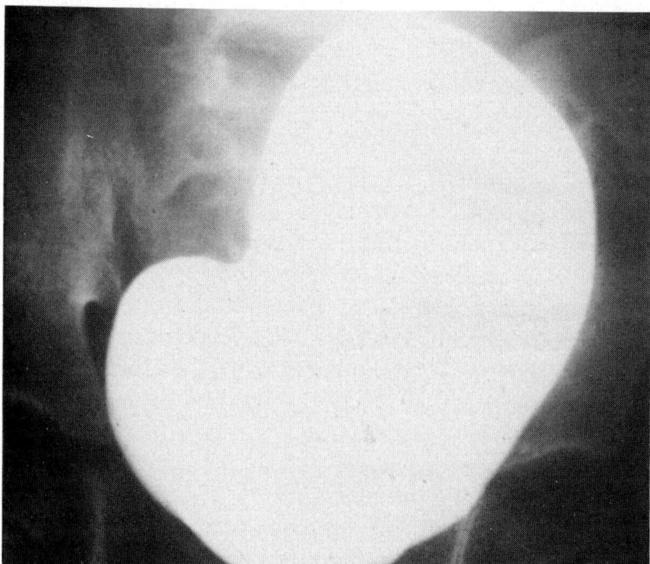

Fig. 45.5 Hour-glass bladder.

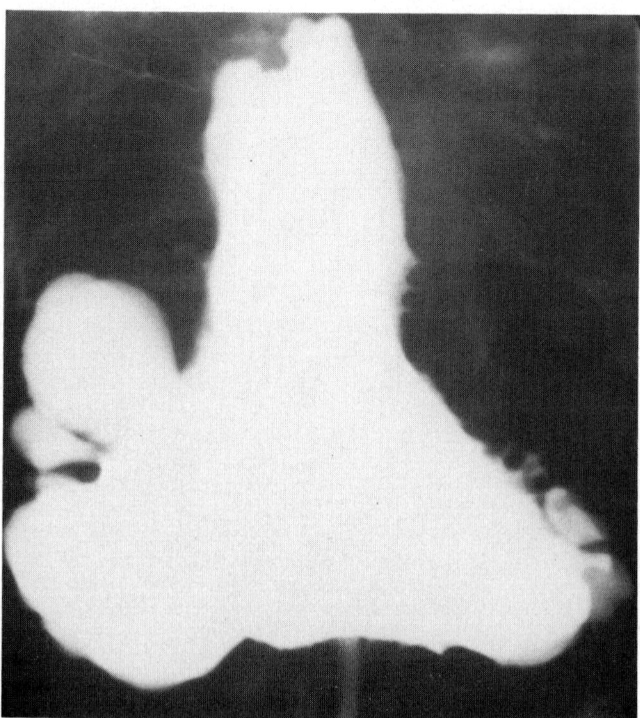

Fig. 45.6 'Pine tree' bladder.

neurone lesions. If only the sensory pathways are affected the bladder is usually large with smooth thin walls.

The micturating cystogram may demonstrate a large atonic smooth-walled bladder with a large residue. Bladder contractions are completely absent, voiding being produced by manual or abdominal expression. Upward and downward movement of the bladder produced by contraction and relaxation of the abdominal wall and diaphragm is seen to persist throughout micturition and is not, as in the normal, confined to the onset of micturition. In these cases the small amount of contrast medium passed demonstrates a normal bladder neck and urethra.

In another variety the bladder is reduced in capacity, its wall is thickened and trabeculated and sacculation is present. It commonly assumes a 'pine tree' shape and the bladder neck is narrowed (Fig. 45.6). Such cases may simulate bladder neck obstruction but they are always associated with abnormal neurological signs and, in the congenital variety, anomalies of the spine or sacrum.

The bladder neck may also be widely open and the urethra filled at rest, producing a funnel-shaped urethra tapering down to a narrow segment at the level of the external sphincter (Fig. 45.7). Less commonly, the widening of the posterior urethra may be confined to its proximal portion (Fig. 45.8).

Dilatation of the upper urinary tract with impairment of renal function is often present and is frequently associated with vesico-ureteric reflux. Upper tract dilatation may also occur in the absence of reflux when it is presumably due to obstruction by a narrowed bladder neck or urethra, or possibly by the hypertrophied bladder wall.

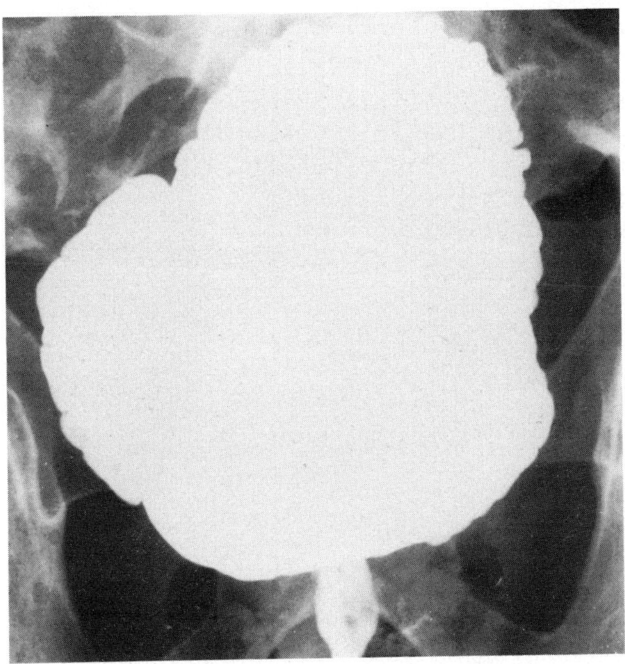

Fig. 45.8 Bladder neck open at rest, urethral dilatation confined to proximal posterior urethra.

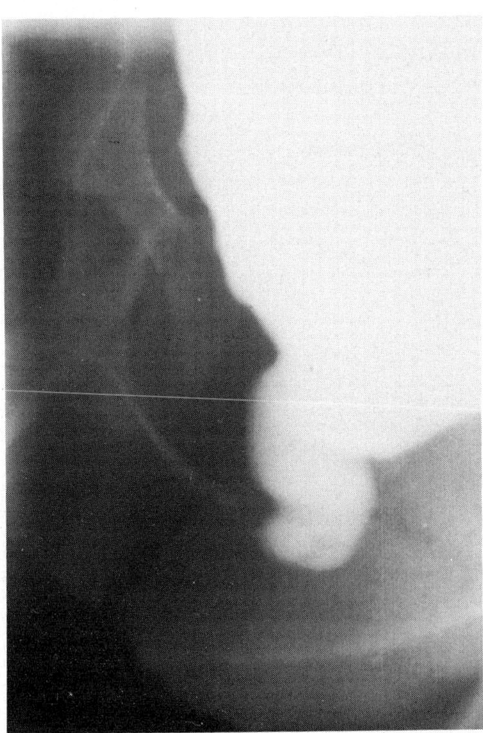

Fig. 45.7 Funnel-shaped urethra tapering down at the external sphincter.

BLADDER TRAUMA

Spontaneous rupture of the bladder is extremely rare but rupture may occur as a result of apparently minor blows to the abdominal wall. Bladder rupture may occur as a result of penetrating wounds and it may also follow instrumentation but it is more commonly due to a fracture dislocation of the pelvis. The bladder contents may leak into the peritoneal cavity or into the extraperitoneal tissues.

Plain films of the abdomen and pelvis will demonstrate any associated fracture or fracture dislocation and extra peritoneal rupture may produce a soft-tissue mass with obliteration of the psoas outline. A paralytic ileus may be seen in both intra- and extraperitoneal rupture. Penetrating wounds may produce an air-fluid level within the bladder on erect or lateral decubitus films.

Intravenous urography is essential to demonstrate the normality or otherwise of the upper tract, the urogram may also reveal deformity and displacement of the bladder shadow by a pelvic haematoma or extravasated urine. Extravasation is not excluded by a normal urogram, but before proceeding to retrograde cystography it is essential that a urethral injury is excluded by retrograde urethrography. If the urethra is normal the bladder may be safely catheterized and water-soluble contrast medium injected

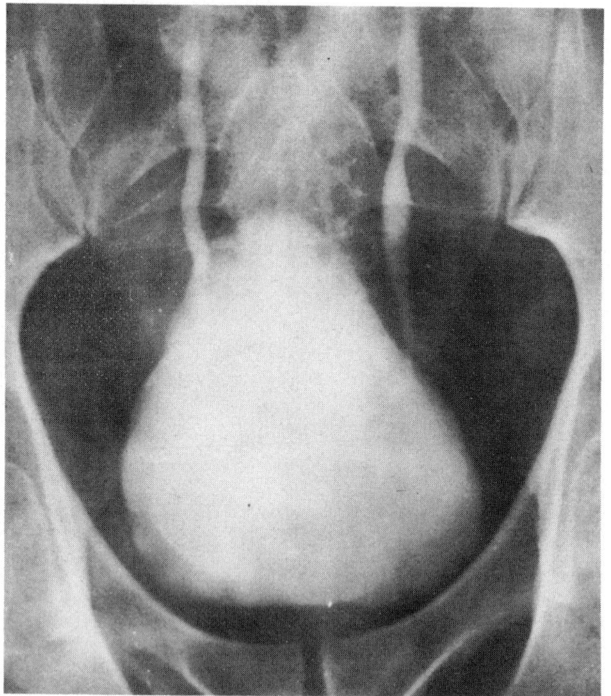

Fig. 45.9 Pear-shaped bladder with medial deviation of the ureters in a muscular Negro.

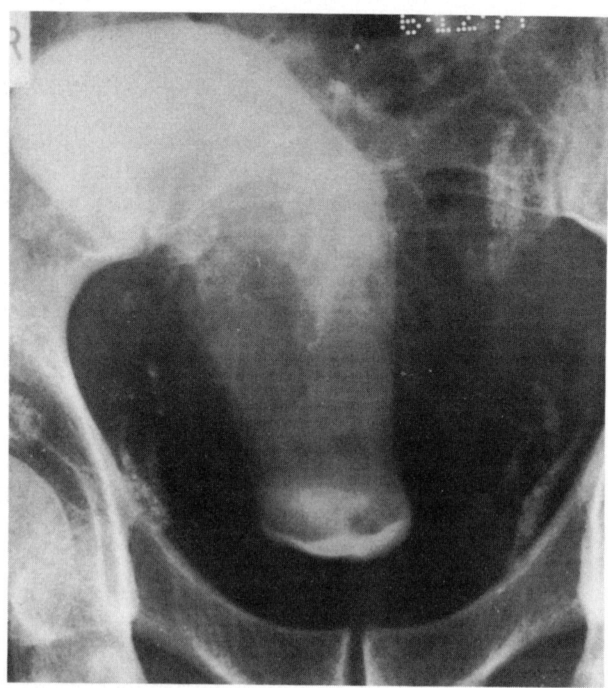

Fig. 45.10 Pear-shaped bladder in lymphoma. A lymphogram has been performed.

under fluoroscopic control, minor degrees of extravasation may only be visible when the bladder contracts during micturition.

If the leak is intraperitoneal the contrast gravitates to the most dependent part of the abdominal or pelvic cavity and loops of gut produce characteristic rounded filling defects, the contrast medium may also be seen below the diaphragm. With extraperitoneal rupture the extravasated contrast produces streaky shadows tracking along tissue planes and may even extend into the thighs.

PELVIC FIBROLIPOMATOSIS

This is an asymptomatic benign condition in which there is an excessive accumulation of fibro-fatty tissue within the bony pelvis. The bladder is elevated and elongated assuming a characteristic pear shape. The ureters may be displaced medially and increased radiolucency of the pelvic wall may be visible on plain films. The retrorectal space is increased in depth, the rectum and sigmoid colon are elevated, elongated and tubular in shape. An identical appearance can also be seen in muscular Negroes when it appears to be due to hypertrophy of the iliacus and psoas muscles (Fig. 45.9). The appearances on computerized tomography are characteristic.

Diffuse pelvic growth, venous and lymphatic obstruction may produce similar appearances (Fig. 45.10).

PROSTATIC ENLARGEMENT

Prostatic enlargement is the commonest cause of lower urinary tract obstruction in the male. It usually presents in late middle age or in the elderly and may be the result of benign hyperplasia or carcinoma.

Benign hyperplasia

The presence of a residual urine may be demonstrated on the plain film by enlargement of the bladder shadow, and prostatic calculi, when present, may be seen to extend beyond the confines of a normal-sized gland.

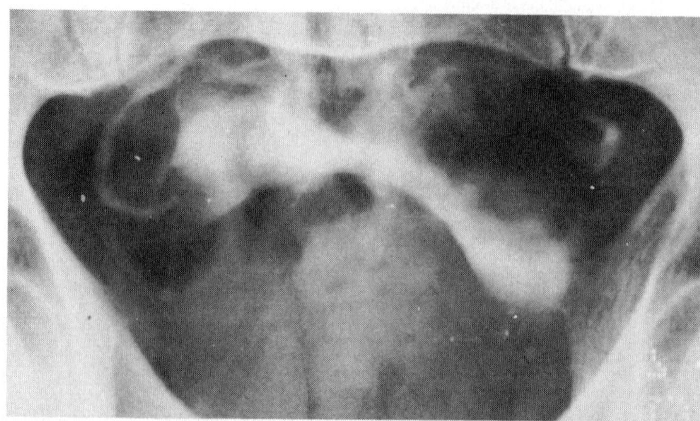

Fig. 45.11 Elevation of the bladder base with 'fish hook' deformity of the lower ureters.

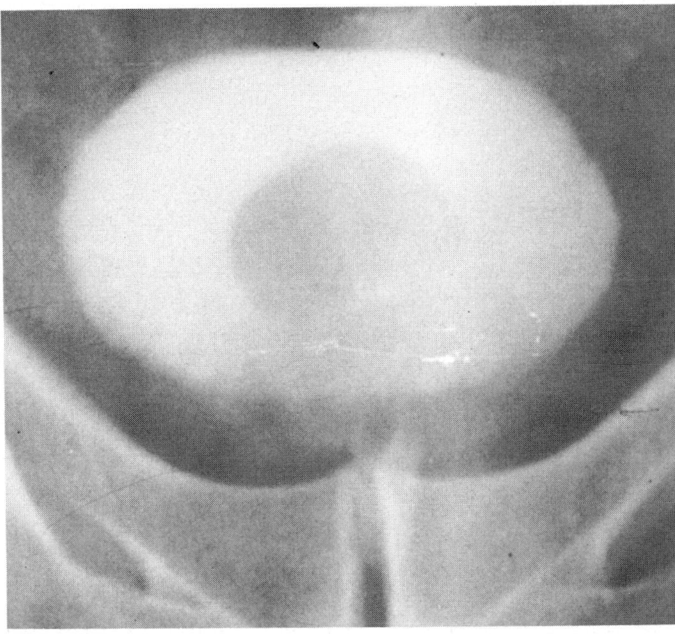

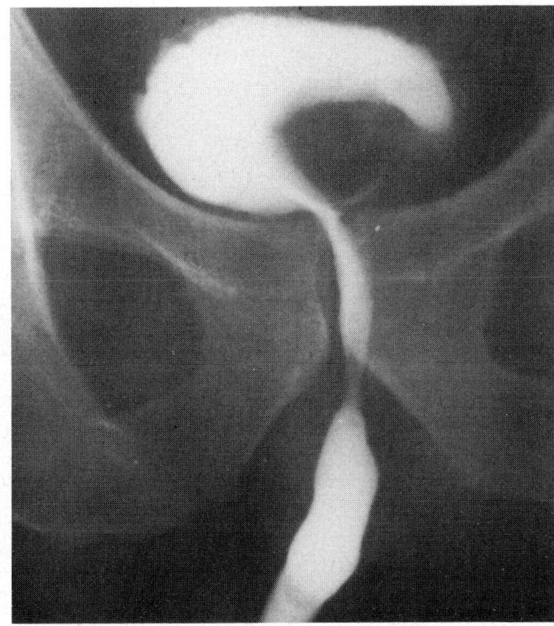

A B

Fig. 45.12 Intravesical filling defect produced by enlargement of the 'median lobe' of the prostate: (A) I.V.U. (B) Retrograde urethrogram.

Intravenous examination may show obstructive changes in the upper urinary tract and with marked enlargement the lower ureters may be elevated, to give a 'fish hook' appearance or show lateral separation. The bladder base is frequently elevated above the symphysis pubis (Fig. 45.11), its wall is thickened with trabeculation and diverticula may be present. Protrusion of the enlarged prostate into the bladder base produces a large smooth rounded (Fig. 45.12A and B), or less commonly lobulated, filling defect, and dense contrast medium may gravitate into a posterior recess behind the intravesical glandular protrusion. A residue is present on the after micturition film.

On the micturating cystogram or injection urethrogram the posterior urethra is lengthened beyond its normal 3 cm and its normal curvature may be increased (Fig. 45.13A and B). Lateral deviation occurs with asymmetrical enlargement and prostatic nodules protruding into the urethral lumen will produce rounded filling defects. The

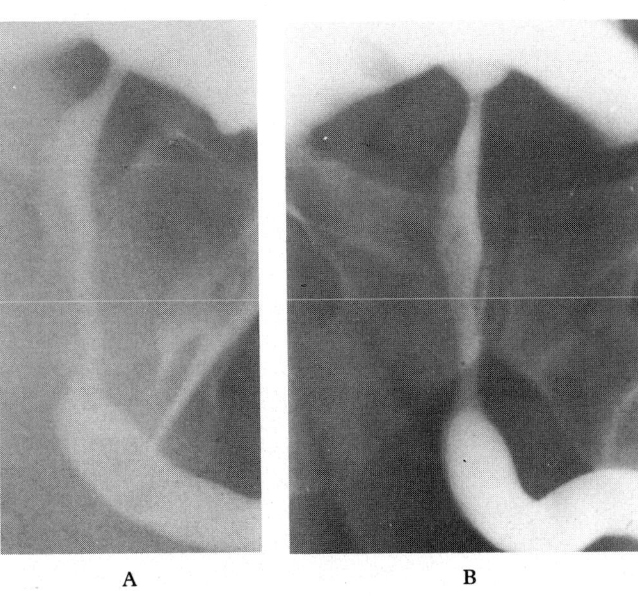

A B

Fig. 45.13 (A and B) Retrograde urethrogram. The posterior urethra is elongated and there is a large prostatic impression on the bladder base.

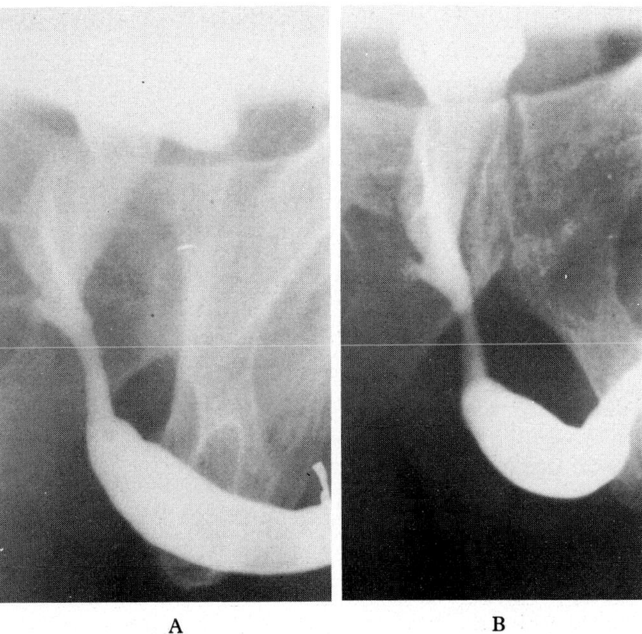

A B

Fig. 45.14 Asymmetrical prostatic enlargement. The urethral lumen is displaced and widened over the surface of the enlarged gland.

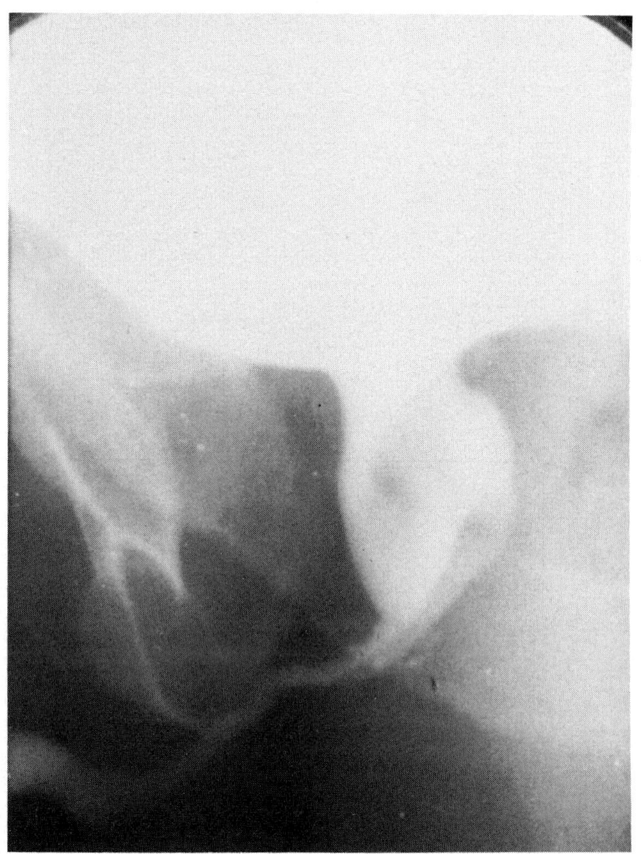

Fig. 45.15 Filling defect in the posterior urethra which is also splayed over the enlarged prostate.

lumen of the urethra may be stretched over the surface of the gland so that although appearing narrowed in one view another view at right angles shows it to be widened (Figs 45.14 and 45.15).

Carcinoma

Prostatic carcinoma produces similar changes to benign hyperplasia and it is not often possible to distinguish between the two (vesiculography has been used for this purpose). Plain films may show evidence of metastases and intravesical protrusion is not as common in carcinoma; when it does occur, the protrusion may have an irregular outline. The posterior urethra is elongated and it may have a narrow, irregular, tubular lumen unlike the stretched slit of benign enlargement. A reduction of the normal urethral mobility may be demonstrated when the patient intermittently contracts the external sphincter.

Sarcoma. See page 901.

Prostatic abscess

Prostatic abscess may be the result of gonococcal or abacterial urethritis and may also occur in tuberculosis, schistosomiasis and following instrumentation.

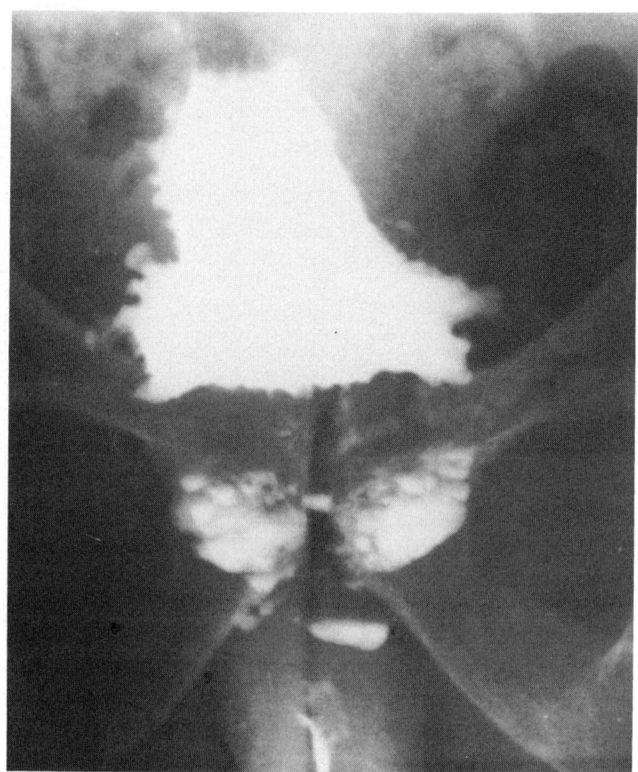

Fig. 45.16 Prostatic abscess with dilated ducts and abscess cavities.

The abscess rarely reaches such a size as to deform the bladder base. The posterior urethra is elongated, its lumen may be deformed and its mobility reduced. The prostatic ducts are dilated and may communicate with irregular cavities which may contain calculi. Fistulous communications may be demonstrated with the rectum, perineum and bladder.

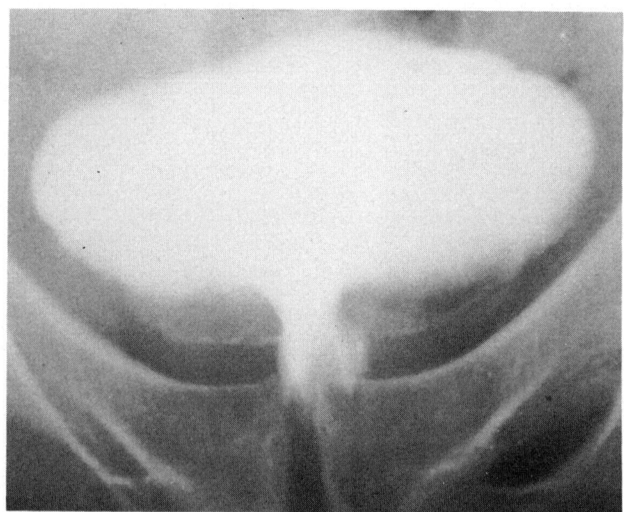

Fig. 45.17 Post-prostatectomy cavity filled through an incompetent bladder neck.

Post-prostatectomy appearances

The normal appearances following prostatectomy are of two types. Commonly there is a residual prostatic cavity which on the cysto-urethrogram is seen to fill with contrast medium through the incompetent bladder neck (Fig. 45.17). Less frequently the prostatic cavity is almost completely obliterated and the bladder neck regains its normal competence so that contrast medium remains confined to the bladder until micturition is initiated.

Post-operative strictures may occur at the bladder neck and in the posterior urethra or, following instrumentation, in the anterior urethra.

Prostatic calculi

Primary prostatic calculi are commonly seen in late middle age and in the elderly. They form multiple small round densities within the prostate gland. Secondary calculi occurring within prostatic cavities are larger in size, fewer in number and may produce urethral obstruction.

REFERENCES AND SUGGESTIONS FOR FURTHER READING

BOJSEN, E. & NILSSON, J. (1962) Angiography in the diagnosis of tumours of the urinary bladder. *Acta radiologica.* **57**, 241–258.

CAINE, M. (1954) The late results and sequelae of prostatectomy. *British Journal of Urology*, **26**, No. 3, 205–226.

ERICSSON, N. O., HELLSTROM, B., NEGARDH, A. & RUDHE, U. (1971) Micturition urethrocystography in children with meningomyelocoele. *Acta radiologica (Diagn.)* **11**, 321–336.

FRIEDMAN, N. B. & ASH, J. E. (1959) Tumours of the urinary bladder. *Atlas of Tumour Pathology*, Section 8, Fascicle 31A, pp. 7–82. Armed Forces Institute of Pathology, Washington, D.C.

NEY, C. & DUFF, J. (1950) Cysto-urethrography. Its role in diagnosis of neurogenic bladder. *Journal of Urology*, **63**, 64–6652.

CHAPTER 46

LOWER URINARY TRACT OBSTRUCTION; STRESS INCONTINENCE

LOWER URINARY TRACT OBSTRUCTION

Obstruction at or below the bladder neck may be produced by:

1. Bladder neck obstruction.
2. Prostatic enlargement.
3. Ectopic ureter (p. 846).
4. Urethral valvular obstruction.
5. Polyp of the verumontanum.
6. Urethral stricture.
7. Urethral diverticula.
8. Urethral tumour.
9. Meatal stenosis.
10. Neurogenic defect (p. 902).
11. Urethral calculi.

All these conditions produce similar changes in the upper urinary tract either as a result of vesico-ureteric reflux (p. 876) or back pressure. The changes produced in the upper tract as a result of back pressure are:

1. *Dilatation and increased tortuosity of the ureters.* Both sides are usually, but not necessarily equally, affected and in the early stages the changes may be confined to one side (Fig. 46.1).

2. *Dilatation of the renal pelvis* with, in the absence of secondary chronic pyelonephritis, a uniform calyceal dilation and narrowing of the renal substance thickness.

3. *Progressive impairment of renal function* with excretion of a dilute contrast medium.

When well established, characteristic signs are produced in the lower urinary tract:

1. Urethral dilatation proximal to the site of obstruction.
2. Vesical residue.

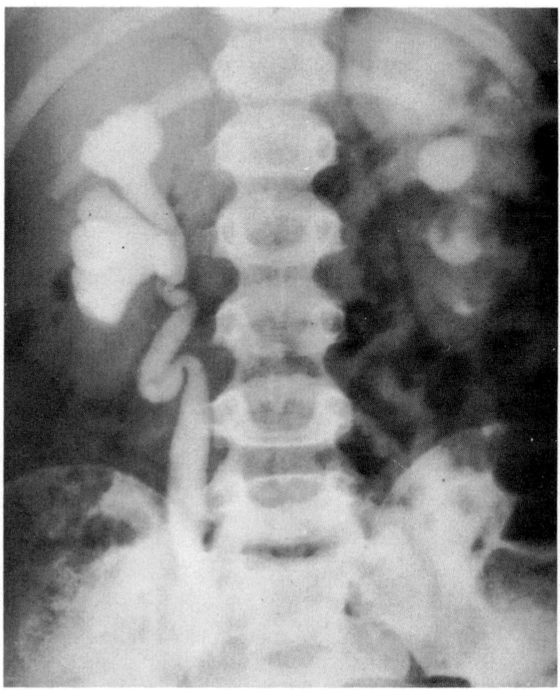

Fig. 46.1 High dose urogram. Back pressure changes due to lower urinary tract obstruction.

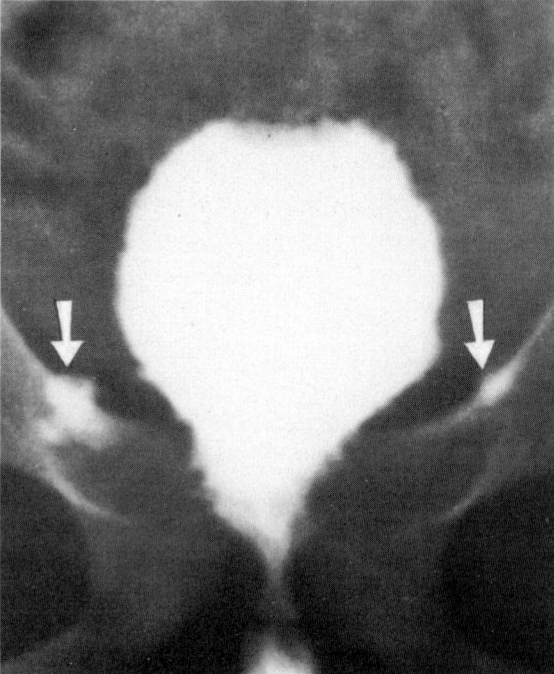

Fig. 46.2 Normal crenation of the contracting bladder outline and normal lateral pouches.

3. Vesical trabeculation, sacculation or diverticulum formation.
4. Bladder neck hypertrophy.
5. Vesico-ureteric reflux, unilateral or bilateral.

The one essential sign of urethral obstruction is the presence of urethral dilatation above the site of obstruction. If the diagnosis is delayed until all the signs are present the disease may have reached an advanced stage with, possibly, extensive renal damage.

The presence of a vesical residue on catheterization or on the after micturition film of the intravenous pyelogram does not necessarily indicate lower tract obstruction. Inability of the bladder to completely empty can be due to paralysis of the detrusor muscle as a result of a neurological lesion and is also not infrequently seen with an atonic bladder after relief of chronic obstruction. A false vesical residue is produced in the presence of reflux, or vesical diverticula. In these cases the bladder empties completely not only via the urethra but also into the diverticula or ureters. On completion of micturition the bladder relaxes and the contents of the ureters or diverticula empty back into the bladder with the production of a false residue. This false residue is readily recognized on fluoroscopy of the micturating cystogram.

The finely crenated outline of the normal contracting bladder must not be confused with trabeculation, and small lateral pouches similar in appearance to saccules are not infrequently seen towards the end of micturition in the normal female bladder (Fig. 46.2). Single or multiple saccules are also frequently seen at the base of the normal contracting bladder in both sexes (Fig. 46.5).

BLADDER NECK OBSTRUCTION

Hypertrophy of the bladder neck may be secondary to an urethral obstruction, the hypertrophy of the bladder neck musculature being part of the general detrusor hypertrophy. The whole length of the urethra must be demonstrated in all cases of apparent primary bladder neck hypertrophy in order to exclude any urethral obstruction.

Primary bladder neck obstruction may present in childhood or in late middle age. In the adult it produces symptoms identical to those produced by prostatic enlargement but the prostate is normal in size. In childhood it is very rare, is almost certainly congenital in origin and usually presents with urinary infection, retention or retention with overflow and renal failure. Histological examination of the bladder neck has produced conflicting results, muscular hypertrophy, submucous fibrosis and overgrowth of fibro-elastic elements have all been described whilst others believe the condition is due to spasm or neuromuscular inco-ordination

The cysto-urethrogram demonstrates vesical trabeculation with sacculation and not infrequently diverticulum formation. In severe degrees of obstruction bladder contractions may appear to be absent, voiding being produced by abdominal expression. The bladder neck is narrowed and the hypertrophied neck may protrude into the bladder base to produce a distinct intravesical impression. The distal urethral lumen is narrowed but this is merely due to the poor flow through the obstructing bladder neck (Fig. 46.3).

Vesico-ureteric reflux is commonly seen and obstructive changes may be present in the upper urinary tract.

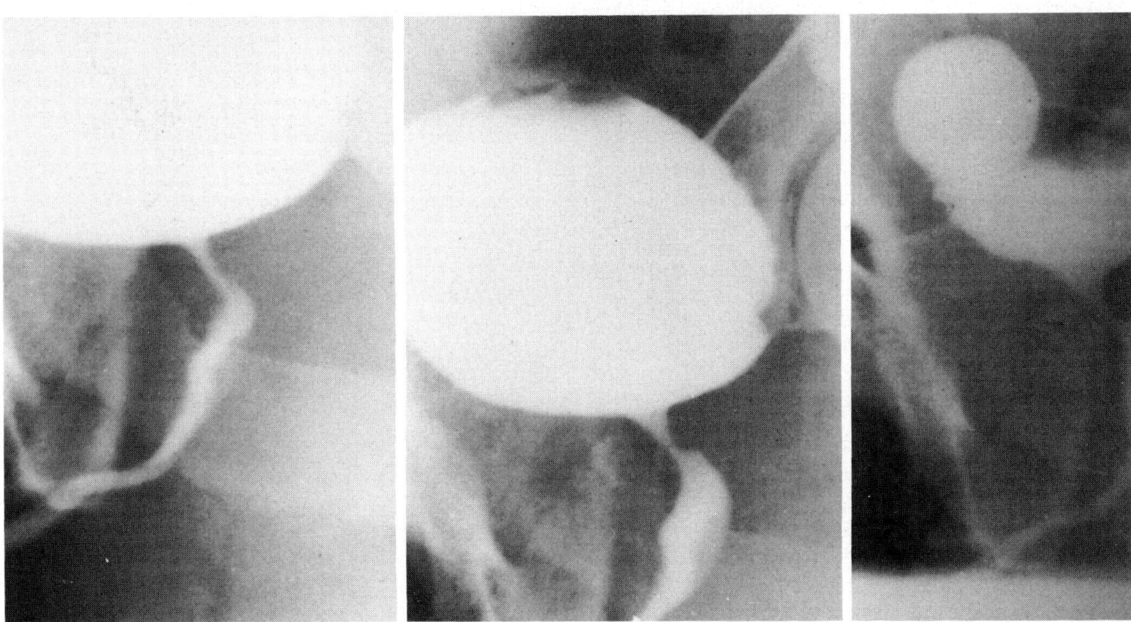

Fig. 46.3 Bladder neck obstruction with diverticulum formation.

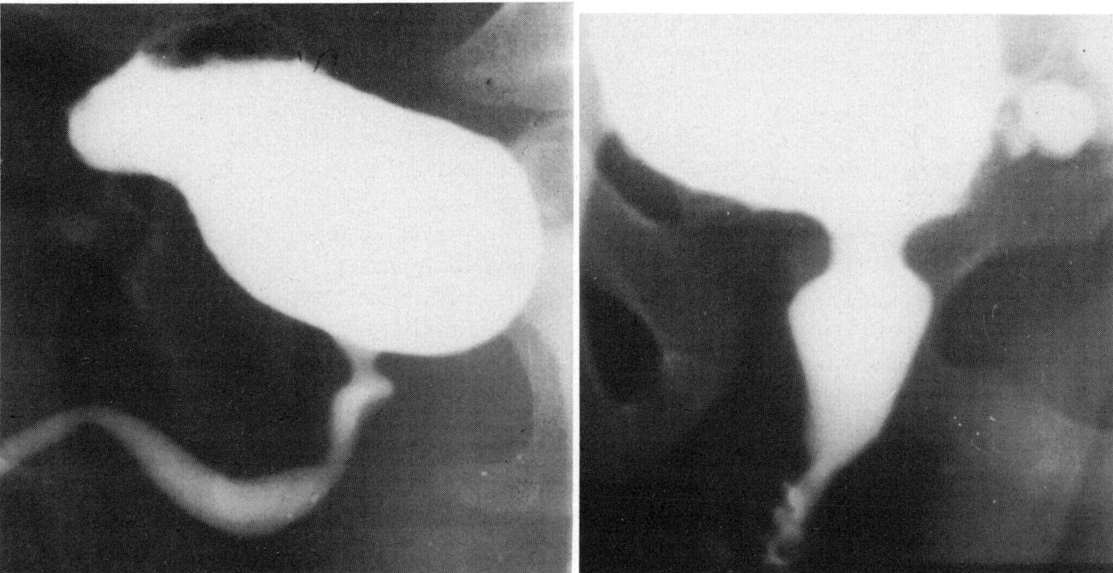

Fig. 46.4 *Fig. 46.5*

Fig. 46.4 Normal bladder neck impression with a good urethral flow.

Fig. 46.5 'Spinning top' urethra with a normal basal saccule.

Neurogenic disorders may produce an identical appearance, but these are associated with abnormal neurological signs and, in the congenital forms, gross defects of the lumbar or sacral spine.

A prominence of the bladder neck is not infrequently seen in the normal cysto-urethogram but there is no other evidence of obstruction and a good urethral flow is preserved (Fig. 46.4).

An appearance aptly described as the *'spinning top urethra'* has been said to be due to both bladder neck hypertrophy and also *Distal Urethral Stenosis* but we believe that this is a normal appearance produced by a high flow rate. The readily distensible normal urethra contrasts with the less distensible bladder neck and external sphincter (Fig. 46.5).

URETHRAL STRICTURE

Congenital urethral strictures are rare, the majority of so-called congenital strictures are the result of urethral instrumentation or the introduction of foreign bodies into the urethra. True congenital strictures are only seen in boys and are usually located at the junction of the bulbous with the membranous urethra. They may also occur as part of the prune belly syndrome (p. 850) and in association with anal atresia (p. 850). The vast majority of urethral strictures are acquired and may be traumatic, inflammatory or carcinomatous in origin.

Traumatic strictures are usually the result of pelvic fracture and occur in the membranous urethra; they may also occur as a result of direct injury, instrumentation and, in the prostatic urethra, following prostatectomy. Inflammatory strictures of the anterior urethra are usually gonococcal or syphilitic in origin, posterior urethral inflammatory strictures may be the result of infection by the gonococcus, tuberculosis, *Schistosoma haematobium* or non-specific infection.

Strictures can be demonstrated by retrograde injection urethrography with a viscous medium (Umbradil U) or, if catheterization is possible, by the micturating cystogram. It should be remembered that strictures producing only minor degrees of narrowing may be missed on the retrograde examination but, owing to dilatation of the proximal urethra, will be demonstrated on the micturating cysto-urethrogram. Associated urethral fistulae, which may occasionally not be demonstrated on the injection urethrogram, will be seen on the micturating cystogram.

Strictures are generally easily recognized as narrowed segments which may be multiple (Fig. 46.6). When very short they may be missed unless several 'spot' films are taken in varying degrees of rotation. Their localization relative to the membranous urethra can only be established by instructing the patient to 'hold back' as if interrupting the stream when the lumen of the membranous urethra will be obliterated and the whole urethra pulled upwards.

Post-inflammatory changes may produce filling of para-urethral glands, Cowper's ducts and glands, prostatic cavities, ejaculatory ducts and seminal vesicles. Para-urethral glandular filling presents as small cavities 1 to 2

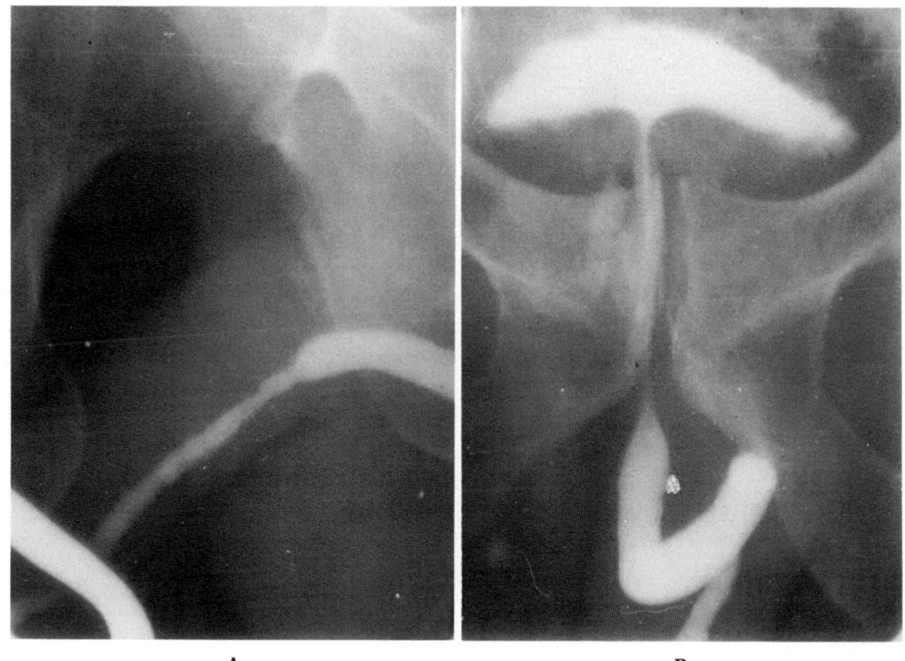

Fig. 46.6 Retrograde urethrogram. Long anterior urethra stricture. The elongation of the posterior urethra and elevation of the bladder base is due to prostatic enlargement.

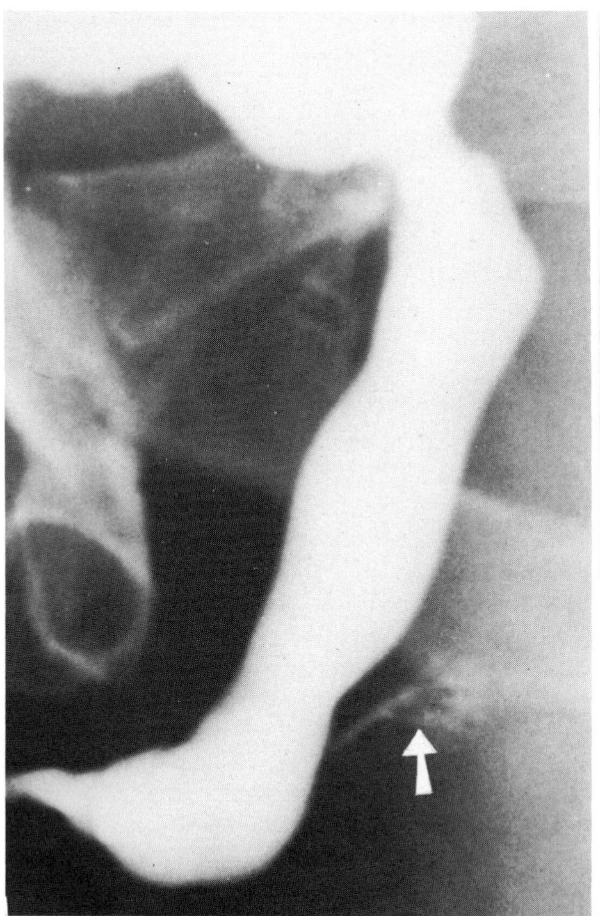

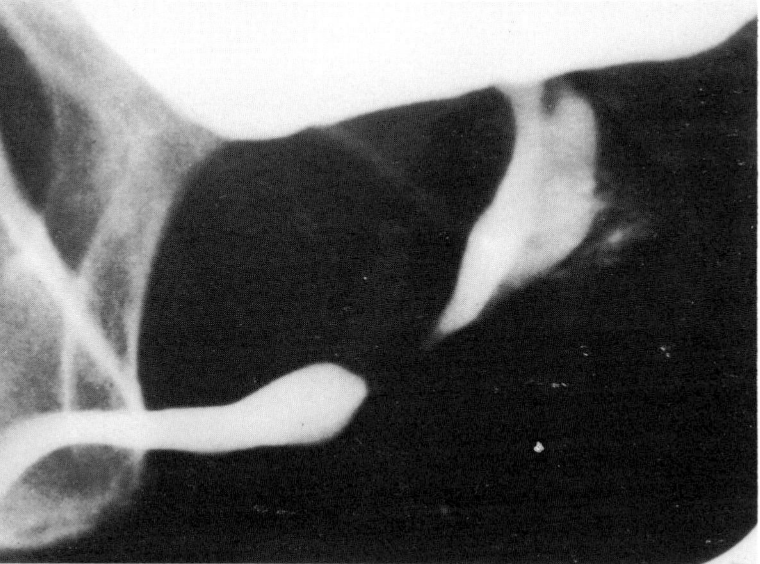

Fig. 46.7 Micturating cysto-urethrogram. Anterior urethral strictures with dilatation of the posterior urethra and reflux filling of Cowper's gland in (A) and prostatic ducts in (B).

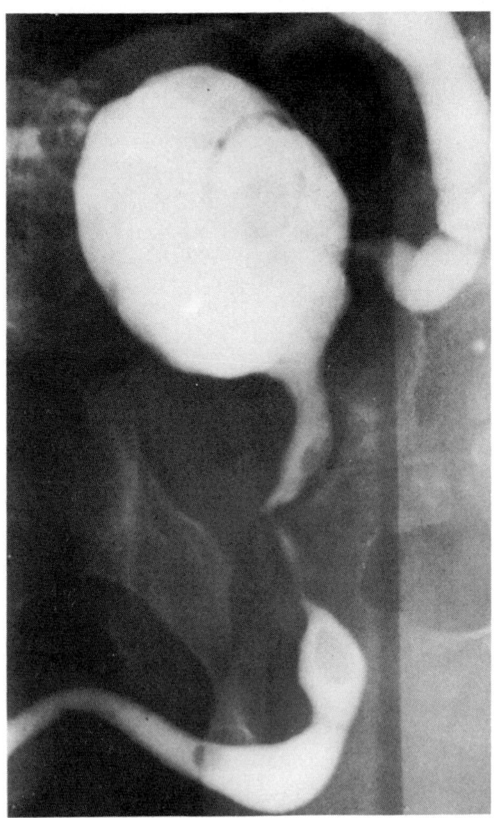

Fig. 46.8 Urethral rupture with wide separation of the posterior and anterior urethra and reflux.

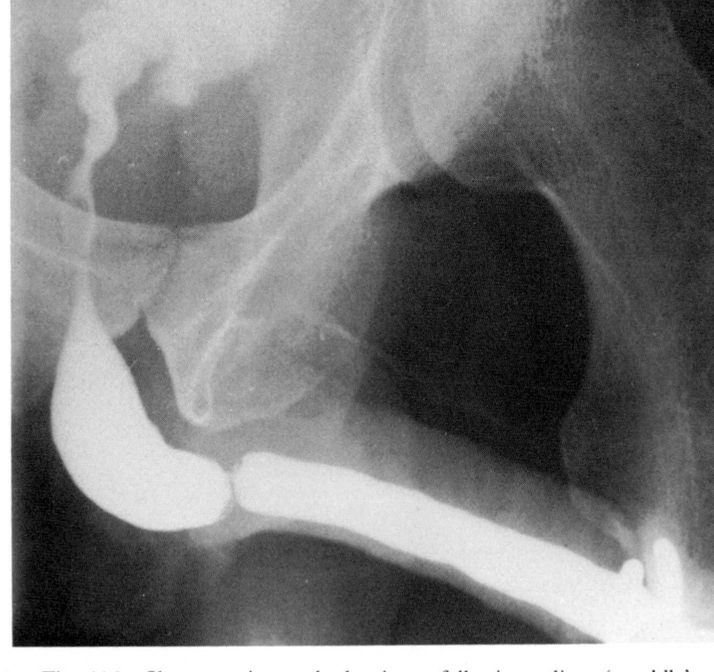

Fig. 46.9 Short anterior urethral stricture following a direct 'straddle' injury.

mm in diameter alongside the urethral lumen and the paired Cowper's glands and ducts are seen as short narrow channels arising from the posterior part of the bulb of the urethra and diverging from the mid line as they pass backwards (Fig. 46.7A and B).

URETHRAL TRAUMA

Urethral injury is usually associated with fracture dislocation of the pelvis and then involves the posterior or membranous urethra. Following complete urethral rupture the two ends may retract and become widely separated (Fig. 46.8). Straddle injuries and direct blows to the perineum involve the anterior and membranous urethra (Fig. 46.9). Urethral injury is rare in women.

An urethral catheter must never be introduced when an urethral injury is suspected; retrograde urethrography will clearly demonstrate rupture of the urethra and urethral mucosal injuries may be revealed by a localized para-urethral extravasation. In the case of complete

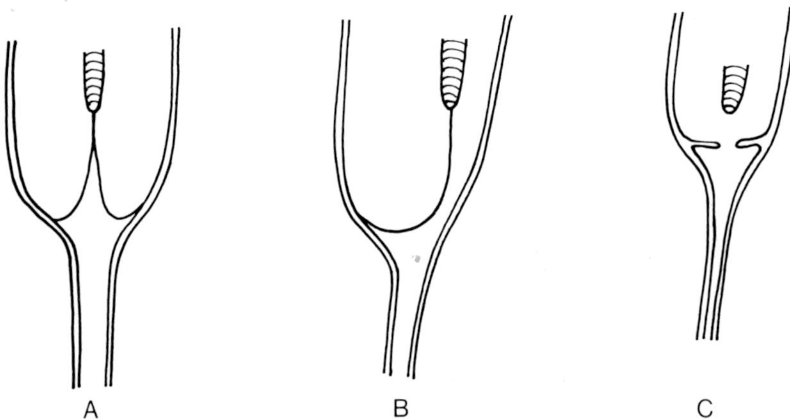

Fig. 46.10 (A) Bicuspid posterior urethral valve; (B) unicuspid posterior urethral valve; (C) urethral diaphragm.

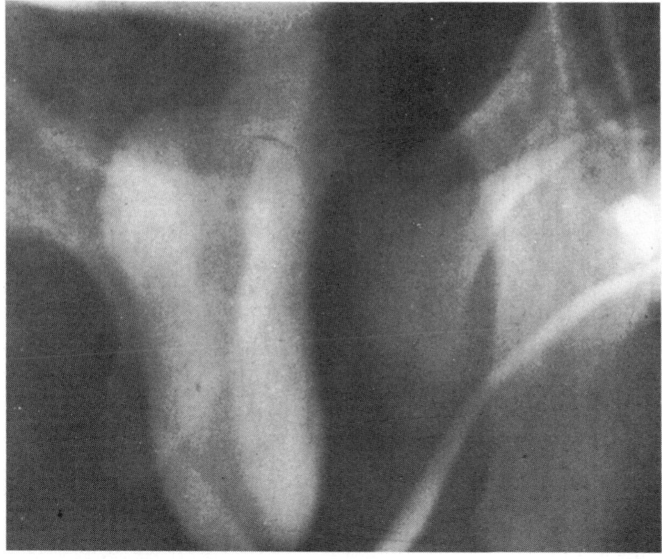

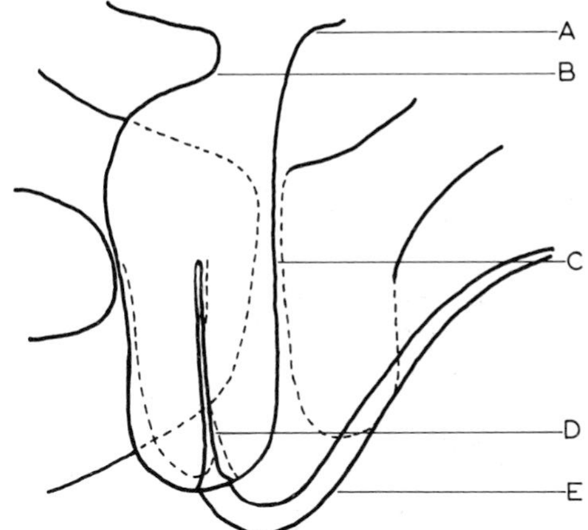

Fig. 46.11 Congenital posterior urethral valves and explanatory diagram. A = bladder base; B = bladder neck; C = dilated posterior urethra; D = valve margin; E = anterior urethra.

urethral rupture the proximal urethral segment can only be demonstrated by micturating cysto-urethrography following suprapubic catheterization.

URETHRAL VALVULAR OBSTRUCTION

Congenital urethral valves give rise to the most severe obstructive uropathies of infancy which may be associated with urinary ascites. They may also present later in childhood and even in early adult life with renal failure, urinary infection or incontinence. The majority take the form of bicuspid or unicuspid mucosal folds at the level of the verumontanum, less commonly an incomplete diaphragm traverses the posterior urethra (Fig. 46.10). They are only rarely seen in the anterior urethra and do not occur in girls. The mucosal valves do not obstruct the retrograde flow of fluid and thus cannot be demonstrated by retrograde injection urethrography.

The micturating cystogram shows evidence of hypertrophy of the vesical musculature with trabeculation of the bladder wall, sacculation and possibly diverticulum formation. Vesico-ureteric reflux may or may not be

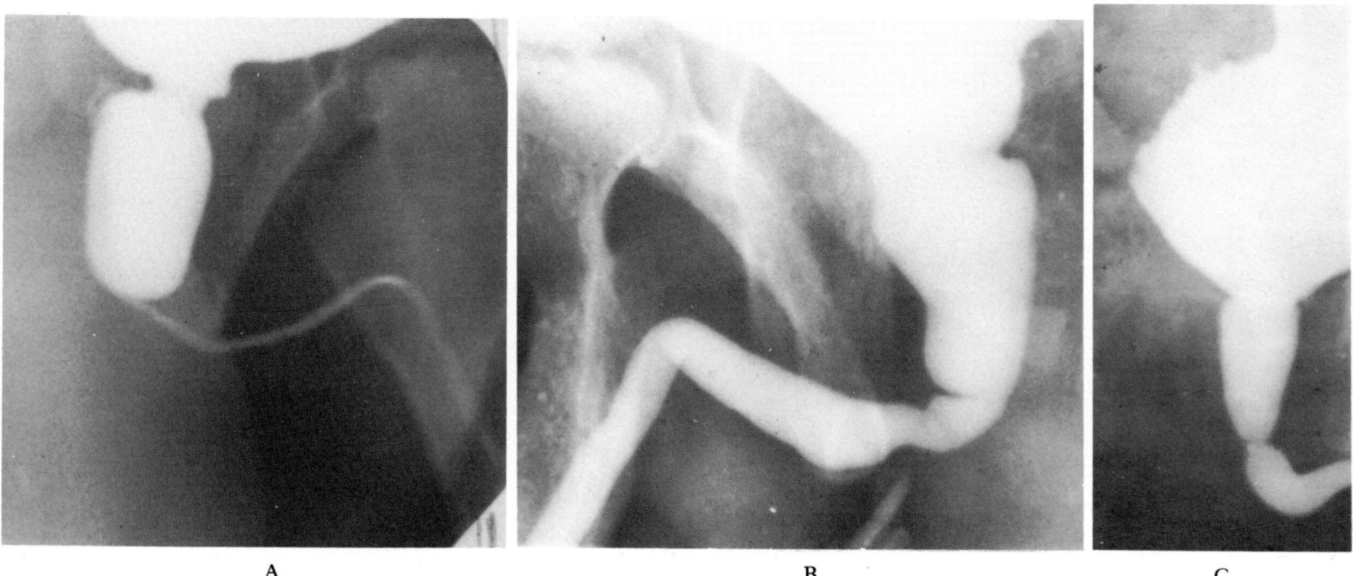

Fig. 46.12 Varieties of posterior urethral valves. (A) Bicuspid; (B) unicuspid; (C) diaphragmatic.

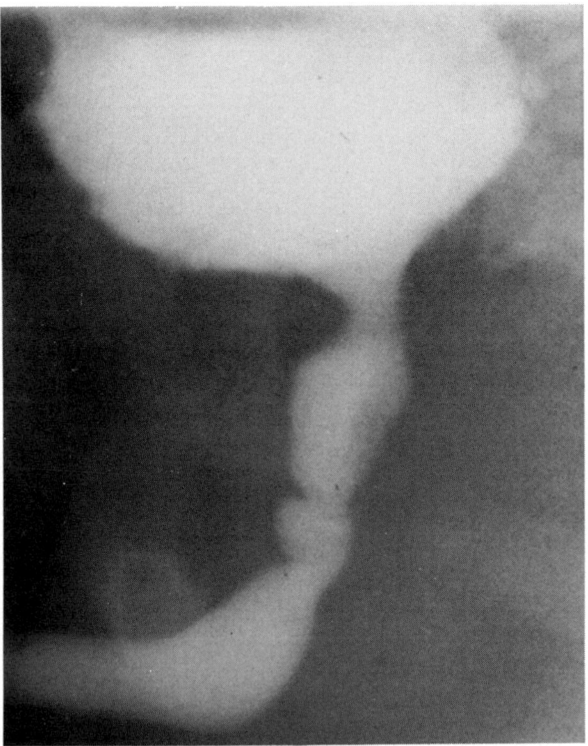

Fig. 46.13 Incomplete non-obstructive urethral folds.

present. During micturition the posterior urethra is seen to be dilated and elongated, the dilatation ending abruptly with usually, but not invariably, a convex lower border bulging downwards. The free valve margins may be visible as linear filling defects within the dilated urethra (Fig. 46.11).

In another, less common variety, an incomplete diaphragm traverses the posterior urethra just distal to the verumontanum (Fig. 46.12A, B and C).

Distally there is a poor stream into a narrow anterior urethra. The increased pressure above the site of valvular obstruction may lead to reflux filling of the prostatic utricle, ejaculatory ducts and even the seminal vesicles. The hypertrophied bladder neck forms a distinct impression on the urethral lumen but this appearance of hypertrophy is exaggerated by the presence of posterior urethral dilatation.

Incomplete non-obstructive folds are commonly seen in the posterior urethra of male children (Fig. 46.13). There is no obstruction to the urethral flow and they are of no clinical significance.

URETHRAL TUMOUR

Carcinoma is the only common primary malignant tumour of the urethra, the urethra may also be involved by extension of a carcinoma arising primarily in the prostate or bladder.

Benign tumours, transitional cell papilloma, fibroma, myoma and angioma are rare.

Urethral condylomata are the result of a viral infection. Retention cysts of the peri-urethral glands and inflammatory polypi may occur as a result of urethritis.

Urethral carcinoma presents radiological appearances identical to those seen in an inflammatory stricture, it usually occurs in the anterior urethra and peri-urethral extension may lead to fistula formation. The diagnosis is usually established on a history of urethral bleeding and

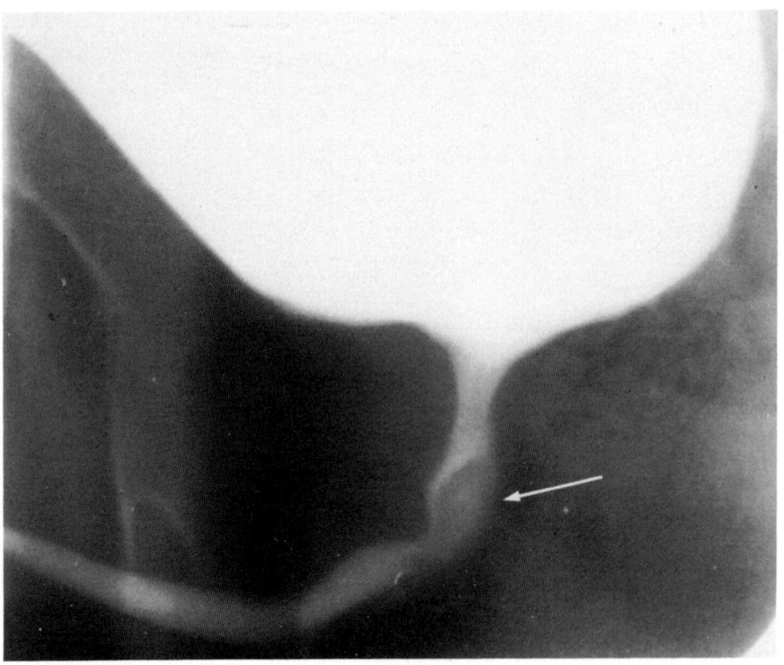

Fig. 46.14 Normal prominent verumontanum.

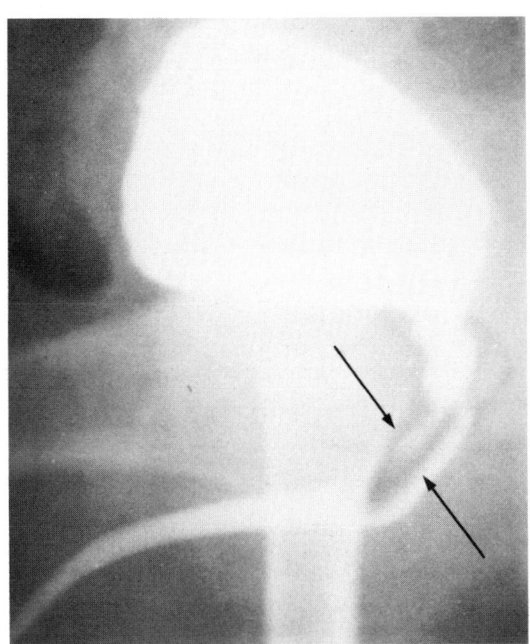

Fig. 46.15 Polyp of the verumontanum.

the presence of clinical evidence of peri-urethral extension with glandular involvement.

Benign and inflammatory tumours produce a well-defined smooth, frequently pedunculated filling defect in the urethral lumen which when large will obstruct the lumen with consequent dilatation of the proximal urethra.

Polyp of the verumontanum consisting of connective tissue covered with transitional epithelium is a rare cause of urethral obstruction in male children which must not be confused with a prominent but normal verumontanum (Fig. 46.14). A polyp is single and usually on a long stalk attached to the verumontanum. In the resting state the polyp may be seen as a filling defect within the bladder close to its base and during voiding it prolapses into and obstructs the urethra (Fig. 46.15).

CONGENITAL MEATAL STENOSIS

Narrowing of the urethral meatus may be congenital in origin and may be associated with hypospadias. Meatal stenosis may also be acquired as a result of surgical

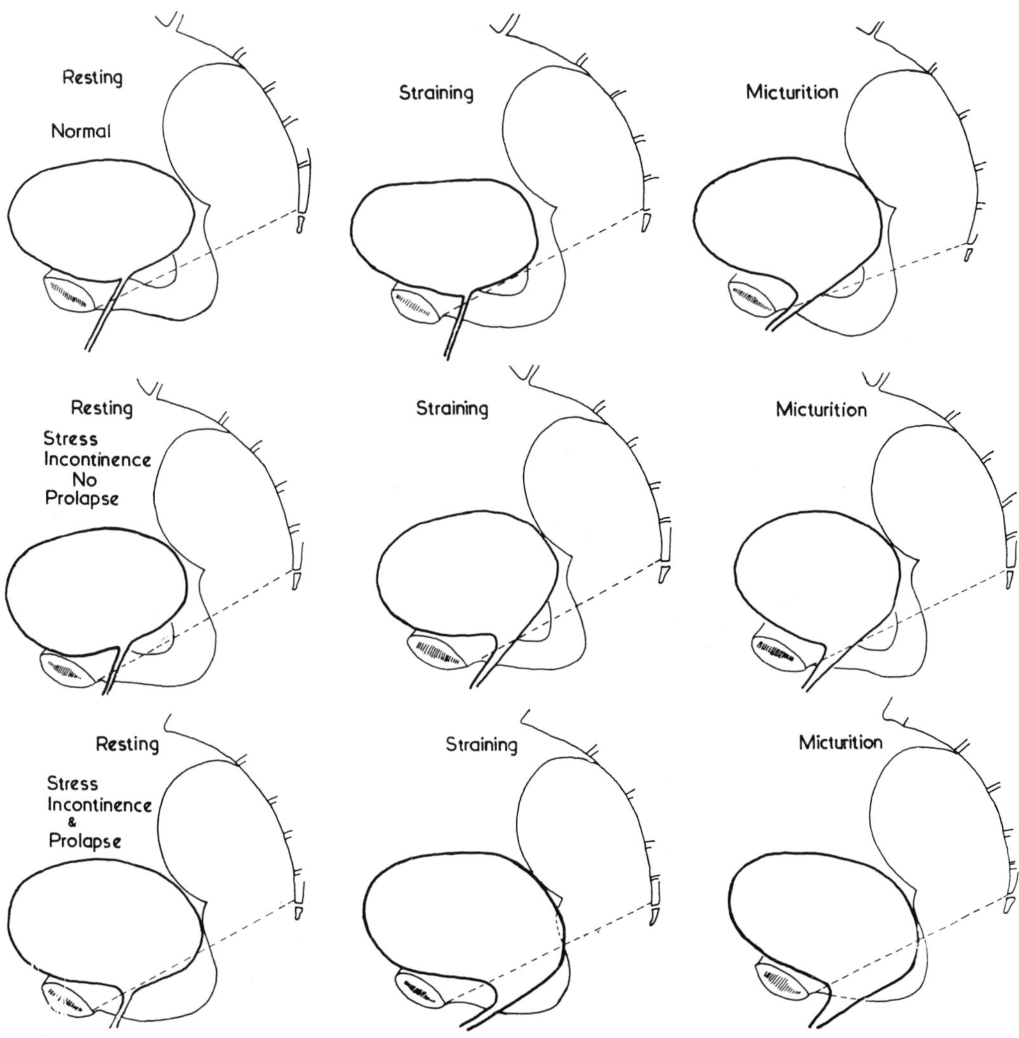

Fig. 46.16 The lateral cystogram.

operations on the external meatus or as a result of meatal ulceration superimposed on a napkin rash. The diagnosis is usually obvious on clinical examination and back pressure effects on the urinary tract are uncommon. Cysto-urethrography demonstrates urethral dilatation down to the external meatus, the dilated urethra terminating abruptly at the meatus.

STRESS INCONTINENCE

Stress incontinence in women is almost invariably due to injury to the pelvic floor during childbirth and is usually, although not invariably, associated with prolapse.

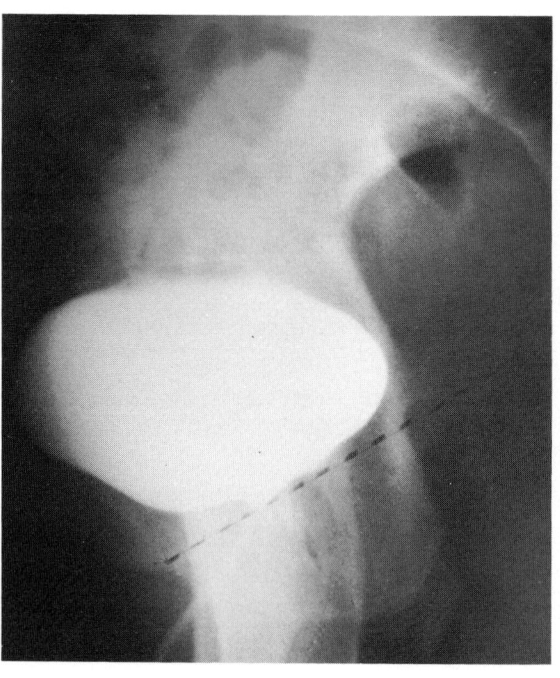

A

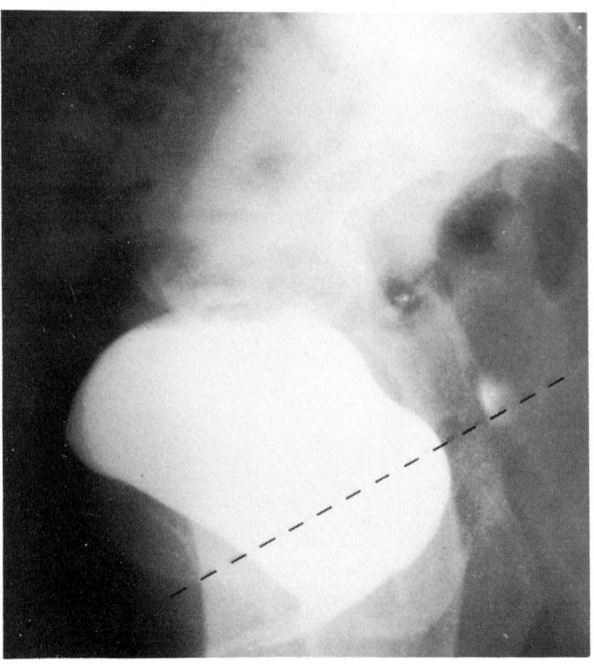

B

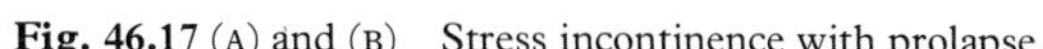

Fig. 46.17 (A) and (B) Stress incontinence with prolapse.

The technique of stress cystography is described on page 837.

The lateral cystogram with normal control of micturition. In the resting state the bladder lies 1 to 2 cm above a line joining the inferior margin of the symphysis to the tip of the last piece of the sacrum. The urethral catheter forms an angle of about 100° with the bladder base and there is often a minor degree of 'beaking' at the bladder neck. On straining, the bladder base and urethra descend but do not pass below the line joining the symphysis to the sacrum, the cysto-urethral angle is preserved and there is no increased 'beaking' at the bladder neck. On micturition descent occurs as on straining and the cysto-urethral angle is obliterated, the urethra and bladder base forming a straight line (Fig. 46.16).

The lateral cystogram in stress incontinence without prolapse. The cysto-urethral angle is obliterated on straining and may also be obliterated at rest. Excessive beaking of the bladder neck is produced on straining and may also be seen on the resting film resulting in a variable degree of urethral filling. The bladder base is normal in position. On micturition the urethra is normal in appearance but retrograde emptying of the urethra into the bladder which normally follows interruption of the stream is delayed, incomplete or abolished.

The lateral cystogram in stress incontinence with prolapse. The appearances are the same as those described above but abnormal descent of the bladder base is also demonstrated (Fig. 46.17A and B).

The lateral cystogram in prolapse without stress incontinence. Abnormal descent of the bladder base is associated with preservation of the cysto-urethral angle and normal retrograde urethral emptying. There is no excessive beaking at the bladder neck.

POST-PROSTATECTOMY INCONTINENCE

In the normal subject voluntary interruption of the urethral stream is produced by an abrupt contraction of the external sphincter. Immediately following the sphincteric contraction the urethra empties distally towards the external meatus and also proximally towards the bladder.

Following prostatectomy in the continent patient the mechanism is similar; external sphincteric contraction is followed by reflux emptying of the remaining segment of

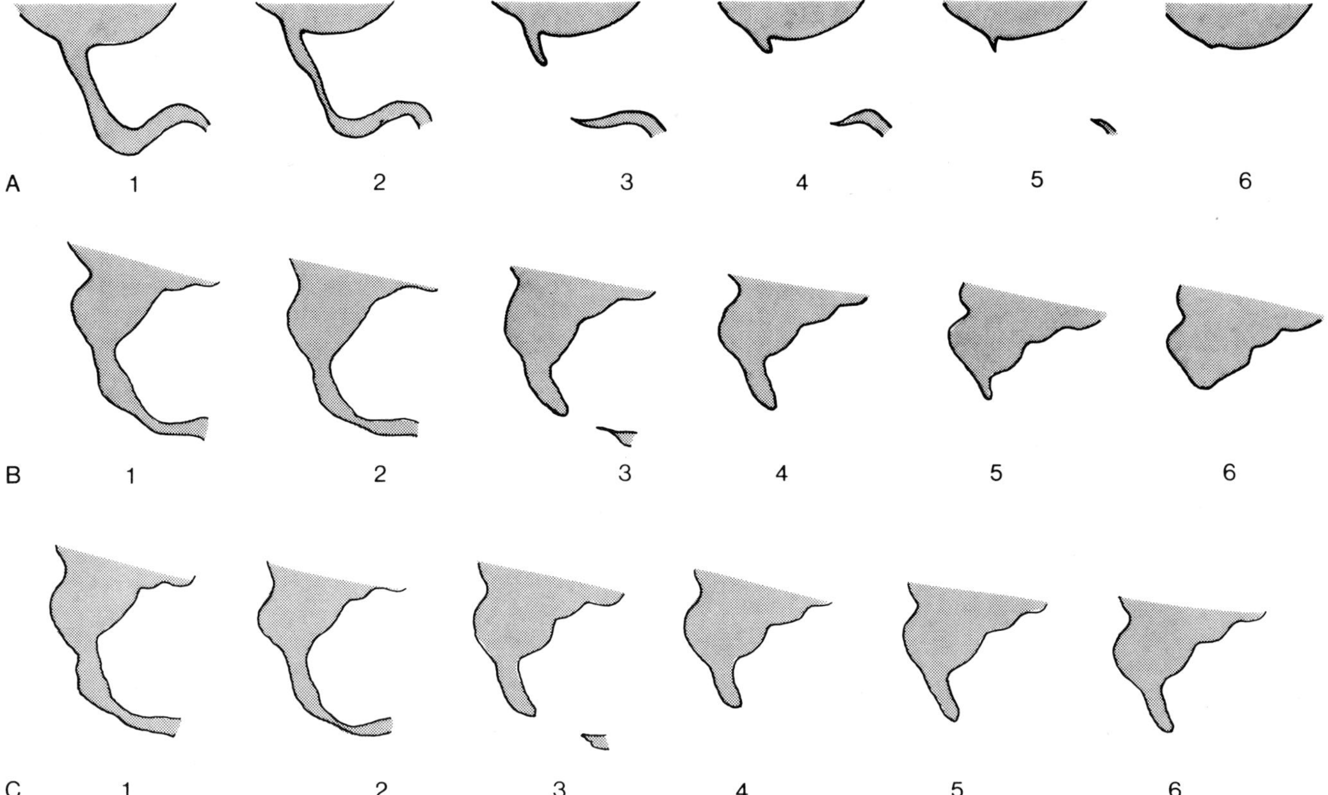

Fig. 46.18 Peripheral control of micturition.
(A) Normal subject: (i) voiding; (ii) to (v) interruption of stream, contraction of external sphincter, reflux emptying of posterior urethra and emptying of distal urethra; (vi) urethra empty.
(B) Post-prostatectomy, normal control, residual prostatic cavity and incompetent bladder neck: (i) voiding; (ii) to (v) interruption of stream, contraction of external sphincter, reflux emptying of posterior urethra into the prostatic cavity, emptying of distal urethra.
(C) Post-prostatectomy incontinence: (i) Voiding, (ii) to (vi) Interruption of stream, contraction of external sphincter, emptying of distal urethra. *No* reflux emptying of posterior urethra into the prostatic cavity.

posterior urethra into a residual prostatic cavity. Where there is no residual prostatic cavity the reflux emptying takes place into the bladder and the appearances are virtually the same as in the normal.

Incontinence following prostatectomy usually consists of a leakage of urine when the patient is relaxed but the leakage can be stopped by voluntary contraction of the external sphincter. Ciné cysto-urethrography in these cases shows that the external sphincter is able to contract normally, but the normal reflux emptying of the posterior urethra does not occur. The column of contrast medium remains down to the external sphincter and when this voluntary sphincteric contraction relaxes incontinence occurs (Fig. 46.18). The damage in these cases is to the smooth muscle layer of the posterior urethra proximal to the external sphincter, the striated muscle of the sphincter being unaffected.

REFERENCES AND SUGGESTIONS FOR FURTHER READING

CAINE, M. & EDWARDS, D. (1958) The peripheral control of micturition. *British Journal of Urology*, **26**, 205.

HERTZ, M. (1969) Pedunculated polyp of the posterior urethra in a three-year-old boy, demonstrated by voiding cysto-urethrography. *British Journal of Radiology*, **42**, 543–544.

JEFFCOATE, T. N. A. (1958) Urethrocystography in the female. *Journal of the Faculty of Radiologists*, **9**, 127–134.

KELLBERG, S. R., ERICSSON, N. D. & RUDHE, U. (1957) *The Lower Urinary Tract in Childhood.* Stockholm: Almquist & Wiskell, Year Book Publishers, Inc.

MORALES, O. & ROMANUS, R. (1952) Urethrography in the male: the boundaries of the different urethral parts and detail studies of the urethral mucous membrane and its motility. *Acta radiologica*, Suppl. 95.

STEPHENS, F. D. (1963) *Congenital Malformations of the Rectum, Anus and Genito-urinary Tracts.* Edinburgh: Churchill Livingstone.

WILLIAMS, D. I. (1968) *Paediatric Urology.* London: Butterworths.

CHAPTER 47

OBSTETRIC RADIOLOGY

The subject of obstetric radiology will be considered under the following headings:

1. Radiation hazards to the fetus
2. Abnormalities of the urinary tract in pregnancy
3. The developing fetus
4. The demonstration of placental site
5. Pelvimetry.

1. RADIATION HAZARDS

The hazards to the fetus attributable to radiation are those of fetal death, malformation of the fetus, and childhood neoplasia (carcinoma and leukaemia). Most attention has been directed to the possible induction of neoplasia in the child as a result of irradiation *in utero*. The early paper of Stewart *et al.* (1956) appeared to show a relation between leukaemia and uterine radiation. This work was based on retrospective questioning of mothers whose children had died from leukaemia and determining how many of the mothers had been radiologically examined during the relevant pregnancy. A further report found other factors apparently associated with an increased incidence of childhood leukaemia. These included threatened abortion, viral infections and excessive age in the mother, and pulmonary infections and severe injuries in the child. These additional factors added confusion to the original findings. On the other hand a review by Brown *et al.* (1960) of 39 166 mothers known to have had irradiation in pregnancy could find no evidence of an excess of childhood leukaemia in their offspring. Recently it has been suggested that the maximum danger to the fetus is in the first trimester of pregnancy. Because of this and also the radiation hazard to the recently impregnated ovum at a stage when the pregnancy may not have caused even one period to be missed, the following recommendation was made in the 1966 report of the International Commission on Radiological Protection: 'Therefore it is recommended that all radiological examinations of the lower abdomen and pelvis of women of reproductive capacity that are not of importance in connection with the immediate illness of the patient be limited in time to this period (i.e. the 10-day interval following the onset of menstruation) when pregnancy is improbable. The examinations that it will be appropriate to delay until the onset of the next menstruation are the few that could without detriment be postponed until the conclusion of a pregnancy or at least until its latter half.' It will be noted that this is only a recommendation, not a rule. Also the second sentence implies that the need to examine the mother, when properly indicated, will take precedence over the possible risk to the fetus unless the need for the examination is such that it can reasonably be delayed until late in the pregnancy. It should further be noted that the irradiation of the mature ovum prior to fertilization may not be without hazard (*British Medical Journal*, 1979), so that it may reasonably be claimed that there is no period when there is no risk to an actual or potential fetus from irradiation. The recommendation of the International Commission was repeated in 1977.

One must consider that there is a natural incidence of about 3 per cent of all live births which have severe defects and that the incidence of major defects due to diagnostic irradiation (up to 5 rads) is under 1 per 1,000 live births. The effect of diagnostic irradiation here is virtually negligible. Diagnostic levels of irradiation appear to have a more profound effect in the induction of neoplasia. The natural rate of leukaemia and carcinoma in childhood is between 0·5 and 1 per 1,000 live births. A dose of 5 rads might increase the incidence 10-fold, or less with decreasing radiation doses.

The matter of radiation hazard is complex, but for a critical review of the subject the reader should consult the article by Mole (1979). From this review it appears reasonable to regard the '10-day recommendation' as reflecting outdated opinions. Mole regards this advice as being excessively restrictive and based on uncertain facts. In this respect he agrees with the advice given in North America by the American College of Radiology (Brown, 1976) and in the recent leading article in the *British Medical Journal* (1979). This suggests that the radiological examination of the abdomen of a woman of reproductive capacity should be conducted without delay or 'scheduling' but that the clinical indications should be well founded and the examination should be carried out with full regard to the requirements of limitation of radiation dose. The Royal College of Radiologists in Britain (1978), however, still recommend the retention of the '10-day principle'.

Diagnostic irradiation is not regarded as an indication for the termination of pregnancy either by the American College of Radiology or by the Radiation Protection and Medical Committees of the British Institute of Radiology as it would be possible to sacrifice 1,000 normal fetuses in order to spare 1 from the hazards of deformity or leukaemia.

2. THE PYELOGRAM IN PREGNANCY

The pyelographic appearances in pregnancy may differ considerably from the accepted normal, but with such frequency as to be considered 'physiological' rather than an indication of disease. The changes consist of a dilatation of the calyces and pelves, and also of the ureters, which show elongation and kinking (Fig. 47.1). The pelvic (lower) spindle of the ureter usually escapes. The changes of dilatation, when they occur, are always seen on the right, and if bilateral, are more severe on the right. There is no evidence of renal functional impairment, as the density of the excreted contrast medium remains normal. However, ureteric atony may lead to slow clearing of contrast into the bladder. Apart from showing a fundal impress from the enlarged uterus, the bladder itself appears normal.

The appearances described may be present at the 8th week of pregnancy and are seen in most cases by the 6th month. After delivery the changes regress over a variable period of weeks, and by 10 to 12 weeks after delivery, the appearances should be normal. If they are not, there is strong evidence of a truly pathological hydronephrosis.

Because of the possible radiation hazards just discussed, pyelography is now rarely undertaken during pregnancy. However, the performance of an excretory pyelogram may occasionally be justified to visualize any possible structural abnormality in the urinary tract and to determine whether there is impairment of renal function in cases presenting as acute pyelonephritiis. The pyelogram in pregnancy may also give valuable information on the presence and position of calculi, and it may indicate a possible renal cause for hypertension found in pregnancy. When possible however, the clinician should be advised to withhold the examination until a suitable time (10 to 12 weeks) after delivery. If a pyelogram is performed during pregnancy the number of films taken should be kept to an absolute minimum.

3. THE DEVELOPING FETUS

DIAGNOSIS OF PREGNANCY

The fetus can usually be visualized radiographically at about the 16th week of gestation, although occasionally visualization is obtained two or three weeks earlier. Early visualization is assisted by a 'bone free' projection of the pelvis in which the tube is angled 15° towards the feet thus

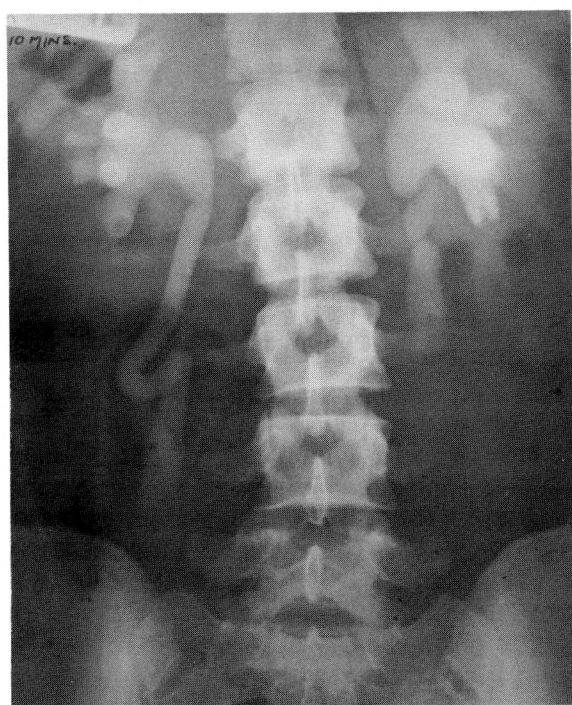

Fig. 47.1 Excretion pyelogram in early (16-week) pregnancy. Note the dilated calyces and ureters.

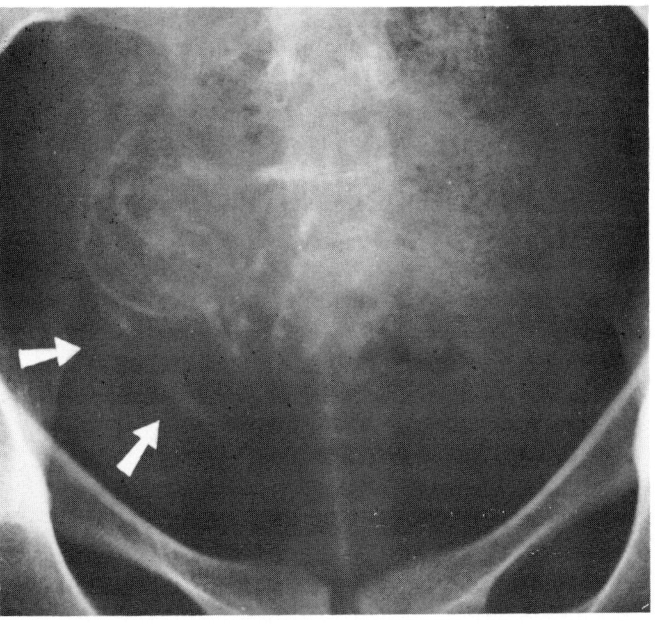

Fig. 47.2 Sixteen-week pregnancy. The foetal skeleton is just visible.

showing the pelvic cavity clear of any incursion of the bony walls (Fig. 47.2). In obese patients the fetus may not be identifiable till about the 20th week. Thereafter absence of fetal parts is a certain indication of the absence of normal pregnancy.

The fetus at an early stage appears as a series of fine calcific opacities; the skull vault, ribs and limb bones are seen as linear opacities and the spine as a series of dots. At this early stage only parts of the skeleton may be seen and a full visualization of cranium, thorax, spine and limbs is not to be expected.

Since the fetus is particularly at risk from radiation in the earlier part of pregnancy, radiology is no longer used to confirm pregnancy and ultrasound is now the investigation of choice. Occasionally the radiologist is called upon to exclude pregnancy in cases of diagnostic difficulty, such as suspected hydatiform mole. Here again ultrasound is now the investigation of choice (see Chapter 68).

ESTIMATION OF FETAL MATURITY

Estimation of fetal maturity may be requested in the later stages of pregnancy to assess the duration of gestation in cases requiring induction of labour or Caesarian section before term and also in cases of possible post-maturity. It is also helpful in cases where there is an apparent discrepancy between the uterine size and the period of amenorrhoea or when the duration of amenorrhoea is uncertain. Estimation of fetal maturity is also indicated in possible retardation of fetal growth.

The obstetrician has a variety of techniques on which he can call for assessment of gestational age and ultrasound has now become the method of choice. It is only where this is not available that conventional radiology may still be required. The main radiological methods available are: (1) those attempting to relate maturity to an exact measurement of a fetal part and (2) those based on particular features of the fetus shown either (a) on the plain film or (b) on amniography.

1. Maturity by bone measurement. This assessment is made by taking a cranial diameter or a limb bone length measured on the film which is then compared with a table or graph of standards to obtain gestational age. A variety of methods have been described using the femur, skull, radius, ulna or tibia. These measurements may be used directly or corrected for magnification using a nomogram.

2*a*. The most common method of assessing fetal maturity is from a plain film of the maternal abdomen. A single prone, oblique P.A. view is used. This view is quite feasible even in late pregnancy as long as the patient is well supported with pillows under the thighs and chest. The prone P.A. projection avoids relative magnification of the fetal head which can easily lead to the mistaken diagnosis of cephalopelvic disproportion or hydrocephalus. The oblique position almost always results in the fetal knees being projected clear of the maternal spine and allows any epiphyses in this region to be more easily seen. The best oblique projection results if the mother takes up the position which she finds most comfortable.

The features to be noted are the general size and stature of the fetus, the density of calcification of the

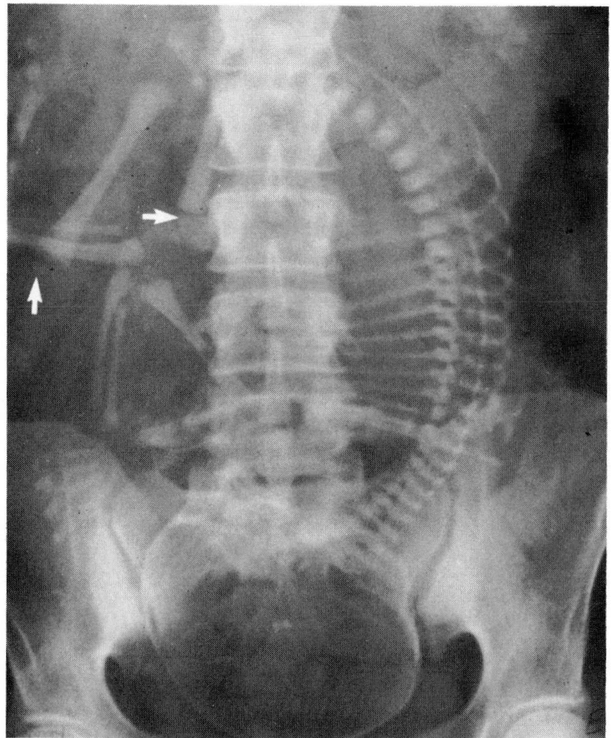

Fig. 47.3 The maturity of the fetus is at least 37 weeks as the lower femoral epiphyses are visible (arrows). The fetal subcutaneous fat line is seen over the back.

fetal cranium and the appearance of certain epiphyses. At 16 weeks the fetus is entirely contained in the pelvis and can just be seen as previously described, while at 36 weeks the uterus and fetus occupy the greater part of the abdomen and project into the epigastrium. Estimation of maturity is rendered more accurate as various epiphyses appear. Thus, the calcaneum appears at 26 weeks, the talus at 28 weeks, the lower femur at 37 weeks (Fig. 47.3) and the upper tibia at 38 weeks. Of these it should be noted that the talus and calcaneum can often be difficult to see and the upper tibial epiphysis is occasionally delayed. This leaves the lower femoral epiphysis as the most reliable criterion of assessment. The cuboid whose appearance has sometimes been recommended as indicating term is probably too variable to be of real use. In the last month of pregnancy the translucency of the fetal subcutaneous fat becomes visible as a dark line outlining the trunk. In a post-mature fetus all the epiphyses mentioned above should be visible, the cranial vault appears particularly well ossified and in a primagravida the head should be engaged in the pelvis.

Whenever a report assessing fetal age is made it is important that the clinical estimation of the duration of pregnancy both from the last menstrual period and the size of the uterus should be available. This enables the radiologist not only to think in terms of absolute figures but in terms of 'compatibility' or 'incompatibility' with the clinical findings. Assessment of maturity therefore rests on the general impression of size and development, certainly as far as the sixth or seventh month of pregnancy and a series of more definite indications of maturity which appear in the last 10 to 14 weeks. Accuracy of assessment is much greater in the last four weeks of pregnancy and whenever possible radiological examination should be delayed until this time. In spite of criticism which is mainly centred on the inevitable biological variation this method is well-proven to be of clinical value. It is wise, however, to allow a margin of two weeks in reporting fetal maturity owing to the approximation inherent in this method.

Variation in epiphyseal appearance in particular situations has been found by Russell and Rangecroft (1969). Twins and fetuses with spina bifida may show some delay in epiphyseal appearance while fetuses of diabetic mothers and anencephalic fetuses both show about one to two weeks acceleration of bone development. They noted that maternal toxaemia, hypertension and urinary infection had little effect.

2*b*. A rough estimate of maturity was at one time possible if amniography was performed. Approximately 6 ml of oily contrast (Myodil) were injected. A single film of the abdomen was taken between 8 and 24 hours after an injection and the extent to which the contrast outlined the fetus was noted. Before 38 weeks the skin of the trunk, head, limbs, fingers, toes and genitalia are shown. Between 38 and 40 weeks the outlining of the limbs and abdomen was patchy, while at term the contrast only adhered to the back and head. This method was of interest if an amniocentesis was to be performed for other examinations (chemistry, cytology, spectrometry). However, amniography is now obsolete as amniocentesis is preferably performed under ultrasound control.

FETAL POSITION AND PRESENTATION

The position of the fetus is described in the following terms:

1. **Lie.** The relationship of the fetus to the maternal axis; the fetal lie can be longitudinal, oblique or transverse (Fig. 47.4). A lie other than longitudinal may indicate a maternal pelvic mass, or placenta praevia.

2. **Presentation.** The fetal part nearest the internal os; the vertex usually presents (Fig. 47.5).

3. **Position.** The relationship of an arbitrary point on the presenting part to the maternal pelvis. Thus in a vertex presentation the position describes the relationship of the fetal occiput to the maternal pelvis. In the most common presentation the fetal occiput lies in the left anterior quadrant of the maternal pelvis (L.O.A.).

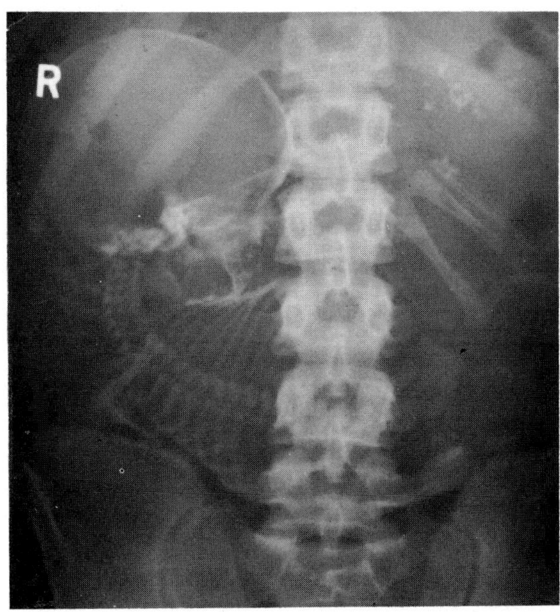

Fig. 47.4 Transverse lie.

4. **Attitude.** The relationship of the fetal parts to each other. The attitude is normally one of flexion. Extension, or extreme flexion in whole or in part, should be looked for. This may be of great importance in the diagnosis of intra-uterine death, and other fetal abnormalities.

The most usual description of the fetus would be a longitudinal lie, vertex presentation, left occipito-anterior position, and an attitude of normal flexion. It is clear that an accurate description of the fetal position, involving as it does a consideration of two planes cannot be obtained from a single film.

Thus from the P.A. film of the abdomen, it can be seen on which side the fetal back lies. A true lateral position is easily identified, but if the position is oblique, it is impossible from the P.A. film to be sure whether the fetal back lies in the anterior or posterior quadrant of that side of the maternal abdomen. The report should merely state in such a case, on which side the back lies or the abbreviation 'X' can be used to indicate that the anterior or posterior position cannot be determined.

Apart from the common variations of presentation, such as occiput to the right, occipito-posterior, or breech,

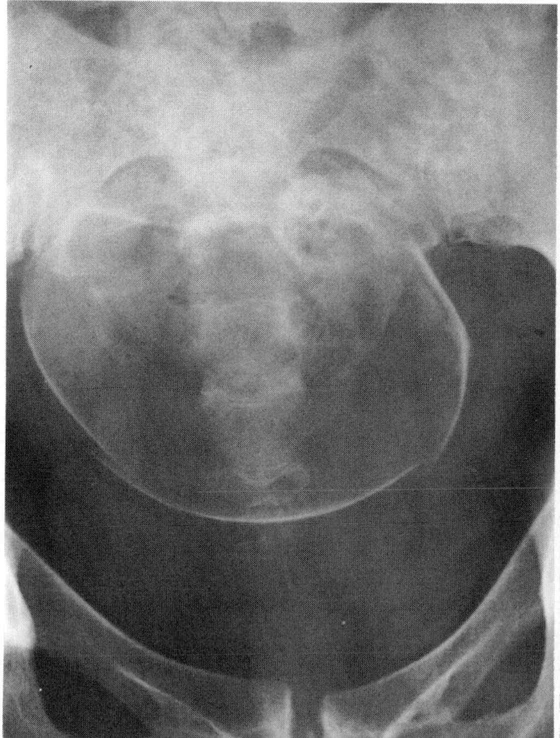

Fig. 47.5

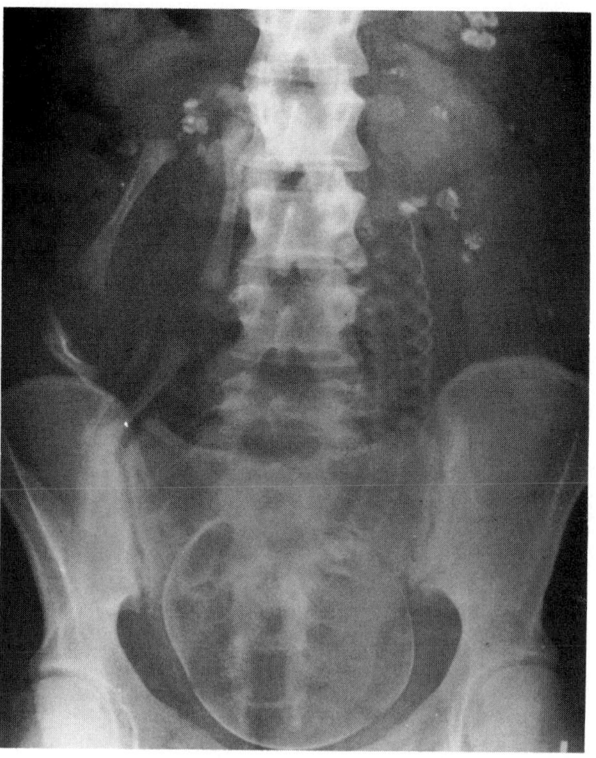

Fig. 47.6

Fig. 47.5 Longitudinal lie, vertex presentation, back to the left. There is a soft tissue shadow of the placenta at the fundus.

Fig. 47.6 Spalding's sign.

any abnormality of lie, attitude or presentation should arouse the suspicion of abnormality of the mother or fetus. A particular scrutiny of the film is then indicated for the following conditions which might be evident:

1. *Maternal.* Ovarian dermoids, uterine fibroids and abnormalities of size and shape of the pelvis.
2. *Fetal.* Placenta praevia, hydramnios, extra-uterine gestation, hydrops, multiple pregnancy, congenital fetal deformities, and fetal death.

FETAL DEATH AND OTHER ABNORMALITIES

The following fetal abnormalities may be demonstrated radiologically:

1. Fetal death
2. Extra-uterine pregnancy
3. Multiple pregnancy
4. Abnormal quantity of liquor amnii: hydramnios: oligamnios
5. Congenital abnormalities of the fetus:
   (*a*) Soft tissues
   (*b*) Cranium
   (*c*) Spine
   (*d*) Limbs
   (*e*) Systemic skeletal abnormalities.

1. Fetal death

Radiology may demonstrate:

1. *Spalding's sign.* This is the 'classical sign' of fetal death and is shown by disalignment and over-riding of the cranial bones (Figs 47.6 and 47.7). This sign may become evident between 4 and 15 days after death of the fetus and the deformity tends to increase with time. For correct interpretation the fetal skull must be reasonably well ossified; therefore the sign is not reliable in early pregnancy. It is important to note that Spalding's sign is often apparently present but of no significance after engagement of the head and particularly during labour, owing to normal moulding. Therefore it must be assessed with the greatest caution after the 36th week. Conversely, it is a most reliable sign in the period from the 26th to the 36th week of pregnancy in vertex presentations, and in breech presentations until term.
2. *Gas translucencies* may be seen in the fetal blood vessels of the chest and abdomen and also in the heart. When present they constitute certain evidence of fetal death (Fig. 47.8). The sign is transient as gas may come out of solution within 12 hours of fetal death, but tends to redissolve after a few days. It can only be identified in the last trimester of pregnancy. Free gas has also been recognized after fetal death under the cranium, in the superior saggital sinus, and in the spinal theca.
3. *An attitude of extreme flexion.* Like Spalding's sign, this may become evident only some days after fetal death and may not be well developed until as much as four weeks

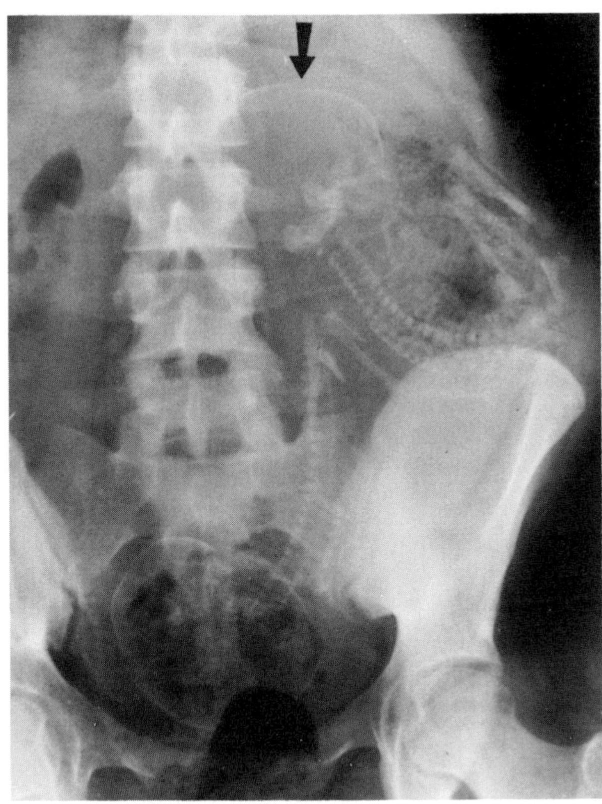

Fig. 47.7 Twins: the upper shows Spalding's sign (arrow).

after death of the fetus. Extreme flexion seen on the P.A. film must be viewed with caution as it can be a purely projectional phenomenon due to the particular lie of the foetus. A lateral view of the abdomen will often confirm or refute the suggestive evidence of the P.A. film. In very doubtful cases an erect film of the abdomen may be necessary to demonstrate either Spalding's sign or the position of flexion and so confirm fetal death. It may be noted that with development of extreme flexion and collapse of the skull, the thorax may collapse as well, these being the signs of macerated fetus (Fig. 47.9).

4. *Deuel's Halo sign.* This is due to elevation of the pericranial fat by underlying soft tissue oedema. The fine translucent fat line which should lie close to the cranium is lifted and so resembles a halo above the fetal cranium. The sign may appear within two days of fetal death but can only be seen in the last month or two of pregnancy. It is not considered to be a reliable sign.

5. *Failure to grow.* This of course requires two examinations at an interval of at least two, and preferably four weeks. It is useful when the evidence of one examination is inconclusive, and particularly in the first half of pregnancy. Placental insufficiency may also manifest itself by retarded growth of the fetus.

6. *A disparity between the clinical and radiological estimations of maturity* may arouse the suspicion of intra-uterine death. However, since the maternal estimate of the

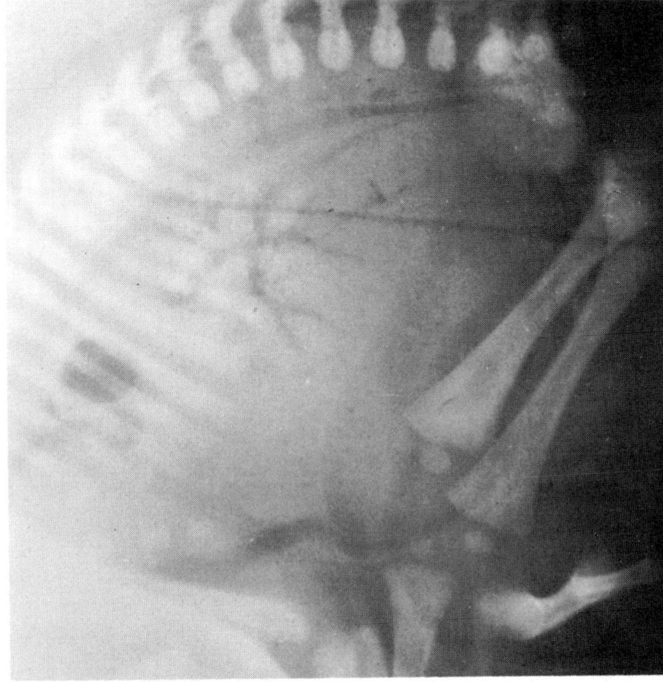

A

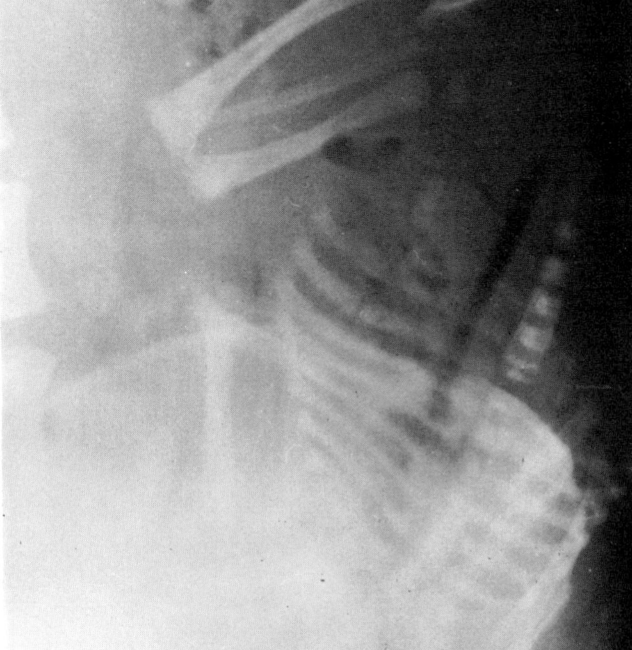

B

Fig. 47.8A and **B** Gas translucencies are seen in the heart, thoracic and abdominal blood vessels.

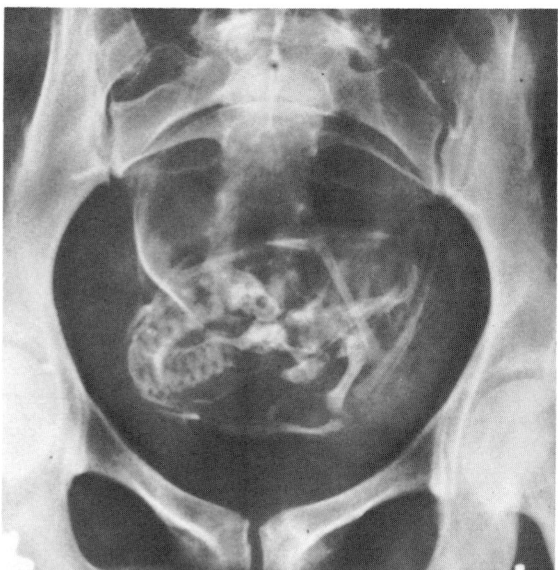

Fig. 47.9 Macerated fetus.

duration of amenorrhoea is frequently inaccurate, additional evidence of fetal death should be sought.

7. *Constancy of fetal position.* This is another sign requiring two examinations separated by an interval. Normally the fetus changes its attitude or position during the course of pregnancy. It is important to note any change of position or even minor changes of the limb attitudes.

2. Extra-uterine pregnancy

Tubal pregnancy usually terminates in rupture of the tube and presents as an acute emergency. Rarely pregnancy can continue outside the uterus even to full term. The radiological signs which may suggest this very rare situation are (Cockshott and Lawson, 1972);

1. An unusual lie, especially transverse
2. An abnormal fetal position, i.e. unusually high or low in the abdomen
3. An unusual fetal attitude; a limb stretched down into the maternal pelvis and a 'swimming' attitude are both said to be characteristic
4. Constancy of fetal attitude and position in repeated examinations and not associated with fetal death.
5. In the lateral view the fetal parts may either overlap the maternal spine or lie unusually close beneath the maternal abdominal wall
6. Unusual clarity of the fetus
7. Absence of the surrounding shadow of the uterus. A spurious shadow can be cast by a thick gestational membrane and omental adhesions
8. On the lateral view maternal gas shadows may overlie the fetus or lie anterior to it. The anterior view may show maternal gas shadows other than the rectum below the presenting part.

Calcification of the fetus (*lithopedion*) is an end result of extra-uterine gestation. Amniography, hysterography and angiography have all been used to confirm the diagnosis.

3. Multiple pregnancy

This is usually easy to recognize on the radiograph. It should be remembered that multiple pregnancy is associated with a higher incidence of fetal abnormalities than single pregnancies. Conjoined (Siamese) twins occur rarely, but may be suggested by (*a*) constancy of position between the fetuses in repeated examination, (*b*) a skeletal defect at the site of union, or (*c*) 'deflexion' of both fetal spines particularly when the fetuses face each other.

A gross discrepancy in size between twins may indicate the death of one. After a prolonged period of intra-uterine death one fetus may collapse and become compressed (fetus compressus) due to the growth of the other. If the dead twin lies low in the uterus it may lead to a persistent malpresentation of the surviving one.

4. Abnormal quantity of liquor amnii

1. *Hydramnios.* This is particularly associated with maternal diseases such as diabetes, toxaemia, twin pregnancy, or fetal abnormalities such as anencephaly and spina bifida. Evidence of fetal abnormality should therefore be sought on the film. The radiological sign of hydramnios is disproportion between the size of the uterus and the fetus. The latter is free to adopt an unusual attitude and position and lacks normal clarity and definition.

2. *Oligamnios.* The uterus appears closely applied around the fetus which may appear excessively flexed. Oligamnios may be associated with placental insufficiency and congenital renal abnormalities in the fetus including absence of the kidneys.

5. Congenital abnormalities of the fetus

(*a*) The soft tissues

Hydrops foetalis (Fig. 47.10), a consequence of erythroblastosis, is often suggested by the characteristic 'Buddha attitude' of the fetus. There is a loss of normal kyphotic curvature; the arms are held at right angles to the body, and the thighs are widely abducted due to the gross subcutaneous oedema. In addition, there may be loss of the normal halo of subcutaneous fat around the fetus, due to the oedema. Elevation of the pericranial fat produces a halo as in Deuel's sign of fetal death. The lower rib cage may be flared due to the hepatosplenomegaly and the skeleton may look frail.

Soft-tissue *tumours of the neck*, *thyroid tumours* and *cystic hygroma* can cause extension of the neck and lead to a face or brow presentation. They are not however

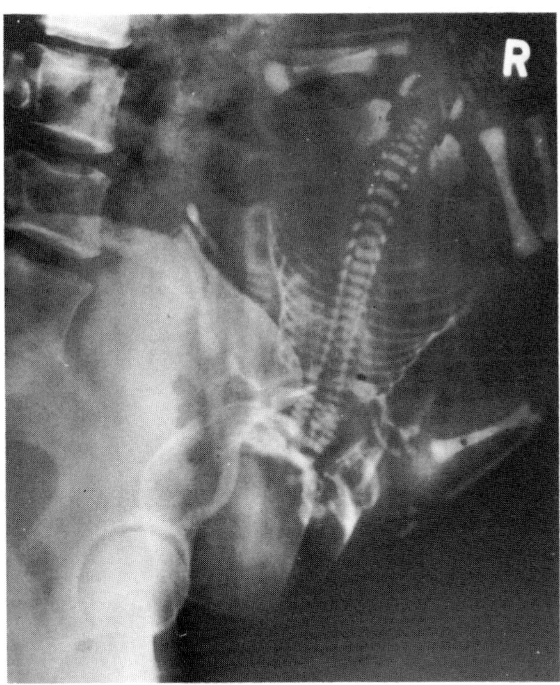

Fig. 47.10 Hydrops foetalis.

associated with bony anomalies of the cervical spine as in *iniencephaly* (see below).

(*b*) **Congenital abnormalities of the cranium**

Hydrocephalus (Fig. 47.11). There is a disproportion between the large size of the cranium and the normal facial bones. The cranial vault is poorly calcified and may even be difficult to see. As already noted, the diagnosis should be made from the P.A. film only.

Anencephaly (Fig. 47.12). The cranial vault fails to develop and the bones of the skull base and the face are often maldeveloped. The cervical spine is also abnormal, often showing shortening with separation of the pedicles. The condition usually occurs in female fetuses.

Craniolacunae. In this condition the cranial vault ossifies irregularly there being scalloped defects on the inner aspect. These may result in the vault being reduced to membrane thickness in parts. This is frequently associated with other congenital abnormalities of the nervous system such as spina bifida and meningocoele, encephalocoele, hydrocephalus and microcephalus.

Cyclops. There is a very rare anomaly in which only one orbit, centrally placed, develops.

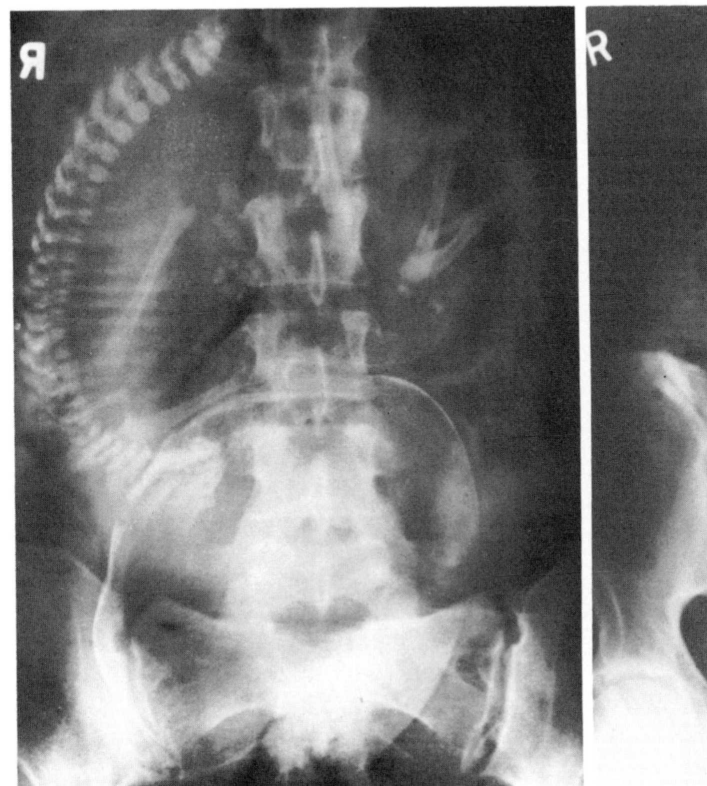

Fig. 47.11 Hydrocephalus.

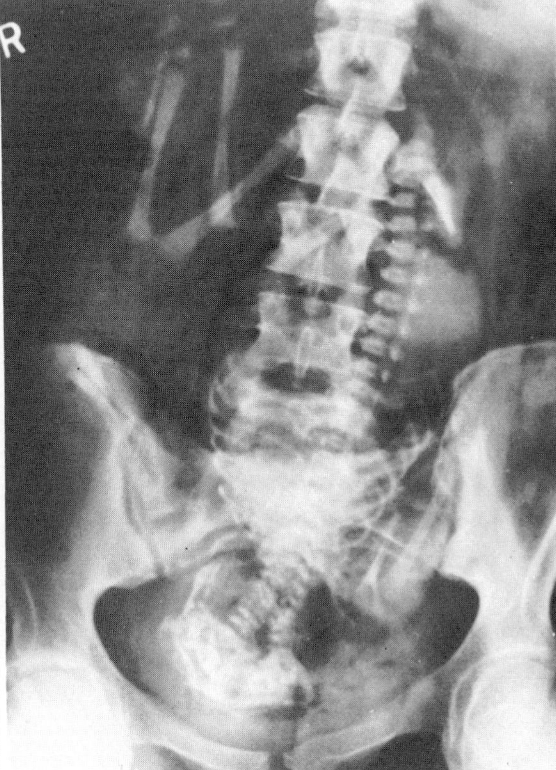

Fig. 47.12 Anencephaly.

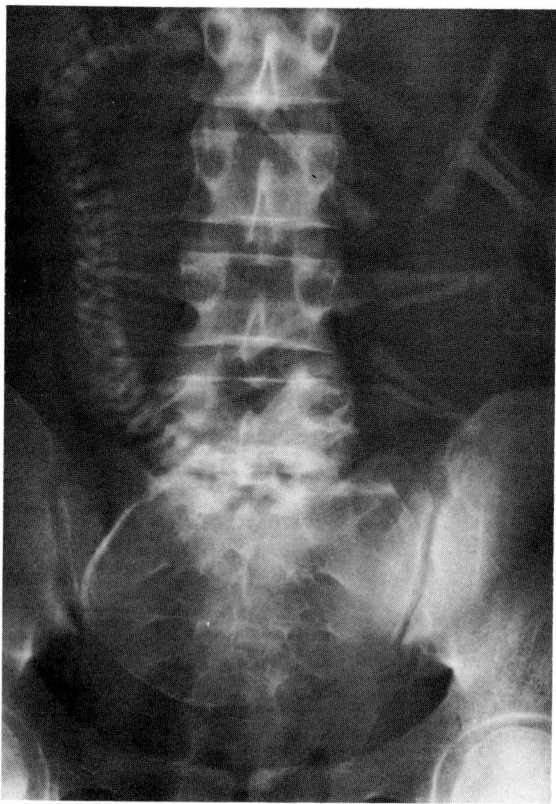

Fig. 47.13 Kyphosis and lumbar myelocele.

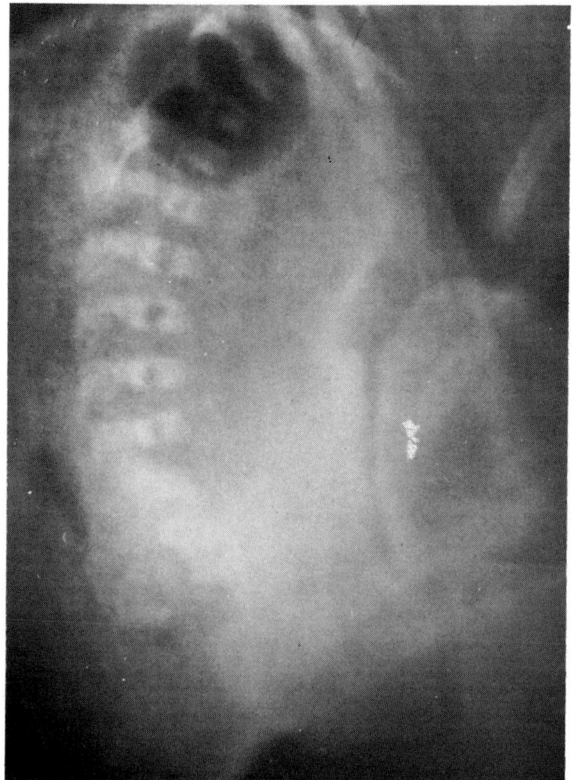

Fig. 47.14 Coronal cleft vertebrae.

(*c*) Congenital abnormalities of the spine

Spina bifida in its more severe degrees can be identified antenatally. At the defect the pedicles are widely separated and there is often a local kyphos (Fig. 47.13).

Iniencephaly. In this condition a cervical spina bifida is associated with a fixed extension of the head. The basi-occiput is abnormally developed and there may be a bony bar connecting it to the cervical spine.

Fetal cervical hyperextension in breech presentation. This posture, the so-called 'star gazing fetus' is associated with Down's syndrome and has also been noted in association with the umbilical cord being wound around the fetus's neck.

Hemivertebra may be suggested by an angular kypho-scoliosis, but accurate identification *in utero* is likely to be difficult.

Coronal cleft vertebra (Fig. 47.14). This is a developmental variation in the ossification of one, or a few, thoracic or lumbar vertebral bodies. Failure of fusion of the primary ossification centres leads to the presence of a translucent longitudinal band in the calcific density of the vertebra as seen in lateral view. The major interest of the condition lies in its being almost completely confined to males thus enabling an antenatal diagnosis of sex to be made. Subsequently ossification continues normally.

(*d*) Abnormal development of limbs

Projectional distortion and foreshortening makes the accurate diagnosis of these deformities difficult on a single film. Critical evaluation of films taken in more than one plane are therefore required. The main types of congenital abnormalities are:

Symmelia: fusion of the limbs in whole or in part (Mermaid).

Amelia: the absence of a limb.

Hemimelia: the absence of the distal segment of a limb.

Phocomelia: the absence of the proximal segment of a limb. This was the characteristic thalidomide defect.

(*e*) Systemic skeletal abnormalities

Osteogenesis imperfecta, osteopetrosis and achondroplasia may occasionally be recognized by their characteristic appearances. Lesions showing characteristic changes at the metaphyses may also be occasionally recognized with fortunate projections and high quality films. These conditions include congenital syphilis and severe hypophosphatasia. In the latter, bony defects in the cranium also occur.

Cleidocranial dysostosis can be diagnosed from the lack of density of the cranium and the absence of clavicles.

(*f*) Fused (Siamese) twins

The radiological features in the diagnosis of Siamese twins have already been noted under multiple pregnancy. The condition is described by the site of fusion thus:

Craniopagus: fusion of the head, usually parietal region.
Thoracopagus: fusion at the thorax, usually on the anterior aspect.
Xiphopagus: fusion at the sternum.
Omphalopagus: fusion at the umbilicus.
Pyopagus: fusion at the buttocks.

INTRA-UTERINE BLOOD TRANSFUSION

This is a technique devised in an attempt to save fetuses in whom a severe haemolytic process has developed before the 34th week and therefore in whom survival is unlikely following induction of labour. The indications depend on the maternal anti-Rh titre and the bilirubin concentration in the amniotic fluid obtained by amniocentesis.

As a preliminary, the fetal gut is opacified by injecting 10 ml of 65 per cent Hypaque into the amniotic cavity 12 hours prior to the transfusion. The mother should be heavily sedated (by intramuscular morphine and Phenergan) prior to the procedure. Metal markers are attached to the maternal abdomen and a preliminary A.P. film taken for general orientation using the overcouch tube. The introduction of the needle is carried out under intensifier screening. A 16 s.w.g. needle and stilette is then introduced vertically through the maternal abdomen and is aimed at the opacified fetal gut. When it is thought that the needle tip is in the fetal peritoneal cavity 2 ml of Hypaque are rapidly injected. If the needle tip is correctly sited the contrast medium will be seen to spread around the coils of gut. It is an advantage next to substitute the needle by an epidural catheter which is threaded through the lumen of the needle. After withdrawal of the needle the position of the catheter tip is similarly checked by another rapid injection of 2 ml of contrast. The transfusion is then given through the epidural catheter and may be up to 120 ml of Group O Rh-negative blood.

The best results are obtained when initial transfusion is carried out between the 28th and 32nd week of gestation. The method itself has a high mortality, between 15–25 per cent of fetuses dying within 48 hours of transfusion, and the results are worst when transfusion is carried out on a fetus before the 28th week.

Results of the technique are questionable. The use of plasma-phoresis to reduce maternal antibodies and prophylactic Rh-immunoglobulin may reduce the frequency with which intra-uterine transfusions are indicated (*British Medical Journal*, 1977).

4. THE DETERMINATION OF PLACENTAL SITE

The indications for determination of placental sites are (1) the occurrence of an antepartum haemorrhage and (2) prior to amniocentesis. The latter indication is to prevent possible penetration of the placenta by the amniocentesis needle.

Antepartum haemorrhage is classified as 'unavoidable' when there is placenta praevia and 'accidental' when it occurs with normal implantation of placenta. The knowledge as to whether the haemorrhage is associated with placenta praevia would affect the obstetrician's management of the case.

Placenta praevia is defined as implantation of the placenta, in whole or in part, into the lower uterine segment. The lower uterine segment extends upwards for about 6 cm (3 in) from the internal os during late pregnancy and undergoes dilatation in labour, thus disturbing the placenta and leading to haemorrhage. Four types of placenta praevia are described:

I. The placental margin just encroaches on the lower segment
II. The placental margin reaches the internal os
III. The placenta covers the internal os when it is closed only
IV. The placenta covers the internal os even when the os is fully dilated.

Type I is sometimes known as *lateral*, and types III and IV as *central* placenta praevia.

Since the placenta, uterus and liquor amnii all cast a similar soft-tissue density on the radiograph, the radiographic demonstration of the placental site can prove difficult. Nevertheless, a high degree of accuracy is essential if the procedure is to be useful to the clinician. Radiology, if successful, may avert the somewhat hazardous procedure of digital examination through the internal os, but it must also be accomplished with the minimum number of radiographic exposures.

The methods available are:

1. Plain films
2. Techniques not using conventional X-rays:
   (*a*) Ultrasound;
   (*b*) Radio-isotopes;
   (*c*) Thermography.

Other methods which have been used in the past included cystography, arteriography and amniography. These are now obsolete being invasive methods. Among the pararadiological imaging techniques listed above neither radio-isotopes not thermography can approach the accuracy of ultrasound which is now without question the method of choice.

1. Plain films (soft-tissue technique)

The determination of placental site by plain films may be by the positive demonstration of the placental site (Fig.

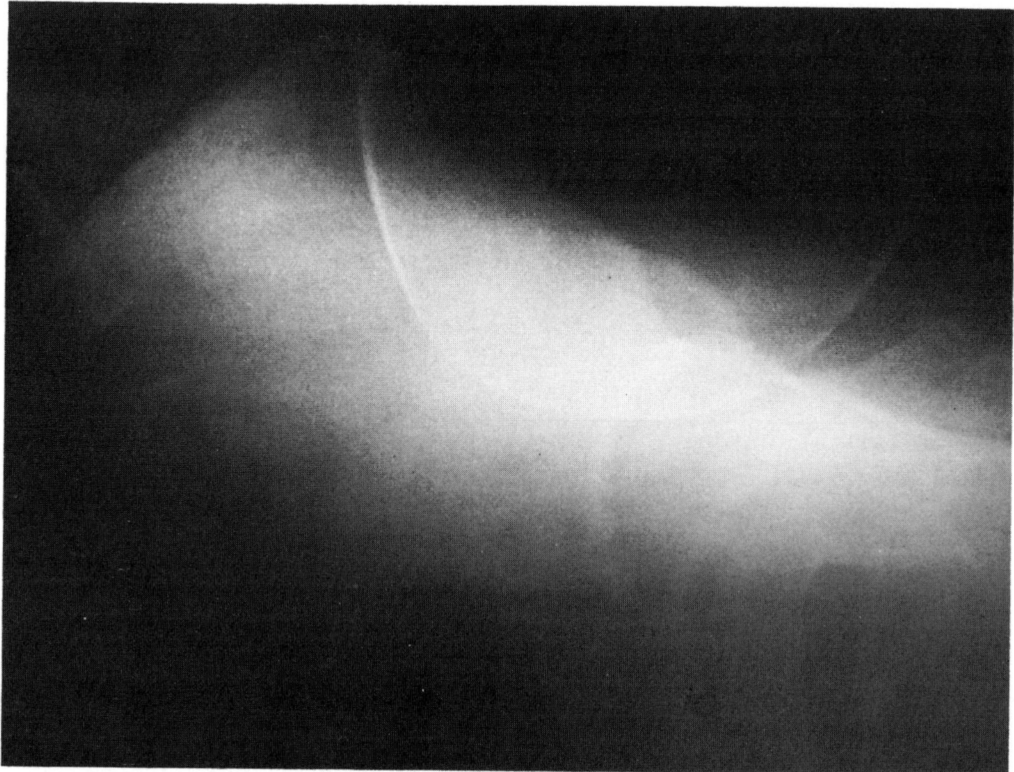

A

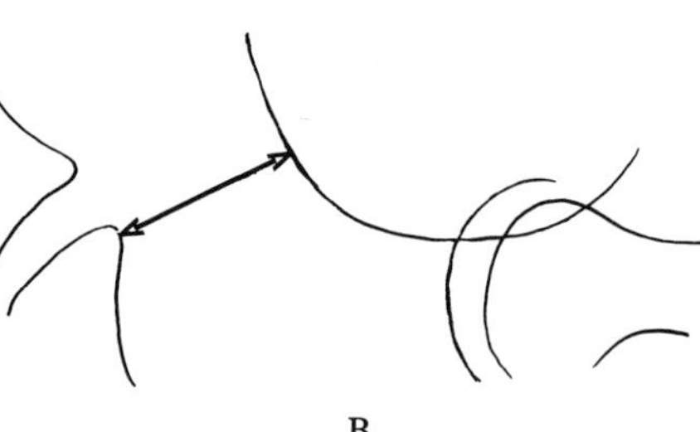

B

Fig. 47.15 Posterior placenta praevia shown on lateral film. (B) Diagram of (A). The arrows indicate the enlarged, irreducible gap between the fetal head and the sacral promontory.

47.16) and by the exclusion of placenta praevia from a consideration of the relationship of the presenting head to the maternal pelvis. These methods are complementary and either, or both, may be applicable in any individual case.

The demonstration of the placenta. Although the various soft-tissues cast a similar density radiographic shadows, the presence of translucent lines such as fetal subcutaneous fat, and gas and faeces in the maternal colon, often give quite a good outline to the pregnant uterus. The general thickness of the uterine wall is about 1 cm while it thickens in the region of the placenta to become approximately 5 cm thick in the last eight weeks of pregnancy. Calcification in the placenta may occur in 20 per cent of patients near term and thus help localization.

Head-pelvis relationships. In the P.A. view the presenting head occupies the mid-plane as it engages in the pelvis. A placenta praevia will hinder engagement and displace the head away from its normal mid position. In order to be sure that the engagement is prevented by placenta praevia only, the rectum and bladder should be empty before the examination begins. Specific enquiries should be made and the examination delayed if necessary till after the patient has been to the toilet for this purpose.

An erect or semi-erect film should be taken with the patient placed on a tilting table at approximately 45° so that gravity may most effectively aid engagement of the head. Assistance can be given by means of a binder or pressure with a gloved hand.

The following possibilities may emerge:

1. The head is engaged: this almost entirely excludes placenta praevia.

2. There is a gap of over 2 cm between the sacral promontory and the fetal head which is not engaged. This is in favour of a posteriorly sited placenta praevia (Figs 47.15A and B).

3. There is a gap of over 2 cm between the symphysis pubis and the fetal head which is not engaged. This is in favour of an anteriorly sited placenta praevia.

4. The issue remains in doubt.

2. Techniques not using conventional X-rays

1. *Ultrasound.* Ultrasonic placentography is now generally accepted as the method of choice, wherever available (see Ch. 68 for a full description).

2. *Radio-isotopes.* The placental sinuses accumulate larger quantities of injected radio-isotope (e.g. 0·5–1·0 mCi Tc^{99m}-human serum albumin) than the surrounding uterus and the method has proved reasonably accurate in placental localization with minimal radiation risk.

Anterior and lateral projections taken on a gamma camera or rectilinear scanner will demonstrate the placental site. Point source markers placed in the vagina

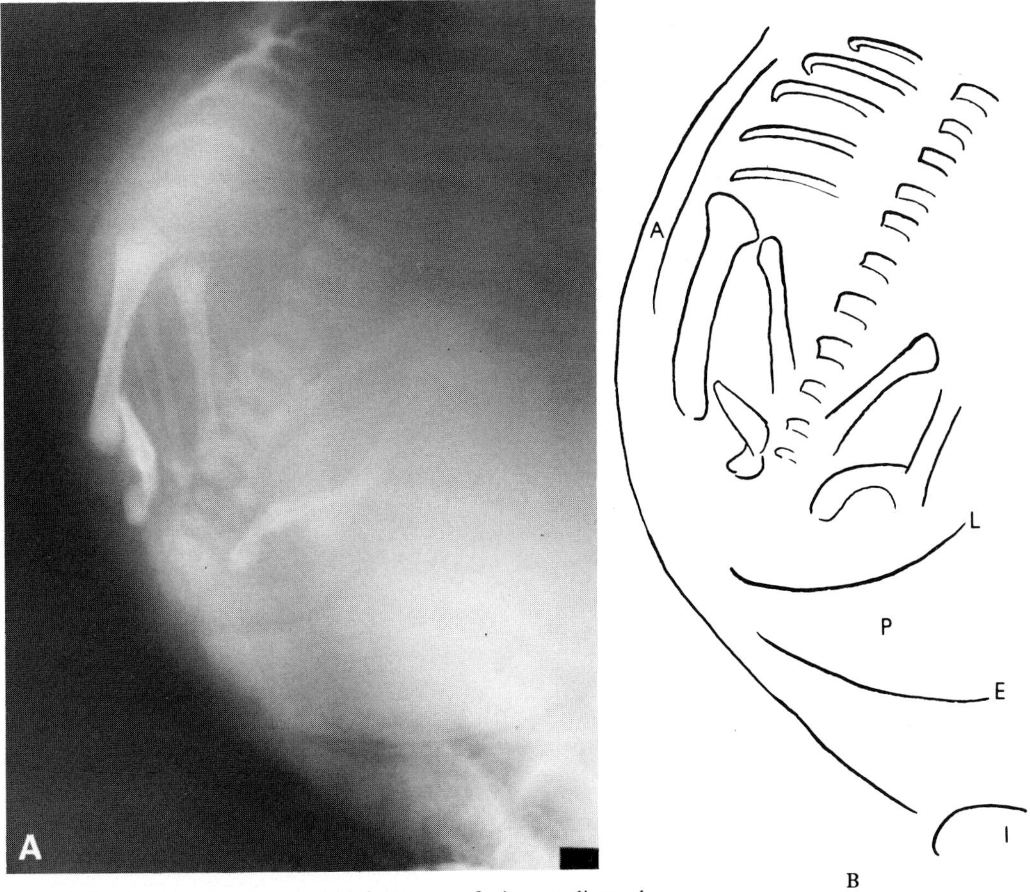

Fig. 47.16 Anterior placenta praevia shown on soft-tissue radiograph. (B) Diagram of (A). I = iliac crest. A = anterior wall of uterus. P = placenta outlined by foetal subcutaneous fat line (L) and the maternal extraperitoneal fat (E).

and on the symphysis pubis make localization more accurate.

3. *Thermography*. The natural emission of infra-red radiation from the body can be detected by an appropriate receiver and recorded on a scan. The placenta being more vascular than the surrounding tissue gives a larger infra-red emission, but to date the results of thermographic placentography have been disappointing.

5. PELVIMETRY

The subject of pelvimetry is considered under the following headings:

1. Clinical indications.
2. The obstetric features of the pelvis.
3. The radiographic technique.
4. The interpretation of results.
5. Additional methods.

1. Clinical indications

The clinical indications for pelvimetry arise when the obstetrician considers there is some likelihood of cephalo-pelvic disproportion. The specific indications in order of importance are:

1. Persistent breech presentation, particularly in primigravidae.
2. Following difficulties during a previous delivery which terminated in a difficult forceps or a non-elective Caesarian section. Pelvimetry is performed as a post-natal examination prior to any ensuing pregnancy.
3. During prolonged labour to assess progress.
4. Failure of the head to engage in a primigravida after the 36th week.
5. Women in whom pelvic deformity is suspected, e.g. patients with old fractures of the pelvis, congenital or rachitic deformity, or deformity in association with spinal or hip abnormality.

2. Obstetric features of the pelvis

The model female pelvis has been described as showing an inlet with smooth, well-curved margins, the transverse diameter lies well forward to give a moderate depth to the posterior segment, the fore pelvis is wide and smooth.

The ratio of the conjugate diameter to the transverse

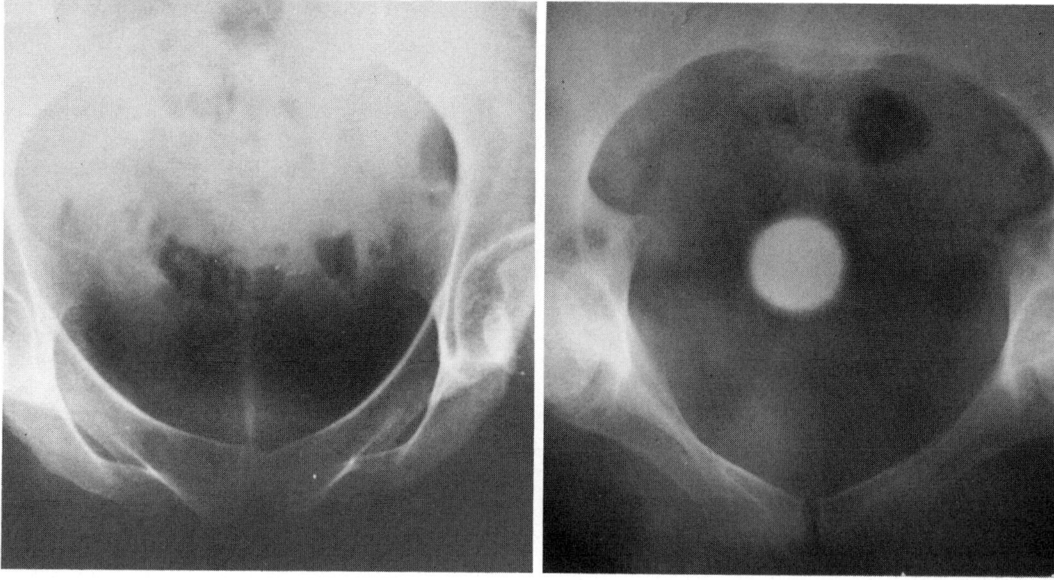

Fig. 47.17 Gynaecoid inlet.

Fig. 47.18 Android inlet. The round opacity is an artefact.

diameter is approximately 11 : 13. The subpubic arch has the shape of a wide Norman arch and its angle measures 80° to 90°. The pelvic side walls are straight and show only a minor convergence from above downwards.

The ischial spines are not large and they point somewhat posteriorly. The sacrum presents a substantial anterior concavity, longitudinally and transversely: five segments only should be present. The sacrococcygeal shelf is not unduly prominent and continues the smooth curve of the sacrum without an abrupt forward deviation. The sacrosciatic notches are moderately wide and smooth.

Numerous attempts have been made to classify the large variety of pelves that are encountered. The terminology of Caldwell and Moloy (1938) is widely used. They endeavoured to classify pelves into four main groups depending on their anatomical characteristics. Their system became cumbersome, since the four primary inlet types had to be subdivided in order to accommodate the varieties encountered in practice, and because the lower part of the pelvis did not necessarily conform with the upper. Since their terms are widely recognized they can be used to describe inlet shapes concisely, providing it is

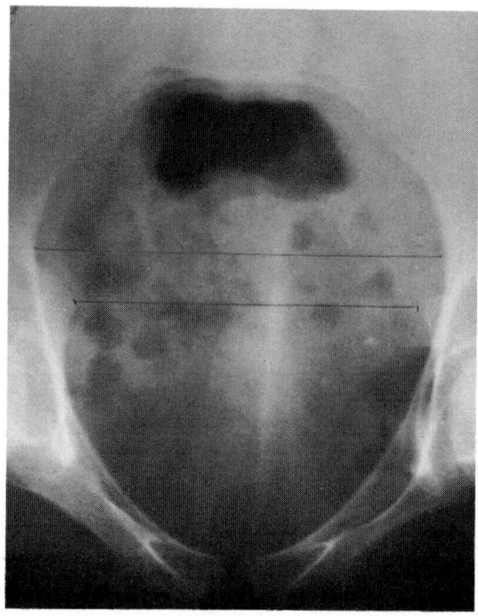

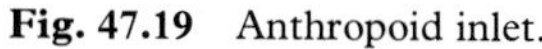

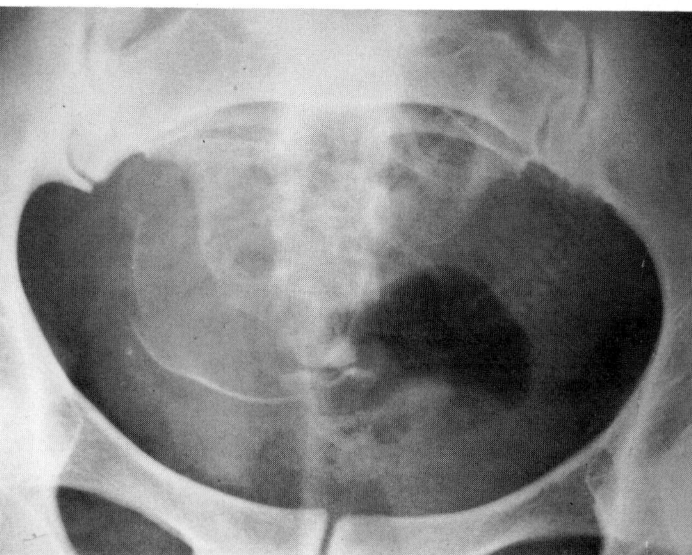

Fig. 47.19 Anthropoid inlet.

Fig. 47.20 Platypelloid inlet.

made clear that the term is restricted to the inlet, while the other major pelvic features are described in terms of variation from the ideal.

The four basic pelvic inlets are:

1. *Gynaecoid* (Fig. 47.17): the optimum round pelvic brim;

2. *Android* (Fig. 47.18): a triangular brim shape said to be characteristic of the male pelvis. The inlet diameters are not necessarily any different from the gynaecoid, but the maximum transverse diameter is displaced posteriorly, thus flattening the posterior segment and causing the anterior segment to take on a triangular or wedge shape.

3. *Anthropoid* (Fig. 47.19): the inlet is of a long oval shape and the conjugate is greater than the transverse. If the dimensions are small overall, the inlet is described as transversely contracted.

4. *Platypelloid* (Fig. 47.20): broad or 'flat' at the inlet, the transverse diameter being well in excess of the conjugate.

The fact that a pelvic inlet is not of gynaecoid shape does not imply that difficulty will occur at the inlet for an obstetrically adequate pelvis may have any of these inlet shapes. The actual measurements must be taken into account in assessing pelvic inlet capacity. The shape does sometimes determine the mode of engagement of the fetal head whose sagittal plane tends to engage parallel to the long diameter of the pelvic inlet.

The qualitative evaluation of the pelvis would therefore consist of a description of the inlet shape, possibly in one of the above terms, and relevant comments on the shape of the sacrum and lumbosacral and sacrococcygeal promontories: the shape of the sacrosciatic notches; the prominence and major direction of projection, posteriorly or medially of the ischial spines; the parallelism of the pelvic side walls and the shape of the subpubic arch.

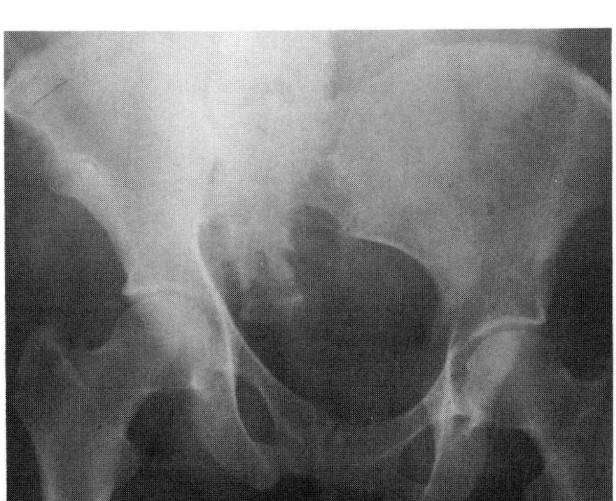

A

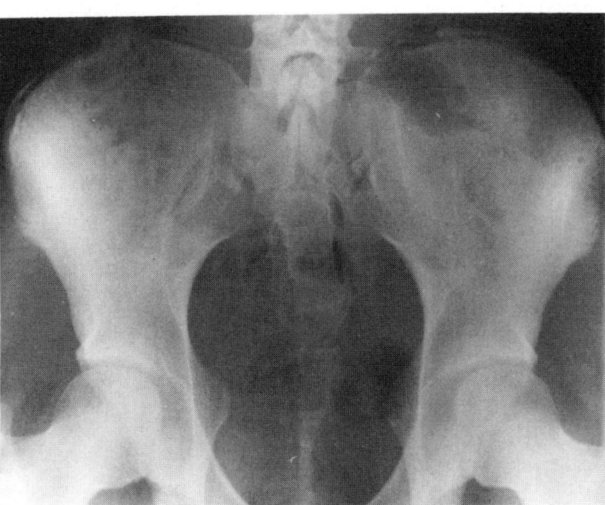

B

Fig. 47.21 (A) Nagele pelvis: there is asymmetrical deformity of the inlet. (B) Robert pelvis; note the hypoplasia of the sacral alae.

The abnormal pelvis

The shape of the pelvis may become abnormal as a result either of congenital or of acquired disease.

Congenital abnormalities

Achondroplasia. The pelvis in achondroplasia usually has a severely contracted conjugate, while the invariable lordosis results in a prominent lumbo-sacral promontory and a steep inclination of the pelvic inlet. These features hinder engagement, although the fetal head is of normal size, and an elective Caesarian section is often indicated.

The Nagele pelvis (Fig. 47. 21A). One sacral ala is aplastic which results in a small and asymmetric pelvis. The condition is rare.

The Robert pelvis (Fig. 47.21B). Here, both sacral alae also fail to develop, and the pelvic inlet is reduced to a narrow ellipse.

Acquired abnormalities

Trauma. Severe pelvic trauma may lead to pelvic deformity which may affect the cephalo-pelvic relationship. The result depends on the nature and severity of the injury.

Metabolic diseases (rickets: osteomalacia). The bone softening allows the weight-bearing areas (that is, the sacrum and the hip joints) to come together. Minor degrees of deformity may reduce only the conjugate, but in severe osteomalacia the cavity can be reduced to a triradiate slit, and an absolute obstruction to labour.

Spondylolisthesis. Minor degrees are of little importance, but when severe, the luxated lumbar vertebral body may impinge on the pelvic inlet. In such cases the conjugate should be measured from the antero-inferior angle of the displaced vertebra, in order to assess the functional reduction of this diameter. In addition, the deformity distorts the normal axis of descent, which may retard progress.

Hip disease (septic and tuberculous arthritis, congenital dislocation (Fig. 47.22) etc.). In association with the diseased hip, the bony pelvis on the same side often appears small and atrophic. The pelvic cavity, however, is usually unaffected, and may even be capacious.

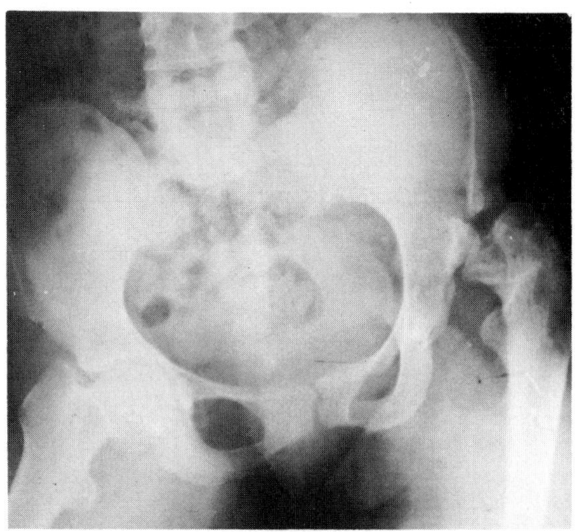

Fig. 47.22 Pelvis showing asymmetry as a result of congenital dislocation of hip.

Poliomyelitis. This may affect the pelvis in two ways, depending on the distribution of the paralysis. Paralysis of the hip muscles produces a unilateral pelvic atrophy as with hip disease. Spinal paralysis results in a lumbar kyphoscoliosis. The pelvic inlet may become quite asymmetric with a relative smallness of the cavity on one side. The sacrum may adopt a relatively vertical position as a result of the kyphosis, so that the axes of the sacrum and pubis converge. The pubosacral dimension may be so reduced as to cause significant outlet contraction.

Tuberculosis and osteomyelitis of the spine. These give rise to a kyphotic deformity which if in the lumbar region may affect the pelvis. The sacrum is drawn upwards and rotated in relation to the innominate bone so that the pubosacral diameter is reduced while the inlet conjugate remains adequate.

3. Radiographic technique

The radiographic objectives are:

1. To produce films which will show the main anatomical features and
2. To allow measurements to be taken which, after the appropriate correction, will give an accurate measurement of the pelvic dimensions.

Thus both a qualitative and quantitative assessment can be carried out. These two aspects of pelvic assessment must be stressed for they are essential to form a useful radiological obstetric opinion.

The measurements taken directly on the films are subject to a geometric enlargement which must be reduced by an appropriate correction factor. This is:

$$\frac{\text{Distance of appropriate plane of pelvis from focal spot}}{\text{Focus film distance}}$$

The denominator (i.e. the F.F.D.) in the correction factor is arbitrarily fixed at 100 cm. To obtain the numerator a direct measurement is taken from an appropriate landmark to the film cassette or table top. In the latter case an allowance of 5 cm (2 in) must be added to the patient–table top distance to allow for the distance from the table top to the film in the Bucky tray. The patient–film distance is then subtracted from the F.F.D. to give the patient–focus distance, i.e. the numerator.

The widespread use of pocket calculators has made the labour of constructing correction charts superfluous.

Four views may be of use in pelvimetry:

1. Erect lateral view of the pelvis
2. Supine A.P. of pelvis
3. Thom's inlet view
4. Outlet view of the sub-pubic arch.

1. The *erect lateral view* (Fig. 47.23A) is taken with the patient standing against the vertical Bucky or a vertical film holder with a grid cassette, and positioned to give a true lateral projection. The distance from natal cleft to film is measured and checked against the symphysis pubis to film distance. Both measurements should be the same. The X-ray beam is centred 5 to 8 cm above the greater trochanter and coned to cover a 30 cm × 40 cm film, vertically placed.

2. A *supine* (Fig. 47.24A) view of the abdomen is obtained with a vertical beam centred 5 cm to 8 cm (2 to 3 in) above the pubis and coned to cover a 30 cm × 40 cm film (12 in × 15 in). The symphysis–table top distance between the patient's thighs should be measured.

3. The *inlet* view is obtained by sitting the patient on the horizontal table. She should be in a semi-reclining position, well supported and arch her back. A proper back rest is a useful accessory. The inlet plane should be parallel to the film and checked by obtaining equal distances for symphysis pubis to table top and posterior superior iliac spine (skin dimple) to table top. The tube is centred 5 cm to 8 cm (2 to 3 in) above the symphysis and coning should permit the whole of the pelvic brim to be seen on a 30 cm × 40 cm (12 in × 15 in) film.

4. The *outlet* view requires the patient to sit directly on a transversely placed 24 cm × 30 cm (10 in × 12 in) grid cassette with thighs drawn well apart and leaning well forward so that the lower part of the symphysis

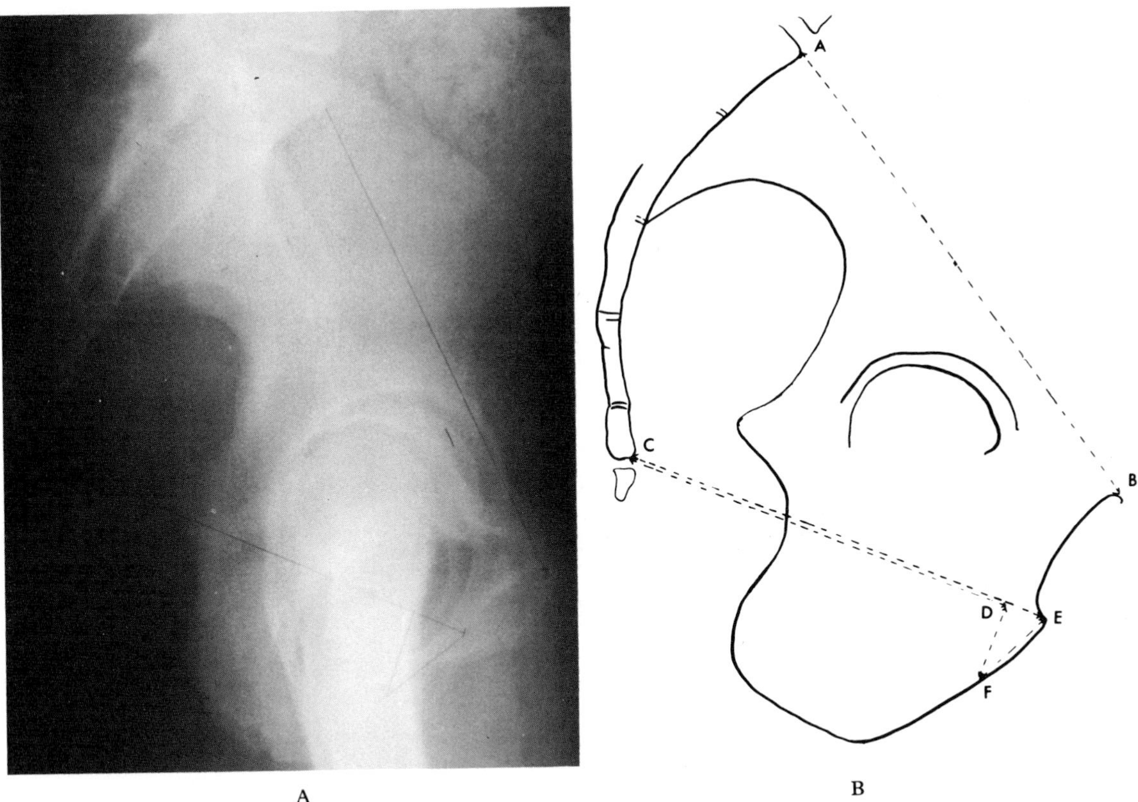

Fig. 47.23 (A) Lateral pelvimetry showing measurement lines. (B) Tracing of A. The letters refer to the lines described in the text.

comes in close proximity to the film. The vertical beam is centred over the middle of the sacrum and the coning should allow the full extent of the inferior ischiopubic rami to be seen.

In the first and last projections the inherent contrast range involved and the super-imposition of other structures may mean that the important structures are a little difficult to see. However, with the use of a bright viewing light it is possible to see all the necessary end points in properly produced radiographs.

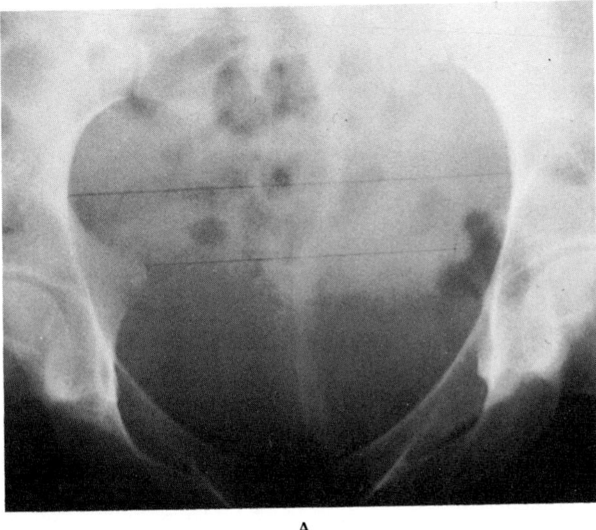

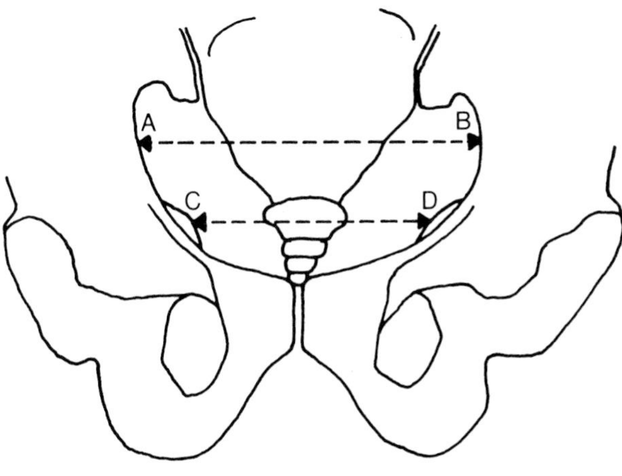

Fig. 47.24 (A) Supine pelvimetry film showing measurement lines. (B) Tracing of supine film showing the measurement lines. The side walls of the pelvis are heavily marked.

Observations

Erect lateral film (Fig. 47.23A and B). The prominence of the lumbosacral and sacrococcygeal junctions are well seen. Any reduction of the conjugate due to spondylolisthesis can be seen and measured, and the form of the sacral curvature should be clearly projected.

The overall inclination of the sacrum relative to the pubic body should be assessed; that is, does the sacrum incline away from the pubis so that the A.P. dimensions increase down through the pelvis from the inlet to the outlet, or do the sacrum and pubis tend to converge to cause outlet narrowing and 'funnel pelvis'. The sacral inclination is reflected in the sacro-sciatic notches. With backward inclination of the sacrum the sacrosciatic notches are wide and rounded, the angle subtended by the limbs of the notch being over 90°. When the sacral inclination is towards the pubis the notches become narrower and the subtended angle is acute. Backward pointing ischial spines are seen in this film.

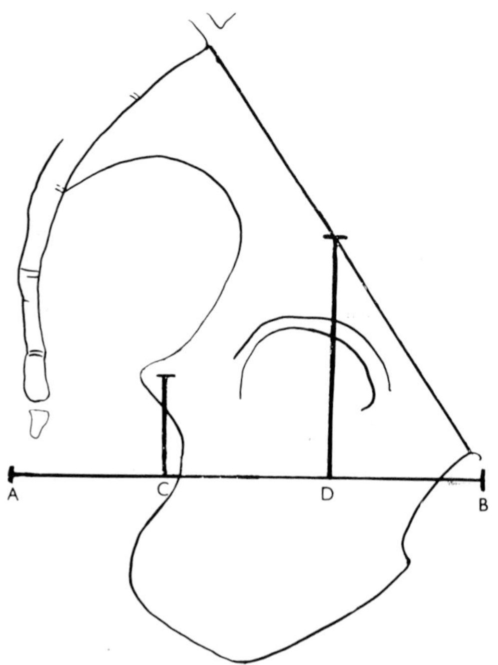

Fig. 47.25 Tracing of lateral view showing the ischial spines and the maximum transverse diameter of the inlet to lie at approximately two thirds (AC) and one third (AD) of the symphysis-film distance (AB) as measured for the supine film measurement correction.

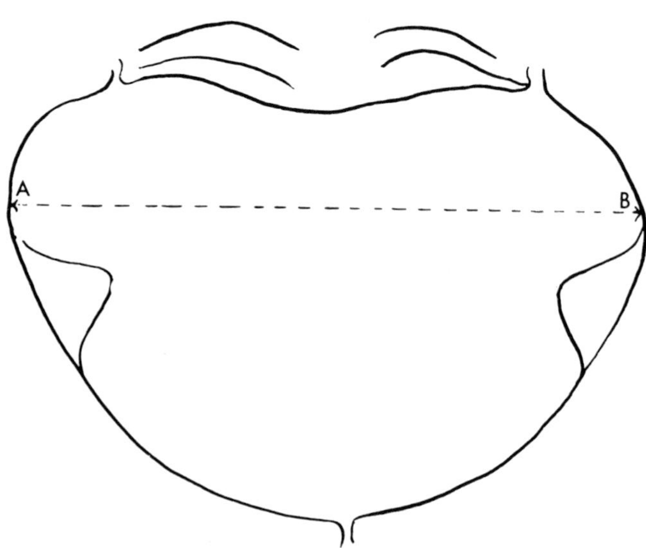

Fig. 47.26 Tracing of inlet view showing measurement for inlet transverse diameter.

The following measurements are taken. The *true conjugate* from the upper and posterior part of the body of the pubis to the sacral promontory, i.e. A.B. in Fig. 47.23B and the distance of the lower part of the body of the pubis to the lowermost fixed point of the sacrum (C.E.). This *pubosacral* diameter is referred to by some authors as the A.P. of the cavity, and by others as the A.P. of the outlet. As will be explained later, this view is also used to determine the 'available A.P. of the outlet'. When the fetal head is engaged, it is on this film that the biparietal dimensions can usually be measured with the greatest accuracy. The same reduction factor is applied to this as is used for the other dimensions in this midplane.

The Supine A.P. view (Fig. 47.24). This is used for a general appreciation of the pelvis and to show any gross deformities. The pelvic side walls show as dense cortical lines. In a good obstetric pelvis they converge just perceptibly towards the outlet. Obvious convergence suggests 'funnelling' at least in the transverse plane. The fetal presentation is well shown on this film and the degree of head flexion may sometimes be better appreciated here than in the former film. The placenta can often be seen in normal implantation as a thickening of the uterine shadow.

The reduction factor for measuring both the transverse diameter of the inlet and the ischial bispinous diameter can be obtained by assuming that the former lies at one third of the symphysis to table top distance and the latter at one third of the symphysis to table top distance (Hartley & Fisher, 1966) (Fig. 47.25).

The inlet view (Figs 47.18 and 47.26). This demonstrates the inlet shape without distortion and from it a description of the inlet type can be derived. The transverse diameter of the inlet (A.B.) can be measured and its situation seen so that the relative capacities of the rear and front segments of the inlet can be estimated. This view should not be used to measure the conjugate as the posterior 'end point' cannot be clearly defined. The conjugate is best measured in the lateral view. The ischial spines are seen on the inlet view and any tendency to point unduly inwards can be seen. The ischial bispinous diameter should be obtained using the supine film as described above.

The outlet view (Fig. 47.27). This demonstrates the shape of the angle between the inferior pubic rami. These should subtend an angle of 80° to 90° but a mere measurement of the angle is not an adequate guide to outlet capacity as a narrow angle may be associated with a large pelvis and plenty of reserve capacity posteriorly. The shape should be assessed qualitatively and the architectural concepts of either a wide round Norman arch, or a narrow pointed Gothic arch form a useful guide. It is easily appreciated that both the shape of the arch and the subtended angle affect the outlet capacity by virtue of the amount of space between the fetal head and the symphysis pubis that cannot be utilized by the 'spherical' head passing the apex of the outlet 'triangle'. This space is sometimes known as the '*waste space of Morris*' and is easily estimated.

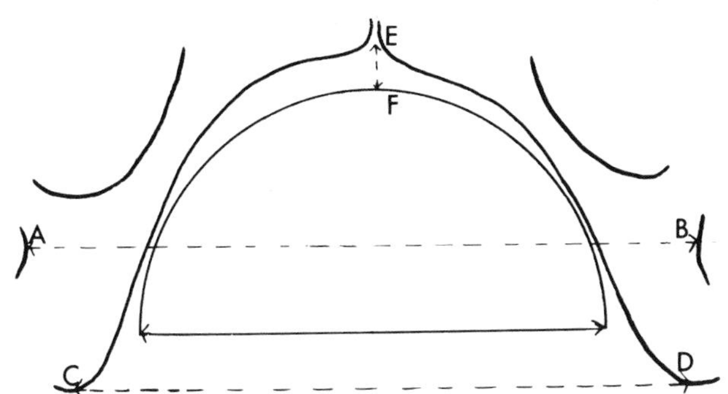

Fig. 47.27 Tracing of outlet view. Letters refer to the lines described in the text.

A circular disc of clear X-ray film 9·5 cm in diameter is used as a model of the engaged fetal head, and is placed on the outlet view so that the bony margins form tangents to the disc. The space between the lower part of the symphysis and the disc is the waste space (E.F.). Williams and Arthure (1949) have utilized the waste space measurement to derive the 'available A.P. of the outlet' by transferring the waste space as measured on the outlet film to the inferior pubic rami as seen in the lateral view (E.F.). A perpendicular (F.D.) is dropped to join the line of the pubosacral diameter (C.E.). The reduced pubosacral diameter (C.D.) represents the projection of the waste space on this plane and indicates to what extent the subpubic angle affects the sagittal dimension usefully available. Further, in an adequate pelvis the line of the horizontal diameter of the 9·5 cm disc as placed on the outlet view should be level with, or anterior to, a line drawn across the base of the ischial tuberosities (C.D.). The intertuberous diameter (A.B.) is the other measurement to be obtained in the outlet view. Accurate end-points are difficult to visualize, but on most films an arc of cortical density is seen on each ischial tuberosity and may be used as an index of the intertuberous diameter. An arbitrary reduction of 0·5 cm can be used in an average sized pelvis, as in this instance the object-film distance is small and variations have a very small effect on magnification.

The following figures indicate the minimum acceptable dimensions of a pelvis:

Inlet plane	Conjugate 11 cm
	Transverse 12·5 cm
Pubosacral	11·5 cm
Interspinous	10 cm
Waste space of Morris	1 cm
Intertuberous	11 cm

4. Interpretation of results

For proper interpretation of a pelvimetry examination it is necessary to understand the course of normal labour and the progress of the fetus in various malpresentations. Moulding of the fetal head and the maternal pelvis are other factors which may influence delivery but they are difficult to quantitate.

Moulding of the fetal head. In fetal head moulding the parietal bones swing towards each other reducing the biparietal diameter. At the same time the parietal bones elevate towards the vertex allowing the frontal and occipital bones to swing under them and reduce the occipitofrontal diameter. Thus the circumference is reduced but at the same time the head undergoes elongation on a base to vertex diameter. Although moulding helps the fetal head to accommodate to the pelvis it is limited in that if excessive in degree or in speed of accomplishment it will lead to intracranial injury.

Moulding of the maternal pelvis. A reserve capacity of the maternal pelvis due to movement between the pelvic bones exists in labour. The sacrum moves in a wedge- and hinge-like manner at the S.I. joints, descending relative to the iliac bones and the coccyx being swung posteriorly. As a result the pubosacral and interspinous diameters are increased. This movement of the sacrum relative to the rest of the pelvis may result in a significant increase in the outlet diameters, particularly in a borderline pelvis (Russell, 1969).

The course of normal labour (occipito-anterior engagement). The fetal head lies above the pelvic brim in a cephalic lie till engagement occurs. This is about 36 weeks in a primigravida, but may not occur till the onset of labour in subsequent pregnancies. With good flexion of the head, the biparietal and sub-occipito-bregmatic diameters engage so that the oncoming head presents as a disc of approximately 9·5 cm diameter. As the fetus descends through the pelvis, the whole fetus assumes an attitude of flexion and moulding of the head occurs as described. As engagement usually occurs in a transverse or oblique plane, the head must undergo internal rotation to bring the occiput immediately under the symphysis. This rotation occurs as the largest cranial circumference passes the plane of the pubis, ischial spines and the sacral tip. A little further descent causes the occiput to pass the symphysis and the head now extends to be delivered. The final movements of descent are limited by the subpubic arch anteriorly, the ischial tuberosities laterally and the tip of the sacrum posteriorly.

The occipito-posterior engagement (Fig. 47.28). In about 15 per cent of cases the occiput engages posteriorly in the pelvis and this is associated with poor flexion of the head. At the level of the ischial spines internal rotation can cause the occiput to rotate through nearly half a circle to become anterior. If flexion is inadequate delivery continues as persistent occipito-posterior. It is evident that in either situation a pelvis of greater than minimum dimensions will be required as the engaging diameters are the occipito- or suboccipito-frontal of 11·5 cm and 10 cm respectively and the biparietal of 9·5 cm. For the long rotation forward the plane of the ischial spines must be able to accommodate the rotation of the poorly flexed head and any prominence of the spines impeding the rotation will lead to the condition of deep transverse arrest. If descent continues as an occipito-posterior then the true outlet will need reserve space to accommodate the poorly flexed head and the less advantageous presenting dimensions.

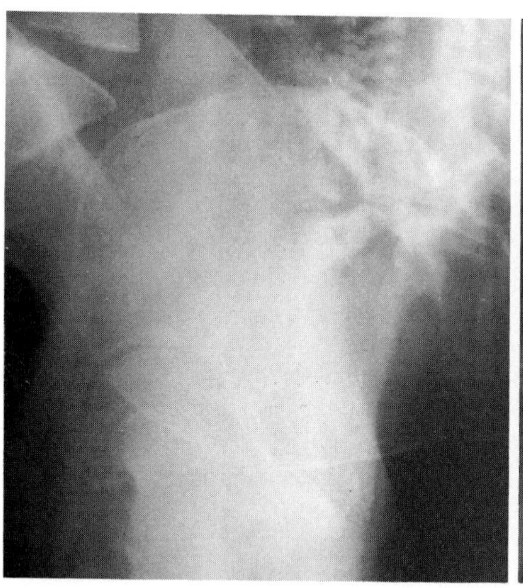

Fig. 47.28

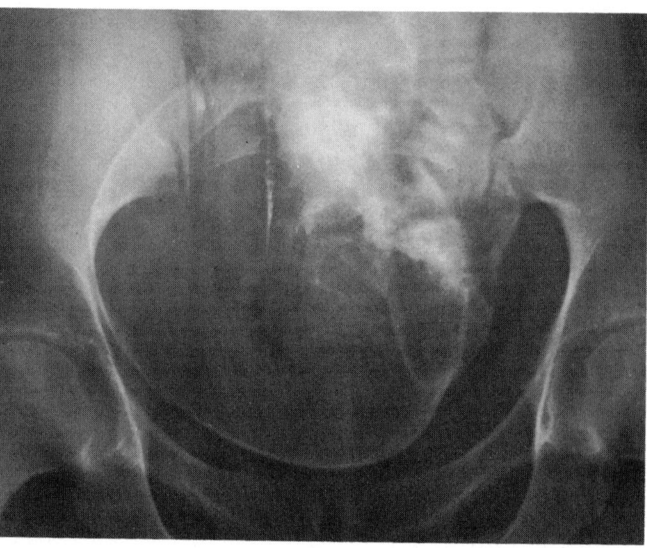

Fig. 47.29

Fig. 47.28 Occipito-posterior engagement. Note the extended position of the head.

Fig. 47.29 Extended head. The brow is the presenting part.

Engagement with extended head (Fig. 47.29). Delivery in brow presentation is almost invariably impossible as the mento-vertical diameter of 13·5 cm is one of the presenting dimensions. Delivery can only proceed if further extension to a face presentation or flexion to a vertex occurs. In either case a smaller antero-posterior diameter is substituted for the originally presenting mento-vertical.

The breech. This is classified as complete when the feet lie alongside the buttocks with legs flexed (Fig. 47.30), or incomplete when its legs are extended (Fig. 47.31). In breech delivery the fetal bitrochanteric diameter (10 cm) engages at the brim and descent is accompanied by lateral flexion of the trunk. The fetal head engages at a late stage of labour in the transverse diameter and passes rapidly through the pelvis, undergoing internal rotation to bring the occiput forwards. Thus moulding cannot be done gradually as in a vertex presentation and the risk of intracranial injury, tentorial tearing in particular, is high. It is for this reason that breech delivery holds dangers to the fetus and is to be avoided if there is any pelvimetric doubt as to the capacity of the pelvis at any plane.

For quantitative assessment the inlet and outlet planes can be considered separately. A dimension of 1 cm below the figures given earlier indicate pelvic contraction in that plane but compensation may result from a large diameter at right angles. A diameter reduced by more than 1 cm compared with the above figures or a reduction in both the conjugate and transverse dimensions of the same plane indicate a great likelihood of dystocia with a normal-sized fetus.

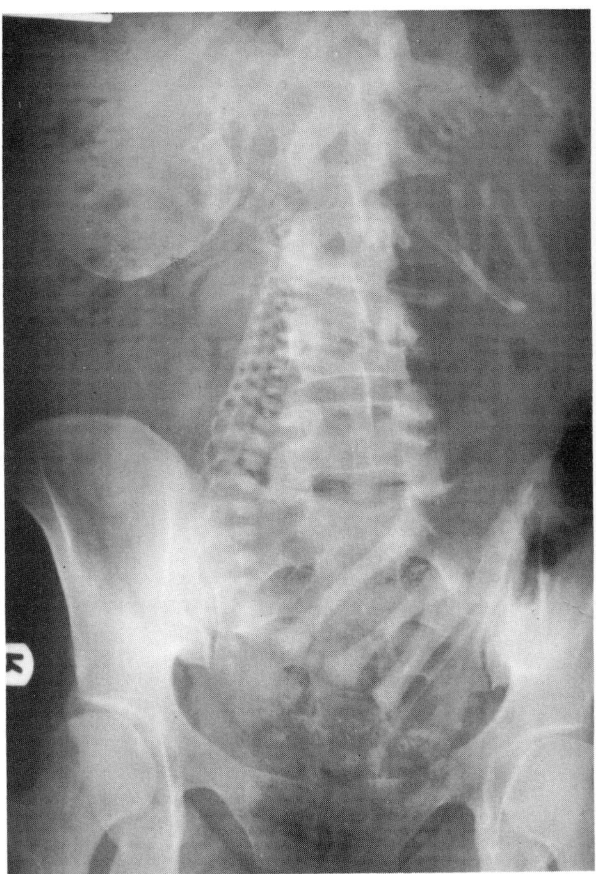

Fig. 47.30

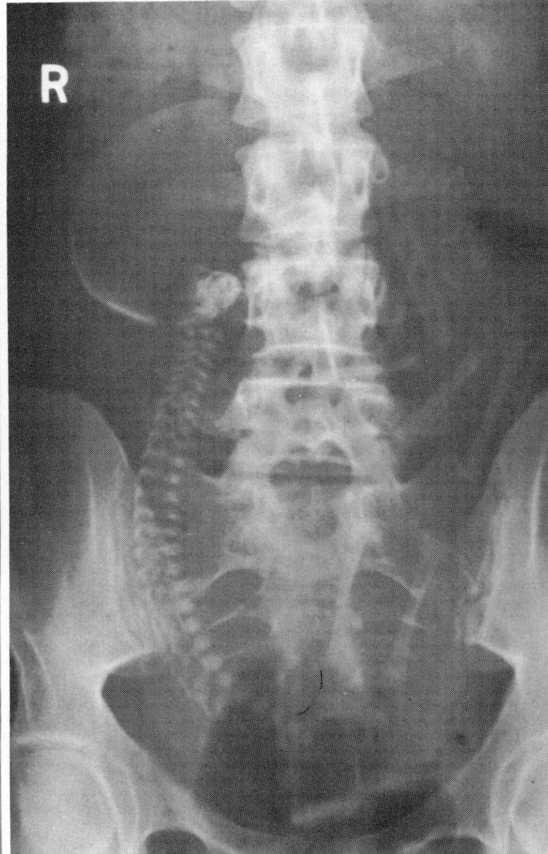

Fig. 47.31

Fig. 47.30 Breech presentation, with flexed legs.

Fig. 47.31 Breech presentation with extended legs.

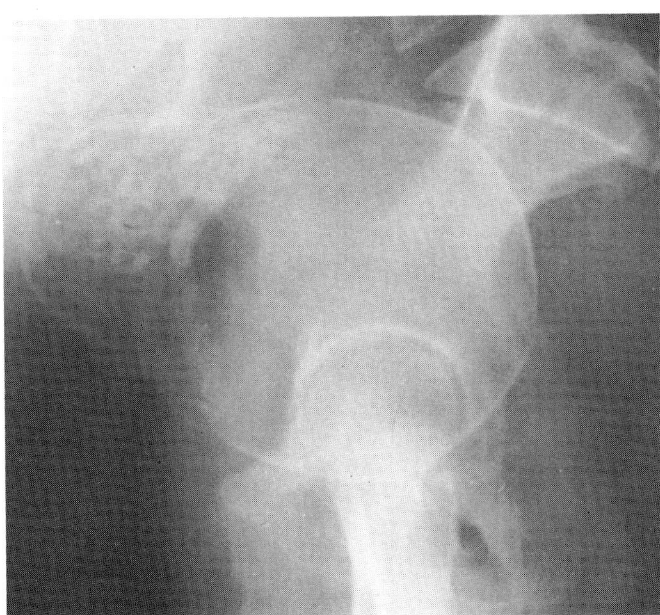

Fig. 47.32 Lateral pelvimetry view. The head is engaging and an accurate biparietal measurement is possible.

When interpreting any pelvimetry, ante- or post-natal, the type of presentation and delivery should be borne in mind and the mechanism of each type assayed against the features of the pelvis. For example an occipito-anterior presentation may be accommodated in a particular pelvis but prominence of the ischial spines in such a pelvis may obstruct a persistent occipito-posterior presentation or lead to deep transverse arrest due to the less favourable dimensions presented by the fetal head. As indicated, a capacious pelvis is required to transmit the aftercoming head in a breech presentation as there is little time for adequate moulding. A post-mature fetus is more resistant to moulding and thus maturity must also be considered in the interpretation of results.

In many cases the cephalopelvic disproportion is marginal and it must be remembered that radiology cannot estimate imponderables such as strength of uterine contraction, the thickness of the soft tissues of the pelvis, and the moulding of the fetal head and maternal pelvis.

The conduct of pelvimetry. Antenatal pelvimetry should, if possible, be undertaken in the last four weeks of pregnancy when there is a reasonable chance of measuring the biparietal diameter (Fig. 47.32). Appropriate allowance can thus be made for final growth in the remaining weeks. In some cases an erect lateral film only may suffice, particularly where an unsuspected occipito-posterior position of the head or extension of the fetal head is preventing engagement of the head in spite of normal pelvic and cranial dimensions. The lateral view will not disclose any transverse contraction at any level in the pelvis and therefore will usually have to be supplemented with a supine A.P. view of the pelvis. The great majority of cases can be adequately assessed on these two films, the erect lateral and the supine A.P. The inlet view is usually contra-indicated on account of the high radiation dose to the fetus with a vertex presentation. It may be indicated in cases of distorted inlet shape (see below). The subpubic arch view is of limited use as this part of the pelvis can be satisfactorily assessed by clinical examination.

5. Additional methods of pelvimetry

For completeness the following additional methods are recorded:

1. The reconstruction chart
2. The assessment of the free space of the outlet
3. Orthodiagraphic pelvimetry (high KV technique).

1. Reconstruction charts. (Gage, 1942; Williams, 1943). A method particularly useful for the asymmetrical pelvis where the conventional measurements may not convey the whole problem inherent in such a pelvis.

2. The free space of the outlet. Gillanders (1959) logically takes the outlet of the pelvis to be two triangles at an angle to each other sharing a common base, the intertuberous line. The apices are the symphysis pubis anteriorly and the sacral tip behind. Any inadequacy of the subpubic arch can only be compensated by backward displacement of the fetal head. This method has been particularly evolved to evaluate the capacity of the posterior part of the outlet.

3. Orthodiagraphic pelvimetry. Orthodiagraphic pelvimetry implies that the required measurements are taken directly from the film and no correction factor for magnification is needed. The reader should refer to Templeton (1965) and Borrel and Radberg (1964) for details. The latter also include a tube shift method with close beam coning for determining the transverse diameter of the inlet, and interspinous and intertuberous diameters. In each paper it has been shown that the techniques markedly reduce the radiation dose to the abdomen and they should be considered where suitable high output equipment is available.

REFERENCES AND SUGGESTIONS FOR FURTHER READING

Borrel, U. & Radberg, C. (1964) Orthodiagraphic pelvimetry with special reference to capacity of distal part of pelvis and pelvic outlet. *Acta radiologica* (Diagnosis), **2**, 273–282.

British Medical Journal (1977) Intra-uterine transfusions. **i**, 990.

British Medical Journal (1979) Radiation and the embryo. **i**, 1380–81.

Brown, R. F. (1976) Prepared remarks for the October 20, 1976 American College of Radiology Press Conference.

Brown, W. M. C. *et al.* (1960) Incidence of leukaemia after exposure to diagnostic irradiation *in utero*. *British Medical Journal*, **ii**, 1539–1545.

Cockshott, W. P. & Lawson, J. (1972) Radiology of advanced abdominal pregnancy. *Radiology*, **103**, 21–29.

Gage, C. (1942) *Recent Advances in Obstetrics and Gynaecology*, 5th edn, edited by Bourne & Williams. London: Churchill.

Gillanders, L. A. (1959) Radiological evaluation of the pelvic outlet. *British Journal of Radiology*, **32**, 371–377.

Hartley, J. B. & Fisher, A. S. (1966) *A Plan for Radiography in Obstetrics*. Manchester: St Mary's Hospital.

I.C.R.P. (1966) Recommendations of the International Commission on Radiological Protection. ICRP Publication 9. Oxford: Pergamon Press.

I.C.R.P. (1977) ICRP Publication 26. Oxford: Pergamon Press.

Mole, R. H. (1979) Radiation effects on prenatal development and their radiological significance. *British Journal of Radiology*, **52**, 89–101.

Royal College of Radiologists (1978) Newsletter, October 1978.

Russell, J. G. B. (1969) Moulding of the pelvic outlet. *Journal of Obstetrics and Gynaecology of the British Commonwealth*, **76**, 817–820.

Russell, J. G. B. & Rangecroft, R. F. (1969) The effect of foetal and maternal factors on radiological maturation of the foetus. *Journal of Obstetrics and Gynaecology of the British Commonwealth*, **76**, 497–502.

Templeton, A. W. (1965) High kilovoltage pelvimetry. *American Journal or Roentgenology*, **93**, 943–947.

Williams, E. R. (1943) The radiological diagnosis of disproportion. *British Journal of Radiology*, **16**, 173–181.

Williams, E. R. & Arthure, H. G. E. (1949) Further radiological studies in the investigation of obstetric disproportion with special reference to the contracted pelvic outlet. *Journal of Obstetrics and Gynaecology of the British Commonwealth*, **56**, 533–575.

CHAPTER 48

GYNAECOLOGICAL RADIOLOGY

PLAIN FILM EXAMINATIONS

Abdomen. A plain film of the abdomen and pelvis is often of assistance in attempts to determine the nature of a pelvic mass, or even in confirming the presence of a mass in an obese patient. A pelvic mass may cause a homogeneous soft-tissue density shadow within the pelvis, or it may extend upwards into the abdomen and displace gas-filled bowel. When small, it may be difficult to differentiate a pelvic mass from a full bladder, and for this reason the patient should be requested to empty her bladder prior to radiological examination. However it is often possible to see a translucent fat-line between the bladder and the uterus making distinction possible.

In addition to scrutiny for a pelvic mass, note should be made of any radiological evidence of ascites. This includes loss of clarity of the visceral outline, overall haziness and increase of density, centrally placed bowel gas shadows and lateral bowing of the body wall lines. The spine and pelvis should also be examined for evidence of neoplastic involvement (Fig. 48.1). Usually uterine masses lie in the midline, whereas ovarian tumours, unless very large, tend to remain on their own side.

Calcification may be present and help to identify the nature of a pelvic abnormality.

Uterine fibroids. These frequently undergo patchy calcification which is diagnostic on the X-ray film. Less commonly, or in association, mural calcification may occur (Fig. 48.2).

Ovarian dermoid. The characteristic diagnostic feature is the presence of teeth, properly formed or merely rudimentary (Fig. 48.3). Mural calcification may occur but is uncommon. The high fat content sometimes renders the tumour relatively radiolucent and is also a diagnostic feature when present.

Ovarian fibroma. These are uncommon tumours but they may undergo dense calcification. When associated

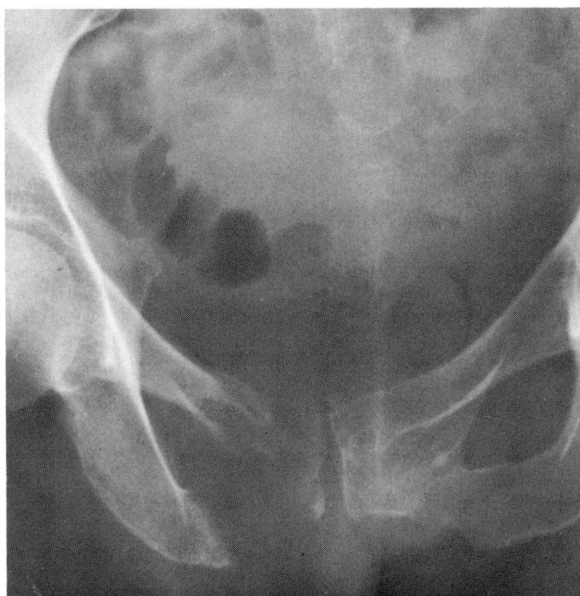

Fig. 48.1 Destruction of pubis and adjacent rami by extensive uterine carcinoma.

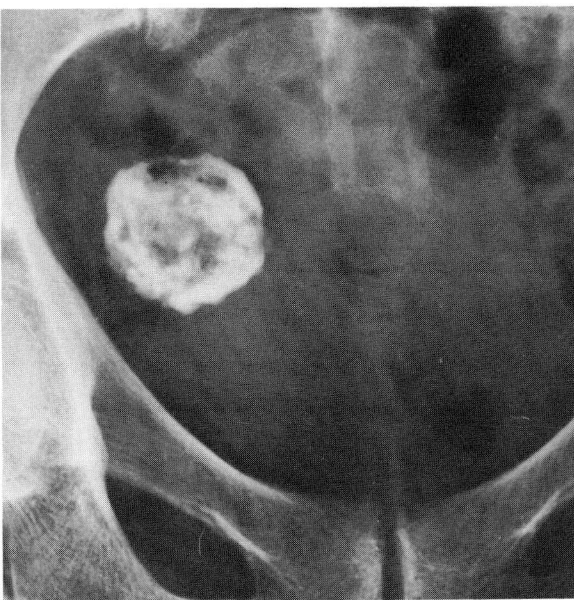

Fig. 48.2 Calcified fibroid.

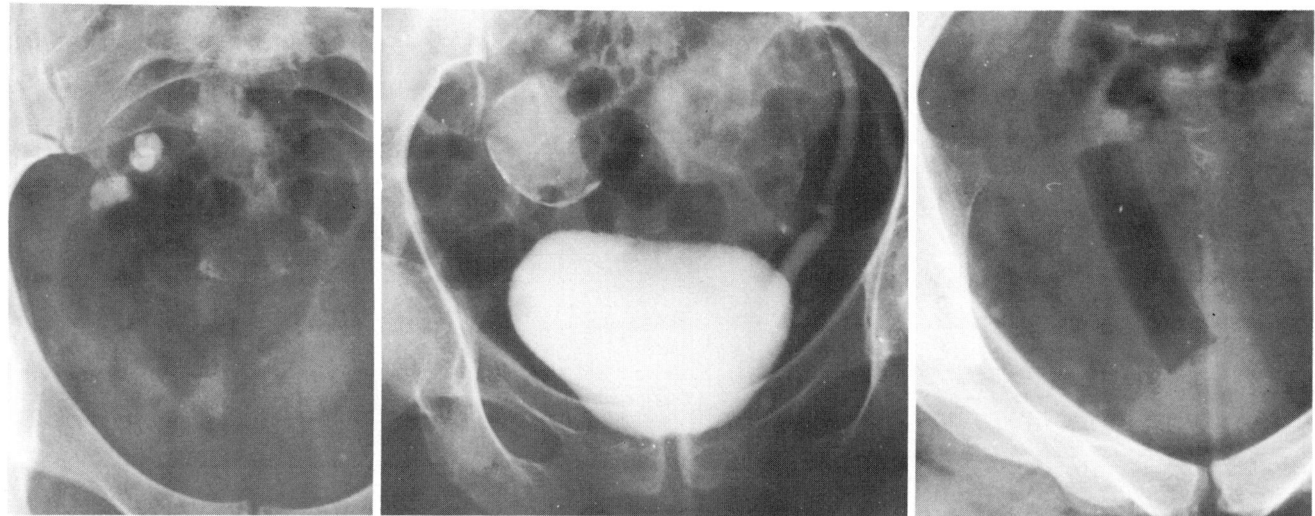

Fig. 48.3 *Fig. 48.4* *Fig. 48.5*

Fig. 48.3 Dental rudiments in an ovarian dermoid.

Fig. 48.4 Calcification in bilateral tuberculous pyosalpinx (contrast in bladder from I.V.P.).

Fig. 48.5 Characteristic translucency of an intravaginal sanitary pad.

with pleural effusion and ascites these constitute Meigs' syndrome.

Ovarian carcinoma. Calcification can occur in omental and peritoneal deposits from ovarian cystadenocarcinoma.

Tuberculous pyosalpinx. Amorphous calcification may form in a tuberculous pyosalpinx (Fig. 48.4). The diagnosis is aided by salpinography.

A broad translucency approximately 1 cm × 4 cm may be seen in the lower part of the pelvis just above the symphysis pubis. This is characteristic of an intravaginal sanitary pad (Fig. 48.5).

Intra-uterine contraceptive devices (IUCD): These are made of radio-opaque material for localization and identification. Three are illustrated (Fig. 48.6). The presence of an IUCD is usually checked by the gynaecologist as the device has fine threads which project through the cervix to facilitate its removal. Sometimes the threads become drawn into the uterine cavity when it may be uncertain whether the IUCD is present or lost. In this case a film of the whole abdomen should be obtained to show whether the device is still present or not or if, as sometimes occurs, it has silently penetrated the uterine wall and migrated to a distant site (Fig. 48.7).

A lateral film may help to show the position of the device relative to the uterus but is unreliable owing to the variable position (anteversion or retroversion) of the uterus. Ultrasound provides a more certain method of localization.

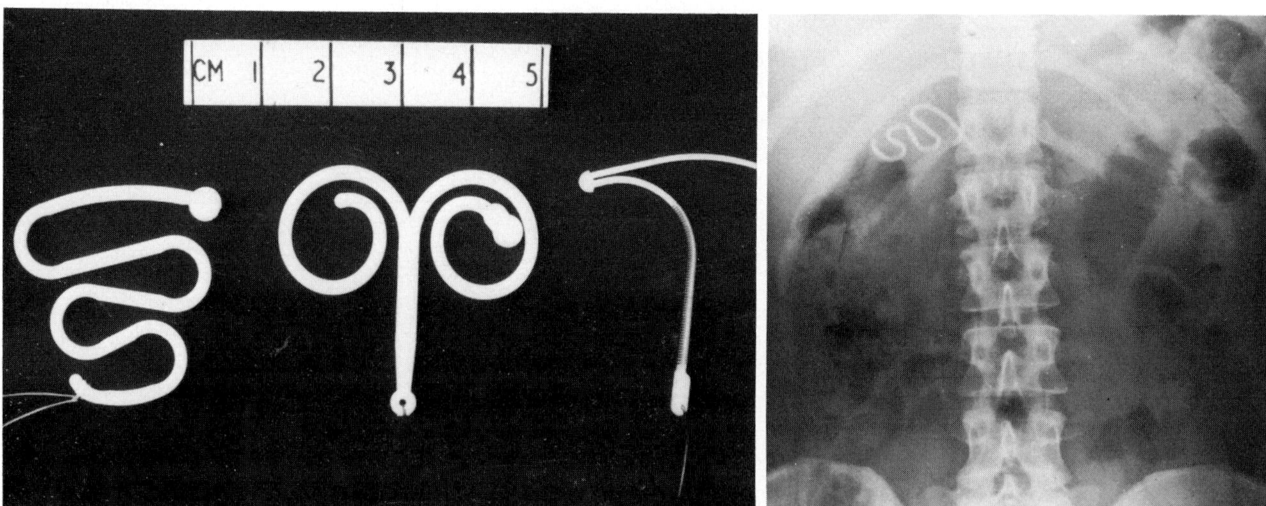

Fig. 48.6 Intra-uterine contraceptive devices: left, Lippes loop; middle, Saf-T; right, copper seven.

Fig. 48.7 An intra-uterine contraceptive device which has silently migrated to the region of the liver.

Chest. A film of the chest may be requested in the investigation of infertility. The infertility may be a toxic effect of active pulmonary tuberculosis, or result from a tuberculous endometritis or salpingitis.

In cases of ovarian and uterine carcinoma, pulmonary metastases and pleural effusion may occur; a chest film is therefore indicated to assess the possibility of such spread.

Trophoblastic tumours (chorion-epithelioma) produce three main types of chest metastases (Bagshawe and Garnett, 1964):

1. Discrete masses, single or multiple
2. Multiple, ill defined metastases producing a 'snowstorm' or miliary appearance

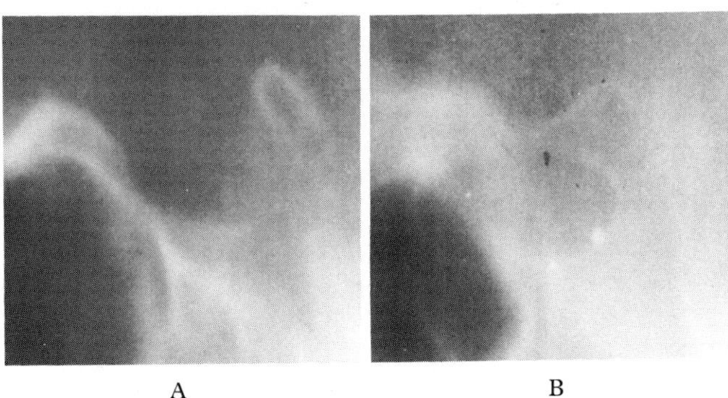

Fig. 48.8A and B Tomographic cuts 1 cm apart showing change of fossa outline associated with a small prolactin secreting tumour.

3. Arterial emboli producing the changes usually associated with pulmonary infarction, or less commonly the changes of 'primary' pulmonary hypertension.

Skull. The investigation of infertility should include a radiograph of the pituitary fossa as a pituitary or suprasellar tumour may affect endocrine function. In particular, minor alterations of the contour of the fossa such as a 'double floor' may be associated with the small prolactin secreting tumours. Tomography may be necessary to clarify the shape of the fossa in some cases (Fig. 48.8). However about 15 per cent of the normal population have such asymmetrical fossae. Serial radiography may be required in pregnancy after the administration of bromocriptine as these microtumours are then liable to undergo quite rapid expansion.

THE URINARY TRACT IN GYNAECOLOGY

The I.V.P. for gynaecological purposes is performed to demonstrate distortion, deviation or obstruction of the urinary tract in the pelvis, and to show any resulting hydronephrosis. Compression is best avoided so that the effect of any pelvic obstruction may be clearly demonstrated. An adequate dose of contrast medium by modern standards should be given. A table allowing head down tilt is also an advantage. In order to assess the effects of abnormality upon the whole of the urinary tract, full length films should be taken from the beginning of the examination. A post micturition film will demonstrate any urinary residue.

A pelvic mass usually causes a fundal impression on the bladder and if large enough may deviate the ureters and give clear evidence of ureteric obstruction. Ureteric obstruction may also occur with procidentia, when the descent of the bladder results in compression of the lower segments of the ureters. Actual invasion of the bladder or ureters by uterine carcinoma is unusual until a late stage, when there is extensive spread in the pelvis.

It has been shown that tomography of the pelvis after a large dose of urographic contrast medium may demonstrate pelvic masses more clearly and indicate their nature (Peck, Yoder and Pfister, 1975) by the total body opacification phenomenon.

Certain complications of hysterectomy may be demonstrated by I.V.P. and include (Whitehouse, 1977):

1. Partial or complete ureteric occlusion by a suture. On the affected side the kidney may fail to excrete, or in the case of incomplete occlusion it may rapidly become hydronephrotic.

2. Division of the ureter. Extravasation of contrast into the pelvic fascia may be seen. Occasionally a vaginal fistula follows and contrast may be visualized in the vagina. In some cases spontaneous closure of the ureteric opening occurs and serial I.V.P. examinations may demonstrate the return to normal.

3. Vesicovaginal fistula. Contrast can be identified in the bladder and the vagina, the ureters appearing normal. If the fistula is large very little contrast may be retained in the bladder as it passes rapidly into the vagina, particularly when the patient is lying in the supine position as she would be during an I.V.P. examination (Fig. 48.9).

4. Pelvic accumulation of blood (haematoma) or lymph (lymphocyst). These accumulations, if large enough, may manifest themselves on the I.V.P. by distorting the shape of the bladder (Fig. 48.10), deviating the course of the ureters and causing dilatation of the renal pelvis and calyces. The presence of a lymphocyst may be confirmed by lymphography.

Cystography. Cystography may be used to investigate stress incontinence and to demonstrate vesico-ureteric reflux in patients with urinary symptoms.

In addition a modified technique is useful for the investigation of vesicovaginal fistula. The patient is set up as for a micturating cystogram with an in-dwelling catheter connected to a bottle of contrast via a disposable irrigation set. The patient is screened in a lateral position and the contrast is run in under screen control with the patient lying on her side. In this way the fistulous connection is often visible (Fig. 48.11) and contrast can be

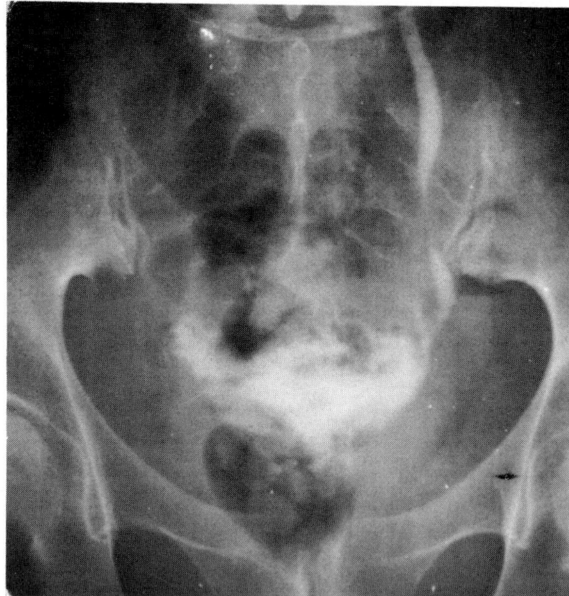

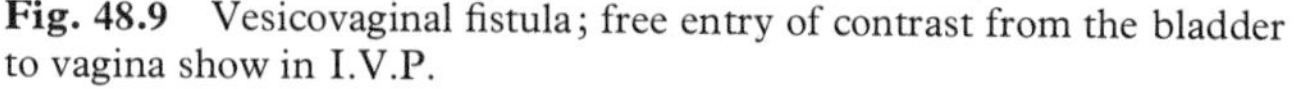

Fig. 48.9 Vesicovaginal fistula; free entry of contrast from the bladder to vagina show in I.V.P.

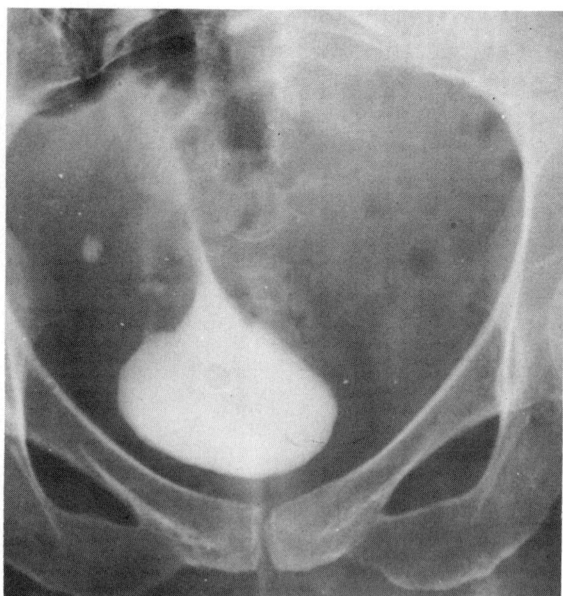

Fig. 48.10 Distortion of the bladder due to large postoperative haematoma on the left.

siphoned back by lowering the bottle so that optimum pictures can be taken with the patient in the most suitable degree of rotation and with the bladder sufficiently filled so as not to obscure the vital field. Occasionally the lateral films during micturition may also be useful.

Barium enema. Routine barium enemas may be helpful to illustrate bowel involvement by spreading pelvic carcinoma or endometriosis or to show irradiation colitis which can occur after pelvic radiation therapy.

Rectovaginal fistulas are often more easily demon-

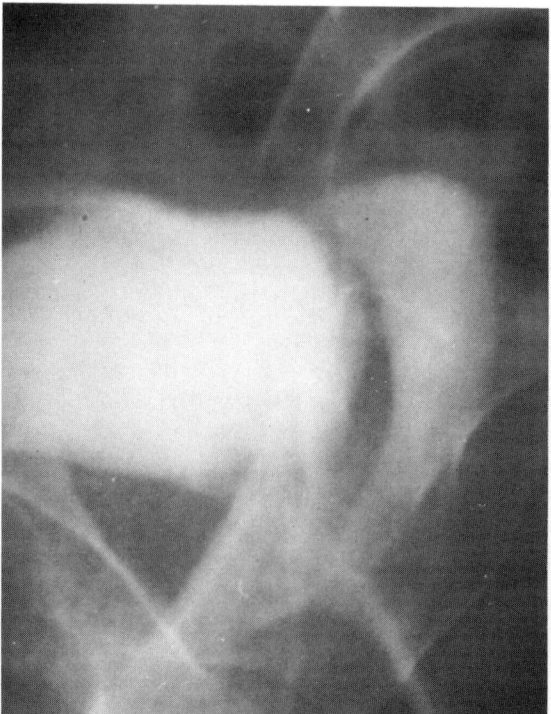

Fig. 48.11 Vesicovaginal fistula shown by 'siphonage' cystography (oblique view).

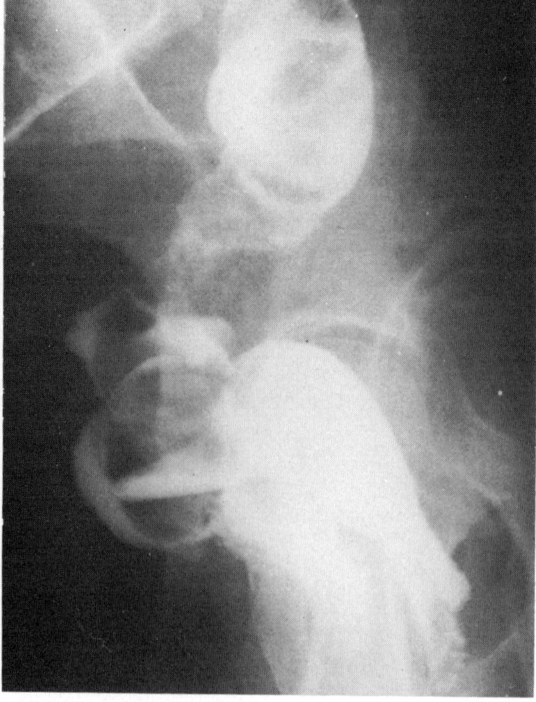

Fig. 48.12 Lateral view of rectovaginal fistula shown by diodone enema (self-retaining catheter in rectum).

strated using water-soluble contrast than barium. Screening and films should be taken in the lateral projection (Fig. 48.12).

HYSTEROSALPINGOGRAPHY

The examination outlines the uterine cavity and Fallopian tubes. The indications are:

1. Infertility: to demonstrate normal patency of the Fallopian tubes and their communication with the peritoneal cavity.
2. Recurrent abortion: to demonstrate congenital abnormalities of the uterine cavity or incompetence of the internal os of the uterus.

The procedure of hysterosalpingography was used more extensively in the past and the appearances of a large variety of gynaecological conditions have been described (Barnett, 1955–56; Foda *et al.*, 1962). Since the indications for the examination are now almost entirely restricted to those given above only a brief description of other abnormalities which may be encountered incidentally are given.

The contra-indications to this examination are:

1. Active pelvic sepsis. The examination may result in spread of infection.
2. Severe renal or cardiac disease.
3. Sensitivity to contrast media.
4. Recent dilatation and curettage.
5. Pregnancy.
6. The week prior to, and the week following menstruation. It is best performed at about the middle of the menstrual cycle.

Timing of the examination. It has just been noted that the examination should be avoided in the week following menstruation to avoid the complication of venous intravasation. This almost excludes the 10-day period recommended for the radiological examination of women in the reproductive period (p. 918). Although these patients are more or less infertile, one method of avoiding accidental foetal irradiation is to advise them to abstain from intercourse or to use some contraceptive method in the interval from the last menstrual period to the examination. If the examination is then carried out late in the cycle a diagnostic curettage can usefully follow the salpingogram.

Technique

The examination is usually conducted in association with a gynaecologist. Although in some clinics the examination is performed without any anaesthesia, or sedation, we consider the examination to be more satisfactory both from the patient's point of view and as an accurate diagnostic procedure if done under a general anaesthetic. At the same time the salpingography can be combined with full bimanual pelvic examination and followed by diagnostic curettage if necessary.

The injection of contrast is made through a cannula or suction device attached to a 20 cc syringe. The cannulae are placed in the cervix and two kinds are available. The Leech-Wilkinson pattern has a screw-threaded 'olive' at its distal end which enables a water-tight fit to be made easily with the cervix and thus prevents the reflux of contrast into the vagina. It has some liability to produce cervical laceration. The Everard-Williams pattern has a smooth 'olive' near the distal end and the tip of the cannula is bent to allow easy introduction into the cervical canal. This is a satisfactory cannula, but requires some care on the operator's part to maintain a good seal at the cervix, to prevent reflux of contrast. More recently a plastic suction cap device has been produced. This is placed on the cervix and suction is applied by a syringe fixed to one end of a plastic tube, which at its other end communicates through the cap to the space between the cervix and cap. A second tube terminates in a short nozzle in the centre of the cap and protrudes into the cervical canal. The injection of contrast is made from the syringe through this latter tube. In patients with a lacerated cervix a suction cap may be difficult to apply but in general this method has the advantage of showing the cervical canal and isthmus more clearly.

The patient is placed in the lithotomy position at the end of the screening table. An operating speculum is introduced into the vagina and the cannula or suction device is applied. The speculum is then removed and the patient carefully moved up the table so that she lies in a supine position and the contrast is injected under image intensifier control. This enables the radiologist to warn the gynaecologist if any contrast is refluxing into the vagina and not entering the uterus. It also allows films to be taken at the most opportune time. One or two films may be necessary to show the cervical canal, the body of the uterus, the Fallopian tubes and the spread of contrast on to the peritoneum.

The contrast media now used are all of the water-soluble variety and the old oily contrast media are now almost entirely superseded. It is preferable for the contrast medium to be rendered a little viscous; 'Salpix' contains polyvinylpyrrolidone as a thickening agent but this has the objection that it is retained in the body if venous intravasation should occur. 'Diaginol viscous' contains dextran which is broken down and then excreted. This is therefore probably the medium of choice.

Complications

Pain. Two types of pain can occur. The first is a hypogastric colic and is probably related to distension of the uterus. The second is a more continuous generalized lower abdominal pain most likely due to peritoneal irritation. Both are transient and are usually of nuisance value only with unanaesthetized patients.

Venous intravasation. The contrast medium is acci-

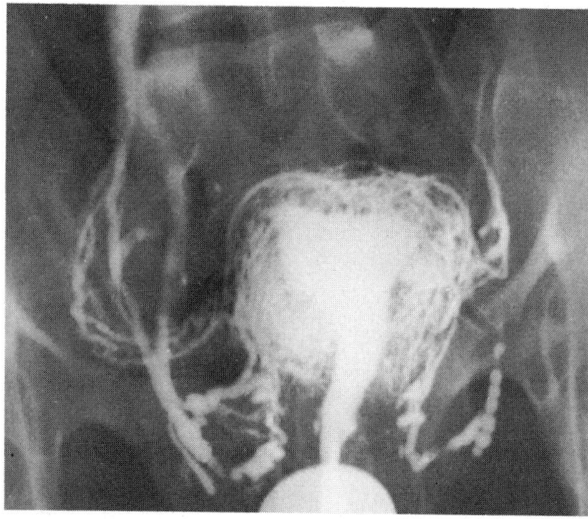

Fig. 48.13

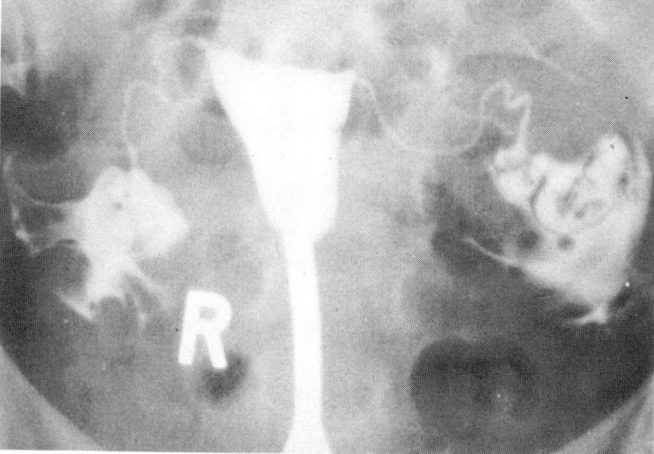

Fig. 48.14

Fig. 48.13 Venous intravasation. The ovarian veins are shown and the is seen in the peritoneal cavity.

Fig. 48.14 Normal salpingogram; both Fallopian tubes fill and contrast is seen in the peritoneal cavity.

dentally injected through the endometrium and taken up by the interstitial veins which outline the thickness of the uterine wall and are seen draining through the iliac and ovarian veins (Fig. 48.13).

Intravasation is said to occur (i) due to excessive injection pressure, (ii) due to traumatization of the endometrium by the tip of the cannula, and (iii) if the examination is performed when the endometrium is deficient as after curettage or menstruation.

Intravasated water-soluble contrast is entirely harmless. The main objection is that it obscures the picture. It is suggested that should venous intravasation occur a delayed picture is taken after a few minutes when the intravasated contrast has cleared, in the hope that tubal filling and any spill of contrast onto the peritoneum may then be visible.

Exacerbation of pelvic infection. Care should be taken not to perform the examination in the presence of any active inflammatory process. It is considered advisable to give prophylactic antibiotics after a hysterosalpingogram in a patient with chronic pelvic infection.

THE NORMAL HYSTEROSALPINGOGRAM

The normal uterine outline is approximately triangular, with sides of 3·7 cm (1·5 in). The cervical canal has a length of about 2·5 cm (1 in) or less. The cornua of the uterus are often seen to have a constriction, possibly a sphincter, at each cornuotubal junction. Under the screen the Fallopian tubes may be difficult to identify but their broader fimbrial ends are usually clearly seen. When spill occurs the contrast takes on an amorphous shape around the end of the tube. The medium then smears the pelvic peritoneum producing a series of curvilinear opacities in the recesses (Fig. 48.14). The pouch of Douglas is often identifiable and the elliptical outlines of the ovaries can sometimes be distinguished. Care should be taken not to confuse residual contrast lying in the vaginal fornices (Fig. 48.24).

Failure of contrast to pass through the tubes to the peritoneum may occasionally be due to cornual or tubal spasm. Inhalation of amyl nitrite used to be recommended to relieve the spasm but its effect is dubious. Gentle injection pressure and patience, giving the spasm time to relax are probably the most important factors in overcoming the tubal spasm.

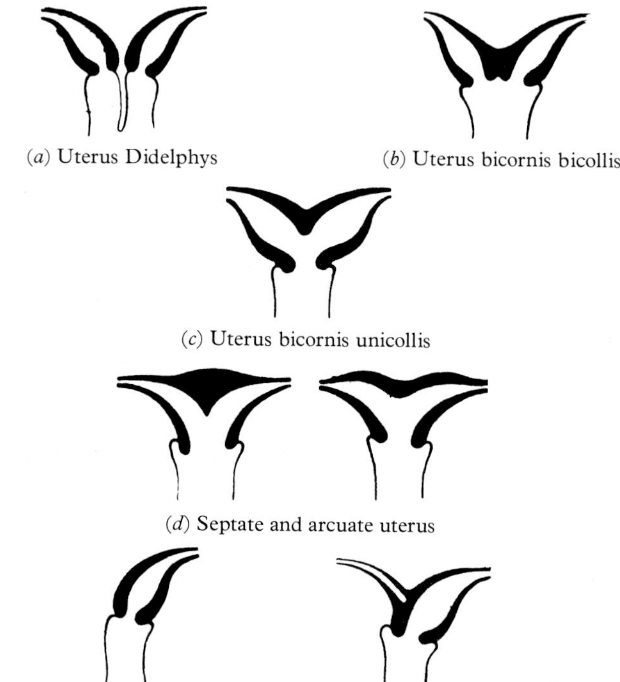

Fig. 48.15 Diagrammatic representation of important congenital abnormalities of the uterus.

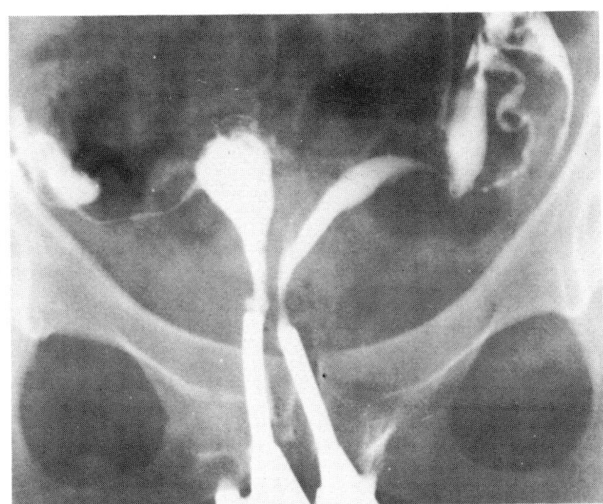

Fig. 48.16 Uterus bicornis bicollis.

THE ABNORMAL SALPINGOGRAM

Congenital anomalies of the uterus

Varying degrees of failure of fusion of the Mullerian ducts lead to a corresponding series of congenital abnormalities of the uterus. These are:

Uterus didelphys (Fig. 48.15A). This is a very rare duplication affecting the whole of the uterus, cervix and the vagina. To each half-uterine body there is a single Fallopian tube.

Uterus bicornis bicollis (Fig. 48.15B and Fig. 48.16). This is similar, but there is a close connection of the moieties in the cervical region.

Uterus bicornis unicollis (bicornuate uterus) (Fig. 48.15C and Fig. 48.17). Each half-uterine cavity has a spindle shape and inclines away from its fellow to communicate with its Fallopian tube. The isthmus is often short and broad. The two uterine moieties share a single cervix.

Septate uterus: arcuate uterus (Fig. 48.15D). These represent minor degrees of division. The dividing septum, varying in length and breadth, protrudes from the fundus and gives rise to these anomalies. The lateral borders of the uterine compartments are more or less straight; the spindle shape is not a feature and the division rarely extends to the isthmus which may again be short and broad. Arcuate uterus is characterized by the shape of the fundus, which projects moderately into the uterine cavity.

Unicornuate uterus (Fig. 48.15E and 48.18). A single spindle-shaped uterine cavity lying to one side of the midline is demonstrated with a single Fallopian tube. A rudimentary opposite horn may be shown if it has any communicating cavity. The differential diagnosis between unicornuate uterus and uterus bicornis bicollis depends on the explicit exclusion of a second moiety after carefully examining the cervix for a second external os.

Infantile uterus. This is small in size, but the cervical canal is long relative to the uterine body.

Abnormalities of position of the uterus

As described above, the normally sited and structurally normal uterus presents an approximately triangular shape. When it becomes anteflexed or retroflexed it is seen radiographically in an almost axial projection on the P.A. film and the cavity presents an elliptical shape. The uterus may be displaced laterally by tumour masses or adhesions. Displacements in either plane can result from the instrumentation and this should be observable on the screen, particularly if the gynaecologist is asked to alter the position of the syringe and cannula.

Uterine fibroids

The hysterographic appearances will be affected by the situation of the fibroids, whether submucous, interstitial or subserous. Although isolated tumours may give charac-

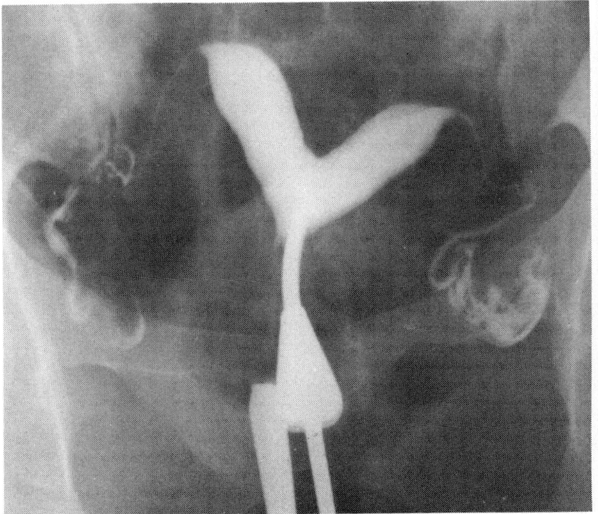

Fig. 48.17 Bicornuate uterus. Note early peritoneal smearing.

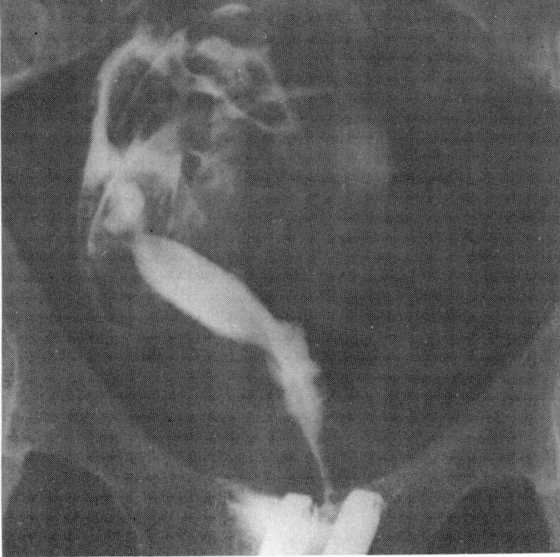

Fig. 48.18 Unicornuate uterus.

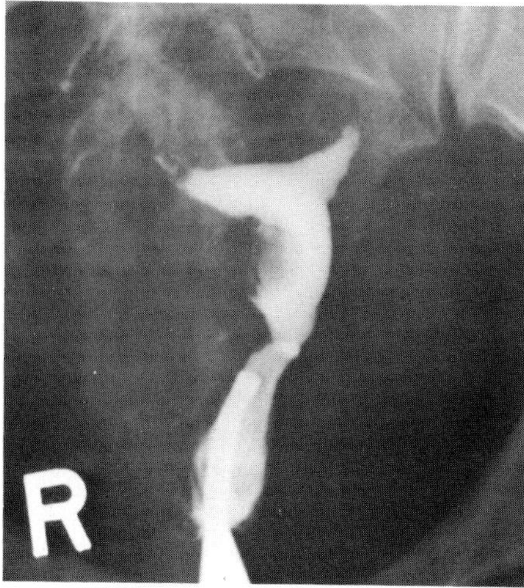

Fig. 48.19 Submucous fibroid.

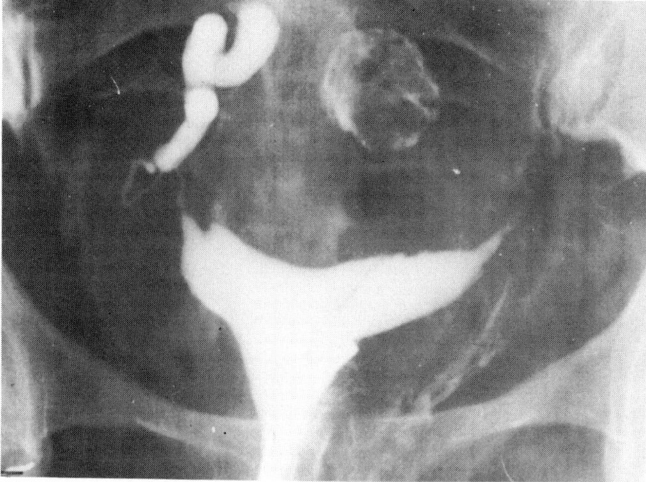

Fig. 48.20 Calcified interstitial fibroid causing generalized enlargement of uterine cavity.

teristic appearances, it must be remembered that fibroids are often multiple and generally enlarge and distort the whole uterine cavity.

Submucous fibroids will appear as sessile or polypoid filling defects in the contrast filled cavity (Fig. 48.19). It may be impossible to differentiate them from other smooth masses in the cavity such as mucosal polyps or an early pregnancy. Interstitial fibroids cause a general enlargement or distortion of the uterine cavity (Fig. 48.20). The effect of subserous masses depends on their position. One at the fundus may cause little or no abnormality or cause the uterus merely to lie in an abnormal position. If situated laterally in the parametrium, the mass will deviate the uterus to the opposite side and the ipsilateral tube will be stretched over the mass.

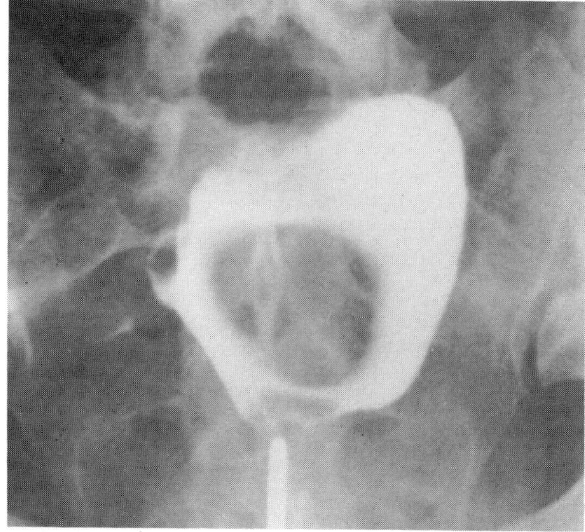

Fig. 48.21 Six weeks pregnancy.

Pregnancy

The gestation sac appears as a smooth or smoothly lobulated filling defect in a generally enlarged uterine cavity (Fig. 48.21).

Missed and incomplete abortion. The disintegrating products of conception may form an irregular filling defect in some cases. In others there may be a smooth filling defect similar to those of a normal pregnancy.

Extra-uterine pregnancy. Hysterosalpingography may be used to confirm this diagnosis. The uterine cavity may be slightly enlarged but is clearly separate from the fetus and its gestational sac.

Tubal pregnancy. The affected tube is dilated and terminates sharply against the gestation sac.

Tumours

Carcinoma of the body. This gives rise to a shaggy and irregular filling defect. A diffuse infiltration causes a general, fine irregularity of the uterine contour.

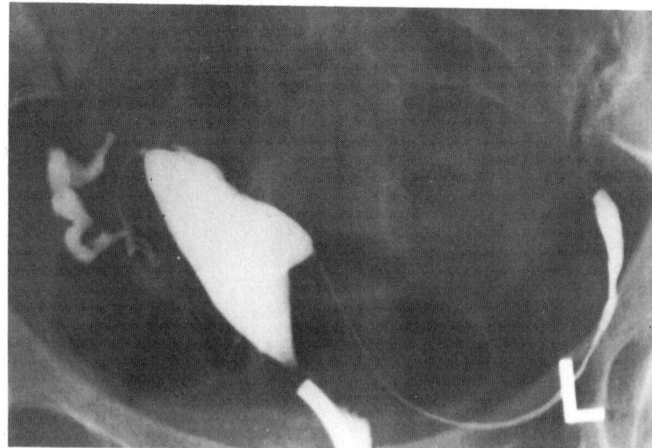

Fig. 48.22 Ovarian cyst displacing left tube.

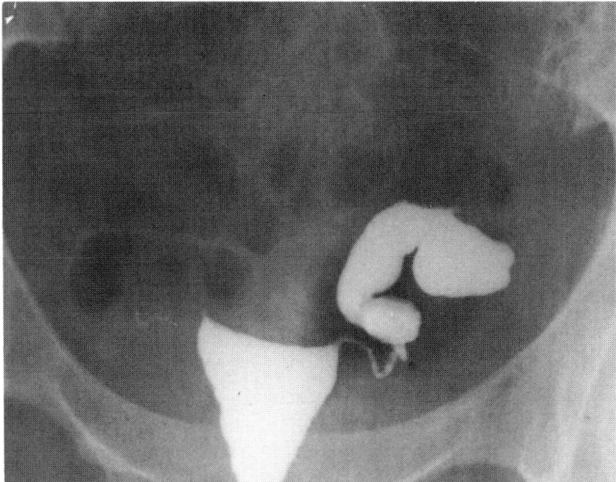
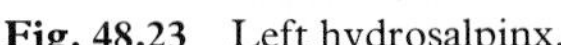

Fig. 48.23 Left hydrosalpinx.

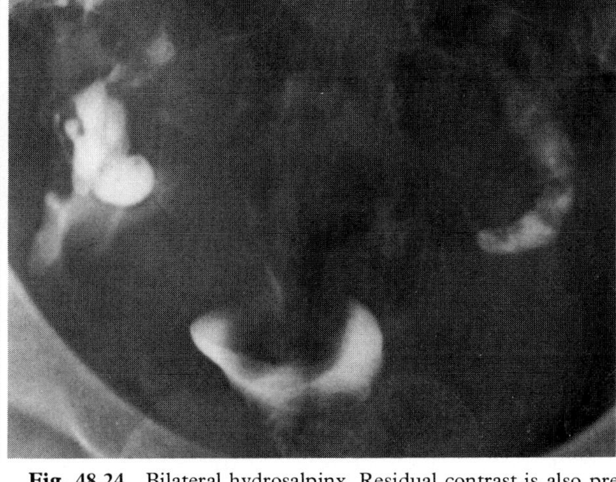

Fig. 48.24 Bilateral hydrosalpinx. Residual contrast is also present in the vagina and outlines the fornices.

Hydatidiform mole. The contrast may seep between the vesicles and a series of irregular curvilinear opacities result outlining the grape-like groups of small filling defects. An alternative method of demonstrating a hydatidiform mole is by transabdominal injection of the uterus using a needle introduced percutaneously a few centimetres below the umbilicus (Greenbaum, Padolak and O'Loughlin, 1969).

Ovarian tumours (Fig. 48.22). Usually these cannot be distinguished from a laterally lying fibroid, the appearances being those of any parametrial mass. Rarely the ovarian mass may be outlined by the spilled contrast and be identifiable.

Abnormalities of the Fallopian tubes

Salpingitis: hydrosalpinx. The examination is contraindicated in acute infection. In some cases previous infection results in blockage of the tube but in others contrast will enter the distended hydrosalpinx and reveal its extent (Figs 48.23 and 48.24). Contrast medium which emerges from a patent tube but which is surrounded by peritoneal adhesions tends to remain in discrete loculi and not spread freely in the general peritoneal cavity.

Tuberculous salpingitis. Tuberculosis of the Fallopian tubes usually results in obstruction of their distal ends but the tubes frequently fill and tuberculous infection is characterized by the irregular calibre of the tubes with small filling defects and some dilatation of their peripheral parts. The contrast may be retained in the small dilatation of the tubes. Occasionally calcification is seen in a tuberculous pyosalpinx (Fig. 48.4). When the uterine cavity is involved in a tuberculous endometritis the result may be a very small irregular contracted uterine cavity (Fig. 48.25).

Salpingitis isthmica nodosa. Sometimes tiny fragments of contrast are seen apparently lying outside the main lumen of the isthmic part of the tubes. This condition of salpingitis isthmica nodosa is uncommon. It is

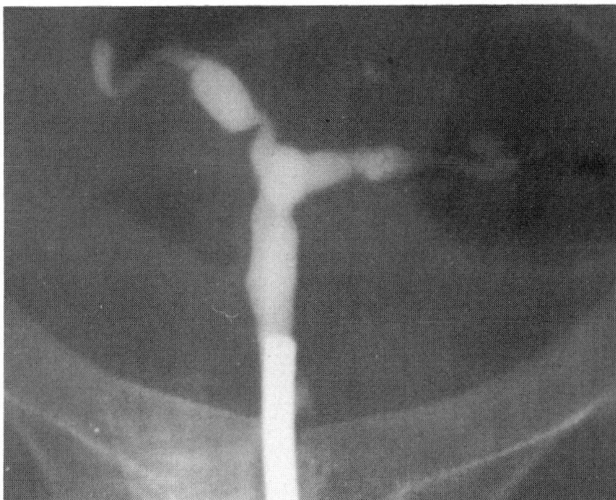

Fig. 48.25 Marked constriction of uterine cavity following tuberculous endometritis.

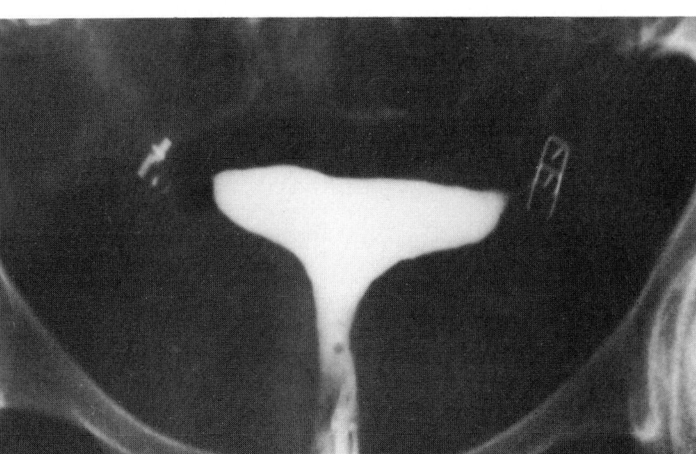

Fig. 48.26 Laparoscopic clip sterilization. A salpingogram has been performed to check the effectiveness of the procedure. Two clips are present on the left side.

due to small tubal diverticula and may be related to endometriosis.

Tubal blockage. The commonest abnormality found on salpingography in cases of infertility is tubal blockage, no evidence of contrast spill on the peritoneum being seen. The obstruction, real or apparent, may be due to a number of causes. Most have already been described, but it is convenient to consider them together under one heading. They are:

1. *Poor operative technique.* If the cannula is not held firmly against the cervix to form a tight seal, much of the contrast medium will leak back into the vagina. The uterus and tubes are poorly filled and a false impression of tubal obstruction is obtained. During screening a watch should be kept on the vaginal vault around the cannula and any leakage reported to the gynaecologist.

2. *Tubal spasm.* This may occur at the cornuotubal junction or along the length of the tube. When no tubal filling or only sparse filling is noted on screening during the injection, gentle injection pressure should be maintained for a few minutes. Tubal spasm usually relaxes if given time.

3. *Obstruction following tubal infection or operation.* Salpingitis may cause obstruction of the lumen of the tubes by inflammatory adhesions. The obstruction may be at the cornu or at a variable distance along the tube, the proximal segment appearing normal. A similar appearance is unfortunately usually seen after salpingostomy as persistent patency of the tube is rare after the operation. It is also seen after tubal amputation. A hydrosalpinx is another sequel to salpingitis; on salpingography the contrast enters and outlines a club-shaped dilatation of the lateral part of the affected tube, the proximal part of which may be of normal calibre.

4. *Fimbrial adhesions.* Pelvic peritonitis or salpingitis may cause adhesions to form around the lateral ends of the tubes and involve the fimbria. The salpingogram demonstrates the whole length of the tube, but the contrast instead of spreading freely over the peritoneum is retained in small loculi at and around its lateral end.

Fimbrial adhesions, hydrosalpinx and normal calibre tubal blockage are the commonest abnormal findings on salpingography in the examination of infertile women.

5. *Tubal pregnancy, tumours, etc.* Obstruction may be demonstrated in association with tubal pregnancy or tumours arising in the wall of the tube or the parametrium; these are relatively rare findings.

6. *Sterilization procedures.* Sterilization procedures include ligation of the Fallopian tubes, with or without tubal division; laparoscopic diathermy of the tubes; laparoscopic clip sterilization, i.e. compressing the tubes with plastic clips placed on the tubes through a laparoscope (Fig. 48.26). Salpingography is sometimes undertaken to confirm that the occlusion is complete.

Cervical canal

The cervical canal is best shown when the contrast is injected through a suction cap device rather than with an 'olive' tipped cannula (Asplund, 1959; Youssef, 1958).

The cervical canal extends from the external os upwards from 1 to 2 cm to the internal os, above which there is a short narrow isthmus which opens into the general uterine cavity. The width of the cervical canal varies with the menstrual cycle, being widest in the proliferative than in the secretory phase.

Distensibility of the canal is of importance in cases of habitual mid-term abortion (incompetent cervix). A method of demonstrating this is by fixing a rubber finger-stall over the olive tip of the cannula. This is then introduced into the cervix and the contrast injected. The fingerstall is blown up by contrast and undue distension of the cervix is clearly shown (Fig. 48.27). A routine hysterosalpingogram injection can then follow.

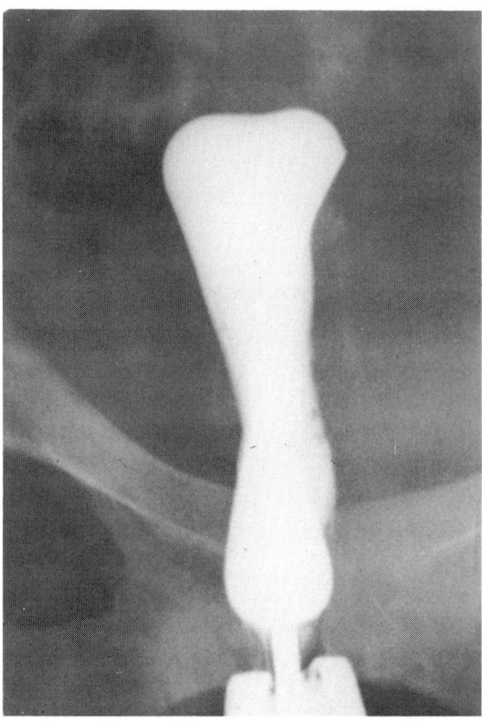

Fig. 48.27 Cervical distensibility shown by use of a finger-stall fixed over injection cannula.

PELVIC ARTERIOGRAPHY

A standard intra-arterial catheter technique is employed. The catheter tip should be placed just below the level of the renal arteries so that both the ovarian and the uterine vessels are filled. Injection of 20–30 ml of contrast medium and serial films taken over a period of 6–8 seconds commencing at the end of injection provides adequate films.

The uterine arteries in the parametrium are usually well seen and the course of the arteries along each lateral uterine wall are shown. A fine artery supplying the Fallopian tube and anastomosing with the ovarian artery can also be seen.

Uterine fibroids are demonstrated with a high degree of accuracy. They cause displacement and stretching of adjacent vessels. They may be avascular but often contain an intrinsic vascular supply which is opacified at angiography.

Trophoblastic tumours are well demonstrated in almost every case. *Hydatidiform mole* is a relatively avascular tumour although the main uterine arteries may show considerable hypertrophy and dilitation. The intervillous spaces in the tumour may cause the contrast within to take on a fine crescentic curvilinear pattern. *Chorionephithelioma* on the contrary is highly vascular and early filling of the drainage veins occurs resembling that seen in angiomas. The examination will often confirm the tumour when clinical and immunological information is inconclusive. It is also an easy method for following the results of surgery or chemotherapy.

The presence of an *ectopic pregnancy* can also be confirmed arteriographically. Placental sinuses have been identified as soon as 35 days after the previous normal menstrual period and are seen to be separate from the normal intrinsic vessels of the uterus. Before embarking on arteriography for the demonstration of ectopic pregnancy, normal pregnancy must be carefully excluded on clinical grounds (Fernstrom, 1955).

LYMPHOGRAPHY

Using an oil-based medium it is possible to demonstrate many of the lymph nodes to which uterine carcinoma metastasizes. Bilateral injection into the dorsum of the feet by the now standard technique demonstrates the inguinal and external iliac groups of glands and the para-aortic glands. Lymphography can demonstrate the extent to which lymphatic spread has occurred without being clinically manifest. Since the internal iliac groups of glands rarely fill with contrast in the absence of proximal lymphatic obstruction, the early spread of carcinoma of the cervix may not be visualized. With oily medium, the glands remain radiologically visible for some months and follow-up films enable assessment of the completeness of surgical excision or the response to radiotherapy to be made.

Pelvic lymphocysts which occur quite frequently after radical hysterectomy can be well shown by lymphangiography as the contrast medium enters the cystic spaces. These spaces may be large and exert pressure effects on the ureters, bladder or bowel and cause venous compression.

Ovarian carcinoma may also spread to the para-aortic and paracaval nodes, in which sites these metastases may be seen by lymphography.

ILIAC PHLEBOGRAPHY

The object of this examination is to demonstrate occlusion, deviation or compression of the pelvic veins and lower vena cava by enlarged lymph nodes.

The veins may be demonstrated by bilateral femoral injection or by the intra-osseous method. The latter, being very painful, requires a general anaesthetic but does show the venous plexuses around the uterus and bladder and the sacral venous plexus more clearly. If the femoral vein method is used better filling can be obtained if abdominal compression is applied just prior to injection causing reflux filling of the internal iliac veins.

Comparative work on the various radiological methods for assessing spread of uterine carcinoma has shown that venography can be more informative in stage I carcinoma when the spread is close to the uterus and lymphography fails to demonstrate the affected nodes. As extension occurs, involved nodes along the common iliac vein are in the line of the injected contrast and lymphography becomes more informative. Venography is also valuable for demonstrating posterior nodes lying between the vena cava and the spine, and the degree of enlargement is sometimes better shown by the filling defect produced on the vena cava. Excretion pyelography is essential in the assessment of the extent of the disease by virtue of its demonstration of obstruction to the urinary tract (Lee *et al.*, 1971).

PELVIC PNEUMOGRAPHY
(P.P.G.; gynaecography)

The P.P.G. is an elegant means of demonstrating the uterus, its adenexa and the adjacent viscera (Lagarde *et al.*, 1962).

Apart from acute pelvic infection and pregnancy there are no contra-indications. Prior to the examination the colon should be cleared by an aperient given 24 hours before and by an enema given 2 to 3 hours before, since a loaded colon can obscure anatomical outlines. In addition the bladder should be emptied: some workers advocate catheterization which also permits air to be injected into the bladder. Under light sedation a pneumoperitoneum is now induced in the standard manner.

Air has been used for many years to induce and maintain the pneumoperitoneum but carries a very small risk of air embolism. For this reason some workers prefer to use CO_2, which however has the disadvantage of rapid absorption. Between 1200 cc and 2000 cc of gas are injected into the peritoneum depending on the patient's size and tolerance. The patient is conscious of abdominal distension and some interscapular pain. The patient now

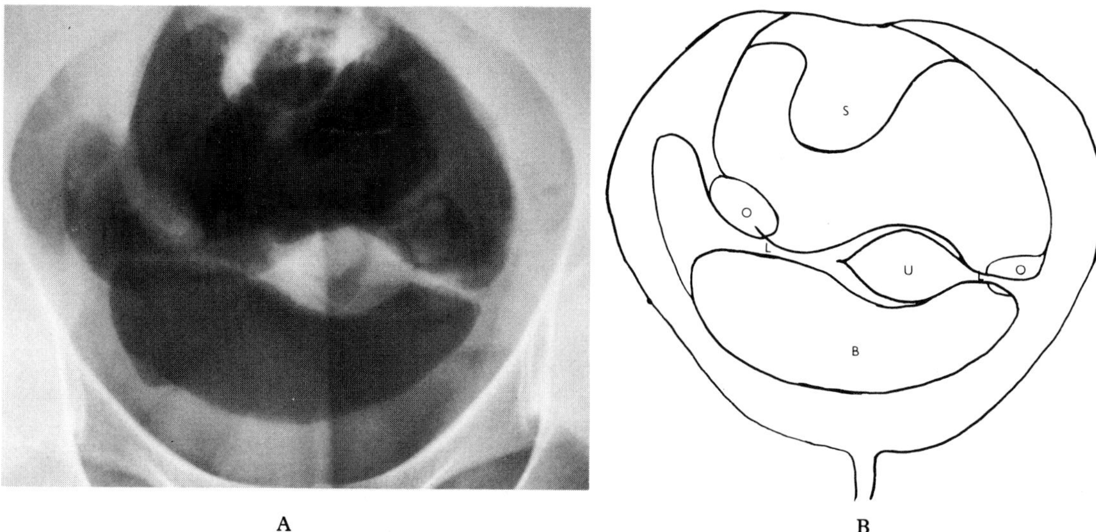

Fig. 48.28 (A) Normal pneumopelvigram. (B) Tracing of (A). B = Injected air in bladder; L = broad ligament; O = ovary; S = sigmoid colon; U = uterus.

lies prone on a tilting table and placed in about 35° of head-down tilt, thus causing the gas to rise into the pelvic cavity. Films are taken with the over-couch tube directed vertically down and centred on the upper part of the natal cleft. Oblique views, which often render the ovaries more clearly visible are obtained by rotating the patient 15° to 20° to either side.

The resulting picture shows the uterus as a double oval contour, the large oval (5–7 cm × 3–5 cm) representing the body and the small oval the cervix. The broad ligaments containing the Fallopian tubes (3–6 mm diameter) extend laterally from the uterus to the pelvic side walls and the round ligament can often be seen in the anterior part of each broad ligament shadow. The ovaries are shown on each side, their long axes lying obliquely across the pelvis. Normally they measure between 2–4 cm × 1·5–3 cm. Anteriorly the shadow of the bladder may be distinguished.

The rectosigmoid lies behind the uterus and occasionally loops of small bowel are seen in the pelvis (Fig. 48.28A and B).

This technique can demonstrate the origin of a pelvic mass, whether uterine, tubal or ovarian (Fig. 48.29A and B). Extension of uterine carcinoma into the broad ligament

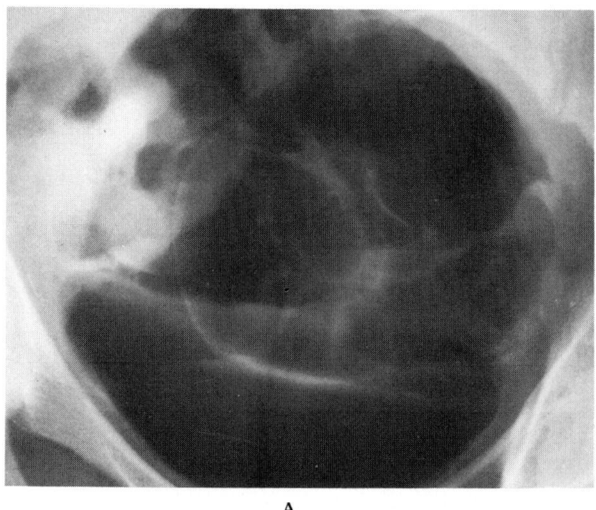

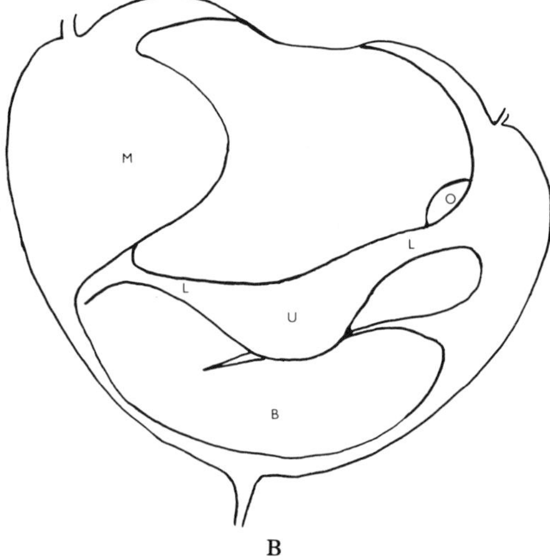

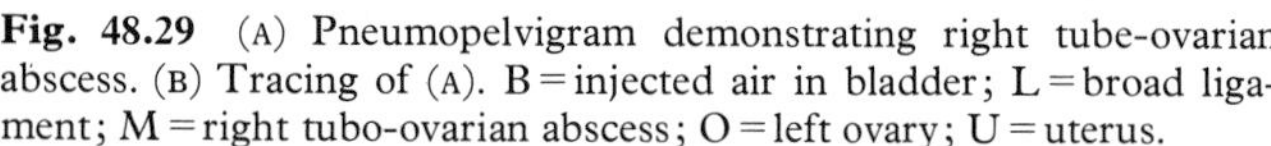
Fig. 48.29 (A) Pneumopelvigram demonstrating right tube-ovarian abscess. (B) Tracing of (A). B = injected air in bladder; L = broad ligament; M = right tubo-ovarian abscess; O = left ovary; U = uterus.

may be seen even before lymphatic metastases can be demonstrated while masses due to endometriosis can also be shown. The procedure has been most frequently used to show the ovarian enlargement in the Stein-Leventhal syndrome (hirsuties, oligomenorrhoea and infertility associated with enlarged polycystic ovaries). It has also proved of use in the investigation of primary amenorrhoea, gonadal dysgenesis and premature ovarian failure.

REFERENCES AND SUGGESTIONS FOR FURTHER READING

ASPLUND, J. (1959) The cervix as a factor in fertility—some radiological considerations. *Acta obstetrica gynecologica scandinavica*, **38**, Suppl. 1, 26–38.

BARNETT, E. (1955–56) The clinical value of hysterosalpingography. Part I. *Journal of the Faculty of Radiologists*, 7, 115–129.

BARNETT, E. (1955–56) The clinical value of hysterosalpingography. Part II. *Journal of the Faculty of Radiologists*, 7, 184–196.

FODA, M. S. *et al.* (1962) Hysterography in diagnosis of abnormalities of the uterus. Part I. *British Journal of Radiology*, **35**, 115–121.

FODA, M. S. *et al.* (1962) Hysterography in diagnosis of abnormalities of the uterus. Part II. *British Journal of Radiology*, **35**, 783–792.

FODA, M. S. *et al.* (1962) Hysterography in diagnosis of abnormalities of the uterus. Part III. *British Journal of Radiology*, **35**, 836–842.

FERNSTROM, I. (1955) Pelvic arteriography. *Acta radiologica*, Suppl. 122.

GREENBAUM, E. I., PODOLAK, G. & O'LOUGHLIN, J. (1969) The use of hysterography in the detection of hydatidiform mole. *American Journal of Roentgenology*, **105**, 885–889.

LAGARDE, C. *et al.* (1962) *La Pneumopelvigraphie.* Paris (VIe): Masson et Cie.

LEE, K. F. *et al.* (1971) The value of pelvic venography and lymphography in clinical staging of carcinoma of the uterine cervix. *American Journal of Roentgenology*, **111**, 284–296.

PECK, A. G., YODER, I. C. & PFISTER, R. C. (1975) Tomography of pelvic abnormal masses during intravenous urography. *American Journal of Roentgenology*, **152**, 322–330.

WHITEHOUSE, G. H. (1977) The radiology of urinary tract abnormalities associated with hysterectomy. *Clinical Radiology*, **28**, 201–210.

YOUSSEF, A. F. (1958) The uterine isthmus and its sphincter mechanism. A radiological study. *American Journal of Obstetrics and Gynecology*, **75**, 1305–1332.

PART 6

E.N.T.; EYES; TEETH; SOFT TISSUES

CHAPTER 49

THE PHARYNX AND LARYNX

The contrast provided by the air content of the pharynx and larnyx makes these structures eminently suitable for examination by X-rays. Radiological investigation has none of the discomfort associated with indirect or direct endoscopy although its accuracy is considerably inferior to that of endoscopy. Nevertheless, particularly in young children and nervous subjects, radiological investigation is invaluable and may be the only method of examination possible without recourse to general anaesthesia. Radiological studies of the pharynx and larynx using contrast material are more accurate than plain radiography but they demand a greater degree of co-operation from the patient and are more time-consuming to perform.

PLAIN RADIOGRAPHY

Plain radiography of the nasopharynx is best performed in a lateral position when the pharynx and larynx are thrown clear of the overlapping shadows of the cervical spine. With the film placed against the shoulder, the incident beam centred on the angle of the jaw and with a tube-film distance of 6 feet, distortion is minimal. Accurate coning avoids scatter and the air content of the pharynx and larynx enables the soft shadows of the pharyngeal walls and the vocal cords to be accurately delineated. When the larynx is examined in the lateral position the incident beam should be centred on the midpoint of the thyroid cartilage. The lower jaw is kept in the normal resting position and the tip of the tongue slightly protruded, whilst the film is taken.

Antero-posterior views are less satisfactory as the overlying shadows of the cervical spine largely obscure the soft-tissue shadows of the pharynx and larynx. Films taken during a modified Valsalva manoeuvre, with the lips closed distending the pharynx, enable the soft tissues to be more readily seen.

Antero-posterior tomographic studies of the larynx with the patient phonating ēe allow the ventricular bands and vocal cords to be seen. The laryngeal ventricle, separating the ventricular bands and vocal cords, because of its air content can also be seen. The incident beam is centred on the larynx with the patient in the supine position and the lower jaw tucked in. The patient's head and shoulders are arranged so the larynx is as far as possible parallel to the film (Fig. 49.1).

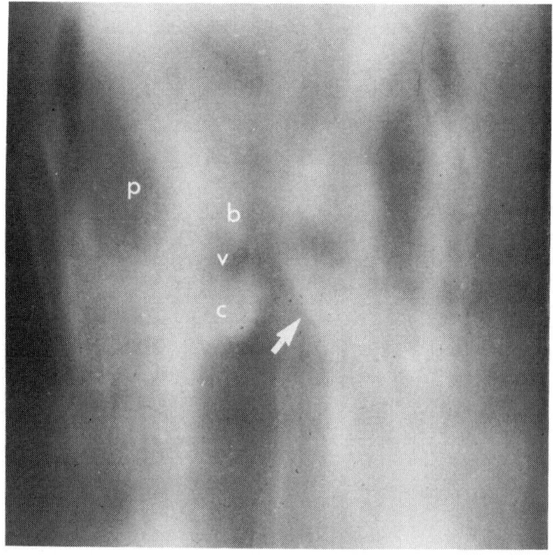

Fig. 49.1 Tomograph of larynx showing the appearances with a recurrent laryngeal palsy. The loss of the sharp angle consequent on the falling-in of the arytenoid cartilage is characteristic. This is seen immediately below the left vocal cord (*arrow*). p = pyriform fossa; b = ventricular band; v = ventricle; c = vocal cord.

Xerograms taken in the lateral position greatly improve the detail seen by the conventional method.

CONTRAST METHODS

Nasopharyngograms. Instillation of 10 ml of oily Dionosil through a polythene catheter introduced through the nostril with the head hyper-extended over the end of the radiographic table allows the contrast medium to pool in the nasopharynx. This enables the outline of the walls of the nasopharynx to be seen. Submento-vertical views with the patient in the same position enable the filled lateral recesses of the nasopharynx to be visualized (Fig. 49.2).

Films taken after a modified Valsalva with the lips closed, before and immediately after swallowing the contrast medium, enable a double contrast examination to be obtained and early mucosal changes in the lateral nasopharyngeal walls to be recognized.

Laryngograms. Instillation of oily Dionosil through a polythene nasal catheter with its tip above the epiglottis after local anaesthetization of the larynx allows the larynx to be coated with contrast material. Preliminary instruction of the patient to enable him to breathe with the larynx open during instillation, and the intramuscular injection of Atropine before commencing the procedure, are measures which greatly improve the quality of the laryngogram.

Films taken on a serial fluoroscopy device with spot films, with the patient phonating or performing a Valsalva manoeuvre, enable the outlines and movements of the vocal cords to be seen. Contrast laryngograms have proved of great value in assessing the outline of tumours of the larynx and in determining the lower extent of tumours, information which cannot be obtained by endoscopy (Fig. 49.3). Oblique views of the contrast outlined larynx are particularly valuable in evaluating spread of cord tumours anteriorly across the anterior commissure, a factor which is of the greatest importance in estimating the prognosis of the growth. Laryngography is also of great value in evaluating laryngeal trauma, and in preoperative assessment of laryngeal strictures (Fig. 49.4).

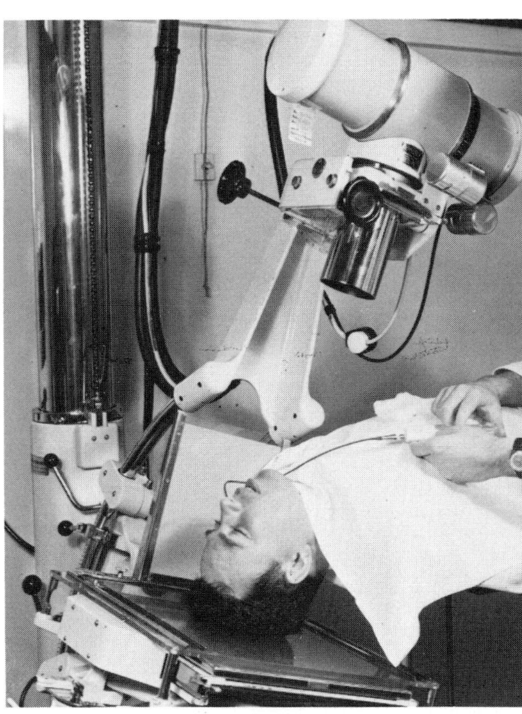

A

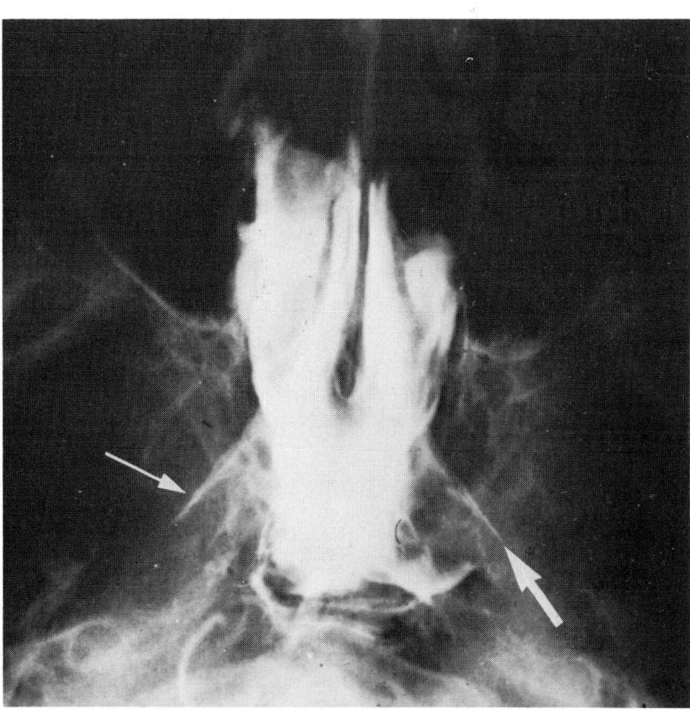

B

Fig. 49.2 A Technique of nasopharyngogram showing the nasal catheter inserted and head held in a submento-vertical position until the nasopharynx is filled. Films are immediately taken and then with forced expiration against a closed nose and mouth. B Normal nasopharyngogram showing filling of Eustachian tubes (*arrows*) and the Eustachian fossa around its origin. The posterior end of the nasal septum is seen as a filling defect in the midline.

PHARYNX

The pharynx is best investigated by a barium swallow. Serial films and cine films during swallowing enable the passage of the bolus of barium to be seen and films taken immediately afterwards show good mucosal relief. The postero-anterior and oblique projections are more valuable than the lateral view in assessing the early changes in the mucosa which occur with neoplasm.

Radiological anatomy. The pharynx is subdivided into the nasopharynx, oropharynx and hypopharynx. The *nasopharynx* lies above the level of the lower margin of the soft palate, the oropharynx being the portion of the pharynx between the soft palate and the root of the tongue, and the hypopharynx that portion of pharynx below this level.

The posterior wall of the nasopharynx is shown on the lateral film as a thin soft tissue shadow lying anterior to the cervical vertebrae (Fig. 49.5). The thickness of this soft tissue shadow varies; it averages 2 to 3 mm in the nasopharynx and 5 mm in the hypopharynx. On the lateral wall of the nasopharynx a dark slit-like shadow

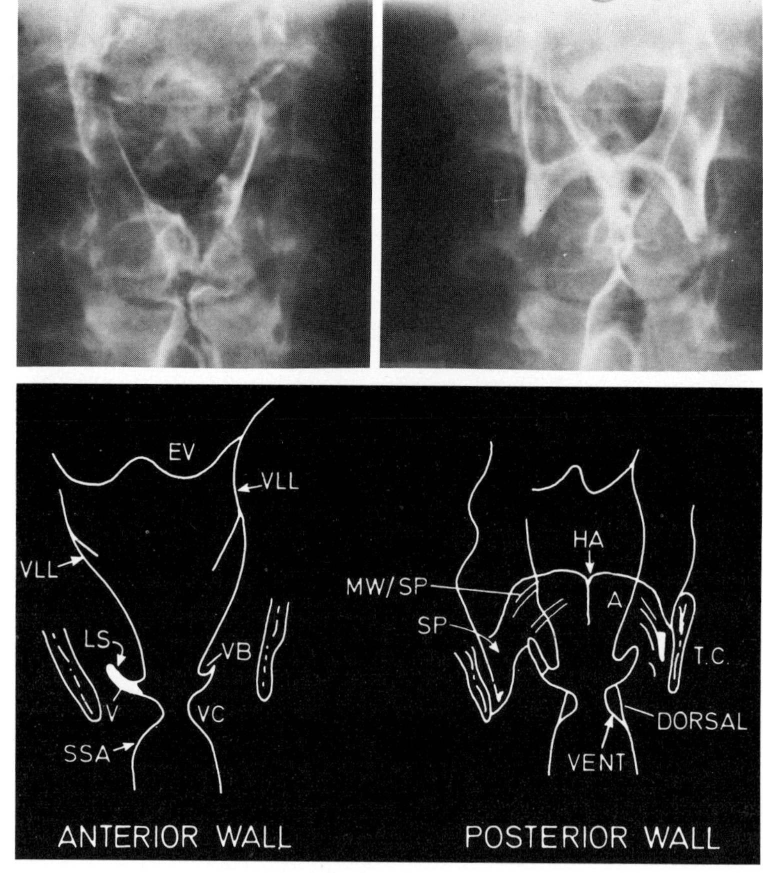

Fig. 49.3 Normal laryngogram, A.P. view. EV—vallecula. VLL—lateral pharyngeal wall. VB—ventricular band. VC—vocal cord. V—ventricle. SSA—subglottic area. HA—mucosa covering posterior wall of larynx. A—arytenoid. SP—pyriform sinus. LS—laryngeal saccule. MW/SP—medial wall pyriform sinus.

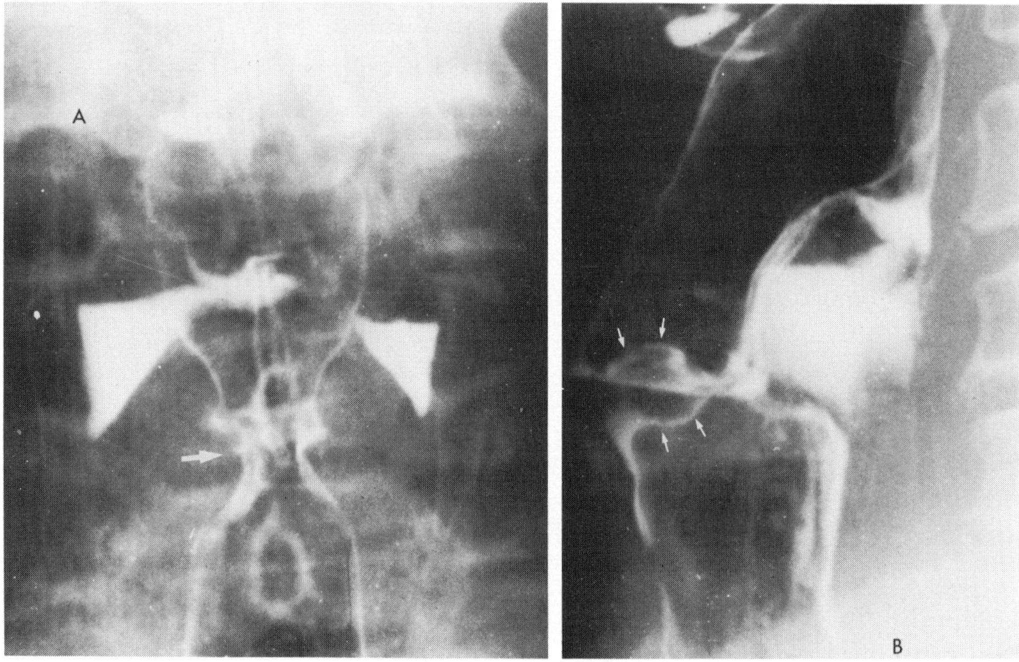

Fig. 49.4 (A and B) Antero-posterior and lateral views of laryngogram showing an intrinsic tumour of the right vocal cord. The tumour is coated with contrast medium (*arrows*) and is far more readily appreciated in the lateral film (B) than in the A.P. film.

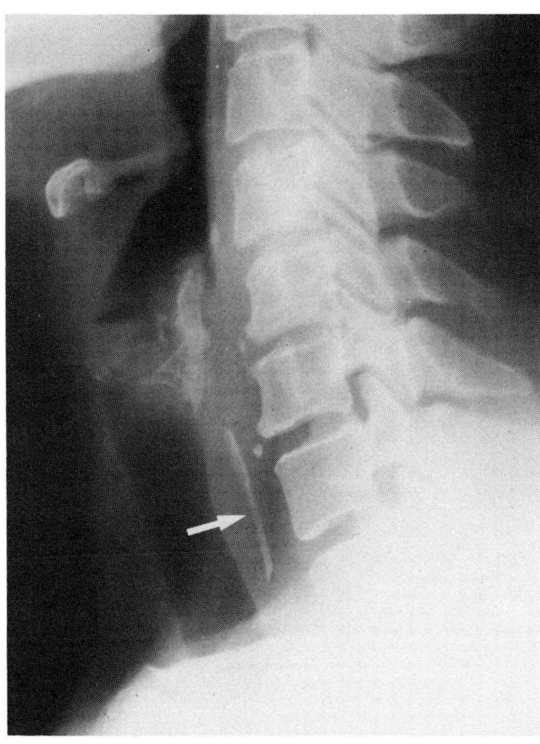

Fig. 49.5 Foreign body—a fishbone impacted in the post-cricoid region seen in the lateral film. The normal markings of the ventricle are seen and the small ossicles of bone in the anterior longitudal ligament of the spine must not be mistaken for a radio-opaque foreign body.

approximately $\frac{1}{2}$ inch long indicates the orifice of the Eustachian tube and a slightly increased density is due to the tubal eminence around the origin of the tube. Anteriorly the nasopharynx is bounded by the posterior choanae with their bone outlines and below by the soft palate.

The *oropharynx* is bounded by the posterior portion of the upper surface of the tongue and the mucosal folds on the back of the tongue vary considerably with the degree of protrusion. With the tongue indrawn the mucosal ridges on the back may show a crenated appearance mimicking a tumour.

The anterior wall of the *hypopharynx* is bounded laterally by the aryepiglottic folds with the valleculae separated by a central median fold and the pyriform fossae lying lateral to the aryepiglottic folds.

LARYNX

Radiological anatomy. The larynx can be clearly seen in the lateral view with the beak-like soft tissue shadow of the epiglottis separating the valleculae in front from the laryngeal entrance behind.

The aryepiglottic folds form linear shadows crossing the entrance of the larynx obliquely (running upwards and forwards) and the soft tissue shadows of the ventricular bands and vocal cords can be seen separated by the triangular increased translucency of the laryngeal ventricle running horizontally across the middle of the thyroid cartilage which surrounds the larynx.

It must be realized that the cartilages of the larynx actually form bone, that is, they ossify and form regular bone patterns. The commonly used term of 'calcification' is completely erroneous.

The thyroid cartilage and cricoid cartilage surround the larynx and show varying degrees of ossification which appear to be genetically determined but which advance in degree with increasing age. This ossification does not appear to be wholly degenerative as the bony pattern shows some regularity; it is seldom seen in younger age groups.

Ossification in the laryngeal cartilages begins in the inferior aspect of the thyroid cartilage and less frequently in the superior and inferior cornua; later patchy ossification occurs in the lateral thyroid laminae.

Ossification also begins in the posterior lamina of the cricoid cartilage, frequently at the same age as when the process starts in the thyroid cartilage. Dense ossification may occur in the arytenoid cartilage (before any ossification has appeared in the thyroid or cricoid cartilage) and superimposition of both arytenoid cartilages may sometimes mimic foreign body. Ossification in the curved horns of the cricoid and in the corniculate and cuneiform cartilages also may be mistaken for swallowed foreign bodies lying in the cervical oesophagus. The epiglottis, being composed of yellow elastic cartilage, ossifies only rarely.

The hyoid bone also ossifies and ossification in the body of the hyoid bone occurs at an early age. Both cornua of the hyoid bone also ossify, the greater cornua being involved to a greater degree than the lesser cornua. Occasionally ossification in the stylo-hyoid ligament may virtually fuse the hyoid bone to the styloid process of the temporal bone.

The soft tissue shadows of the adenoid lymphoid pad can be seen in the nasopharynx arising from the postero-superior wall and radiology forms an easy means of detecting enlargement of this structure in young children. The tonsils when enlarged may also cast soft tissue shadows in the lateral film.

Congenital lesions

Congenital deformities of the larynx are a cause of stridor in infancy. Web formation and under-development of the larynx are the commonest malformations. Radiological examination of the larynx is valuable and differentiation of these two conditions is important as congenital web persists, whereas with the under-developed larynx this deformity gradually disappears as the infant grows and the laryngeal stridor clears *pari passu* with increase in laryngeal size.

Papillomata and congenital laryngeal cysts are less common causes of infantile stridor, but can equally be recognized in lateral views as soft tissue masses with well-defined outlines projecting into the laryngeal air space. The papilloma can sometimes be differentiated from the cyst by the presence of air entrapped between the papillary folds.

Traumatic lesions

Major injuries to the larynx generally result in rapid asphyxiation unless life-saving measures to restore the airway are immediately instituted. Radiological investigation is seldom needed in the acute stage.

The recognition of fractures of the hyoid or thyroid cartilages may cause some difficulty owing to the variability of ossification in these structures and gaps in the ossific pattern may be confused with fractures. Laryngography has enabled dislocations of the arytenoid bone to be recognized. Such dislocations are associated with hoarseness and alterations in the voice quality and loss of the arytenoid swelling is shown.

Necrosis of any part of the laryngeal cartilages may follow infection or radiotherapy treatment for malignant disease, and stricture formation of the larynx with stenosis may be a sequel.

Injuries involving the pharynx are rare but may occur as the result of stab wounds in the neck, or may follow surgical intervention or endoscopy. The commonest cause of injury in both the pharynx and larynx is, however, a sequel of a swallowed or inhaled foreign body or following its attempted removal. Swallowed radio-opaque foreign bodies may lodge in the pharynx or in the cervical portion of the oesophagus at any age. In infants and the very elderly they may regurgitate into the nasopharynx, where a foreign body of considerable size may remain without producing symptoms for an appreciable time. The commonest ingested foreign body is a fish or meat bone and it is important to distinguish the calcification in the foreign body from the normal ossification in laryngeal cartilages already described (Fig. 49.5). A barium swallow with barium mixtures of different thicknesses usually locates the foreign body. Barium soaked pledgets of cottonwool may cause some fibres to be held up in a foreign body and indicate its site when conventional barium swallows fail. The extensive use of plastic for dentures, buttons and other common objects which may be swallowed makes it imperative that a barium swallow be undertaken in any case of suspected foreign body. These objects are relatively radiolucent and cast little or no shadow on the plain radiograph.

Infections

Laryngitis, either acute or chronic, does not produce any radiological signs, and tuberculous laryngitis, even when there is considerable mucosal ulceration, seldom shows more than a generalized swelling of the laryngeal soft tissues with partial obliteration of the air spaces. All cases of chronic laryngitis should have a chest radiograph as cases of tuberculous laryngitis still occur, particularly in the elderly.

Infections of the pharynx may spread to the retropharyngeal space or from abscesses around the tonsils. Retropharyngeal abscesses can be readily appreciated in the lateral film by an increase in the width of the soft tissue space anterior to the cervical vertebrae. Laterally placed pharyngeal abscesses around the tonsillar bed may give no signs in the lateral film, and submento-vertical films which show an indentation of the lateral wall may be difficult to take owing to muscle spasm associated with the abscess. Axial zonograms may help in these circumstances.

Perforation of the pharynx by a swallowed foreign body, e.g. a fish bone, may give rise to retropharyngeal abscesses and extensive swelling and surgical emphysema of the prevertebral soft tissues may occur. These changes are particularly clearly demonstrable in the lateral film and a fluid level may be visible. Less commonly, retropharyngeal infection occurs from a focus in the vertebral body and still more frequently from breakdown of the lymphatic glands in the retropharyngeal spaces. Infection in these two sites may be tuberculous.

Laryngoceles

An air-filled sac arising from a congenital pouch at the upper end of the ventricle of the larynx constitutes a laryngocele and gives a characteristic radiological appearance (Fig. 49.6).

Laryngoceles may be internal or external depending on whether they lie inside or outside the thyroid lamina. Internal laryngoceles may cause obstructive respiratory symptoms whereas the external laryngoceles produce soft tissue swellings visible in the subcutaneous tissues of the neck. Films taken in the antero-posterior position with forced expiration are more useful than lateral films in outlining the laryngocele. In the lateral position a small laryngocele may be superimposed on the normal laryngeal air shadow and may be overlooked. Tomographic studies in the antero-posterior plane are essential for the clear demonstration of small laryngoceles (internal) which have not extended outside the thyroid cartilage.

Congenital deformities of pharynx

Pharyngeal pouches, although thought to be the sequel of congenital weaknesses in the posterior pharyngeal wall (between oblique and transverse fibres of the inferior constrictor muscle) do not develop or present symptoms until well into adult life. Their radiological features are described in Chapter 32.

Strictures of the pharynx are seldom congenital as, if complete, they are not compatible with life. Web formation when it occurs is really in the cervical portion of the oesophagus and is almost invariably acquired and frequently associated with an iron-deficiency anaemia. Thus web formation is frequently associated with the Plummer-Vinson (Patterson-Brown-Kelly) syndrome and the condition is a probable precursor of malignant disease in the post-cricoid region.

These web-like shadows are most readily demonstrated when a barium swallow is carried out in the supine position and the passage of the barium bolus is considerably slowed. They usually arise in the upper 2 inches of the cervical oesophagus. They must be differentiated from deformities produced by a pharyngeal plexus of veins. Cineradiography or 100 mm films at six exposures per second are of great value in detecting small pharyngeal webs and are also invaluable in analysing any abnormalities of swallowing.

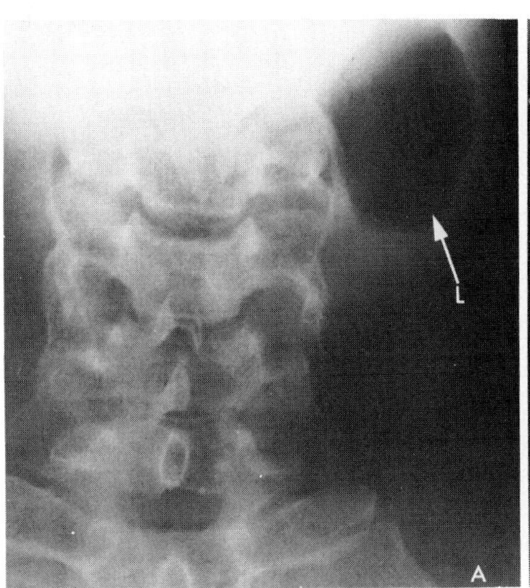

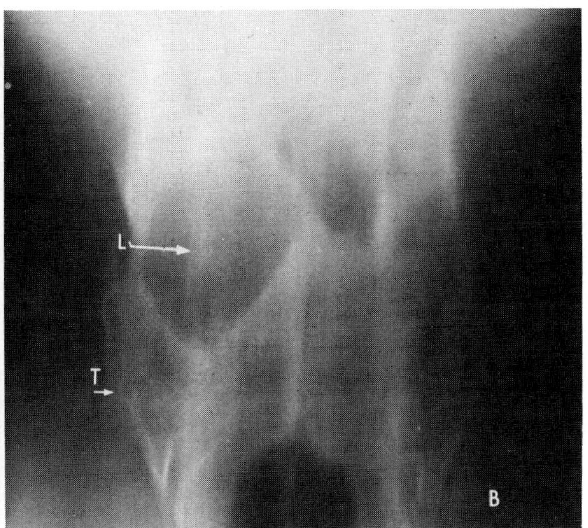

Fig. 49.6 A External laryngocele. Antero-posterior view showing distended air-containing sac. B Internal laryngocele. The air sac has remained within the confines of the thyroid cartilage (A.P. tomogram). L—laryngocele. T—thyroid cartilage.

TUMOURS OF THE PHARYNX AND LARYNX

NASOPHARYNX

Adenoid enlargement obliterating the nasopharyngeal air space to a varying degree and appearing as a soft tissue mass can be seen in the conventional lateral view of Antro-choanal polypi produce soft tissue masses of the same density, but can be seen to protrude through the posterior choana. In long-standing cases nasal polypi may produce bony atrophy of the choanal walls.

Benign tumours. A special type of tumour occurs in the nasopharynx in adolescent males, the *nasopharyngeal fibroma* (angiofibroma). These tumours, which are claimed to undergo spontaneous regression at puberty, have the radiological appearances of a large nasal polyp but attempts at removal may result in exsanguinating haemorrhage.

Nasopharyngeal fibroma may cause pressure atrophy and expansion of the bony nasal fossae, and this radiological feature allows the differentiation of these tumours from antro-choanal polypi which only produce bone changes in the elderly. The pressure atrophy associated with nasopharyngeal fibromata must be differentiated from destruction associated with malignant bone infiltration by the patchy nature of the latter process (Fig. 49.7).

Malignant tumours. Malignant tumours of the nasopharynx most frequently occur in the middle-aged or elderly and are usually adenocarcinoma. *Carcinoma* may arise in the ethmoid cells or in the nasopharynx and the appearance of metastatic malignant nodes in the neck may be the first sign of the disease. Paralysis of the cranial nerves is usually a late sign but represents extension of tumour into the foramina at the base of the skull.

Carcinoma occurring in the lateral wall of the nasopharynx may not be seen in the lateral film, and submentovertical views and nasopharyngograms are needed to demonstrate the tumour (Fig. 49.8A and B). As already stated, nasopharyngeal carcinoma frequently presents as metastatic enlargement of the glands in the cervical region and in such cases the detection of the primary tumour may be considerably assisted by careful radiography of the nasopharynx.

Other tumours arising in the sphenoidal region are *chordoma* and *carcinoma of the sphenoid sinus*. *Rathke's pouch tumours* also occur in this region and may protrude downwards into the nasopharynx, presenting a nasopharyngeal soft tissue mass. The destruction of the

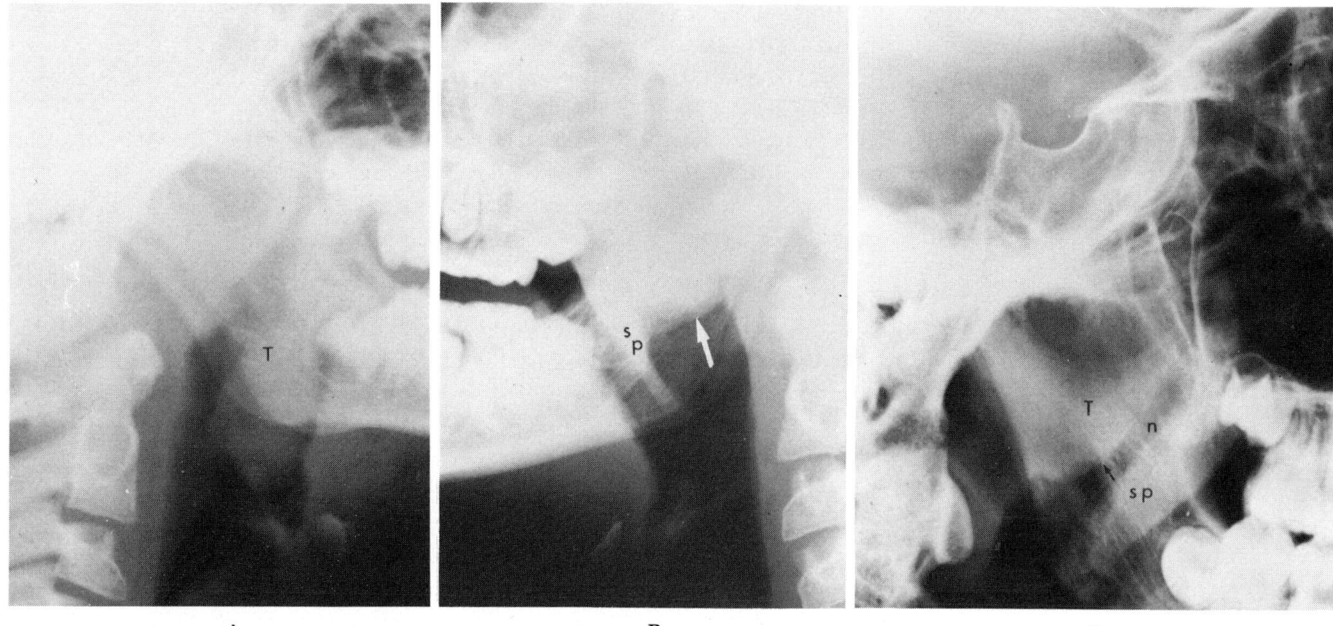

A B C

Fig. 49.7 A Adenoid pad. Lateral view of nasopharynx showing the soft tissue shadow of the adenoid arising from the postero-anterior part of the nasopharynx. Note also the large tonsillar shadows (T). B Fibrosarcoma in a child of 10 years. The lower border of the mass (*arrow*) is seen projecting into and obliterating the nasopharynx. The soft palate (sp) is displaced anteriorly. C Angiofibroma of nasopharynx (↖) in boy of 14 years. Lateral view of nasopharynx. T—tumour. n—nasopharyngeal air space compressed by tumour. sp—soft palate.

sphenoid bone may be extensive in all these types of tumour and it may not be possible to arrive at a definite diagnosis by radiological means alone.

Computerised axial tomography (C.A.T.) has provided a valuable new technique for the assessment of nasopharyngeal tumours and is extremely valuable in demonstrating the extent of spread and bone invasion (see. Ch. 65).

Oro- and Hypopharynx

Malignant tumours of the oro- and hypopharynx are almost invariably carcinomatous in origin and present

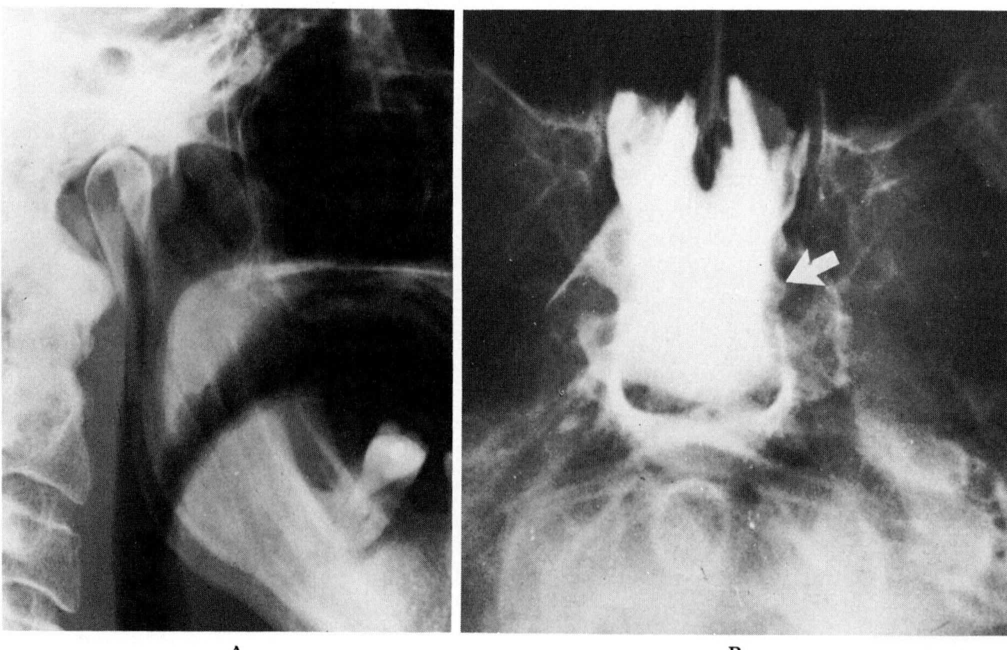

A B

Fig. 49.8 A Lateral view of nasopharynx showing no evidence of a carcinoma arising on the lateral wall of the nasopharynx. B Nasopharyngogram showing the displacement of the body of the oil inwards by the mass on the lateral wall of the nasopharynx (*arrow*).

as either *ulcerative* or *proliferative* lesions. Ulcerative tumours tend to occur on the anterior wall of the oropharynx around the base of the tongue (Fig. 49.9). Proliferative tumours, on the other hand, are more frequently found along the aryepiglottic folds.

Radiologically tumours of the oro- and hypopharynx present as:

(*a*) Soft tissue tumours encroaching on normal air-filled spaces, e.g. vallecula or pyriform fossa.

(*b*) Filling defects in a barium swallow when the lesion is advanced. However, antero-posterior studies to show mucosal relief are far more valuable in detecting early growths.

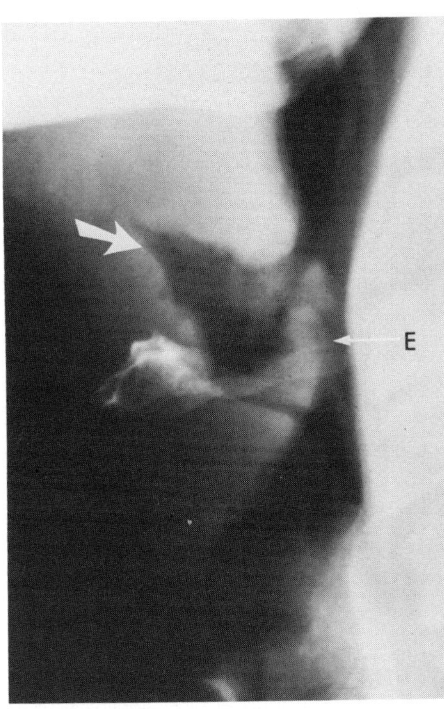

Fig. 49.9 Ulcerating cancer of base of tongue involving vallecula and destroying epiglottis (E). The ulcer crater with irregular outlines is clearly seen (*arrow*).

(*c*) Changes in the mucosal relief pattern. Contrast pharyngograms and laryngograms using oily Dionosil dropped over the back of the tongue on to an anaesthetized pharynx allow coating of the mucosa with the possible demonstration of early changes in mucosal pattern associated with malignant disease.

Growths in the hypopharynx usually occur in the post-cricoid region. Their relationship to oesophageal webs and the possible precancerous nature of such webs has already been described in Chapter 32. Predominantly, these growths are adenocarcinomata and occur in middle-aged females.

The radiological features are:

(*a*) Widening of the post cricoid space. Determination of what can be accepted as normal is the greatest problem in diagnosis, but an increase of the post-cricoid space of over 1 cm must be regarded with suspicion.

(*b*) Irregularity and hold-up in the barium swallow. The outline of the pharynx is irregular, the mucosal folds are destroyed and filling defects etc. are noted in the barium swallow.

(*c*) In the more advanced growths plain films may reveal that the cricoid and thyroid cartilages are both displaced forwards and tilted forward. Reflux and oesophageal contents into the trachea may occur with advanced growths, and suppurative broncho-pneumonia is a frequent complication.

LARYNX

The early diagnosis of tumours of the larynx is of greatest importance as early recognition can achieve a high cure rate. The common benign tumours of the larynx are cysts or papillomata, but in comparison with malignant disease they are uncommon.

Laryngeal cysts. Laryngeal cysts are either retention or congenital in origin. The congenital type are of utmost importance as they cause symptoms of laryngeal obstruction and stridor in the neonatal period and in infancy. They may also present as feeding problems in infancy.

The cysts can be recognized in plain lateral films of the larynx by the following signs:

1. The air cavity of the larynx is obliterated by the soft tissue swelling and the normal markings, e.g. the ventricle, are obliterated.
2. The oropharynx above the larynx is distended as a result of the laryngeal obstruction.
3. The upper outline of the cyst may be visible as a smooth rounded border visualized against the air-distended hypopharynx.

Laryngeal papilloma. Papilloma of the larynx may occur in infants or in adults. Laryngeal papillomata occurring in infancy do not predispose to malignancy and they are of importance because of the respiratory distress that they may produce.

They can be shown in lateral films of the larynx by the soft tissue mass which sometimes shows air trapped in the interstices of the papilloma and presents a characteristic speckled appearance. The papilloma may, however, present as a full, smoothly rounded shadow which cannot be differentiated from a laryngeal cyst. It may be associated with similar lesions in the bronchial tree.

Papilloma in the adult is premalignant and early recognition is of importance. Papilloma is best seen in the postero-anterior tomographs and in laryngograms and it may be impossible to differentiate such a tumour from papillary carcinoma.

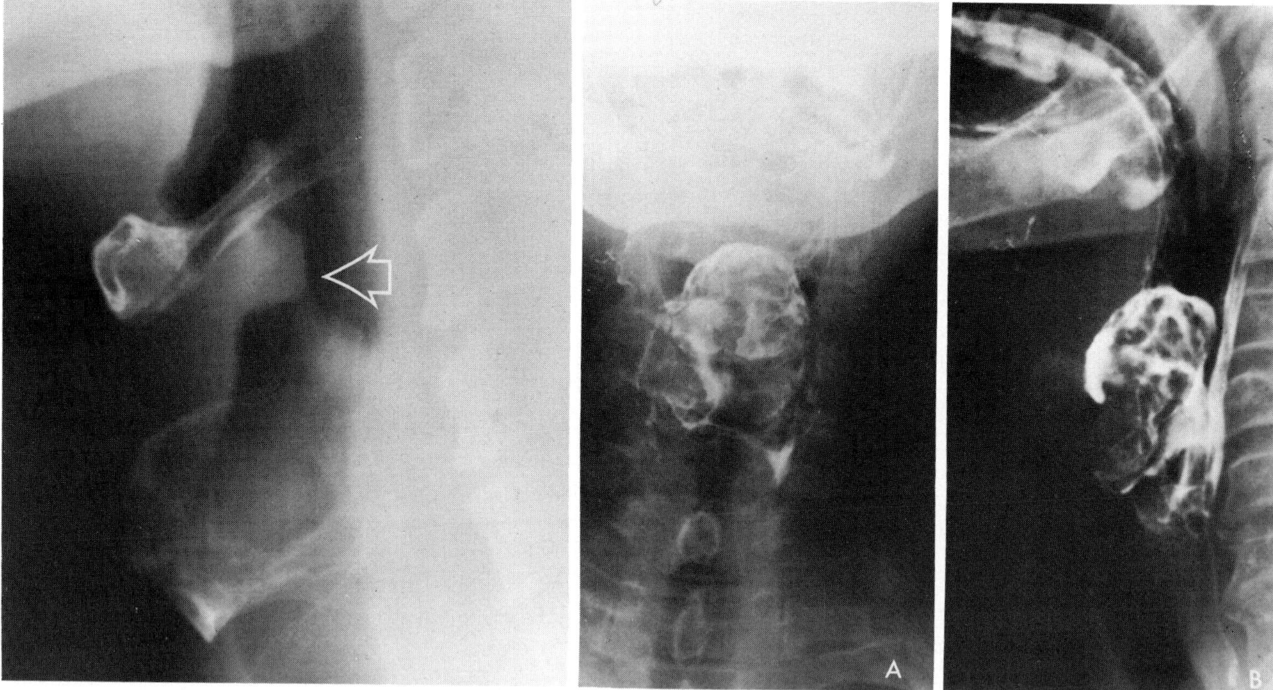

Fig. 49.10 Carcinoma of epiglottis. Soft tissue mass involving and destroying the epiglottis (*arrow*).

Fig. 49.11 (A and B) Carcinoma of pyriform fossa. Antero-posterior and lateral views after barium swallow. The mass is seen to project posteriorly into the midline having arisen in the right pyriform fossa. The outline of the tumour mass is covered with barium.

Malignant growths

The majority of malignant growths are carcinomata; sarcomata are extremely rare. Carcinomata are customarily classified into *supraglottic* (Figs. 49.10 and 49.11), *glottic* and *subglottic* growths depending on the site of origin of the tumour.

Glottic tumours. Just over two-thirds of carcinoma arising in the larynx occur in the vocal cord. Growths most frequently arise in the anterior two-thirds of the cord, less frequently on the anterior commissure, and still more rarely in the cartilaginous portion of the cord.

They are usually *proliferative* or *infiltrative* (*ulcero-erosive*) in type. The growth, especially in the latter type, may extend into the thyroid cartilage in the later stages but in the anteriorly situated tumour spread across the commissure occurs early and indicates a poor prognosis.

Growths of the vocal cord are best seen in the antero-posterior tomogram when a soft tissue tumour may be seen; spread across the anterior commissure is more difficult to detect in this view.

The lateral film is of more importance in estimating the forward spread of tumour when widening of the space behind the thyroid cartilage is more readily appreciated. These changes are more readily appreciated in the laryngogram.

Invasion of the thyroid cartilage by growth is difficult to diagnose as the irregular nature of ossification of the cartilage makes recognition of invasion difficult. The part

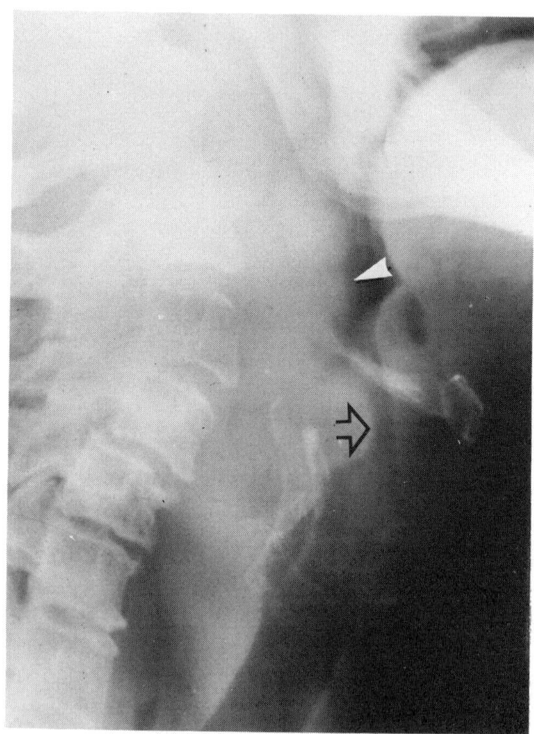

Fig. 49.12 Carcinoma of the hypopharynx arising from the posterior wall and almost obliterating the laryngeal entrance. The soft tissue mass (*hollow arrow*) projects into the laryngeal air space and there is a considerable upward (*solid arrow*) and downward extension of the growth. An extrinsic growth of the larynx spreading anteriorly may be difficult to differentiate.

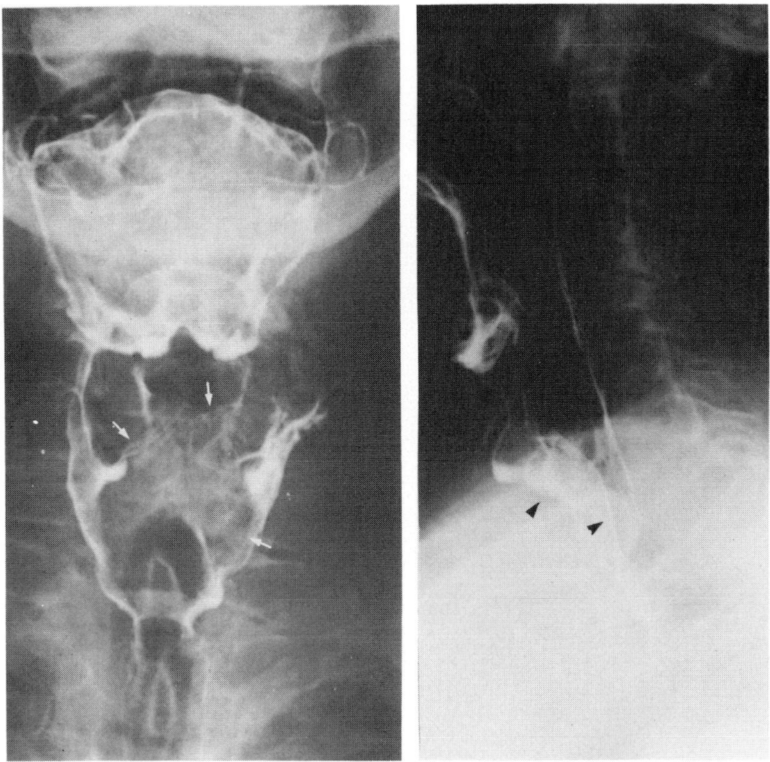

Fig. 49.13 Carcinoma of larynx (*arrows*)—showing invasion posteriorly into hypopharynx and mimicking carcinoma of oesophagus. A.P. and lateral projections with barium swallow.

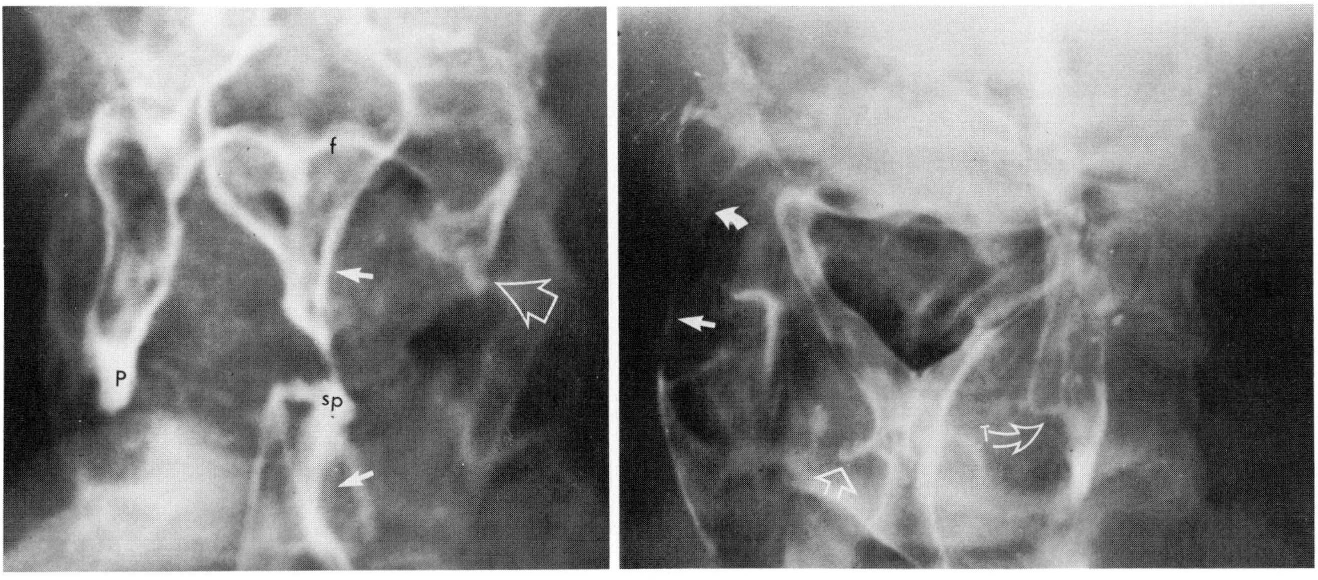

Fig. 49.14 A Laryngogram showing laryngeal cancer extending laterally and involving the left pyriform fossa (*hollow arrow*) and bulging the antero-lateral wall of the larynx (*solid arrow*) and also the subglottic space (sp). P = right pyriform fossa normally filled with contrast medium f = posterior mucosal folds at laryngeal entrance. B Valsalva in same case with distension of larynx (right lateral wall is shown by thick arrows). Straight hollow arrow indicates right ventricle. Curved hollow arrow indicates invasion of left pyriform fossa.

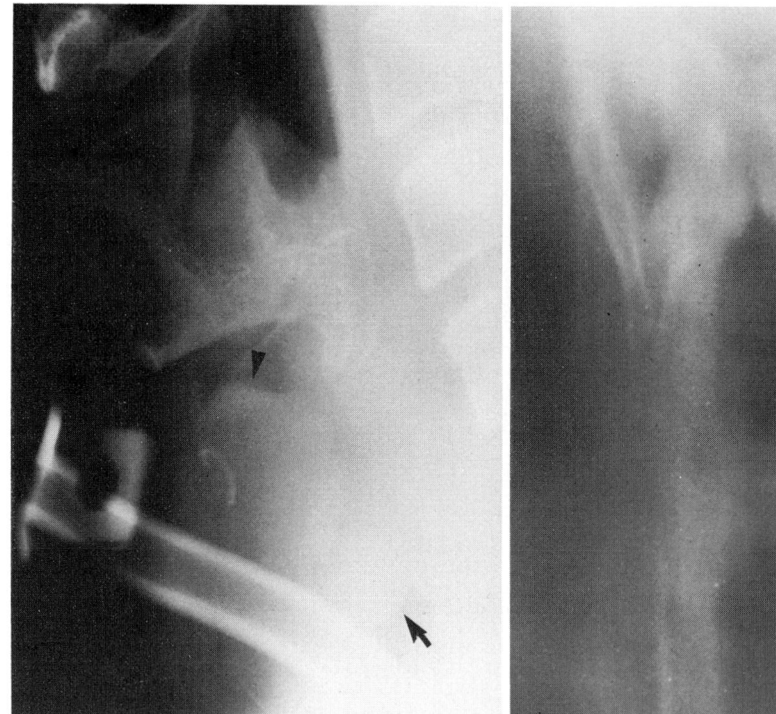

Fig. 49.15 *Fig. 49.16*

Fig. 49.15 Plasmocytoma of trachea—an extra-medullary plasmocytoma (*arrows*). Note the well-defined outline lying above the tracheostomy which was performed for tracheal obstruction.

Fig. 49.16 Secondary invasion of trachea (←) from a thyroid carcinoma. Note the absence of constriction of the trachea.

of the cartilage invaded depends on the site of origin of the growth. The appearance of mottling and irregularity in the anterior and inferior portion of the larynx usually implies anterior spread of the growth.

Supraglottic growths. Growths arising from the epiglottis usually arise from the posterior surface and tend to infiltrate deeply into the root of that structure. They have to be differentiated from growths arising in the superolateral part of the vestibule. The pharynx may be involved by direct spread of these growths (Fig. 49.13).

Growths arising in the ventricle of the larynx may penetrate deeply and may be difficult to distinguish from other supraglottic growths (Fig. 49.14).

Infraglottic growths. Growths arising in the subglottic space are far less frequent than supraglottic growths although extension downwards of supraglottic growths is not an unusual occurrence. They can be readily appreciated by the relative ease with which they show against the air-filled trachea (Figs. 49.12 and 49.13).

Tracheal tumours are uncommon and cylindroma is the commonest variety, and like infraglottic laryngeal growths they are easily seen in tomographs and plain films.

Plasmacytoma. One of the commonest sites for the development of extramedullary plasmacytoma is in the larynx or upper air passages. To the naked eye these tumours appear as grey or yellowish-grey masses. They may be the only manifestation of the disease but, although they may remain solitary for many years, the disease usually becomes generalised and ends with a diffuse multiple myelomatosis.

The tumour mass appears radiologically as a smooth rounded tumour, homogeneous in consistency and often indistinguishable from carcinoma of the larynx. The presence of a large, relatively asymptomatic mass should suggest the possibility of a plasmacytoma (Fig. 49.15). Invasion of the trachea may occur from a malignant thyroid growth (Fig. 49.16).

Recurrent nerve paralysis

The detection of the paralysed vocal cord can usually be made by simple laryngoscopy but in some circumstances the vocal cord cannot be seen.

Tomographic films in the antero-posterior position during phonation will demonstrate the failure of the cord to move and the generalized thickening of the affected side of the larynx with thickening of the subglottic tissues consequent on the falling forwards of the arytenoid cartilage associated with the nerve paralysis (Fig. 49.1). The ventricle on the affected side is enlarged and normal subglottic right angle becomes obtuse.

The same features can be seen after contrast laryngograms, and the general thickening of the soft tissues on the lateral wall is clearly seen in the subglottic region.

REFERENCES AND SUGGESTIONS FOR FURTHER READING

ARDRAN, G. M. & KEMP, F. H. (1967) The mechanism of the larynx, Parts I and II. *British Journal of Radiology*, **40,** 372–389.

CAVANAGH, F. (1965) Congenital laryngeal web. *Proceedings of the Royal Society of Medicine*, **58,** 272–277.

EPSTEIN, B. S. & WINSTON, P. (1957) Intubation granuloma. *J. Lar. Otol.*, **71,** 37–48.

HEMMINGSON, A. (1973) Corrugated vocal cords. *Acta radiologica Stockholm Diagnosis*, **14,** 289–294.

OWSLEY. W. C., Jr. (1962) Palate and pharynx: roentgenographic evaluation in the management of cleft palate and related deformities. *American Journal of Roentgenology*, **87,** 811–821.

POWERS, W. E., HOLTZ, S. & OGURA, J. (1964) Contrast examination of larynx and pharynx: inspiratory phonation. *American Journal of Roentgenology*, **92,** 40–42.

RIDEOUT, D. F. (1975) Appearances of the larynx after radiation therapy. *Canadian Journal of Otolaryngology*, **4,** 98–101.

STOUT, A. P. & KENNEY, F. R. (1949) Primary plasma cell tumours of the upper air passages and oral cavity. *Cancer*, N.Y., **2,** 261–278.

TUCKER, G. F. (1962) A histological demonstration of the development of laryngeal connective tissue compartments. *Transactions of the American Academy of Ophthalmology and Otolaryngology*, **66,** 308–318.

VALVASSORI, G. E. & GOLDSTEIN, C. (1970) Radiographic evaluation of the larynx. *Otolaryngologic Clinics of North America*, **3,** 465–481.

CHAPTER 50

THE PARANASAL SINUSES

ANATOMY

The paranasal sinuses consist of frontal sinuses, sphenoid sinuses, maxillary antra and the ethmoid complex of air cells. These sinuses lie within the facial bones and are grouped around the nasal cavities which contain the superior, middle and inferior turbinate bones on their lateral walls. The nasal cavities are separated by a septum which is partly cartilaginous and partly bony. The paranasal sinuses are lined by columnar-celled mucosa continuous with that of the nasal cavities with which they all communicate. The precise function of the paranasal sinuses is still not understood.

The *frontal sinuses* lie within the frontal bone and are separated by a bony or less frequently a fibrous septum which is seldom exactly midline in position. Occasionally the intersinus septum is completely or partly absent. Each frontal sinus consists of a vertical portion and a horizontal (supra-orbital) extension. The roof of the sinus is grooved by bony ridges from which fibrous septa extend into the sinus giving it a scalloped outline. Occasionally these fibrous septa are complete and the frontal sinus becomes loculated. The wall of the sinus has a thin bony cortex on which the mucosal lining lies and which produces a sharply defined pencil-like outline on the radiograph. Each frontal sinus drains via a fronto-nasal duct which runs vertically and slightly posteriorly to open into the anterior end of the hiatus semilunaris in the middle meatus.

The *maxillary antra* are the largest of the paranasal sinuses and are pyramidal-shaped cavities occupying the maxillae, each having three extensions into the surrounding facial bones, namely the zygomatic, tuberosity and alveolar recesses. The roots of the premolar and molar teeth, embedded in the maxilla, project upwards into the floor of the antrum. With loss of teeth the alveolus absorbs and the floor of the antrum frequently becomes separated from the mouth by only a thin bony layer. Each antrum opens via an ostium (halfway up its medial wall) into the hiatus semilunaris in the middle meatus.

The *sphenoid sinuses* are paired and occupy the body of the sphenoid bone and are separated by a thin bony septum. They may extend laterally into the pterygoid plates and occasionally into the greater wings of the sphenoid bone. Each sinus drains anteriorly into the superior recess of the nasal cavity. Normally the posterior limit of the sinus is approximately at the junction of the anterior two-thirds and posterior third of the sphenoid bone.

The *ethmoid sinuses* are a complex of small air cells lying in the lateral wall of the nasal cavity between its upper part and the medial wall of the orbit. The cells extend into the middle and superior conchae and drain individually into the middle or superior meatus. They have been grouped into anterior and posterior ethmoid groups but they are extremely variable in distribution. They may extend laterally into the maxillary antrum forming the ethmoidal bulla.

RADIOGRAPHIC TECHNIQUE

Radiographic views of the paranasal sinuses must be standardized as far as possible to facilitate reproducibility and subsequent comparison. Technical factors which are essential for good radiography of the sinuses are accurate coning of the incident beam, fine focal spot X-ray tubes and a Potter Bucky or fine grid to obtain maximum contrast. Some workers dispense with grids and consider that accurate coning is sufficient to obviate scatter; the resulting film however has less contrast which frequently makes it difficult to interpret the significance of minor loss of translucency in a sinus.

The standard radiographic projections usually employed are:

1. **Occipito-mental.** The subject sits facing the film and the radiographic base line is tilted to 45°. The incident beam is tilted 10° caudally and centred on the occipital bone 3 cm above the external occipital protuberance (Fig. 50.1).

In young subjects a tube tilt is unnecessary as they can readily extend the head to obtain the necessary tilt, but in older persons it may be necessary to increase the tube

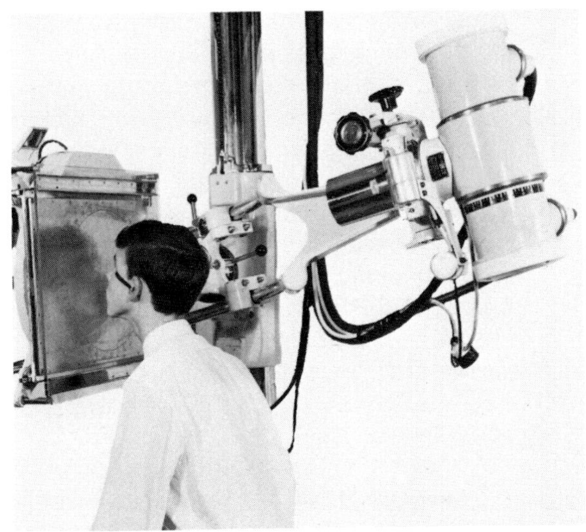

Fig. 50.1 Occipito-mental view showing the radiographic base line tilted to an angle of 45° and the incident beam angled caudally to 10° and centred 3 cm above the occiput.

tilt to 10° or 20° to compensate for the restricted extension of the head.

This view shows the maxillary antra free of any overlap of the petrous bones and if the mouth is kept open during the examination (particularly if the patient is edentulous), the sphenoid sinuses and nasopharynx can be seen through the open mouth.

The frontal sinuses are foreshortened in this view.

2. **Occipito-frontal.** The subject sits facing the film with his forehead in contact with the table top so that the base line is at right angles to the film. The incident beam is tilted 10° towards the feet and centred 3 cm above the external occipital protuberance (Fig. 50.2).

This projection demonstrates the fine detail of the frontal sinuses and also the lateral walls of the antra are seen, although the overlapping petrous temporal bones largely obscure the antra.

3. **Lateral.** The subject sits with the radiographic base line horizontal and the sagittal plane parallel to the film. The incident beam is centred through the antrum. the superimposition of the frontal sinuses and also of both maxillary antra detracts somewhat from the value of this projection.

4. **Submento-vertical.** The head is extended so that the vertex rests against the table top and the incident beam is centred between the angles of the jaw so that it is at right angles to the base line (Fig. 50.3).

In middle-aged and elderly patients the tube has to be considerably tilted upwards as few patients in this age group can attain the degree of extension necessary to bring the skull base parallel to the film. This projection demonstrates the sphenoid sinuses and also the maxillary antra and orbital walls.

5. **Oblique.** Rotation of the sagittal plane of the skull through an angle of 39° and angulation of the base line cranially to 30° will enable the posterior ethmoid cells to be projected through the orbit and will show these cells largely clear of overlap shadows. The optic foramen is seen end-on in this projection.

Examination of the sinuses should always, if possible, be made in the erect position to allow the demonstration of fluid levels within the sinus. Fluid in the sinus may be pus or mucopus occurring as a sequel of infection or allergy, but on occasion may be frank blood as a result of trauma. These different types of fluid cast shadows of identical density on the radiograph and the nature of the fluid cannot be recognized.

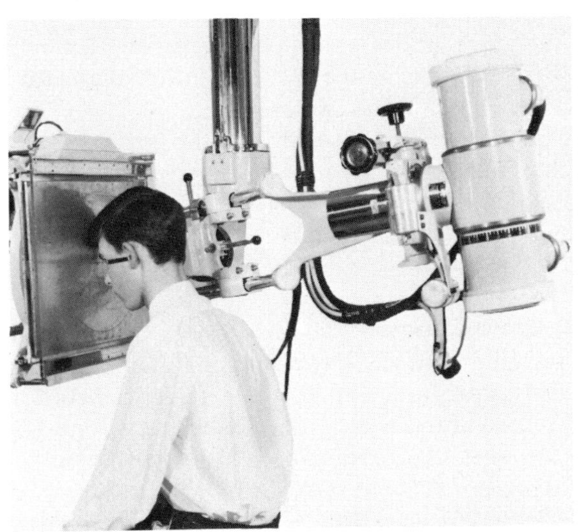

Fig. 50.2 Occipito-frontal view with a horizontal base line and the incident beam angled caudally by 10° and centred 3 cm above the occipital protuberance.

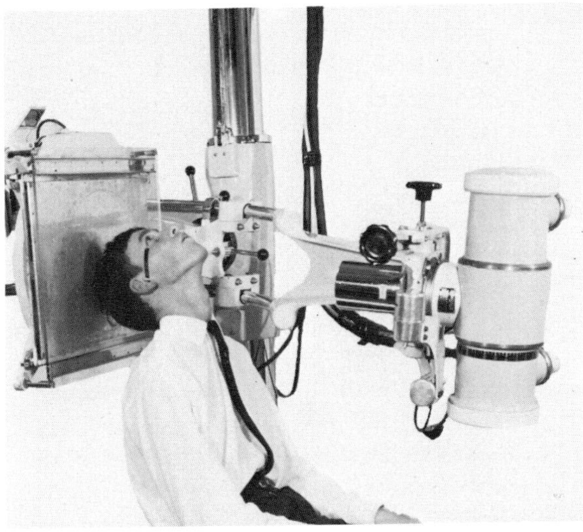

Fig. 50.3 Submento-vertical view with the base line parallel to the film and the incident beam centred at a point midway between the angles of the mandible and at right angles to base line.

Several types of specialized equipment are now in use for radiography of the sinuses, replacing the older type of sinus stand. These modern units operate by aligning the central beam on the film regardless of the position of the tube, and allow a wide range of radiographic projections to be carried out with minimum disturbance to the patient.

Specialized radiographic procedures such as *tomography* are of the greatest value in detecting fractures, foreign bodies and bone destruction of the sinus wall in malignant disease. A less commonly used radiographic procedure is the introduction of opaque medium by displacement (*Proetz technique*) to allow the mucosa of the sinus to be investigated. It has been claimed that this method can be used to assess the functional capacity of the antrum by demonstrating the ability of the ciliated lining mucosa to clear the sinus of the contrast medium.

COMPUTERISED TOMOGRAPHY

Computerised tomographic scanning has provided an important addition to the radiographic investigation of the paranasal sinuses. The size and extent of ethmoidal mucoceles and the extent of orbital invasion are far more readily assessed by this method.

Spread of tumour and recurrent growths of the nose and paranasal sinuses are more readily appreciated as are the extent of the soft tissue mass and the degree of bone erosion (see Ch. 65).

TRAUMA

Fracture of the facial bones is a common occurrence, and in motor vehicle accidents when the passengers are thrown forward, such fractures almost invariably affect one or more of the paranasal sinuses as a sequel of fracture of the facial bones. Fractures of the facial bones involving the paranasal sinuses may be grouped into:

1. Lateral face fractures
2. Mid-face fractures—
   (*a*) upper third
   (*b*) middle third
   (*c*) lower third
3. Nasal bone fractures

In the commonest fracture—the lateral fracture of the zygoma (tripod fracture)—the fracture lines involve the zygomatic arch, the lateral wall and the roof of the maxillary antrum (Fig. 50.4), and the fracture is associated with widening of the fronto-zygomatic synchondrosis (see p. 223). The fracture through the roof of the maxillary antrum may or may not cross the inferior orbital canal involving the inferior orbital nerve and producing anaesthesia in the distribution of the nerve.

The radiographic changes in the antra vary with the degree of trauma but are usually one of the following:

1. Complete loss of translucency. This may be caused by mucosal thickening due to traumatic oedema and may be associated with haemorrhage into the antrum.

2. Localized opacities due to mucosal or submucosal haematoma—which generally in the case of the maxillary antrum appear as clear-cut swelling of the mucosa along the roof or lateral wall in relation to the fracture line.

3. The antral translucency may be normal despite involvement of its walls by the fracture line.

Fractures of the middle third of the face are the result of force directed to the midline and may be grouped into upper, middle and lower mid-third facial fractures depending on the relation of the lines of fracture to the nasal and maxillary bones.

The *upper third* fractures involve the nasal processes of the frontal bones and the medial walls of the orbit. The fracture line extends along the floor of the frontal sinus and the cribriform plate and consequently is frequently associated with dural tears and cerebrospinal rhinorrhoea. Orbital emphysema may also be associated with upper third fractures and in fractures involving the ethmoid bones it may be the only indication of a fracture. Orbital emphysema must not be confused on the radiograph with the translucency which is associated with fat in the eyelid. In such cases the symmetry of the radiolucent fat line enables it to be differentiated from orbital emphysema. Intracranial pneumatocele or spontaneous ventriculography may be seen after this type of fracture. Tomography is invaluable in detecting the extent of the fracture line and in demonstrating unexpected extensions of the fracture, and is most informative in the postero-anterior rather than the lateral position.

Fractures of the *middle third* of the face involve the medial walls of the maxillary antra. They are frequently associated with backward displacement of the fractured segment, giving rise in the lateral view of the face to a 'dish face' appearance. The planes of fracture are such that the whole of the middle third of the facial bones is pushed backwards and impacted.

Lower third fractures extend through the dense bone of the maxilla and separate the hard palate and the tooth-bearing alveolus. They are especially prone to produce malocclusion and may be more readily appreciated from an inspection of the dental occlusion than on the radiograph.

Lateral views of the facial bones are of importance in assessing the displacement, and stereoscopic views in occipito-mental and the 30° occipito-mental positions are also useful in assessing the degree of displacement.

Occasionally a fracture of the roof of the antrum (floor of orbit) may occur without injury to the orbital margin—*blowout fracture*. The trauma is transmitted through the intact globe to the floor of the orbit and fracture of the floor of the orbit is associated with a loss of orbital tissue, muscle and fat, which is displaced downwards into

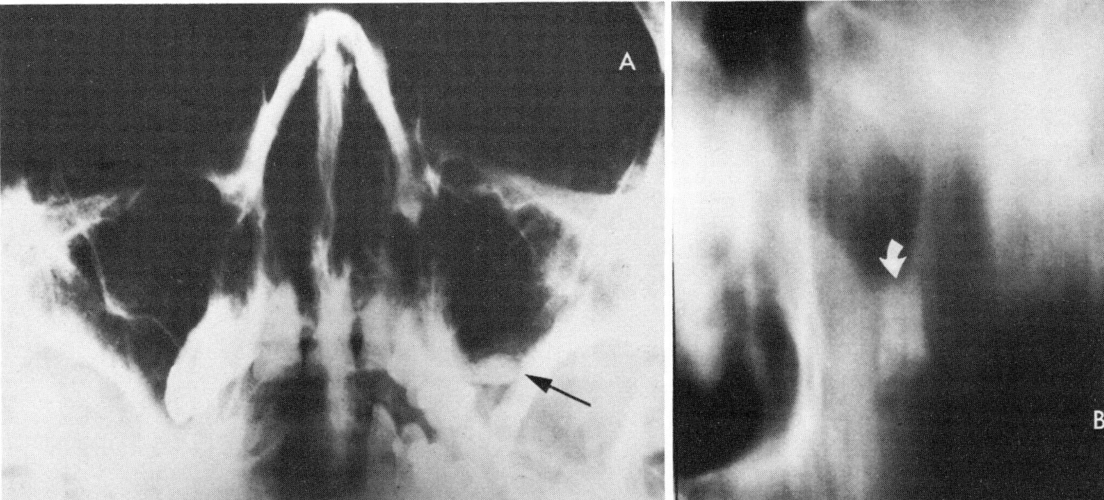

Fig. 50.4 Traumatic antro-oral fistula. A Occipito-mental view showing root lying below mucosa of left antrum. B P.A. tomograph demonstrating root lying in left antrum. Tomography is necessary to show root when covered by mucosal thickening.

the antral cavity. The globe sinks as a consequence of loss of support from the orbital floor and diplopia may result in some cases.

Barotrauma

A special form of trauma affects the paranasal sinuses as a result of alterations in atmospheric pressure. These changes were noted originally during flying in unpressurised aircraft. Barotrauma changes today are more commonly seen in divers or sub-aqua swimmers.

In barotrauma obstruction of the ostium of the antrum or fronto-nasal duct, usually due to a flap of mucosal thickening or polypoid mucosa, causes a failure of pressure equalization between the atmospheric pressure and that of the sinus. The altered pressure within the sinus may cause an outpouring of secretion and a thickening of the lining mucosa.

Occasionally the changes may be sufficiently severe to cause submucosal bleeding which gives rise to a localized polypoid swelling of the lining mucosa.

The radiological appearances of barotrauma may be complete opacification of the antrum due to generalized mucosal swelling, or localized mucosal thickening simulating a polyp. Barotrauma changes are more prone to occur in a sinus if there is pre-existing disease such as allergy or antral polypi present.

Traumatic antro-oral fistula

Fracture of the tooth socket may occur during extraction with displacement of a tooth root into the antrum. The root may lie below the mucosa and produce few and localized changes in the antral mucosa (Fig. 50.4) or more commonly may enter the antral cavity proper producing a completely opaque antrum. In such cases postero-anterior tomograms may be needed to demonstrate the tooth root through the opaque antrum.

INFLAMMATORY AND ALLERGIC CHANGES

Allergic, vasomotor and infective changes all produce oedematous swelling of the mucosa which may be associated with varying degrees of exudation into the affected sinus. In the case of the allergic or vasomotor changes the exudate is usually clear of mucopurulent (Fig. 50.5). In infective conditions of the sinuses, which are almost invariably a result of spread of infection from the nasal cavities after an upper respiratory infection, the secretions may become mucopurulent or frankly purulent (Fig. 50.6).

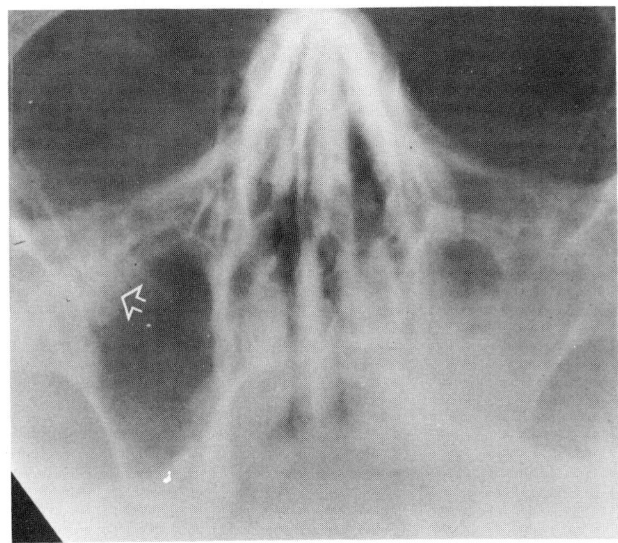

Fig. 50.5 Mucosal thickening in left maxillary antrum and to a lesser extent in right antrum. Note polypoidal thickening of the mucosa over the lateral wall of the right antrum (arrow).

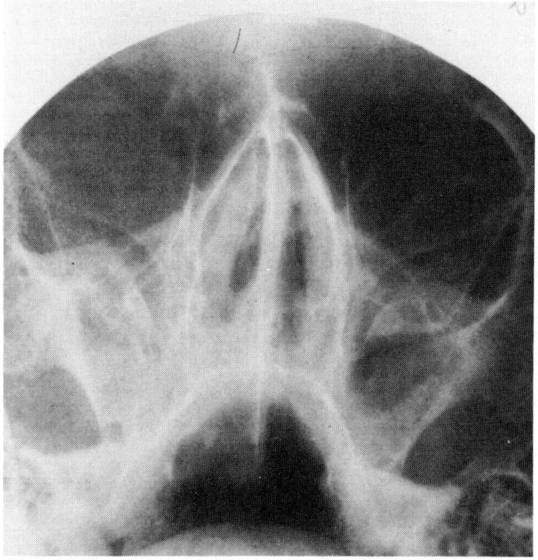

A

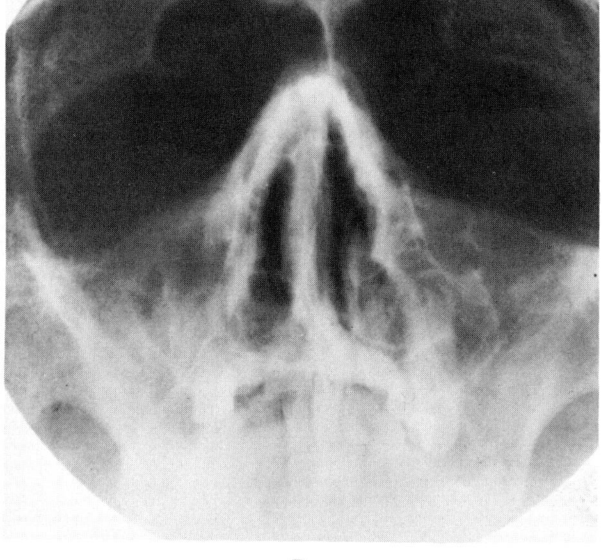

B

Fig. 50.6 (A and B) Mucosal thickening—occipito-mental views. A. shows an air space in left antrum while the right is completely opaque. B. Both antra are opaque.

The organisms responsible for paranasal sinus infection are almost identical with those responsible for upper respiratory tract infections, namely streptococci and, less frequently, staphylococci. Bacterial infection frequently may be a secondary invasion after a virus infection of the upper respiratory passages.

Allergic and vasomotor changes affecting the mucous membranes also predispose to infection with the consequence that pathological processes of both allergy and infection become superimposed.

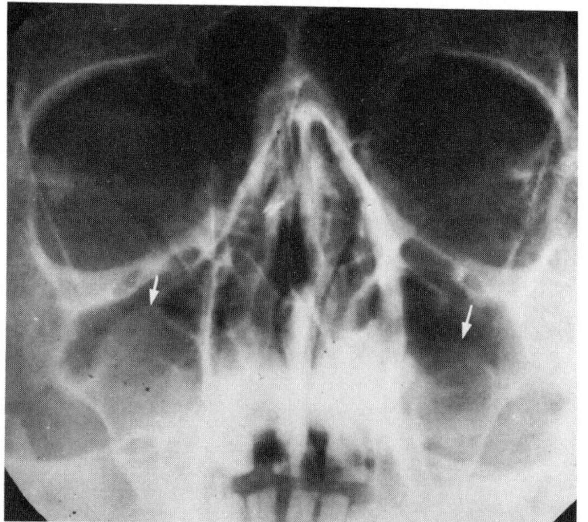

Fig. 50.7 Non-secreting cysts of both maxillary antra (*arrows*). The remaining mucosa in both maxillary antra is unaffected. These cysts have to be differentiated from polyps and localized areas of mucosal thickening.

While it may be possible in some instances to differentiate between allergic and vasomotor changes from the radiograph, far more frequently such a differentiation is not possible (Fig. 50.7). The radiological signs which may enable differentiation to be made are as follows:

Allergic	*Infective*
Mucosal thickening tends to produce a scalloped lining to the antral cavity.	Mucosal lining tends to parallel the antral walls.
Fluid levels are uncommon.	Fluid levels are common.
The turbinates are usually swollen and thickened.	The nasal turbinates may not be altered radiologically.
Polypus formation is common.	Polypus formation is less frequently seen.
Diffuse involvement of the sinuses is more common.	Involvement of more than one sinus is less common.

With marked thickening in the mucosa due to either cause the whole sinus may be completely opaque and differentiation is impossible. This is usually due to the central cavity being compressed to a thin slit by the swollen mucosa (Fig. 50.8). In other instances the central cavity is wholly or partly occupied by mucopurulent fluid. Only if the central cavity remaining in the sinus is sufficiently large and there is sufficient air and fluid present will a fluid level form in the antrum.

Fluid levels. Fluid levels are most easily demonstrated in the maxillary antrum. In the occipito-mental position the fluid runs into the deepest part of the sinus and forms a level. Small quantities of fluid may, however, be insufficient to form a recognizable fluid level.

It may be necessary to allow some lapse of time with the head in the tilted position before the radiographs are taken to allow the more viscous types of exudate to

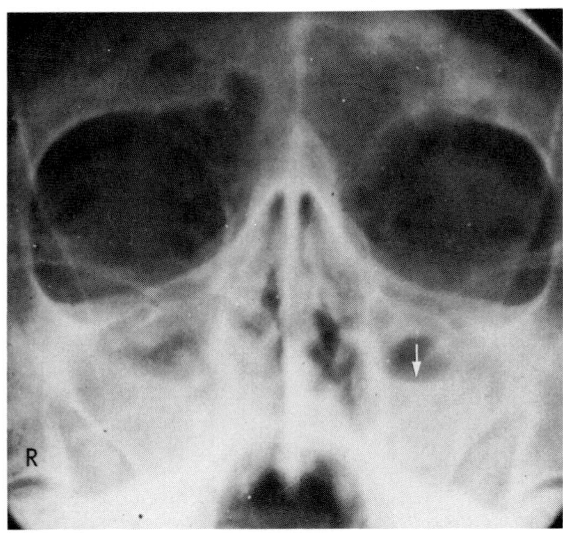

Fig. 50.8 Fluid level shown in left maxillary antrum (arrow). Right maxillary antrum shows gross mucosal thickening and at first sight the thickened mucosa over the floor simulates a fluid level although it can be seen not to be truly horizontal.

achieve a horizontal fluid level. Fluid in the maxillary sinus can be shown by tilting the head 45° to the affected side with the head in the occipito-mental position. It must be remembered that a fluid level is dependent on a horizontal beam and an upwards or downwards tilt in relation to the fluid interface may result in a blurred and indistinct level.

Small quantities of fluid in the frontal sinus are best demonstrated by taking films in the occipito-frontal position with the patient lying on his affected side and using a horizontal beam. In this position small quantities of fluid will gravitate to the lateral portion of the sinus and form a fluid level.

Polypi. Nasal polypi arise as a sequel of allergic or infective changes in the nasal mucosa and consist of fleshy, watery-looking mucosal outgrowths with a varying-sized pedicle. Occasionally an isolated polypus can be shown as a smooth, round soft tissue swelling in the nasal cavity (Fig. 50.9). More frequently the associated mucosal thickening causes a diffuse loss of translucency giving the whole nasal cavity or sinus a 'ground glass' appearance.

Less frequently an allergic polypus may arise from the lining membrane of a sinus, notably the antrum, and may project into the nasal cavity occluding the nasal passage. Increase in size may cause the polyp to project into the nostril or posteriorly into the choana, forming an antro-choanal polyp.

Antro-choanal polypi may be recognized through the open mouth in the occipito-mental view. The polypus can also be seen in the lateral position but must be differentiated from the soft tissue shadow of the soft palate (Fig. 50.11). The soft tissue outline projecting into the nasopharynx is less clearly seen if the polypus is large and completely occludes the posterior nasopharyngeal air space. Large polypi of long-standing may produce pressure atrophy of the nasal cavity walls and nasal septum, and such destruction has to be differen-

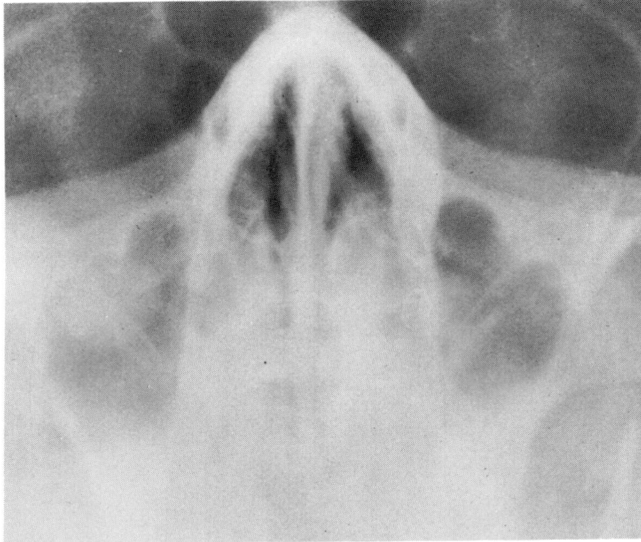

Fig. 50.9 Polyp arising from roof at right side of antrum. Mucosal thickening is present in left antrum.

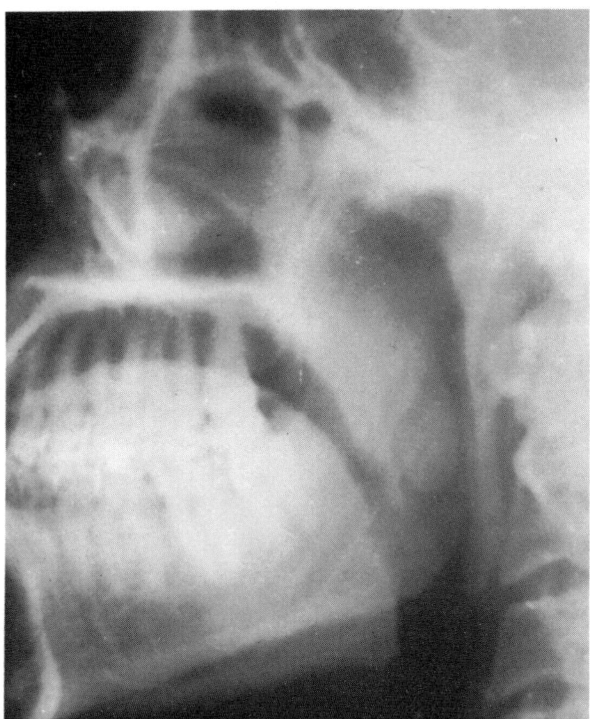

Fig. 50.10 Antro-choanal polyp. Lateral view showing soft tissue mass of polyp projecting above soft palate into nasopharynx.

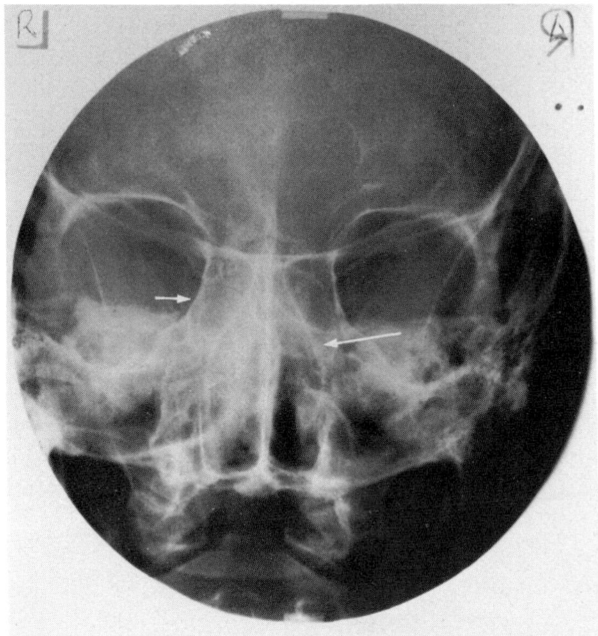

Fig. 50.11 Bone thinning associated with nasal polypi (*arrows*).

tiated from malignant invasion (Fig. 50.11). The patchy nature of the bone change in the latter condition aids differentiation.

When the infection subsides or the allergic process resolves, the mucosal swelling gradually shrinks and as the ostium of the sinus again becomes patent, the air-containing space in the sinus reappears. These changes can be followed on the radiograph as, when the central air-containing space reappears and the mucosal outline shrinks, the translucency of the sinus reappears. The fluid level disappears as the contents of the sinus are absorbed or are discharged into the nose. Complete return to normal may not occur and the thickened mucosa may remain as a line parallel to the sinus wall. It is important to recognize that such appearances may persist indefinitely.

After antral operations on the sinus, e.g. radical antrostomy, loss of translucency of the affected sinus may remain permanently and flare-up of infective changes may be difficult to detect by radiological means for this reason.

COMPLICATIONS OF SINUS INFECTION

Osteomyelitis. Spread of infection into the bone around the sinus seldom occurs nowadays, although prior to the advent of antibiotics it was not an infrequent sequel. The frontal bone is most frequently involved by such a spread and often follows surgical operation on the frontal sinus. Osteomyelitis of the maxilla after antral infection is less common, but as in the frontal sinus, it occurs more frequently after surgery has been performed on the maxillary antrum. Osteomyelitis of the maxilla in infancy may follow infection of the tooth buds.

During the acute stage radiological signs of osteomyelitis, namely (*a*) decalcification of bone, (*b*) loss of bone trabeculation and (*c*) blurring of bony sinus outlines, usually lag several days after the appearance of clinical signs. Treatment should therefore not be delayed until the appearance of these radiological signs. In acute frontal sinusitis with associated osteomyelitis, there is loss of the thin pencil-like outline of the sinus as well as the opacity of the sinus.

Persistent infection of a sinus with spread of infection to the surrounding bone may result in thickening and sclerosis of the surrounding bone with the loss of the delicate pencil-like outline of the sinus. In the frontal bone the bone sclerosis results in the intersinus septa becoming thickened and the ridges of the sinus roof more pronounced. Associated with these changes there is invariable thickening of the sinus mucosa and a loss of translucency of the sinus.

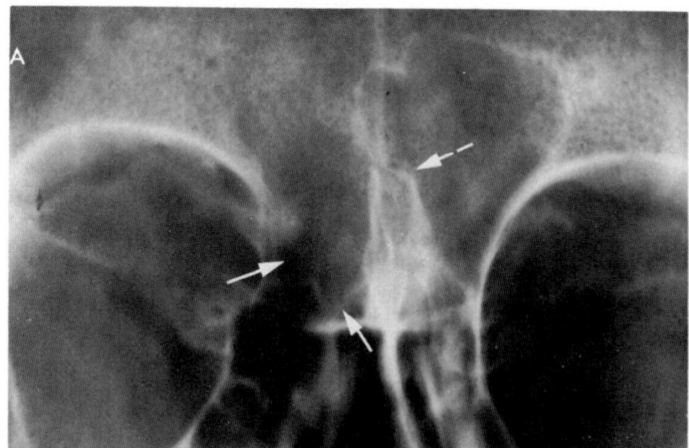

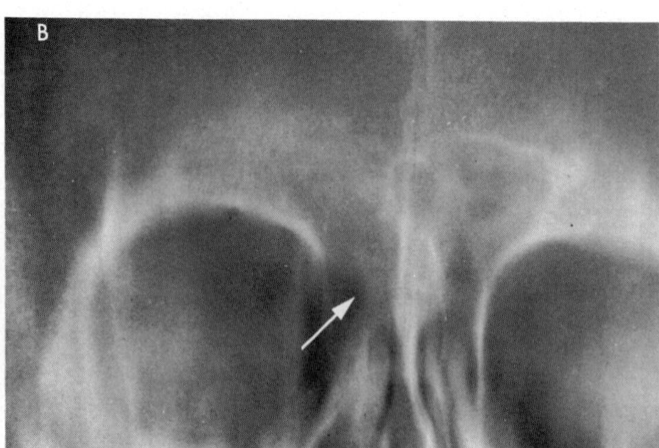

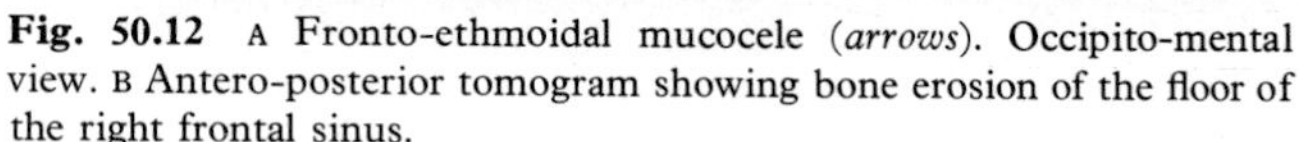

Fig. 50.12 A Fronto-ethmoidal mucocele (*arrows*). Occipito-mental view. B Antero-posterior tomogram showing bone erosion of the floor of the right frontal sinus.

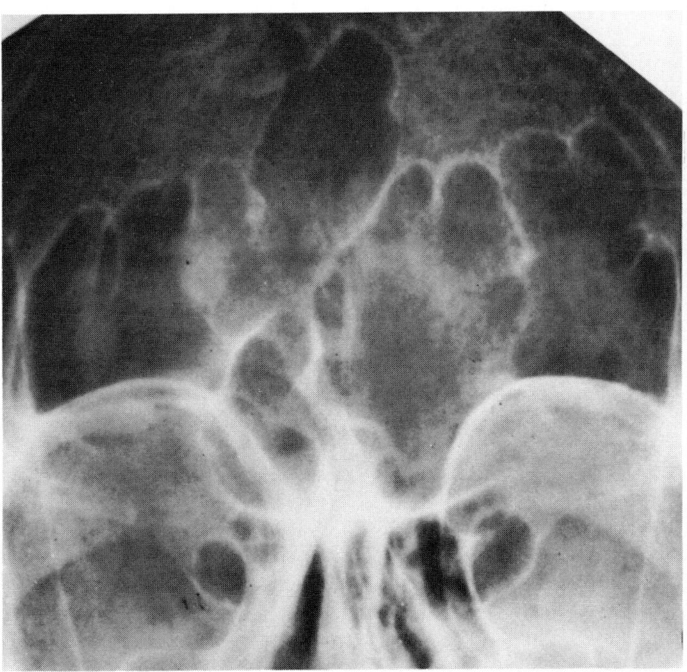

A

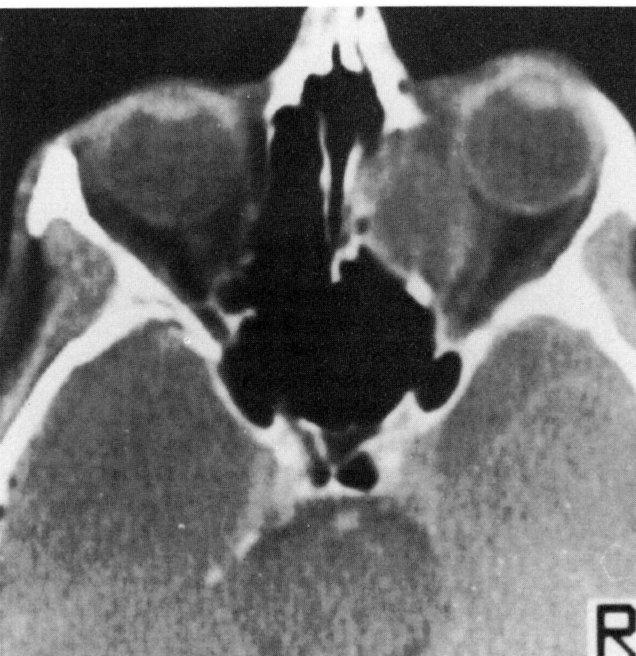

B

Fig. 50.13 Secondary ethmoid mucocele.
A Occipito frontal view showing extensive pneumatization of the frontal sinuses in a patient with a history of a previous external frontal operation and a complaint of diplopia. No significant radiological changes can be seen. B C.T. scan demonstrates posterior ethmoidal mucocele displacing internal rectus and producing slight exophthalmos. (Courtesy of Dr. W. A. Kerr and Dr. P. de Villiers.)

These bone changes of chronic osteomyelitis are most frequently seen in the bone surrounding the frontal sinus, but less frequently they may be seen in the maxilla and sphenoid bone. They have to be distinguished from the bone thickening seen in localized fibrous dysplasia.

Empyema and mucocele. Empyema of a sinus occurs when the ostium is blocked and infection persists within the sinus, giving rise to a sinus filled with pus. The frontal and sphenoid sinuses are most frequently the sites of empyema and the maxillary sinus is only infrequently the site of an empyema. Empyema of the sphenoid and frontal sinuses is particularly dangerous because of potential spread of infection to intracranial structures usually associated with venous thrombosis of the veins adjoining the sinuses.

Empyema of a sinus may show relatively little difference radiologically from the appearance of a sinus completely opacified by simple mucosal thickening or filled with mucopurulent fluid. In some cases decalcification of the bony sinus wall and surrounding bone may suggest the diagnosis, but in most instances it is the severity of the constitutional signs, rather than the radiographic signs, that indicates the diagnosis of empyema as opposed to simple infection of a paranasal sinus.

Mucoceles of the sinus develop when the infection subsides and the ostium remains closed and the retained aseptic fluid produces changes by pressure erosion of the bony walls of the sinus. Mucoceles are especially prone to occur in the frontal sinus where the erosion of the thin bony septa on the roof of the sinus is the first sign, and bulging of the intersinus septum points to the development of a mucocele. The increased translucency, which is perhaps a surprising finding, results from a thinning of the bony wall so that despite the increased density from the fluid contents, which should opacify the sinus, the sinus appears more translucent because of the overlying bony loss (Fig. 50.12).

The frontal mucocele may extend down into the ethmoidal region and produce orbital proptosis by the spread of the mucocele into the orbital cavity (Fig. 50.13B). The pressure erosion of bone by the mucocele must not be mistaken for bone destruction associated with an infiltrating neoplasm of the sinus.

Ethmoidal mucoceles may be difficult to recognise on conventional radiographs. Tomographic examination in the submento-vertical view may succeed in showing them well, but C.T. scanning if available is a more certain method of showing them clearly (Fig. 50.13).

CYSTS AND TUMOURS OF THE SINUSES

Cysts occurring in the paranasal sinuses may be derived from the antral lining or from an inward extension from adjoining structures. The latter type particularly affect the maxillary antra, where cysts of dental origin are particularly liable to spread into the maxillary antrum and mimic lesions arising from that structure.

Cysts arising from the sinus mucosa proper are *false cysts* as no secreting glands are present in the antral mucosa. Non-secreting cysts of the antrum are thought to arise by dehiscence of the lining membrane with the formation of a degenerative cyst and do not have a lining membrane, consequently they are not true cysts. These cysts contain a high proportion of cholesterol fluid and as such are doubly refractile to light. Sinuses containing such cysts consequently appear opaque to X-rays but may appear clear on transillumination.

If the maxillary sinus, which is the sinus most frequently involved, is completely occupied by such a cyst that sinus appears uniformly opaque. More frequently the cyst appears as a smooth rounded opacity projecting into its lumen. These cysts are not under tension and consequently tend slightly to alter their convex borders when the head is tilted. As they are not tense they do not erode bony walls of the antrum.

Cysts of dental origin. Cysts of dental origin are either of developmental origin, e.g. dentigerous cysts, or infective such as radicular cysts or primordial cysts (keratocyst).

Dentigerous cysts are usually associated with maldevelopment of a tooth bud and frequently extend upwards into the floor of the maxillary antrum. Pathologically they enclose the crown of the unerupted tooth and are attached to the neck. In later decades they most commonly involve the canine tooth. They produce expansion of the antral walls and may be associated with a uniform opacity of the maxillary antrum. When they increase in size they may produce pressure atrophy of the bony walls of the maxillary antrum and may occupy the whole antrum. The bony atrophy must be differentiated from the changes of bone invasion by malignant tumours (Fig. 50.14).

Radicular or primordial cysts of infective origin may equally spread upwards into the maxillary antrum, but seldom produce the degree of expansion produced by dentigerous cysts. Radicular cysts are commoner than primordial in the maxilla; the latter may have a scalloped outline suggesting multiple cysts.

Congenital cysts. The complex development of the maxilla and premaxilla gives opportunity for the development of inclusion cysts at the sites of fusion of tissue planes, e.g. implantation dermoids, globulo-maxillary, or incisive canal cysts, and such cysts may produce opacities in the maxillary antrum.

Globulo-maxillary cyst is a fissural cyst at the site of fusion of the premaxilla with the maxilla and lies in the region of the canine fossa. It may extend upwards into the antrum. There is some doubt as to whether globulo-maxillary cysts are true fissural cysts or whether they are odontogenic in origin. In the latter case they may be either lateral periodontal cysts or a residual radicular cyst if there is a missing tooth in that area.

SIMPLE TUMOURS

Osteomata. The commonest benign tumours of the sinuses are usually of bony origin and may be dense (ivory) or cancellous. The frontal sinuses are most frequent site for osteomata. Osteomata may be pedunculated or sessile and in the frontal sinus frequently occur in the region of the origin of the fronto-nasal duct.

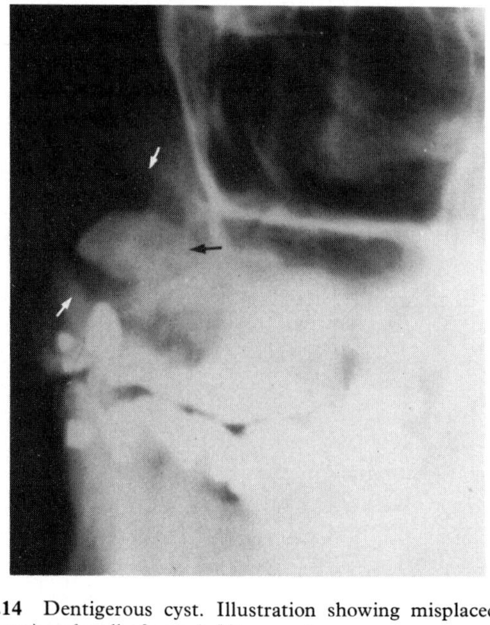

Fig. 50.14 Dentigerous cyst. Illustration showing misplaced canine (*black arrow*) and wall of cyst (*white arrow*).

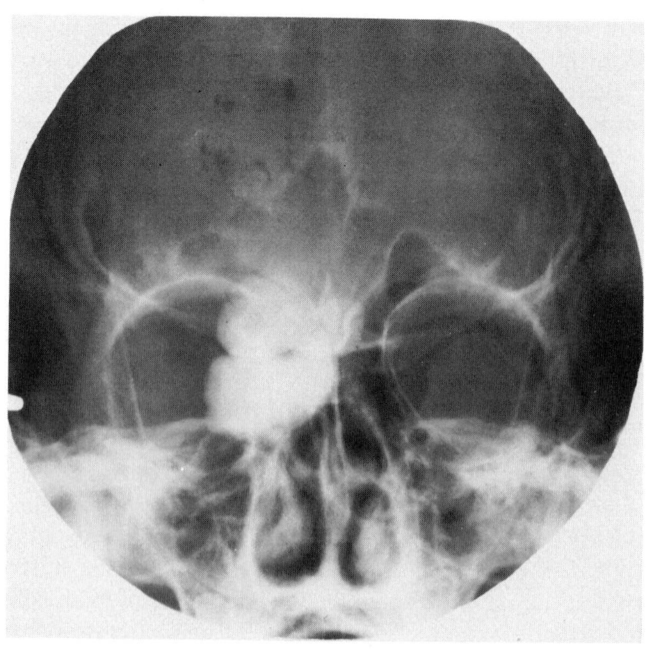

Fig. 50.15 Ivory osteoma of the right frontal sinus extending down into the ethmoid sinuses.

Osteomata arising in this site are especially liable to obstruct the fronto-nasal duct, which almost invariably leads to obstruction to the drainage and the development of infective changes. Osteomata may produce dense shadows (ivory osteomata) (Fig. 50.15) but in other instances they may be poorly calcified producing a relatively soft shadow on the radiograph. Indeed, some of the relatively poorly calcified cancellous osteomata may be difficult to distinguish from the shadow of an ossifying fibroma.

Fibro-osteoma is a less common type of benign tumour which occurs in the maxilla in young adolescents and is characterized by an expansion of the maxilla, the expanded maxilla bearing a strong resemblance to an osteosarcoma. Fibro-osteoma is associated with a pressure atrophy of the antral wall which further increases its resemblance to an osteosarcoma. New bone is seldom associated with this type of tumour, which enables it to be differentiated from an osteosarcoma. Fibro-osteoma has also to be distinguished from a *localized fibrous dysplasia* of bone, but the differentiation of these two conditions on radiological grounds alone may not be possible.

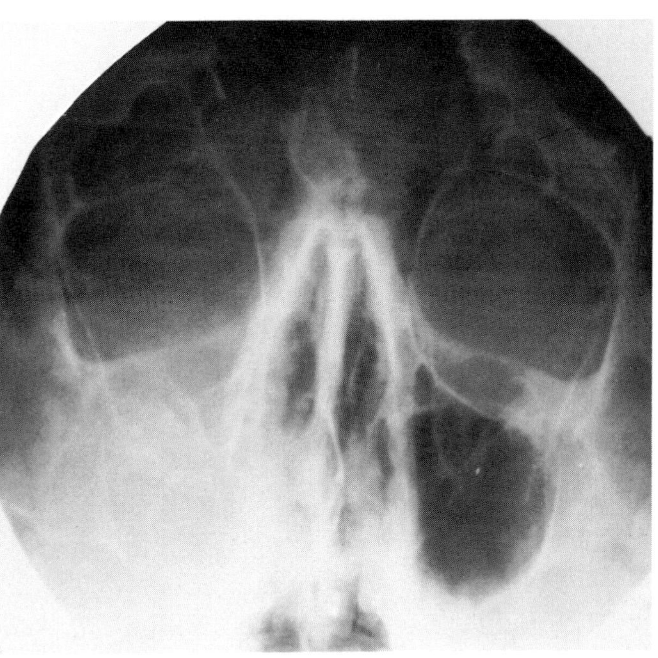

Fig. 50.16 Carcinoma of right antrum showing erosion of lateral wall.

MALIGNANT TUMOURS

Malignant growths of the paranasal sinuses are most commonly *carcinomata* and most frequently arise in the ethmoid or in the maxillary antrum. The growths are usually of the columnar celled variety; if squamous metaplasia occurs a squamous celled carcinoma may develop Carcinoma of the frontal and sphenoid sinus also occurs but is relatively rare. Carcinoma of the paranasal sinuses tends to occur in the middle-aged patients and the symptomatology depends on the sinus involved. Males predominate over females.

Antral carcinomata present with pain along the maxillary division of the fifth cranial nerve, whereas ethmoidal carcinomata usually present with nasal obstruction and a bloody nasal discharge; local pain develops later in the course of ethmoidal carcinoma.

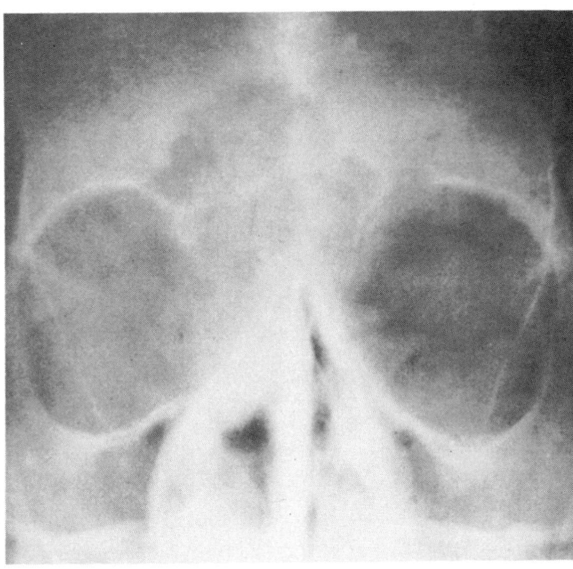

A

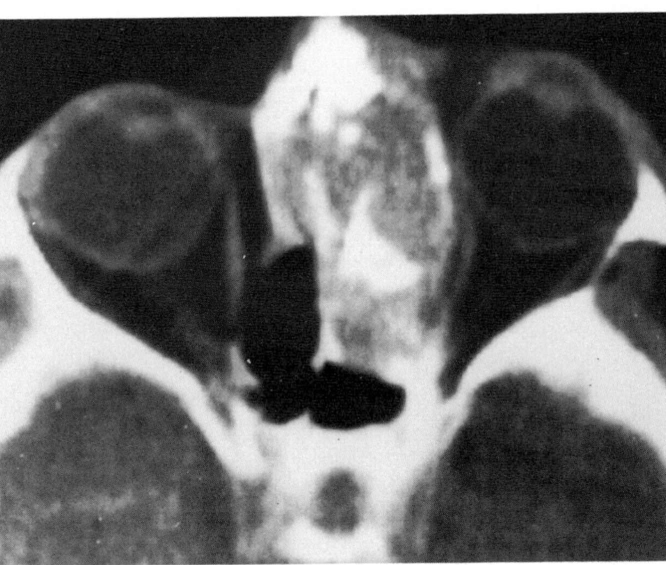

B

Fig. 50.17 Fibrosarcoma of nose (recurrent).
A Occipito frontal view in 72-year-old man who had a fibroma removed 10 years previously. Destruction of ethmoidal plate and floor of right frontal sinus. The frontal sinus is opaque due to infective change.
B C.T. scan showing soft tissue mass with destruction of ethmoidal bone and bulging of mass into right orbit.

Carcinomata of the sphenoid sinus on the other hand present with signs of involvement of the cranial nerves (ocular paresis, etc.) as a consequence of lateral spread of the growth.

The radiograph shows the basic characters of malignant tumour formation common to all sinus growths, namely opacity of the sinus due to the growth and infiltration and destruction of the wall due to an extension of the growth into the bony walls of the sinus (Fig. 50.16).

In carcinoma of the maxillary antrum the lateral or medial wall of the antrum are most frequently destroyed, but in advanced cases there may be extension downwards with bulging of the head palate, or upwards into the orbital cavity with the development of proptosis. Evaluation of destruction of the medial wall of the maxillary antrum is a difficult radiological problem as due to the thinness and obliquity of the wall it may apparently be lost in normal individuals.

In the case of carcinoma of the sphenoid sinus, the lateral extension of the growth causes destruction of the floor of the middle cranial fossa. Carcinoma of the sphenoid sinus has to be differentiated from *chordoma* occurring in the basisphenoid which equally can produce extensive areas of bone destruction, as can tumours arising in Rathke's pouch, *craniopharyngioma*. These tumours which are probably in the group of adnexial celled tumours, extensively infiltrate the sphenoid sinus and surrounding bone without any marked degree of soft tissue swelling. Tumours arising from the pituitary gland and nasopharynx extending secondarily into the sphenoid sinus have also to be differentiated from primary sphenoidal sinus tumours. In both types of growth the sphenoid sinus is completely opaque.

Ethmoidal carcinomata extensively infiltrate the ethmoidal cells. Destruction of the thin bony walls in this region is extremely difficult to assess but tomographic sections in the postero-anterior plane may be of great assistance. C.T. scanning is invaluable in assessing the spread of carcinoma of the paranasal sinuses.

Sarcomata of the paranasal sinuses are far less common than carcinoma (Fig. 50.17). Osteosarcoma of the maxilla occurs in the young age group and may show the typical 'sunray' appearance. The majority of sarcomata occurring in the older age group are usually called 'fibrosarcomata'. Many of the cases originally reported as such are found on more detailed histological examination to be forms of anaplastic carcinomata.

REFERENCES AND SUGGESTIONS FOR FURTHER READING

BRUNNER, H. (1953) Primary tumours of the frontal bone. *Archives of Otolaryngology*, **57**, 2.

CHIDEKEL, N., JENSEN, C., AXELSSON, A. & GREBELIUS, N. (1970) Diagnosis of fluid in the maxillary sinus. *Acta Radiologica*, **10**, 433.

FRIEDMAN, I. (1971) *J. Lar. Otol.*, **85**, 631.

HARRISON, D. F. N. (1974) Non-healing granulomata of the upper respiratory tract. *British Medical Journal*, **4**, 205.

JEFFERSON, A. & LEWTAS, N. (1963) Value of tomography and subdural pneumography in subfrontal fractures. *Acta Radiologica*, **1**, 119.

LLOYD, G. (1975) *Radiology of the Orbit*. Philadelphia: Saunders.

LLOYD, G., BARTRAM, C. I. & STANLEY, P. (1974) Ethmoid mucoceles. *British Journal of Radiology*, **47**, 646.

MINAGI, H., MARGOLIS, M. T. & NEWTON, T. H. (1972) Tomography in the diagnosis of sphenoid sinus mucocele. *American Journal of Roentgenology*, **115**, 587.

POTTER, D. G. (1972) Tomography of the orbit. *Radiologic Clinics of North America*, **10**, 21.

RADCLIFFE, A. (1949) Fractures involving air sinuses. *Journal of Laryngology and Otology*, **63**, 453.

CHAPTER 51

THE TEMPORAL BONE

The petrous temporal bone contains and forms a bony covering (bony labyrinth) for the membranous labyrinth comprising the semicircular canals, the utricle, saccule and cochlea.

The conducting mechanism of hearing, namely the external auditory meatus, tympanum, middle ear and auditory ossicles, also lies in the confines of the temporal bone. Extending throughout the temporal bone and into the mastoid process is a system of air cells which are contiguous with each other and with the mastoid antrum. The function of the mastoid air cells, like the paranasal sinuses, is not clearly understood.

The middle ear communicates with the nasopharynx via the Eustachian (tympanic) tube. Physiologically the Eustachian tube serves to equalize pressure between the middle ear and the atmosphere. Its patency is essential for the proper functioning of the middle ear. When disease or infection of the nasopharynx occurs it unfortunately forms a potential route for spread of infection to the middle ear.

Embryologically the middle ear is developed from the tubo-tympanic recess of the primitive pharynx, and the mastoid antrum is developed as an outgrowth from the middle ear. The mastoid cells later occur as outbuddings from the mastoid antrum, and this is the route by which infection of the mastoid process occurs from the middle ear. At birth no mastoid cells are developed, but by the age of 5 years the mastoid antrum is already well formed.

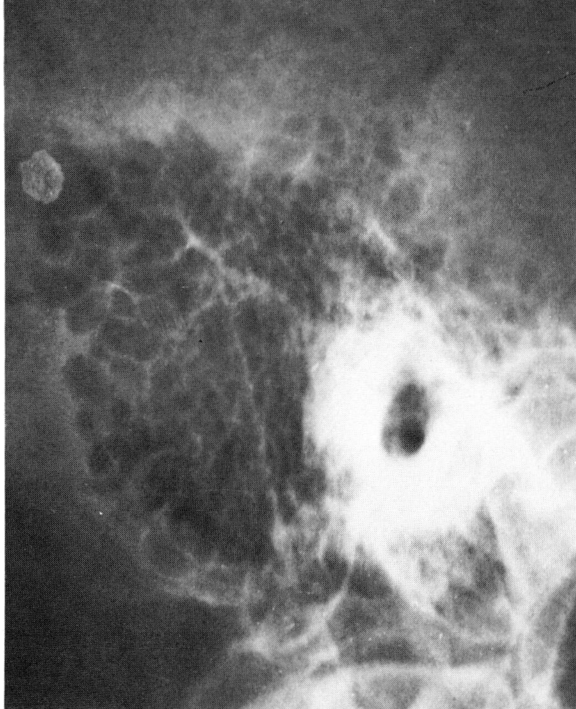

Fig. 51.1 Normal cellular mastoid on the lateral oblique view. The extensive cell system with spread of cells to the tip of the mastoid process and to the squamous temporal is seen.

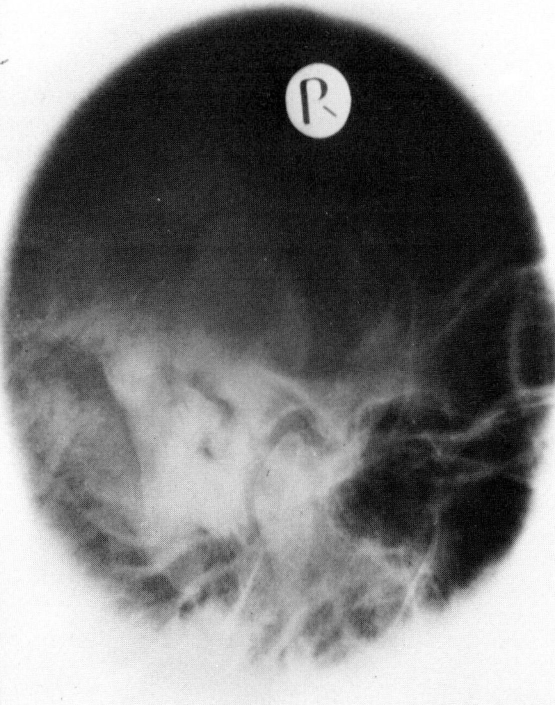

Fig. 51.2 Sclerotic mastoid process. No cells visible but erosion of bone in the region of the mastoid antrum is shown in cholesteatoma.

Pneumatization then proceeds with age until the mastoid antrum is fully developed towards the end of adolescence and an extensive cell system is then present.

The adult mastoid may be one of three varieties:

1. **Cellular mastoid**—where normal cell development has occurred and the mastoid process and the apex of the petrous bone are fully pneumatized (Fig. 51.1).

2. **Diploic mastoid** (infantile mastoid)—where cellular development has not occurred or has been arrested at an early stage of development with the consequence that the temporal bone is filled with diploic-like structure.

3. **Sclerotic mastoid**—when a sclerotic process, developing as a sequel of infection, has obliterated a once cellular mastoid; or sclerosis had developed in an infantile mastoid, the mastoid appearing accellular and surrounded by dense bone. Some authorities consider that sclerotic changes may develop as the result of failure of pneumatization of the mastoid process (Fig. 51.2).

RADIOGRAPHIC TECHNIQUE

Many of the standard X-ray projections still used in the examination of the mastoid process are relics from the pre-antibiotic days when acute and chronic mastoiditis was a far commoner problem and the emphasis of radiological investigation was on the detection of infection and a determination of its extent in the mastoid process. The development of conservative surgery in the restoration of hearing has reorientated the main radiological emphasis to the middle ear and its contained structures. No standard set of positions can therefore be recommended for the investigation of the mastoid process; these positions must vary with the clinical problem under review. The rigid adherence to one standard set of positions for every mastoid examination will inevitably produce inadequate radiological coverage in many cases.

Specialized X-ray equipment for mastoid radiography which centres the X-ray beam to the centre of the film regardless of the angle used has been developed and this equipment certainly simplifies the radiographic positioning. The basic essentials in the production of good mastoid radiographs are similar to those for the paranasal sinuses and consist of accurate coning of the incident beam and a proper understanding of the anatomy and pathology of the area being investigated.

A scheme for the radiographic investigation of the mastoid process dependent on the pathological condition under investigation is as follows:

Survey views

1. *Lateral oblique*. The sagittal plane of the skull is rotated to form an angle of 15° (Schuller), 30° (Owen), or 45° (Mayer) (Fig. 51.3A and B) with the radiographic base line being kept horizontal. The incident beam is inclined caudally to the same angle as the rotation of the skull in each projection. The incident beam is centred so that it emerges through the external meatus of the affected mastoid. These views give a general survey of the mastoid process which enables the cell system, the middle ear and attic to be seen.

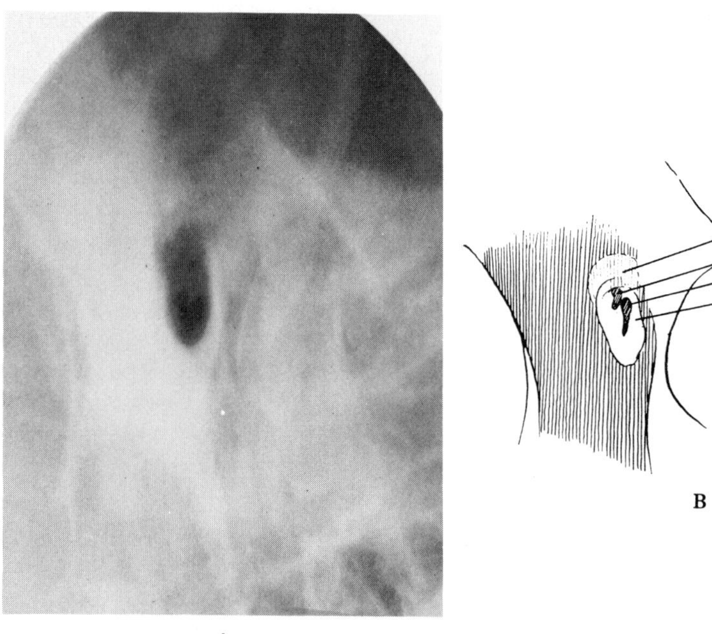

Fig. 51.3 (A and B) Mayer's projection showing the attic, malleus and incus projected through the external auditory meatus.

2. *Submento-vertical position.* This is taken with the incident beam angled through the middle ear at right angles to the base line of the skull. Coned views of each middle ear taken separately greatly improve the detail of the middle ear structures.

Middle ear views

1. *Chaussé III projection.* In this projection the incident beam is inclined along a line drawn from the outer end of the eyebrow to the midpoint of the external meatus. The centring point is midway between these two points (Fig. 51.4A and B). The sagittal plane of the skull is rotated between 5° and 10° towards the opposite side (Fig. 51.4B). This position, whilst demonstrating the middle ear, has the disadvantage of projecting the ossicular shadow over the horizontal semicircular canal as the incident beam is not strictly tangential to the medial wall of the middle ear (Fig. 51.5A and B).

2. *Transorbital projection (Guillen).* The radiographic base line is horizontal and the incident beam centred on the medial canthus of the eye on the side to be examined and the sagittal plane is rotated 5° to 10° towards the mastoid examined. The incident beam passes through the orbit along and tangential to the medial wall of the middle ear and the ossicular shadow is projected lateral to the horizontal semi-circular canal. The middle ear is seen through the orbit (Fig. 51.6A and B). This view should be performed in the P.A. position as the radiation dose to the lens is reduced by a factor of 6 (Fig. 51.7).

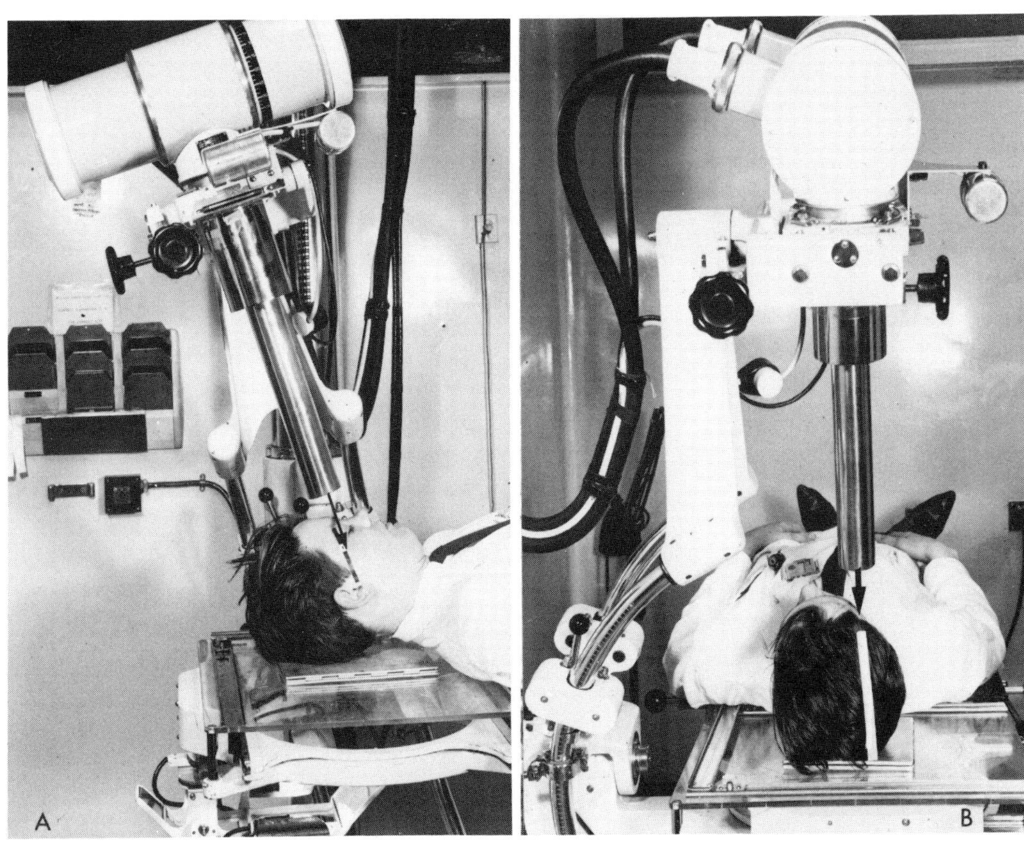

Fig. 51.4 (A and B) Chaussé III projection demonstrates the middle ear. The line of the incident beam is shown by the white line.

Apex and posterior surface of petrous bone views

1. *Stenvers' view.* The sagittal plane of the skull is rotated 30° away from the side to be examined, the radiographic base line is tilted cranially to 20°, and the incident beam centred at a point 1 inch medial to the tip of the mastoid process and inclined cranially at an angle of 8°. A clear view of the apex of the petrous bone and the internal meatus is obtained. The middle ear cannot be clearly seen and only gross changes in the mastoid process can be seen in this view.

2. *70° occipito-mental view.* This is taken with the base line tilted cranially to 35° and the incident beam inclined caudally to the same angle and centred on the external occipital protuberance. This position is of value in demonstrating the jugular foramen and the posterior surface of the petrous temporal bone.

In all views where maximum detail is required it is essential that the incident beam is coned to a circle of

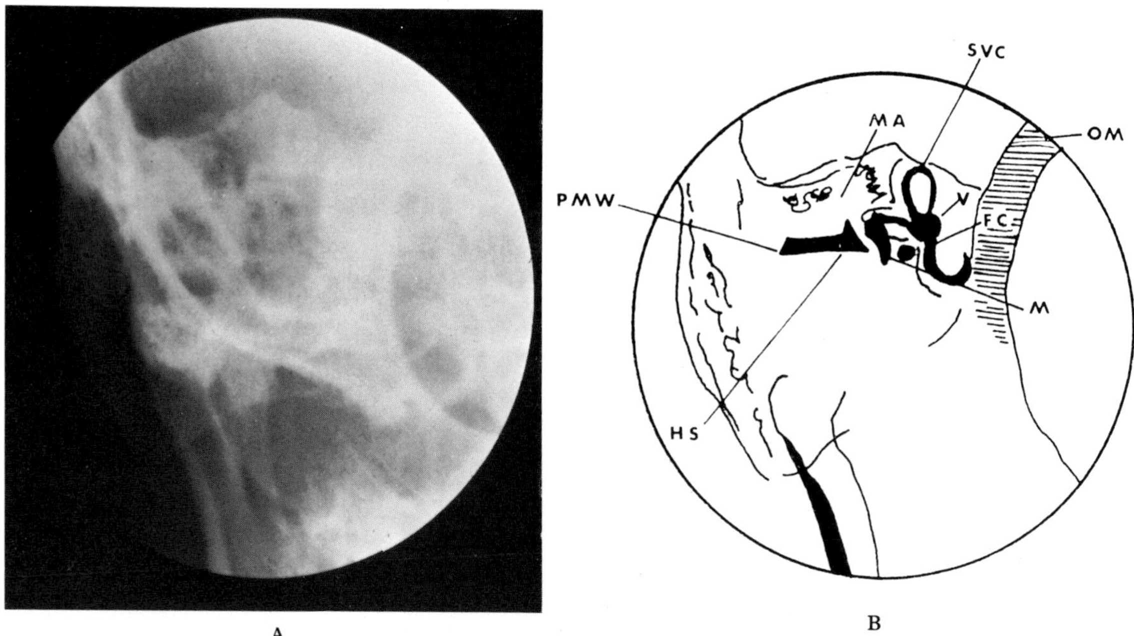

Fig. 51.5A Radiograph taken in Chaussé III. B Diagram showing structures—M, malleus; OM, orbital rim; SVC, superior semicircular canal; PMW, posterior meatal wall; HS, post-meatal spur; V, ventricle; MA, mastoid antrum; FC, facial canal.

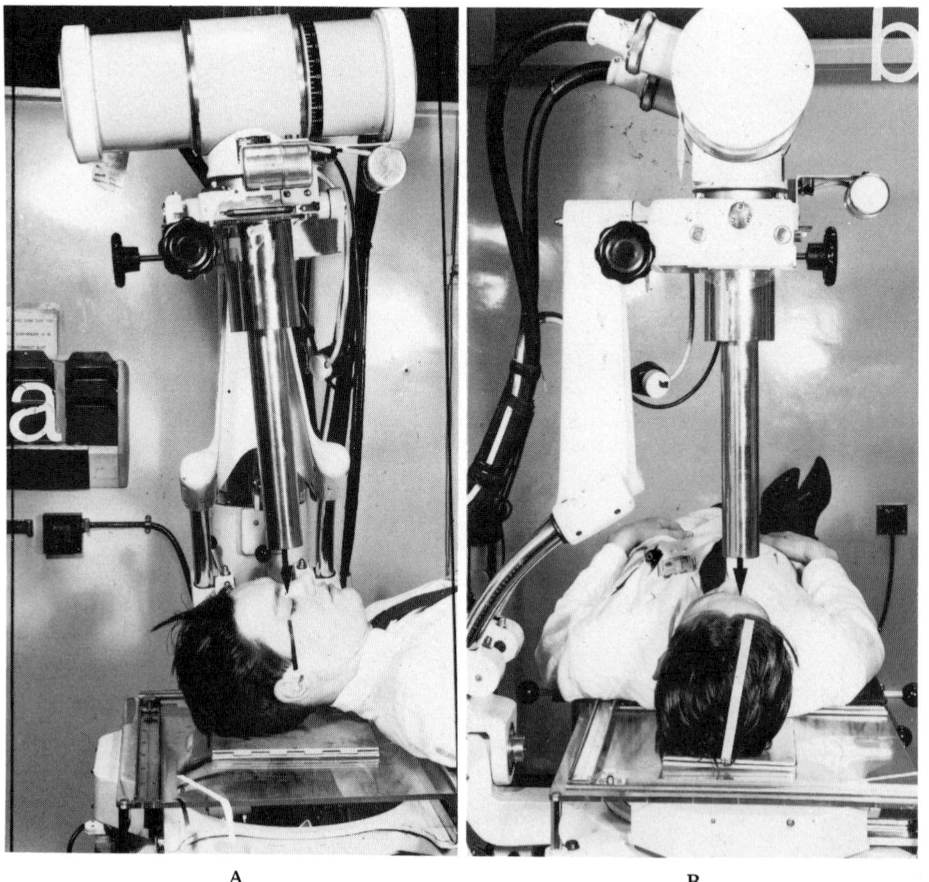

Fig. 51.6 (A and B) Transorbital projection (Guillen). The line of the incident beam is indicated by the lines on the patient's face and skull.

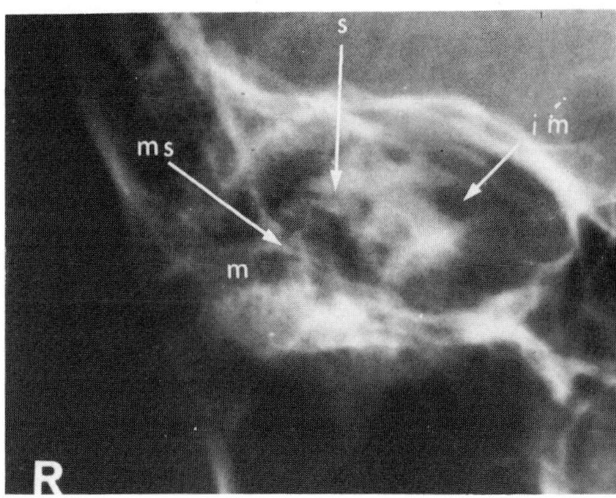

Fig. 51.7 Radiograph taken in transorbital projection. im = internal meatus. ms = postero-meatal spine. m = external meatus. s = lateral semicircular canal.

diameter of 5 to 8 cm and this dispenses with the need to use a grid. If the area covered is greater than 8 cm a Potter Bucky diaphragm or fine stationary grid should be used to improve contrast and eliminate scatter.

Tomography

Tomographic studies using the hypocycloidal, spiral or linear, cuts are essential in investigating middle ear disease and are especially necessary in the diagnosis of fractures and congenital deformities of the middle ear and temporal bone. Tomographs are also particularly useful in evaluating bony changes in the internal auditory meatus (Fig. 51.8A–C) and in detecting bone destruction in and around the middle ear.

Contrast examination

After intrathecal introduction of Myodil (Pantopaque) carefully tilting the patient under fluoroscopic control will permit the contrast medium to be brought to the posterior cranial fossa and the internal auditory meatus to be filled with oil. This is by far the most accurate method of diagnosing small auditory nerve tumours. Spot films taken under fluoroscopic control are usually adequate but tomographic films with oil *in situ* are a further sophistication.

The contrast medium should not be allowed to run into the middle cranial fossa and should be run backwards down to the lumbar region and re-aspirated.

CAT scanning

Computerized axial tomography has its major use in temporal bone disease in detecting the extent of bone involvement and destruction in the various tumours. For the diagnosis of diseases of the middle ear or labyrinth its full potential has yet to be explored.

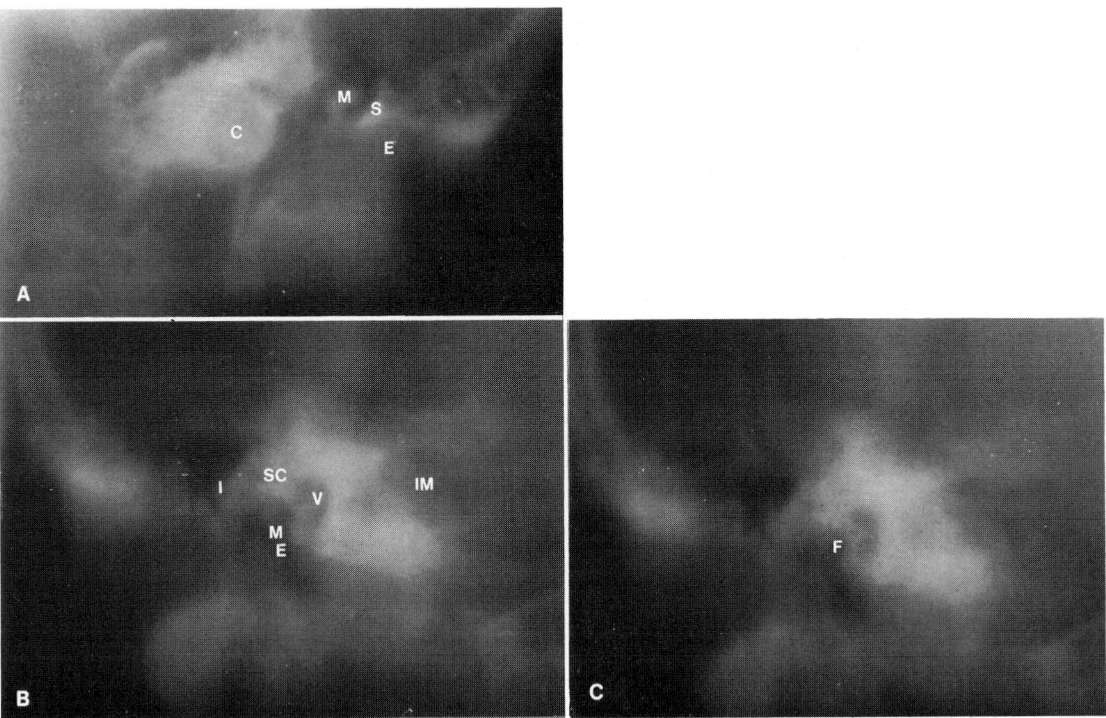

Fig. 51.8A Postero-anterior tomograph at level of cochlea (cochlear cut). M—malleus, S—meatal spur, E—external meatus, C—cochlea.
B Cut 2 mm posterior to Figure 51.8A (vestibular cut). SC—external semicircular canal. V—vestibule. I—incus. IM—internal meatus.
C Cut 2 mm posterior showing the genu of the facial canal (F).

CONGENITAL ABNORMALITIES

Since the middle ear and inner ear are derived from embryologically different structures developing at different times, their congenital abnormalities are not frequently associated, with the exception of Thalidomide-induced deformities.

The commonest and the most easily recognized deformity is the *Mundini deformity* in which the normal $2\frac{1}{2}$ turns of the cochlea is replaced by a basal turn and a single cavity above. More severe forms of aplasia may be associated with complete *absence of the cochlea* (Fig. 51.9B and C).

infrequently associated with varying degrees of maldevelopment of the external meatus. The commonest malformation is *complete* or *partial atresia* of the meatus.

Other more complex embryological maldevelopments involving the branchial arches such as the *Treacher Collins syndrome* and *cranio-facial dysostosis* result in malformations of the middle ear as well as those affecting the external meatus. The commonest is the development of a *bony bridge* attaching the ossicles to the medial wall of the attic, but other deformities such as *displacements*, *fusions*, or *malformations of the ossicles* frequently occur.

Other generalized skeletal deformities, such as

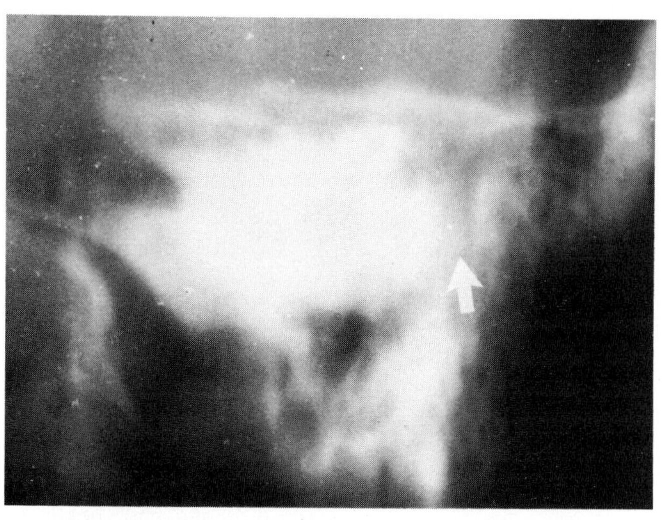

A

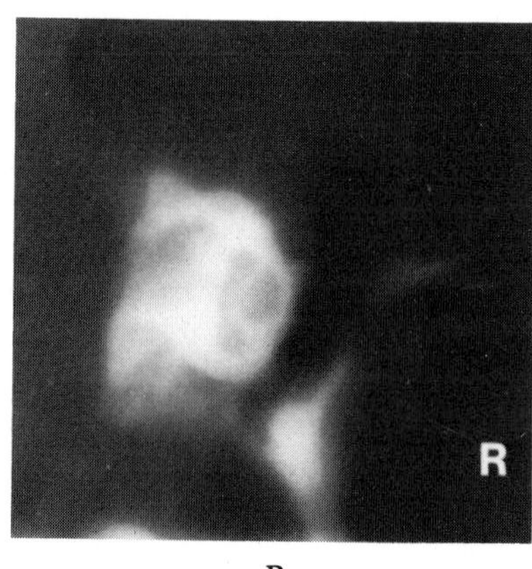

B

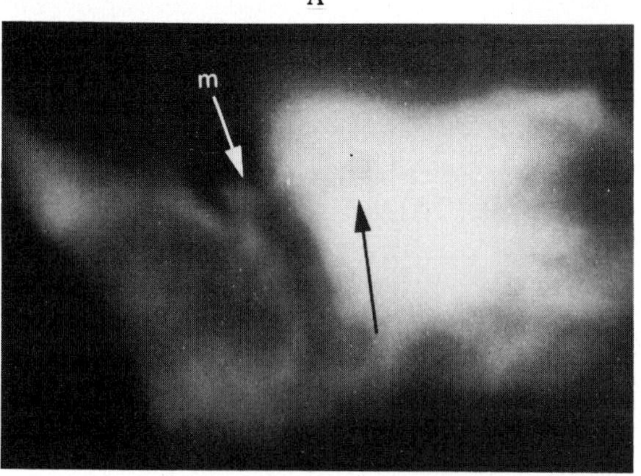

C

Fig. 51.9 A Atresia of external meatus. P.A. tomogram showing complete absence of the external meatus (*arrow*). The middle ear is deformed and the ossicles displaced medially—the inner ear is normal. B Mundini deformity showing $1\frac{1}{2}$ turns instead of the normal $2\frac{1}{2}$. C Atresia of the labyrinth showing complete absence of the internal labyrinth in the P.A. tomogram. A female aged 21 years who complained of vertigo, deafness in right ear and a facial palsy. m = malleus (*white arrow*). Black arrow indicates dense temporal bone and absence of labyrinth.

Aplasia and *malformations of the semicircular canals* may also occur and the *internal meatus* may be grossly atretic and narrowed. Perhaps more important is the extreme *dilatation of the internal meatus* which may be seen on rare occasions, as this may be mistaken for expansion by a tumour.

The external auditory meatus is developed from an ectodermal source and consequently generalized ectodermal dysplasias such as *onycho-osteodystrophy* are not

chondro-osteodystrophy, achondroplasia and Klippel-Feil syndrome, may be associated with deformities of the middle ear. In some of these cases the deformity of the middle ear is usually secondary to the deformity of the base of the skull. As a result the distortion of the middle ear results in *malposition* and *dislocation of the ossicles.*

Atresia, either partial or complete, *of the external meatus* with or without associated deformities of the auricle is undoubtedly the commonest congenital malformation affecting the ear. The radiological investigation in such cases is of inestimable value and the following information should be obtained (Fig. 51.9A):

1. The extent of loss of the external meatus and the presence or otherwise of a bony block.

2. The degree of development of the mastoid process and the middle ear.

3. The presence of ossicles, their shape and deformities.

4. The presence of a bony labyrinth and internal auditory canal.

Tomography is essential in estimating the deformities of the middle ear, as the distortion of normal anatomical landmarks associated with the deformity of the base of the skull renders recognition of anatomical landmarks on conventional radiographs difficult.

Tomography is best carried out with a hypocycloidal movement in the postero-anterior position (lead eye shields are used for lens protection in the A.P. position) and sections taken at 2 mm intervals posteriorly from 1 mm posterior to the anterior wall of the external meatus. This most anterior plane (Fig. 51.8A) is the '*cochlear plane*' and shows the cochlea, facial canal (genu), the ossicles, postero-meatal spur and external meatus. The carotid canal is situated below the middle ear.

The '*vestibular plane*' lies about 4 mm posterior to the cochlear plane and shows the external semicircular canal, incus, mastoid antrum and vestibule, the lateral and superior semicircular canals, the internal auditory canal, and the jugular fossa below (Fig. 51.8B).

Semi-axial planes (with the sagittal plane rotated 20° to the opposite side) and axial cuts made across the length of the petrous bone are necessary for the detailed investigations of the changes seen in the petrous bones in congenital diseases and otosclerosis.

Tomographic cuts in the lateral plane extending from the middle ear inwards to the internal auditory meatus are invaluable in assessing the relationship of fracture lines to the facial canal. They may also be useful in detecting early signs of bone thinning associated with acoustic nerve tumours.

Recognition of abnormalities of the labyrinth can only be achieved by tomography in the P.A., lateral and axial planes. Developmental defects of the labyrinth range from *complete absence* (Fig. 51.9C) to sac-like deformities of the vestibule and cochlea (*Michel deformity*), and to lesser degrees of malformation of the cochlea (*Mundini deformity*) where the normal $2\frac{1}{2}$ turns are replaced by $1\frac{1}{2}$ turns of the cochlea.

TRAUMATIC LESIONS

Barotrauma may produce an exudate in the middle ear, opacifying the middle ear and blurring the ossicular shadows. The detection and estimation of the extent of fractures involving the petrous temporal bone is, however, the main problem in trauma.

Fractures involving the temporal bone may be isolated ones or an extension of fractures of the base or vertex of the skull. The fracture lines may be (*a*) *vertical* (*b*) *oblique* or (*c*) *transverse* (Fig. 51.10A and B).

Radiological investigation of suspected fractures of the temporal bone is of value in detecting the relationship of the fracture line to the facial canal and to the labyrinth. These findings are of importance in assessing the possible recovery from facial palsy or deafness

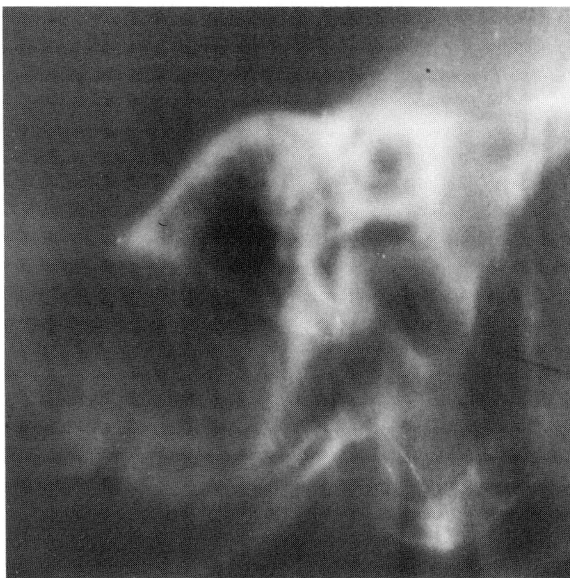

A

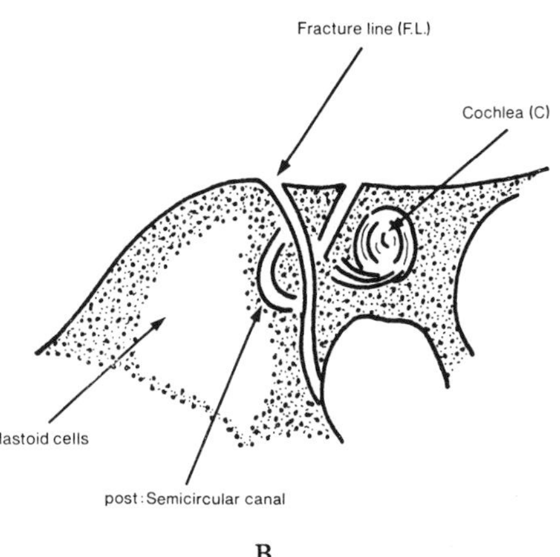

B

Fig. 51.10 (A and B) Fracture of temporal bone involving labyrinth.

following injury, as fracture lines involving the facial canal below the genu may require surgical treatment. Likewise, post-traumatic deafness shown as being due to dislocation of the ossicles rather than to a fracture involving the inner ear has the potentiality of surgical treatment with restoration of hearing.

If the fracture line involves the mastoid cells, exudation and haemorrhage into the cells may result in opacification of the cells surrounding the fracture line. Later if infection supervenes the whole of the mastoid cells may become opaque.

INFECTIONS

Acute mastoiditis. Infective changes involving the mastoid processes are usually the result of a spread of infection from the nasopharynx via the Eustachian tube and the middle ear to the mastoid cells (Fig. 51.11). In children infection frequently occurs as a complication of the exanthemata and in adults following nasopharyngeal infection. More rarely blood-borne infection may occur as part of a septicaemic process, and tuberculous infection is considered to be blood-borne. Less frequently acute mastoiditis may follow traumatic rupture of the tympanic membrane and the spread of infection from the external meatus into the middle ear. Acute mastoiditis usually occurs in cellular mastoids, but since the use of antibiotics in the treatment of middle ear infections acute mastoiditis is now less frequently seen.

Radiological appearances. The radiological findings of acute mastoiditis are:

1. Opacity of the middle ear with blurring of the ossicular shadows. This can be best appreciated in the submento-vertical projection.

2. Blurring of the outlines of the mastoid antrum and cells with a loss of translucency of the cells occurs with the spread of infection into the mastoid process. These changes are most marked in the cells surrounding the mastoid antrum and gradually extend into the peripheral cells of the mastoid process. The change is most easily seen in the lateral oblique position.

3. Breakdown of mastoid cell walls with abscess formation is more difficult to interpret as simple decalcification associated with infection may result in an apparent loss of cell outlines.

4. Abscess formation results from the breakdown of cell walls and is particularly liable to occur around the sinodural angle, less frequently in the tip of the mastoid process.

Antibiotic mastoid. The administration of antibiotics may mask the clinical symptoms of acute mastoiditis, but unless correct and adequate dosage is given the infection may proceed insidiously.

The radiological changes lag behind the clinical symptoms in their appearance and as a consequence reliance on radiological signs only may give a false sense of security. Equally, resolution of the radiological changes may be delayed and complete clearing of opaque cells may take several weeks after the infection has subsided. In other instances bone destruction may proceed stealthily without any clinical signs of infection and large abscess cavities full of necrotic material may develop without any grave constitutional disturbance.

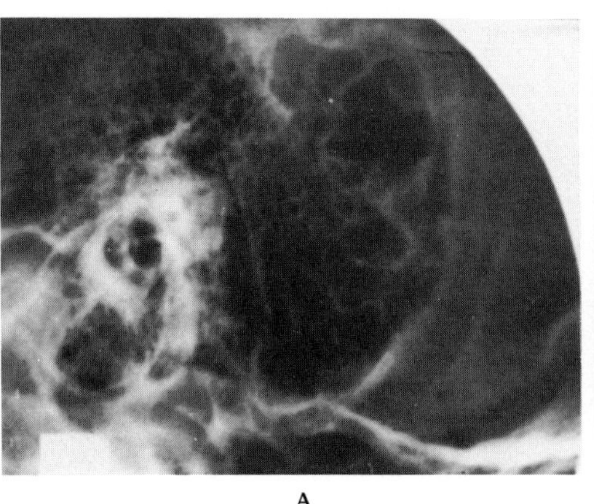

A

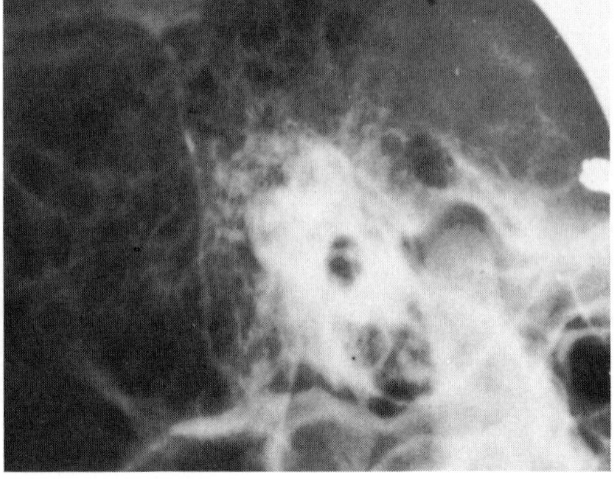

B

Fig. 51.11A Normal radiograph showing cellular mastoid. B Acute mastoiditis in a cellular mastoid. The cells show a loss of translucency and blurring of cell outlines in the left mastoid process.

Chronic mastoiditis. Chronic mastoiditis occurs as a sequel of acute mastoiditis when the infection fails to resolve completely or may be chronic from its onset. Inadequate antibiotic therapy may result in persistence of low grade infection with the ultimate development of chronic mastoiditis. Certain specific bacterial infections such as tuberculosis may be chronic from inception.

The combination of destruction of cell walls and reactive sclerosis accounts for the radiological appear-

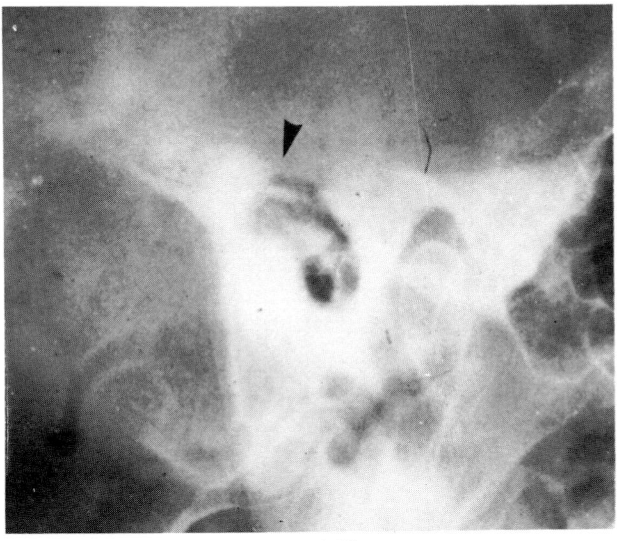

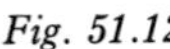
Fig. 51.12

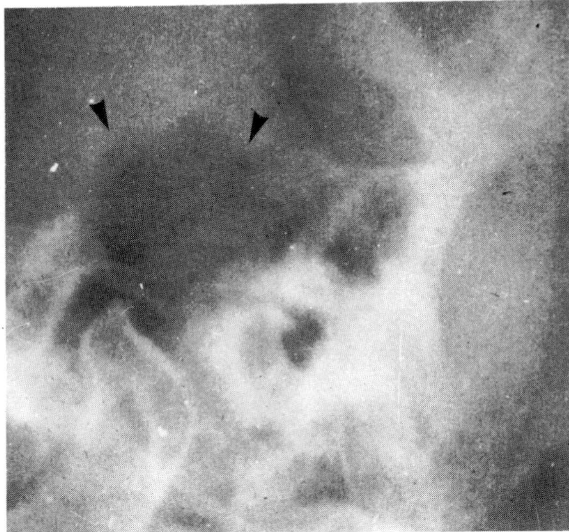

Fig. 51.13

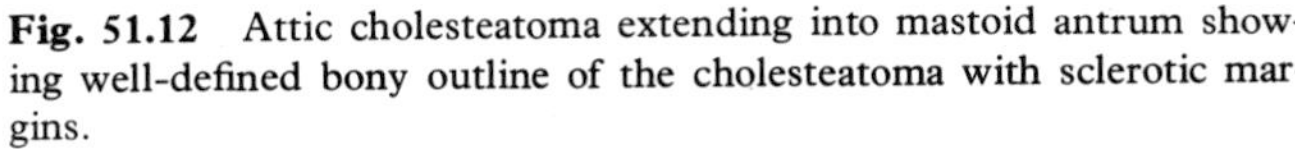
Fig. 51.12 Attic cholesteatoma extending into mastoid antrum showing well-defined bony outline of the cholesteatoma with sclerotic margins.

Fig. 51.13 Lateral oblique view of cholesteatoma showing extensive destruction of bone in the mastoid antrum and an extensive forward spread into the squamous temporal bone (*arrows*). The outlines of the cholesteatoma cavity are clear-cut but show no sclerosis.

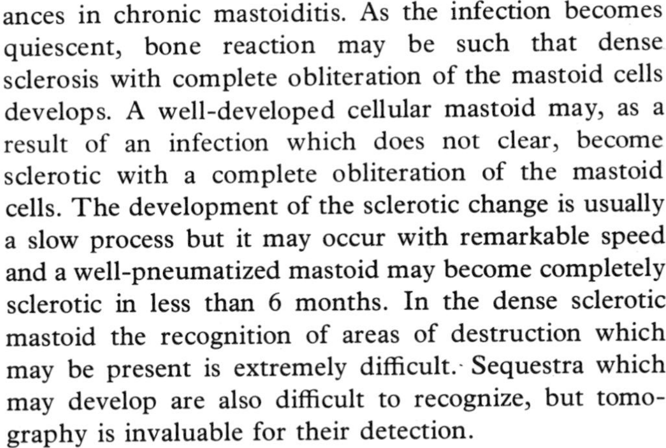
ances in chronic mastoiditis. As the infection becomes quiescent, bone reaction may be such that dense sclerosis with complete obliteration of the mastoid cells develops. A well-developed cellular mastoid may, as a result of an infection which does not clear, become sclerotic with a complete obliteration of the mastoid cells. The development of the sclerotic change is usually a slow process but it may occur with remarkable speed and a well-pneumatized mastoid may become completely sclerotic in less than 6 months. In the dense sclerotic mastoid the recognition of areas of destruction which may be present is extremely difficult. Sequestra which may develop are also difficult to recognize, but tomography is invaluable for their detection.

Complications

Abscess formation. Localized destruction of cell walls with confluence may result in abscess formation. The abscess cavity may be surrounded by an area of bone sclerosis. Bone destruction in chronic mastoiditis may be caused by granulation tissue rather than frank pus and many of the abscess cavities at operation are found filled with granulation tissue or even fluid-containing cholesterol crystals.

Cholesteatoma. The development of a cholesteatoma, composed of a mass of sequestrated epithelial cells, is one of the most serious sequelae of chronic infection of the middle ear or mastoid process. Considerable discussion has ranged around the origin of the epithelial cells constituting the cholesteatoma. They were at one time thought to be derived from the epithelium of the external meatus which had grown inwards through a perforation in the drum, and at other times considered to be derived from epithelial cell rests in the mastoid process. It has recently been shown that epithelial cells can migrate

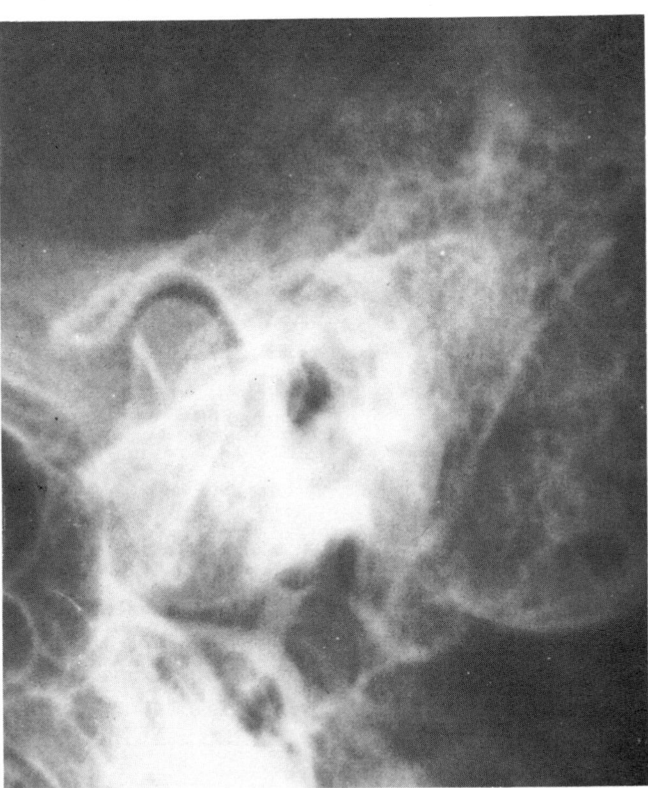

Fig. 51.14 Cholesteatoma in a cellular mastoid process. The cell outlines are partly blurred and hazy. Cholesteatoma seldom occurs in a cellular mastoid, and the bone destruction in a cellular mastoid is less easily recognised.

through an intact drum. The epithelial cells are stimulated to proliferate as the result of infection and erode the bony walls of the attic, antrum or middle ear and destroy the ossicular chain. Upward spread of a cholesteatoma may erode the tegmen tympani and open up into the middle cranial fossa, whilst posterior spread of the cholesteatoma may occur towards the sinodural angle. Whether the cholesteatoma in the infective process is responsible for the bone destruction has yet to be resolved.

Cholesteatoma more commonly occurs in the epitympanic recess (attic) than in the middle ear or mastoid antrum. The well-developed cholesteatoma with a large bony erosion is relatively easy to recognize, but the more superficial bone erosion associated with a cholesteatoma spreading along the bone surface may be overlooked. Other cholesteatoma may degenerate and form cholesteatomatous cysts rather than solid tumours. These cysts produce destructive changes indistinguishable from solid tumours. The signs of cholesteatoma relate to their sites of origin, e.g. middle ear, attic, etc., but basically may be recognized by the following signs:

1. An area of bone destruction in the attic or mastoid antrum associated with a smooth clear-cut outline and little sclerosis around the bone destruction (Figs. 51.12 and 51.13).

2. The mastoid process is usually sclerotic although not invariably so. In cellular mastoids quite extensive destruction of cell walls may occur (Fig. 51.14).

3. Erosion of the attic is best recognized in the lateral oblique or submentovertical projections (Fig. 51.15) and they are particularly useful in evaluating the presence of cholesteatoma in this region.

4. Postero-anterior and lateral tomographs are essential for evaluating the extent of bone destruction. Minimal bone erosion particularly in the region of the aditus ad antrum is one of the earliest signs of cholesteatoma formation.

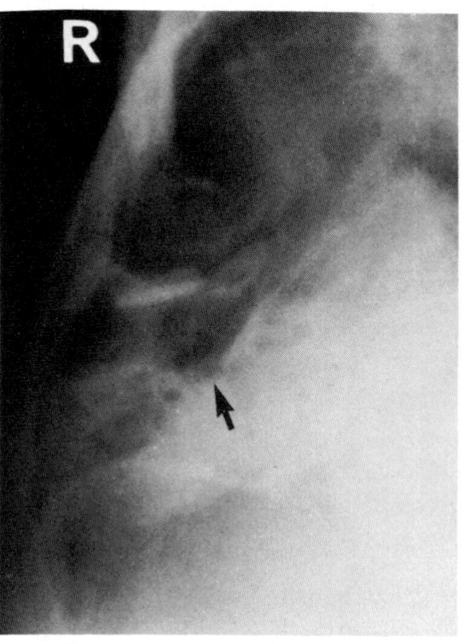

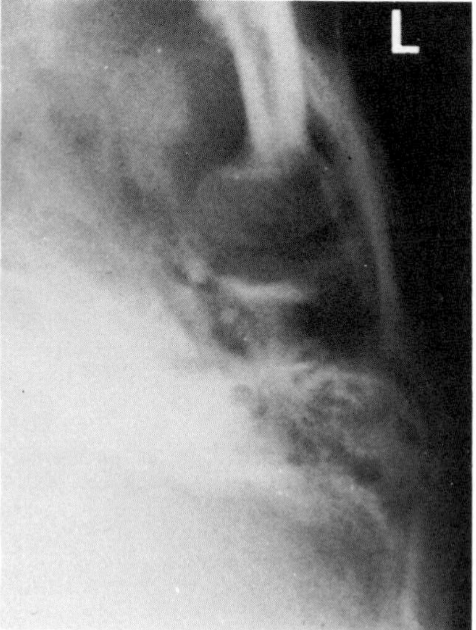

Fig. 51.15 Attic cholesteatoma. SMV view showing bone erosion in right attic region (*arrow*) and loss of outline of ossicles. Extension backwards through the aditus ad antrum has occurred with widening of that opening.

Owing to the fact that some cholesteatoma may cause no or only superficial bone erosion, approximately 25 per cent of all cholesteatoma cannot be diagnosed by radiological methods alone.

Congenital cholesteatoma (epidermoid) involves the apex of the petrous bone, and extensive destruction with no bony sclerotic changes is seen. This type of tumour has to be distinguished from acoustic neuromas, xanthomata and other lesions causing bone erosion of the apex of the petrous bone. They are unassociated with any infection and may present as an intracranial tumour.

Tuberculosis. Tuberculous disease of the mastoid process occurs on rare occasions often unassociated with tuberculous infection in other areas. It is characterized by extensive destruction of the cell system with little or no bone reaction. The radiological appearances of extensive destruction with little or no bone reaction are not dissimilar to carcinoma of the middle ear, but whereas the clinical symptoms of tuberculous disease are relatively slight, with carcinoma of the middle ear severe pain is a constant and prominent feature.

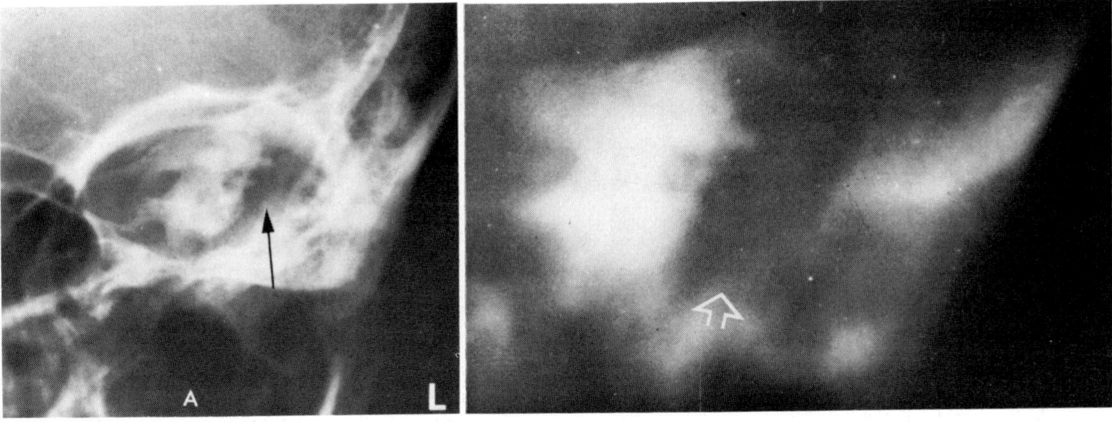

Fig. 51.16 Carcinoma of the middle ear. A Transorbital view showing destruction of bone in the middle ear and along its floor (*arrow*). B Postero-anterior tomogram showing extensive destruction of the bone. Arrow shows bone erosion in hypotympanic region.

TUMOURS

Tumours involving the **external meatus** are usually *benign exostoses*. They can best be seen in the lateral view when the meatus is narrowed to a slit. Tomography in the lateral position may be invaluable in demonstrating the exostosis. Cold-water swimming is a specific factor in the development of exostosis of the external meatus.

Frequently they almost completely occlude the external meatus and when occlusion is completed by wax, infective changes arising behind the wax may give rise to an acute mastoiditis and the exostoses in the external meatus may be overlooked.

Malignant tumours involving the external meatus are usually a sequel of an overlying *rodent ulcer* or *squamous celled carcinoma* of the pinna or adjoining skin which secondarily invades the bone. Such bone invasion is characterized by destruction with little or no reactive sclerosis.

Tumours of the **middle ear** are usually *carcinomata* and usually develop as a sequel to chronic infection of the middle ear. In some instances, however, the reverse

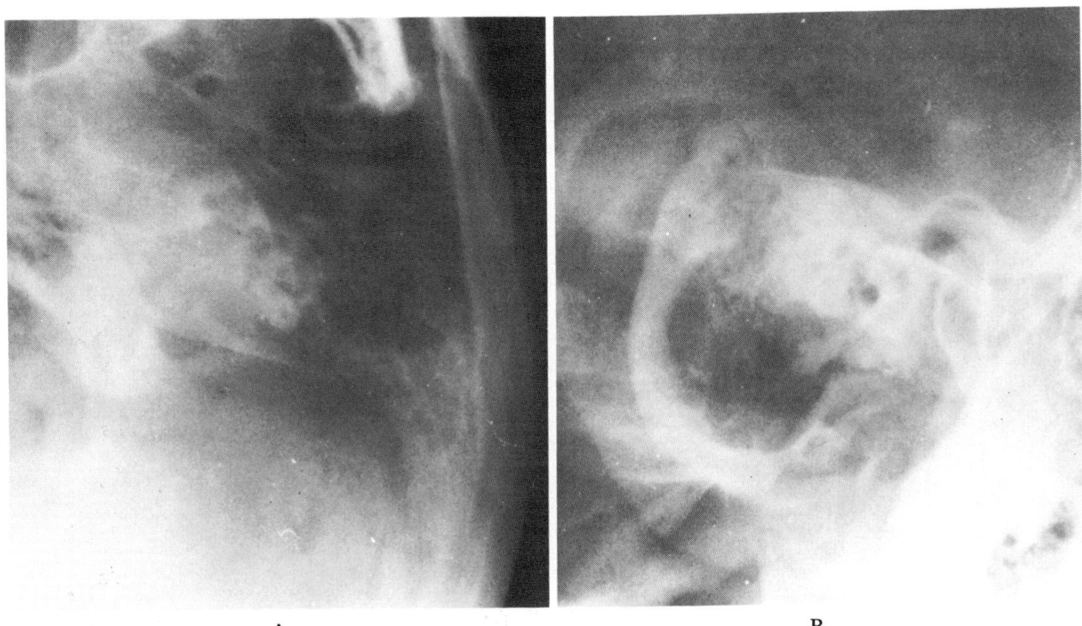

Fig. 51.17 Glomus tumour of middle ear showing extensive destruction of the bone. A Basal view. B Lateral oblique view. The extent of bone sclerosis depends on the degree of associated infection.

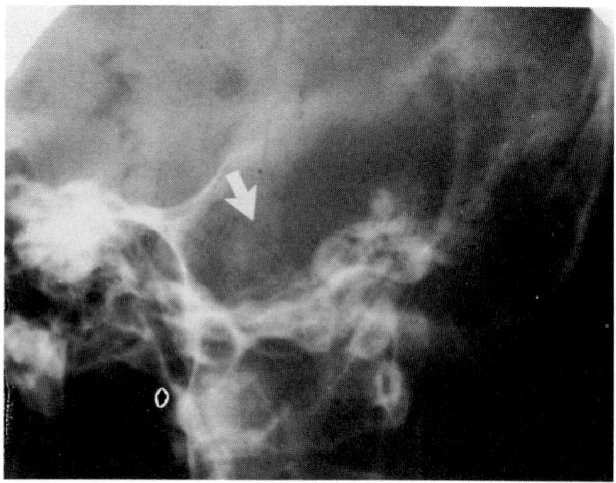

Fig. 51.18 Secondary deposit in apex of petrous bone producing gross erosion (from primary carcinoma of breast).

occurs and infection may develop as a sequel of tumour formation.

Carcinoma of the middle ear is associated with extensive bone destruction (Fig. 51.16A and B), but as infective changes are frequently present sclerosis of the petrous bone may also be present.

Other tumours which cause extensive destruction of the petrous bone and mastoid process and are locally malignant but seldom metastasize are *chemodectomata* (*tympanic body* and *glomus jugulare tumours*) (Fig. 51.17A and B). These tumours, arising from the chemoreceptor system along the internal jugular vein and from Jacobson's nerve, cause extensive bone destruction. They have a marked predominance in females and are relatively slowly growing. As these tumours have a large vascular component they can be well shown by carotid angiography and jugular phlebography.

Sarcomata seldom occur in the temporal bone and they are usually osteosarcomata. *Metastatic tumours*, however, are not uncommon and usually have their primary tumour in the breast or lung. Facial palsy may be the first symptom (Fig. 51.18).

Eighth nerve tumours

Tumours of the eighth nerve are usually of two types, the common *Schwannoma* derived from the nerve sheath, and the exceptionally rare *neurofibroma* which may be associated with a generalized neurofibromatosis and may be bilateral and familial. These tumours may present with a relatively long clinical history, but radiological changes in the early stages may be only slight and may be easily overlooked.

Radiologically the features are:

1. Disappearance of the crista transversalis in the internal auditory meatus. The crista transversalis is a thin ridge of bone which separates the termination of the facial nerve from the acoustic nerve. The crista may be seen in routine projections and can almost always be seen in good A.P. tomograms. Disappearance of this bony ridge must be regarded as an early diagnostic sign before expansion of the internal meatus has occurred.
2. Widening of the internal auditory meatus. There is considerable variability in the width and length of the internal auditory meatus and only about 40 per cent of internal meati are symmetrical in the postero-anterior view. It must be rememberd that the inner end of the auditory meatus normally has a bulbous appearance (Fig. 51.19).
3. Erosion and shortening of the internal meatus.

Radiologically these tumours have to be differentiated from congenital variations of the internal meatus, decalcification due to apical petrositis, cholestaetoma, meningioma, and glomus jugulare tumours.

Contrast filling of the cerebello-pontine angle with air after encephalography or with Pantopaque after the performance of a lumbar myelogram may detect these tumours when they are still intra-canalicular.

CT scanning only visualizes medium-sized neuromas (2–3 cm) even with contrast enhancement and should follow polytomography in the investigation of these tumours. Negative CT scans in clinically suspicious

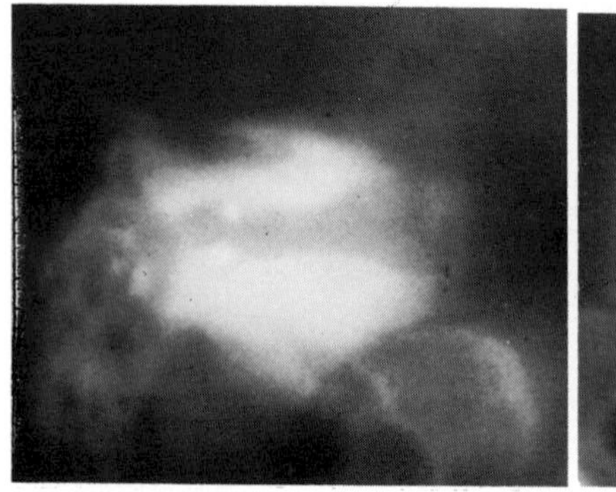

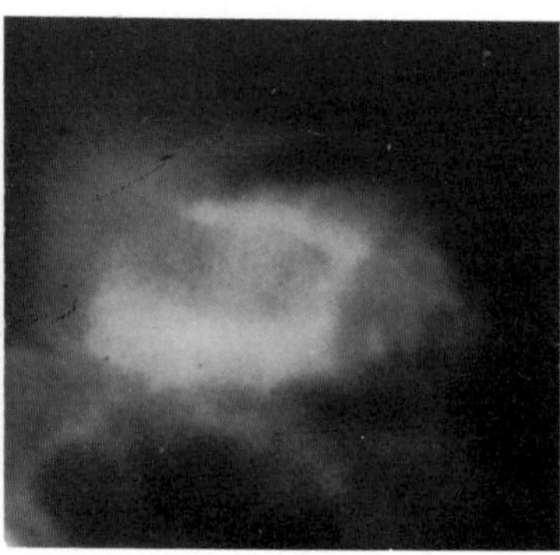

Fig. 51.19 Acoustic neuroma. P.A. tomograms showing enlargement of Rt. internal meatus. A Normal left side. B Enlarged right meatus.

cases should be followed by positive contrast myelography.

OTOSCLEROSIS

Radiological examination has two functions in otosclerosis, one to exclude other causes of deafness, e.g. chronic infection, and secondly to demonstrate specific changes of otosclerosis in the petrous bone.

In the great majority of otosclerotic subjects the disease commences around the oval window and the round window is less frequently involved. Changes in fenestral otosclerosis can be shown when good quality tomograms show the oval window. The thickening of the edges of the foramen and the blurring of the outlines of the window can be identified in 75 to 80 per cent of cases. Retrofenestral otosclerosis when the cochlea is involved is less critical and only about 50 per cent of such cases show any radiological change.

REFERENCES AND SUGGESTIONS FOR FURTHER READING

Britton, B. H. & Hitselberger, W. E. (1968) Iophendylate examination of posterior fossa in diagnosis of cerebellopontine angle tumours. *Archives Otolaryngology*, **88,** 608.

Guinto, F. C., Jr. & Himadi, G. M. (1974) Tomographic anatomy of the ear. *Radiologic Clinics of North America*, **12,** 405.

Jensen, J. (1974) Congenital anomalies of the inner ear. *Radiologic Clinics of North America*, **12,** 473–482.

Jensen, J. & Rovsing, H. (1968) Tomography in congenital malformations of the middle ear. *Radiology*, **90,** 268.

Pendersen, G. B. & Brünner, S. (1970) Tomographic examination of cholesteatomas in the middle ear. *Acta Otolaryngologiea*, **70,** 167.

Potter, G. D. (1973) Trauma of the ear. *Otolaryngologie Clinics of North America*, **6,** 401.

Samuel, E. & Lloyd, G. A. S. (1978) *Clinical Radiology of the Ear, Nose and Throat*. 2nd Ed. London: Lewis.

Schuknecht, H. F., Allam, A. F. & Murakami, Y. (1971) Primary and metastatic tumours of the temporal bone. *Laryngoscope*, **81,** 1273.

Zizmor, J. & Noyek, A. M. (1969) Tumours and other osseous disorders of the temporal bone. *Seminars in Roentgenology*, **4,** 151.

Zizmor, J. & Noyek, A. M. (1974) Inflammatory diseases of the temporal bone. *Radiologic Clinics of North America*, **12,** 491.

CHAPTER 52

THE ORBIT AND EYE

RADIOGRAPHIC TECHNIQUE

Plain X-ray examination of the orbit should consist, in the first instance, of standard skull projections—that is a P.A. projection, lateral and half axial (Towne's) view. When the patient examined has a *unilateral proptosis* then the standard projections should be augmented by views of the optic foramina. The radiographic position for these projections is obtained by tilting the orbito-meatal base-line of the skull 30 degrees upwards from the occipitofrontal position, and rotating the head 39 degrees away from the affected side, thus projecting the optic canal into the inferolateral quadrant of the orbit. A modification of the optic canal view is also a useful additional projection for patients suspected of having an enlargement of the superior orbital fissure. This projection is achieved by using slightly less angulation of the orbito-meatal line, i.e. 25 degrees instead of 30 degrees, and using less obliquity of the head than normally employed for optic canal projections. The film obtained affords better visualization of the apex of the orbit and surrounding structures and is the optimum method of demonstrating erosion of the optic strut by plain X-ray.

An occipito-oral view should also be used routinely in an orbital skull series. The radiographic position for this is similar to that of the standard occipito-mental view used in the radiography of the para-nasal sinuses, but with the orbito-meatal line tilted 35 degrees to the film instead of 45 degrees, as in the latter projection. A similar projection may be obtained by placing the head in the position for a standard postero-anterior view with 35 degree angulation of the tube caudally. The central ray is thus directed along the plane of the horizontal axis of the orbit so that the roof is more completely seen than in the standard postero-anterior view, with less foreshortening, and the petrous bones are projected below the inferior orbital margin.

A routine series of radiographs of the orbit should, therefore, include the following:

1. Standard lateral view,
2. Standard postero-anterior view,
3. Towne's projection,
4. Occipito-oral view,
5. Standard optic canal projections,
6. Apical views of the orbit, if enlargement of the superior orbital fissure is suspected.

Plain X-ray changes

Alterations in the general radiographic density of the orbit are dependent upon a decrease or increase of the soft tissue contents; thus, in the presence of a space-occupying lesion causing proptosis, oedema of the soft tissues or ecchymosis, a decrease in orbital translucency is to be expected. Conversely, enophthalmos resulting from a decrease in the contents of the orbit, will produce a slight hyper-translucency. These changes in the soft tissue density of the orbit are of little practical diagnostic significance and simply reflect a change which is obvious clinically. Alterations in the size of the orbit are a common accompaniment of long-standing orbital pathology. *Decrease in size* may occur after early enucleation of the eye before the orbit has reached adult size; it may also be seen in congenital microphthalmos and anophthalmos. *Enlargement* is normally the result of raised intraorbital pressure producing changes in the orbit analogous to those seen in the calvarium in raised intracranial pressure. Any growing tumour may produce these X-ray changes if sufficient time has elapsed, but the response of the orbit to a space-occupying lesion is more rapid in a child than an adult, and whilst orbital enlargement usually denotes a benign lesion of long standing, this rule is not applicable to children.

Invasion and erosion of the walls of the orbit may take the form of *osseous destruction* and is then usually due to a malignant primary or secondary neoplasm. Rarely it may be due to an infective process such as tuberculosis. A local indentation of the orbital wall with clear-cut edges is characteristic of a benign tumour such as a dermoid cyst or epidermoid. Increased bone density or hyperostosis in the orbit may occur in a number of conditions, principally a pterional or sphenoid ridge *meningioma*, but it may also be due to osteoblastic *metastases, fibrous dysplasia, Paget's disease* and *chronic periostitis*.

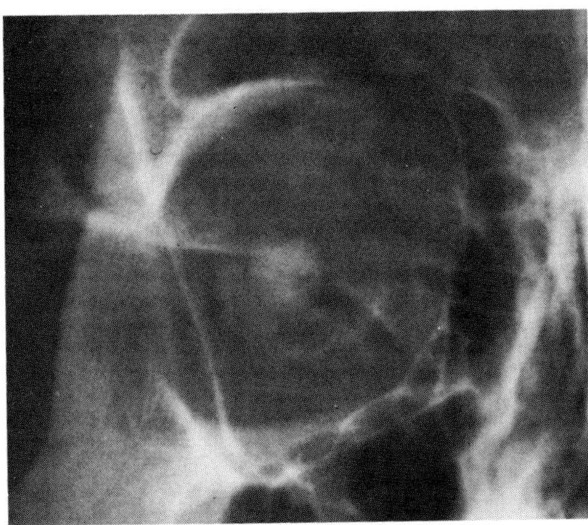

Fig. 52.1 Phthisis bulbi. Calcification in the lens and vitreous.

Calcification within the soft tissues of the orbit is uncommon. Within the globe it may be present in the lens in *senile cataract*, and ossification may occur in the vitreous and choroid as a result of degenerative changes following injury or infection (Fig. 52.1). Finely stippled calcification may be demonstrable in cases of *retinoblastoma,* and Taybi (1956) has reported macroscopic global calcification in 14 of 22 children with *retrolental fibroplasia*. Calcinosis oculi has also been reported in *hyperparathyroidism* (Heath, 1962). Calcification in the retro-orbital structures may be seen in *meningiomas* of the optic nerve. This may take the shape of calcification within the sheath of the optic nerve, or a finely stippled calcification may be present in the tumour mass, usually located towards the apex of the orbit. The identification of phleboliths in the orbit is an important observation in the differential diagnosis of patients presenting with proptosis and it indicates the presence, either of a *venous malformation,* or a *cavernous haemangioma* (Fig. 52.2). In the author's experience the former diagnosis is by far the more likely. However, histologically verified haemangiomas containing phleboliths have been reported in the orbit by several authors including Lombardi (1967).

Changes in the optic foramina and in the sphenoidal fissure may also indicate the presence of an intraorbital lesion. This is discussed elsewhere (see Ch. 58).

Tomography of the orbit

Tomography is an essential part of the X-ray investigation of the orbit and related paranasal sinuses. Abnormalities not readily visualized on plain X-ray may be demonstrated by means of tomographic section, and changes seen on standard films are frequently better delineated in size, extent and relationship to adjoining structures, by this means. Complete tomography of the upper part of the facial skeleton requires films taken in three planes: *viz.* coronal, lateral and axial. For tomographic studies of the optic canal a 39-degree oblique projection may also be needed.

Tomography in the coronal plane has its most important application in the demonstration of expanding processes and bone destruction, either inflammatory or neoplastic, in paranasal sinus disease, and in the demonstration of fractures involving the orbit and sinuses. An important example is a 'blow out' fracture of the floor of the orbit, in which it is the best method of showing both the herniation of orbital contents in the upper part of the maxillary antrum and the fragments of displaced and depressed bone from the orbital floor (Fig. 52.3). Elsewhere in the orbit it has its most important application in the demonstration of lacrimal fossa enlargement

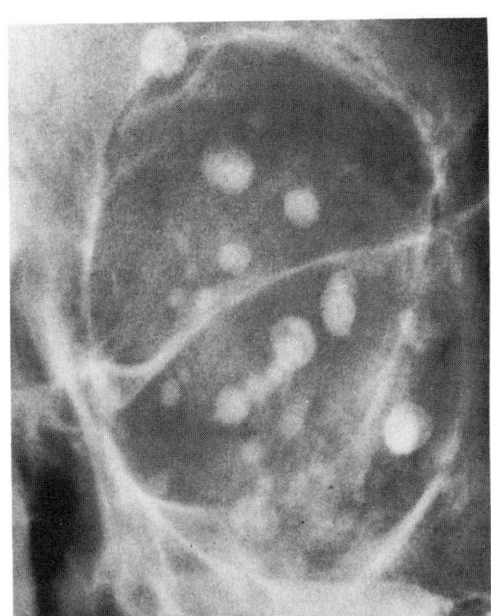

Fig. 52.2 Venous malformation. Multiple phleboliths in an enlarged left orbit.

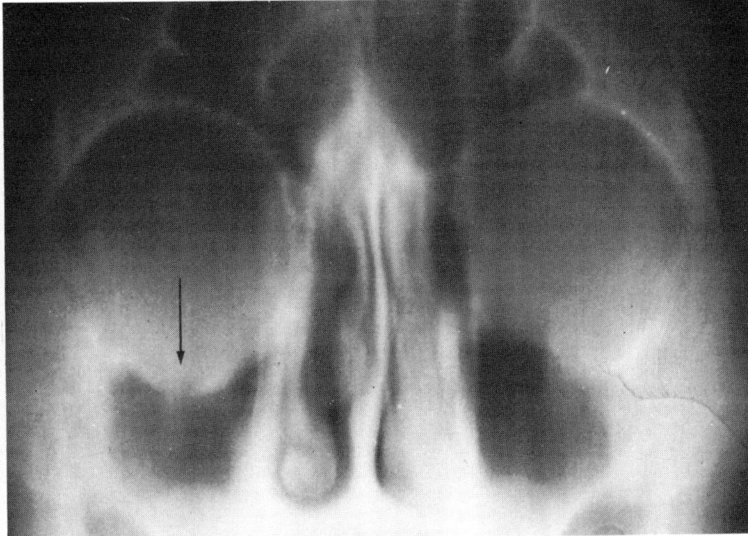

Fig. 52.3 Coronal tomogram showing blow-out fracture of the orbital floor (right).

and bone erosion in the presence of a lacrimal gland tumour.

Lateral orbital tomography is also used to demonstrate 'blow out' fractures of the orbital floor and is a useful procedure preoperatively to estimate the posterior extent of the fracture. Other applications of lateral tomography include the demonstration of mucocoeles of the frontal sinus invading the orbital roof. It is sometimes possible to demonstrate a thin rim of expanded bone forming the inferior border of the mucocoele on these lateral films. In frontal sinus mucocoeles it is also important to determine whether the posterior wall of the frontal sinuses is intact or not, since the sac of the mucocoele may be in contact with the dura if erosion of the posterior wall is complete.

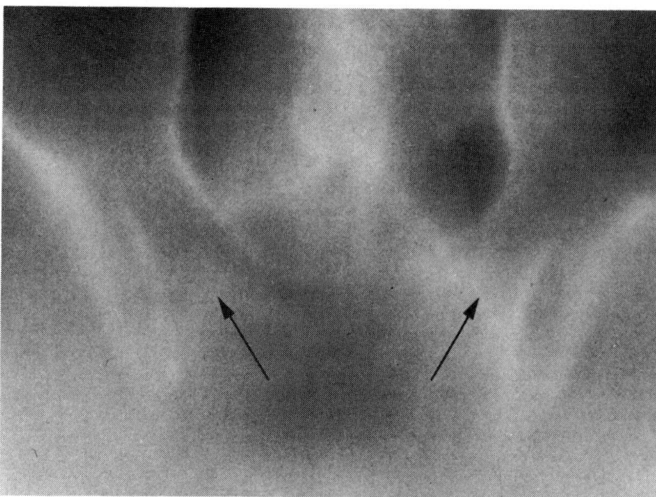

Fig. 52.4 Axial hypocycloidal tomography of the optic canals (*arrows*). The anterior clinoid processes are shown in plan view lateral to the canals, and the normal decrease in width of the canals anteriorly is apparent.

In the technique evolved for axial tomography of the orbits (Lloyd, 1971), the Philips Massiot polytome has been used exclusively. The hypocycloidal movement has been found to produce the best results, but other rotational tomographic movements will give adequate results in most instances. In the author's experience axial tomography is the most informative method of tomographic examination of the orbit and paranasal sinuses and has become a special technique in its own right (Lloyd, 1975). It should be used routinely for the investigation of unilateral proptosis. There are three principal applications:

1. The demonstration of tumours and expanding lesions in the paranasal sinuses involving the orbit.
2. The demonstration of tumours and other space occupying lesions in the orbit.
3. Tomography of the optic canal in the axial plane.

Using this technique, positive evidence of the presence of a space-occupying lesion in the orbit may be shown by the following X-ray changes:

1. Bone destruction or hyperostosis in the walls of the orbit.
2. Generalized enlargement of the orbit in the transverse plane.
3. Indentations of the orbital walls.
4. The demonstration of a tumour as a soft tissue mass (Lloyd, 1975).

The technique of axial tomography has added a new dimension to roentgenographic studies of the optic canal. By this method it is possible to produce a complete plan view of both canals (Harwood-Nash, 1970) (Fig. 52.4). On the tomograms the effect is as if the observer were looking at the deroofed canals from above, and it is possible to appreciate the normal widening of the transverse diameter of the canal posteriorly. Axial tomography has the advantage of showing both canals on a single projection so that an accurate comparison of the two sides can be made. The pathological changes occurring in this view in optic nerve glioma have been described by Harwood-Nash (1972).

COMPUTERIZED AXIAL TOMOGRAPHY

This technique is now widely used in orbital diagnosis and is described in more detail in Chapters 63 to 65. It is now the dominant method of orbital investigation after plain X-ray.

Technique. The optimum apparatus for CT Scanning of the orbit is one that allows scans to be made in at least two planes and if possible, three. In effect this means discarding the original head scanning format and using a body scanning machine in which the scanning aperture is large enough to allow the head to be manipulated into the required positions to produce, not only axial scans, but also coronal scans and sometimes sagittal sections. Coronal sections in addition to the normal axial scans are now highly desirable for the routine investigation of the orbit and should be obtained as routine. This particularly applies to pathology in the paranasal sinuses, extending into the orbit (Fig. 52.5). As in conventional tomography the main skin port for computerized tomography should be through the back of the head, whether the scanning X-ray tube is positioned over or under couch. For CT Scanners with an over couch gantry, this means that the patient must be positioned prone. In this way the incident beam of X-rays is directed for the most part through the back of the skull reducing the radiation dose received by the lens and cornea to less than one-sixth of that received when the patient is supine. The attitude of the patient's head is important so that the optimum scanning plane can be obtained through the orbits. Satisfactory scans should include the globes and show the lens, optic nerve, lateral and medial rectus muscles on

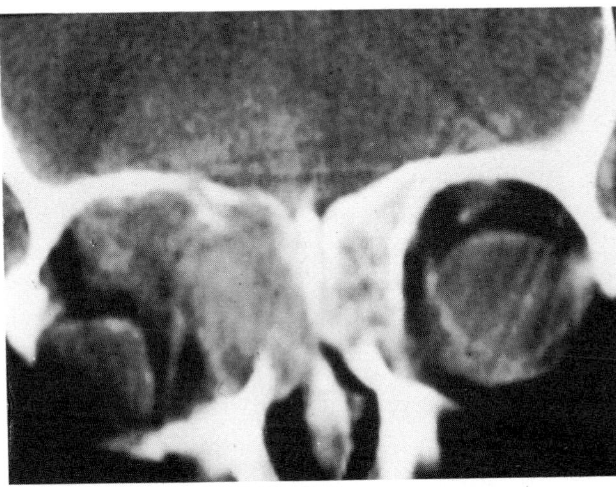

Fig. 52.5

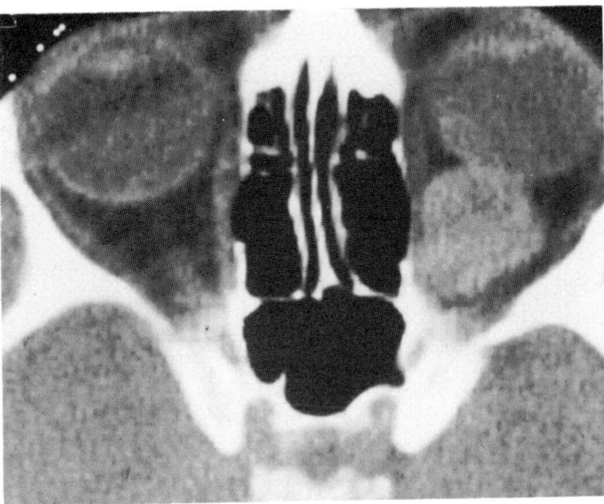

Fig. 52.6

Fig. 52.5 Coronal CT Scan showing primary sarcoma of the frontal sinus invading the right orbit and extending upwards into the anterior fossa.

Fig. 52.6 Rounded encapsulated tumour in the intra-conal space of the left orbit, shown at surgery to be a cavernous haemangioma.

the same cut. To do this the position of the head should be adjusted so that the scanning plane forms an angle of 16° caudally from the orbito-meatal line. This line should be marked out on the skin prior to scanning. Optimum orbital scans will be obtained if the posterior clinoids are shown on scans which also include the optic nerves and clearly show the globes on both sides.

For coronal scans the patient lies prone with the chin elevated so that the radiation port is again principally through the skull vault. A similar position can be obtained by placing the patient supine with the head hyper-extended but this incurs an unacceptable level of radiation to the lens and cornea and is therefore to be avoided.

Diagnosis

For CT diagnosis orbital disease may be divided into *primary*, originating within the orbit, and *secondary*, by extension of pathology from neighbouring structures, i.e. the cranium, paranasal sinuses or nasopharynx.

Primary orbital disease. The aetiology of a mass in the orbit may, in some instances, be determined by its site of origin. Most *optic nerve tumours*, whether gliomata or meningiomata show as enlargements of the optic nerve. The location of a mass with respect to the rectus muscle cone is also a guide to the possible aetiology. The commonest tumour in this category is a *lacrimal gland neoplasm*. These are as a rule readily palpable; and computerized tomography is not needed to make the diagnosis, but is useful to show the soft tissue extent of the tumour prior to surgery. Malignant disease may also be located extraconally, for example *metastases* and *lymphomata*. *Dermoids* are usually found in the roof of

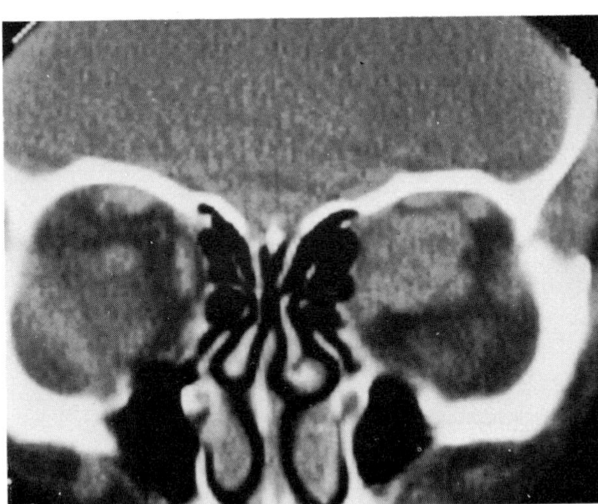

Fig. 52.7 Coronal CT Scan showing cavernous haemangioma in the left orbit located in the upper part of the muscle cone and displacing the optic nerve downwards.

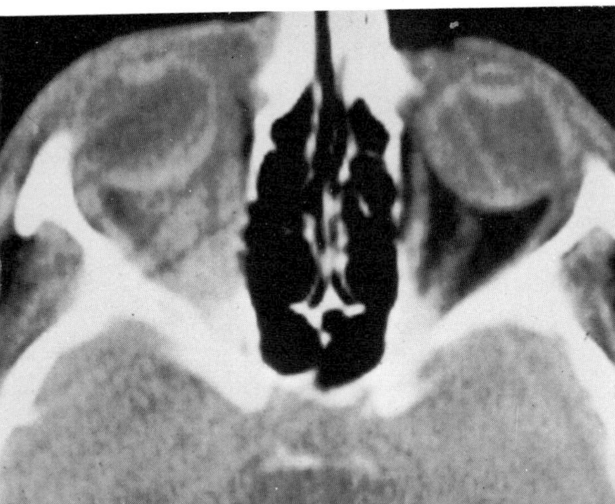

Fig. 52.8 Diffuse mass in the intra-conal space of the right orbit due to a pseudotumour.

the orbit outside the muscle cone. Another tumour which is found extraconally is an *orbital haemangiopericytoma*.

Some differentiation of the common intraconal space-occupying lesions found in the orbit is possible on the basis of their shape and density (CT morphology). Benign encapsulated tumours are readily identified on this basis. The commonest is a *cavernous haemangioma* (Fig. 52.6); these show a mass of rounded contour and even density sometimes almost completely circular in outline. Their exact location can be determined by coronal studies (Fig. 52.7). These benign encapsulated tumours may be clearly differentiated from infiltrative processes occurring within the orbit. Typical of the latter are the *pseudotumours* or *granulomas*; these may be distinguished from the clearly defined tumours described above, by their ill-defined edge and uneven density (Fig. 52.8). Pseudotumours may extend both inside and outside the muscle cone; they may involve the lacrimal gland; they may sometimes be bilateral; and they may cause local muscle enlargement. This latter sign is by no means specific however, since it may occur in a variety of other conditions, most commonly *dysthyroid exophthalmos* (see below). Local rectus muscle enlargement has also been recorded in *venous* and *arteriovenous malformations* in the orbit, and enlargement has also been observed affecting the lateral rectus muscle in three patients with lacrimal gland neoplasms. Another feature which may be present on computerized tomograms of a pseudotumour or granuloma is an apparent thickening of the posterior coats of the globe—probably the result of inflammatory tissue being contiguous with the posterior surface of the sclera. In some instances the abnormal tissue may fill the whole of the intraconal space obliterating the outline of normal structures by an isodense mass. Another lesion which may give an appearance indistinguishable from a pseudotumour is a lymphoma; and some metastases may show as a diffuse mass within the rectus muscle cone. Hence, it is not always possible to make a clear distinction of the CT morphology between an inflammatory process and malignant infiltration in the orbit.

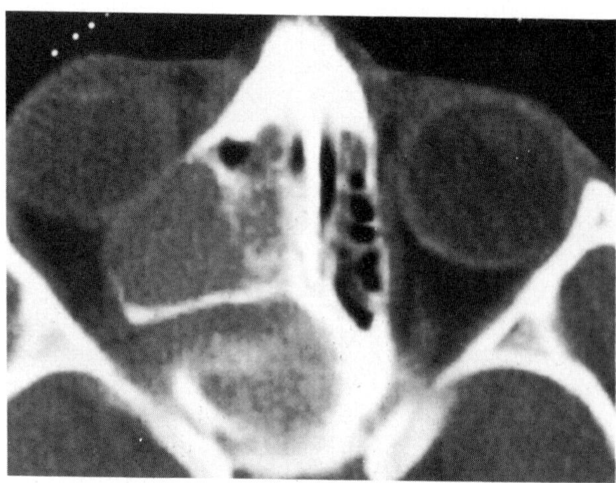

Fig. 52.9 Right spheno-ethmoidal mucocele demonstrated by axial CT.

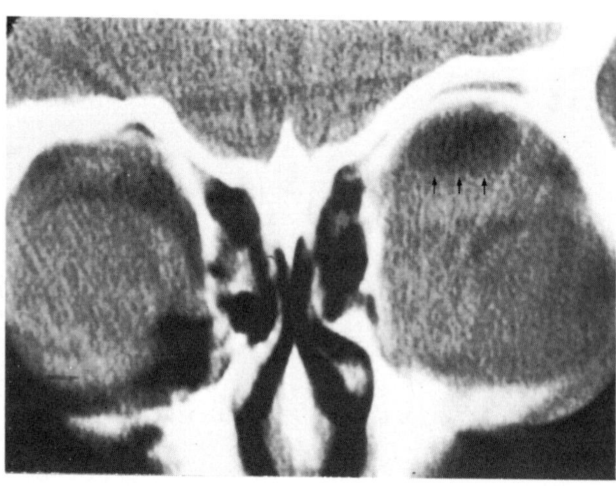

Fig. 52.10 Coronal CT Scan showing area of low attenuation in the roof of the orbit (arrows) due to a dermoid cyst.

Attenuation values and intravenous contrast medium. Possible tissue recognition by means of the attenuation values and their behaviour after intravenous contrast medium has been investigated by Lloyd and Ambrose (1977). In this study consideration of the attenuation values from three common types of tumour found in the orbit (meningioma, haemangioma and lymphoma) showed that there was no means of differentiating these on the evidence of the initial values, or on the degree of enhancement following intravenous contrast medium. The only observable difference was found in the granulomata, some of which showed values in the negative range of the EMI scale. It was concluded however that the most probable explanation for this was the incorporation of normal fat cells found in the muscle cone within the inflammatory tissue. In other words the presence of negative attenuation values simply indicated the infiltrative nature of the abnormality present and was not tissue specific. The work of Ambrose *et al.* (1977), has shown that it is unlikely that the contrast agents normally used such as Conray are taken up by the cells of tumours to any significant degree, and that the increased X-ray attenuation observed in cases of tumours following administration of these agents, probably reflects increases in the vascularity and interstitial fluid mass in the region of the lesion. Thus the more highly vascular orbital tumours, those which can be expected to show a strong tumour blush on arteriography are, likely to show most attenuation enhancement. Haemangiopericytomas and some meningiomata are the tumours which most often fall into this category. Conversely very low attenua-

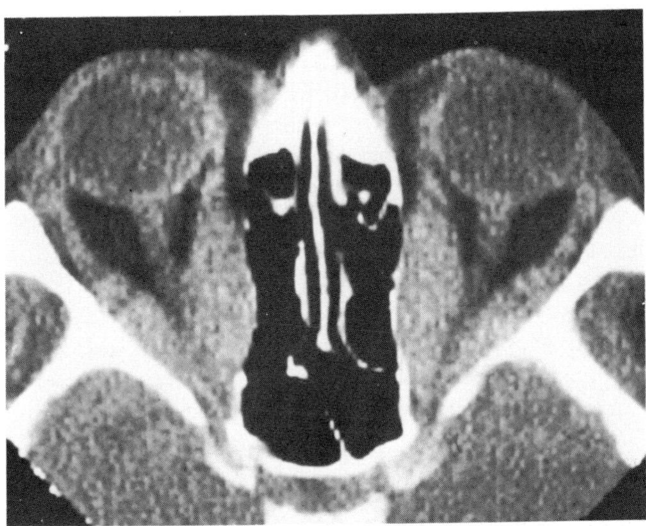

Fig. 52.11 Dysthyroid exophthalmos. Axial CT Scan showing muscle enlargement and bilateral indentation of the ethmoid labyrinth by the enlarged medial recti.

tion values within a tumour mass indicate the presence of fat or oil and are diagnostic of a dermoid cyst (Fig. 52.10).

Secondary orbital lesions. Tumours and other lesions in the middle fossa invading the orbit and causing proptosis may be clearly demonstrated by computerized tomography. A *meningioma* is the commonest tumour in this category. Other lesions such as *neurofibromatosis* or an *infraclinoid aneurysm* may also be shown, and the presence of a *carotico-cavernous fistula* may be inferred, if the superior ophthalmic vein is unusually conspicuous in a patient with clinical evidence of a shunt.

In the majority of patients, *paranasal sinus disease* invading the orbit is diagnosable by plain X-ray and conventional tomography. Computerized tomography may act as a substitute for conventional tomography in sinus disease (Fig. 52.9), but its main contribution in this respect, is its ability to show the exact soft tissue extent of a tumour or granuloma invading the orbit, anterior fossa, or infratemporal fossa. *Neoplasms and other expanding processes arising in the frontal sinus and ethmoids* are optimally demonstrated in their extent and spread by computerized tomography (Fig. 52.5). For these studies coronal sections are clearly essential. Frontal sinus pathology cannot be adequately demonstrated on axial scans alone. By its ability to show the soft tissue extent of disease in the paranasal sinuses. computerized tomography has a unique and vital role to play in diagnosis and radiotherapy field planning.

Dysthyroid exophthalmos. The enlargement of the extra-ocular muscles which occurs in this condition may be clearly demonstrated by computerized tomography. In addition to muscle enlargement the intraconal space may appear enlarged, probably due to mucopolysaccharide infiltration. In dysthyroid patients the degree of muscle swelling, as depicted on computerized tomography is often uneven, and in some instances may be due to selective enlargement of individual or groups of muscles, particularly when the exophthalmos is unilateral. Enlargement of the medial rectus muscle may also cause a characteristic 'waisting' of the ethmoid labyrinth due to symmetrical pressure on the medial orbital wall by enlarged medial recti (Fig. 52.11). Brismar, *et al.* (1976), have recorded a pitfall in the differential diagnosis of endocrine exophthalmos by computerized tomography. Due to the enlarged rectus muscles in the apex of the orbit, simulated tumour formation may be shown on the scan. This is explained by the tomographic section intersecting obliquely one of the enlarged muscles (usually the inferior rectus), thus producing a false tumour like structure on the scan (Fig. 52.12). The problem has been largely overcome by

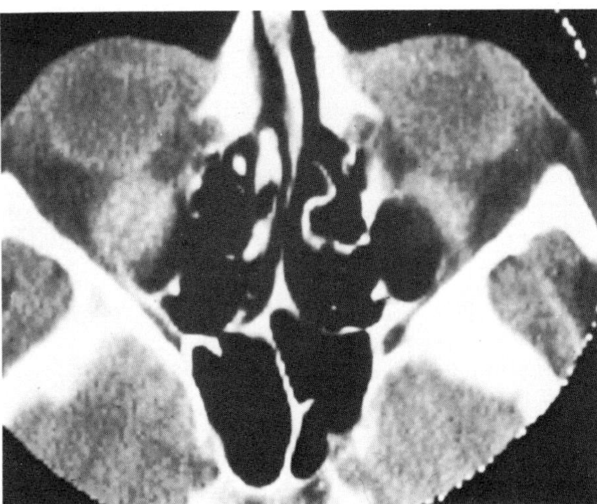

Fig. 52.12 Dysthyroid exophthalmos. False tumour formation on axial CT due to bulbous enlargement of the inferior rectus muscles.

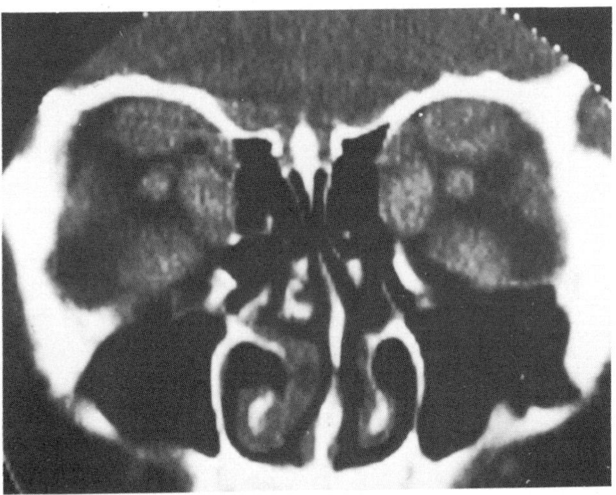

Fig. 52.13 Same patient as Figure 52.12. Coronal scan shows gross and generalized enlargement of the rectus muscles including the inferior recti.

the application of coronal CT Scanning (Fig. 52.13), which clearly shows the origin of the abnormality.

Ultrasound

Initially A mode ultrasonography was used for orbital diagnosis and a very high degree of diagnostic accuracy has been claimed by some authors for this method. Most centres now employ B scan systems for ophthalmic examination, the advantage being that they provide an anatomically arranged pattern of the soft tissues in which both normal and abnormal configurations may be recognized and recorded photographically. The introduction of a mechanically operated transducer for holographic imaging of ophthalmic ultrasound also allows the recording of C scan ultrasonic images (Lloyd, 1977).

The normal echo pattern in the orbit is demonstrated by the high reflectivity of the fat cells in the muscle cone, and the majority of space-occupying lesions are recorded as areas of lower reflectivity within the pattern of fat echoes. Similarly the optic nerve is shown as a linear filling defect on B scan (Fig. 52.14) and as a central acoustically negative area on C scan (Fig. 52.15) (Lloyd, 1977).

The use of ultrasonography for orbital soft tissue diagnosis has become less necessary with the development of CT scanning, which generally shows the location

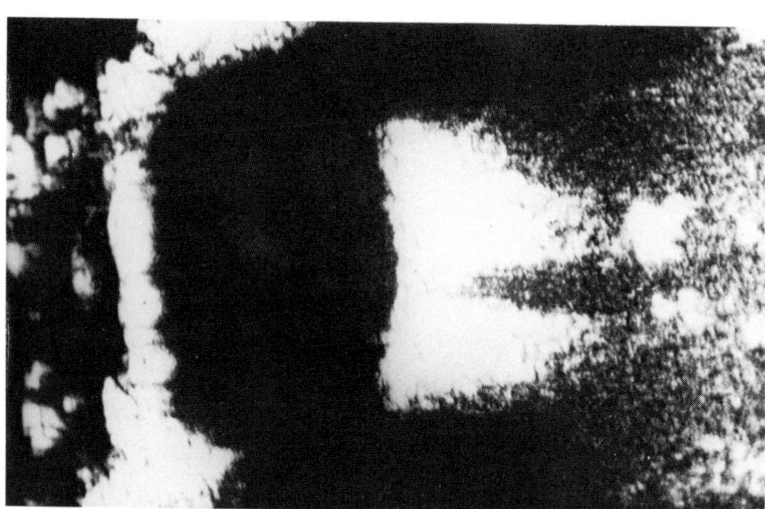

Fig. 52.14

Fig. 52.15

Fig. 52.14 Normal B Scan showing optic nerve as a linear filling defect

Fig. 52.15 Normal C Scan of the retrobulbar structures. The optic nerve is represented as a central negative area.

and shape of soft tissue masses more obviously. However, B and C mode ultrasonography is an easy examination to perform, has the merit of being without radiation hazard, and may carry the second stage of diagnosis as far as computerized tomography, in that it can differentiate between an infiltrative process in the orbit and an encapsulated tumour. In practice the method is used for the demonstration of small retrobulbar tumours and especially for optic nerve lesions (Fig. 52.16).

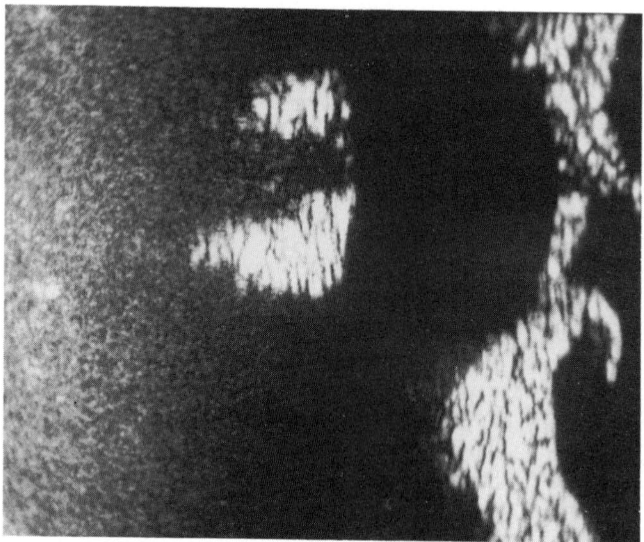

Fig. 52.16 B Scan. Enlargement of the optic nerve impression by a sheath meningioma.

Tissue recognition by A scan ultrasonography has been described by Ossoinig and Blodi (1974). These authors claim a high detection rate for their technique (98 per cent) and base the differential diagnosis of orbital mass lesions on (a) quantitative echography which differentiates orbital lesions by their capacity for reflecting ultrasound, or their reflectivity, and (b) by their topography, i.e. whether they are diffuse, poorly outlined, or well-delineated lesions. Jackson Coleman (1972) also divides mass lesions in the orbit by their ultrasonic characteristics recorded by B scan. Lesions are divided first into either rounded or irregular according to their outline. Rounded lesions showing poor ultrasonic transmission are characteristic of solid tumours such as neurofibromas and meningiomas, while those showing good transmission are usually cystic, for example a dermoid. Mass lesions exhibiting an irregular surface are again divided into those showing good ultrasonic transmission and those showing poor transmission. The former combination is characteristic of angiomatous tumours, while the latter usually denotes an infiltrative lesion such as a lymphoma, metastasis or granuloma.

CONTRAST STUDIES OF THE ORBIT

In addition to the plain X-ray examination of the orbit and the non-invasive tests described, several contrast techniques have been used in the investigation of orbital space-occupying lesions. These include carotid angiography and orbital phlebography.

Carotid arteriography

The recent introduction of non-invasive techniques such as ultrasonography and Emiscan has made carotid arteriography less necessary for the routine investigation of unilateral exophthalmos. CAT has largely taken over the role of carotid angiography in the exclusion of intracranial lesions causing proptosis; and these new methods, in combination with established techniques such as orbital venography, have made intra-orbital diagnosis far more exact preoperatively, so that in the majority of patients surgery may be safely undertaken without the risk of the morbidity which attends carotid puncture. This investigation should therefore only be carried out on selected patients, principally those with suspected vascular anomalies either in the orbit or middle fossa; for example a dural ateriovenous malformation or infraclinoid aneurysm. In the orbit it should be remembered that approximately 25 per cent of space-occupying lesions may be classified as vascular anomalies and these are by their nature best demonstrated by angiography—by venography in the case of a venous malformation and by arteriography when there is an arteriovenous shunt. Arteriography may also be needed to define the blood supply to a vascular tumour in the orbit prior to surgery.

Technique. In a patient with proptosis the essential requirement of arteriography is that it should combine an adequate study of the intracranial vessels with a detailed investigation of the orbit; and to do this some elaboration of normal technique is needed. For the injection of the contrast medium straight needle puncture is not to be recommended because of the manipulation of the head required for the modified axial projection (see below). Displacement of the needle may result with the inherent danger of an intramural injection. Some form of catheterization or cannulation is therefore needed and also should provide a means of selective injection of both the internal and external carotid arteries.

For the angiogram series three projections are used. These are all magnified geometrically using a high energy X-ray tube (0.3 mm focus or less).

1. A standard lateral arteriogram series of the skull and a series of lateral macro-angiograms coned to the orbit.
2. An antero-posterior series.
3. A modified axial view to provide a plan view of the orbital vessels (Lloyd, 1969) (Fig. 52.17).

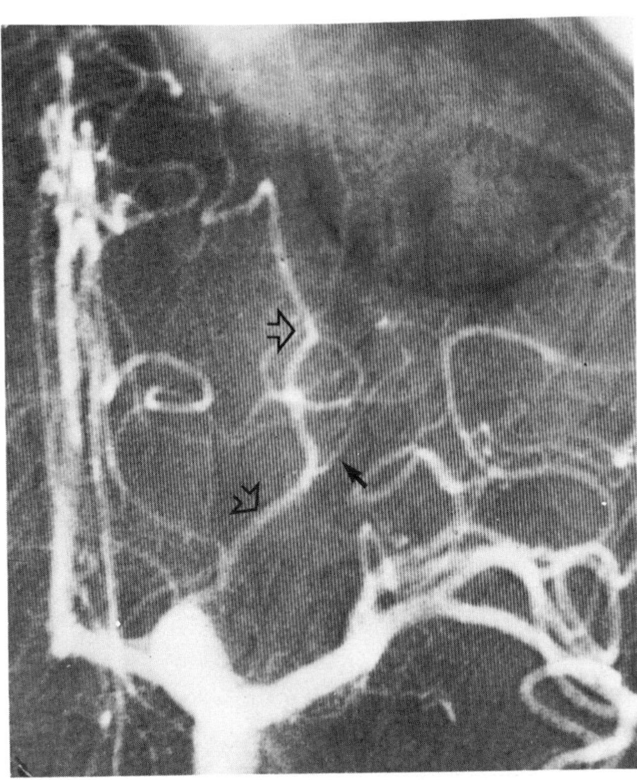

Fig. 52.17 A modified axial projection showing plan view of the orbit with ophthalmic artery (*open arrows*) and lacrimal branch (*closed arrow*). The subtraction has been made using the first and second films of the series so that the choroid is identified as a black crescent.

Diagnosis. Orbital tumours may be shown by carotid angiography in three ways: (1) by displacement of vessels; (2) by the demonstration of a pathological circulation; and (3) by deformation of the choroid crescent.

Displacement of the ophthalmic artery. To understand the displacements of the ophthalmic artery which may occur and their significance in terms of the presence and location of a space-occupying lesion in the orbit, it is necessary to bear in mind the normal course of the ophthalmic artery in relationship to other structures within the orbit. In its intra-orbital course the vessel in its first part is closely applied to the undersurface of the optic nerve and is attached to the dura covering the nerve by loose connective tissue. A similar attachment exists between the dura and the artery in the second part of the vessel as it crosses above the optic nerve. It is only in the third part of the ophthalmic artery, as it passes above the medial rectus, that the vessel is not closely related to the optic nerve; and here it is usually anchored to the medial wall of the orbit by the short stout branch of the anterior ethmoidal artery. It follows therefore that displacements of the ophthalmic artery, for the most part, simply reflect displacements of the optic nerve within the orbit; only in the more distal part of the artery does this not apply, and here the extraconal position of the artery, closely applied to the medial orbital wall, makes displacements difficult to appreciate and of little diagnostic value.

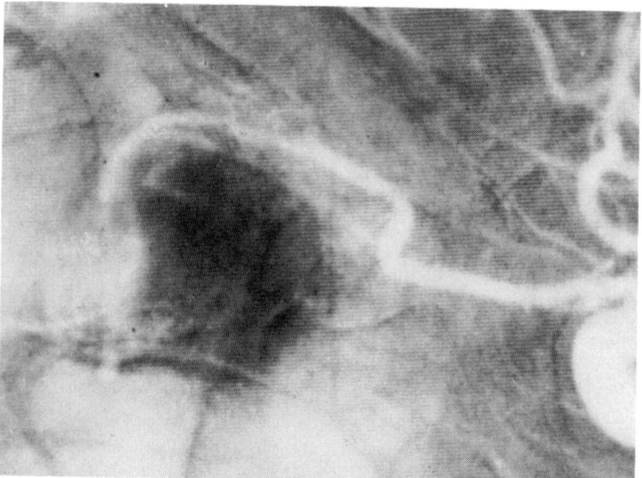

Fig. 52.18 Hemangiopericytoma. Tumour blush shown on lateral subtraction arteriogram.

In assessing displacement of the ophthalmic vessels subtraction studies in the lateral and plan views are necessary—assessments of ophthalmic artery displacements from the antero-posterior projection are difficult to appreciate. Displacements may be observed in all four directions, lateral, medial, superior and inferior, the first two being naturally best demonstrated on the plan view and the last two in the lateral projection.

One characteristic displacement may be seen in the presence of an expansion of the optic nerve from whatever cause, but most often due to a glioma or meningioma. Expansion of the dural sheath causes a stretching of the loop of the second part of the ophthalmic artery as it ascends above the optic nerve, which may be observed on the axial view. By the same expansion on the lateral view, the first part of the artery is depressed downwards with increased angulation of the junction of the first and second parts and apparent elongation of the loop.

Pathological circulation. The demonstration of a well-defined pathological circulation in the orbit is the most emphatic X-ray evidence of an orbital tumour (Fig. 52.18). The lateral view is usually the best projection to show this change, since there is no overlap of intracranial circulation as in the antero-posterior or plan view of the orbit. Subtraction studies are absolutely necessary and should be combined with macro-angiography; it has been possible to show, by magnification, pathology which was either less obvious on standard size films or not adequately demonstrated at all. Using these techniques, it should be possible to show a pathological circulation in over 30 per cent of patients with proven tumours in the orbit. One further point of technique needs mention: some tumours, notably the haemangiomas, are fed from vessels derived from the external carotid artery, usually via the maxillary or infra-orbital branches. It is therefore necessary to make sure that films are obtained with good external carotid filling either from a common carotid puncture or from a selective external carotid injection.

Choroid crescent. The position of the posterior coats of the eye may be shown at arteriography by the pooling of contrast medium in the choroid plexus. This is seen as a thin crescent of contrast in the lateral and plan views. It is rarely visible in the frontal projection but when it does show, it is seen as a circle corresponding with the outline of the globe.

The choroid crescent is visible on lateral films in all normal patients if full subtraction studies are obtained. Filling of the choroid plexus of veins begins in the late arterial phase of arteriography and persists into the early venous phase. Flattening and indentation of the crescent may be seen in the presence of an orbital space-occupying lesion.

Orbital phlebography

In the original technique the superior ophthalmic vein was filled from an injection into the angular vein either by cut down or by percutaneous puncture. This technique has now been superseded as the first approach to orbital venography by the method of frontal vein injection originally described by Vritsios (1961). In this method the injection of contrast is made into a frontal vein or main tributary. Immediately prior to injection a rubber band is placed around the forehead at the hairline (Fig. 52.19), to prevent reflux of contrast medium over the scalp, and the facial veins also need to be occluded either by a compression bandage or by finger pressure applied by the patient (Fig. 52.13). In some patients the most prominent forehead vein is the anterior temporal branch, and it can be used successfully to make the injection provided the temporal vein is occluded above the angle of the jaw by finger pressure. A 23-gauge scalp vein needle is normally used for the injection unless the veins are large enough to employ a 21-gauge needle which will allow a more rapid injection.

10 to 12 cc of 280 Conray or equivalent contrast medium are used to make the injection and films are taken after delivery of 5 cc and immediately prior to the end of the injection. A preliminary control film is also obtained for subtraction studies. Both orbital venous systems normally fill provided sufficient contrast medium is used, and this is an advantage of the frontal vein approach since minor degrees of displacement of the veins on the abnormal side may be detected by comparison with the opposite, normal side. In over 90 per cent of patients frontal venography can be performed without anaesthesia and on an out-patient basis. In children, and in adults with difficult veins, in whom venipuncture has failed initially, a general anaesthetic may be required.

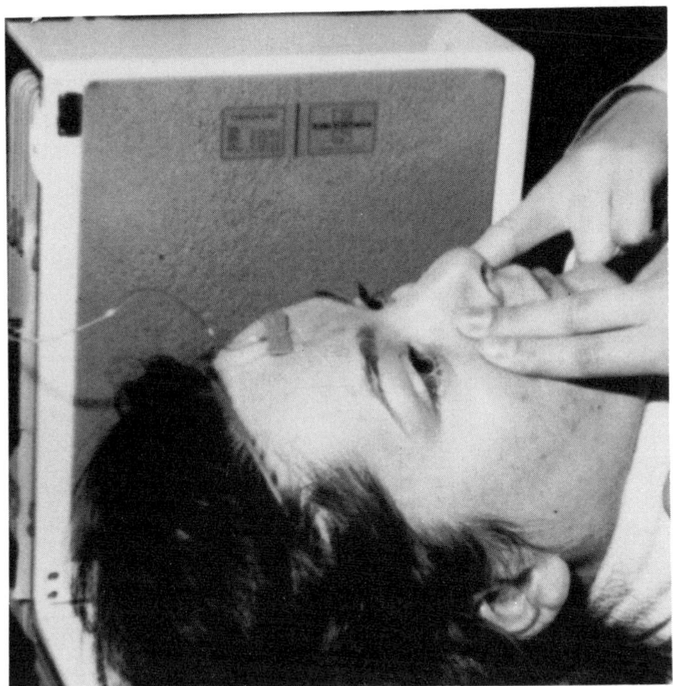

Fig. 52.19 The technique of frontal venography. A 23-guage scalp vein needle is used to make the injection, and the facial veins are compressed so that the contrast medium is forced into the orbital venous system. A rubber band is placed around the hairline to prevent loss of contrast over the scalp and to ensure that there is no superimposition of scalp veins on axial projections of the venograms.

Diagnosis. A tumour or other space-occupying lesion in the orbit may be demonstrated by venography in three ways: it may cause displacement of veins; it may obstruct the venous system in the orbit; or it may be revealed by the presence of a pathological venous circulation. These changes are often found in combination, but the type of change does indicate to a very great extent the likely pathology present; displacement is usually caused by a benign tumour, obstruction by an inflammatory or malignant process and pathological veins by a venous malformation.

Displacement of veins

The recognition of venous displacement to determine the presence of an orbital space-occupying lesion has become less necessary with the introduction of the soft tissue imaging techniques mentioned above, i.e. CT scanning and ultrasound. These are far more emphatic in their demonstration of a mass lesion, and a knowledge of the relationship of venous displacement to the location of a tumour in the orbit has largely become of academic interest only. For details of the various types of venous displacement encountered in the orbit, the reader is referred to a previous publication (Lloyd, 1975).

Obstructions of the orbital venous system

These may be divided according to the site of obstruction in relation to the rectus muscle cone and can be described as pre-conal, intra-conal or post-conal blocks. Thus the location of the obstruction may be either a total non-filling on one side, or an obstruction in the first part of the superior ophthalmic vein (pre-conal block); or obstruction in the second or third parts of the superior ophthalmic vein (intraconal block); and lastly obstruction at the superior orbital fissure or in the cavernous sinus (post-conal block).

Pre-conal obstruction. Total non-filling of the orbital veins on frontal venography may occur in any patient with unilateral exophthalmos, whatever the cause, particularly if the natural flow of the venous system is towards the non-proptosed side. Before recognizing a true obstruction, therefore, it is necessary first to occlude all collateral venous channels particularly drainage into the normal orbit and temporal veins. A history of previous orbital surgery with possible venous ligation also needs to be excluded. Unilateral total non-filling of the orbital veins is characteristically seen in patients with a carotico-cavernous fistula, and bilateral non-filling may occur if both superior ophthalmic veins are involved in the shunt.

The other major cause of pre-conal venous obstruction is dysthyroid disease, which may produce either total non-filling on the abnormal side or obstruct the first segment of the superior ophthalmic vein. Obstructions proximal to this site within the muscle cone are unusual in dysthyroid exophthalmos.

Intraconal obstruction. A high proportion of patients showing obstruction in the second and third parts of the superior ophthalmic vein as it traverses the intraconal space have an inflammatory process or granuloma in the orbit (Fig. 52.20), the obstruction either being the result of external compression or due to an associated thrombophlebitis. This change whilst being non-specific is nevertheless highly suggestive of a granuloma (pseudotumour). Of the non-inflammatory causes of venous obstruction in the intraconal space the most common is a secondary malignant tumour extending to the orbit, either from adjacent structures (carcinoma of the sinuses, sphenoid ridge meningioma) or from a distant primary site. Most of these will show obvious bone destruction or osteosclerosis on plain X-ray and may be distinguished from an inflammatory process by this means, prior to venography. It is evident therefore that venous obstruction in this part of the orbit is nearly always due to an infiltrative process, either inflammatory or neoplastic. Benign intraconal tumours (haemangioma, optic nerve meningioma, neurilemmoma) seldom cause obstruction of the veins: the veins to a large extent accommodate to the presence of a slow growing encapsulated mass and simply displace as the tumour enlarges. Venous obstruction only occurs when there is gross displacement of the superior ophthalmic vein.

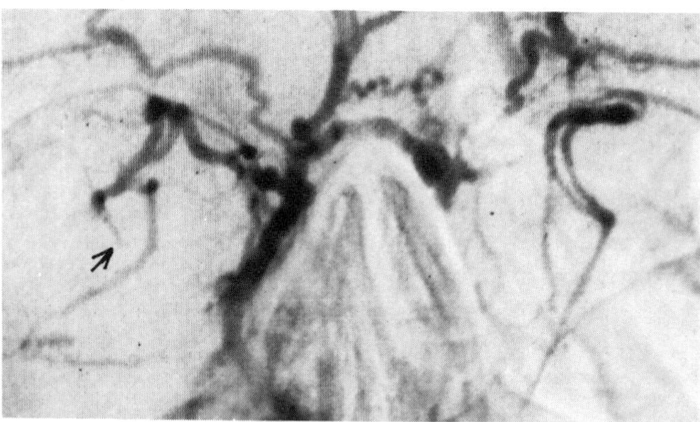

Fig. 52.20 An obstruction of the third part of the superior ophthalmic vein (*arrow*) in a pseudotumour (granuloma) of the orbit.

Post-conal obstruction. Conditions causing obstruction of veins at the superior orbital fissure or in the cavernous sinus include infraclinoid aneurysm, naso-pharyngeal tumours, pituitary tumours, parasellar meningioma and Tolosa-Hunt syndrome.

Pathological veins.
Collectively orbital varices (*vide infra*) form the major subgroup of conditions associated with abnormal veins on frontal venography, but pathological veins may be demonstrated in the orbit in association with both malignant and benign tumours. Although malignant neoplasms, particularly metastases, are more commonly associated with abnormal veins, some benign tumours, for example a cavernous haemangioma, may also show this change. An abnormal venous circulation has also been seen in one patient with an intraconal neurofibroma, and in a granuloma or pseudotumour of the lacrimal gland. A hypervascular collateral circulation in the orbit may also follow surgical ligation of the superior ophthalmic vein or result from a venous thrombosis, and examples of thrombi demonstrated as filling defects may sometimes be shown by venography.

UNILATERAL EXOPHTHALMOS

The causes of this condition can be divided for convenience of diagnosis into four main categories:

1. Dysthyroid disease.
2. Intracranial lesions giving rise to unilateral proptosis.
3. Causes arising in the paranasal sinuses and nasopharynx.
4. Intraorbital space-occupying lesions.

Dysthyroid exophthalmos does not show any plain X-ray abnormality apart from that caused by an increase in the orbital soft tissues which will produce increased radiographic density on the affected side, but distinctive changes may be shown on axial tomography, frontal venography, ultrasonography and CT scan. The changes depend upon the general enlargement of the orbital muscles which occurs in this condition. On axial tomography it may sometimes be possible to identify thickening of the lateral rectus muscle. As a rule because of the more contrasty soft tissue definition, the CT scan will show this change more emphatically and will demonstrate thickening of all rectus muscles. Phlebography gives a characteristic appearance: the second part of the ophthalmic vein may be displaced downwards with an exaggerated upward concavity. This selective displacement of one part of the venous system is caused by the combined increased bulk of the levator palpebrae and superior rectus muscles lying immediately above this part of the superior ophthalmic vein.

In a small proportion of patients proptosis may be due to an *intracranial lesion.* A *sphenoid ridge meningioma* is the commonest intracranial lesion to cause unilateral exophthalmos. More frequently the cause of the proptosis is to be found in the paranasal *sinuses* or *nasopharynx,* usually the result of a *tumour, infection* or *mucocoele.* The final group of patients are those in which the cause of the proptosis arises primarily within the orbit. These may be sub-divided into (a) vascular anomalies, (b) tumours and (c) inflammatory processes.

Vascular anomalies

Vascular anomalies in the orbit may be classified into (1) ophthalmic artery aneurysms, (2) arteriovenous malformations, (3) haemangiomas and (4) orbital varices.

Ophthalmic artery aneurysm. Saccular aneurysms arising from the intra-orbital course of the ophthalmic artery are extremely rare and there are less than six authentic cases in the literature (Henderson, 1973). The majority of ophthalmic artery aneurysms arise from the junction of the internal carotid and ophthalmic arteries and are designated carotid ophthalmic aneurysms.

Arteriovenous malformation. The orbit is a relatively uncommon site for an arteriovenous malformation but because of the use of angiographic techniques the condition is being increasingly reported in the literature. The lesion may occur as a congenital anomaly or follow trauma to the anterior orbit (Dilenge, 1974). Clinically the anomaly may present either as a pulsating exophthalmos, sometimes associated with an audible bruit, or as a simple proptosis. Carotid angiography is the essential investigation, both to show the nature of the lesion and its blood supply. Studies of the internal and external carotid vessels may be needed, since some of these malformations are fed in part from the external carotid artery.

Haemangioma. The orbital haemangiomas are divided into capillary and cavernous types. Capillary haemangioma is a lesion which occurs in infants and may give rise to unilateral proptosis. It is often associated with a superficial capillary naevus and may be demonstrated as a fine vascular network on carotid angiography or sometimes as a diffuse and extensive pathological circulation in some patients fed from the external carotid (Dilenge, 1974). Cavernous haemangioma, on the other hand, is a disease of adult patients, and some authors regard the condition as a more developed form of infantile capillary haemangioma. Orbital cavernous haemangioma is a benign encapsulated neoplasm or hamartoma which is typically found within the muscle cone and gives rise to an axial proptosis. The incidence of cavernous haemangioma is undoubtedly less than that normally reported. This is mostly because of the confusion in the literature between the cavernous haemangioma on the one hand and a venous malformation on the other. The latter condition is about twice as common as cavernous haemangioma and there is little doubt that many of the reported examples of cavernous haemangioma are in fact entirely venous and therefore should be classified with the venous malformations.

The commonest change on plain X-ray is enlargement of the affected orbit. The cavernous haemangioma being a slow growing tumour produces moderate degrees of orbital enlargement which can be demonstrated both by plain X-ray and by tomography. These tumours are well demonstrated prior to orbitotomy by CT scan, the lesion showing as a well demarcated tumour mass with even density values and a rounded margin. This investigation has made arteriographic studies unnecessary in most patients with this condition. Nevertheless the most positive evidence of a cavernous haemangioma is often provided by angiography. On phlebography an associated venous malformation is sometimes demonstrable (*vide infra*) and on arteriography it may be possible to demonstrate 'venous pools' within the muscle cone in the capillary and venous phase of the examination, and these may be fed by contrast medium from the external carotid circulation (Lloyd, 1975).

Orbital varices

These may be primary or secondary and a classification based on this division is given in Table 52.1.

Table 52.1 Classification of orbital varices

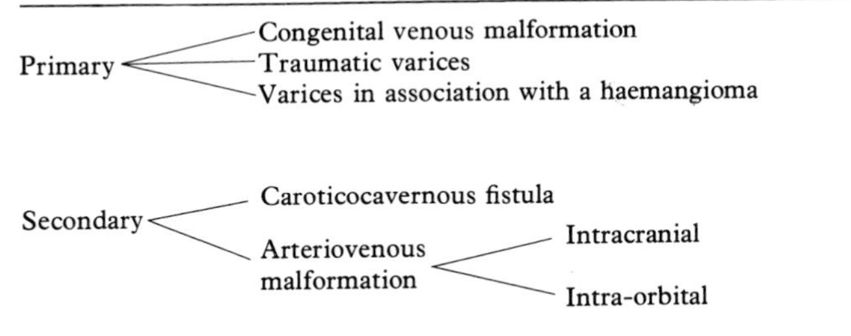

Primary	Congenital venous malformation	
	Traumatic varices	
	Varices in association with a haemangioma	
Secondary	Caroticocavernous fistula	
	Arteriovenous malformation	Intracranial
		Intra-orbital

Congenital venous malformation. A detailed description of this anomaly has been given by Lloyd *et al.* (1971) and by Wright (1974). These patients usually give a history of proptosis dating from birth or early childhood and characteristically the proptosis is provoked or made worse by an increase of venous pressure in the head. Orbital varices may be accompanied by venous abnormalities elsewhere in the head and neck, particularly on the scalp of the affected side. Cases have also been recorded of associated venous malformations in other parts of the body and the condition may also be associated with the Klippel-Trelauney syndrome.

The characteristic plain X-ray features which may be present in these patients are (a) enlargement of the orbit: this is often a gross enlargement since the venous anomaly is present from birth; (b) the presence of phleboliths in the orbit or in adjacent structures (Fig. 52.2); (c) prominent vascular markings and venous 'lakes' in the frontal bone of the same side corresponding to the venous dilatations in the scalp.

By venography it is usually possible to identify two types of venous abnormality; either a local saccular dilatation of the veins in the orbit resembling a venous aneurysm, or a whole system of abnormal venous channels throughout the orbit (Fig. 52.21). Ultrasonography is a good ancilliary means of identifying orbital varices and by jugular compression it is possible to show enlargement of the filling defects caused by the varices in the retrobulbar fat pattern (Lloyd, 1975).

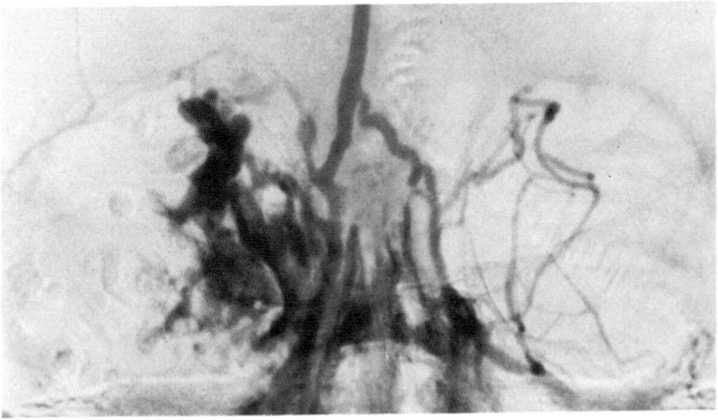

Fig. 52.21 Antero-posterior venogram showing an extensive system of abnormal venous channels in the right orbit of a 14-year-old male patient.

Traumatic varices. Hanafee (1972) has described venous lakes occurring in the orbit after trauma originating from a tear of the superior ophthalmic vein at the superior orbital fissure and demonstrated by venography. In the author's experience it would seem likely that the most probable cause for so-called traumatic varices is the rupture of a pre-existing varix with extravasation into the muscle cone. This may occur spontaneously without trauma.

Varices in association with a haemangioma. Lloyd (1974) has described three patients in whom it was possible to show an abnormal venous circulation by frontal venography in patients with an intraconal cavernous haemangioma. In one patient small local draining vessels from the site of the tumour were demonstrated but in two other patients an abnormal collection of venous channels was outlined remote from the site of the haemangioma, the varices principally affecting the deep temporal venous system.

Secondary varices. The venous system in the orbit may dilate secondarily as a result of a carotico-cavernous fistula or dural arteriovenous shunt in the middle fossa. Secondary dilatation of the ophthalmic veins may also be caused by an arteriovenous malformation, either in the middle or anterior fossa of the skull or to an intraorbital arterio-venous malformation. These lesions are best demonstrated by carotid arteriography.

visual impairment and may show the following features on plain X-ray:

1. Enlargement of the optic foramen. This may be a slightly irregular enlargement.
2. Hyperostosis affecting the apex of the orbit and anterior clinoid process.
3. Calcification. This is either a granular or cloudy area of calcification in the apex of the orbit, or in some instances it may take the form of a diffuse calcification in the optic nerve sheath causing parallel lines of calcification on the radiographs. On optic canal projections this is seen as a circular opacity within the outline of the optic foramen (Lloyd, 1971).

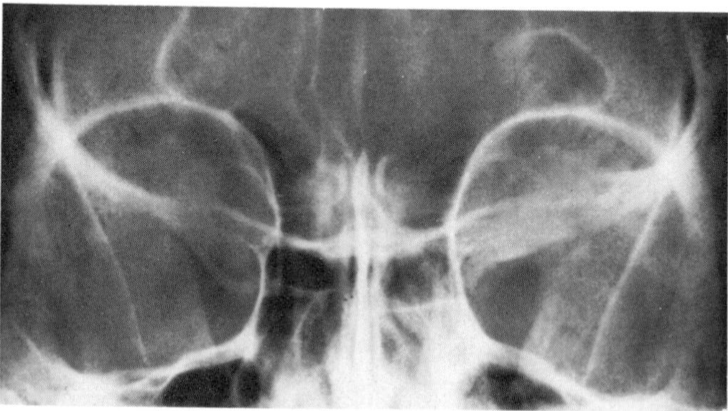

Fig. 52.22 Hyperostosis of the greater and lesser wings of the sphenoid with enlargement of the superior orbital fissure (left) due to a meningioma.

TUMOURS OF THE ORBIT

Orbital meningioma. Meningioma in the orbit may occur as a primary tumour or it may be present as the secondary extension of a growth originating in the anterior or middle fossa of the skull. Primary intra-orbital meningiomata may be classified as:

1. Extradural: arising within the orbit remote from the optic nerve.
2. Sheath meningioma: arising from clusters of arachnoid cap cells found in the meningeal sheath covering the optic nerve.

The sheath meningioma may be further subdivided into foraminal tumours, and tumours arising from the retro-bulbar part of the optic nerve. These distinctions are important since the clinical and radiological presentation depends to a large extent upon the site of the tumour. The extradural meningioma usually presents as an intraorbital space-occupying lesion causing proptosis and sometimes giving positive plain X-ray changes, of which hyperostosis affecting the walls of the orbit is the most characteristic sign when present. On angiography displacement of the ophthalmic vessels is usually the only evidence of a tumour but a minority may show a pathological circulation on carotid angiography.

The foraminal meningiomata normally present with

The meningioma arising from the retro-bulbar part of the optic nerve sheath may give no evidence of their presence either on plain X-ray or on angiography, but optic nerve enlargement can be demonstrated by the non-invasive techniques of computerized tomography and ultrasonography (see above).

Secondary meningioma. These occur as an extension of a meningioma arising in the middle fossa of the skull or less commonly in the anterior fossa. Meningioma en plaque, affecting the greater and lesser wings of the sphenoid and taking origin in the region of the pterion, is the most common variety to affect the orbit secondarily (Fig. 52.22). In these patients the cause of the proptosis is the result of a hyperostosis on the lateral wall and roof of the orbit, provoked by the meningioma affecting the inner surface of the greater wing of the sphenoid. The degree of hyperostosis and its extent is best assessed by tomography, particularly in the axial plane, and is often much more extensive than suspected on plain X-ray.

Dermoids and epidermoids. These tumours result from sequestration of the primitive ectoderm in the region of the orbit. Epidermoids occur when epidermal elements are solely concerned, and a dermoid when the deeper dermal layer is also involved (Pfeiffer and Nicholl, 1948). Strict differentiation of the two types of tumour is to a large extent academic and many are of transitional type, but the dermoids are cystic and may contain oil, sebum, cholesterol and hair whilst the epidermoids are solid tumours consisting of a mass of desquamated cells containing keratohyaline, encased in a capsule of well-differentiated stratified squamous epithelium. Both may arise in the diploe of the skull and bones of the orbit and in their growth expand both inner and outer tables, thus producing sharply demarcated bone defects on the radiographs, with well-defined and in some cases slightly sclerotic margins. They occur in characteristic locations in the orbit, more commonly in the superolateral quadrant, but they frequently occur in the medial part of the orbital roof, and sometimes in the greater wing of the sphenoid or lateral wall of the orbit, where they produce a very characteristic cyst-like appearance in the bone (Fig. 52.23). Rarely, they may occur in the inferior part of the orbit.

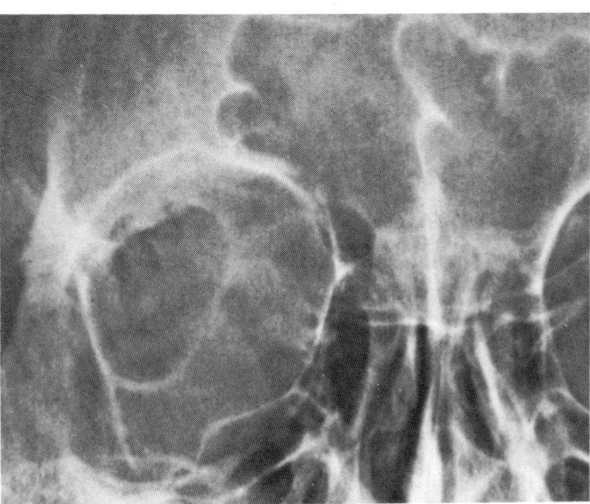

Fig. 52.23

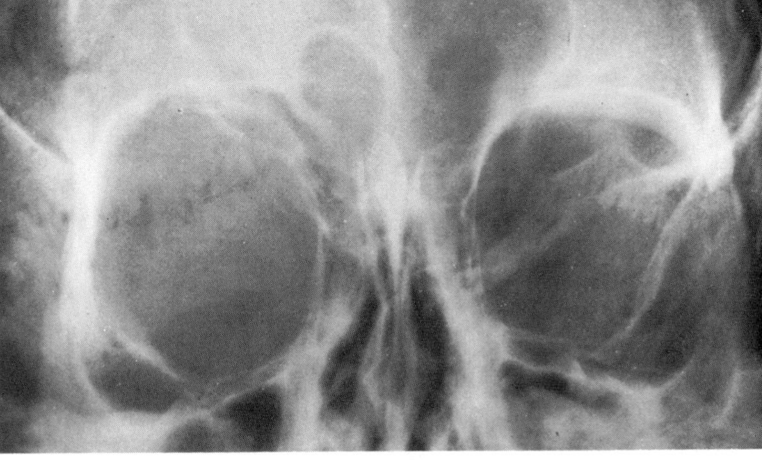

Fig. 52.24

Fig. 52.23 Clear-cut cystlike area in the greater wing of the sphenoid due to a dermoid.

Fig. 52.24 A postero-anterior view showing 'bare' orbit of neurofibromatosis (right).

The superficially placed peri-orbital dermoids may also show minor X-ray changes. The most common locality for these tumours is the outer part of the upper eyelid and they may cause a shallow localized indentation on the orbital rim at its superolateral angle.

Neurofibromatosis. The changes in the orbit and adjacent parts of the skull which can occur in this condition are striking and characteristic. Typically, the orbit is enlarged, the sphenoid ridge elevated to the level of the orbital roof and there may be a large defect in the greater wing of the sphenoid forming the posterior boundary of the orbit. This allows the cranial pulsation to be transmitted directly to the eye and orbital contents, thus producing a pulsating exophthalmos. The result of these changes is the so-called 'bare' orbit of neurofibromatosis seen on the P.A. radiograph (Fig. 52.24).

Associated changes which may be present in the skull are (a) enlargement of the middle fossa, (b) enlargement of the optic canal due to the presence of an optic nerve glioma and (c) enlargement of the pituitary fossa.

Rhabdomyosarcoma. Rhabdomyosarcoma of the orbit, although a rare tumour in absolute terms, is nevertheless the most common cause of malignancy in the orbit of children, and the majority of these tumours occur in the first decade of life. Three histological types are recognized: (1) embryonal rhabdomyosarcoma; (2) differentiated rhabdomyosarcoma; and (3) alveolar rhabdomyosarcoma, which is the most malignant variety with an invariably poor prognosis. Clinically the condition presents with exophthalmos with rapid and even alarming progression (Jones, Reese and Kraut, 1966) and this is often accompanied by a superficial swelling in the eyelids, canthi or fornices.

Radiologically these tumours produce progressive enlargement of the orbit and later they may cause bone destruction with extension to extra-orbital structures including the temporal fossa and cranial cavity. Enlargement of the orbit may be appreciated on plain X-ray but is shown at an earlier stage by axial tomography; the first evidence of enlargement is usually a positive 'medial wall' sign—an incurvation of the medial wall (Lloyd, 1975). Elaborate techniques of orbital investigation are seldom necessary in the management of these patients; straight skull films, hypocycloidal tomography to show bone involvement, and a chest radiograph to exclude metastases are generally all that is required, prior to orbit exenteration.

Glioma of the optic nerve. (See Ch. 58).

Lacrimal gland tumours. Epithelial tumours of the lacrimal gland are similar to those found in the salivary glands and are classified by Reese (1956) into: (1) *mixed* *types*; (2) *carcinomas*, which may be adenocystic or miscellaneous types. In addition *lymphomas* may occur as a primary tumour in the lacrimal gland. The prognosis of lacrimal gland tumours depends upon the histology and whether there is extension of the tumour outside the capsule. Benign mixed tumours, if completely removed with capsule intact, have a favourable prognosis but in contrast the carcinomas, even after total exenteration of the orbit, result in a fatal outcome in almost all cases.

Radiological features. Plain X-ray features depend upon the histological type of tumour to some extent and in general the mixed cell type of tumour, of relatively slow growth and long duration, produces more obvious changes in the underlying lacrimal fossa. The most common change is a local enlargement of the lacrimal fossa without invasion of bone. However, many malignant tumours also show this change and there are no absolute X-ray criteria which will identify the type of histology present.

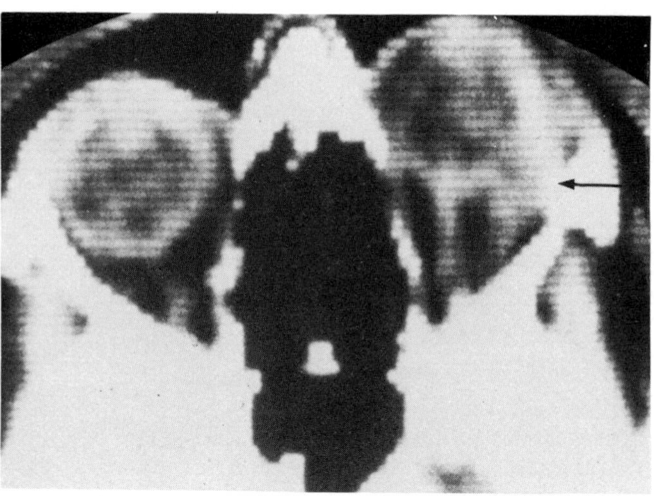

Fig. 52.25 A lacrimal gland tumour (left) (*arrow*) shown by CT.

In *carcinoma* bone invasion is shown by irregular osteolysis in the adjacent frontal bone or in some instances a local reactive change may occur producing osteosclerosis and increased bone density on the radiograph. Tomography can be very helpful in doubtful cases and may show a more obvious bone erosion than plain X-ray studies. Coronal tomograms are usually most informative but it is possible sometimes to show a soft tissue mass, i.e. the tumour on axial tomography. Of the new techniques for soft tissue demonstration ultrasonography has not been found to be of any great value in delineating these tumours, because of their extraconal location; but computerized tomography clearly demonstrates the soft tissue mass in the axial plane (Fig. 52.25) and is a complementary procedure to hypocycloidal tomography in showing the tumour extension in the orbit preoperatively.

Lymphoma of the lacrimal gland characteristically cause little change in the underlying bone, but it may sometimes be possible to show minimal enlargement of the lacrimal fossa either on plain X-ray or more often by tomography.

INFLAMMATORY DISEASES IN THE ORBIT

Orbital and retro-orbital pseudotumours (granulomas).

The name of pseudotumour has been given to a group of cases which are difficult to differentiate clinically from an orbital tumour but which on pathological investigation have proved to be granulomas of chronic inflammatory origin. Pseudotumours of the orbit present a difficult nosological problem as they are a spectrum of different conditions rather than a single entity (Garner, 1973). They occur throughout the orbit from the region of the lacrimal gland to the orbital apex and present very different signs and symptoms according to their position (Levy, Wright and Lloyd, 1973). Plain X-ray examination seldom shows any significant abnormality in the affected orbit but enlargement may be demonstrable on axial tomography. Significant enlargement was shown by this technique in 60 per cent of patients in a series reviewed by Lloyd (1973). One other feature that may occur in the more posteriorly placed granulomas is an enlargement of the sphenoidal fissure. This has been observed in three patients and has been recorded by other authors (Lombardi, 1967). In one instance it was associated with slight enlargement of the optic canal. Some patients with pseudotumours show an associated clouding of the nasal sinuses due to infection or nasal polyposis.

On orbital venography, pseudotumours may produce a displacement of the venous system in the orbit, but the most characteristic venographic feature is a venous block usually in the second or third part of the superior ophthalmic vein. Positive evidence of the presence of a pseudotumour may be demonstrated on B-scan ultrasonography. Coleman (1972) has described a characteristic appearance in which the pseudotumour presents an irregular edge in the retrobulbar echo pattern. Positive evidence of an increased soft tissue density within the orbit may also be obtained by CT scan. Characteristically the changes are those of an infiltrative lesion, with an irregular ill-defined edge and variable density values, but occasionally a pseudotumour may present features closely resembling an encapsulated tumour with a well defined border and even density.

The Tolosa-Hunt syndrome

This syndrome is characterised by an ophthalmoplegia, usually of rapid onset and preceded by pain in the back of the orbit and in the distribution of the first division of the trigeminal nerve. In the full condition there is a complete superior orbital fissure syndrome, with involvement of the III, IV, V and VI cranial nerves. In some of the patients described by Hunt *et al.* (1961) there was also optic nerve involvement although this would imply that the cause in these patients was in the orbital apex rather than the superior orbital fissure. As in the case of pseudotumours in the orbit, the condition usually responds dramatically to steroid therapy and the aetiology is generally considered to be due to a non-specific inflammatory process with the presence of granulation

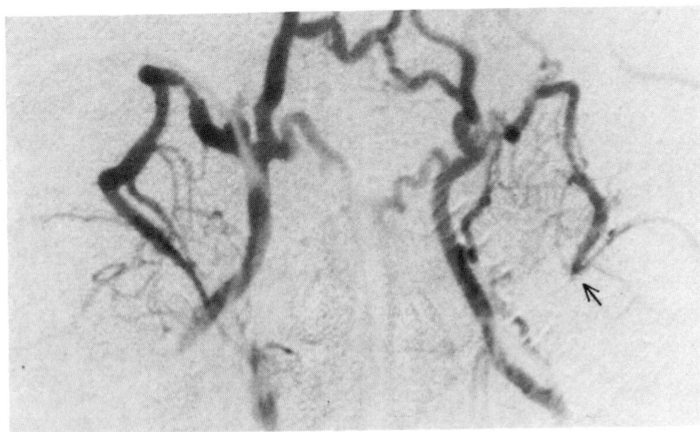

Fig. 52.26 Tolosa-Hunt syndrome. Obstruction of the superior ophthalmic vein (*arrow*) immediately anterior to the superior orbital fissure.

tissue in the superior orbital fissure (Laake, 1962) or in the cavernous sinus. In Tolosa's (1954) case, which came to autopsy, granulation tissue was found within the cavernous sinus surrounding the internal carotid artery and causing narrowing of the vessel by extrinsic pressure; adjacent nerve trunks were found to be included in the inflammatory mass. A similar autopsy report has also been described by Levy, Wright and Lloyd (1973). The X-ray changes which accompany the syndrome may be characteristic, and consist of:

1. Venous obstruction at the superior orbital fissure (Fig. 52.26) or in the cavernous sinus on orbital venography. This is usually not accompanied by any significant displacement of the vein, and it may be possible to demonstrate re-canalization of the superior ophthalmic vein following successful steroid therapy (Lloyd, 1972).

2. On carotid angiography a smooth narrowing of the intracavernous segment of the internal carotid artery may be demonstrable. This corresponds to the narrowing, which has been shown at autopsy (see above) to be caused by the extrinsic pressure of granulation tissue in the cavernous sinus.

DACROCYSTOGRAPHY

Dacrocystography was first described by Ewing (1909) using bismuth subnitrate as contrast medium to outline a lacrimal sac abscess cavity. The conventional method derived from Ewing's original technique consists of cannulation of the inferior or superior canaliculus, injection of contrast medium into the duct system, followed by postero-anterior and lateral films taken after withdrawal of the metal cannula. Campbell (1964), using this method of injection, introduced a radiographic enlargement technique and showed the advantages of the improved detail on the radiographs by macro-dacrocystography. Iba and Hanafee (1968) reported a method of distension dacrocystography, drawing attention to the advantages of making the X-ray exposure while the contrast medium was being injected. The technique advocated is a combination of these two methods, and when combined with subtraction studies is the optimum way of demonstrating the lacrimal duct system radiographically. The greater detail of the canalicular system provided by this technique is especially important in deciding the surgical approach to abnormalities of the common canaliculus. Geometrical enlargement of the radiographic image is obtained by placing the X-ray film some distance from the patient's head, and by using an X-ray tube fitted with a 0.3 mm focal spot, linear magnification of 1.6 x to 1.9 of the image can be achieved. The exposure of the films is made during the actual injection of contrast medium through the catheter. This is important if optimal filling of the duct system is to be obtained and in most instances will produce an image of the contrast medium which is continuous throughout the duct system. Before catheterization of the inferior canaliculus, a drop of local anaesthetic (Amethocaine) is instilled into the conjunctival sac and any mucus in the duct system is expressed by pressure over the inner canthus. A non-viscous contrast medium is preferred, since the bore of the catheter is too small to allow a brisk injection of the more viscous variety of Lipiodol generally used in dacryocystography. Two ml Lipiodol ultrafluid are drawn up into a syringe which is then connected to a 12-inch intravenous catheter (outside diameter 0.63 mm) and any air bubbles are expressed. The punctum is first dilated with a Nettleship dilator and the tip of the catheter is introduced into the canaliculus. The catheter is held in place by sticking plaster applied to the cheek. The lower canaliculus is usually catheterized as this is more convenient and functionally more important. It is usual practice to carry out bilateral intubation macrodacryocystograms simultaneously, because of the high incidence of bilateral abnormalities, and the useful information that can be obtained by comparison with the normal macrogram. It is wise to take an upright lateral film subsequently to make sure that the contrast medium

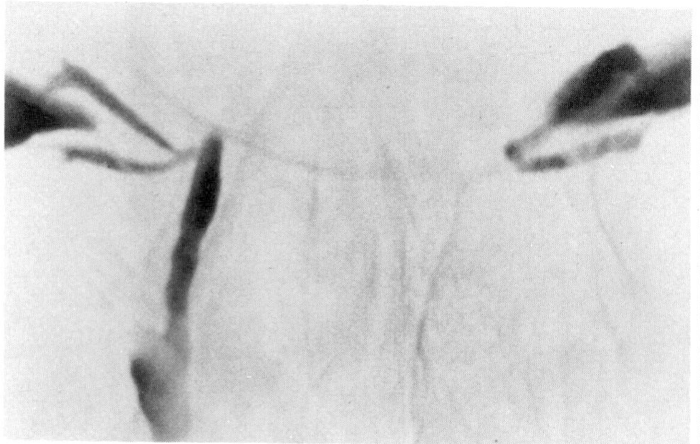

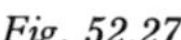

Fig. 52.27

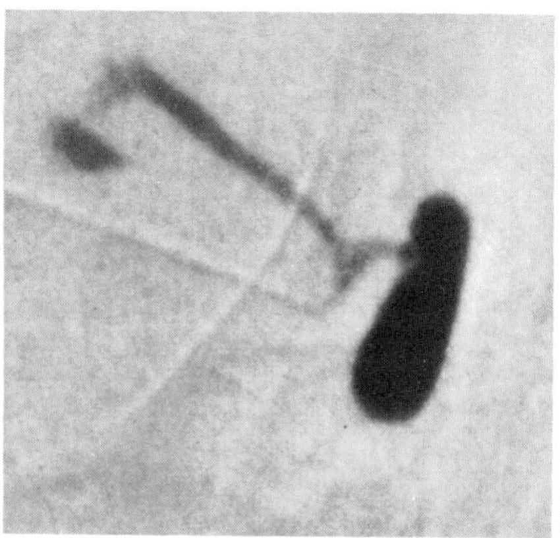

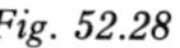

Fig. 52.28

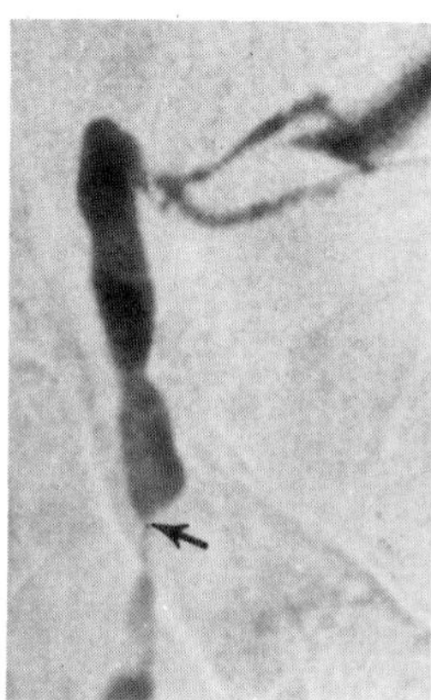

Fig. 52.29

Fig. 52.27 Left common canaliculus block (proximal end). Normal right side for comparison.

Fig. 52.28 Subtraction macrodacryocystogram showing a lacrimal sac mucocoele.

Fig. 52.29 General dilatation of the lacrimal sac and duct due to an incomplete obstruction at the lower ostium (*arrow*).

has had an opportunity to gravitate to the nasopharynx and so confirm the patency of the system. If bilateral macrodacryocystograms have been carried out, the same information can be obtained from an oblique film.

Demonstration of the site of stenosis. Blocks in the upper and lower canaliculi are indicated, when contrast regurgitates through the punctum injected and on the radiographs the injected canaliculus is outlined as far as the stenosis, no contrast entering the common canaliculus. Common canaliculus blocks are characterized by regurgitation of contrast through the upper punctum and outlining of both upper and lower canaliculi on the radiographs, without filling of the lacrimal sac if the obstruction is complete or with partial filling of the sac if the obstruction is incomplete. Subtraction studies are particularly useful for demonstrating the common canaliculus. Partial filling of the common canaliculus usually denotes an obstruction at its medial end at the level of the lacrimal sac mucosa. Non-filling of the lumen of the common canaliculus suggests a block involving its whole length (Fig. 52.27) or, in a partial occlusion, narrowing may be demonstrated either throughout the whole length of the canaliculus, or for part of its course. The most frequent site of obstruction in the lacrimal passages is at the neck of the sac and this may result in a mucocoele (Fig. 52.28). The sac is seen to be dilated and no contrast has entered the lacrimal duct below. Blocks in the nasolacrimal duct itself are commonly found at the entrance of the bony canal or at the lower ostium (Fig. 52.29). They are characterized by dilatation of the duct proximal to the obstruction and failure of the contrast to enter the nasal cavity.

LOCALIZATION OF FOREIGN BODIES IN THE EYE

Since the discovery of X-rays many methods have been described for the radiological localization of foreign bodies in the eye, and more than 60 special techniques have been described in the literature (Erkonen and Dolan, 1972). In the author's opinion the limbal ring method is the most foolproof of these and is recommended to the inexperienced radiologist who is only called upon to make the occasional localization. This, however, does involve the co-operation of an ophthalmologist and is an extra minor surgical procedure for the patient.

The use of contact lenses, some of which involve the application of a negative pressure to the anterior surface of the cornea, is unnecessary for accurate foreign body localization and cannot be entirely devoid of clinical hazard in patients who have received a perforating injury to the globe. The Bromley localizer (1943) uses a method in which a metal pointer is placed 1 cm in front of the cornea and the foreign body related to it in three planes. In practice the placement of the pointer and its accurate location along the central axis of the eye cannot be relied upon. The method also requires two exposures with an intervening tube shift, during which time the patient must maintain the injured eye in a fixed position. Only with first class patient co-operation, therefore, can accurate results be expected. The same drawback is also inherent in the Sweet method of intraocular foreign body localization.

The account which follows is based on the procedure normally carried out by the author, when the case of suspected foreign body is referred to the X-ray department. As will be evident complete reliance is not placed upon a single localization technique nor is the method stereotyped but is modified according to the particular problem at hand and the proposed route of extraction of the foreign body. In this respect close co-operation between the radiologist and the ophthalmic surgeon is important so that the clinical and radiological findings can be evaluated together. This will not only lead to more accurate results but frequently may spare the patient unnecessary X-ray procedures. It should be remembered that when visible to the ophthalmoscope an intra-ocular foreign body can be localized accurately by this means alone and in these circumstances there is often no need for full X-ray localization.

The localization procedure may be considered under the following headings:

1. Preliminary radiographs to determine if an intra-ocular foreign body is present, and localization of the foreign body from these films.
2. The use of a special procedure to confirm the localization.
   (*a*) Multisection tomography.
   (*b*) Limbal ring method.
3. Localization by radio-opaque marker.
4. Bone free technique.
5. Ultrasonic technique.

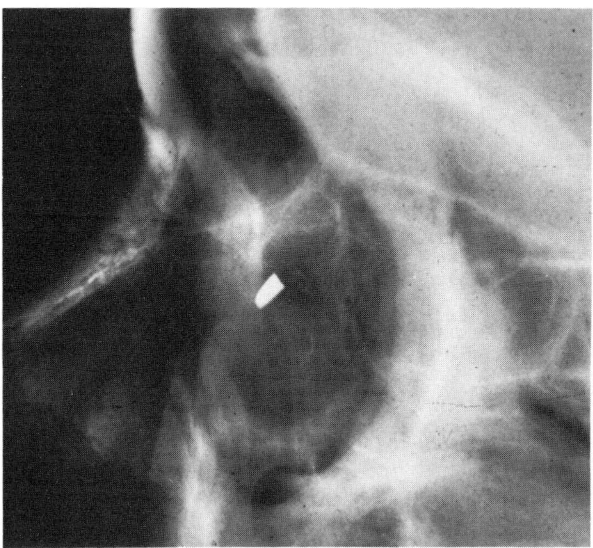

Fig. 52.30

Fig. 52.30 Standard lateral view used to establish the presence of a foreign body and its approximate position in relation to the anterior surface of the cornea.

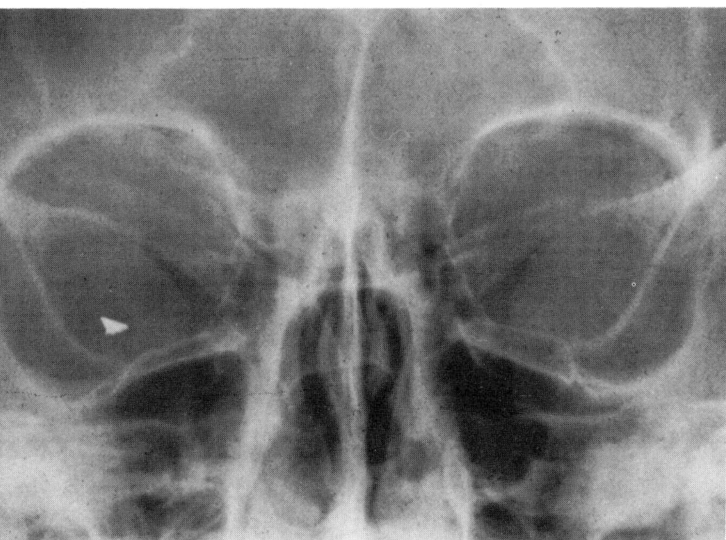

Fig. 52.31

Fig. 52.31 Postero-anterior (nose-chin) view showing position of the foreign body. If the intra-ocular location of the foreign body has been confirmed by an eye-moving film, it is apparent that the foreign body lies in the 6 o'clock meridian.

Preliminary films and localization

The first step in localization is to establish that there is a radio-opaque foreign body present in the region of the globe. To do this a straight lateral film is taken using non-screen film. This is centred to the outer canthus of the eye with the affected side close to the film and the eyes fixed on a spot at eye level immediately in front of the patient (Fig. 52.30). If this film gives positive evidence of a foreign body in the orbit, two further views are then taken to show whether the foreign body is intra- or extra-ocular. These are (1) a postero-anterior projection, taken in the nose/chin position (orbito-meatal line tilted cranially 35 degrees) (Fig. 52.31), and (2) an eye moving lateral view using two exposures, the eye first looking upward and then downward while the head remains still. From these views it will be possible to establish that there is a definite intra-ocular foreign body present, if in the postero-anterior view there is an opacity within the outline of the orbit, and if the foreign body shows on the eye moving view the typical displacement of an intra-ocular foreign body: namely a movement of the foreign body in the arc of a circle around the central axis of rotation of the globe. Having determined that there is an intra-ocular foreign body present by examination of these films it is often possible to make an accurate localization without further procedure. The postero-anterior view is first examined to check that the positioning is correct: firstly there should be no rotation of the head on the radiograph, and secondly the degree of tilt of the head should be such as to project the upper border of the petrous ridge through the upper half of the maxillary antrum. Once these positioning criteria have been satisfied, it is possible to place the foreign body accurately into its correct meridian with respect to the eyeball by simply looking at the film and relating the foreign body to the outer rim of the orbit as a simulated clock face. This provides half the essential information required by the ophthalmologist for the recovery of the foreign body. The remainder may be obtained from examination of the lateral film. Provided this is accurately centred it is possible in most patients (using non-screen film) to visualize the anterior surface of the cornea. The distance back from the anterior surface of the cornea to the foreign body can then be measured directly, allowance being made for radiographic magnification. This completes the data required for localization. Figure 52.32 shows a plan view of the eye in which the various meridia may be plotted as seen from above. It is apparent that the position of the foreign body will be placed at the point where the plot, representing the known meridian in which the foreign body lies, intersects the line representing the distance back from the anterior surface of the cornea as measured on the lateral film. This method of localization assumes that the foreign body lies within or attached to the coats of the globe, and while this is true for the vast majority of foreign bodies in the eye there is a small minority in which this is not so. The location of these is for the most part easily diagnosible, however, from the standard films (Lloyd, 1975). The data obtained from the preliminary films thus allows an accurate plot to be made on a localization chart of the position of the foreign body and the limbus to foreign body measurement can then be obtained (see below, Charting the Foreign Body).

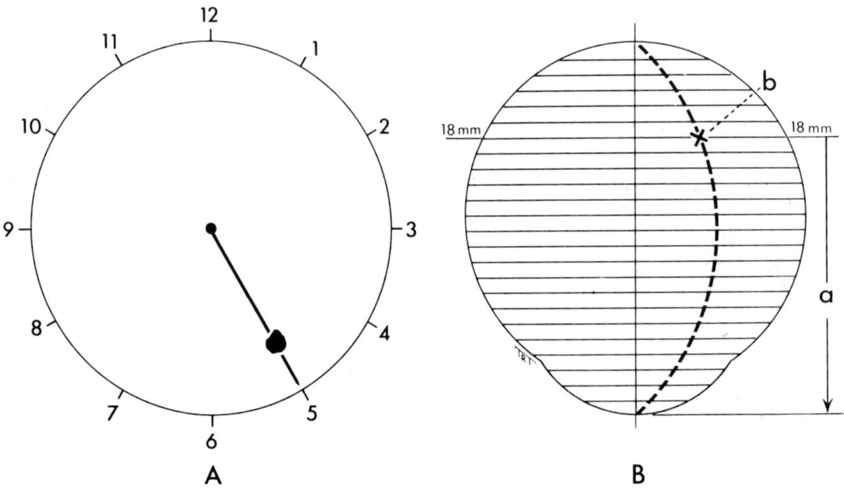

Fig. 52.32 Method of foreign body localization from plain radiographs. The foreign body is placed in its correct meridian by examination of the postero-anterior film (A) (in this case 5 o'clock). The line of the 5 o'clock meridian is then plotted on the plan view of the eye (B). The distance (a), i.e., anterior surface of the cornea to the foreign body, is measured from the lateral film. The foreign body must then lie at the position where the 18 mm line intersects the line of the 5 o'clock meridian (b).

Multisection tomography. This technique does not involve instrumental contact with the eye or depend upon the accurate placement of a pointer in relation to the anterior surface of the cornea. The patient co-operation required is minimal and the method does not need any additional apparatus other than a simple linear tomograph and a Perspex set square arranged on a leaded base, which serves as a step wedge or calibrater for the tomograph. (For a full description of the apparatus and technique see Lloyd, 1973.) Since in this method measurements are made directly from the anterior surface of the cornea shown as a soft tissue structure on the tomograms, the measurements in the long axis of the eye and in the vertical plane are extremely accurate. The measurement to the nasal or temporal side of the vertical corneal axis is less accurate (within 1–2 mm) but will produce good localizations, if used in conjunction with properly taken plain X-rays as described above.

In addition to its use as an ancillary means of localizing solitary foreign bodies in the eye, multisection tomography is indispensible when making localizations in the presence of multiple foreign bodies such as those found in injuries caused by explosions and shotgun wounds; and the technique was originally devised for this purpose. In the presence of multiple metallic fragments, the image of a foreign body in one plane cannot be accurately related to another image in a plane at right angles to it on plain X-rays. since there are multiple opacities present; for the same reason an eye moving lateral film is equally difficult to interpret. Tomography overcomes this difficulty by blurring out the image of the metallic fragments in the opposite orbit or in the same orbit but outside the globe, thus allowing an accurate assessment of the exact number and site of the intraocular foreign bodies.

Limbal ring localization

This is a very simple and foolproof method of localization and is to be recommended to the radiologist who is not routinely called upon to localize many foreign bodies. Rings of 12 mm diameter are used and fixed to the limbus by three or four conjunctival sutures. The rings should be carefully fitted since if they are off-centred, inaccurate results may be obtained. After the ring is

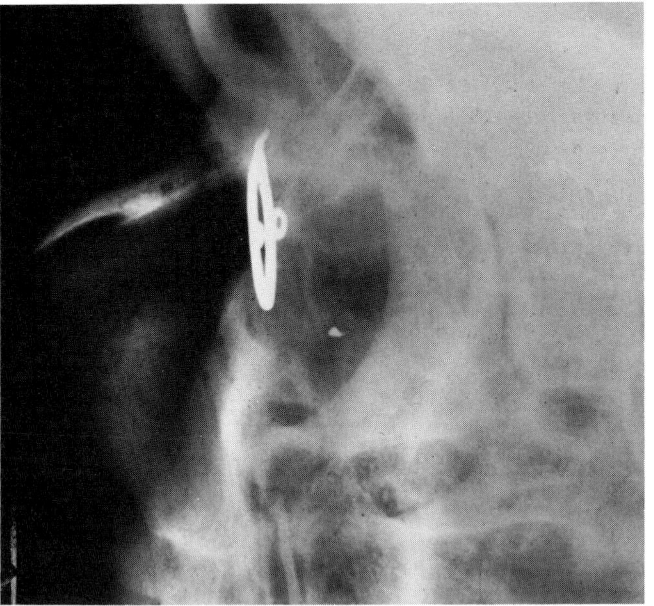

Fig.52.33 Standard lateral film with limbal ring *in situ*.

fixed in place, the patient is sent to the X-ray department, where a postero-anterior, a lateral, and in some instances an eye-moving lateral film are taken exactly in the manner already described. The lateral view should be carefully centred so that the image of the ring appears as a straight line rather than an ellipse (Fig. 52.33). By drawing a line on this film backwards from the central point of the limbal ring shadow and at right angles to it, the following measurements can be obtained: (a) the distance of the foreign body deep to the plane of the limbus, or, if 3 mm are added, deep to the plane tangential to the centre of the anterior surface of the cornea and (b) the distance in millimetres of the foreign body above or below the horizontal corneal axis. From these two measurements the position of the foreign body in two dimensions may be very accurately determined and can then be plotted on a suitable localization chart of the eye (Fig. 52.34). The third measurement, that is, the

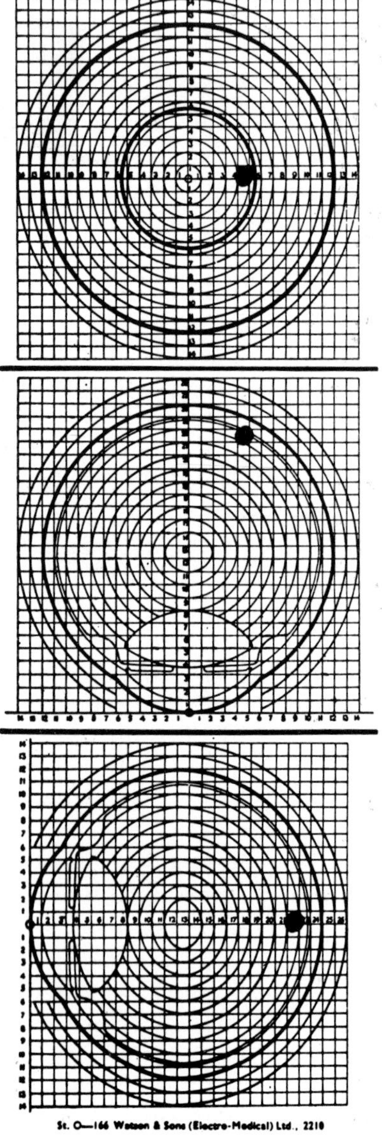

Hospital ....

Ward ....

Patient W.R.

Age 45 X-Ray No. 2105 Date 22.5.75.

Eye to be examined Left

The F.B. is present in the left ~~right~~ orbit

LOCALISATION.

(A) 4.5 mm. to the ~~nasal~~ temporal side of the vertical corneal axis

(B) 21.5 mm. deep to the plane tangential to the centre of the anterior surface of the cornea.

(C) 0 mm. above/below the horizontal corneal axis

It is intra ~~extra~~ globular.

The foreign body lies in the coats of the globe in the 3 o'clock meridian, 20mms. back from the limbus by caliper measurement.

Signature of Radiologist ....

Date ....

Fig. 52.34 Specimen localization chart.

distance of the foreign body to the nasal or temporal side of the vertical corneal axis, is obtained from the postero-anterior film. To obtain this measurement, the central point of the circular image formed by the limbal ring is determined and plotted on the radiograph. If a vertical line is drawn through this point it will represent the vertical corneal axis and direct measurements may then be made of the position of the foreign body relative to this line, either to the nasal or temporal side.

Localization by radio-opaque marker

There is an additional method which is mandatory when the foreign body is found to be non-magnetic. It is obvious that in these patients the scleral incision for removal of the foreign body must be placed with pin-point accuracy. To do this, the position of the foreign body is first localized as accurately as possible by the methods described, and the surgeon then attaches a small opaque body such as a needle point or wire suture at the calculated point of scleral incision. Standard lateral and postero-anterior views are then taken in the operating theatre, and the position of the foreign body related to the marker. This allows any error in the original localization to be corrected when the scleral incision is made, and it can be appreciated that this will also correct for the other possible sources of error: for the anatomical variation in the size of the eye in different individuals, and possible surgical error in determining the position of the meridian.

Bone free technique

Very small metallic foreign bodies may not always be visible on standard postero-anterior and lateral films, but they may sometimes be demonstrated by bone free radiographs if they are located anteriorly in the globe. For this method of examination a dental film is placed in the inner canthus of the eye to be radiographed and the tube centred just behind the lateral canthus. In this way as much as possible of the anterior part of the globe is projected onto the dental film with complete absence of overlapping bone shadows. The obvious limitation of this technique is that little more than a quarter of the globe can be visualized by this means; nevertheless, it is a very useful procedure and should always be carried out if a foreign body is clinically suspected in the forward part of the eye and cannot be seen on preliminary radiographs.

Ultrasonic localization

Ophthalmic ultrasound is a very useful ancillary method of localizing foreign bodies in the eye, and to a very large extent is complimentary to X-ray methods. A scan ultrasonography can give an exact measurement of the axial length of the eye, so that individual variations can be recognized and allowed for in the X-ray localization. An estimation of the axial length of the globe is also important in dealing with foreign bodies situated close to the posterior pole of the eye, when their position, either intra- or extra-ocular, may be hard to determine. Foreign bodies are difficult to recover surgically from this location and if it can be definitely established by measurement or eye moving films, that they are extra-ocular, they are best left alone.

B scan ultrasonography records a cross sectional representation of the eye and can be used to make very accurate localizations of intraocular foreign bodies when a clear echo is received from them (Fig. 52.35). This is particularly important in the search for non radiopaque fragments which are readily identified by ultrasound. A mechanically operated B scan capable of registering scans in two planes (lateral and plan view) is ideal for intraocular foreign body localization. In the equipment used by the author, linear B scans can be made at one millimetre intervals in both sagittal and transverse directions over the whole aperture of the scanner. The position of the transducer is calibrated to an accuracy of one millimetre, so that the transducer position, registering optimum echoes from the foreign body, can be directly related to the central corneal axis in two planes. These measurements, combined with the cornea to foreign body measurement derived either from A scan or B scan, will allow an accurate localization of the foreign body.

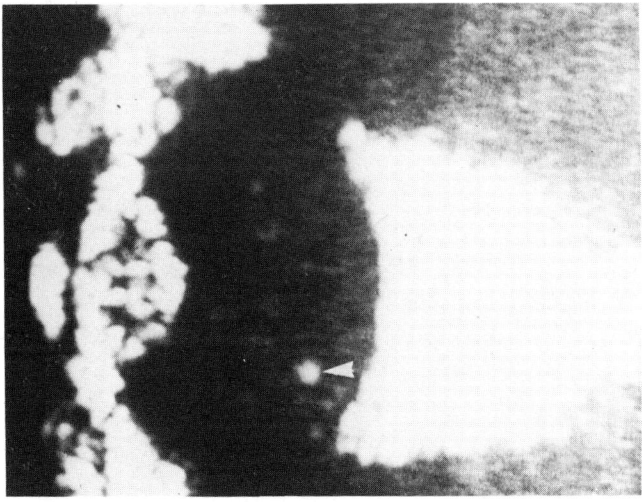

Fig. 52.35 Foreign body demonstrated by ultrasonic B scan (*arrow*).

In practice the majority of foreign bodies are best localized by X-ray. Ultrasound is only needed to make the localization when the foreign body is non radiopaque, or too minute to show by X-ray. It is also needed to verify the radiological localization in selected cases: these are usually patients with multiple intraocular

foreign bodies, in whom the complexity of the localization problem requires both multisection tomography and B scan ultrasonography for total accuracy.

Charting the foreign body

The final stage in the process of localization is to plot the position of the foreign body on a suitable localization chart. This is needed whatever method of localization is used, in order to get a true measurement of the distance of the foreign body from the limbus. The measurement can only be obtained from the charts whatever method of localization is used. For example, with the limbal ring technique, direct measurements (taken from the lateral film) of the limbus-foreign body distance will be accurate if the foreign body lies in the 6 or 12 o'clock meridian but not at 3 or 9 o'clock or in intermediate positions if it is close to the equator. To get an accurate measurement from the charts, the foreign body should be plotted in three planes and the limbus-foreign body distance taken from the appropriate projection of the globe depending upon the position of the foreign body. For instance, this measurement is best obtained from the plan view of the eye if the foreign body lies at 2, 3 and 4 o'clock, or at 8, 9 and 10 o'clock. For foreign bodies in other locations the distance should be measured from the lateral projection of the globe. A specimen localization chart is illustrated in Figure 52.34.

REFERENCES AND SUGGESTIONS FOR FURTHER READING

BROMLEY, J. F. & Lyle, T. K. (1943) An apparatus for localising foreign bodies in the orbit. *Trans. Ophth. Soc. U.K.*, **63**, 164.

BRISMAR, J., DAVIS, K. R., DALLOW, R.L. & VBRISMAR, G. (1976) Unilateral Endocrine Exophthalmos. Diagnostic problems in association with C.T. *Neuroradiology*, **12**, 21–24.

CAMPBELL, W. (1964) The radiology of the lacrimal system. *British Journal of Radiology*, **37**, 1.

COLEMAN, D. J. (1972) Reliability of ocular and orbital diagnosis with B-scan ultrasound (orbital diagnosis). *American Journal of Ophthalmology*, **74**, 704.

DEJEAN, C. & BOUDET, C. (1951) Du diagnostic des varices de l'orbite et de leur complications par la phlebographie. *Bull. Soc. Fr. Ophth.*, **64**, 374.

DILENGE, D. (1974) Arteriography in angiomas of the orbit. *Radiology*, **113**, 355.

ERKONEN, W. & DOLAN, K. D. (1972) Ocular foreign body localization. *Radiol. Clin. North Am.*, **10**, 101.

EWING, A. E. (1909) Roentgen ray demonstration of the lacrimal abscess cavity. *Am. J. Ophth.*, **26**, 1.

GARNER, A. (1973) Pseudotumours of the orbit. In *Modern Problems in Ophthalmology*. Basel: Karger.

HANAFEE, W. N. (1972) Orbital venography. *Radiol. Clin. North Am.*, **10**, 63.

HARWOOD-NASH, D. C. (1970) Axial tomography of the optic canals of children. *Radiology*, **96**, 367.

HARWOOD-NASH, D. C. (1972) Optic gliomas and pediatric neuroradiology. *Radiol. Clin. North Am.*, **10**, 83.

HEATH, P. (1962) Calcinosis oculi. *Am. J. Ophth.*, **54**, 771.

HENDERSON, J. W. (1973) *Orbital Tumors*. Philadelphia: Saunders.

HUNT, W. E., MEAGLIER, J. M., LEFEUR, J. E. & ZEMAN, W. (1961) Painful ophthalmoplegia: its relation to indolent inflammation of the cavernous sinus. *Neurology*, **11**, 56.

IBA, G. M. & HANAFEE, W. N. (1968) Distension dacryocystography. *Radiology*, **90**, 1020.

JONES, I. S., REESE, A. B. & KRAUT, J. (1966) Orbital rhabdomyosarcoma: An analysis of 62 cases. *Am. J. Ophth.*, **61**, 721.

LAAKE, J. P. W. (1962) Superior orbital fissure syndrome. *Arch. Neurol.* **7**, 289.

LEVY, I. S., WRIGHT, J. E. & LLOYD, G. A. S. (1973) *Proceedings of the 2nd International Symposium on Orbital Disorders (Amsterdam, 1973)*. Basel: Karger.

LLOYD, G. A. S. (1969) A technique for arteriorgraphy of the orbit. *British Journal of Radiology*, **42**, 252.

LLOYD, G. A. S. (1971a) The radiology of primary orbital meningioma. *British Journal of Radiology*, **44**, 405.

LLOYD, G. A. S. (1972) The localisation of lesions in the orbital apex and cavernous sinus by frontal venography. *British Journal of Radiology*, **45**, 405.

LLOYD, G. A. S. (1973) Radiographic measurement in the diagnosis of orbital space occupying lesions. *Trans. Ophth. Soc. U.K.*, **93**, 301.

LLOYD, G. A. S. (1973b) Multisection tomography as an aid to the localisation of intraocular foreign bodies. *British Journal of Radiology*, **46**, 34.

LLOYD, G. A. S. (1974) Pathological veins in the orbit. *British Journal of Radiology*. **47**, 570.

LLOYD, G. A. S. (1975a) *Radiology of the Orbit*. Philadelphia: Saunders.

LLOYD, G. A. S. (1975) Axial hypocycloidal tomography of the orbits. *British Journal of Radiology*, **48**, 460.

LLOYD, G. A. S. (1977) The impact of C.T. scanning and ultrasonography on Orbital Diagnosis. *Clinical Radiology*, **28**, 583–593.

LLOYD, G. A. S. & AMBROSE, J. (1977) An evaluation of C.A.T. in the diagnosis of Orbital space occupying lesions. In *Computerised Axial Tomography in Clinical Practice*, 154–160. Berlin: Springer-Verlag.

LLOYD, G. A. S., AMBROSE, J. & WRIGHT, J. E. (1975) New techniques in investigation of the orbit. *Trans. Opth. Soc. U.K.*, **95**, 233.

LLOYD, G. A. S., WRIGHT. J. E. & MORGAN, G. (1971) Venous malformations in the orbit. *British Journal of Ophthalmics*, **55**, 505.

LOMBARDI, G. (1967) *Radiology in Neuro-ophthalmology*. Baltimore: Williams and Wilkins.

OSSOINIG, K. C. & BLODI, F. C. (1974) Pre-operative diagnosis of Tumours with Echography. Part IV. Diagnosis of Orbital Tumours. *Current Concepts in Ophthalmology*, **17**, 313.

PFEIFFER, R. L. & NICHOLL, R. J. (1948) Dermoids and epidermoid tumours of the orbit. *Arch. Ophth.*, **40**, 639.

TAYBI, H. (1956) Ocular calcification and retrolental fibroplasia. *American Journal of Roentgen*, **76**, 583.

TOLOSA, E. (1954) Periarteritis of carotid siphon with clinical features of carotid infraclinoid aneurysm. *J. Neurol. Neurosurg. Psychiat.*, **17**, 300.

VRITSIOS, A. (1961) Methode de phlebographie des veins ophthalmiques des veins de la face et des vaisseaux superfices du crane. *Arch. Soc. Ophth. Grèce de Nord*, **12**, 223.

WRIGHT, J. E. (1974) Orbital vascular anomalies. *Trans. Am. Acad. Ophth. Otol.* **78**, 606.

YASARGIL, M. G. (1957) *Die Röntgendianostik des Exophthalmus Unilateralis*. Basel: Karger.

CHAPTER 53

TEETH

Teeth may be affected by many diseases. There are two infectious lesions which, besides threatening the teeth themselves, can lead to systemic disease. Developmental errors occur and there are cysts and neoplastic diseases peculiar to the mouth. Bone dysplasias can produce striking changes in the jaws and skull and these bone changes are very well shown in the fine detail of dental films.

Anatomy

The bulk of a tooth is formed of *dentine* which is sensitive to temperature change and other stimuli. In the centre of the tooth crown and down the root to the tooth apex is a hollow space occupied by the *pulp* which is soft tissue containing nerves and vessels. The crown projects from the gum and is protected by a layer of *enamel* in the form of a thimble or cap (Fig. 53.1). Enamel is insensitive and hard like ivory but is susceptible to caries. Beyond the crown there is a thin layer of *cementum* covering the dentine of the root and this layer forms the anchorage for the *periodontal membrane* or *ligament* which slings the tooth in its bony socket. The bony anchorage for the fibres of the periodontal membrane is a thin layer of compact bone lining the socket called the *lamina dura.* Beyond the lamina dura is the cancellous bone of the *alveolar process* (the tooth-supporting bone) of the jaw and this is covered with a thin layer of compact bone beneath the gum.

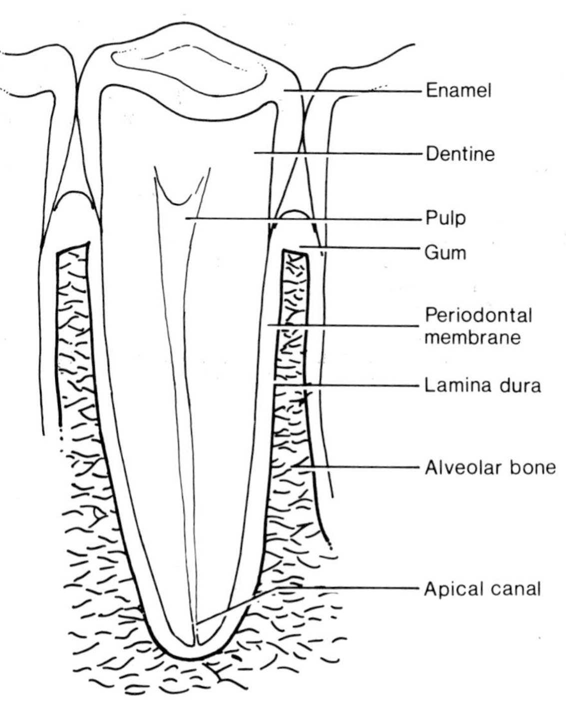

Fig. 53.1 Diagram of a lower premolar in its socket as shown in a dental film.

Enamel is denser to X-rays than dentine which is comparable in density to compact bone while the pulp space is darker than dentine.

The thin layer of cementum covering the root beneath the gum is radiographically indistinguishable from dentine. The cancellous bone forming the alveolar process surrounds the sockets on at least three sides and so the shadow of its trabecular network is superimposed on the periodontal membrane and on the roots of the teeth.

INFECTION

Caries is a bacterial invasion of the tooth which first liquefies a narrow track through the enamel and then causes more extensive softening and staining of the adjacent dentine. It attacks the occlusal surface of molars, the neighbouring surfaces, especially of the cheek teeth, and the necks of the teeth where carbohydrate food residues have been allowed to remain. Interstitial caries of the cheek teeth is shown in its earliest stages by the bitewing film when it is still clinically obscure. It appears as a dark track through the enamel just above the contact point in upper teeth and below in lower teeth with a larger darker area in the underlying dentine (Fig. 53.2).

Caries is by far the commonest cause of pain near the mouth and a bitewing film of the appropriate side will often show interstitial caries which can be obscured clinically by a filling. The pain of toothache may be referred to the ear but not across the midline and is

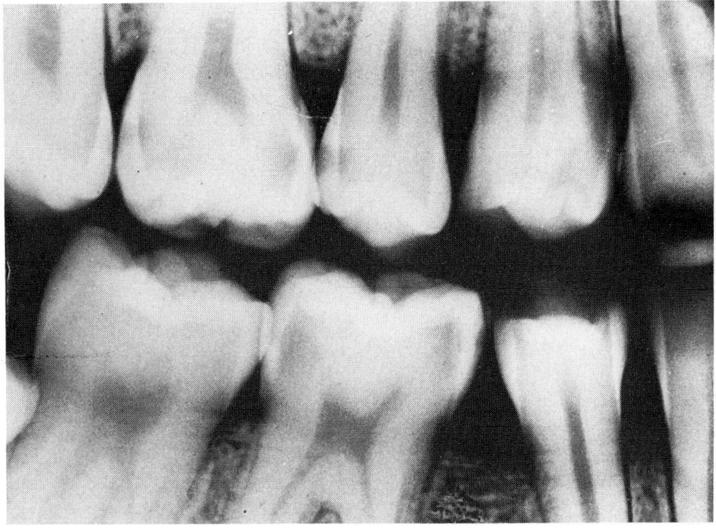

Fig. 53.2

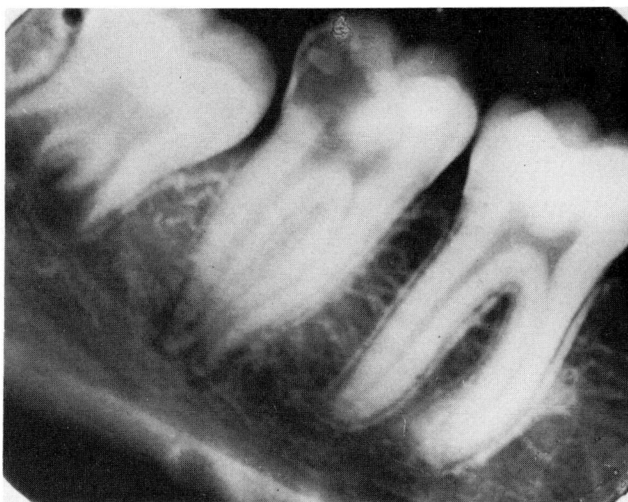

Fig. 53.3

Fig. 53.2 Bite-wing film showing typical interstitial caries of both first molars and the upper second premolar and some occlusal caries of the upper first premolar. The darkening at the necks of many of the teeth is a normal effect resulting from the space between the enamel thimble covering the crown and the bone surrounding the root.

Fig. 53.3 Early periapical infection beneath the lower second molar in a youth of 16. The lamina dura is destroyed round the apical thirds of its roots with widening of the dark line around the roots. Compare with the normal first molar and the incompletely formed roots of the third molar.

often not well localized to the decayed tooth. An apical film, the common dental projection, will show the whole tooth and the bone beyond its apex but the view of the crown is often oblique and so unreliable to eliminate caries.

Deep caries will kill the pulp which tends to be strangled by the inflammatory exudate in the rigid space in the tooth. In young teeth before the apex is closed and for some years after this while the apical canal is still wide, the pulp is more tolerant of carious involvement. Once the pulp has died infection may spread to the periapical region. Root treatment after removal of all infected and dead pulp tissue is aimed to avoid this or to enable the periapical infection to heal.

When infection has spread beyond the apex, the effect depends on the severity of the inflammation. An acute abscess is the most marked reaction with throbbing pain and a very tender (periostitic) tooth. There is swelling of the gum and of the face and, if the tooth is related to the antrum, of the antral mucosa also. There are no bone changes unless this acute lesion is superimposed on a previous chronic infection.

A *sub-acute abscess* or gumboil will show X-ray evidence of bone destruction around the apex and present clinically with a swelling of the gum, usually on the outer side and near the root of the affected tooth. There will be a sinus with a purulent discharge and the opening is often on a rather sac-like projection of the oral mucosa. The bone destruction shows a diffuse area of darkening at the tooth apex including the lamina dura of the socket in this region. The lamina dura is the thin layer of compact bone lining the socket and is the first bone to be destroyed near the tooth apex when infection has spread to this region (Fig. 53.3). Darkening due to natural thinning of the bone or to superimposition of a foramen (like the mental foramen—which is usually just anterior to the apex of the lower second premolar) is associated with an intact lamina dura round the normal tooth apex (Fig. 53.4).

Chronic apical infection may be present without clinical signs. The X-ray changes then are those of a discrete periapical darkening sometimes outlined by a white line which is continuous with the lamina dura of the socket at

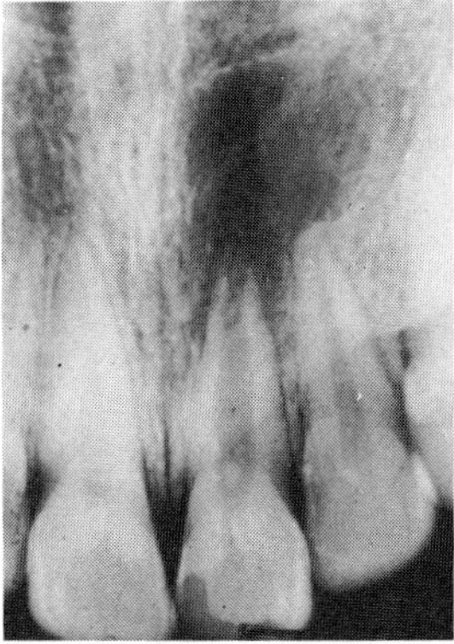

Fig. 53.4

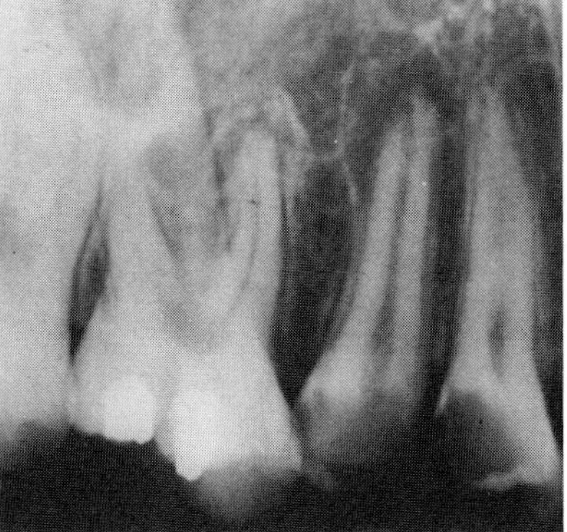

Fig. 53.5

Fig. 53.4 A large discrete area of bone destruction above the left incisors but arising from the central which has lost the lamina dura round its apical third. This tooth was killed by trauma at age 8 and its root is incomplete. There is some darkening above the right incisors due to less thick overlying bone but the lamina dura is intact here.

Fig. 53.5 There is a granuloma at the apex of the second premolar surrounded by a thin halo of bone formed by the antral mucoperiosteum. There is a similar pattern over the mesial root apex of the first molar.

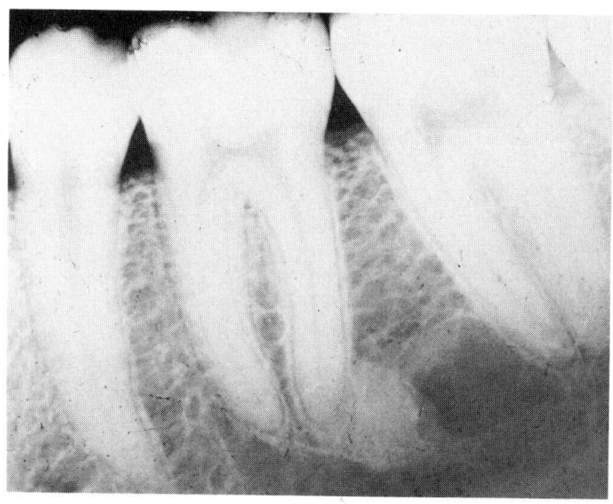

A

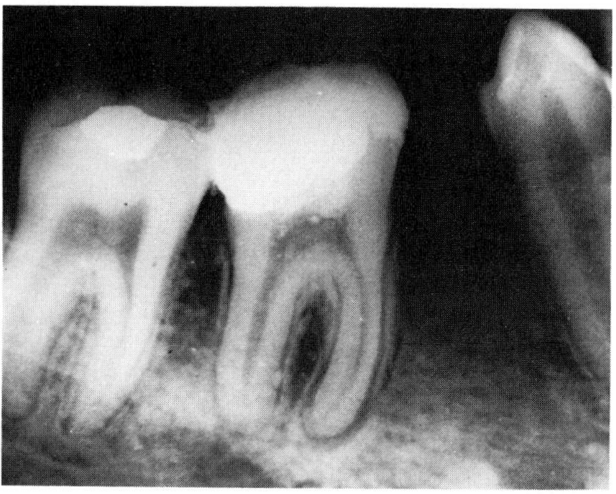

B

Fig. 53.6A A compact bone island at the distal apex of this lower left first molar. It merges with the lamina dura but the periodontal membrane shadow remains uninterrupted. B Inflammatory sclerosis beyond small areas of bone destruction at the apices of this lower right first molar.

the margin of the lesion (Fig. 53.5). Chronic infection on a tooth at the antral floor lifts the mucoperiosteum over the granuloma and this can develop a bony halo surrounding it. Commonly, recurrent sub-acute infection leads on to chronic infection but there may be a return to a more active clinical manifestation.

Inflammatory sclerosis of bone beyond the tooth apex occasionally occurs, particularly from dead lower molars. Also in this region are found developmental *compact bone islands* which appear in many other bones. These are often close to a socket or to the mandibular canal margins, whereas sclerosing osteitis is centred on one or both apices with a small area of bone destruction at the apex (Fig. 53.6A and B).

Root treatment is used to preserve accessible teeth whose pulps would otherwise die or are already dead. Sometimes *apicectomy* is performed to remove the chronic periapical granuloma and infected apex after treatment of the root canal but efficient modern root canal treatment will also lead to eradication of such an apical area. The periapical bone, including the lamina dura, will be re-formed over a period of one or two years once all the necrotic pulp tissue has been removed. Root fillings are almost always radiopaque due to zinc oxide or other metal salts. Inadequately treated dead teeth can be a source of acute or chronic infection and still lower grade infection can cause the formation of a periodontal (dental) cyst (p. 10).

Periodontal disease is initially a gingivitis and this can be acute as with a Vincent's infection. If the inflammation persists, resorption of the peaks of the underlying interdental bony papillae can result and this may be demonstrated radiologically (Fig. 53.7). The interdental bony papilla is blunted and shortened and has a broader top, while its edge will be ragged and poorly defined in the active stage of the disease. There are often deposits of calculus (tartar) around the neck of the tooth and this opaque material will show in the films (Fig. 53.8). It will also aggravate the chronic or sub-acute gingival inflammation, of course. Cervical caries can occur beyond the edge of the enamel after gum and bone have receded.

The pattern of bone loss in periodontal disease takes two forms, horizontal loss and vertical loss. In horizontal loss (Fig. 53.8) there is general all round recession and this is a slow but steady progression of the disease, with

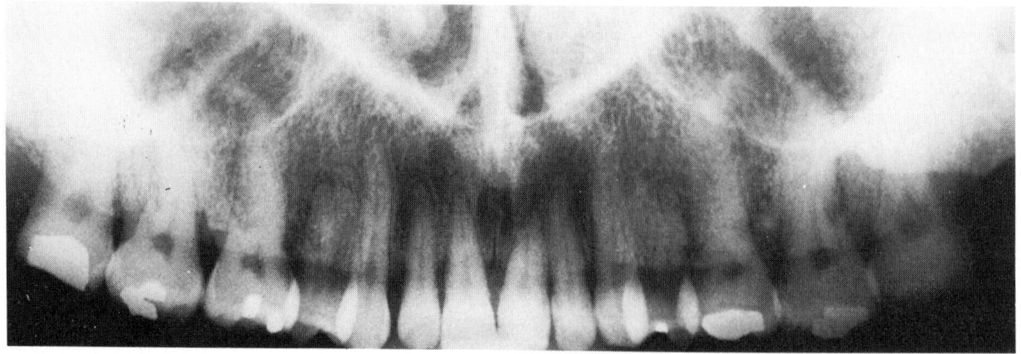

Fig. 53.7 A film of the maxilla taken with the Panagraph, an example of the static panoramic machine, which shows early loss of tooth-supporting bone especially round the upper left second molar.

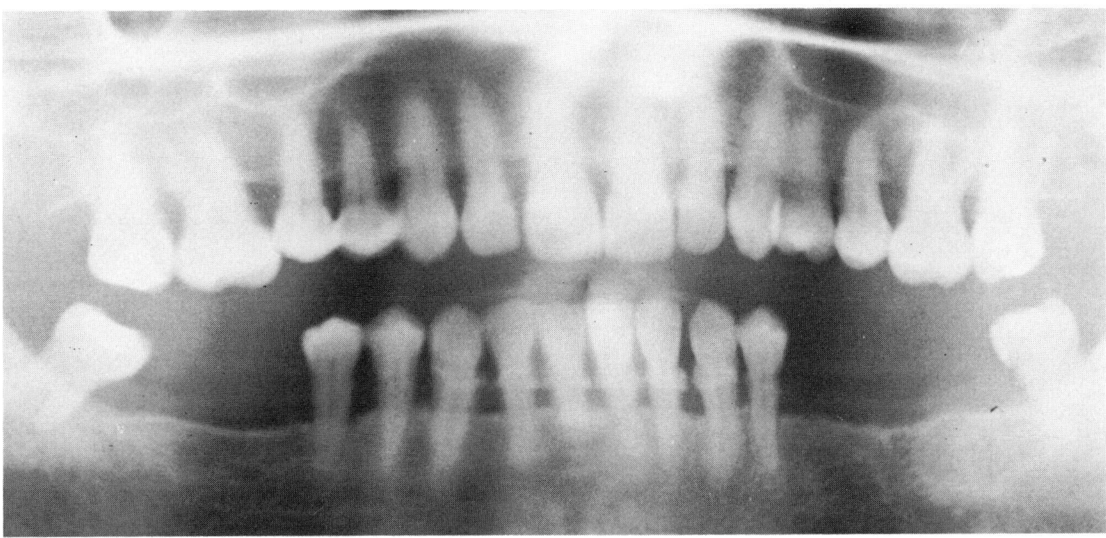

Fig. 53.8 A Panelipse film showing general horizontal loss of supporting bone with deposits of calculus.

deeper loss of the supporting bone than in the normal recession with age. In vertical loss, there is irregular and deep local loss which may reach the tooth apex in some regions and thus some teeth are lost. This implies a deficiency and susceptibility to periodontal disease which is sometimes familial and also racial in origin.

Chronic dental infection both periapical and periodontal used to be blamed for a number of diseases and teeth were too easily condemned and removed. A transient bacteraemia can result from ordinary masticatory forces on inflamed gums or on teeth with apical infection. In moderation and in otherwise fit people, this does not cause trouble but it can give rise to sub-acute bacterial endocarditis in hearts with previous damage or in those who have had operations involving the endocardium. In these subjects dental infection must be eliminated and this may mean condemning teeth unless the infection can be cleared by treatment. Extensive dental sepsis can also cause pyrexia with a raised E.S.R. and constitutional upset yet with little by way of local symptoms (Berry and Silver, 1976).

Panoramic dental machines are extensively used in hospital practice and they are of two types, the *orbiting* and the *static*. In the orbiting machines, a vertical slit of X-rays passes through the head and traverses from behind one ramus of the mandible all round to the other exposing a narrow strip of both jaws at a time. The beam is only roughly perpendicular to that part of the jaws being X-rayed and there is a degree of tomographic effect which blurs out much of the unwanted shadows. In the static machines, the source of rays is 0·1 mm focal spot on a projection from the tube which is placed in the mouth and each jaw is exposed separately. The radiation dose in this machine is very low.

Bone detail in the orbiting machines is usually quite good in the molar regions, angles and rami but rarely good in the anterior part of the jaws (Fig. 53.8). The condyles can be shown with the jaw extruded or the mouth wide open. The static machines, on the other hand, give good detail definition round to the first molars and sometimes further back (Fig. 53.7). The two together are supplementary for complete coverage of the teeth and jaws and the total dose of radiation is much less than that from a full mouth of dental films. The maxillary antra can be seen in both types of panoramic machine and the antral floor may be well shown. With the orbiting machines spurious shadows arise from earrings and from inherent structures and an occipito-mental projection is necessary as well or instead to demonstrate the condition of the antra.

More widespread infection of bone may occur in the mandible. It is mostly limited in extent and only rarely affects the maxilla. This *subacute osteomyelitis* usually extends from a tooth socket, either after extraction or from an apical abscess, when conditions are unfavourable. The early radiographic pattern, from about three weeks after onset, is of patches of darkening with islands of normal looking bone between them (Fig. 53.9). The lamina dura is early included in this destructive process.

Some but not all of these patches of normal-looking bone will develop into sequestra, and sooner or later there will be evidence of sub-periosteal new bone formation. This appears as a soft fusiform opacity along the lower border or on the outer or inner margin of the jaw (Fig. 53.10). The sequestra are either portions of cortex, which may be confirmed by an occlusal film, or else fragments of socket or bony papilla. In the later stages, the area of bone destruction becomes sharply defined and the periosteal new bone becomes consolidated (Fig. 53.11). More acute and extensive osteomyelitis of the mandible is rare nowadays but is sometimes of blood-

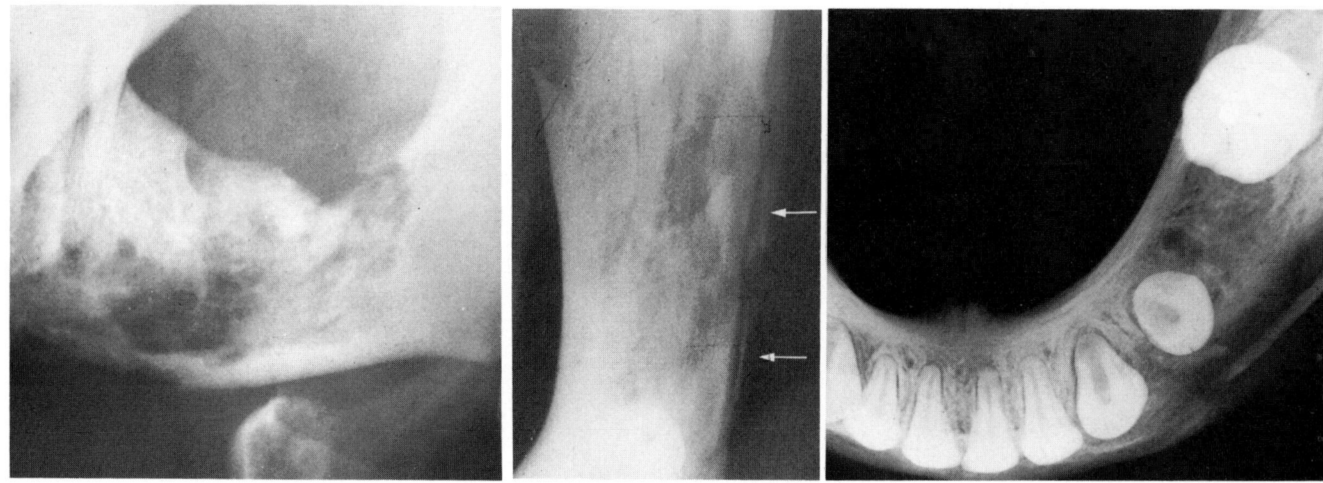

Fig. 53.9 *Fig. 53.10* *Fig. 53.11*

Fig. 53.9 Irregular bone destruction in the mandible of a man of 41 some 6 weeks after onset of osteomyelitis.

Fig. 53.10 A few weeks later than Figure 53.9, there is periosteal new bone formation on the buccal aspect of the jaw (arrow).

Fig. 53.11 A sequestrum from the buccal plate separating at about 6 weeks after the acute phase in a boy of 9 years. His symptoms had rapidly improved with cloxacillin intramuscularly and by mouth and now he had only slight local signs. The periosteal bone had already consolidated—much more rapid progress than in an adult.

borne origin particularly in those rare examples which occur in infancy before the teeth have erupted. In childhood the condition can arise without a dead tooth from periodontal infection. Alternatively, a well localized osteomyelitis in childhood without sequestrum formation is relatively common (Fig. 53.12).

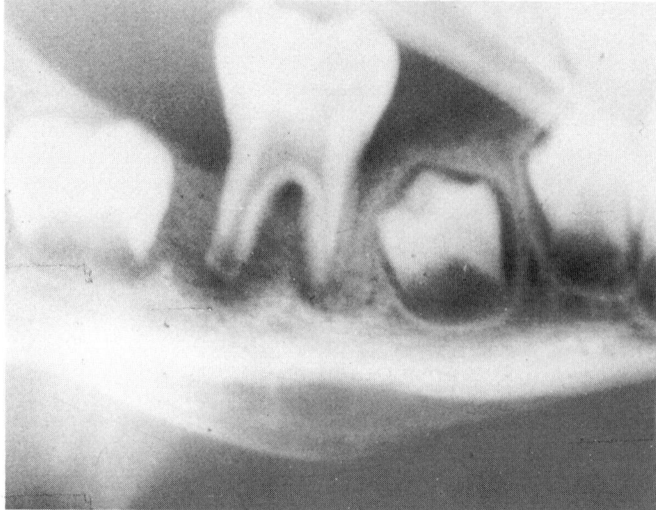

Fig. 53.12 An abscess beneath the first molar in a child of 7 years with considerably more than the immediate periapical bone involved. There is a multilayered periosteal bone response along the lower border of the jaw stimulated by recurrent inflammatory exudates.

Radionecrosis occurs in the jaws when the bone has been damaged by radiotherapy some years before. This misfortune is less likely to arise after modern irradiation techniques have been employed. The pattern is of destruction and sequestrum formation with no periosteal new bone. The lesion is more likely to develop in the presence of teeth, by which infection is introduced, but it also occurs in the edentulous jaw and is early complicated by infection from the mouth (Fig. 53.13). It often arises as a sequel to tooth extraction when penicillin cover has not been used to protect the susceptible bone where endarteritis from radiation injury has reduced its vascularity. The condition frequently proceeds to fracture, partly due to its inexorable extension and partly to the lack of any splinting by callus from the periosteum. Extensive excision is often necessary to relieve the pain and to eradicate the lesion.

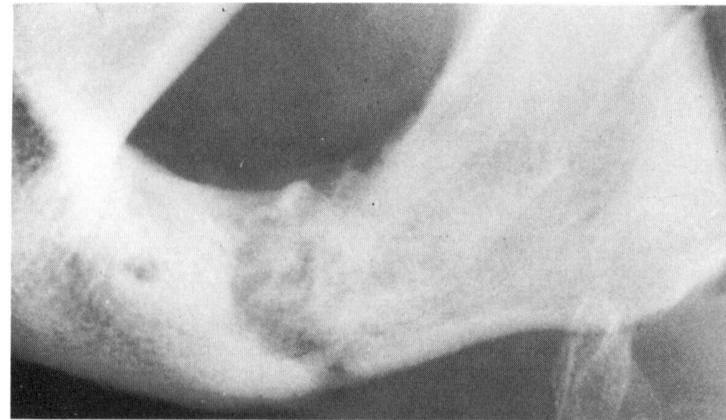

Fig. 53.13 Radionecrosis 3 years after irradiation for an anaplastic carcinoma of the nasopharynx and the cervical nodes in a man of 68. Three months after onset the bone infection has reached the lower border of the jaw and it proceeded on to fracture a month later.

TRAUMA

A blow on a tooth may cause no disruption of the X-ray pattern and yet the blood supply to the pulp may have

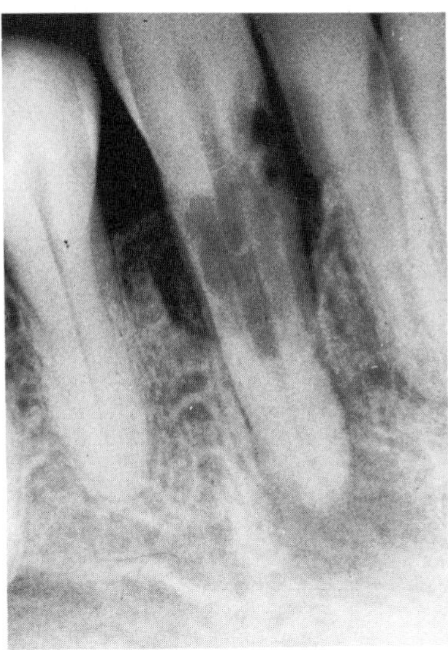

Fig. 53.14

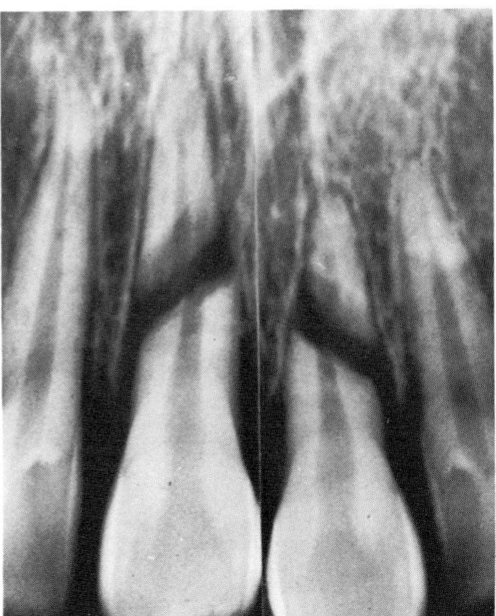

Fig. 53.15

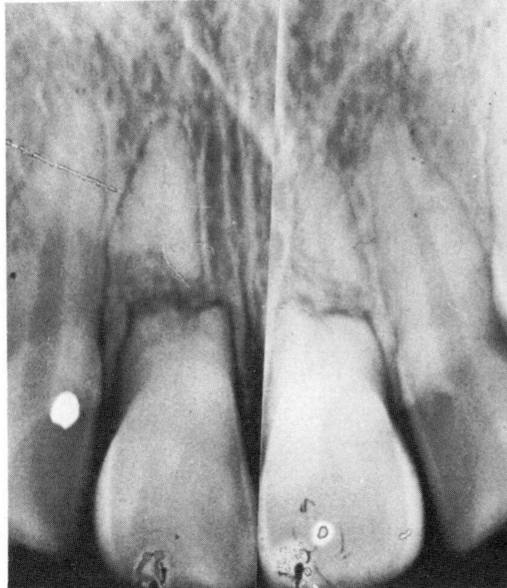

Fig. 53.16

Fig. 53.14 Extensive external root resorption in a man of 62. This erosion reaches into the crown as well as halfway down the root but the outline of the pulp persists although it must have been breached. Infection from the gum margin has reached the pulp and led to an apical abscess.

Fig. 53.15 Fracture of both upper central incisor roots 1 week before this film in a girl of 14. The pulp survived in both portions of each tooth as it often will in young jaws.

Fig. 53.16 Two years later, the vital but damaged pulps have partly calcified up in root as well as in crown portions of the teeth. A layer of bone has formed between the root ends separated by a dark line like periodontal membrane from the root and with an intact lamina dura beyond this.

been interrupted. The pulp may then die and become infected from the blood stream or periodontal lymphatics, with the effects already described. Less commonly, the pulp vessels are only damaged and the response is obliteration of the pulp space by dentine over a period of perhaps a year. In either case, the crown can become darkened clinically by blood pigments in the dentine.

A less common effect of pulp damage by trauma or even by caries is a *pulp granuloma*—internal resorption of the dentine. External resorption of the root at the neck of the tooth also occurs sometimes following trauma and also when the pulp is dying from carious infection (Fig. 53.14).

The tooth may be dislodged from the depth of its socket without escaping from the mouth. With dislocation or subluxation of a tooth, the dark line of the periodontal membrane is widened on the radiograph to resemble a space surrounding the root while the lamina dura remains intact. On the other hand the root or the crown may be fractured across by the injury (Fig. 53.15). In either event, the pulp may be killed but, in young teeth with a still large apical foramen or a frankly incomplete root, it has a better chance to survive. The damaged pulp of such a severed tooth will react by becoming partly obliterated (Fig. 53.16).

When an upper first molar is removed from a patient with a large antrum, the bony floor of the sinus may be fractured. Sometimes the tooth instead is broken. A root may remain in the socket with the lamina dura intact around it or, in an attempt to remove it, the root may be pushed up through the socket into the bony space of the antrum. It usually comes to lie beneath the antral mucosa and above the level of the remaining teeth. An *oro-antral fistula* may be formed from a large bony breach, but in either event, suppuration can be avoided and the socket can heal with little trouble.

The mandible and the other facial bones are liable to fracture. The mandible may suffer a direct fracture at the site of a blow at any point round to the angle. There is very often also an indirect fracture at the neck of the condyle on the opposite side. The indirect fracture may be at the base of the condylar process, in the ramus or a vertical split of the condyle head. The midline mandible is displaced towards the side of the condyle neck fracture and the occlusion will be deranged. Bilateral fracture of this region can occur from a blow on the chin.

DEVELOPMENTAL ERRORS

Lower third molars are fairly commonly misplaced. There is usually insufficient room for them to erupt completely and they may impact against the second molar or backwards against the bone of the ramus. Even if they become vertical, they frequently fail to erupt clear of the gum and so inflammation starts from this site of stagnation round the crown. Thus arises the common trouble with wisdom teeth—pericoronitis. Caries may also occur in inaccessible places on second and third molars because of an impaction and this similarly causes pain. The impaction itself is only a very rare cause of pain.

Unless teeth have been lost earlier so that there is space for the third molars, most lower wisdom teeth give trouble in the early twenties and have to be removed. The dental surgeon needs X-ray films to show the shape of the complete roots and the relationship to the second molar, to the jaw bone and to the mandibular canal and the orbiting panoramic machines usually give an adequate view of the third molars.

If the upper canine has failed to erupt by about 14 years of age, its position has to be determined by radiography.

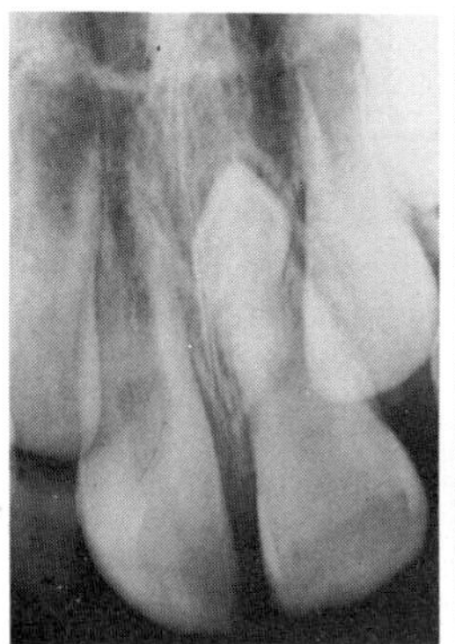

Fig. 53.17

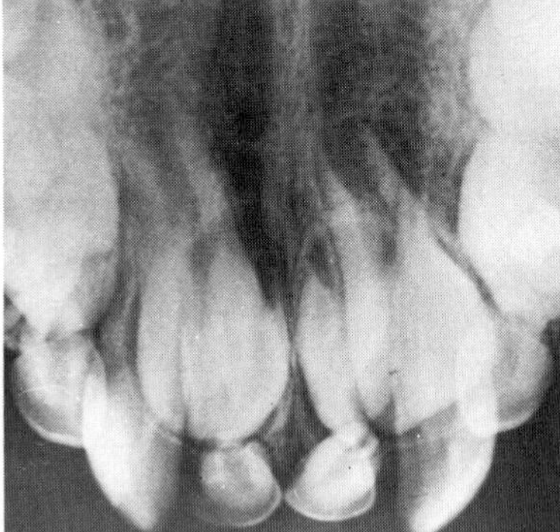

Fig. 53.18

Fig. 53.17 A mesiodens overlying the left central root in a girl of 7. The central incisors are erupted although their roots are only half formed and the laterals are still unerupted. The mesiodens is small and inverted with its crown upwards but its root is already complete.

Fig. 53.18 There are two late supernumerary teeth, one on each side, obstructing the eruption of each permanent central incisor in a boy of 9. The temporary centrals are retained still but the laterals have erupted normally. The permanent centrals are high, more horizontal than usual and still enclosed in bone while the supernumeraries are in the ridge in their place. Their roots are not yet formed at all and the dark space of each tooth germ above the crown overlaps the shadow of each buried central.

True lateral and occipito-frontal films taken in a craniostat are most widely used by orthodontists to confirm their clinical impressions. Most unerupted upper canines are palatal to the incisors though some are merely late erupting and correct in position. If they are labial, that is, in correct position for normal eruption, the crown is usually palpable high in the sulcus. Parallax shift with two occlusal films is also used, one centred at the midline and the other in the canine region.

Three types of *supernumerary tooth* arise in the upper incisor region. The most common is the mesiodens which develops close to the midline and at a time between the first and second dentitions (Fig. 53.17). It may deflect one or both permanent centrals as they erupt, or it may appear in the palate behind them or it may pass unnoticed up to the floor of the nose. Quite often two mesiodentes develop and one may point back while the other's crown is forwards.

The supplemental, the most rare of the supernumerary teeth, is a near copy of a normal tooth bone in shape and stage of development, usually the permanent upper lateral incisor.

The late supernumerary develops after the permanent teeth, but frequently obstructs eruption of the permanent central incisor which remains high and labial to the other teeth lying nearly horizontal (Fig. 53.18). The condition is quite often bilateral.

Cleft of the hard palate is a defect in the floor of the nose just lateral to the midline, but it may be bilateral. It usually extends forwards through the alveolar process medial to the canine. The premaxilla between the two canines may be very distorted or rudimentary, containing small misshapen denticles. It is usually necessary to keep all possible teeth as an anchorage for an obturator: they are difficult teeth to radiograph. The static panoramic machine with its focal spot in the mouth usually gives a better display of the teeth and bone in cleft palate than do intra-oral films but the orbiting panoramic film is usually of very little value.

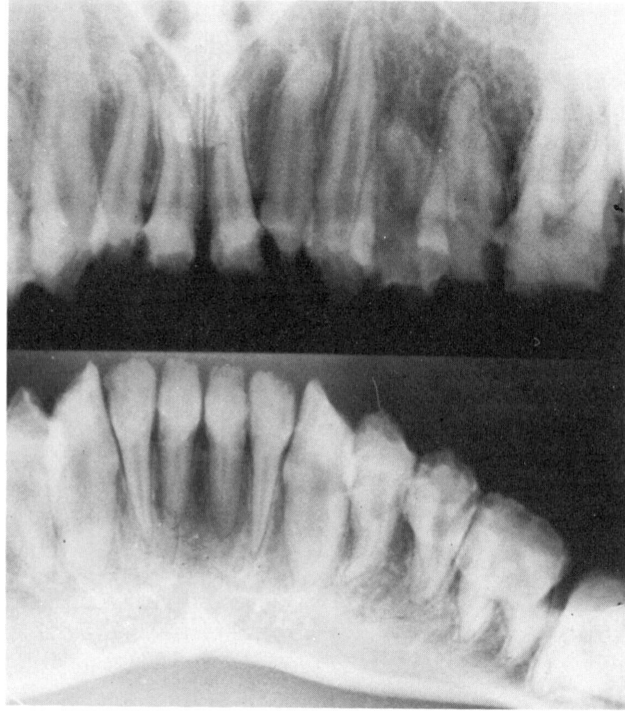

Fig. 53.19 Amelogenesis imperfecta in a boy of 8. Parts of two static panoramic films showing the enamel layer on all crowns to be of reduced and very irregular thickness. The greater deficiency of enamel in the upper anterior region is partly due to added caries.

In *amelogenesis imperfecta*, the enamel is deficient in varying degree. There may be a very thin but even layer of enamel or a very irregular thickness of enamel over the crowns of both dentitions (Fig. 53.19). Caries supervenes and increases the deficiency.

In *dentinogenesis imperfecta*, the grey colour of the abnormal dentine shows through the normal enamel and radiologically the pulp calcifies extensively and the pulp space becomes invisible. Enamel is poorly anchored and tends to flake off; the teeth are small and are liable to be lost early. A proportion of sufferers from osteogenesis imperfecta have this abnormality of their dentine but the two conditions also occur separately.

The *calcified odontomes* are aberrations of the tooth germ in various patterns of deformity. Not all of them are shaped like a tooth but all are at least partly buried in the jaw in the tooth-bearing region. They are nearly always denser than bone and are surrounded by a dark line representing soft tissue with a lamina dura beyond. This surround of a thin dark space and a white line distinguishes these lesions from dense bone.

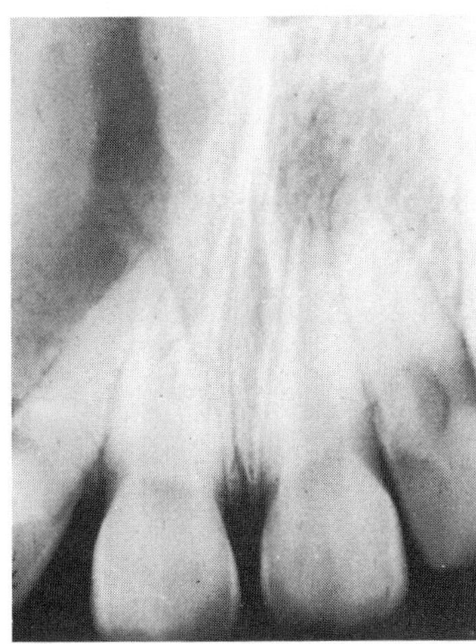

Fig. 53.21 A midline apical film of the maxilla of a girl of 14 who fell 6 years before and chipped both central incisor crowns. They were killed by the blow and their roots remain incomplete. A large cyst developed on the right central extending from the midline to the first molar and separating the roots of the lateral and canine. The lateral pulp has calcified up as a result of the injury. The left central developed a more active infection and there was a sinus from this in the labial sulcus.

CYSTS OF THE JAWS

These may be classified as follows:

1. *Cysts of Dental Origin*

(*a*) Infective—Periodontal (radicular, dental)
Residual

(*b*) Developmental—Dentigerous (follicular)
Primordial (odontogenic keratocyst)

(*c*) Neoplastic—Cystic adamantinoma (ameloblastoma)

2. *Fissural Cysts*

Incisive canal (naso-palatine)
Globulo-maxillary

3. *Non-epithelial cyst*

Simple bone cyst (haemorrhagic, traumatic, extravasation)

The commonest cyst is an *apical*, *periodontal*, or *dental cyst* which arises near the apex of a dead tooth and is lined with squamous epithelium. Almost as common is the residual cyst which remains in the jaw and continues to enlarge when the causative dead tooth has been removed. They arise from epithelial cell remnants in the periodontal membrane which are made to proliferate by irritation from low grade infection. The centre of the resulting mass liquefies and proliferation of the cells continues until the internal tension developed in the cyst is relieved. This may come about from surgical intervention or, when the cyst has expanded beyond the bone, and reached the mucosal surface. Secondary infection with breakdown can then occur but the small opening thus made gives only temporary relief.

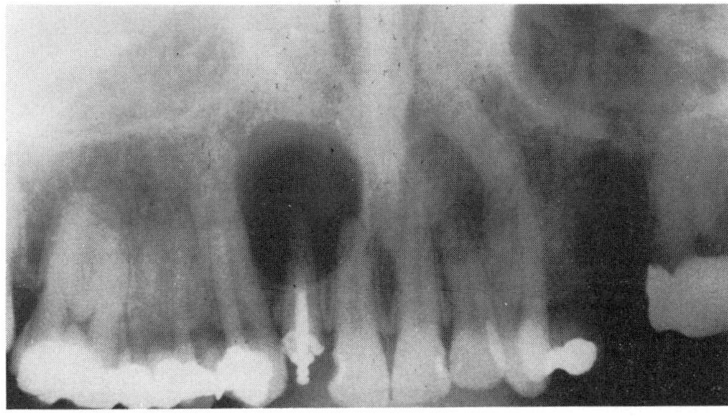

Fig. 53.20 A static panoral film of the maxilla of a man of 29 showing the early stage of a cyst arising on the right upper lateral incisor which had been inadequately root filled and developed a low grade apical infection.

The cyst appears as a rounded translucency in the bone (Fig. 53.20) and continues to enlarge until it reaches the bone surface where typical expansion is produced with a convex linear outer margin, often incomplete and seen best in occlusal films. In the maxilla, the median suture offers resistance to expansion of the cyst (Fig. 53.21), but if the bone cavity of the maxillary antrum is reached, there is ready enlargement up into this. In the mandible, the thick cortex is more resistant and a cyst will extend along the medullary space while causing only moderate expansion (Fig. 53.22A). The lamina dura is eroded from the socket of the causative tooth but also from those of the adjacent vital teeth where the cyst impinges (Fig. 53.22B and C). Tooth roots may be eroded by continued pressure but this erosion occurs much more slowly than erosion and expansion of the bone.

In young jaws, the teeth will drift from the pressure of a cyst, but this effect is late and less widespread in adult jaws. Any dead tooth can give origin to a cyst. In either jaw, an anterior tooth which has died quietly after trauma is commonly the culprit.

The common developmental cyst is the *dentigerous*

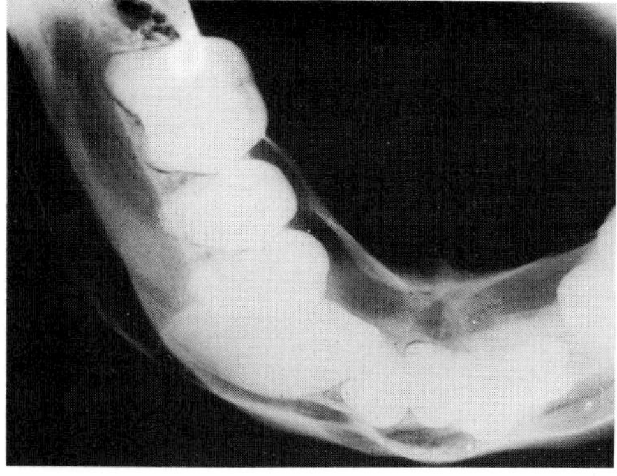

A

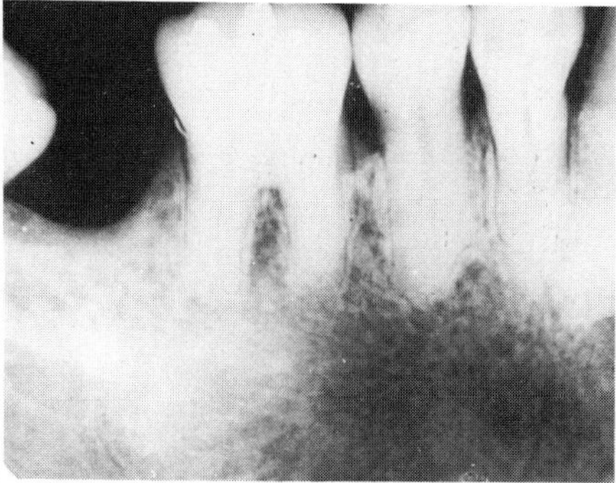

B

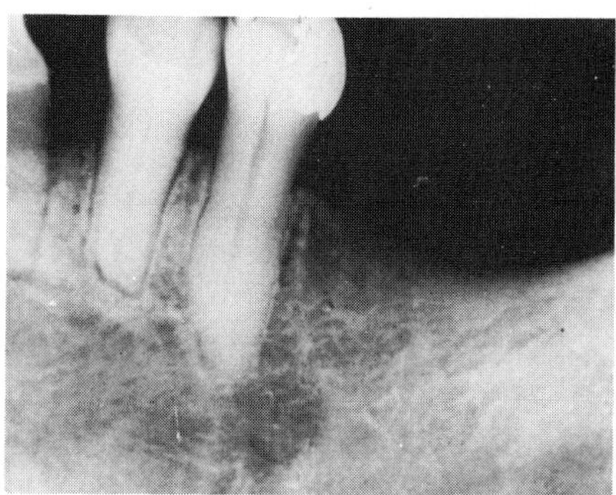

C

Fig. 53.22A A lower occlusal view of a large cyst in a man of 36. This extended from the left second premolar round to the first right molar with mostly only moderate expansion and arose on a dead central incisor.

Fig. 53.22 (B and C) Apical films of the two ends of this cyst at 10 months after operation. The cyst was opened in the labial sulcus below the incisors (marsupialized) and the opening maintained till it had shrunk to a mere dimple. The bone regenerated more slowly but is here shown largely filling the cavity. Many of the vital teeth had their roots truncated by long standing pressure from the cyst but now lamina dura and periodontal membrane shadows have reformed across their root ends.

which develops on an unerupted tooth, usually a third molar (Fig. 53.23). The permanent upper canine, either lower premolar or canine and the lower second molar are less common contenders. The responsible tooth is displaced, pushed away or aside by the cyst which normally includes its crown at least in the cavity. An upper third molar cyst may occupy the whole antrum and the tooth may come to lie close under the orbit before the maxilla is much expanded.

Normal teeth at the antral floor have laminae durae round their roots but when a cyst of dental origin occupies the antrum the roots are partly denuded. Concurrently the thinned antral walls have less substance and less pattern because the cancellous bone has been eroded away by the expanding cyst (Fig. 53.24). The convex expansion will often show in a central anterior occlusal film. The occipito-mental view will show opacity of the whole or lower part of the antrum with expansion of its medial or lateral wall (Fig. 53.25). The cyst arises beneath the antral muco-periosteum and so its rounded upper margin is often partly outlined with bone.

The *primordial cyst* is much less common and develops in place of a tooth and without any inflammatory cause. Most usually it arises in the lower third molar and angle region of the mandible and occasionally it is multicystic. It shows minimal expansion as a rule, has a well-defined margin, and is often found by chance.

A proportion of the developmental cysts, primordial and dentigerous, show hyperkeratosis of the lining squamous epithelium. These hyper-keratotic cysts have a strong tendency to recurrence.

Expansion by all these cysts in the mandible is outwards in the body of the bone but also lingually with further enlargement. Behind the third molar, however, the inner side of the bone is expanded first by odontogenic cysts and lateral expansion comes later. This

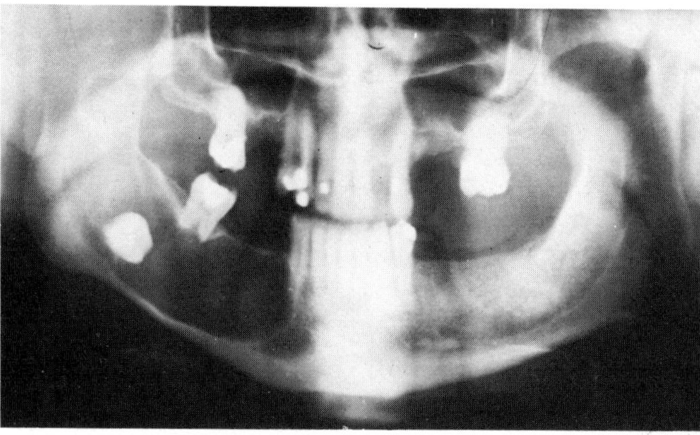

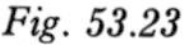

Fig. 53.23

Fig. 53.23 A large dentigerous cyst containing the lower right third molar in a man of 52. It extends from the canine region nearly to the sigmoid notch and the lining was of keratinizing squamous epithelium.

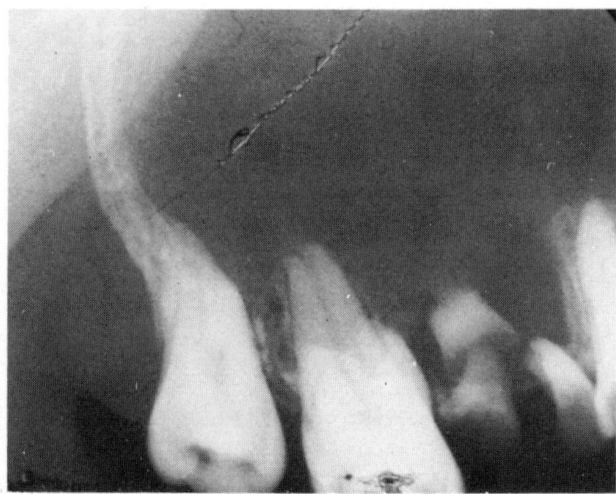

Fig. 53.24

Fig. 53.24 A large periodontal cyst expanding the antral space and arising on the carious first molar roots. The pressure of the cyst has denuded lamina dura from part of the roots of the other teeth and the line of the normal antral floor has gone.

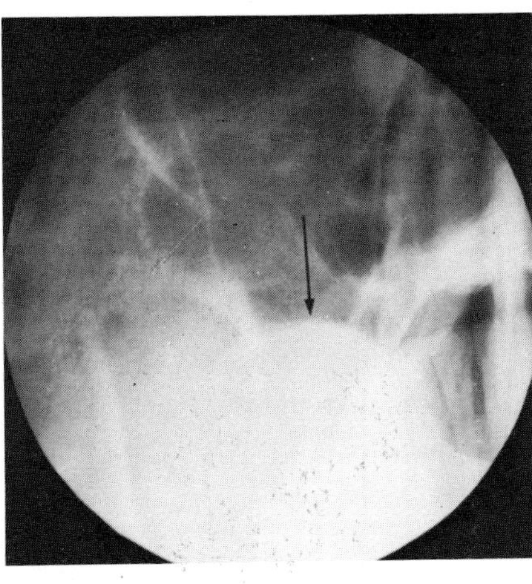

A

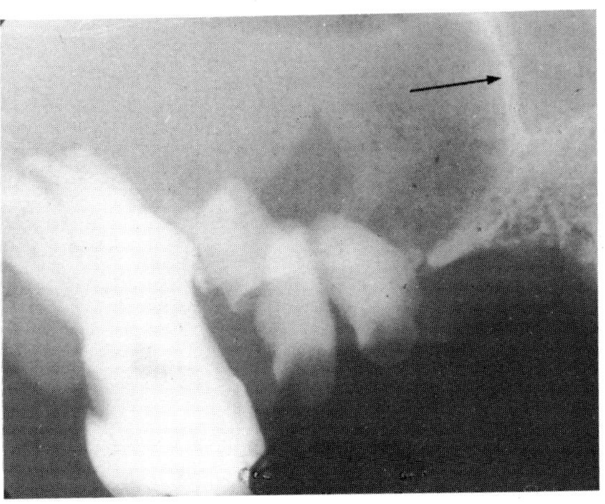

B

Fig. 53.25A The right antrum in an occipito-mental film with a dental cyst in its lower half. The lower lateral maxillary wall has been destroyed by the cyst expanding from the alveolar bone and the mucoperiosteum of the antrum has formed a bony wall between cyst and antral space (arrow). B This cyst arose on the neglected first molar roots and the only antral cavity visible in this film is in the upper right hand corner of the film (arrow).

expansion is best demonstrated by a P.A. film (reversed Towne's) for the ramus and the back of the body of the mandible and by a true occlusal film (Fig. 53.22A) for most of the body.

Some people are more prone to form cysts than others, both infective and developmental. There is marked susceptibility to developmental cysts in Gorlin's syndrome to which there is a familial tendency. This may present in children with multiple dentigerous cysts and there is a liability to other developmental abnormalities. The most severe of these is multiple basal cell carcinomas of the skin of trunk or face. There are often bifid ribs and other minor skeletal or developmental anomalies.

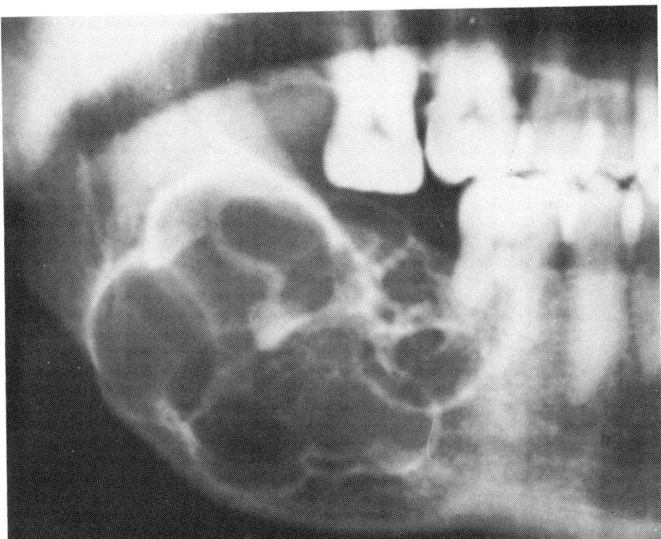

Fig. 53.26 The right side of an orthopantomagraph showing a multicystic adamantinoma in a man of 37. The distal root of the molar has been extensively eroded.

The other important cyst which predominantly affects the lower third molar and angle region is the *cystic adamantinoma*. This is classically multilocular but may be monocystic, and is locally invasive (Fig. 53.26). Expansion of the bone usually calls attention to it and an unerupted third molar may occasionally become involved. The lesion has a sharp margin in the bone but beyond the normal bone contour, the outline is more often incomplete or absent than with a periodontal cyst.

Three types of *non-dental cyst* occur in the jaws. The commonest of these is the *naso-palatine cyst* (fissural cyst) in a fossa astride the median suture of the maxilla behind the central incisors (Fig. 53.27). It is very slow to enlarge, does not involve the teeth and only becomes of significance when it has suppurated. This may not happen until old age when, long after loss of the teeth such a cyst comes close to the gum surface as the alveolar bone of the maxilla shrinks away.

The less common fissural cyst is the *globulo-maxillary* which develops between the upper lateral incisor and canine and is classically pear-shaped when of small or moderate size. If either tooth is dead, a cyst at this site is much more likely to be periodontal, but ciliated epithelium is often found in either of the fissural cysts.

The *simple bone cyst* occasionally occurs in the mandible around the beginning of the second decade (Fig. 53.28A and B), but sometimes appears later on even up to the 30s. There are no dead teeth, it has no epithelial lining and produces only minimal expansion of the jaw. It frequently extends up between the roots of the cheek teeth but often their laminae are largely preserved.

The *mucosal retention cyst* of the antrum may appear in dental films of the upper cheek teeth but is more easily seen in films of the edentulous jaw (Fig. 53.29). It is mucosal in origin and does not involve the bone.

Recognition of the different types of cyst is necessary to avoid condemning teeth which might be saved. It

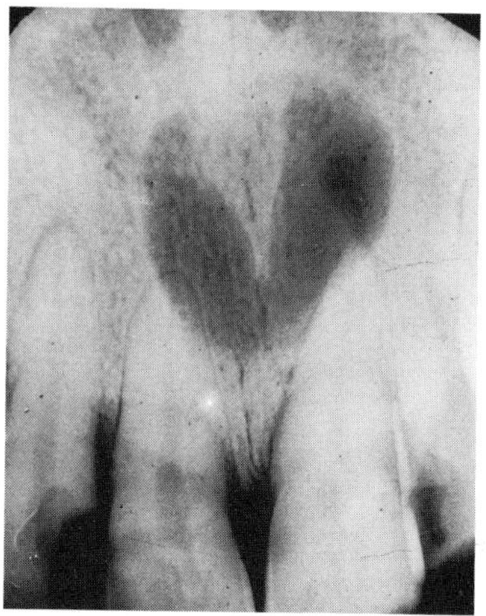

Fig. 53.27

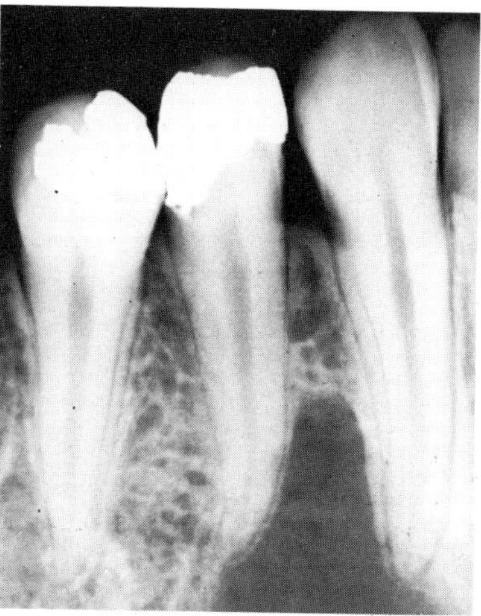

Fig. 53.28A

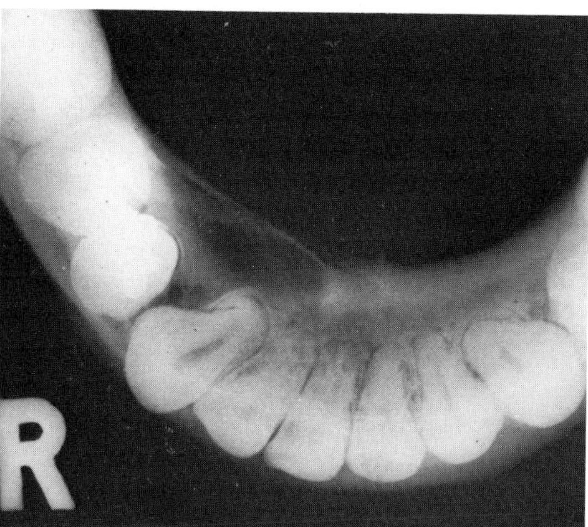

Fig. 53.28B

Fig. 53.27 A typical naso-palatine cyst astride the midline above the upper central incisors. Their lamina dura and periodontal membrane shadows remain intact.

Fig. 53.28A The upper part of a simple bone cyst in the mandible of a girl of 15. It extends up between the teeth and usually thins the lamina dura of sockets though here it is intact. The cyst had remained hardly changed over several years. B The lingual cortex is thinned and expanded and the buccal cortex is less thinned and this accounts for the darkening in Figure 53.28A. The lower cortex of the mandible was also reduced in thickness. A dental cyst would expand buccally first.

should also alert the observer to the possibility that a lesion may be an adamantinoma and so be locally invasive.

NEOPLASMS

The adamantinoma is the common benign neoplasm of the jaws and epithelioma of the floor of the mouth or the gum is the common malignant neoplasm of the region and this may infiltrate the bone. Neoplasms may be classified as follows:

	Benign	*Malignant*
Epithelial	Adamantinoma	Epithelioma
	Adenoma	Adeno-carcinoma
		Metastasis
Mesothelial	Fibroma	Osteosarcoma
	Osteoclastoma	Myeloma

Benign neoplasms

An *adamantinoma* (ameloblastoma) is a solid neoplasm which often becomes cystic and presents as a cystic expansion of the jaw (Fig. 53.26). It is locally invasive so that recurrence after local removal is not uncommon, but it does not metastasize except after repeated surgery. The solid lesion extends very slowly but the cystic one grows more quickly, and this presents with expansion of the

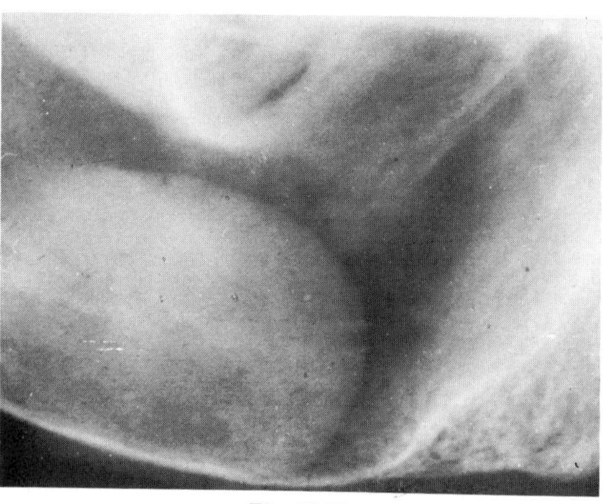
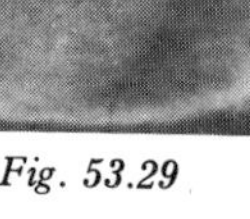

Fig. 53.29

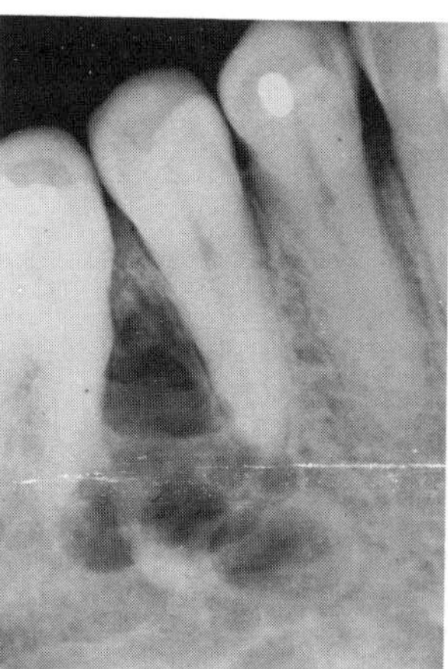
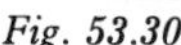

Fig. 53.30

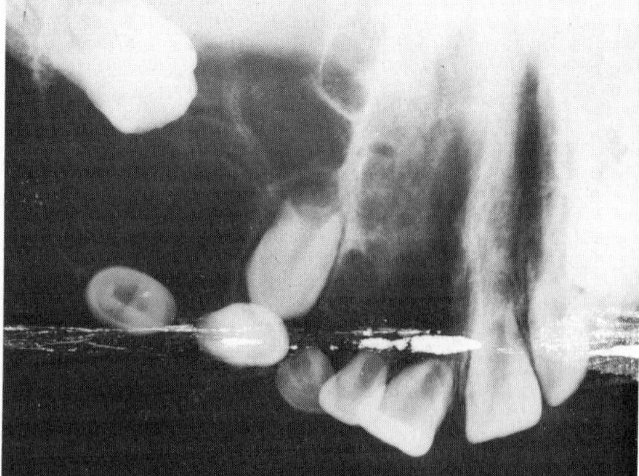

Fig. 53.31

Fig. 53.29 An unusual view of a small mucosal cyst in the large right antrum of an edentulous maxilla. This dental film shows most of the cyst inside the antrum and on its intact bony floor.

Fig. 53.30 A well-circumscribed 'solid' adamantinoma in a woman of 31. There is early erosion of the adjacent tooth roots but the lesion was very slow to change.

Fig. 53.31 An occlusal view of a large giant cell lesion expanding the right maxilla in a boy of 8 which has displaced several teeth.

jaw. Both are very sharply defined in the bone (Fig. 53.30).

The adamantinoma appears as an area of bone replacement or a collection of adjacent small areas with a well-defined margin at the normal bone. Quite dense septa may break up the translucency of the lesion which can look like a group of small cysts. It develops from epithelium derived from the dental lamina which gives origin to the tooth germs and so may arise in either jaw, but it is most often found in the angle or body of the mandible.

A *simple adenoma* or the pleomorphic adenoma (*mixed salivary tumour*) is uncommon in the bone but may occupy the antrum. It presumably reaches either site from the surface mucosa. It appears as a rounded or lobulated translucency when in the bone and the pleomorphic adenoma is prone to recurrence. Cysts can displace teeth in the child's jaw but, if adult teeth are separated by a translucent lesion with no tooth missing, this is strongly suggestive of a solid lesion.

A *fibroma* may be central in the tooth-bearing part of the bone or peripheral, arising on the gum as a pedunculated tumour called an *epulis*. This form is relatively common, and either form may ossify or calcify in part. The central lesion grows very slowly and remains surrounded by a sharp bone margin. The calcified epulis will show up in films. Tooth roots may be eroded by pressure from the solid central lesion and teeth may be moved or separated as it steadily expands.

Some fibromata form dense bone and may be called *fibro-osteomata*, but purely bony lesions are found as projections on the outside of the mandible. They cease to grow when bone growth stops and are better called *exostoses*. A bony prominence on the lingual side in the lower premolar region is the mandibular torus.

A true *osteoclastoma* is rare in the jaws but a giant cell lesion arises in young jaws from 7 years to the early 20s called, after Jaffe, a giant cell reparative granuloma. It is a central soft tissue mass replacing bone and may look clear-cut like a cyst or have a much less well defined margin. It arises in the tooth-bearing part of the jaw, will displace developing teeth and expands the bone (Fig. 53.31).

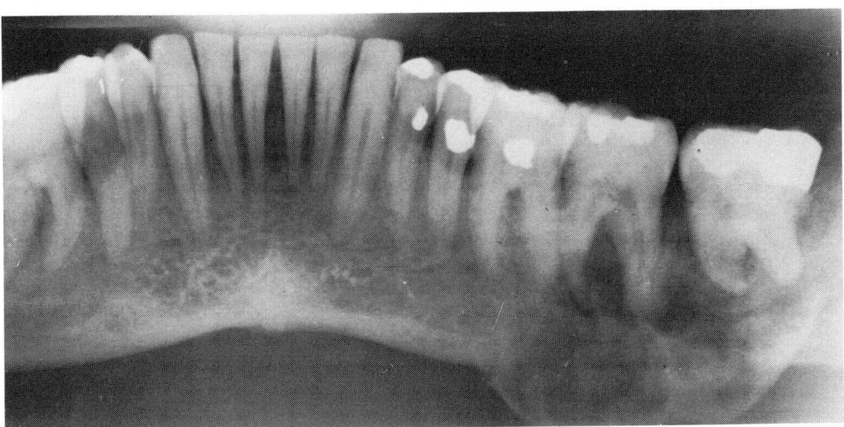

Fig. 53.32

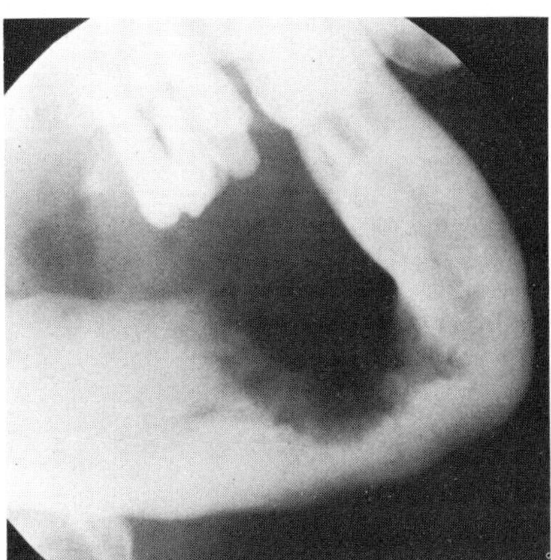

Fig. 53.33

Fig. 53.32 A static panoramic film of a man of 39 who presented with loosening of the lower left second molar and rapid recurrence of calculus deposits round the teeth. There is a giant cell tumour expanding the jaw and the lamina dura is much slighter all round the jaws than normal. He had a parathyroid adenoma.

Fig. 53.33 Typical bone destruction from epithelioma of the gum or floor of the mouth. Many such lesions are adherent to bone and are invading it before X-ray evidence of this is detectable. On the other hand, I have seen half the mandible destroyed when the patient first presented.

Any cyst-like or less well-defined bone-replacing lesion without a clear local cause or explanation may be a manifestation of *hyperparathyroidism*. Although this condition is uncommon, it can present with a local enlargement of the jaw (Fig. 53.32). Apart from such a local lesion, more diffuse mobilization of calcium from the bone in parathyroid hyperactivity may be demonstrated by loss of lamina dura from the tooth sockets and a diffuse, patchy, reduced density of the bone. Small, more discrete areas of bone loss also occur and these are early stages of brown tumours, the giant cell lesions of hyperparathyroidism.

The more generalized severe changes of hyperparathyroidism seem to be secondary to chronic renal deficiency. Localized lesions, even if multiple on a normal basic bone pattern, usually arise from a parathyroid adenoma.

Malignant neoplasms

Epithelioma of the gum, cheek or mouth-floor frequently involves the mandible and rather less often the maxilla. The lesion readily becomes attached to bone, but X-ray evidence of bone destruction by the invading neoplasm is less frequent. The bone destruction has an

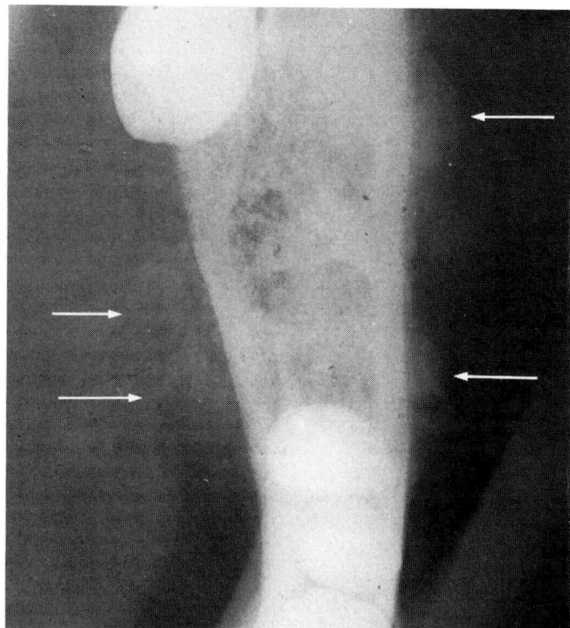

Fig. 53.34 An occlusal view of an osteosarcoma in a man of 36. There was a firm mass surrounding the jaw and soft periosteal new bone extends on the outer side and well across the floor of the mouth (arrows). There was little evidence of bone destruction.

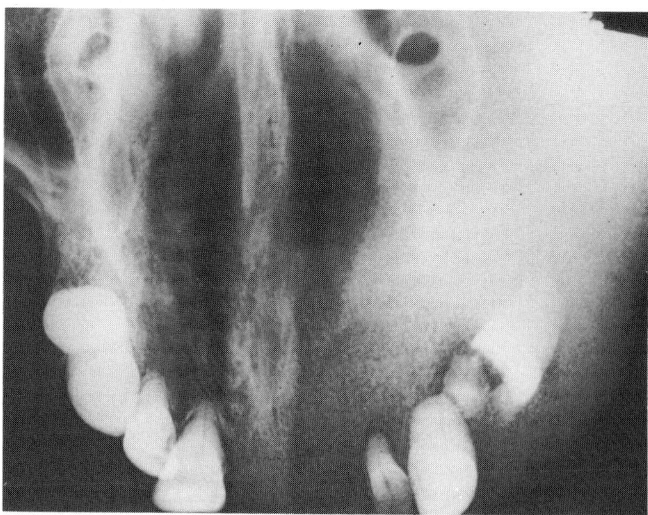

Fig. 53.35 A maxillary occlusal showing enlargement, increased density and a finer than normal pattern in the left half of this jaw. The lamina dura is slighter here because it is replaced by the fine patterned bone but the transition to normal more commonly occurs in the canine region than at the midline. This woman of 51 had had the bony swelling as long as she could remember but attended now with abscesses above her carious roots.

ill-defined irregular margin and can be very extensive or very slight (Fig. 53.33).

Epithelioma also arises in the antral mucosa as does the adenocarcinoma. The radiological manifestations are of bone destruction and air displacement, with swelling, perhaps pain and numbness clinically. Regional lymph nodes may be clinically involved from oral or antral carcinoma making the prognosis poor even when bone destruction is still minimal.

Metastases from a distant carcinoma are rare in the jaws but similar to bone metastases elsewhere. The classical site in the mandible is the angle; bone destruction is apparent radiologically when the cortex is involved.

Osteo-sarcoma is very rare and similar to that occurring in the long bones, except that the patient is usually a decade or so older (Fig. 53.34).

Myeloma is only likely to involve the jaw in the late stages but occasionally presents as an apparently solitary lesion which may occur in the jaws as well as in any other bone. Deposits are clear-cut and often erode the cortex from inside the jaw, as they do in the ribs and other bones.

BONE DYSPLASIAS

There are two bone conditions which occur in the jaws and produce a characteristic local pattern. They are monostatic fibrous dysplasia and Paget's disease.

Localized fibrous dysplasia (regional osteitis fibrosa) occurs typically as an enlargement of one side of the maxilla (less often of the mandible) with an increase in its radio-density. Although bone marrow is replaced with fibrous tissue, in the jaws much new bone is formed as well and the result is a much finer pattern than that of the normal cancellous bone. The lesion is usually homogeneous, fully replacing the normal architecture of the

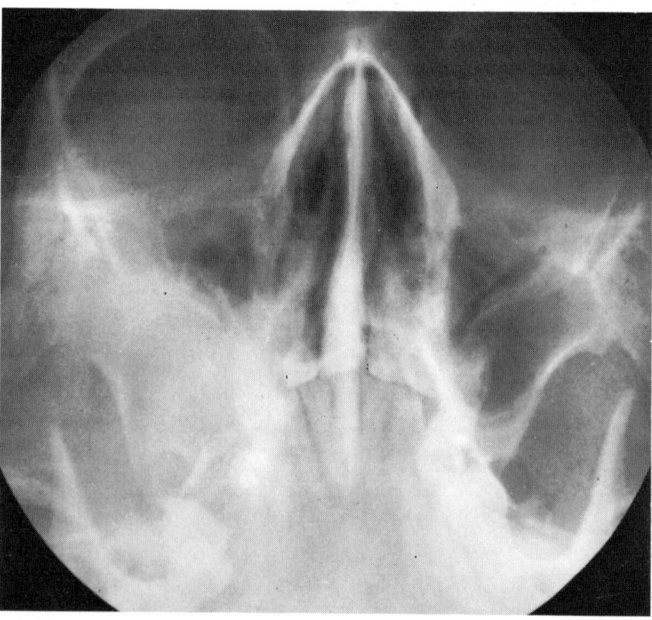

Fig. 53.36 An occipito-mental view of a young adult showing monostotic fibrous dysplasia occupying half the right antral space. There was enlargement outwards also but her dentist observed this before she did.

region and, with enlargement of the affected part of the jaw, the lesion is usually denser than normal (Figs. 53.35 and 53.36).

It arises in the second decade or just before and is painless and easily overlooked, but a developing tooth may be displaced and fail to erupt. Small or moderate-sized lesions are often discovered years later when the dental surgeon finds the gum and the bone are thickened but the phase of active enlargement does not extend much into the third decade.

Paget's disease

Paget's disease (osteitis deformans) is uncommon before 50 years and occurs in two stages. In most regions of the body these are not distinct but they can be so in the jaws and skull. The first stage is osteoporosis and this may occur in the jaws without change in size or shape. Besides the bone being much less dense than normal, it is altered to a much finer pattern. The maxilla is considerably more likely to be affected than the mandible. Usually all the facial bones above the mandible become porotic and the frontal bone may develop osteoporosis circumscripta. By the time these changes are discovered, the second stage is commencing in part of the maxilla and the symptoms calling attention to this, bring the lesion to notice. The patient often has neuralgic pain in the enlarging alveolar ridge of one side and the artificial denture becomes too tight.

With the onset of the second stage in part of the jaw, there is bone enlargement and the development of sclerotic patches (Fig. 53.37). The fine homogeneous pattern all round the maxilla gives place, usually on one side first, to a more irregular patterned and denser bone. Irregular dense sclerotic patches may form on teeth, if any are present, or merely in what had been the tooth-bearing bone.

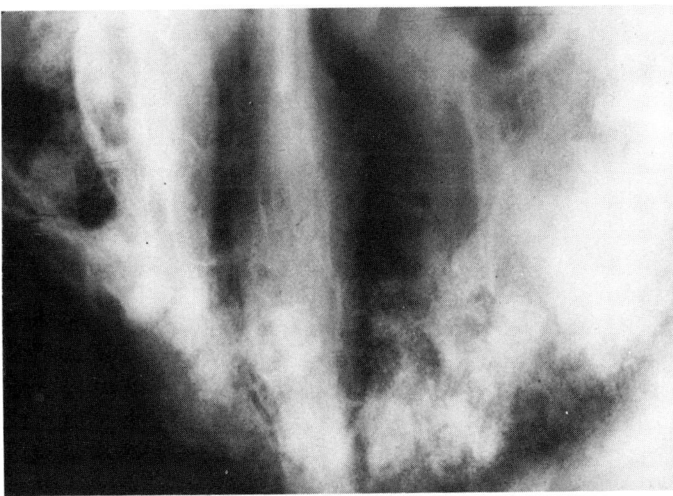

Fig. 53.37 The second stage of Paget's disease in the maxilla of a woman of 54. There is enlargement of the left side of the jaw with irregular dense patches on both sides, more extensive on the left. The bone pattern is fine throughout with no normal cancellous appearance. She had striking osteoporosis circumscripta of frontal and occipital regions.

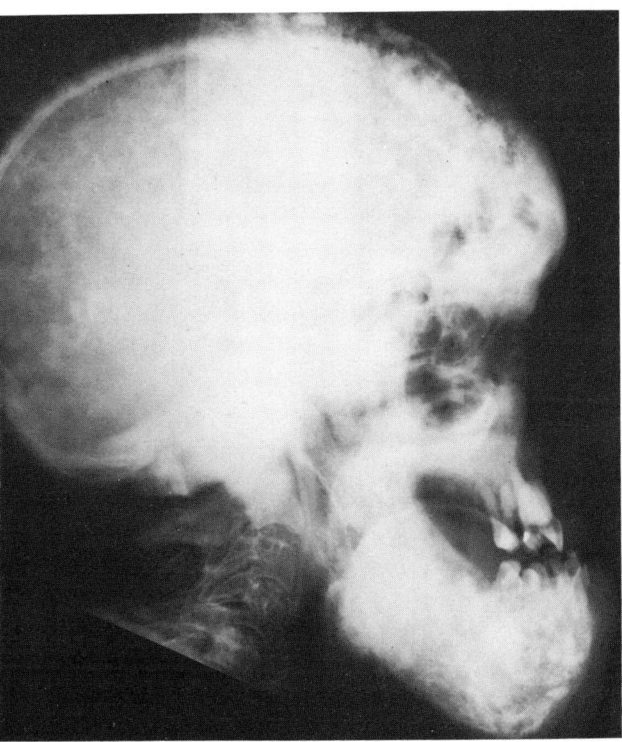

Fig. 53.38 Late Paget's disease of the skull vault and the mandible with the maxilla remaining in the porotic stage. The lamina dura was hardly visible in dental films of the maxilla and lost entirely in the irregular sclerosis of the mandible.

The mandible often remains normal but it may be affected with or without the other bones. Either jaw can become very large indeed as the second stage proceeds (Fig. 53.38).

Of the three complications to which Paget's bone is liable, infection is relatively common and may be the presenting lesion, especially in the mandible. Fracture and neoplasm are rare in the Paget's jaw, but infection from a recent socket, from a dead tooth or perhaps from a denture ulcer finds little resistance in the abnormal bone. A large sequestrum is likely to form and to separate slowly.

REFERENCES AND SUGGESTIONS FOR FURTHER READING

Berry, E. & Silver, J. (1976) Pyorrhoea as cause of pyrexia. *British Medical Journal*, **2**, 1289–1290.

Ingram, F. L. (1965) *Radiology of the Teeth and Jaws*. 2nd edition. London: Arnold.

Stafne, E. C. (1969) *Oral Roentgenographic Diagnosis*. 3rd edition. Philadelphia: Saunders.

Worth, H. M. (1963) *Principles and Practice of Oral Radiological Interpretation*. Chicago: Year Book Medical Publishers.

CHAPTER 54

THE SOFT TISSUES

Every radiograph has a soft tissue component and it is important to pay due attention to this. Careful examination of the soft tissue shadows reveals a wealth of information and helps to avoid numerous traps. Unfortunately, soft tissue shadows are frequently over-exposed on films taken to show bone detail, and it should therefore be an invariable rule to examine such films with a bright light if the soft tissues are over-exposed. Soft tissue detail may be better demonstrated by reducing kilovoltage by about 15 kV. A convenient method of obtaining a similar result consists in placing a non-screen film on top of the ordinary X-ray cassette. A single exposure suitable for the screen film will usually provide acceptable soft tissue detail on the non-screen film without further irradiation. A more sophisticated method for X-raying soft tissues has been described by Deichgräber and

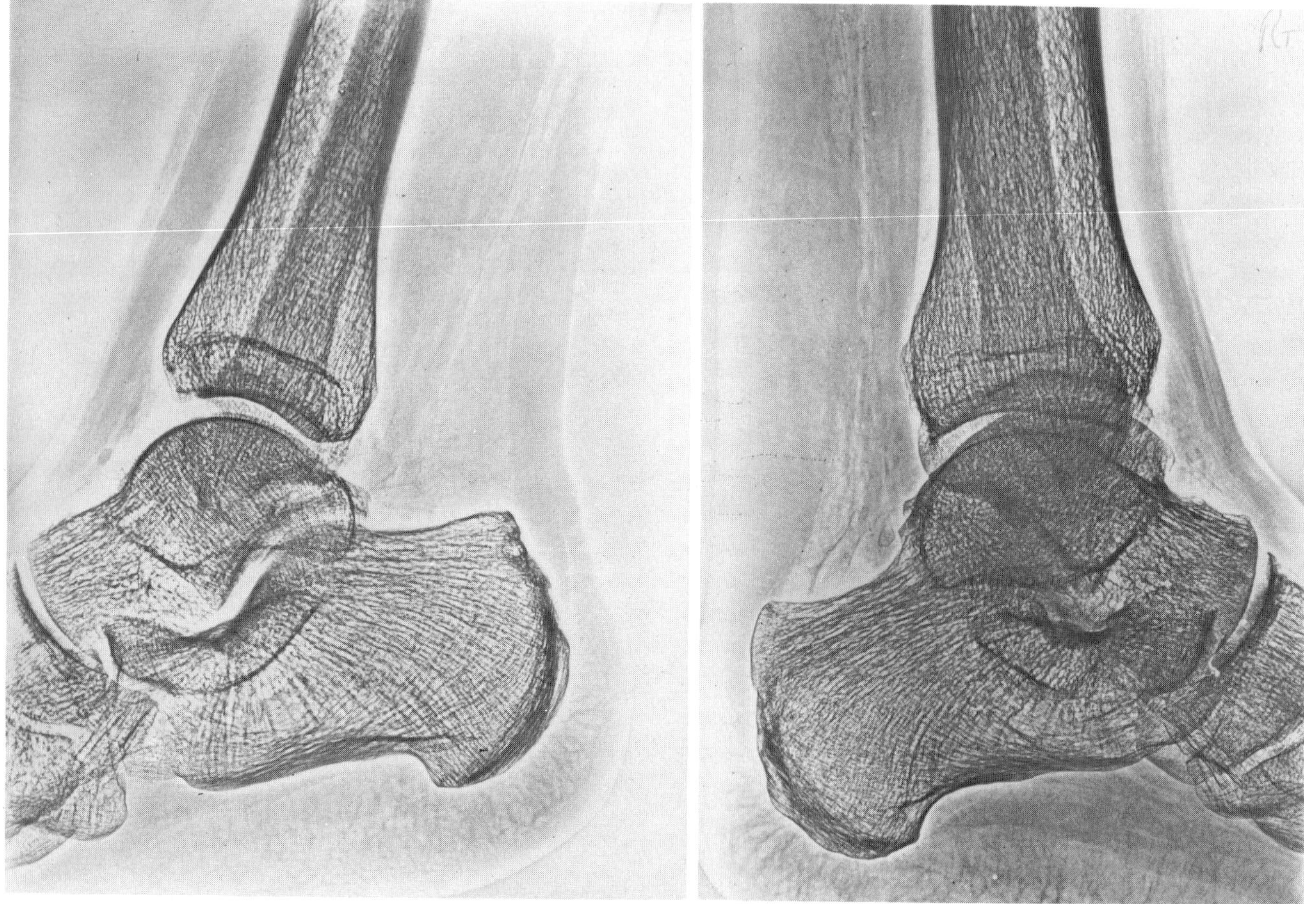

Fig. 54.1A Xerogram of normal ankle. Note intact tendo-Achilles and well preserved fat space. B Partial rupture of tendo-Achilles.

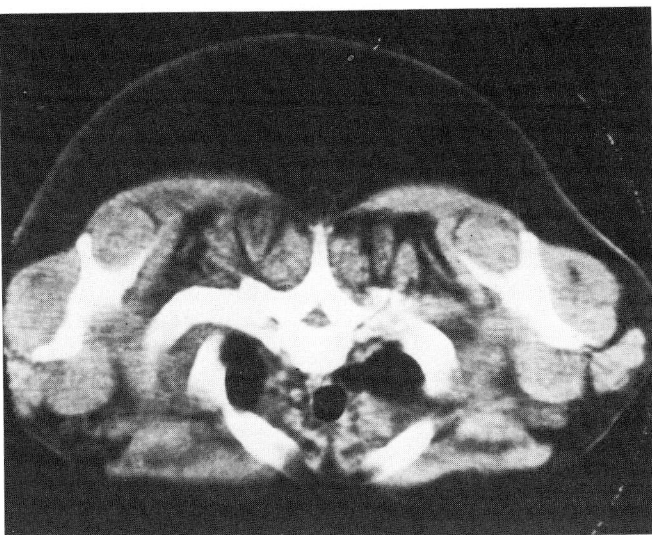

Fig. 54.2 CT scan through lower abdomen. The patient is lying prone. There is a very large lipoma on the back.

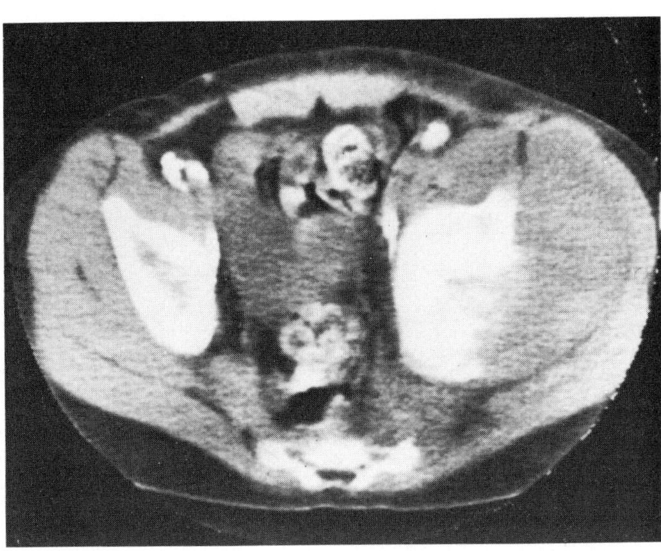

Fig. 54.3 CT scan of upper pelvis. The patient has a Ewing's tumour of the ilium with a large soft tissue component.

Olsson (1975), who applied a modification of a mammographic technique for examining the shoulder and were able to obtain useful diagnostic information.

In recent years two further techniques have been used for this purpose—*xeroradiography* and *computerized tomographic scanning*. Their full contribution has yet to be evaluated.

Xeroradiography is suitable for soft tissue radiography because fine contrast differences are well brought out by the edge effect which is such a characteristic of the xerogram. The advantages have been described by Wolfe (1969). The application of xerography is illustrated in Figure 54.1 (A and B), which shows the appearance of a normal fat space above the os calcis (A), compared with the oedema found after partial rupture of the tendo-Achilles (B). The long head of the biceps is another situation where tendon rupture is not infrequent and where xerography would be useful, but it can also be more widely employed to explore soft tissues.

Computerized tomographic (CT) scanning is even more recent, but clearly will play an increasingly important role. Weinberger and Levinsohn (1978) have reported on CT scanning in the diagnosis of tumours in the thigh and found that it added substantially to a more precise histologic preoperative diagnosis and to accurate anatomic localization. The method is capable of showing subcutaneous tumour nodules as well as deep masses. Figures 54.2 and 54.3 show a superficial lipoma on the back, and the soft tissue component of a deep-seated Ewing's tumour arising from the ilium, respectively.

The radiologist should be aware of various misleading appearances which can be produced by soft tissue shadows. In the chest a pneumothorax may be simulated by a *skin fold* in tiny infants. The *sternomastoid muscle*

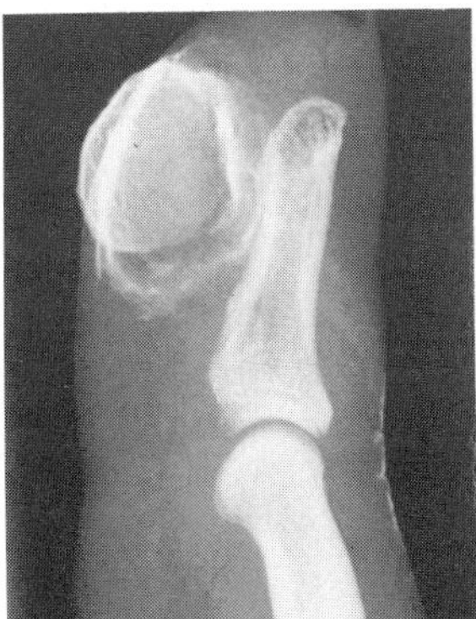

Fig. 54.4

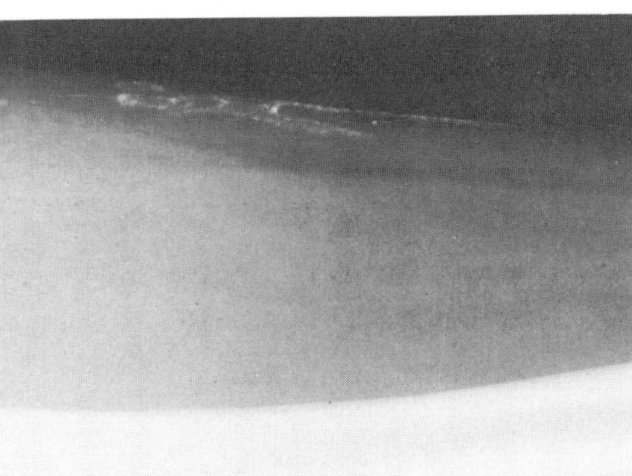

Fig. 54.5A

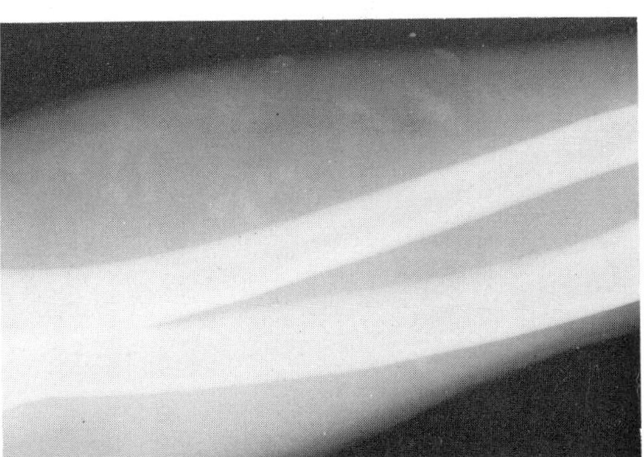

Fig. 54.5B

Fig. 54.4 Silver nitrate paint on wart.

Fig. 54.5 (A and B) Mercury and iron compounds in pigments used for tattooing forearm.

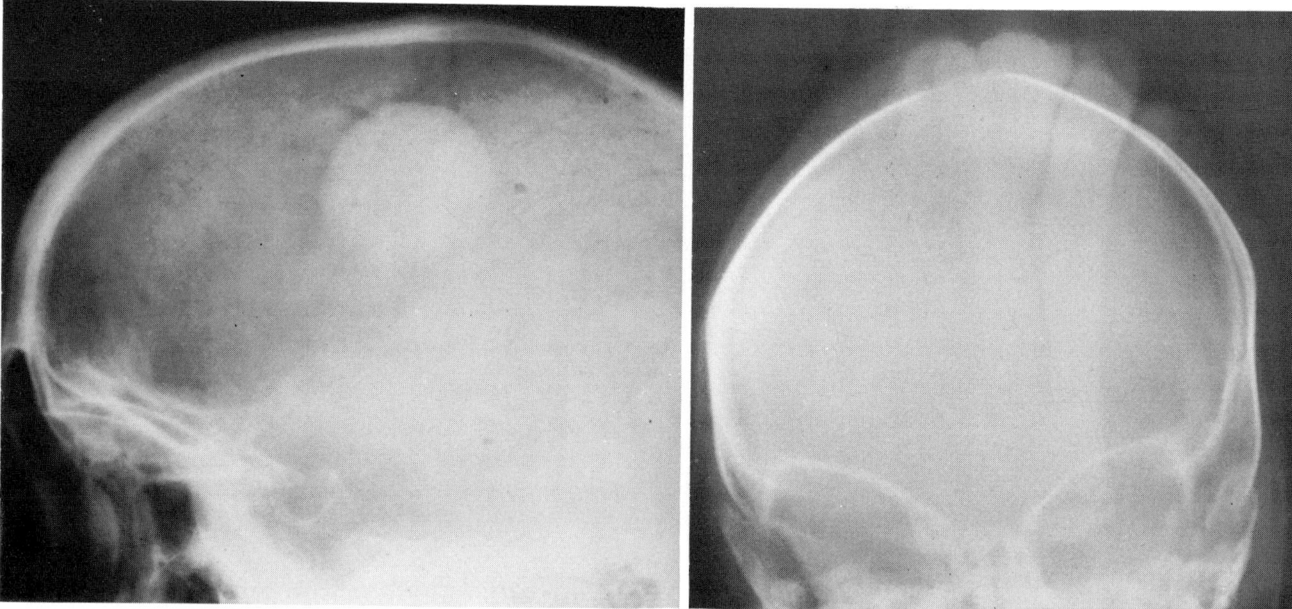

Fig. 54.6 Sebaceous cyst.

Fig. 54.7 Wrinkled skin over skull of a new-born baby.

sometimes produces an opacity over a lung apex, but a more common difficulty is caused by the *nipple shadows.* These shadows are usually bilateral and are found below the anterior end of the fourth and fifth rib; when only one is seen, it may cause real difficulty in interpretation. If in doubt, the patient should be re-examined after metal markers have been placed over the nipples. This particular problem is encountered more frequently in male patients, but the heavy shadows which may be cast by the female breasts raise their own problem by obscuring the lung bases. These can be demonstrated by a heavily penetrated chest film or by elevating the breasts before repeating the radiograph. Incidentally, when examining a 'female' chest radiograph, the radiologist should always make certain that both breasts are present. Marked breast development is seen in men receiving oestrogens in the treatment of carcinoma of the prostate. It also occurs in men with cirrhosis of the liver due to defective break-down of oestrogens, and rarely in male patients with carcinoma of the bronchus.

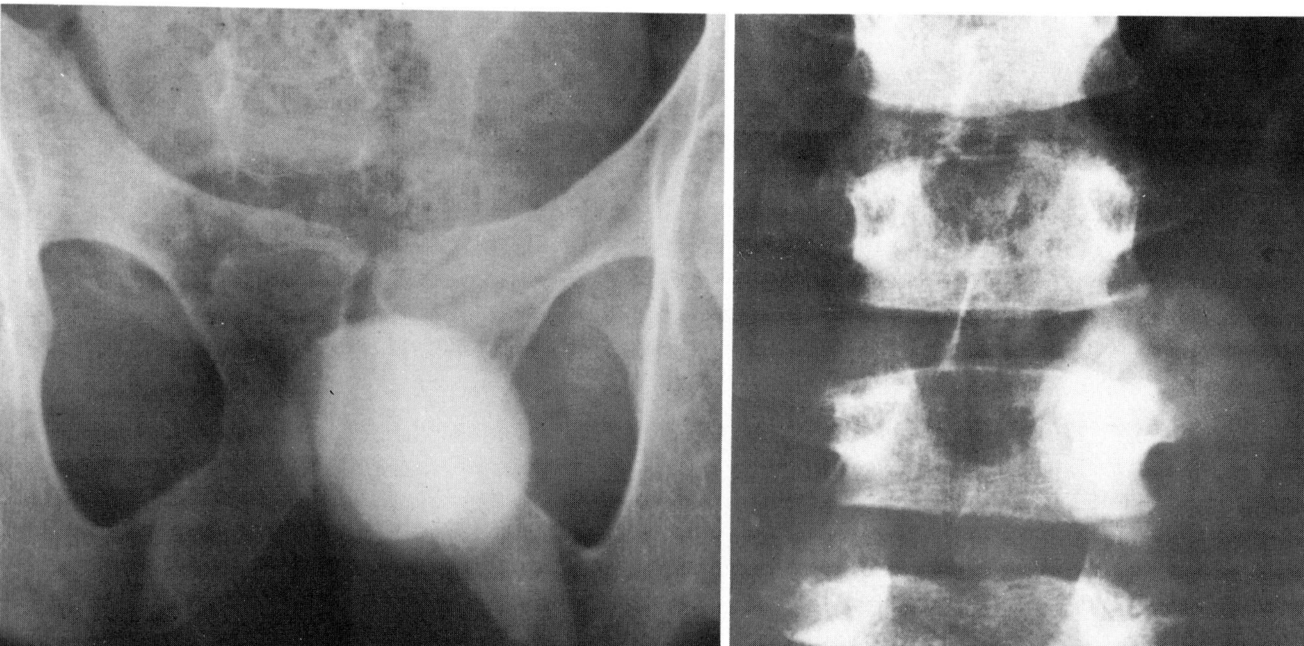

Fig. 54.8 Shadow of penis over lower pelvis.

Fig. 54.9 Round shadow to the left of the spine is due to a colostomy.

Apart from nipple shadows, various *skin tumours* on the chest may cast shadows over the lung field and, before making a diagnosis of a pulmonary abnormality, the radiologist should make certain that an opacity is not due to an extra-pulmonary mass. This mistake is not only highly embarrassing, but could easily lead to an unnecessary thoracotomy. Numerous such opacities may be seen in cases of *multiple neuro-fibromatosis*. A striking, wrinkled appearance of the skin is seen in *congenital ichthyosis*, but this is not of much diagnostic importance. A detailed account of the application of radiology to dermatology can be found in Volume VIII of the *Encyclopaedia of Medical Radiology* (1968). Another trap may be due to the loss of skin. Thus, an ulcer over the medial malleolus can resemble an area of porosis in the lower end of the tibia, and puzzling appearances are caused by traumatic skin evulsion.

Opacities may be due to *substances on the skin*. Lead paint or ointments containing metals or iodine (Fig. 54.4) should be fairly obvious, but the pigments used in tattooing cast shadows which may not be readily interpreted (Fig. 54.5A and B). As so often in radiology, one look at the patient is worth more than any amount of theorizing.

Various errors of interpretation are possible in radiographs of the skull. *Hair* may be visible, particularly when thickly dressed with hair cream; *long hair* may project over the lung apices. *Electrode jelly* on the head after an electro-encephalogram may throw a number of dense shadows and an area of 'increased bone density' may be due to a *sebaceous cyst* of the scalp (Fig. 54.6). The crescentric shadow cast by the *lobe of the ear* on a lateral skull film is well known, but a very puzzling appearance to the uninitiated is caused by *wrinkling of the scalp* in a new-born (Fig. 54.7). Overlapping *folds of skin*, for instance at a flexed elbow, cast dense shadows and a surprisingly dense opacity may be caused by the *glans penis* over the bladder area, resembling a calculus (Fig. 54.8). The cutaneous lip of a *colostomy* is usually well seen (Fig. 54.9) and may be misinterpreted.

FOREIGN BODIES

The recognition of opaque foreign bodies is one of the easiest tasks in radiology, and was amongst the earliest uses of X-rays. Metal fragments show up well and those interested in the forensic aspects of the speciality will find information on the recognition of various types of missile in *Roentgen Diagnosis of Trauma* by Zaztkin (1965). Occasionally, even simple metal foreign bodies may offer a greater challenge to diagnostic acumen. In a case seen by the writer, the diagnosis of drug addiction was first suggested by a film showing several broken needle tips in the soft tissues.

Gravel can frequently be identified in the soft tissues following road traffic accidents. Glass often contains enough lead to render it opaque to X-rays. If a piece of the glass suspected to have entered the body is available,

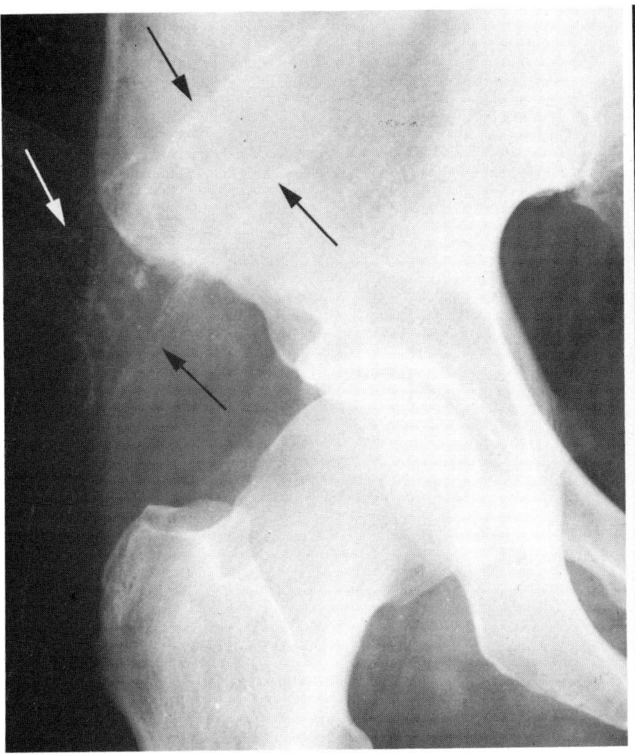

Fig. 54.10 Bismuth injection in buttocks.

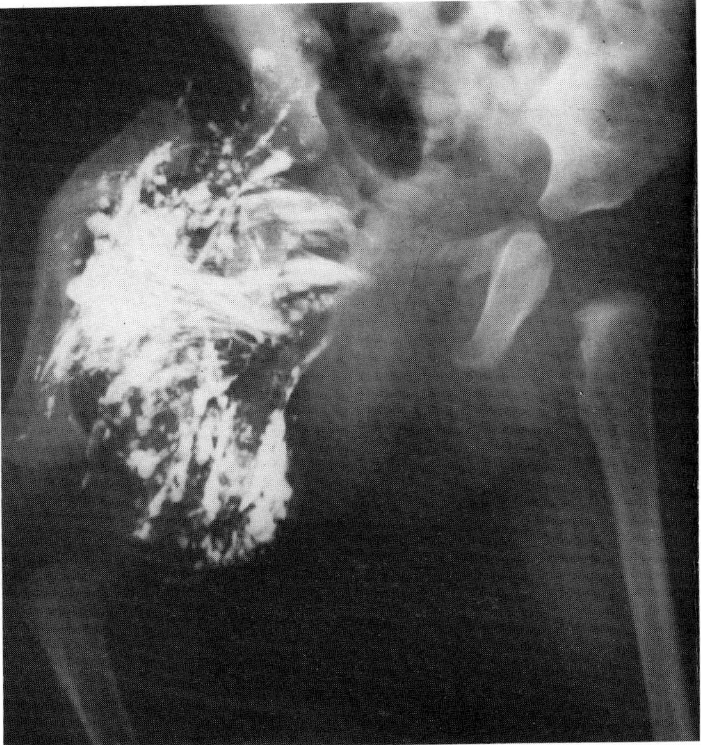

Fig. 54.11 Contrast medium in muscles following a failed arthrogram.

it is sometimes helpful to X-ray it in order to assess its radio-opacity. If it is not opaque, the presence of a similar glass foreign body cannot be ruled out. Wood is not opaque, but may be rendered visible if it happens to be covered with lead paint. Plastic objects are not usually visible.

Localization of a foreign body is a more difficult task. The simplest method, and the one most commonly used, is to obtain two films at right angles to each other. The position of most foreign bodies can be determined in this way. Unfortunately, when dealing with surfaces curving in three planes, for instance the skull and parts of the abdominal wall, films in two planes may not be enough. In such cases a stereoscopic examination may be helpful, provided the radiologist has taken the trouble to train his stereoscopic vision. In Great Britain the method has been largely abandoned, but it is still widely used in the U.S.A. Occasionally tomography may be helpful. Other more complex methods of localization are more rarely used and will not be discussed here.

A practical point sometimes forgotten is the usefulness of having X-ray facilities available in the operating theatre at the time of the attempted removal of a foreign body. Some foreign bodies, particularly needles, may move quite considerable distances due to muscle action or after entering the blood stream. It is therefore a wise precaution to repeat the examination immediately before the incision is made.

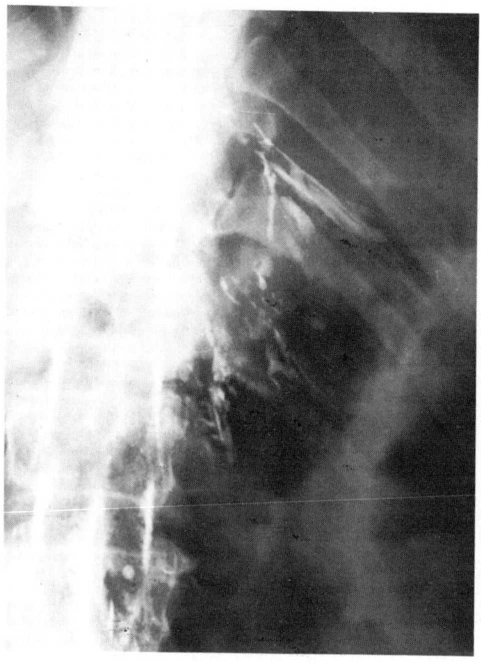

Fig. 54.12

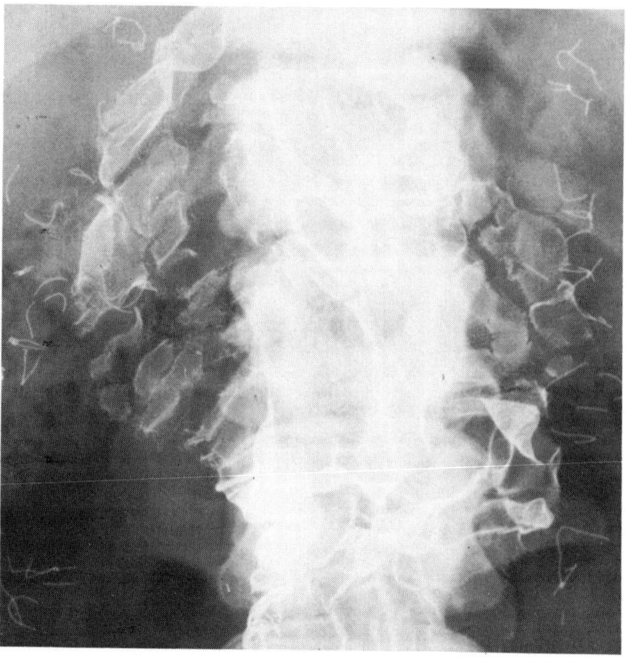

Fig. 54.13

Fig. 54.12 Myodil spreading from theca following a myelogram.

Fig. 54.13 Tantulum gauze used for repair of an incisional hernia. Note fragmented wire sutures which are also present. Fragmentation takes place months or years after the introduction of the suture.

In addition to accidental foreign bodies, a variety of substances may be introduced iatrogenically. Historically, Lipiodol was first used as a treatment for rheumatoid arthritis. Though long abandoned for this purpose, one occasionally encounters patients who have had intramuscular injections of this substance. More commonly, but now in decreasing numbers, one sees patients who have had bismuth injected into the buttocks in the treatment of syphilis; other injections also may leave linear or round opacities (Fig. 54.10). Contrast media are found in the tissues after sinograms; around joints after failed arthrograms (Fig. 54.11); spreading as a number of parallel lines from the spine after injection of Myodil in the course of myelogram (Fig. 54.12). All these substances persist in the tissues for many years after their introduction. A very characteristic appearance of a fine, dense net is caused by tantalum gauze used in the treatment of hernias (Fig. 54.13) and by wire sutures. Thorotrast, once widely used for angiography, is retained indefinitely in the spleen and liver (see Ch. 29).

SOFT TISSUE CALCIFICATION

Arterial. This is a common and almost normal concomitant of ageing. Two forms are recognized: the irregular plaques of *atheroma* and the multiple ring-like calcification of *medial sclerosis* (Fig. 54.14). Arterial calcification is common in the femoral and popliteal arteries and rather less common in the calf vessels; its incidence in this region appears to be higher in diabetics. Arterial calcification is found not infrequently in the carotid artery, but is uncommon in the upper limbs. It is

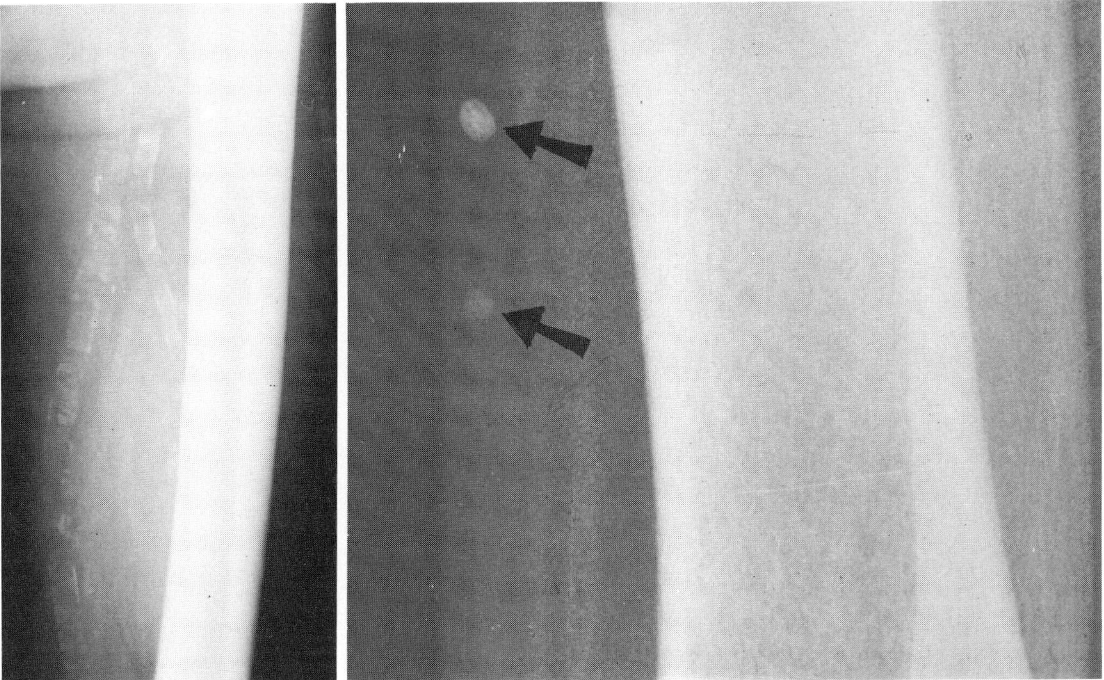

Fig. 54.14 *Fig. 54.15*

Fig. 54.14 Medial sclerosis involving superficial and profunda femoris arteries.

Fig. 54.15 Phleboliths in the soft tissues of the leg.

not a feature of Buerger's disease; occasionally it is encountered in infancy without discoverable cause.

Widespread arterial calcification may be seen in conditions associated with a raised serum calcium, particularly hyperparathyroidism, primary or secondary. It is also a feature of Werner's syndrome, a rare condition associated with premature ageing. Finally, calcification is common in aneurysms in any situation, producing a crescentic opacity which may suggest the correct diagnosis on a plain film.

Venous. It is unusual to be able to demonstrate radiologically calcification in the walls of a vein. On the other hand, calcification in thrombosed veins is extremely common. Usually it gives rise to one or several oval opacities of about 3 mm length, often with a translucent centre. These are known as phleboliths. They are most common in the pelvis in relation to uterine and prostatic veins, but they are also found in the calf in the presence of varicose veins (Fig. 54.15). Rarely, varicose veins may show more extensive calcification (Fig. 54.16), presumably following thrombosis. Phleboliths are common in haemangiomas and may be an important clue to diagnosis when they occur in unusual situations (Fig. 54.17). In addition, these vascular tumours may be visible as a soft tissue mass or a swollen or enlarged limb. Some angiomas which are prominent in childhood tend to disappear as the child gets older, but others persist. Their extent is best demonstrated by angiography, but

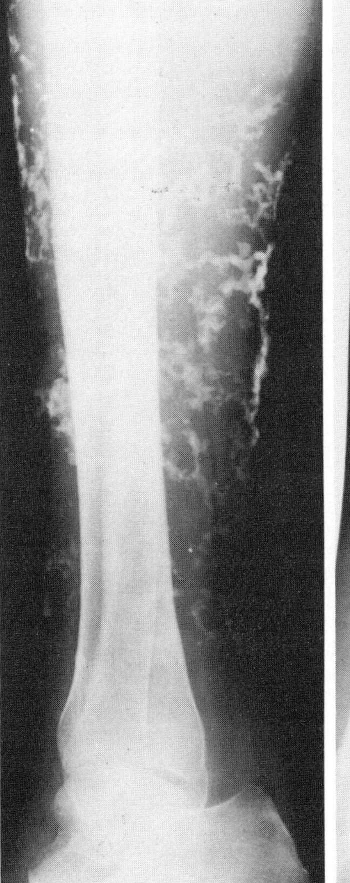

Fig. 54.16

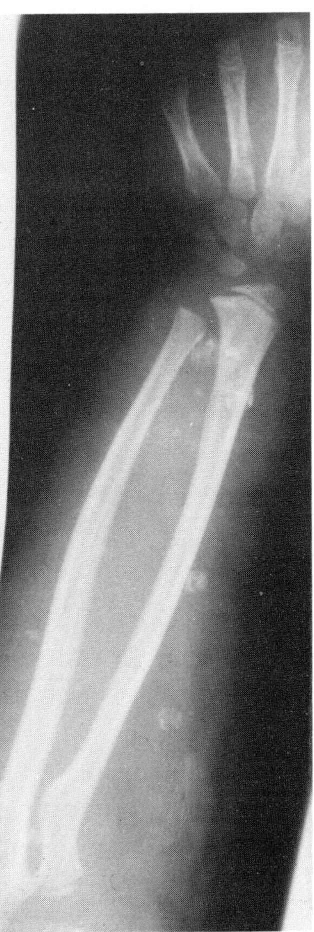

Fig. 54.17

Fig. 54.16 Gross soft tissue calcification complicating varicose veins.

Fig. 54.17 Phleboliths in an angioma in the forearm of a child.

some cavernous angiomas, because of the slow rate of flow through them, appear surprisingly 'avascular', unless the supplying vessels are injected quite selectively, when their extent is often unexpected. Accurate delineation of angiomas has become of importance with the introduction of trans-catheter embolization as a form of treatment. Many, because of the complexity of their blood supply, are unsuitable for surgical treatment and the radiologist may be in a better position to treat the lesion than the surgeon, or at least render surgery more feasible. From a practical point of view it is worth bearing in mind that very large angiomas can sequestrate platelets and, by producing a thrombocytopenia, prolong bleeding after an arterial puncture. Haemangiomas associated with multiple chondromas are found in the condition known as Maffucci's syndrome.

Another, uncommon, type of vein calcification occurs in the femoral veins as a band-like opacity delineating these vessels and is the result of previous femoral vein thrombosis. It must not be confused with a rather similar appearance caused by ossification in the sacrotuberous ligament (Fig. 54.18).

Nerves. Calcification in nerves is very rare and has so far only been recorded in leprosy (Fig. 54.19) and in neurofibromatosis.

Metabolic. Any condition associated with a high serum calcium is a potential cause of soft tissue calcification. It may occur occasionally in *hyperparathyroidism* and has been reported in *vitamin D overdosage.*

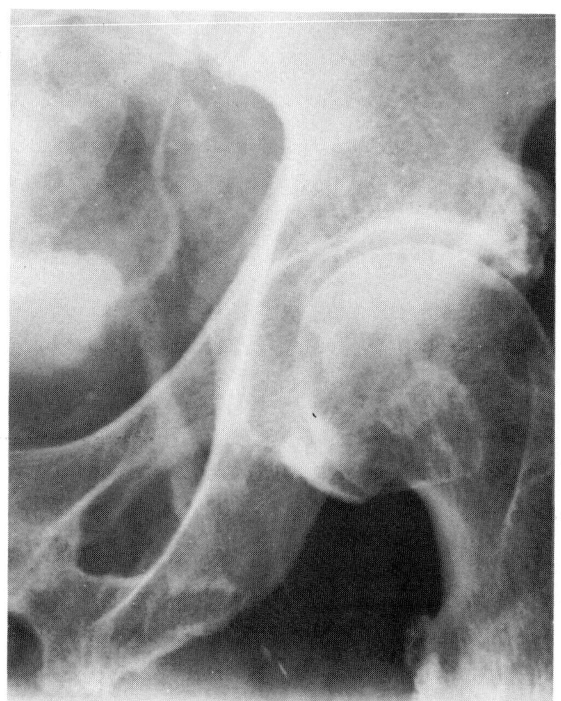

Fig. 54.18 Ossification in the sacro-tuberous ligament. Similar appearances can be caused by calcification in thrombus in the femoral and iliac veins.

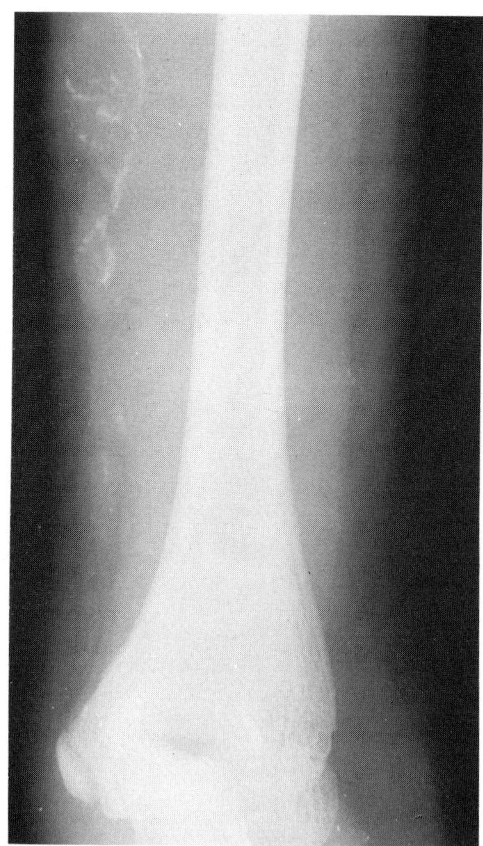

Fig. 54.19 Neural calcification in leprosy.

An important cause of soft tissue calcification is *chronic renal failure* and is seen also in patients on long-term haemodialysis (Fig. 54.20). Calcification occurs particularly round joints and arterial calcification may be a prominent feature. Larger areas of calcification may show layering with changes in body position. These deposits are not necessarily permanent and can disappear with improved treatment. One surprising feature is the difference in the incidence of soft tissue calcification during long-term dialysis reported from different centres round the world. The reason for this is still not clear; one suggested explanation is the difference in the water supply in different areas.

The subject of soft tissue and arterial calcification is complex. Meema, Oreopoulos and de Veber (1976) have made a detailed study of it, and the reader is also referred to *Radiology of Renal Failure* (1976) by Griffiths.

Conversely, soft tissue calcification may be observed in patients with *hypoparathyroidism* and *pseudohypoparathyroidism.* In the latter condition the diagnostic areas are the hands and feet, where soft tissue calcification is associated with characteristic shortening of the fourth and fifth metacarpals and, to a lesser extent, metatarsals (Fig. 54.21).

Calcium urate is deposited in the tophi of *gout* in relation to the peri-articular, punched out bone defects characteristic of that disease (Fig. 54.22). In the ear

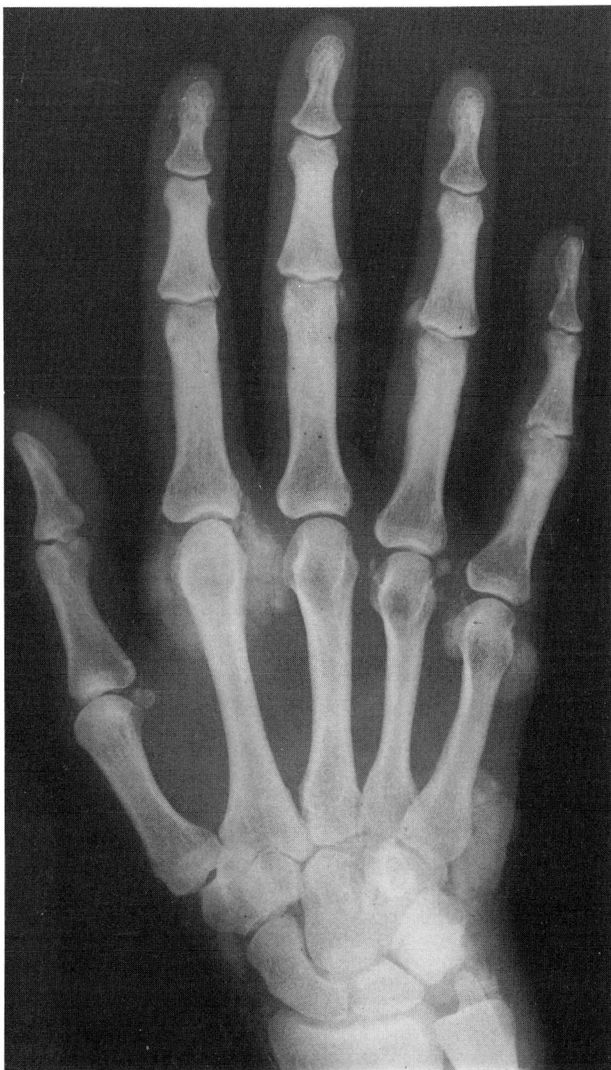

cartilage, calcification occurs in *alkaptonuria* and is some times found in the same situation in *Cushing's syndrome*, *Addison's disease* and *relapsing polychondritis*. It may proceed to ossification (Fig. 54.23). (It also follows *frost bite*—see below.)

Haematomas. Calcification may occur in any haematoma, often circumferentially (Fig. 54.24). It is important and sometimes difficult, to distinguish this appearance from malignant bone disease such as a parosteal sarcoma, particularly when a periosteal reaction is present. An angiogram does not always make the distinction easier, since the capsule of the haematoma is often highly vascular. Close examination of the vessels shows that they do not have the irregularity of outline and arterio-venous shunting that is seen in a malignant tumour. Conversely not all malignant tumours are highly vascular.

Another instance is the *cephalhaematoma*. Shortly after birth a swelling is observed over the baby's skull, usually in the parietal region. This is accurately confined to the limits of the underlying bone. Slowly the swelling regresses, but a radiograph taken about 6 weeks later may show an extensive shell of calcium surrounding the remains of the haematoma. Over the years the calcium shell tends to be absorbed and become invisible. Occasionally the outer table remains irregular for many years and can give rise to a very confusing appearance (Fig. 54.25A and B).

Soft tissue necrosis. Necrosis of the soft tissues is commonly followed by calcification. This takes place,

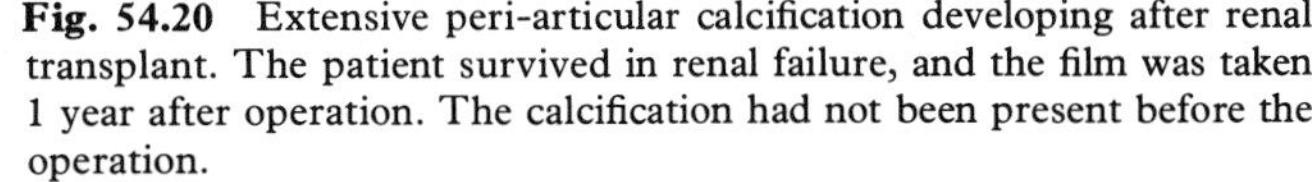

Fig. 54.20 Extensive peri-articular calcification developing after renal transplant. The patient survived in renal failure, and the film was taken 1 year after operation. The calcification had not been present before the operation.

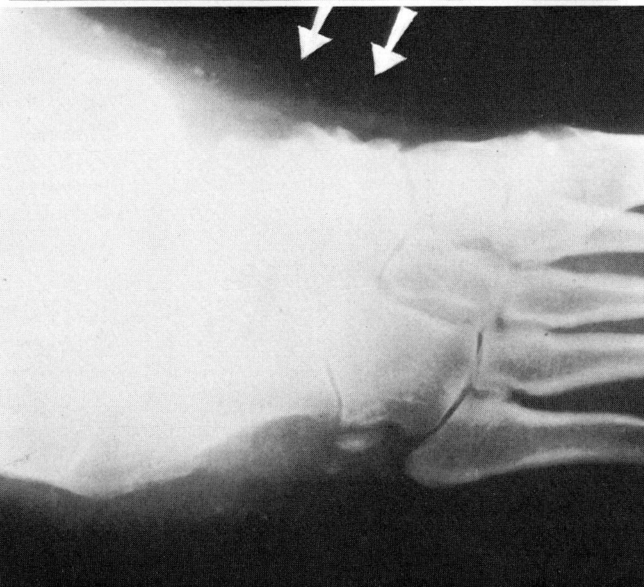

Fig. 54.21 Soft tissue calcification in the foot of a patient suffering from pseudo-hypoparathyroidism.

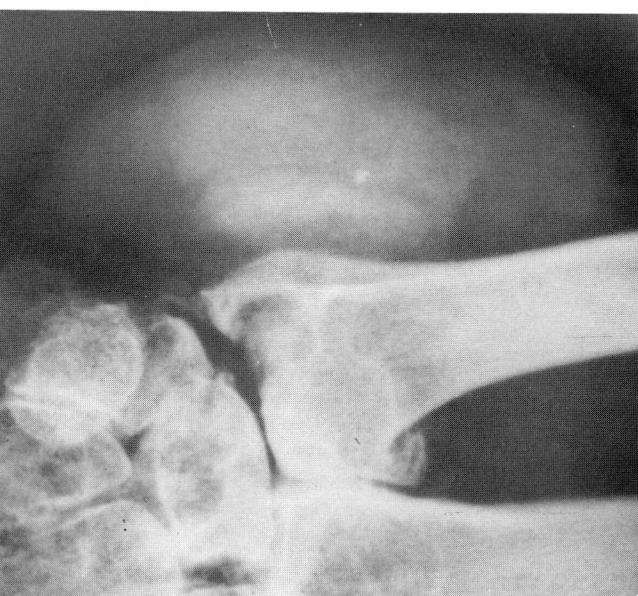

Fig. 54.22 Calcification in a gouty tophus.

for instance, in *tuberculous lymph nodes*, often in the neck, where they must be distinguished from arterial and cartilaginous calcification. Calcification may also follow *intra-muscular injections*; quinine in particular results in oval ring shadows in the gluteal regions, but other injections may have similar results. Tissue necrosis from *frost bite* may lead to calcification—this in fact is the commonest cause of calcification in the pinna. Calcification in the fingers is an important and striking feature of the soft tissue necrosis associated with the Raynaud phenomenon. It is therefore common in patients with *diffuse systemic sclerosis* (*scleroderma*). The calcium deposits are often very dense and sharply localized, particularly near the finger tips and joints (Fig. 54.26). In addition, there may be obvious soft tissue loss of the finger tip or of part of a finger. Rarely, similar calcification is found accidentally in patients with no specific complaints.

Necrosis of subcutaneous fat is probably the basis of the oval, subcutaneous and roughly symmetrical calcification seen in the *Ehlers-Danlos syndrome*. Subcutaneous calcification may also occur in *Christian-Weber's disease* (Fig. 54.27).

Fat necrosis is found round sites of *insulin injections* and in *dermatitis artefacta*.

The most extensive soft tissue calcification, however, occurs in *dermatomyositis* (Fig. 54.28A-C).; in this condition almost the entire body may be encased in a shell of calcium salts which may ulcerate through the skin. This is probably the condition referred to as *calcinosis*

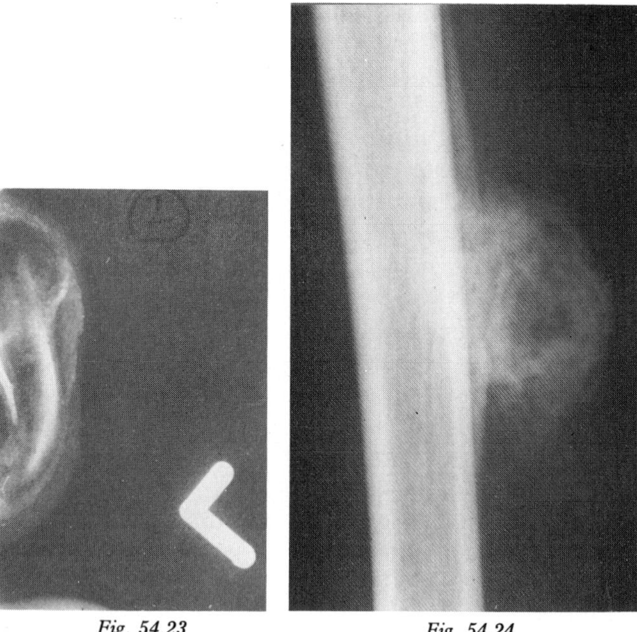

Fig. 54.23 *Fig. 54.24*

Fig. 54.23 Calcification and ossification in the ear in Addison's disease.

Fig. 54.24 Calcification and ossification in an haematoma in the upper arm.

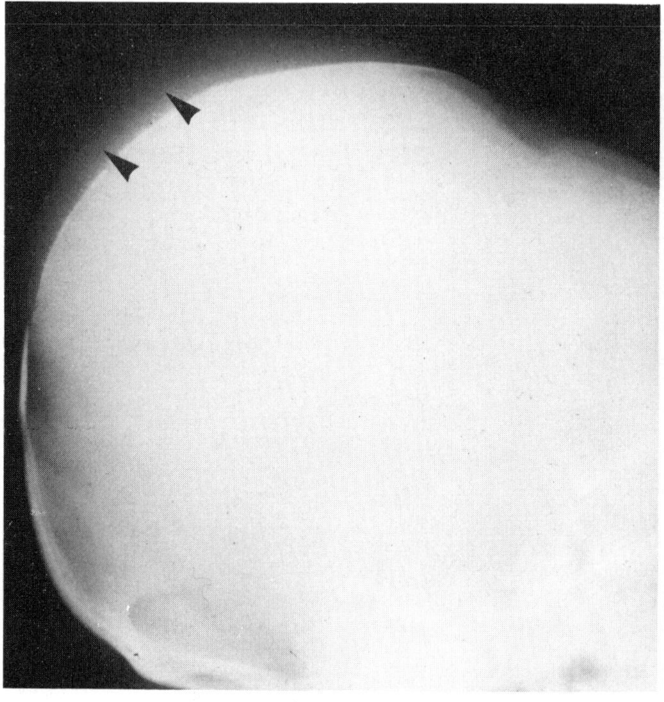

A

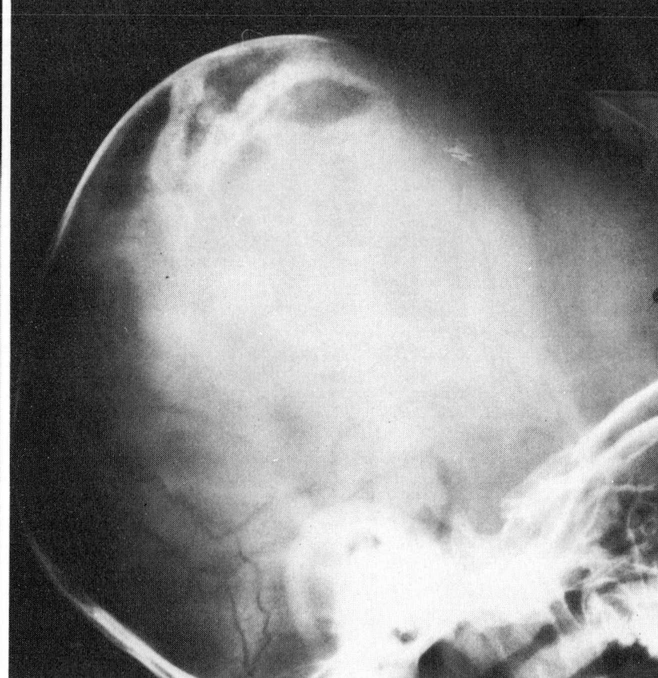

B

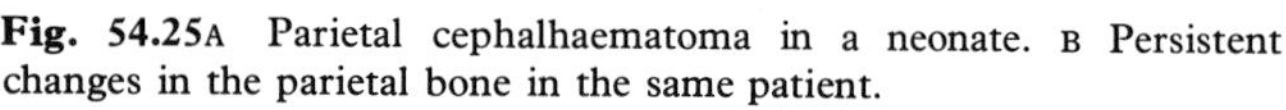

Fig. 54.25A Parietal cephalhaematoma in a neonate. B Persistent changes in the parietal bone in the same patient.

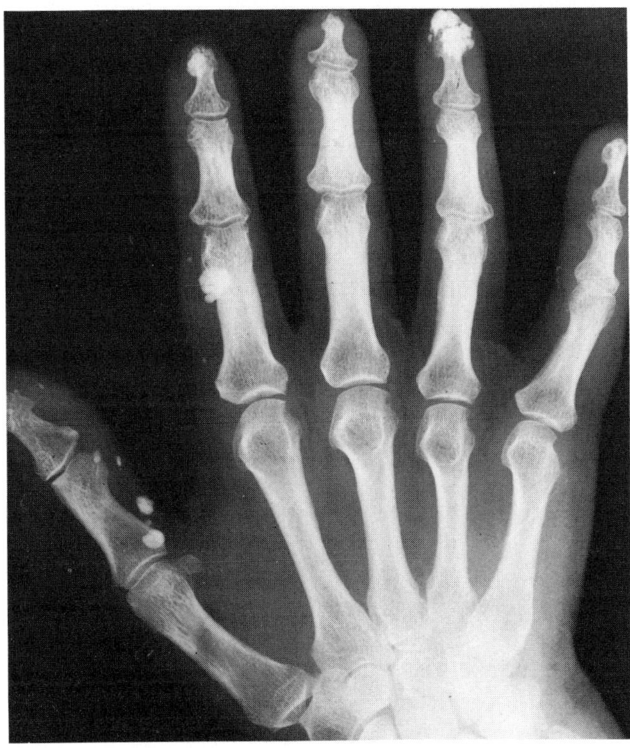

Fig. 54.26

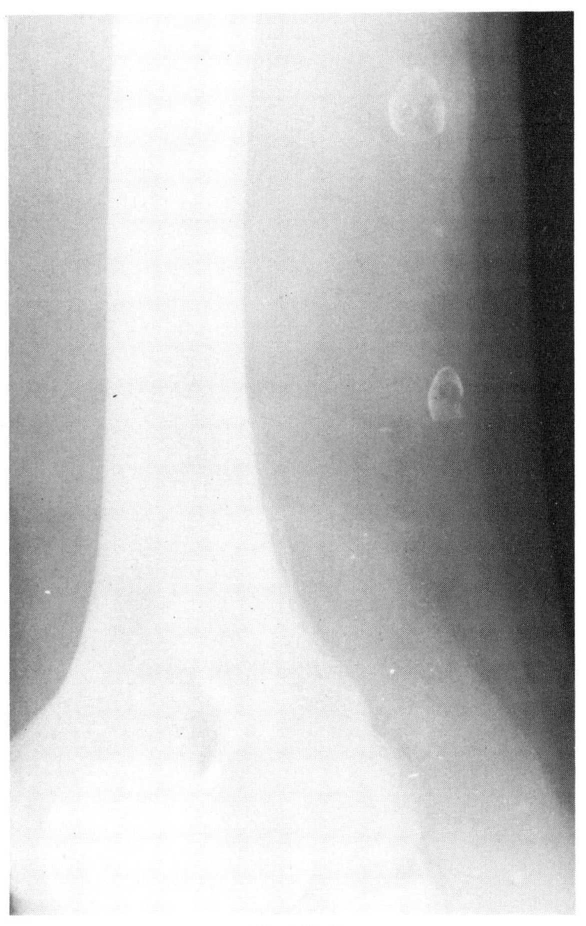

Fig. 54.27

Fig. 54.26 Soft tissue calcification in the fingers in systemic sclerosis. Note also the loss of soft tissues at the tips of the fingers.

Fig. 54.27 Calcification in areas of fat necrosis in Christian-Weber's disease.

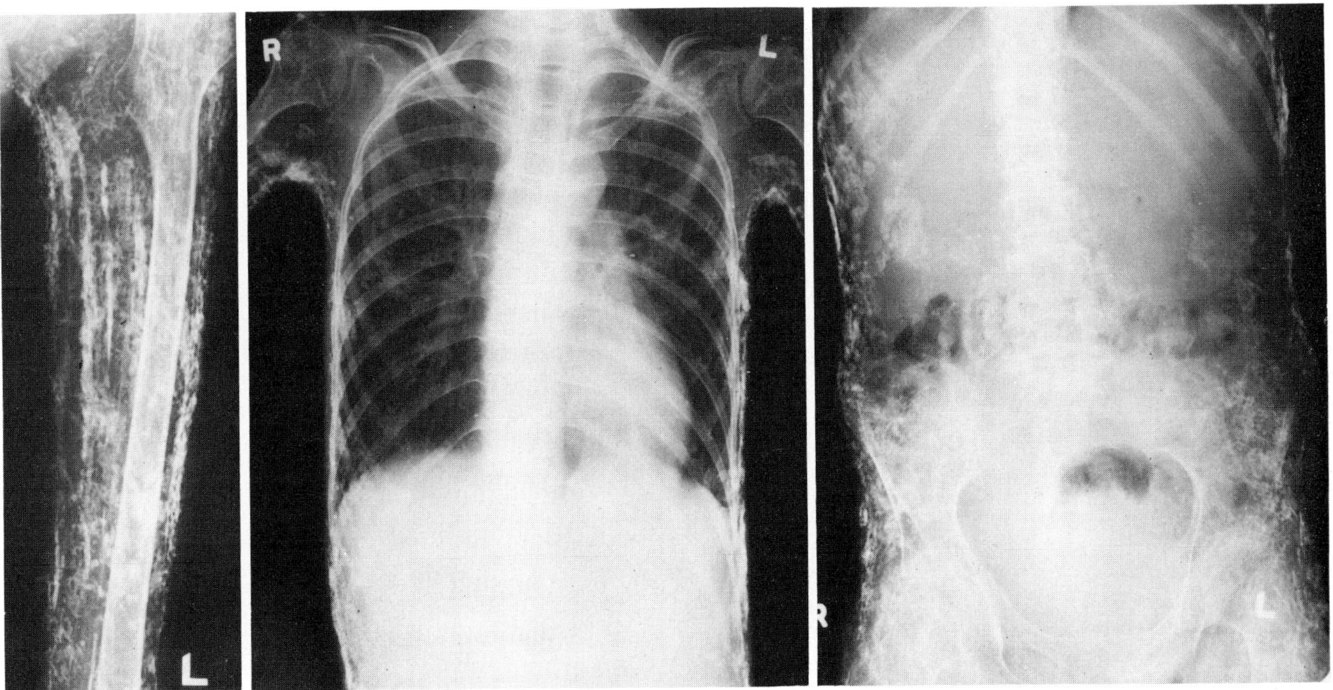

A B C

Fig. 54.28 (A–C) Extensive soft tissue calcification in a 13-year-old boy suffering from dermatomyositis.

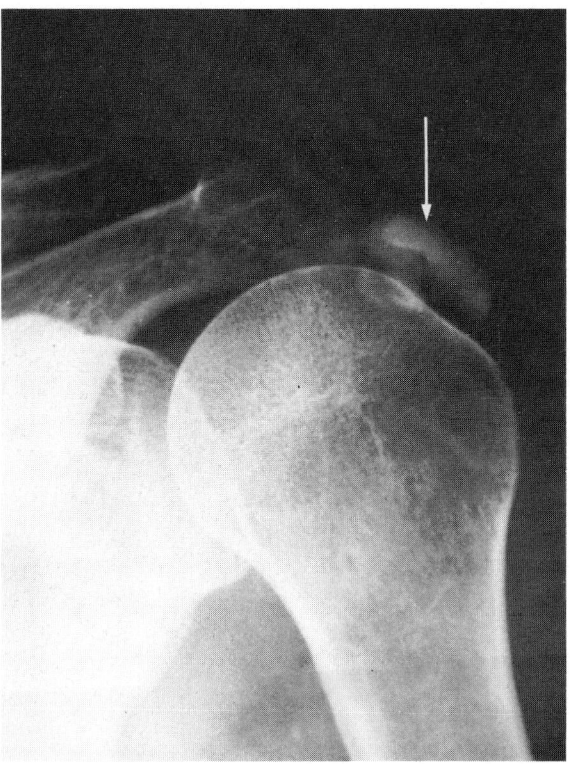

A

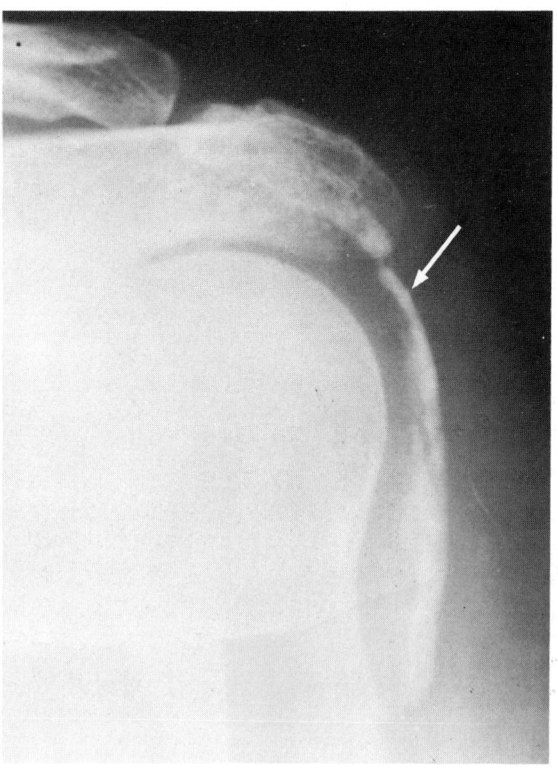

B

Fig. 54.29A Characteristic appearances of calcification in the supraspinatus tendon. The patient had severe shoulder pain. B Same patient; the pain ceased abruptly. The radiograph taken the following day shows that the calcarious matter has ruptured out of the tendon.

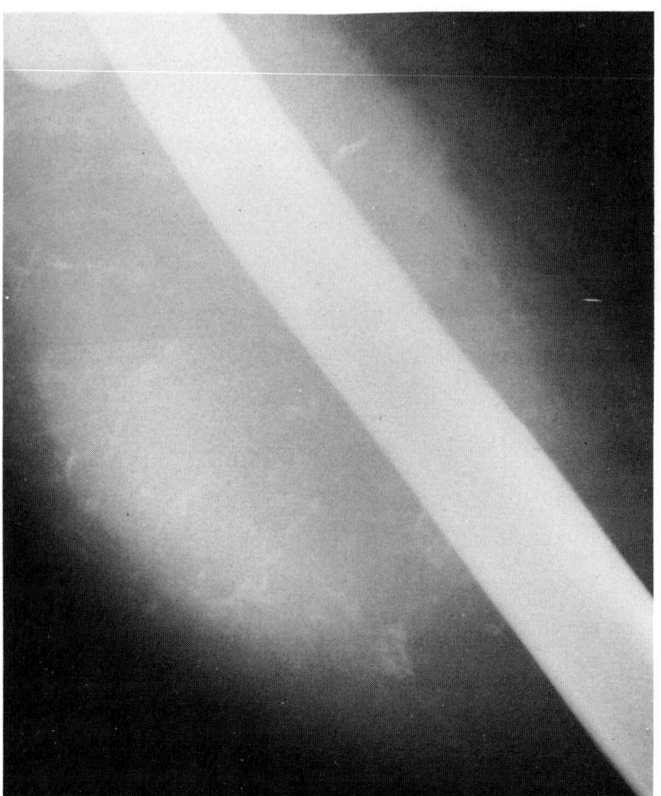

Fig. 54.30 Calcification in a fibro-sarcoma of thigh.

universalis in older text books. The mechanism responsible for calcium deposition is unknown. The disease is rare and it is difficult to gather much experience, but it would seem that extensive calcification is a feature of idiopathic dermatomyositis and is not characteristic of the variety of dermatomyositis associated with malignant disease.

Calcification in tendons. The commonest site is the tendon of the supraspinatus muscle. The cause is unknown, neither is it known why this tendon should be so commonly and almost uniquely affected. The radiograph shows a crescentic, featureless opacity situated above the head of the humerus, its narrow end pointing towards the greater tuberosity. The amount of calcification varies greatly. This lesion is often associated with severe pain in the shoulder; the tendon may rupture and discharge the semi-fluid calcific material into the joint space with instant relief of symptoms (Fig. 54.29A and B). Paradoxically, calcification in the supraspinatus tendon is discovered occasionally in patients with no complaints. It is therefore clear that there is no simple and direct relationship between the calcification and clinical symptoms.

Calcification in tumours. Calcification is sometimes seen in tumours of soft tissue origin. It occasionally consists of irregular, non-specific densities. Its demonstration does not help in deciding on the probable histology of the tumour and, although it is more common in malignant tumours, it is of little value in distinguishing

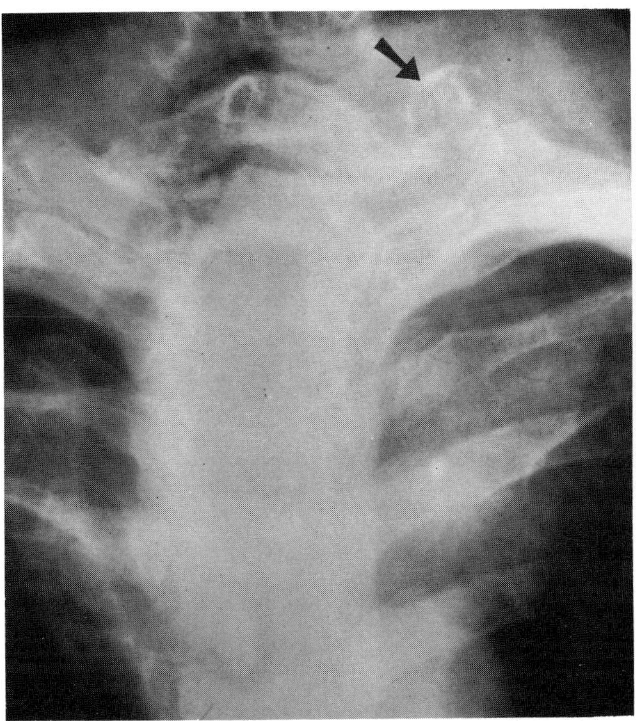
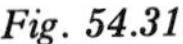

Fig. 54.31

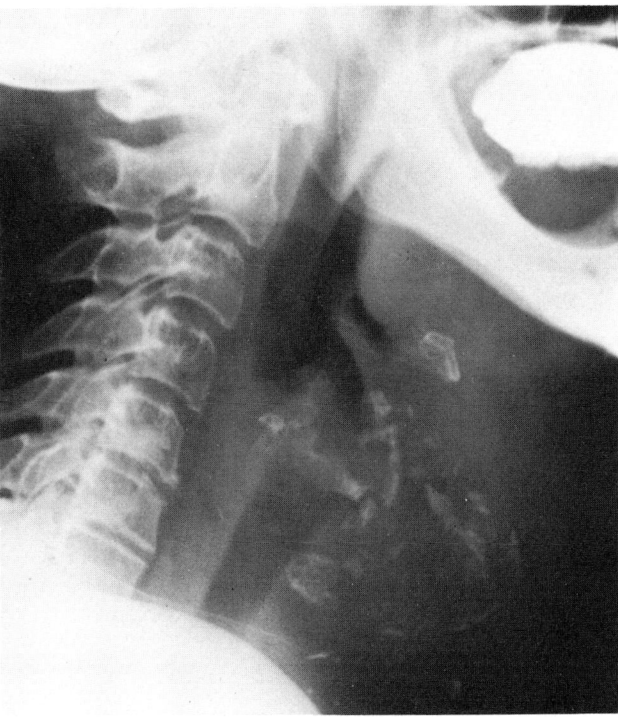

Fig. 54.32

Fig. 54.31 Circumferential calcification in a thyroid adenoma (*arrow*). Note also displacement of trachea to the right.

Fig. 54.32 Irregular thyroid calcification.

between benign and malignant growths (Fig. 54.30). A rather fine type of calcification is said to occur particularly in haemangiopericytomas and medullary carcinoma of the thyroid. Thyroid adenomas often show typical peripheral egg-shell calcification (Fig. 54.31), but sometimes thyroid calcification is quite irregular (Fig. 54.32).

PARASITIC CALCIFICATION

Cysticercus cellulosae. Following ingestion of the ova of *Taenia solium* by man, the embryos develop in the human intestinal tract. They penetrate through the mucosa and enter the bloodstream to become distributed round the body. Some parasites enter muscles, where they may survive for several years in an encapsulated state. When they die, the cysts slowly calcify and only then can their presence be demonstrated radiographically. The calcified cyst produces an oval shadow, 10 to 15 mm long and 2 to 3 mm broad, usually with a translucent centre. The number of cysts varies greatly and may reach the hundreds. If only one cyst is present on a radiograph, its significance is easily overlooked, but the appearance of multiple ones, arranged in the direction of the muscle fibres in which they lie, can hardly be misinterpreted (Fig. 54.33). While the presence of cysts in the muscles is in itself not of great significance, they may be associated with cysts in the brain; the latter only occasionally calcify and are therefore more difficult to demonstrate. Cysticercosis is widespread in the eastern Mediterranean, the Middle and Far East and Australia, but is rarely acquired in the U.K.

Loa-loa (Calabar swelling). This disease is caused by a microfilaria and is common in West Africa. The worm is found in the subcutaneous tissues and may undergo calcification after its death. It is seen most commonly in the hand and produces coiled, thread-like opacities in amorphous calcification (Fig. 54.34). According to Chatres and Cockshott (in *Tropical Radiology*, edited by Middlemiss), this type of calcification is frequently seen in Ibadan, where loiasis is considered to be uncommon and onchocerciasis is common.

Guinea worm *(Dracunculus medinesis)*. This parasite also becomes visible only when it undergoes calcification after its death. It produces an elongated or coiled strip of calcium density (Fig. 54.35). In time this may be crushed by muscular action into a round irregular mass which it is difficult to identify without a proper history. The disease is highly endemic in India, the Middle East and parts of Africa.

Armillifer armillatus. The cyst is curved in one plane and its distribution is confined to the muscles of the chest and abdomen (Fig. 54.36) where the calcification is characteristic. The parasite is a worm-like arthropod living in the respiratory tract of snakes in Africa, but which may be transmitted to man.

One is sometimes requested to X-ray limbs in a search for *Trichinella spiralis*. It is therefore important

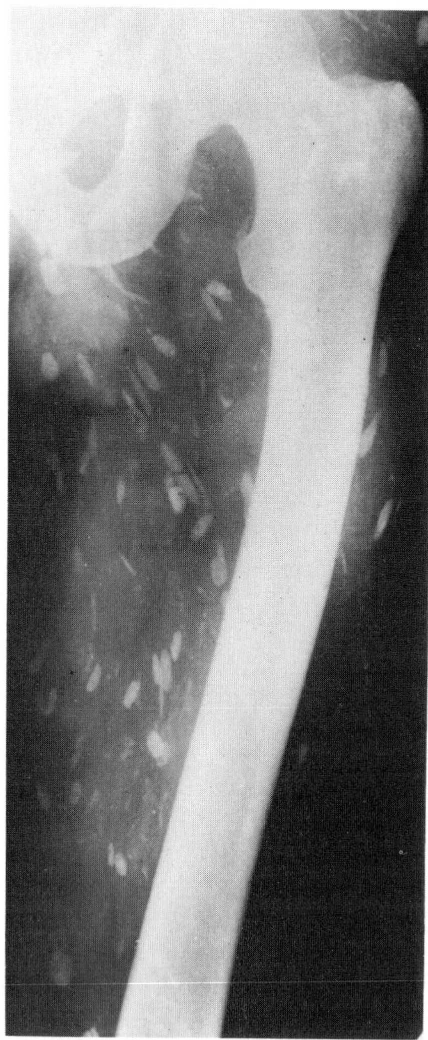

Fig. 54.33 Calcified cysticercosis cysts.

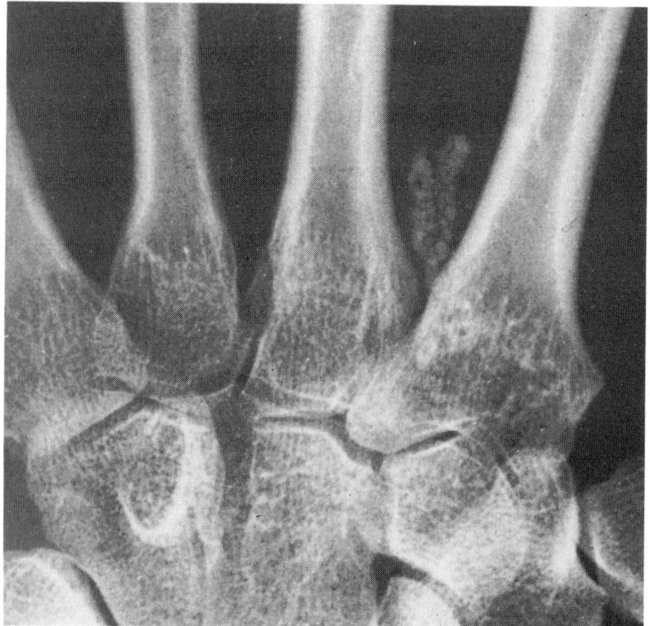

Fig. 54.34 Loa-loa.

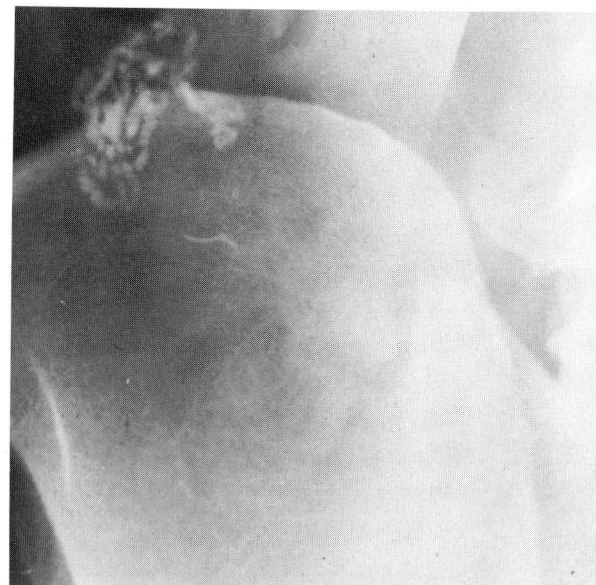

Fig. 54.35 Calcified guinea worm.

to realize that the cysts of this parasite are too small to be demonstrated radiographically.

Ossification in soft tissues

Ossification of various ligaments is seen as a normal phenomenon and must not be confused with the result of disease. It is found not infrequently in the ligamentum nuchae, and rather uncommonly in the ilio-lumbar and sacro-tuberous ligaments in the pelvis.

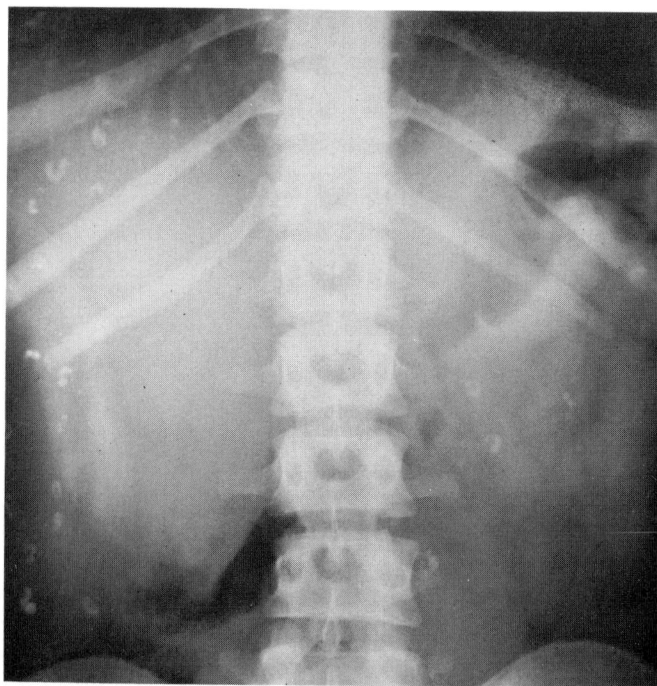

Fig. 54.36 Calcified cysts of *Armillifer armillatus.*

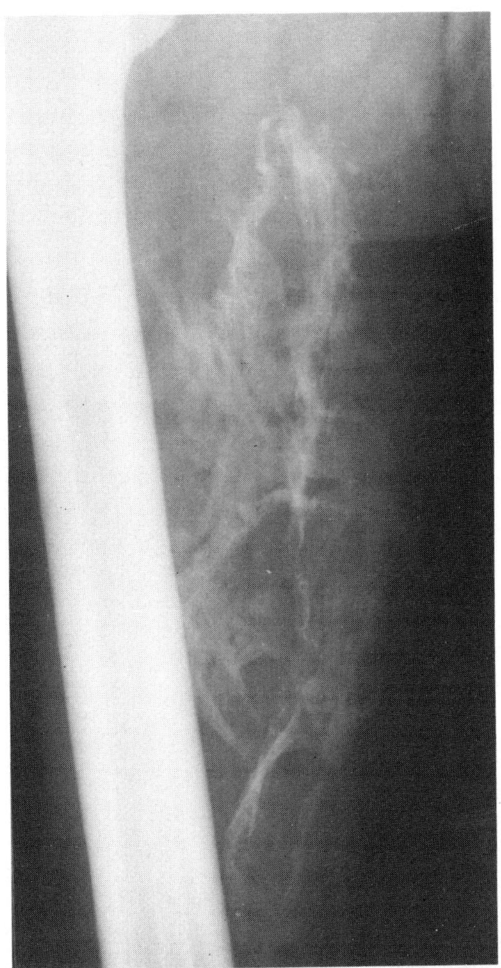

Fig. 54.37 Traumatic myositis ossificans in the medial aspect of the thigh.

Traumatic. Following trauma, usually in association with a fracture, ossification may occur in the soft tissues near the site of the trauma. The amount of bone laid down may be sufficient to interfere with the movement of the limb. The brachialis and quadriceps femoris muscles are especially prone to become the site of traumatic myositis ossificans (Fig. 54.37). It is important that the radiologist recognizes the true nature of the ossification, since histological examination may be misleading; the pathologist may report the presence of a malignant lesion as a result of the very actively growing tissue which he sees under the microscope.

Ossification in relation to joints, most commonly the hips, elbows and shoulders, also occurs after extensive burns. The new bone formation is not a direct result of the burning, since it may develop at sites distal to the injury. The cause is unknown (Fig. 54.38).

Repeated minor traumata may give rise to local areas of ossification, as in the 'rider's bone' in the adductor muscle. Ossification is frequent in the medial collateral ligament of the knee (Pellegrini-Stieda lesion), probably also the result of trauma (Fig. 54.39).

Congenital. Progressive myositis ossificans is a congenital disease quite unrelated to the traumatic variety. Ossification takes place in the fibrous tissues of the muscle planes and not in the muscles themselves. Sheets of bone are deposited in the neck, thorax and limbs (Fig. 54.40), limiting movement severely. The disease manifests itself in early childhood and is usually

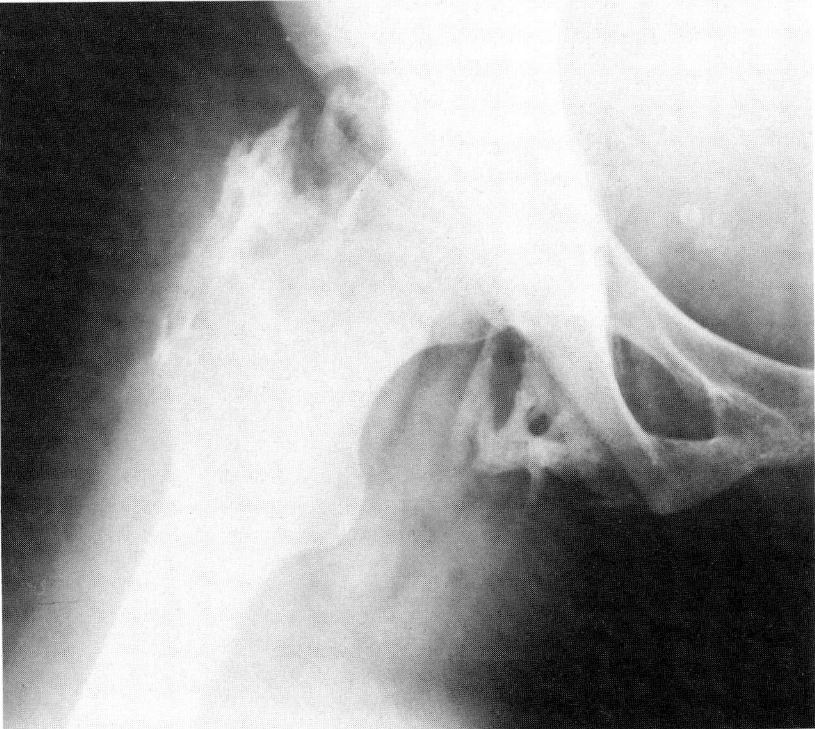

Fig. 54.38 Soft tissue calcification following burns.

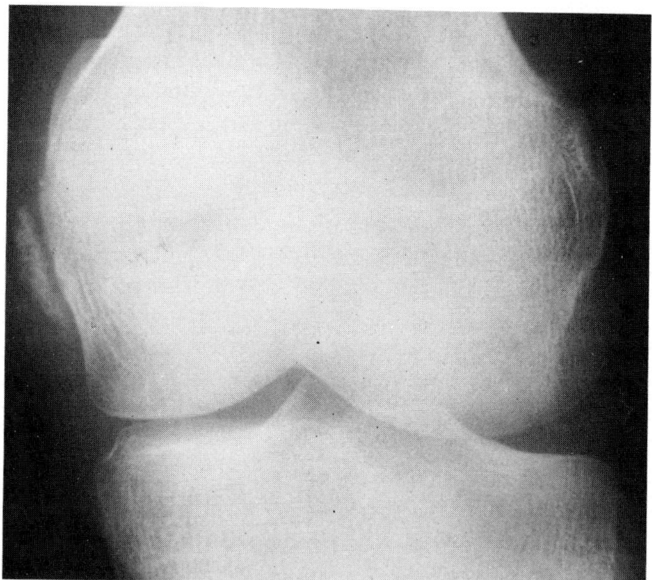

Fig. 54.39 Pellegrini-Stieda lesion.

associated with a mild, but characteristic, skeletal deformity, consisting of a short metacarpal of the thumb and short metatarsal of the great toe (Fig. 54.41).

Paraplegia. Remarkably extensive bone formation in soft tissues is sometimes seen in patients with paraplegia. It occurs in adults with spinal lesions and in children with spinal dysraphism. It is found particularly in relation to the pelvis and the new bone may develop quite rapidly. The abnormal bone has a characteristic woolly appearance: it extends from the normal skeleton into the soft tissues and obscures the normal bone outlines (Fig. 54.42).

A somewhat mysterious condition is *Tumoral Calcinosis.* In this a mass bone is laid down in the soft tissues, often near joints. It is found at any age, and can occur in children. The mass may cause discomfort and possibly limitation of movement, and there is usually no previous history of trauma. It was described, and appears to be more common, in negroes (Palmer, 1966), but can occur in other populations. In a few patients a 'calcium' fluid level in the tumoral mass has been observed (Fig. 54.43).

Heterotopic bone formation. Surprisingly, true bone may form away from any pre-existing bone structure or periostium. This is seen in scar tissue, e.g. after surgical operations.

AREAS OF DECREASED DENSITY

Fat. The transmission of X-rays through fat is somewhat greater than that through muscle. The difference is slight, but sufficient to produce a distinct variation in

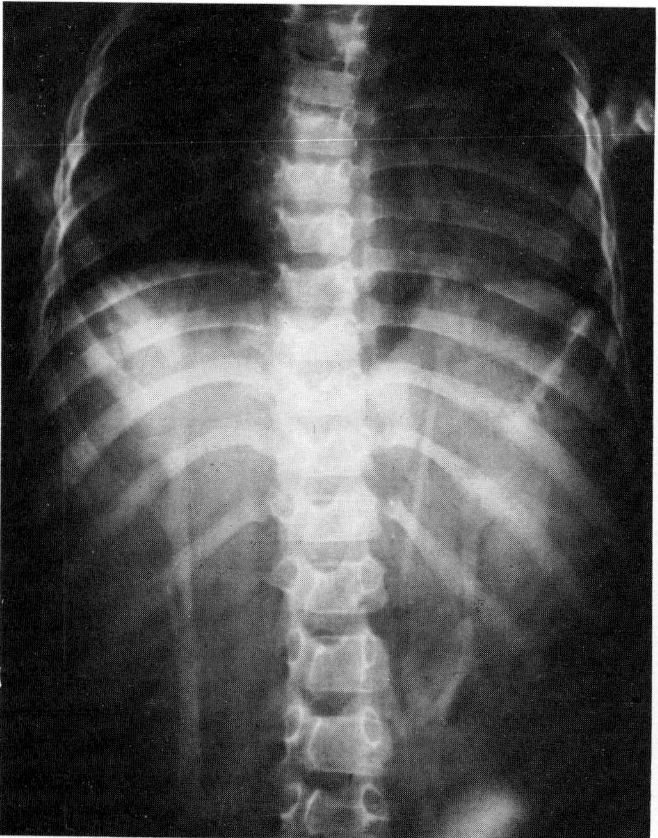

Fig. 54.40 Myositis ossificans congenita. Note bone formation in the soft tissues of the back.

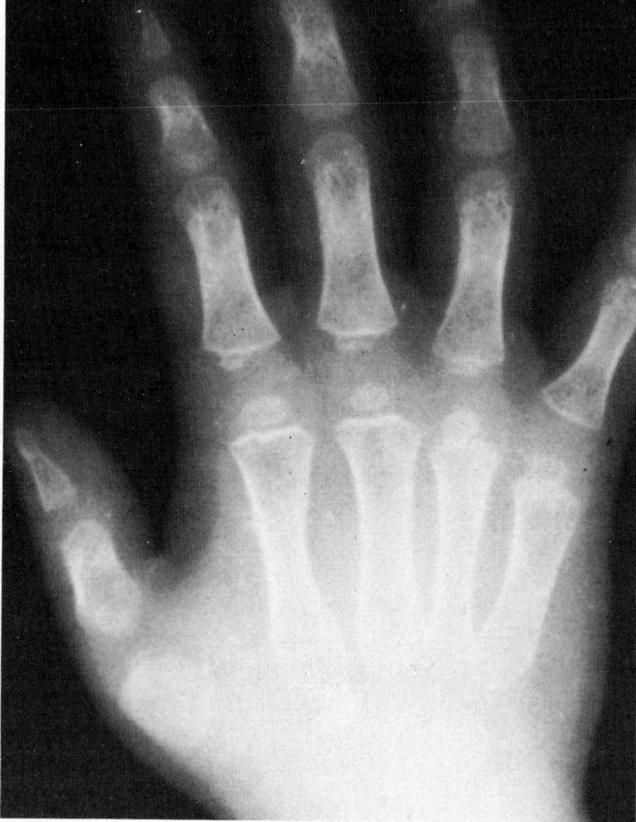

Fig. 54.41 Short first metacarpal in a child with congenital myositis ossificans.

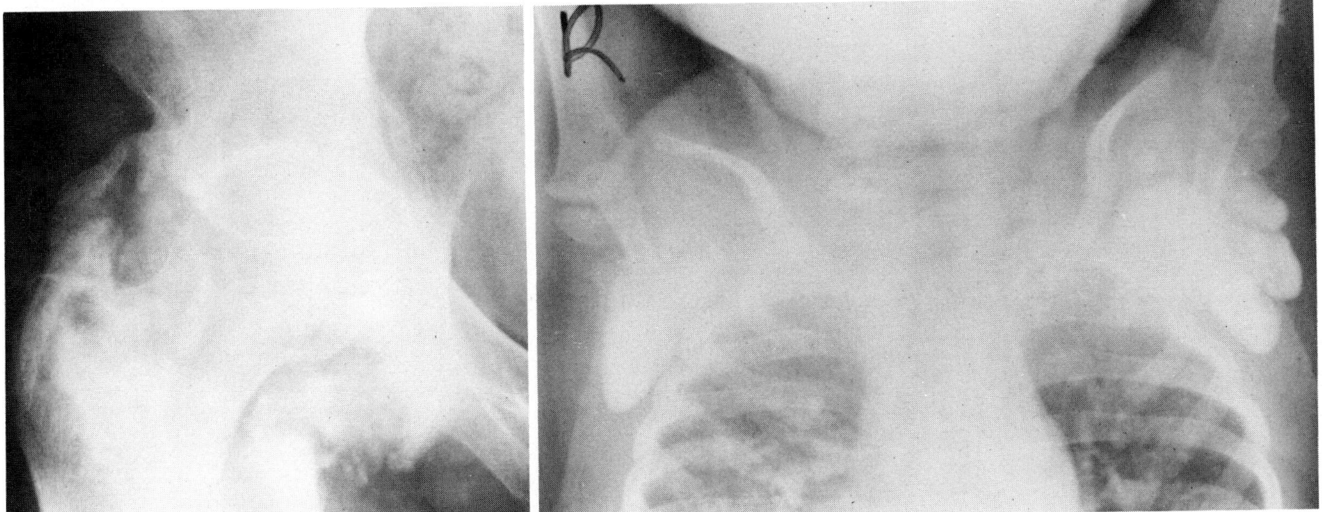

Fig. 54.42 *Fig. 54.43*

Fig. 54.42 Extensive bone formation round hip in a patient with paraplegia.

Fig. 54.43 Tumoral calcinosis.

density on a good radiograph. It is therefore possible to recognize lipomas within muscles as well-defined translucent areas (Fig. 54.44). Usually these lipomas are benign; liposarcomas tend to contain a considerable quantity of non-fatty stroma and are often less clearly defined.

Fat produces translucencies in certain well-defined areas under normal conditions—in front of the lower end of the humerus, below the patella and in front of the Achilles tendon. Obliteration of these translucencies indicates oedema or haemorrhage into the fat. Forward displacement or obliteration of the translucency in front

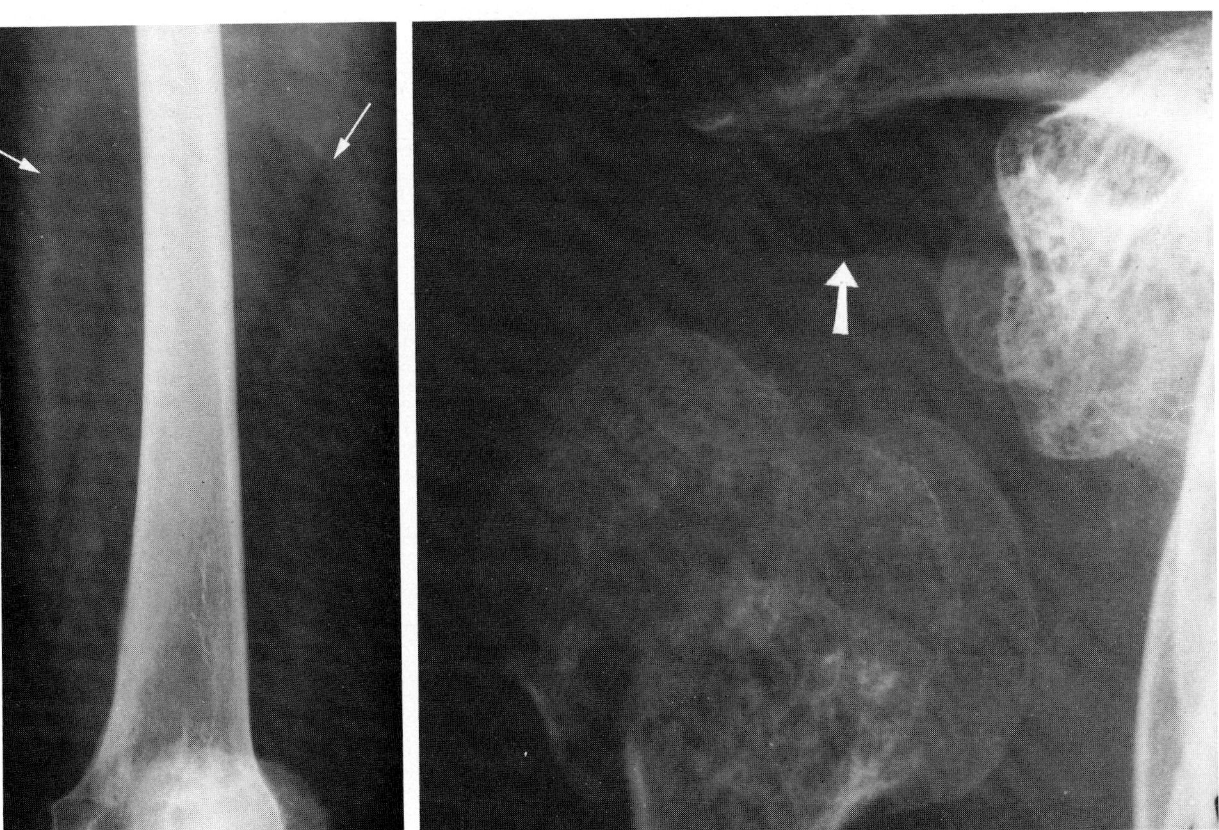

Fig. 54.44 Large lipoma in thigh.

Fig. 54.45 Lipohaemarthrosis of shoulder. Note fracture-dislocation of head of humerus with a fat-blood level.

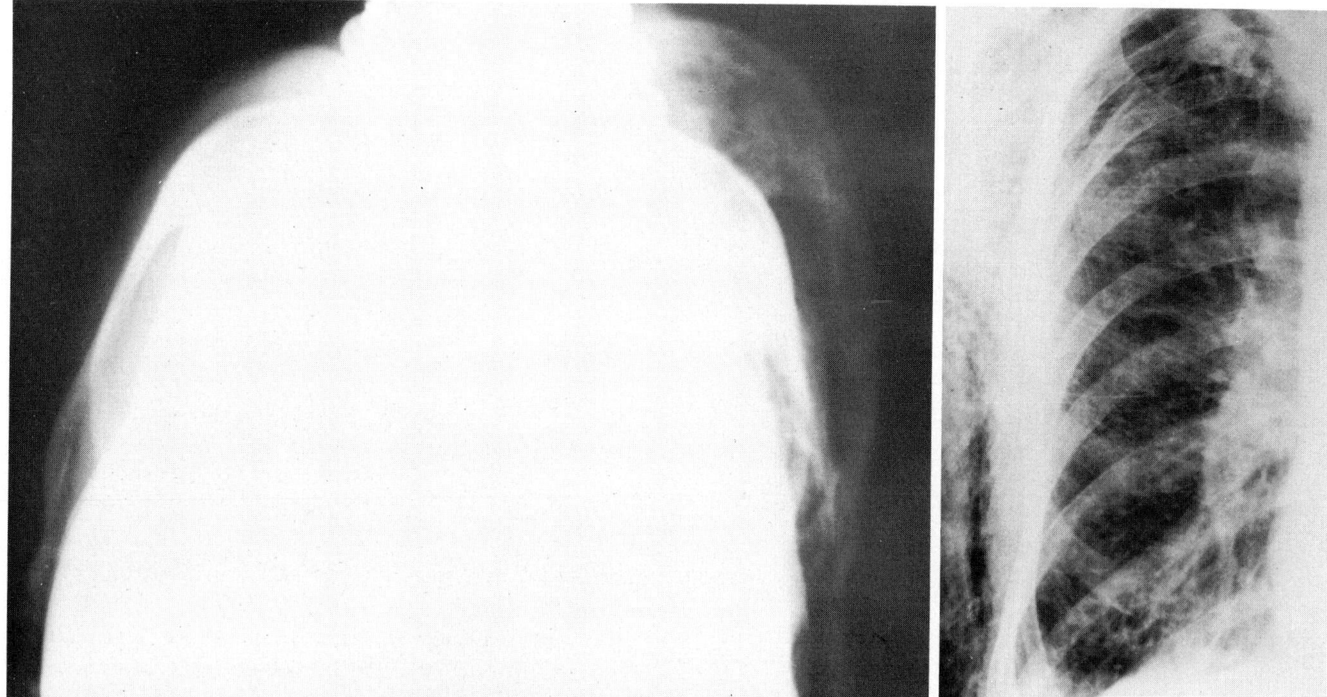

Fig. 54.46

Fig. 54.47

Fig. 54.46 Compound fracture of facial bones on the left. A large quantity of air has reached the subcutaneous tissues through a fracture of the maxillary antrum.

Fig. 54.47 Subcutaneous emphysema of chest.

of the lower end of the humerus is a valuable sign indicating a supracondylar fracture, which otherwise may be difficult to detect. Similarly, displacement of the normal fat lines at the outer end of the clavicle may aid in the diagnosis of dislocations of the acromio-clavicular joint (Weston, 1972).

Although not dependent on fat for its recognition, this is a convenient point, in discussing soft tissue signs of fractures, to mention the increase in the width of the post-nasal soft tissues in fractures of the base of the skull. This type of fracture is notoriously difficult to diagnose, and the sign described by Andrew (1978) may be helpful. The width of the soft tissues at the base of the skull is measured along a line drawn from the middle of the external auditory canal to the back of the hard palate. Normally this is about 10 mm in adolescents and adults but, in the presence of a fracture at the base of the skull, it usually measures more than 20 mm.

Fractures may lead to the release of fat from the marrow cavity and bleeding into a nearby tissue space. The fat floats on the blood and, if a film of the injured area is taken with a horizontal ray, a characteristic horizontal level is demonstrated due to the fat-blood interface. This condition has been termed lipohaemarthrosis (Fig. 54.45). It is seen particularly as a result of fracture-dislocations of the shoulder or fractures round the knee. Even when the fracture is not at once obvious, the unequivocal demonstration of a lipohaemarthrosis is compelling evidence for the presence of bone injury.

Gas may be seen below the inguinal ligament or in the scrotum in the presence of hernias containing intestine. Gas may, however, be present actually within the tissues. It may reach these either by entering from the outside or by being formed locally.

Air entering from outside. Small air bubbles are often seen near compound fractures and disappear rapidly following the injury. Larger quantities of air may be seen in the facial soft tissues after fractures of the paranasal sinuses (Fig. 54.46), or may reach the thoracic soft tissues from the lungs. This condition, termed subcutaneous emphysema, may follow rib fractures with laceration of a lung or thoracentesis and it is almost universal after thoracic surgery. Its sudden development or increase after several days after pulmonary resection indicates that an air leak has developed from the bronchial stump and is therefore worth mentioning in the radiological report. The appearance of a severe case of subcutaneous emphysema is very striking and contrasts markedly with the slight discomfort suffered by the patient with this condition. The skin shadow is separated from the ribs by coalescing translucencies due to air; these may extend into the neck. The changes are more marked on the side of the operation, but in severe cases extend to the other side. Air amongst the muscle bundles of the pectoralis major produces a streaky, fan-shaped pattern over the upper lateral thorax (Fig. 54.47).

Air may reach the soft tissues of the neck in other ways. It may enter through the mediastinal planes. *Mediastinal emphysema*, with or without a pneumothorax, is a rather unusual sequel to a severe asthmatic attack and has been described as a complication of diabetic coma; it is presumably caused by the over-breathing due to the acidosis. It may also follow rupture of the oesophagus (either spontaneous or due to instrumentation). Presacral air or oxygen insufflation almost invariably results in a pneumomediastinum with spread to the neck. This is not the case if carbon dioxide is used, since this gas is absorbed before it has a chance to reach the mediastinum. A diagnostic pneumomediastinum is followed by air in the neck.

Gas bubbles may also be seen in the soft tissues after the application of hydrogen peroxide to wounds, due to the liberation of oxygen to the action of catalase in blood or pus.

Rarely, gas may be found in the lower abdominal wall and thigh following rupture of a pelvic abscess due to diverticulitis or after perforation of a hollow viscus in a hernia. These appearances then resemble those seen in gas gangrene (Fig. 54.48).

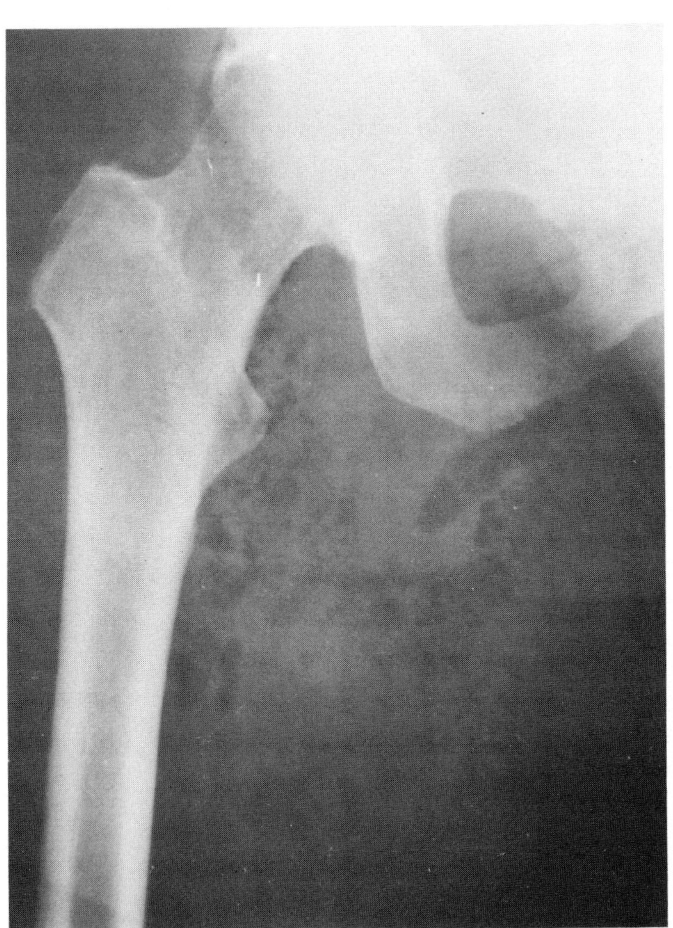

Fig. 54.48 Gas in upper thigh tracking down from the abdomen.

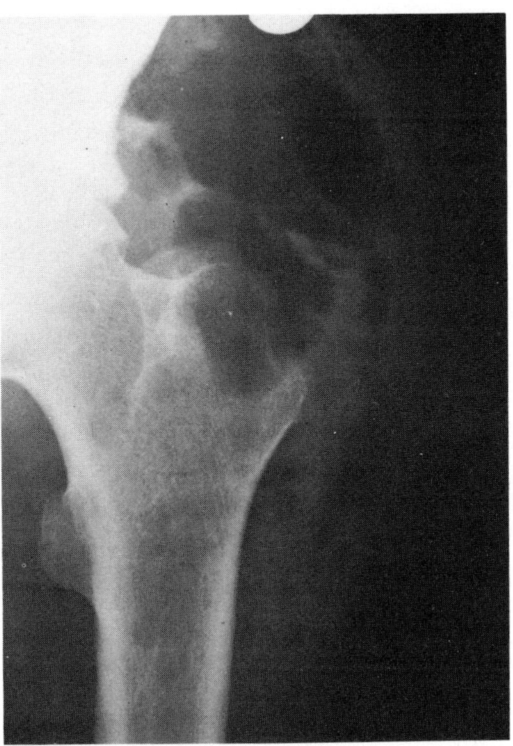

Fig. 54.49 Gas gangrene. Note gas formation in the soft tissues round the hip.

Gas formed within the tissues. This is invariably the result of infection, the gas being produced by the infecting organism. It is particularly liable to occur in uncontrolled diabetes, resulting in a number of small gas bubbles in an area of tissue necrosis.

Of particular interest is infection with gas gangrene organisms. *Clostridium welchii* predominates, but usually there is a mixture of invading organisms and frequently a foreign body is present. Gas may be produced as a number of bubbles in the tissue planes (anaerobic cellulitis). It differs from air bubbles introduced at the time of injury by their later appearance (3 to 4 days after injury) and by the tendency for the amount of gas to increase. Anaerobic myositis is an even more serious condition in which muscle necrosis is associated with profound toxaemia. Its course is rapid and gas may not be detectable till late in the disease. Radiologically the gas can be recognized within the muscles, separating the muscle bundles, but may also be present in other tissue planes, for instance under the skin (Fig. 54.49).

In cases of fetal death, gas may be demonstrated in the fetal vascular system (see Ch. 48).

ABNORMALITIES OF MUSCLES AND SUBCUTANEOUS TISSUES

Atrophy of muscles in the limbs resulting from disuse or lower motor neurone lesions can readily be appreciated

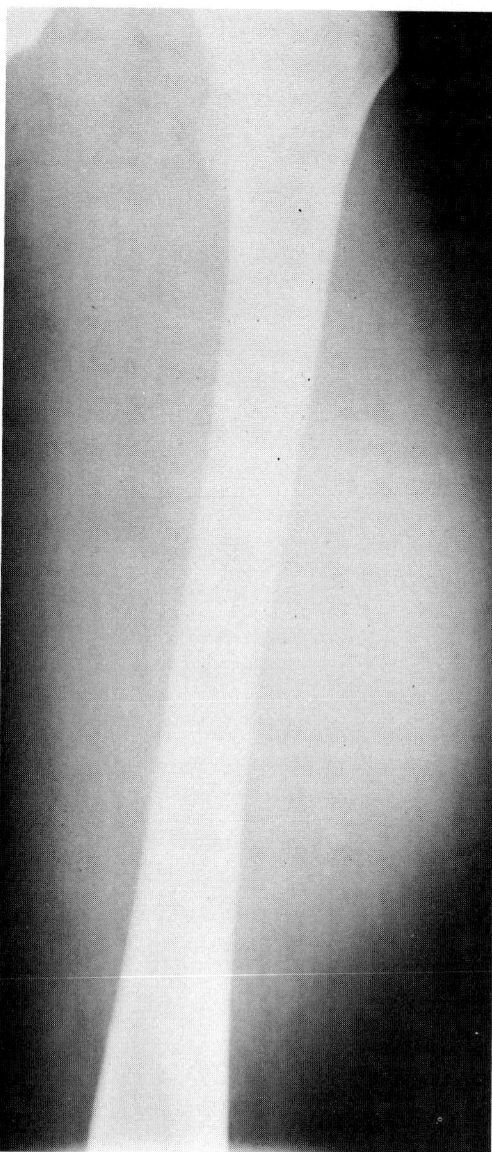

Fig. 54.50 Haematoma of thigh. Note obliteration of the normal muscle planes.

on a good radiograph, but these changes will also be evident clinically. Muscle bulk may be increased by a haematoma (which also obliterates the normal muscle planes) (Fig. 54.50) and in the early stages of pseudo-hypertrophic muscular dystrophy. In this condition there is an increase in the fat content within the muscle planes which can occasionally be recognised as a rather characteristic 'herring-bone' pattern. Abnormal prominence of the intramuscular planes may also be noted in peroneal muscular dystrophy (Fig. 54.51).

Characteristic soft tissue changes, consisting of peri-articular contractures and webbing, is also found in arthrogryposis congenita multiplex (amyoplasia congenita). This condition, which may be grouped with muscular dystrophies, is a congenital disease of unknown origin leading to limb deformities. Bone changes occur, but are non-specific: the bones tend to be thin, poorly tubulated and poorly mineralized (Fig. 54.52).

Oedema of the soft tissues produces widening of their shadow with a rather characteristic thickening and blurring of the soft tissue septa (Fig. 54.53) or thickening of subcutaneous tissues in cellulitis (Fig. 54.54).

As already indicated, tumours of soft tissues may be apparent from their bulk, their fat or calcium content, or displacement of anatomical features. In general it is difficult to suggest histology. Pure lipomas are said to be invariably benign and sometimes angiography may be helpful, more for definite outlining of the extent of the tumour than for recognition of a tissue type. Martel and Abell (1973) carried out a retrospective study of 60 soft tissue tumours. They found more difficulty in distinguishing between malignant tumours and chronic inflammatory lesions than between benign and malignant tumours. Peripheral secondary deposits are rare, and if present often arise from a bronchial primary (Fig. 54.55).

Heel pad thickening. The thickness of the soft tissue between the postero-inferior tip of the os calcis

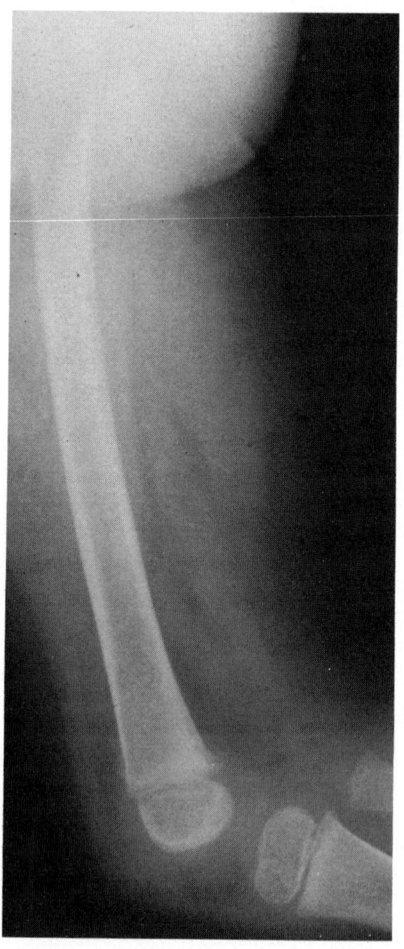

Fig. 54.51 Peroneal muscular dystrophy. Note the prominent separation of muscle in the thigh.

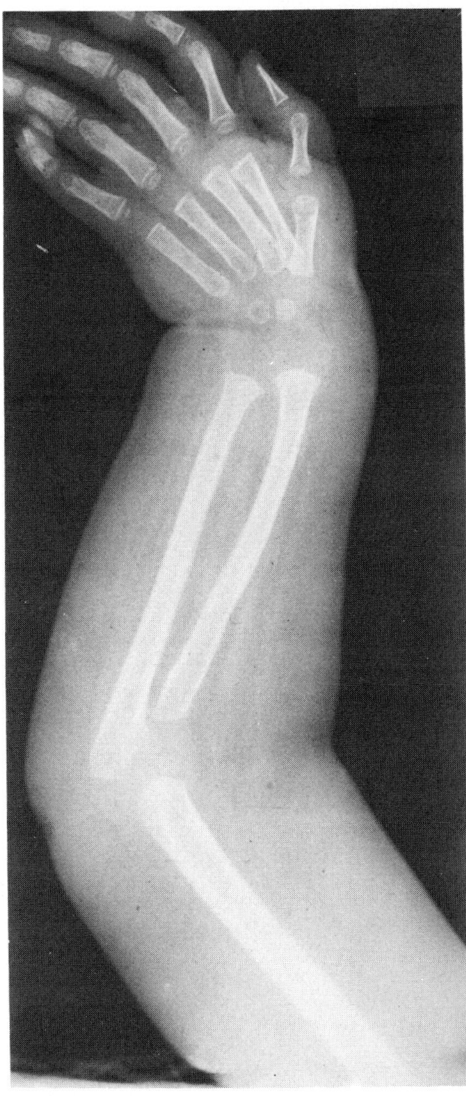

Fig. 54.52 Arthrogryposis congenita multiplex. Note the webbing round the joints.

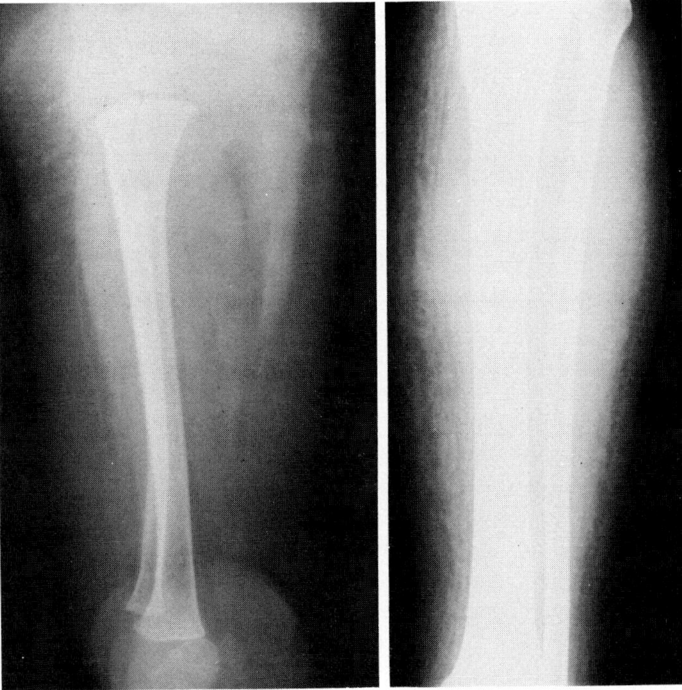

Fig. 54.53 *Fig. 54.54*

Fig. 54.53 Oedema of calf in an infant with spina bifida. The muscles are poorly developed, but the subcutaneous tissues are widened and the fibrous tissue septa are thickened.

Fig. 54.54 Cellulitis of shin.

and the surface of the skin is increased in acromegaly and this has been used as a diagnostic sign. Kho *et al.* (1970) found that the actual measurement is influenced by the patient's sex and weight and, in their paper, provide a graph taking account of this. However, they suggest the upper limit if normal to be 23 mm for males and 21.5 mm for females. In practice this is not a very valuable sign since the diagnosis is more easily made in other ways. These authors have produced evidence that heel pad thickness is related to the level of circulating growth hormone in the serum, and the measurement is of more value for following the course of the disease after treatment.

Apart from acromegaly and obesity, heel pad thickness is also increased after injury or infection, in peripheral oedema, in myxodema, and Kattan (1975) has reported heel pad thickening in patients on Dilantin (Epanutin).

Fat thickness in infants of diabetic mothers. New-born babies of less than 30 weeks' gestational age and with normal mothers do not show any fat along the lower thoracic wall. Kuhns *et al.* (1974) have made the interesting observation that babies of diabetic mothers show an increase in the subcutaneous fat visible on a chest radiograph, even when the baby is not large for the dates. The ratio of subcutaneous fat to transverse thoracic diameter is shown graphically in their paper, to which the interested reader is directed. The observation holds true whether the mother has overt or gestational diabetes. It may sometimes be impossible to establish the diagnosis

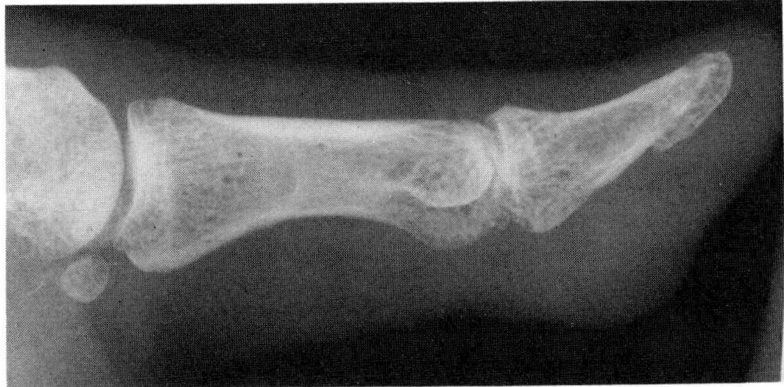

Fig. 54.55 Secondary deposit in thumb. Deposits beyond the elbows and knees are rare. When they do occur, they are frequently from carcinoma of the bronchus.

of gestational diabetes after delivery, since the glucose tolerance curve may return to normal. The observation of increased subcutaneous fat in a neonate may therefore help to explain the findings of symptoms associated with a 'diabetic' gestation in an apparently normal mother after delivery.

SINOGRAPHY

Sinuses may result from bone or soft tissue infections, or follow trauma or surgery. They are often exceedingly complex and for effective treatment an exact knowledge of their extent and ramifications is necessary. For this purpose contrast medium is introduced through the skin opening, the aim being complete delineation of the sinus. If, at the time of the proposed examination, the sinus happens to be closed, it is best to postpone the sinogram until, as will inevitably happen, the sinus reopens.

Contrast medium. Any type of contrast medium can be used, but in general oily, iodine-containing substances are most suitable, e.g. Lipiodol or, if the sinus is very narrow, a less viscous medium such as Myodil may be preferred.

Technique. Strict cleanliness should naturally be observed, but most sinuses are heavily infected and complete asepsis is hardly possible. If a drain is present in the sinus, this is best removed at the beginning of the examination. The sinus is gently explored with a fine probe in order to obtain some information on its length and direction. Contrast medium is injected, using either a rubber nozzle or a syringe or a fine catheter passed into the sinus. If the latter method is used, care must be taken to avoid placing the catheter tip beyond a branch of the sinus, which may then fail to fill. Contrast medium tends to leak back, but this can be prevented by pushing the rubber nozzle firmly into the opening, or pinching the skin round the catheter. When the sinus is full, leak-back can no longer be prevented; the nozzle or catheter is then removed and the mouth of the sinus packed firmly with ribbon gauze to prevent any further escape of contrast. The sinus opening is marked with a metal ring and films are then taken.

Generally, better films are obtained by use of the overhead tube and screening is rarely required. Occasionally, if the sinus is very complex, it may be helpful to follow the course of the contrast medium on the screen It may be necessary to tip the patient in order to fill all parts of the sinus.

Great gentleness is required during the examination. Most sinuses are devoid of pain sensation, but occasionally the examination may prove painful. Moreover, rough handling might cause entry of organisms into the blood stream.

Radiographic technique. Before the contrast medium is introduced, plain films of the area should be obtained in order to exclude any opaque foreign bodies which may be present in the sinus and which may be obscured by the contrast medium. After the introduction of contrast, films at right angles to each other are taken. Occasionally stereoscopic films may be very helpful. The films should include some easily recognizable anatomical landmarks to which the sinus can be related.

REFERENCES AND SUGGESTIONS FOR FURTHER READING

ANDREW, W. K. (1978) The soft tissue sign: a new parameter in the diagnosis of fractures of the base of the skull. *Clinical Radiology*, **29**, 443–446.

DEICHGRÄBER, E. & OLSSON, B. (1975) Soft tissue radiography in painful shoulders. *Acta Radiologica (Diag.)*, **16**, 393–400.

DUNNICK, N. R., SCHANER, E. G. & DOPPMAN (1978) Detection of subcutaneous metastases by computed tomography. *Journal of Computer Assisted Tomography*, **2**, 275–279.

ENCYCLOPEDIA OF MEDICAL RADIOLOGY (1968) Roentgen diagnosis of the soft tissues, Vol. VIII, 124–177, ed. Diethelm, L. Berlin: Springer-Verlag.

GRIFFITHS, H. J. (1976) *Radiology of Renal Failure.* Philadelphia: Saunders.

KATTAN, K. R. (1975) Thickening of the heel pad associated with long-term Dilantin therapy. *American Journal of Roentgenology*, **124**, 52–56.

KHO, K. M., WRIGHT, A. D. & DOYLE, F. H. (1970) Heel pad thickness in acromegaly. *British Journal of Radiology*, **43**, 119–122.

KUHNS, L. R., BERGER, P. E., ROLOFF, D. W., POZNANSKI, A. K. & HOLT, J. F. (1974) Fat thickness in the newborn infant of a diabetic mother. *Radiology*, **III**, 665.

MARTEL, W. & ABELL, M. R. (1973) Radiologic evaluation of soft tissue tumours: restrospective study. *Cancer*, **32**, 352–366.

MEEMA, H. E., OREOPOULOS, D. G. & DE VEBER, G. A. (1976) Arterial calcifications in severe chronic renal disease and their relationship to dialysis treatment, renal transplant and parathyroidectomy. *Radiology*, **121**, 315–321.

MIDDLEMISS, J. H. (Ed.) (1961) *Tropical Radiology.* London: Heinemann.

MURRAY, R. O. & JACOBSON, H. G. (1977) *The Radiology of Skeletal Disorders.* Edinburgh: Churchill Livingstone.

PALMER, P. E. S. (1966) Tumoral calcinosis. *British Journal of Radiology*, **39**, 518–523.

DE SANTOS, L. A. GOLDSTEIN, H. M., MURRAY, J. A. & WALLACE, S. (1978) Computed tomography in the evaluation of musculo-skeletal neoplasms. *Radiology*, **128**, 89–94.

WEINBERGER, G. & LEVINSOHN, E. M. (1978) Computed tomography in the evaluation of sarcomatous tumours in the thigh. *American Journal of Roentgenology*, **130**, 115–118.

WESTON, W. J. (1972) Soft tissue signs in recent subluxation and dislocation of the acromio-clavicular joint. *British Journal of Radiology*, **45**, 832–834.

WOLFE, J. N. (1969) Xeroradiography of bones, joints and soft tissues. *Radiology*, **93**, 583–587.

ZATZKIN, H. R. (1965) *The Roentgen Diagnosis of Trauma.* New York: Year Book Medical Publishers.

CHAPTER 55

MAMMOGRAPHY

A technique of mammography described by Leborgne (1953) has acted as a basis for further developments in the ensuing years. The original method employed a fine focus tungsten anode X-ray tube and *non-screen* film. Modified X-ray tubes with *tungsten* target and thin glass ports were developed for use without additional filtration and with fine grain, industrial type film. The disadvantage of tungsten as the target material is that at the low kilovoltages employed, it emits X-radiation of continuous spectrum. Some radiation of unsuitable wavelength is produced which leads to a reduction in the contrast of the image.

Molybdenum anode tubes were developed to overcome this problem. When molybdenum is exposed to kilovoltages in the 25 to 35 kV range X-radiation of discontinuous spectrum is emitted with two peaks of characteristic radiation at 0·6 to 0·9 Å range. The radiation in this range is nearly monochromatic and is very suitable for soft-tissue radiography of the breast. Various commercial units are available using different methods of filtration and different anode-film distances. Some use the inherent filtration of the glass envelope itself and others have beryllium ports with added molybdenum filters.

The standard procedure is to obtain at least two images of each breast. The basic projections are the *craniocaudal* and *mediolateral* views. The *mediolateral* view is best obtained with the patient in the supine-oblique position. In this way a portion of the chest wall may be easily included on the film so that the whole of the breast and the retromammary space are seen. The axillary tail of the breast is included on the mediolateral projection but as it is only rarely completely seen on the craniocaudal projection an additional *supero-inferior projection, centred over the axillary tail* itself, may be taken. Other additional projections used are an *axillary* view to show more clearly the contents of the axilla and a *lateromedial* projection to highlight lesions in the inner half of the breast. Lundgren (1977) has advocated the use of single-view mammography of each breast for screening purposes. The projection used is an oblique mediolateral view and it is maintained that the glandular portion of the breast is practically always completely demonstrated.

Details of radiographic technique are important in mammography. The use of as fine a focal spot as possible is advisable. Collimation of the beam reduces scatter. Compression of the breast reduces movement and reduces the thickness of the tissues with consequent reduction in scatter and radiation dosage. The breast should be in contact with the wrapped film to reduce geometrical blurring. Hand processing of the film gives better quality images than automatic processing.

With technical advances in recent years it is now possible to use various film-screen combinations for mammography and these lead to varying degrees of reduction of skin dosage. A single fine-grain intensifying screen is used as a backscreen in conjunction with a suitable film. The film and screen are vacuum packed in a plastic envelope thus giving excellent film-screen contact. Asbury and Barker (1975) have measured the mean total skin dosage (the dosage measured in the upper inner quadrant of a breast during the four-exposure sequence for the basic examination of both breasts) with various film-screen combinations. The following mean total skin dosages were obtained. Using a fine-grain film system *without screen* (Kodak Industrex C film) the dose was 4·9rad. A combination of 'Medichrome' film (Agfa-Gevaert) and Kodak High Resolution screen gave a dose of 1·1rad and 'Medichrome' film with Ilford High Definition screen a dose of 0·5rad. By using 'Trimax XD' film (3M Company) and a 'Trimax Alpha 4' rare-earth, phosphor screen the dose was further reduced to 0·18rad. These film-screen combinations have been recommended for use in mass surveys which entail repeated examinations. They are ideally suited for this purpose with respect to the reduced dosage, but some deterioration in image quality is associated with the use of screens.

Xeromammography is a relatively new method of examination. It is an electrostatic process rather than a chemical process. The principles of xerography and its applications in breast examination have been well described by Wolfe (1972). Basically, a charged selenium plate is discharged by X-radiation in proportion to the amount of radiation reaching the plate. This gives rise to an invisible electrostatic image on the plate, which is then developed by the use of charged blue powder. The visible image is transferred and fixed to paper. Either a 'negative' image may be obtained, which is similar to a film radiograph, or a 'positive' image may be obtained. This is the reverse of a film radiograph (Gravelle and Hallett, 1976).

The xeroradiographic image has several characteristics. It has a wide recording latitude enabling the skin, nipple, base of breast and even chest wall to be seen equally clearly on a single image. There is relatively low general contrast, allowing penetration of dense breasts and dense lesions. Local contrast is accentuated due to an 'edge-enhancement effect', so that the margins of lesions and microcalcifications are highlighted. Both tungsten and molybdenum anode tubes may be used for xeromammography. By using a tungsten anode, total filtration of the order of 3 mm aluminium and the negative mode of the xerographic process a total skin dosage of under 2rad may be achieved without significant deterioration of the images.

NORMAL APPEARANCES

In the adolescent the glandular portion of the breast is dense and clearly separated from the subcutaneous fat. The retromammary fat line is also clearly seen separating the breast disc from the chest wall (Fig. 55.1). Structures such as ducts, blood vessels and trabeculae are not well seen due to the density of the glandular portion of the breast. These, however, are well seen on xeromammography.

With increasing age and maturity and especially following pregnancies, an increasing amount of fat deposition occurs within the glandular portion of the breast (Fig. 55.2). Blood vessels and trabeculae are more easily seen and the margins of the breast disc become less well defined.

In the menopausal and post-menopausal age groups the glandular tissue is replaced by fat, eventually giving a fatty, atrophic breast (Fig. 55.3). Vessels and trabeculae are very clearly seen and lactiferous ducts may also be seen beneath the nipple—especially in multiparous women. Very small cancers can be easily seen in such breasts as a result of the natural contrast provided by the fat.

During pregnancy the glandular portion of the breast

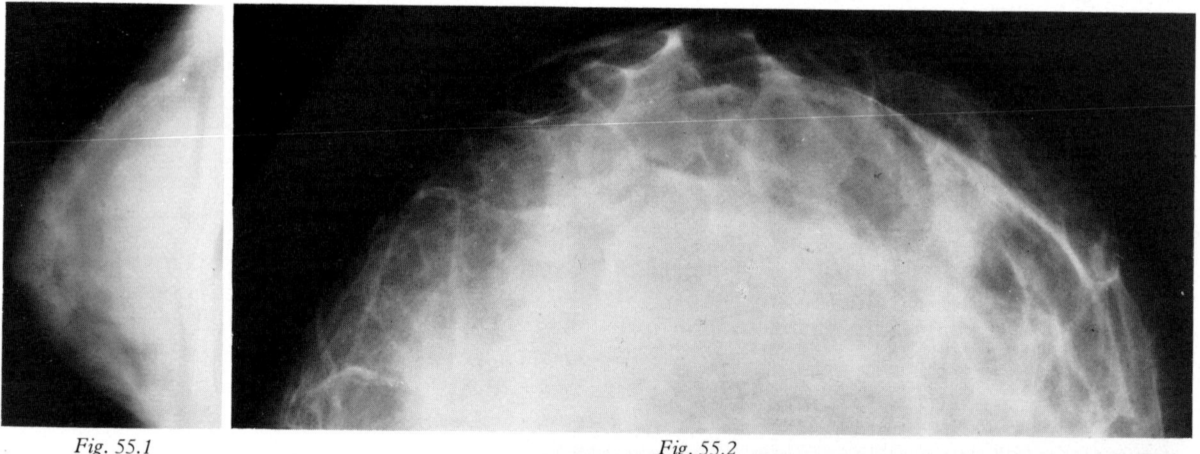

Fig. 55.1 *Fig. 55.2*

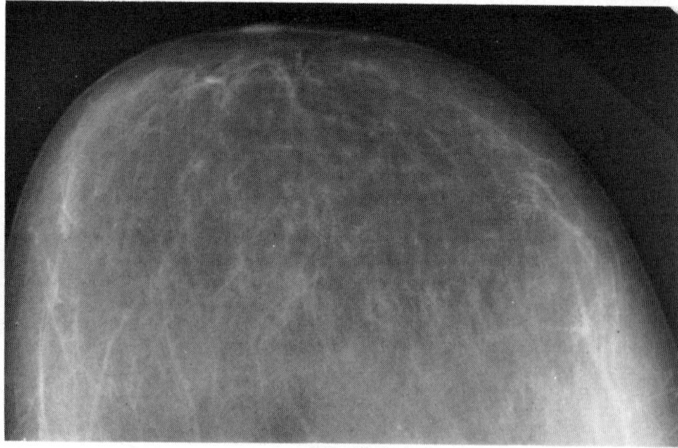

Fig. 55.3

Fig. 55.1 Immature, adolescent breast.

Fig. 55.2 Mature, glandular breast.

Fig. 55.3 Fatty, atrophic breast.

becomes progressively more dense and vascular. In late pregnancy and following parturition enlarged lactiferous ducts are seen.

ABNORMAL APPEARANCES

The various abnormalities found on mammography are superimposed on the normal varieties described. The main clinical problem is differentiation of malignant from benign conditions. Consequently differentiating features will be tabulated and discussed.

Table 55.1 Differentiation of malignant from benign lesions

Malignant	*Benign*
Primary signs	
1. High density, non-homogeneous irregular opacity	1. Relatively low density, homogeneous, smooth opacity
2. Microcalcification	2. Relatively coarse calcification
Secondary signs	
1. Disruption of architecture	1. Distortion of architecture
2. Usually increased vascularity	2. Normal vascularity or occasional hypervascularity
3. Perifocal haziness	3. Rarely perifocal haziness
4. Radiological size smaller than clinical size	4. Radiological size the same or larger than clinical size

PRIMARY SIGNS

The mass

A *malignant* lesion is usually of high density, the opacity nearly always showing a non-homogeneous texture as a result of asymmetric growth of the tumour (Figs 55.4, 55.5 and 55.6). In addition, the margins of a malignant lesion, if not completely irregular, are usually irregular in part. These irregularities may take the form of long thin spicules (Fig. 55.5), or shorter and broader tentacles (Fig. 55.4). Less commonly there are short fine irregularities and occasionally the margins of the tumour are ill-defined rather than irregular (Fig. 55.8). Rarely the tumour is well circumscribed and smooth in outline (Fig. 55.7). This type of change is found in colloid or mucoid carcinoma and in intracystic carcinoma and provides great diagnostic difficulties, as often the lesion shows homogeneous density also. The tumours that morphologically show irregular margins are usually scirrhous in nature. Quite commonly a tumour will be partly smooth and partly irregular (Fig. 55.6). In such a case, when the irregularities are elongated, a 'comet-tail' appearance is found. In advanced malignancy the breast becomes increasingly dense due to infiltration and oedema (Fig. 55.8). The primary breast lesion may be obscured in such cases.

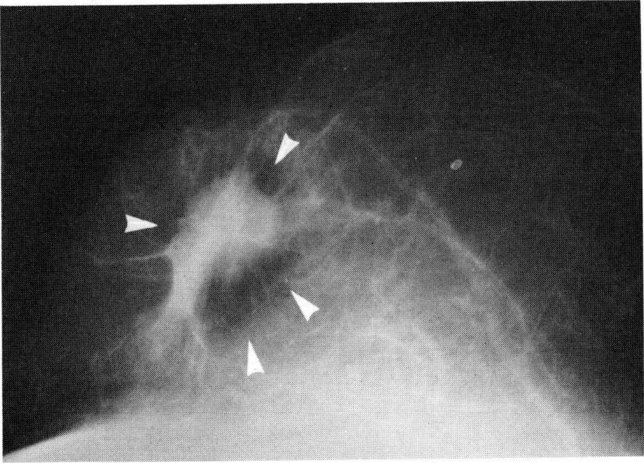

Fig. 55.4 Scirrhous carcinoma with tentacles, spicules and 'pseudo-lipoma' (arrowed).

Benign lesions are of variable but homogeneous density. They usually have low densities compared with malignant lesions and may even be transradiant. A fibroadenoma is usually of similar density to the surrounding glandular tissue, whereas cysts are often a little more dense than the glandular tissue (Fig. 55.16). However, large fibroadenomata and giant fibroadenomata can show great density whereas small cysts may show low density (Fig. 55.18). Lipomata are constantly transradiant (Fig. 55.18) and fat necrosis (Fig. 55.12) and galactocoeles may be transradiant or opaque, depending on the stage of development. Occasionally ducts are seen as transradiant bands when their contents contain a high percentage of fat.

A benign lesion usually has smooth margins and is usually round, ovoid or lobulated. Occasionally fibroadenomata may be partly irregular or partly ill-defined, as they develop from the surrounding fibroadenotic tissue. Acute inflammatory processes and acute abscesses are ill-defined but an abscess tends to become circumscribed with increasing chronicity (Fig. 55.17).

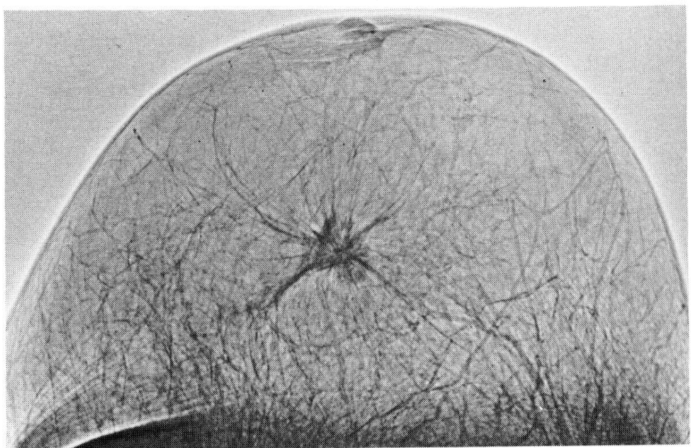

Fig. 55.5 Positive xerogram. Spiculated, scirrhous carcinoma.

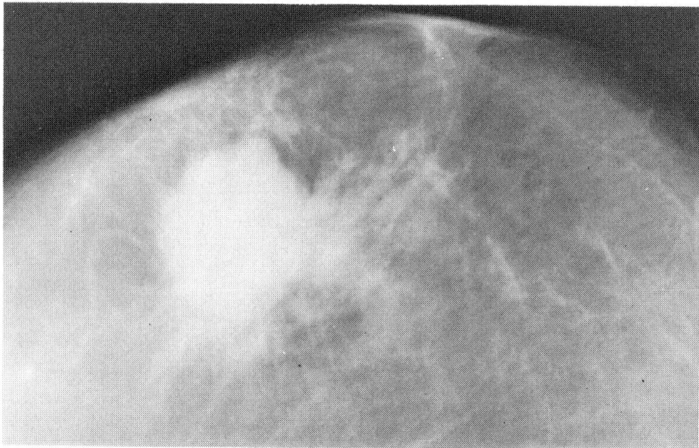

Fig. 55.6 Carcinoma with partly smooth and partly irregular outline. Dilated ducts and nipple retraction. Localized skin dimpling.

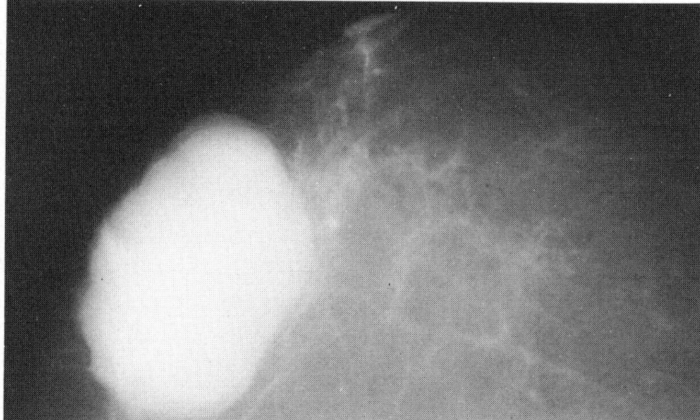

Fig. 55.7 Smooth, dense, lobulated, colloid carcinoma.

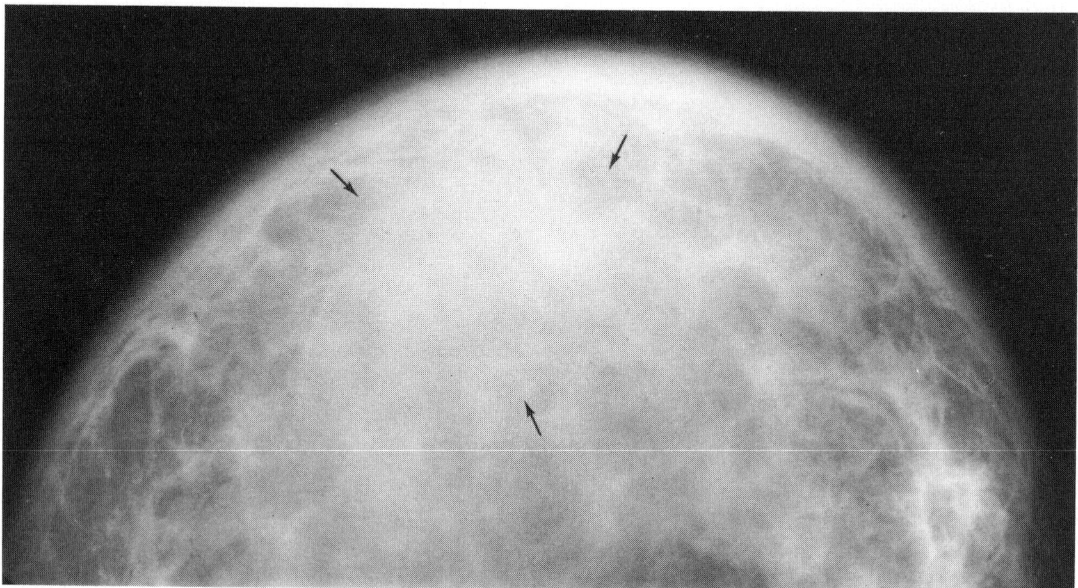

Fig. 55.8 Diffuse malignant infiltration. Ill-defined primary tumour (arrowed).

Calcification

The importance of calcification in the breast is that an accurate, pathological diagnosis can usually be made on the basis of the radiological features and distribution of the calcification. Differentiation between malignant and benign disease is often though not invariably possible. The presence of a particular type of calcification adds weight to the radiological diagnosis. Clinically unsuspected and impalpable cancers may be diagnosed on the basis of microcalcification alone.

The features of the various types of calcification are given in Table 55.2.

The calcification associated with **malignant** disease is usually finer than that found in benign breast disease, hence the term 'microcalcification'. The individual grains of calcification are frequently as small as 0·08 mm to 0·1 mm in diameter. The microcalcifications may be granular in form or elongated. The elongated form may be straight, curved or even branched and occasionally lace-like patterns may be found. On close inspection this fine calcification is seen to be irregular in outline. The microcalcifications may be found within a malignant mass or at a distance from the mass. When situated within a mass the calcifications are usually haphazardly arranged, i.e. without polarity. When separate from the mass they often show polarity as they are within the ducts. Small, individual granules in close apposition within the ducts give rise to the elongated, irregular type of microcalcifications. This fine microcalcification may be found in practically any type of cancer but especially in *intraduct* and *scirrhous carcinoma*. All these features are shown in Figure 55.9.

Table 55.2

Calcification in malignant disease	
1. Fine and irregular (0·1–0·08 mm) Granular Elongated—straight, curved or branched Lace-like	Seen in any type of cancer but particularly in intraduct and scirrhous carcinoma
2. Coarse and irregular (1 mm or over) Flake-like	Mucoid carcinoma and cystosarcoma phylloides
3. Coarse and smooth (1 mm or over)	Following local radiotherapy
Calcification in benign disease	
1. Coarse and smooth (1 mm or over)	
Ring-shaped, elongated, tubular and branched in the line of ducts	Duct ectasia (secretory disease)
Peripheral or central in position	Fibroadenoma
Rounded, ovoid or lobulated Amorphus lumps	Fat necrosis and scars
2. Fine and smooth (0·1–0·5 mm)	
Punctate, spheroidal—localized or scattered	Papilloma, sclerosing adenosis Epithelial hyperplasia
Elongated—localized or scattered	Epithelial hyperplasia
Egg-shell	Fat necrosis. Cysts and galactocoele

A less common, coarse, flake-like irregular calcification is seen occasionally in *mucoid carcinoma* and *cystosarcoma phylloides*.

Following radiotherapy to a breast tumour, existing microcalcifications may disappear or increase in number; microcalcifications may appear for the first time or smooth, coarse calcifications may appear. These latter coarse calcifications may be due to tumour necrosis or fat necrosis. Appearance of fine microcalcifications may be due to tumour necrosis also and disappearance may be due to reabsorption of calcified necrotic debris.

The incidence of microcalcification in malignant disease found on mammography varies with the radiographic technique employed. Quoted figures vary from 30 to 40 per cent for film only and film-screen techniques (Black and Young, 1965; Price *et al.*, 1976). In a personal series of 138 consecutive cancers an incidence of 63 per cent was obtained using xeromammography.

The calcifications found in **benign** breast disease are generally larger than those found in malignancy and also have smooth margins. The size of the calcifications are usually over 1 mm in diameter and in some rare instances

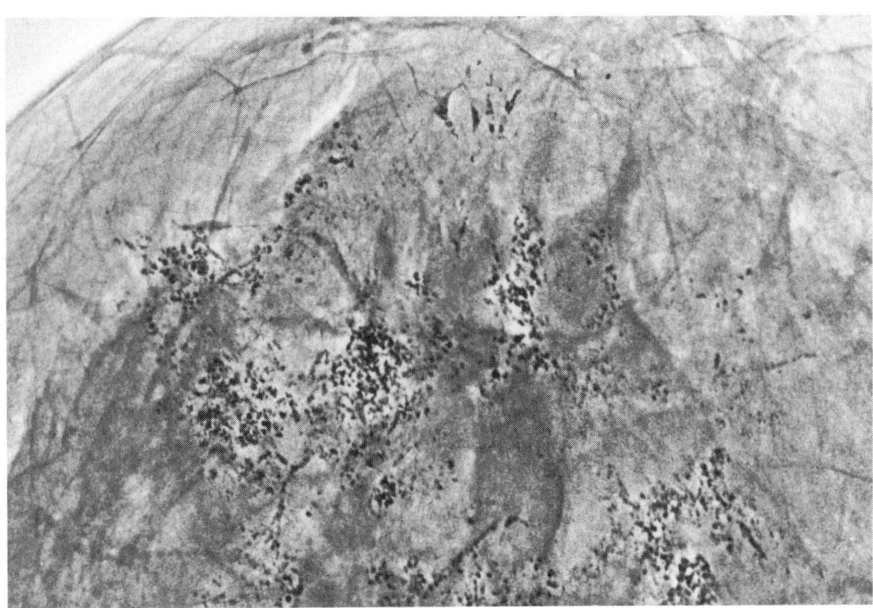

Fig. 55.9 Positive xerogram. Microcalcifications in malignancy. The calcifications are represented as black opacities.

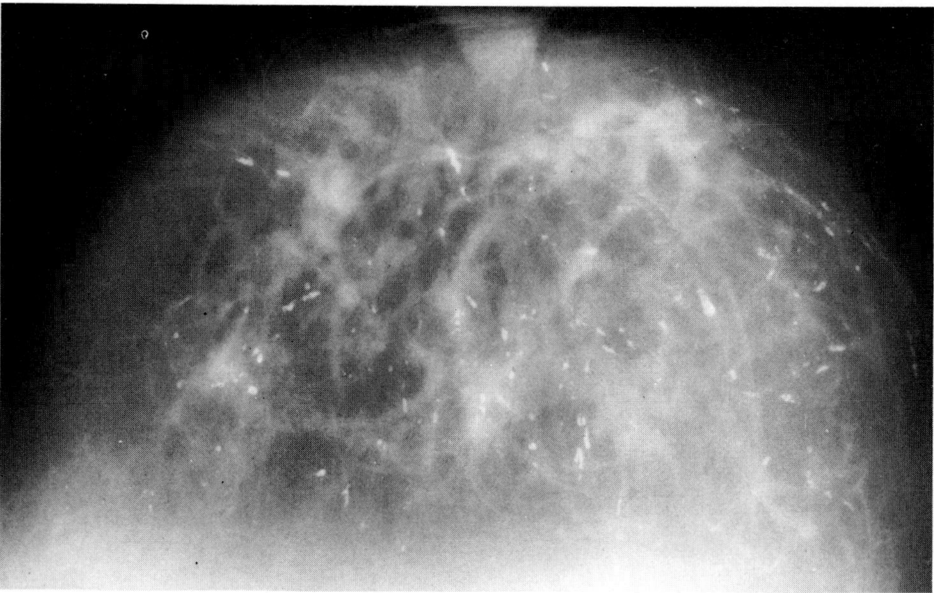

Fig. 55.10 Duct ectasia showing coarse, smooth calcifications (white). There are dilated ducts and nipple retraction.

are over 1 cm in diameter. The important features are the coarseness and smoothness of the calcifications.

The commonest cause of benign calcification is *duct ectasia*, alternatively known as '*secretory disease*'. In this condition the calcification is smooth and ring shaped, i.e. there is often a transradiant centre. The calcification can also be elongated, tubular and branched in the line of the lactiferous ducts in this condition. Even the elongated calcifications may have a transradiant centre. The calcifications in duct ectasia are frequently associated with tubular shadows due to dilated or thickened ducts, and a retracted nipple is often demonstrated (Fig. 55.10).

Coarse, smooth calcifications situated peripherally or centrally in a rounded, ovoid or lobulated soft tissue lesion are a pathognomonic sign of *fibroadenoma* (Fig. 55.11). When the calcification occurs in amorphous lumps without an associated soft tissue lesion the usual diagnosis is calcified *fat necrosis*.

Benign breast disease may give rise to fine calcifications also but usually these are smooth and a little larger than the microcalcifications associated with malignancy. *Papillomatosis*, *sclerosing adenosis* and *epithelial hyperplasia* may give rise to fine, granular, smooth calcifications. These may be localized (Fig. 55.14) or scattered through the breast (Fig. 55.13) and are usually bilateral in sclerosing adenosis and epithelial hyperplasia. Epithelial hyper-

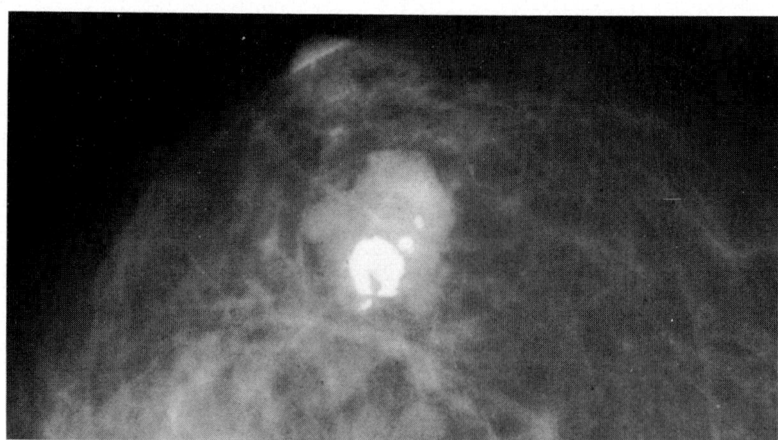

Fig. 55.11 Smooth, lobulated, partially calcified fibroadenoma.

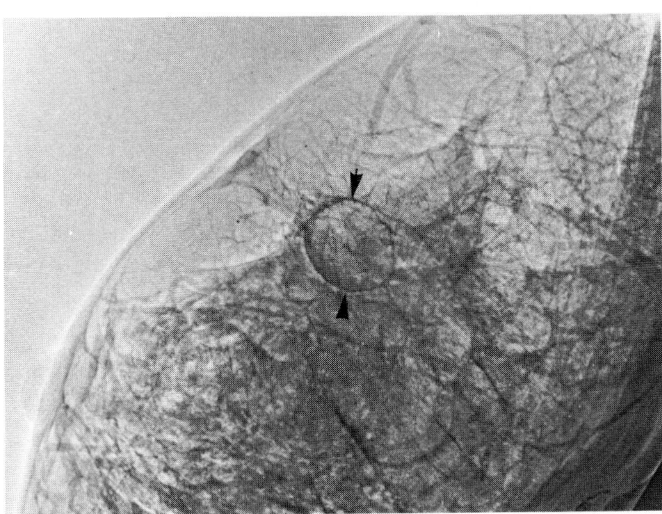

Fig. 55.12 Transradiant lesion with egg-shell calcification. Traumatic fat necrosis following biopsy. Note superficial skin thickening and dimpling.

plasia may give rise to localized or scattered elongated, smooth, fine calcification but this seems to be less of a diagnostic problem than sclerosing adenosis (Fig. 55.14).

Egg-shell calcification may be found in *cysts*, *fat necrosis* (Fig. 55.12) and *galactocoeles*. It always encircles a moderately dense lesion in breast cysts. However, it may encircle a moderately dense lesion or transradiant lesion in galactocoeles or fat necrosis. The fat necrosis may be post-traumatic or the result of plasma cell mastitis.

There is no diagnostic difficulty when the fine calcification is in association with a mass or is as profusely and characteristically distributed as in Figures 55.9 and 55.13. The diagnostic difficulties arise when there is a small group of fine calcifications of 5 to 15 in number, either alone or associated with fine scattered calcifications. In such circumstances radiological diagnosis is only approximately 50 per cent accurate (Fig. 55.14A and B).

When there is no palpable abnormality, localization of the possible malignant lesion is important for the surgeon. Localization to a particular quadrant is inaccurate as the breast is not in comparable position during radiological examination and operation. To overcome this problem 0·5 ml of a mixture of 25 per cent Hypaque and Patent Blue Violet is injected directly into the breast by the radiologist to the site of the calcification. Then cranio-caudal and mediolateral views are taken. The Hypaque is visible radiologically (Fig. 55.15A and B) and the position of the violet dye is visible to the surgeon for many hours following injection. Consequently the surgeon can accurately localize the breast calcifications. The biopsy specimen should always be X-rayed to confirm removal of the suspicious calcifications. The appropriate area should then be separated from the biopsy specimen by the radiologist so that the pathologist can examine the correct area (Preece *et al.*, 1977).

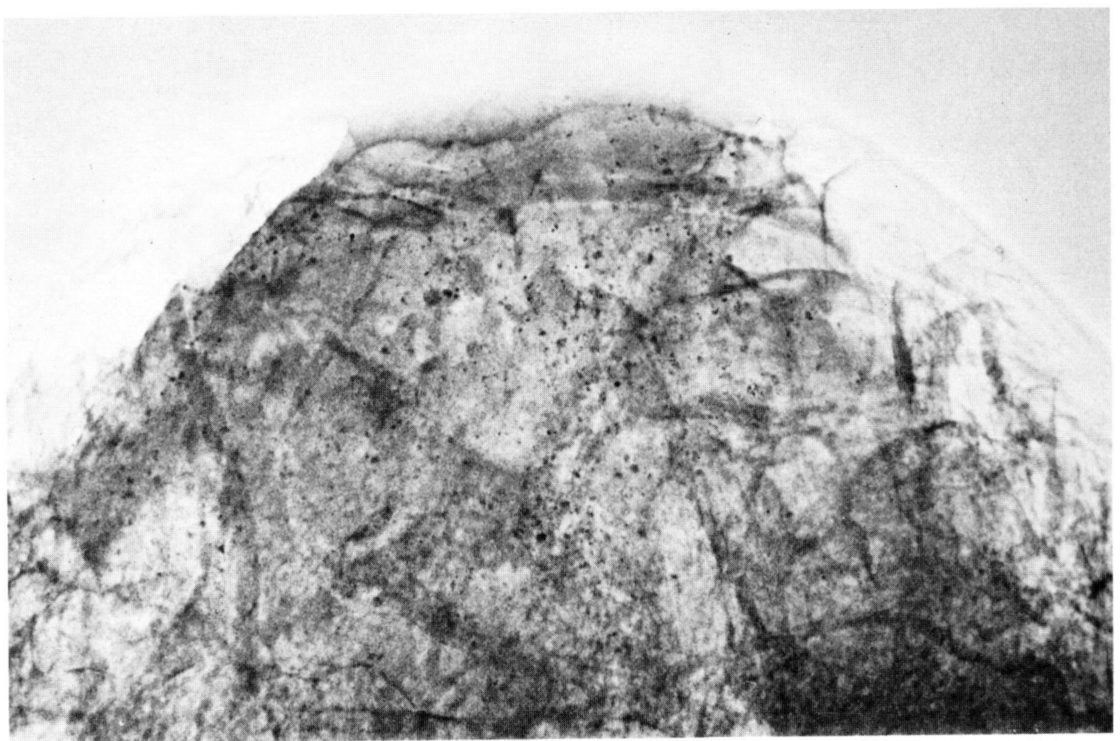

Fig. 55.13 Positive xerogram. Sclerosing adenosis with fine scattered calcifications shown as black dots.

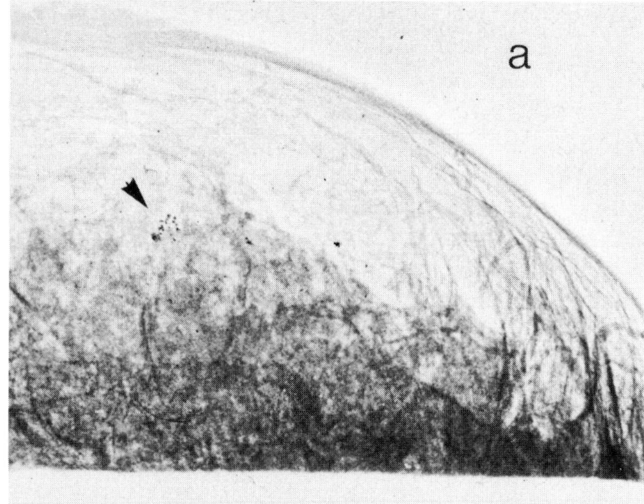

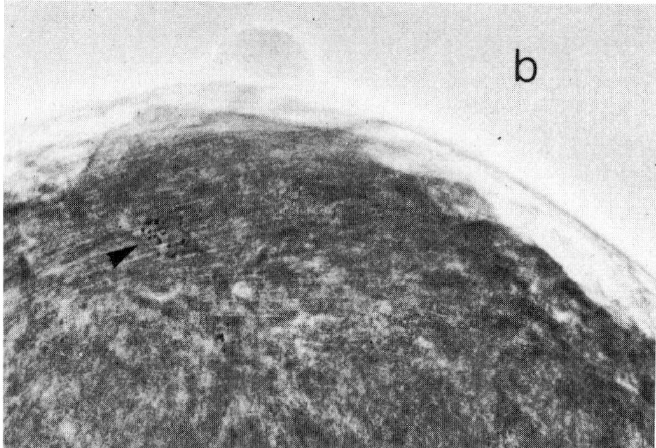

Fig. 55.14 Positive xerograms. (a) Calcifications in sclerosing adenosis (arrowed). (b) Calcifications in intraduct cancer (arrowed).

SECONDARY SIGNS

Changes in breast architecture

Disruption of anatomical structures occurs in malignancy. *Trabeculae* may be partially destroyed and distorted or trabecular thickening may be found. This thickening can be a localized or generalized feature (Figs. 55.6 and 55.8). *Lactiferous ducts* may be straightened or enlargement of ducts may occur (Fig. 55.6). The enlargement may be due to intraduct tumour or distal blockage by the cancer. *Nipple retraction* occurs secondarily to a fibrotic response to the tumour (Fig. 55.6). Deformity of *breast fat* may be seen. This takes two forms. The most common deformity is associated with scirrhous cancers and is due to irregular trabecular disruption and distortion. The fat around the tumour is also distorted giving a 'pseudo-lipomatous' appearance (Fig. 55.4). A rare finding in mucoid or colloid cancers is a smooth 'halo' of compressed fat. *Skin dimpling* over the tumour is a common occurrence (Fig. 55.6). *Skin thickening* may be localized or generalized. When generalized thickening occurs in diffuse infiltration trabecular thickening also occurs and many more trabeculae are visible in the subcutaneous fat than in a normal breast (Fig. 55.8). An early indication of impending diffuse infiltration is often found in thickening of the skin over the lower inner quadrant of the breast (Shukla *et al.*, 1979). Generalized oedema of the breast may be found in lymphoma of the axillary nodes. Enlargement of axillary lymph nodes is often seen in malignancy but this is not absolute proof of malignant involvement.

In benign disease breast architecture is distorted rather than disrupted or destroyed. Trabeculae are frequently seen to be displaced by cysts and fibroadenomata. Trabecular thickening occurs with inflammatory disease. Ducts may also be displaced but the most common duct abnormality is enlargement (Figs. 55.10 and 55.20). The enlargement may be due to dilatation of the duct or to thickening of the duct wall. Differentiation is not possible on plain films but galactography will distinguish the two causes. Duct ectasia is the commonest cause of nipple retraction. Enlargement of ducts is also seen in papillomatosis (Fig. 55.20).

Deformity of breast fat takes the form of compression in benign disease giving rise to a 'halo' around the lesion. This is commonly seen with fibroadenoma and cysts (Fig. 55.16) and is not a distinguishing feature of either. Skin dimpling and thickening may occur with inflammatory disease or following biopsy (Fig. 55.12). Diffuse skin thickening and oedema of the breast may be seen in acute infection or plasma cell mastitis. Axillary node enlargement occurs with inflammatory conditions and nodes may be variably replaced by fat following degeneration.

Vascularity of the breasts

It is important to realise that in about 45 per cent of normal women the left breast is more vascular than the right breast. Therefore it is difficult to assess hypervascularity of the left breast if only marginal changes are present. However, increased vascularity of the right breast should always be regarded as significant.

Increased size and number of veins frequently occur in association with malignancy but the changes are not invariable. The vascular pattern may be normal in slow growing tumours in the elderly and also in some cases of non-invasive intraduct cancers.

Benign inflammatory conditions are associated with hypervascularity and so also are some fibroadenomata and even cysts at times.

Perifocal haziness

Some cancers have a surrounding area of ill-defined haziness which is said by Ingleby and Gershon-Cohen (1960) to be due to oedema and collagenosis. It is usually found in association with aggressive tumours.

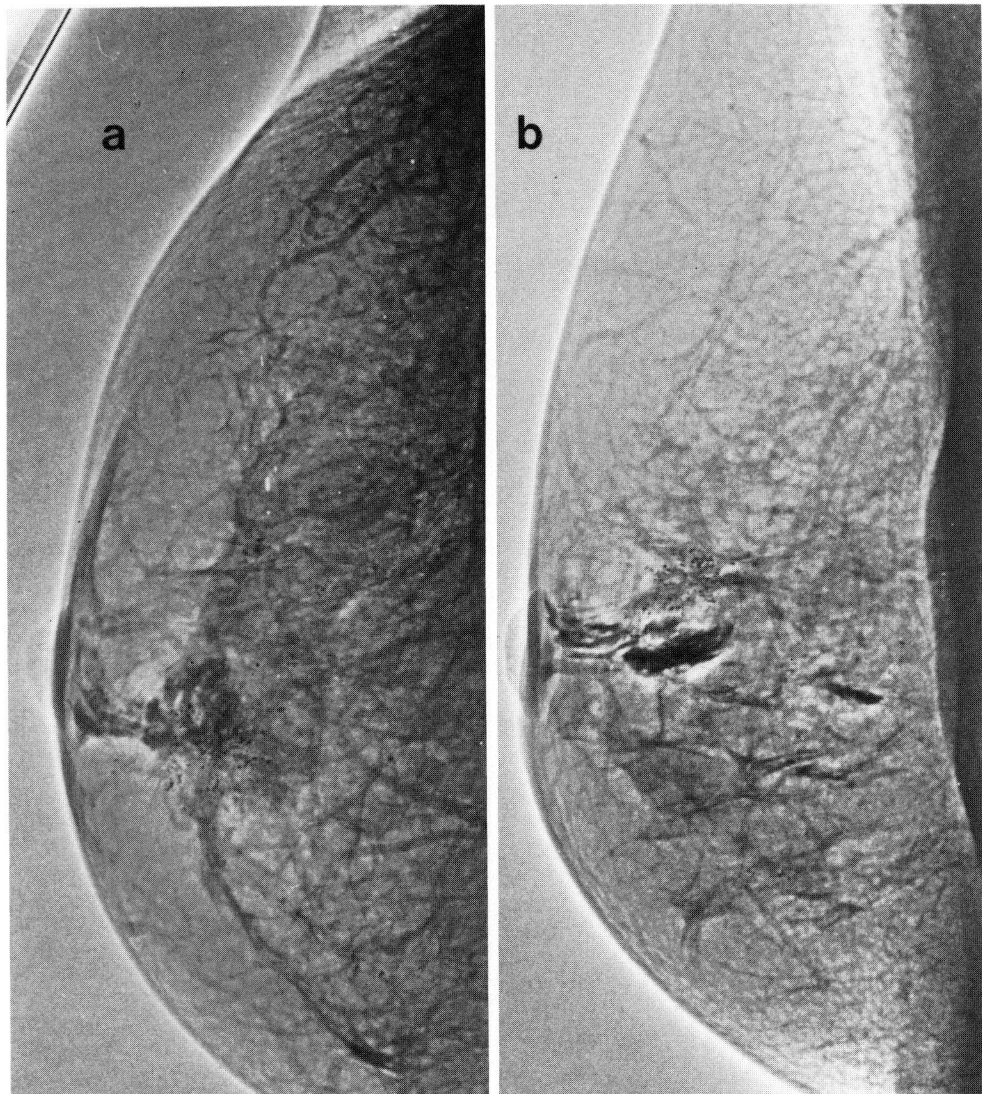

Fig. 55.15 Positive xerograms of localization technique. Note the dense Hypaque adjacent to the microcalcifications. (a) Craniocaudal projection. (b) Mediolateral projection.

A similar change due entirely to oedema may be found in inflammatory breast diseases.

Size of the lesion

The oedema and collagenosis associated with cancer may not be completely visible on a mammogram but they are palpable. Consequently the clinical size of the cancer is often larger than the radiological size. This does not hold for the smooth, circumscribed, colloid cancers, however, as there is little tissue reaction around such tumours. Clinical and radiological size will be the same in these cancers. This is also true of many benign lesions but inflammatory lesions may be larger clinically than radiologically. Lax cysts may be larger radiologically than clinically as they may be flattened out as the result of compression applied during radiography.

These facts regarding tumour size and many of the other features of malignant and benign lesions were described by Leborgne (1953).

MISCELLANEOUS BREAST LESIONS

Carcinoma of the male breast

Cancers of the male breast show identical features to those of the female breast. Microcalcification is rare however, and smooth circumscribed carcinomas are relatively more common in the male.

Paget's disease of the nipples

This condition is associated with breast cancer which may be clinically apparent or impalpable. Radiologically, there

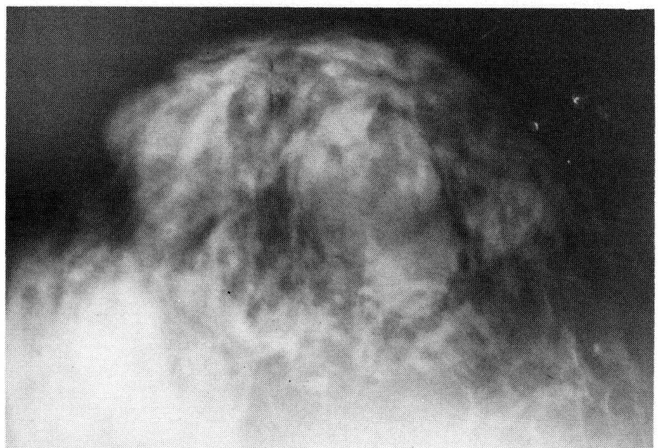

Fig. 55.16 Multiple cysts. Note density of the cysts and associated fat 'haloes'.

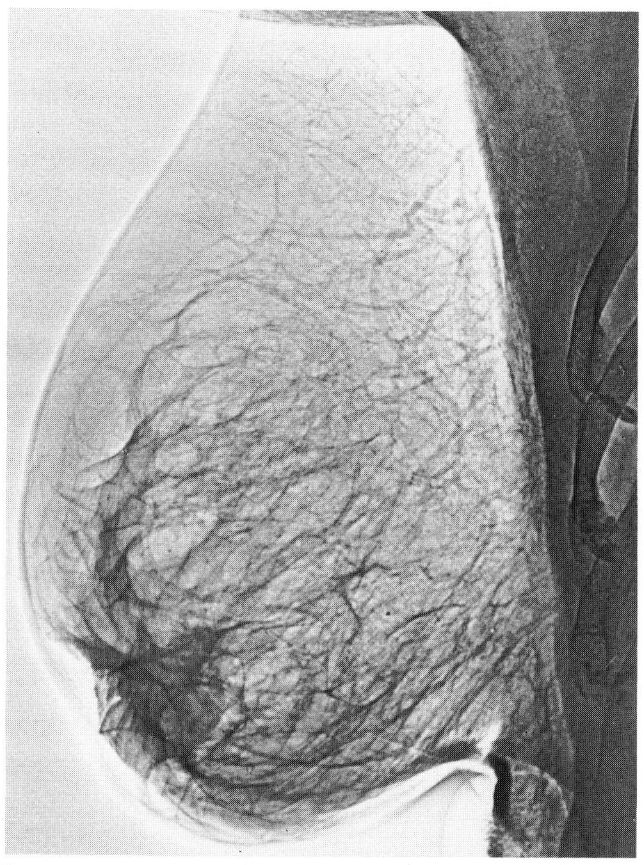

Fig. 55.17 Positive xerogram. Subacute, subareolar abscess.

may be an irregular mass with microcalcification or microcalcification may be the only sign of malignancy.

Cystosarcoma phylloides
As the name implies this is a cystic, fleshy tumour. It may be benign or malignant and may even metastasise. It is usually a large, smooth, dense, lobulated lesion with well defined margins and deep intersticies between numerous cotyledons.

Fibroadenosis (fibrocystic disease; mammary dysplasia) (Figs 55.16 and 55.18)
This benign condition is extremely common. It frequently presents with periodic mastalgia related to the menstrual cycle. Radiologically the diagnosis is made on increased density of the glandular portion of the breast in association with multiple, smooth, rounded lesions which may be either cysts or fibroadenomata (Fig. 55.18).

Wolfe (1976) maintains that women with severe 'mammary dysplasia' are at high risk for the development of breast cancer. This is not a new concept and has also been propounded by Haagensen (1971). Wolfe also maintains that women with a marked 'prominent duct pattern' are also at high risk. Mammary dysplasia and prominent duct patterns are extremely common findings on mammography so that they would be expected to be found often in association with breast cancer. Further investigation

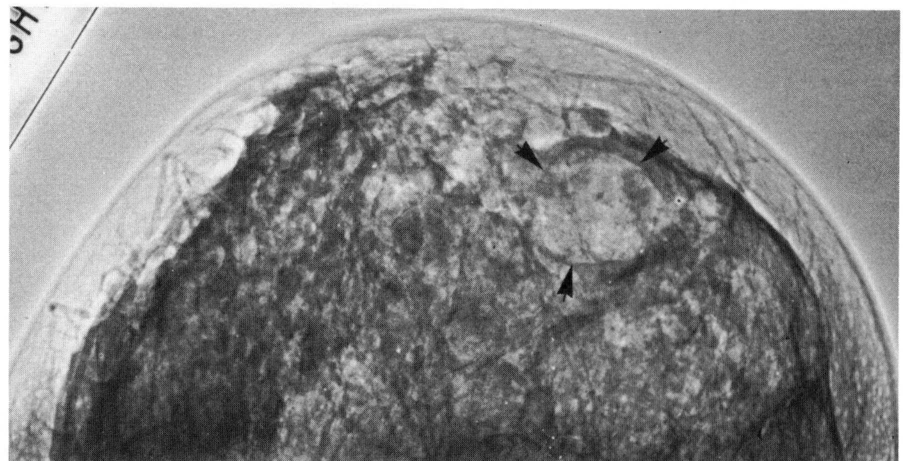

Fig. 55.18 Positive xerogram. Fibroadenosis with many small cysts. Transradiant lipoma (arrowed).

is necessary to elucidate the association of breast cancer with these conditions.

Sclerosing adenosis (lobular fibrosis) (Figs 55.13 and 55.14A)

Sclerosing adenosis mimics carcinoma of the breast in several ways. It may present clinically as a hard mass (sometimes fixed) with or without associated breast discomfort. Radiologically it gives rise to small groups of calcifications often indistinguishable from microcalcification of malignancy. It may present a stellate appearance on radiographs with distorted trabeculae. However, the clinical size is the same as the radiographic size.

Plasma cell mastitis (periductal mastitis)

This inflammatory condition is an association of duct ectasia ('secretory disease'). A painful lump is the usual clinical presentation. Radiologically this is associated with visible, enlarged ducts. The opacities produced are often flame-shaped or conical when peripherally situated but more ill-defined in the subareolar region. There is associated hypervascularity and in severe cases generalized oedema of the breast. Plasma cell mastitis may give rise to fat necrosis.

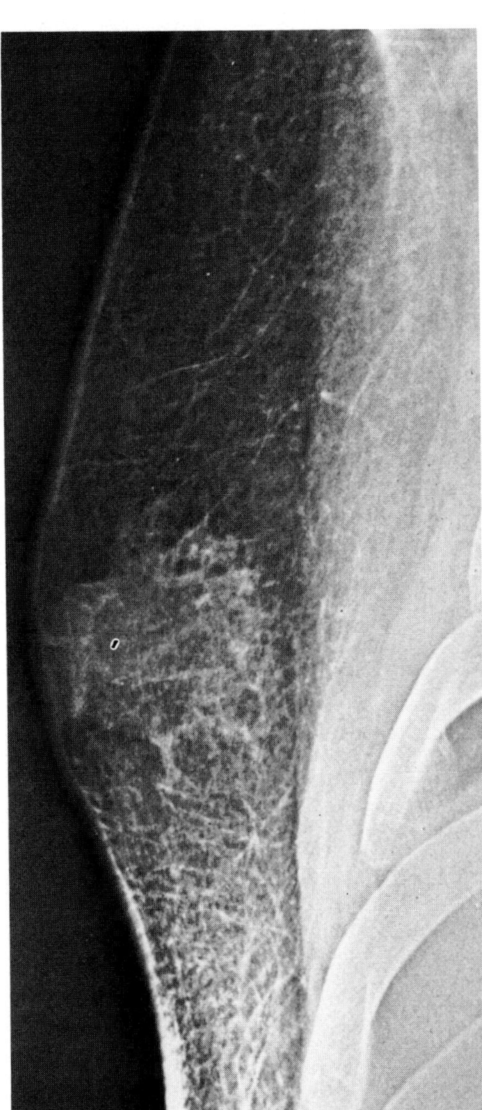

Fig. 55.19 Negative xerogram. Gynaecomastia.

Gynaecomastia (Fig. 55.19)

In the normal male breast the mammogram shows a small faint linear density beneath the nipple. In gynaecomastia a low density opacity of varying size is seen. The changes may be unilateral or bilateral. The importance of the condition is its differentiation from cancer of the male breast and its associations with systemic disease. A good account of this condition is given by Ginsburg (1969). The causes are physiological, pathological and pharmacological. The *physiological* types include neonatal, pubertal and senescent gynaecomastia. The *pathological* causes include endocrine disorders such as feminizing testicular tumours, e.g. chorion-epithelioma, seminoma and interstitial cell tumour; or hypogonadism, e.g. Klinefelter's syndrome. Feminizing adrenal tumours also cause gynaecomastia and occasionally it is seen in association with acromegaly. Carcinoma of the bronchus and chronic liver disease are other causes. *Pharmacological* causes include therapeutic use of oestrogens and digitalis.

CONTRAST EXAMINATIONS OF THE BREAST

Galactography (Fig. 55.20)

Contrast examination of the lactiferous ducts is a well established supplementary method of investigation of breast disease (Leborgne, 1953; Bjørn-Hansen, 1965). Its main value is in the investigation of nipple discharge, particularly a discharge from one duct orifice. The size and margins of the duct are demonstrated and any intraduct lesion shown. The commonest indication is a bloodstained nipple discharge and the commonest cause of this condition is *intraduct papilloma*. It also occurs frequently with *duct ectasia* and during the later stages of *pregnancy* and *lactation*. Less commonly the underlying cause is *carcinoma* of the breast, either invasive carcinoma or non-invasive intraduct carcinoma. It is important to realise that on occasions a serous nipple discharge may be due to carcinoma but usually this is due to *fibroadenosis with cysts*—especially when multiple ducts are involved. Greenish or brownish nipple discharge are associated with duct ectasia and fibroadenosis. Smooth intraductal, filling defects on galactography are usually due to papillomatosis but are indistinguishable from non-invasive, papilliferous, intraduct cancer and granulomata. Irregular, narrowing of the duct with distal dilatation is found with invasive carcinoma.

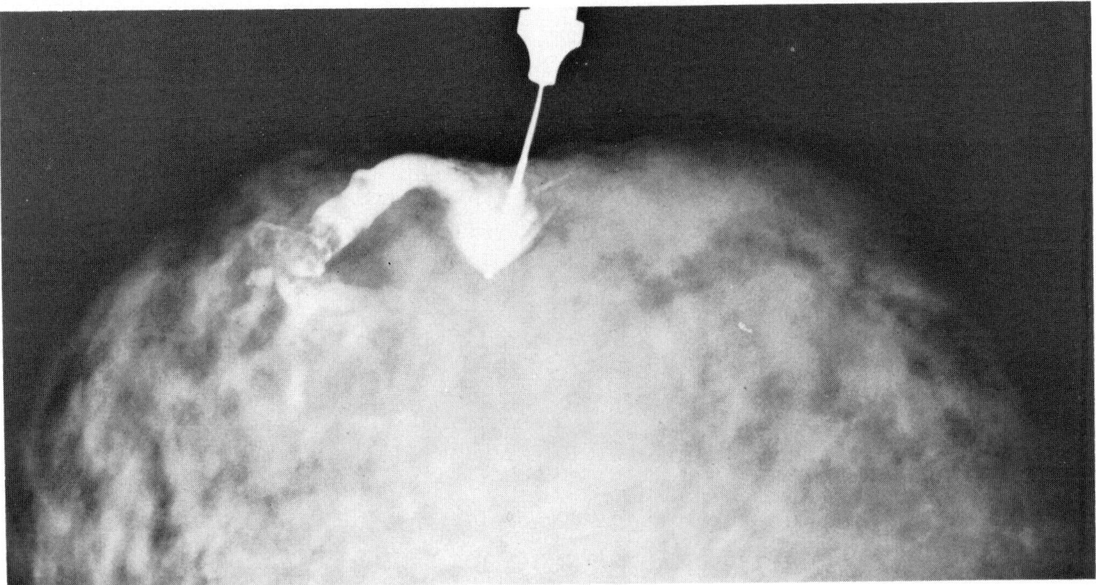

Fig. 55.20 Galactography. A dilated duct containing papillomata.

Nipple discharge of any variety arising from a solitary duct should be thoroughly investigated even in the absence of palpable abnormality.

Pneumocystography (Fig. 55.21)

Aspiration of the contents of a breast cyst with replacement by the same volume of air enables the internal lining of the cyst to be well demonstrated (Haage and Fischedick, 1964). The technique may be employed to demonstrate cysts that recur after aspiration. These frequently do not refill following pneumocystography. The main indication is the finding of blood-stained fluid on aspiration of a cyst. This indicates the presence of an intracystic papilloma or carcinoma. Pneumocystography demonstrates the presence, position and extent of an intracystic tumour pre-operatively and usually a diagnosis of benign or malignant tumour can be made.

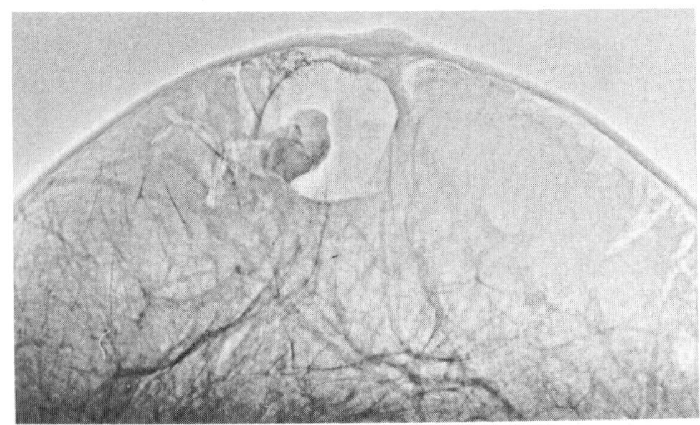

Fig. 55.21 Positive xerogram. Pneumocystography showing intracystic papilloma.

INDICATION FOR MAMMOGRAPHY

The main use for mammography is in the investigation of symptomatic patients as a complementary method to clinical examination. It is useful to confirm or refute the clinical diagnosis in patients with a palpable lesion. It may show an unsuspected impalpable carcinoma in patients with a clinically benign lesion, either in the same breast or in the opposite breast. Similarly it may show an unsuspected carcinoma in the contralateral breast in association with a clinically obvious carcinoma of the breast. It is a useful complementary method of examination in patients with vague breast symptoms, eczema of the nipple or nodular breasts. Accurate assessment of the response of the primary breast cancer is possible in cases treated with radiotherapy or chemotherapy. Finally, unsuspected cancers of the breast may be found on mammographic screening of well women. Whether this is a valuable procedure or not is still questionable (Bailar, 1976; Baum, 1977).

REFERENCES AND SUGGESTIONS FOR FURTHER READING

Asbury, D. L. & Barker, P. G. (1975) Radiation dosage to the breast in well women screening surveys. *British Journal of Radiology*, **48**, 963–967.

Bailar, J. C. (1976) Mammography: A contrary view. *Annals of Internal Medicine*, **84**, 77–84.

Baum, M. (1976) The curability of breast cancer. *British Medical Journal*, **i**, 439–442.

Bjørn-Hansen, R. (1965) Contrast mammography. *British Journal of Radiology*, **38**, 947–951.

Egan, R. L. (1972) *Mammography*. Springfield, Ill.: Thomas.

Evans, K. T. & Gravelle, I. H. (1973) Mammography, Thermography and Ultrasonography in Breast Disease. *Radiology in Clinical Diagnosis* Series. London: Butterworth.

GINSBURG, J. (1969) Gynaecomastia. *The Practitioner*, **203**, 166–170.

GRAVELLE, I. H. & HALLETT, P. (1975) Xeromammography—the process and image characteristics. *Medical and Biological Illustration*, **25**, 93.

HAAGE, H. & FISCHEDICK, O. (1964) Die Solitärzyste der weiblichen Brust im Röntgenbild. *Fortschritte Röntgenstrahlen*, **100**, 639–645.

HAAGENSEN, C. D. (1971) *Diseases of the Breast*. Philadelphia: Saunders.

INGLEBY, H. & GERSHON-COHEN, J. (1960) *Comparative Anatomy, Pathology and Roentgenology of the Breast*. Philadelphia: University of Pennsylvania Press.

LEBORGNE, R. A. (1953) *The Breast in Roentgen Diagnosis*. Montevideo: Impresora Uraguy S.A. and London: Constable.

LUNDGREN, B. (1977) The oblique view at mammography. *British Journal of Radiology*, **50**, 626–628.

PREECE, P. E., GRAVELLE, I. H., HUGHES, L. E., BAUM, M., FORTT, R. W. & LEOPOLD, J. G. (1977) The operative management of sub-clinical breast cancer. *Clinical Oncology*, **3**, 165–169.

PRICE, J. L., DAVIES, P. M. & BUTLER, P. D. (1976) Mammograms on medichrome film. *Clinical Radiology*, **27**, 371–373.

SHUKLA, H. S., HUGHES, L. E., GRAVELLE, I. H. & SATIR, A. M. A. (1979) The significance of mammary skin oedema in non-inflammatory breast cancer. *Annals of Surgery*, **189**, 53–57.

WOLFE, J. N. (1972) Xeroradiography of the breast. Springfield, Ill.: Thomas.

WOLFE, J. N. (1976) Breast patterns as an index of risk for developing breast cancer. *The American Journal of Roentgenology, Radiation Therapy and Nuclear Medicine*, **126**, 1130–1137.

PART 7

THE CENTRAL NERVOUS SYSTEM

CHAPTER 56

PATHOLOGY AND METHODS OF EXAMINATION

A. PATHOLOGY OF INTRACRANIAL TUMOURS

The study of neuroradiology is difficult without a good knowledge of the pathology of intracranial tumours and of tumours involving the skull. It is also important to understand the relative frequency of incidence of such tumours. Large neurosurgical series analysed in the past (Cushing, 1932; Cairns, 1957; Olivecrona, 1952) showed an approximate incidence as in Table 56.1. This is compared with the incidence in a large pathological series (Zimmerman, 1971).

Whilst all neurosurgical series are to some extent selected, the table gives a good idea of the relative proportion of different intracranial tumours encountered in neurosurgical centres. In the neurosurgical series the proportion of secondary or metastatic tumours is underestimated since many patients with known primary tumours and cerebral metastases are referred to radiotherapists rather than to neurosurgeons, and others develop cerebral metastases in the terminal stages of their illness. The proportion of pituitary tumours is also atypically high in the neurosurgical series because of Cushing's special interest and expertise in this field.

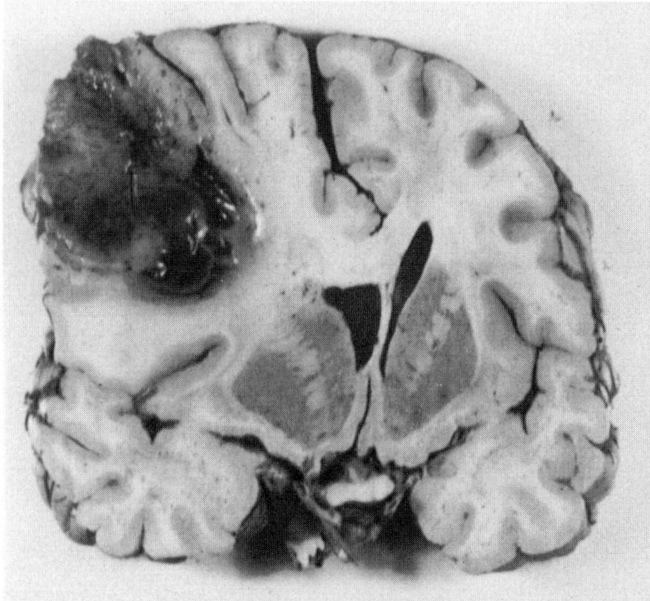

Fig. 56.1 Large malignant glioma in the parietal region. Note the displacement of the lateral ventricles and the downward displacement of the insula.

Gliomas (Fig. 56.1) are the commonest intracranial tumours and comprise between 40 and 50 per cent of the cases in most series. They vary greatly in malignancy. The well-differentiated tumours, e.g. oligodendroglioma or the well-differentiated astrocytoma, are relatively slow growing. On the other hand, the undifferentiated tumours such as glioblastoma multiforme are highly malignant. The classification of gliomas has been a matter of some controversy in the past. Most authors favour grading according to the degree of malignancy, e.g. Kernohan and his colleagues from the Mayo Clinic, whilst other workers have favoured the retention of specific names for the different types of glioma.

Table 56.1

Series	Neurosurgical	Zimmerman (1971)
Total number of cases	6876	5199
	percentage	*percentage*
Glioma	45	31·4
Meningioma	15	15·4
Pit. adenoma	11	4·4
Acoustic tumour	8	1·5
Blood vessel tumour	4·5	5·9
Congen. tumour	4	2·0
Metastatic	4	20·3
Granuloma	1·5	6·4
Miscellaneous	7	12·3

On the whole, gliomas tend to occur more frequently in males than in females and in large series there seems to be a greater incidence in the left hemisphere than in the right. It has also been shown that the temporal lobe is more commonly affected than other lobes. A small but significant proportion of the less malignant gliomas may show calcification on simple X-ray examination.

Meningiomas (Fig. 56·2) are one of the most important intracranial tumours. This is not only because they form between 10 and 20 per cent of the tumours encountered but also because they are usually benign. Thus a correct diagnosis followed by surgical removal may result in a complete cure. Meningiomas are alleged to be derived from rests of arachnoid cells in the dura. Occasionally they occur intracranially, when they are thought to be derived from aberrant cell rests, or from the choroid plexus. Whilst the majority of these tumours are benign, a few appear to be more invasive and malignant. The relationship of so-called malignant meningioma to what were once erroneously called sarcomas of the brain has been a matter for controversy in the past. It is now thought that most cases diagnosed as sarcomas were, in fact, malignant meningiomas. Meningiomas frequently produce characteristic bone changes which permit a pathological diagnosis at simple X-ray (see Chapter 58).

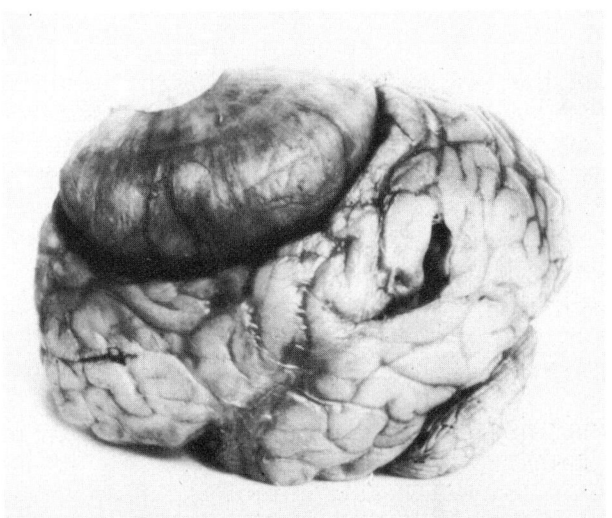

Fig. 56.2 Large parasagittal frontoparietal meningioma. This is entirely extracerebral and is displacing and deforming the brain.

Pituitary tumours. The majority of these tumours are adenomas. In the past these have been classified on microscopy findings into chromophobe, basophil and acidophil. From the neurosurgical point of view, the most frequently encountered were *chromophobe adenomas*. Clinically, these cases usually present with visual failure. A bitemporal field defect indicating chiasmal pressure is frequently present and there may be clinical evidence of hypopituitarism. *Basophil adenomas* (which give rise to Cushing's syndrome) are of little neurosurgical importance, since they are usually microscopic and only on isolated occasions have they been known to give rise to recognizable pituitary enlargement. However, if a patient with Cushing's syndrome is treated by bilateral adrenalectomy, then secondary pituitary hyperplasia may result with recognizable sellar enlargement (Nelson's syndrome). The *acidophil adenoma* (which gives rise to acromegaly in the adult, and to gigantism in the young) produces pituitary enlargement in about 50 per cent of cases. There are also other typical changes in the skull and skeleton which are described in other chapters.

This classification of pituitary tumours based on light microscopy findings into acidophil, basophil and chromophobe and the view that the first two are secretory and the latter non-functioning is no longer valid. Some patients with acromegaly have been found to have purely chromophobe adenomas and some patients with Cushing's syndrome have also been associated with chromophobe adenomas. It is now generally thought better to classify tumours as *functioning* and *non-secretory*. In the past, 80 per cent of pituitary adenomas have been regarded as non-secreting. Recent studies, however, have shown that a high proportion of these have *hyperprolactinaemia*. This leads to gonadal dysfunction in both sexes and to galactorrhea in a proportion.

Prolactin secreting adenoma of the pituitary is now a well recognised entity. It can, as noted above, be associated with large tumours. On the other hand, it may be associated with quite tiny tumours only a few mms in diameter and known as *micro-adenomata*. Some of these tiny tumours can produce small eccentric enlargement of the pituitary fossa which can be diagnosed by tomography. However, great caution is necessary before accepting findings based on slight asymmetry of the pituitary floor since such asymmetry can occur in the normal.

Hyperprolactinaemia can also be drug induced and there are many different drugs which can produce it including chlorpromazine, haloperidol, metaclopromide, reserpine, methyl-dopa, tricyclic antidepressants and some oral contraceptives. It is, of course, important for these drug cases to be excluded before investigating radiologically.

Pituitary *carcinoma* is extremely rare, but is occasionally encountered.

Acoustic neuromas form an important group of posterior fossa tumours. Clinically, classical cases show a depressed corneal reflex and other evidence of 5th nerve involvement, 8th nerve deafness on the affected side, and ipsilateral facial weakness. Raised intracranial pressure may or may not be present, and many cases can present in an atypical manner. Radiological diagnosis is discussed in detail below.

Trigeminal neuroma is a very rare intracranial tumour arising from the 5th nerve in the region of the Gasserian ganglion. It can be dumb-bell in shape, presenting both in the middle and posterior fossa. These tumours can simulate acoustic neuromas if they enlarge mainly in the posterior fossa. The radiological diagnosis is discussed below.

Angiomas (Fig. 56.3). These are not true tumours but are 'angiomatous malformations' of congenital origin. They were once thought to be rare but, since the widespread use of angiography, have been recognized in increasing numbers and are now known to be one of the commoner intracranial lesions.

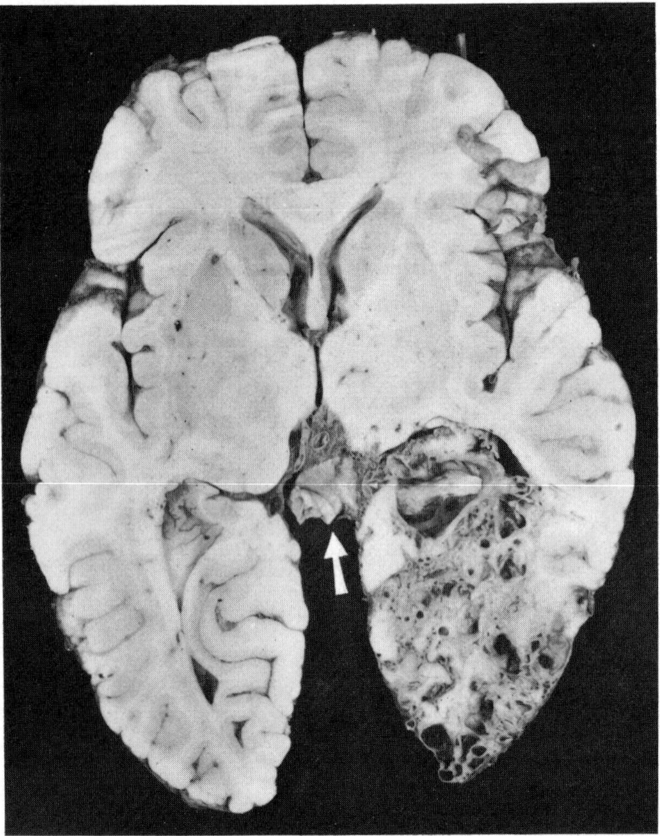

Fig. 56.3 Large angiomatous malformation occupying most of left occipital lobe. Horizontal section of the brain from frontal to occipital poles. Note dilated Vein of Galen (↑).

Metastases. The brain is a common site for secondary deposit, and the commonest primary sites are lung, breast and kidney. On most occasions metastases are multiple, but occasionally solitary metastases are encountered in the brain. Occasionally such solitary metastases have been successfully removed together with, or after removal of, the primary tumour.

Lymphoma can involve the c.n.s. and extradural deposits in the spine may give rise to cord compression. Involvement of the meninges over the brain may also occur, though frank intracerebral masses are rare.

Microglioma is a form of primary lymphoma involving brain which may present as a localised mass or, more frequently, as a diffuse, ill-localised infiltration. There is still considerable controversy as to its relationship to lymphoma in general. There is no doubt that it may occur purely in the central nervous system though some cases may co-exist with unsuspected lymphoma elsewhere in the body. It is malignant but radiosensitive. There is an abnormally high incidence of this lesion in patients undergoing immuno-suppressive treatment, particularly organ transplant patients.

MISCELLANEOUS TUMOURS

Medulloblastomas are highly malignant tumours which, unfortunately, are found most frequently in children. They may occasionally occur in adults when their course seems to be more benign than in children. The tumours usually arises in the posterior fossa near the midline. An unusual feature is that subarachnoid seeding may occur with spread of the tumour along the spinal axis. The tumour is sensitive to radiation but usually recurs eventually. These cases are normally treated by radiotherapy applied to the whole spine and posterior fossa. Surgery is limited to exploration and biopsy, decompression, or a shunt operation.

Rathke pouch tumours (synonyms: craniopharyngioma, suprasellar cyst, epidermoid, adamantinoma). These tumours are thought to arise from remnants of Rathke's pouch and usually grow above the pituitary fossa. A few, however, grow in the sella and produce enlargement and deformity of the pituitary fossa.

Most of these tumours present in children though they are occasionally seen for the first time in adults. They tend to merge with the floor of the 3rd ventricle and with the infundibulum, which makes complete surgical removal difficult or impossible. A high proportion show calcification.

Haemangioblastomas. These relatively rare tumours are found in the posterior fossa, and most frequently in the cerebellum. The association of haemangioblastoma with angioma of the retina has received much prominence in the past and is usually referred to as Lindau's syndrome. This, however, is a very rare entity whilst haemangioblastoma of the posterior fossa is not infrequent, and may be multiple. It usually shows a characteristic appearance at angiography. Haemangioblastoma may also occur in the spinal cord where it presents as an intramedullary tumour.

Pineal tumours are probably teratomas in most cases. They present with abnormalities of occular movement and of the pupils, due to compression of the quadrigeminal plate, or with hypothalamic symptoms which may include precocious puberty.

Colloid cysts (synonym: paraphyseal cyst). These unusual cysts (Fig. 56.4) grow from the roof of the 3rd ventricle and may produce gross symmetrical hydrocephalus when still quite small. They may also produce false, or no localizing signs. They are rewarding tumours to diagnose since they can be removed with complete cure of the patient, or successfully treated by ventricular shunting.

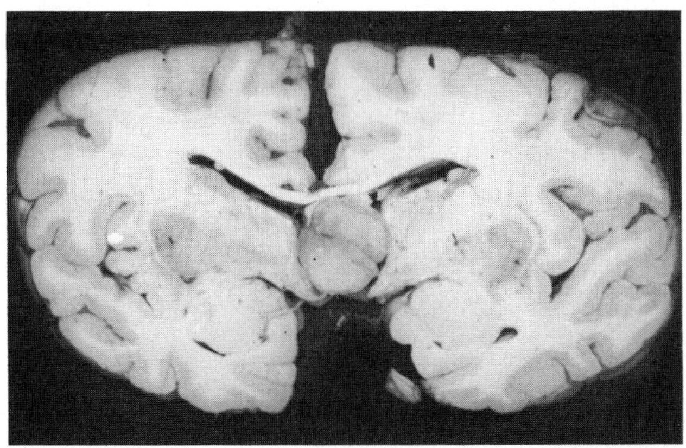

Fig. 56.4 Colloid cyst occupying and completely occluding the third ventricle. Coronal brain section through the lateral ventricles and the cyst.

Papillomas. These rare tumours arise from the choroid plexus and are most commonly seen in the 4th ventricle in children. They may also occur in the lateral ventricle (usually on the left side), or in the 3rd ventricle. Rather surprisingly they can give rise to considerable hydrocephalus although sited in a lateral ventricle. It is thought that this may be due to overproduction of cerebrospinal fluid.

Ependymomas. These tumours, which may be regarded as a form of glioma, can occur within the brain substance, when they are thought to be derived from ependymal rests. They may also grow from the ventricular wall, and they have been encountered in the lateral ventricle and in the 3rd and 4th ventricles. The latter situations usually preclude successful removal.

Intracranial ependymoma is relatively rare, but spinal ependymoma is the commonest spinal intramedullary tumour.

Chordomas are tumours derived from the primitive notochord which extends from the basiphenoid through the spine to the sacrum. They can arise anywhere along the spinal axis though they are commonest at the upper and lower ends, i.e. in the clivus or sacrum. Tumours in the clivus can extend intracranially where they form a large cerebral mass pressing on the brain stem and cranial nerves. Rarely they may be more anterior and involve the parasellar region or even the orbit.

Myeloma presenting as plasmacytoma or so called solitary myeloma can occasionally present in the skull vault as a large lytic lesion expanding the skull vault and pressing on underlying brain.

Glomus jugulare tumours arise in the region of the jugular bulb and extend into the petrous bone and internal ear producing basal erosion. They can also extend into the posterior fossa. They present in adult life and women are affected three times as frequently as men.

Dermoids and epidermoids are rare tumours, particularly the former. Dermoids present mainly in children and young adults and are found particularly in the posterior fossa or at the base of the brain. The commoner epidermoid occurs mainly in the cerebello pontine angle or para-pituitary region and middle fossa. Rarely it may be found in a hemisphere and has been described in the cavity of a lateral ventricle. At operation the nodular capsule may show a mother of pearl sheen which gives rise to the term 'pearly' tumour.

NON-NEOPLASTIC INTRACRANIAL MASSES

The differential diagnosis of intracranial tumours both clinically and radiologically may include certain non-neoplastic lesions, and these will be briefly noted.

Abscesses in the brain arise most commonly by direct spread from infected mastoids or sinuses. An extradural abscess may form or the infection may penetrate into brain tissue. Mastoid infections spread either to involve the temporal lobe or into the posterior fossa.

Brain abscess is less commonly haematogenous in origin and may be related to bronchiectasis or endocarditis, particularly in congenital heart disease with a right to left shunt as in Fallot's tetralogy.

Haematomas

Intracranial haematomas are usually associated with the history of an acute vascular accident. However a large intracranial haematoma will give the same mechanical effects as any other large intracranial pathological mass. If the patient is found unconscious the diagnosis may be in doubt and require special investigation.

Similarly, **extradural haematomas** are readily suspect on the presenting history of severe head trauma. They are generally associated with a fracture in the skull vault involving a meningeal vessel. Again, however, if the patient is found unconscious and there is no clear evidence of trauma, special investigation may be necessary to establish the diagnosis.

Subdural haematomas by way of contrast can present with little or no previous evidence to suggest the diagnosis. For this reason they are particularly easy to miss in alcoholic and psychiatric patients who cannot give an adequate history. With an intelligent patient a history of minor head trauma may or may not be obtained. The clinical signs may be negligible and are often limited to headache, inability to concentrate, and other symptoms with no localizing value. These can easily be mistaken for neurosis. Large subdural haematomas, however, are usually associated with focal signs such as a contralateral hemiparesis.

Aneurysm can occasionally reach a very large size without rupturing and intracranial *aneurysms* of this type, particularly when the basilar artery is involved, may be mistaken for local tumours.

Arachnoid cysts are unusual lesions of the meninges, the aetiology of which is obscure but which may be developmental. They usually contain clear fluid and can reach a large size, when they will act as an intracranial mass or tumour with symptoms, depending on the site. Arachnoid cysts can also occur in the spine.

Granulomas resembling tumours are becoming less common and *tuberculoma* which was once frequent is now very rarely seen except in under-developed countries.

Infestations of the brain occasionally present as tumours. *Cysticercosis* was at one time the type most commonly seen in this country, usually acquired by soldiers who had seen service in India. In certain areas such as South America or South Africa *hydatid cysts* are encountered in the central nervous system and present as local expanding lesions. Cerebral *paragonimiasis* is encountered in the Far East, most cases being reported from Korea and China.

Other non-tumorous conditions which occasionally enter into the differential diagnosis of cerebral tumours include *developmental lesions* such as *epiloia*.

Toxic or otitic hydrocephalus is a condition of obscure aetiology which also enters into the differential diagnosis of some cases of suspected cerebral tumour. Some of these cases are secondary to middle ear disease, and the condition may be associated with sinus thrombosis; in other cases no definite cause is demonstrated. These latter cases are usually children or young females with a few weeks history of headaches and papilloedema. Investigations such as C.T. arteriography and air encephalography show normal ventricles and the cerebrospinal fluid is also normal. The prognosis is good and recovery is accelerated by treatment with steroids.

B. METHODS OF EXAMINATION

The methods of examination available to the neuroradiologist investigating a suspected intracranial lesion include:

1. Simple X-rays
2. C.A.T.
3. Angiography
4. Pneumography
5. Cisternography
   (a) Myodil
   (b) Amipaque
6. Isotope scanning
7. Ultrasound
8. Thermography
9. Stereotaxis
10. Cystography and pyography

Most of these techniques are considered in detail in the following chapters. However, it is pertinent at this stage to include a short discussion of the general place of particular special investigations in neuroradiological diagnosis and the criteria by which different methods are chosen for individual patients. This will be followed by a short description of some of the techniques which are not described in detail in the later chapters.

Simple X-ray examination, and if necessary *tomography*, will be the first radiological method of examination in most patients with suspected intracranial and spinal lesions.

There has always been some degree of controversy as to which of the other special techniques should then be used in particular cases and practice differed from centre to centre.

When the second edition of this text was published in 1975 the revolutionary new technique invented by the British physicist Hounsfield had only recently become available (Hounsfield, 1973) and its impact could only be predicted. Since then the most optimistic forecasts have been more than justified, and the method has become widely available with rapid technical improvement. The impact of this brilliant new conception has dramatically changed the practice of neuroradiology. Computerized axial tomography scanning is now the special technique of choice for the investigation of cerebral tumours and of most other intracranial lesions. Several of the special investigations listed above have diminished in importance and may soon be obsolete. Thus *isotope scanning* which was becoming increasingly important before 1973 is now little practised in the investigation of tumours where C.A.T. is also available. Similarly, *ventriculography* and *encephalography* once so important in the localization of cerebral tumours are now rarely used, being mainly reserved for the demonstration of small lesions where the C.A.T. scan has been equivocal or negative in the presence of strong clinical evidence of a lesion. This applies particularly to the better demonstration of small suprasellar tumours, and brainstem or cerebello-pontine angle tumours where C.A.T. has been inconclusive Pneumography is also still used for confirmation of the 'empty sella' syndrome or other specific problems.

Angiography has also diminished in importance though to a lesser degree and it remains essential in the investigation of many vascular lesions. C.A.T. is now the primary investigation of choice not only in suspected intracranial tumours and in head injuries but also in most suspected vascular lesions. These include subarachnoid haemorrhage, intracerebral haemorrhage and cerebral thrombosis.

In the case of tumours some surgeons now operate purely on the C.A.T. evidence except in special cases. Others still favour angiography to complement the C.A.T. findings. This is particularly so in cases of meningioma where they wish to define the vascular supply and relations of the tumour, or in glioma which may prove excessively vascular at operation, or in cases where specific diagnosis remains controversial on the C.A.T. findings. Angiography is still of course essential in cases of subarachnoid haemorrhage to define the aneurysm or other source of bleeding even though C.A.T. may have already helped to show the site of the bleed and influenced the type of angiogram. C.A.T. may, however, provide little or no help in some of these vascular cases. It may also prove of little help in the investigation of suspected extracerebral vascular disease, e.g. in cases of repeated transient ischaemic attacks (T.I.A.). In these cases C.A.T. findings are usually negative and angiography is usually diagnostic. C.A.T. may also prove unhelpful or equivocal in the case of an isodense haematoma, when angiography is diagnostic. The value of C.A.T. in the various vascular lesions is discussed in detail below (see Ch. 64).

With head injuries and suspected extradural or subdural haematoma *ultrasound* can still be a useful primary procedure which will demonstrate any marked shift of the midline structures. In the same way echo-encephalography can occasionally prove a useful primary investigation in some patients with suspected but poorly lateralized intracranial tumours. However, where C.A.T. is available ultrasound is now little practised since a normal ultrasound does not exclude bilateral haematomas or midline tumours, and an abnormal ultrasound will in any case require C.A.T. for further elucidation prior to surgery.

ISOTOPE BRAIN SCANNING

(See also Chapter 66)

A small tracer dose of the radioisotope is administered intravenously, and the scanning is carried out at a variable time later depending on the isotope used. Di Chiro was the first to establish the value of radioisotopes in the diagnosis of intracranial lesions in a large scale trial. He used radioactive iodinated serum albumen (R.I.S.A.) tagged with ^{131}I.

Since then radioactive mercury in the form of ^{203}Hg and ^{197}Hg has been used and later sodium pertechnetate (^{99}Tc^{m}). This latter radio-isotope has a half-life of only 6 hours compared with 65 hours for ^{197}Hg and 8 days for ^{131}I.

The radiation dose from ^{99}Tc^{m} is very small indeed and from this point of view it was rapidly accepted as the best medium. Nevertheless, every attempt must be made to keep the radiation dose down and patients should not have repeated scans during young adult life. Children, of course, should not be repeatedly scanned without very strong indications.

An even safer isotope has been introduced in the form of ^{113}In^{m} or radioindium. This has a half-life of only 1·7 hours and in this respect is an ideal medium for brain scanning. However, owing to technical problems with its preparation it is not widely used.

Technique. Once the isotope has entered the blood and passed to the brain it appears to be taken up by certain intracranial tumours and other intracranial lesions. The exact mechanism for this is not very well understood but is probably associated with the cerebral lesions affecting the blood-brain barrier locally and allowing permeation of the isotope.

The technique of brain scanning has been rapidly improved in recent years and the so-called 'gamma camera' has largely replaced linear scanners enabling more rapid scans to be obtained.

Further refinements of the techniques which have been studied are methods which enable the rate of uptake and removal of the isotope from brain lesions to be assessed. This time pattern adds considerably to the diagnostic value of the method since different lesions behave in different ways and considerable aid with diagnosing pathology has been claimed. However, the prolonged nature of these investigations which require repeated examinations over a period of time has made them impractical except at special centres.

Dynamic studies are also undertaken with the gamma camera. The isotope is injected into an arm vein as a bolus. Fifteen or 20 millicuries of sodium pertechnetate (^{99}Tc^{m}) are used and sequential images at the rate of 1 per sec. are recorded of the neck and head as the bolus passes up the carotid and vertebral arteries and through the cerebral circulation. The images are recorded on 35 mm film, and although resolution is poor it is adequate to demonstrate gross differences between the two sides on anteroposterior or vertex films. Thus unilateral ischaemia due to *carotid thrombosis or stenosis* can be recognized. The method is also useful for detecting large arterio-venous shunts such as occur in *angiomatous malformations* (Fig. 56.14).

With modern data processing apparatus the passage of the bolus can be recorded on tape with the differing scintillation counts in different areas. This can be played back at leisure and the information analysed in a variety of ways. Thus the uptake in different areas of the brain can be directly compared, and comparative flow studies obtained. The results can be presented either as images or as histograms, or both.

Interpretation. The method has proved of most use in the diagnosis of supratentorial lesions. Diagnosis in the posterior fossa may be confused by the normal increased uptake over the suboccipital muscles. However, positive scans can be obtained even in the posterior fossa. Apart from the suboccipital muscles, increased uptake is normally seen over the sagittal and lateral sinuses and torcula, and over the temporal muscles and face.

Pathological increased uptake will be seen in a high proportion of tumours. However, the findings are not specific since increased uptake is also seen in certain non-tumorous lesions including subdural haematoma, abscess, brain infarct or ischaemia, angiomatous malformation, and large aneurysm.

Among the true tumours *meningiomas* show up very well and produce quite dense well-demarcated areas of increased uptake. This fact together with their characteristic parasagittal or superficial site may strongly suggest the diagnosis (Figs. 56.8 and 56.9).

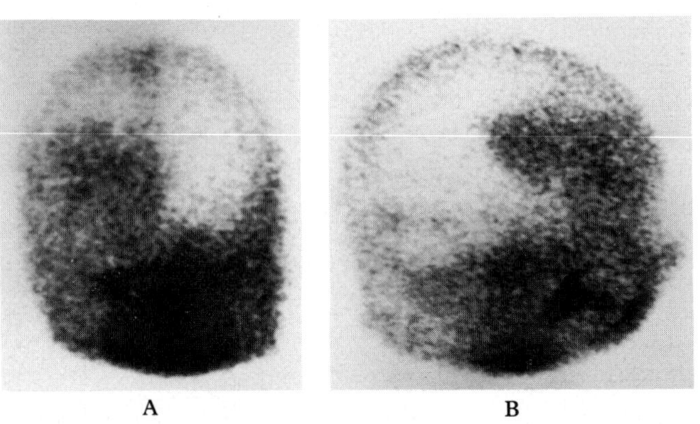

Fig. 56.5 Highly malignant glioma in the frontal region with high uptake. (A) Antero-posterior. (B) Right lateral view.

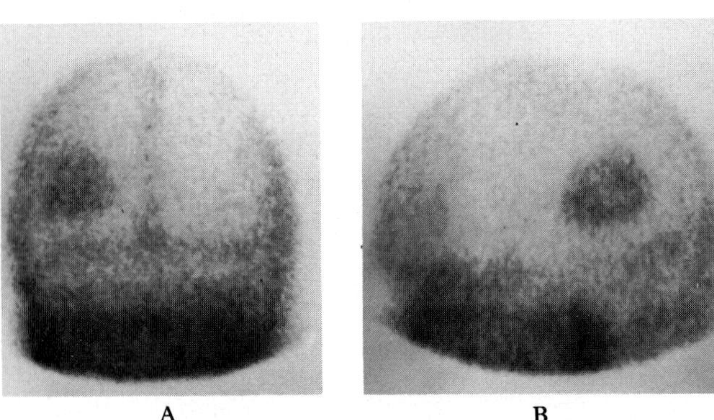

Fig. 56.6 Increased uptake in the occipitoparietal region. Malignant glioma. (A) Postero-anterior. (B) Left lateral view.

Gliomas also show up well, the more malignant ones producing the denser uptake, but even relatively low-grade malignant gliomas can produce very positive findings (Figs. 56.5, 56.6, and 56.7).

Secondary deposits are usually quite well shown and often better than by angiography. The presence of separate discrete areas of increased uptake will of course

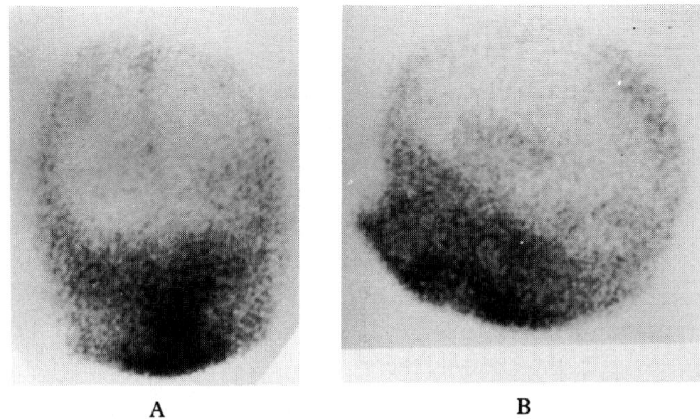

Fig. 56.7 Moderately increased uptake in left frontotemporal glioma. (A) Antero-posterior. (B) Left lateral view.

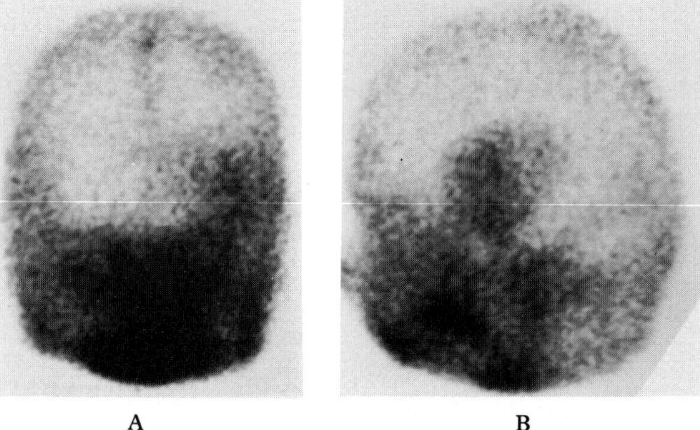

Fig. 56.8 Left pterion meningioma showing high superficial uptake. (A) Antero-posterior. (B) Left lateral view.

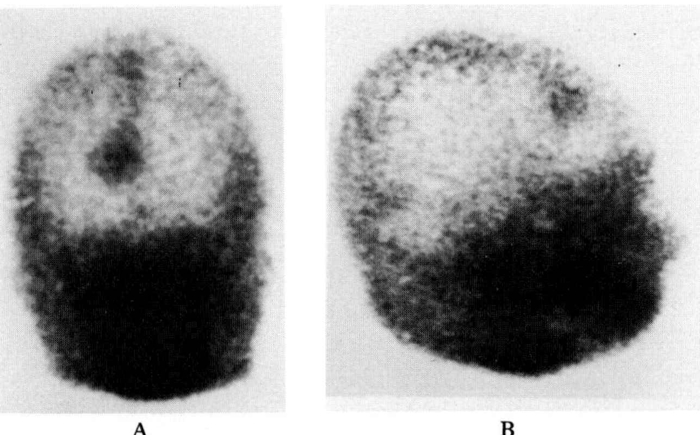

Fig. 56.9 Small parasagittal meningioma in the frontal region. (A) Antero-posterior. (B) Right lateral view.

suggest the diagnosis of deposits because of the multiple nature of the lesions.

Figures 56.5 to 56.15 illustrate typical intracerebral lesions demonstrated by brain scanning with a gamma camera.

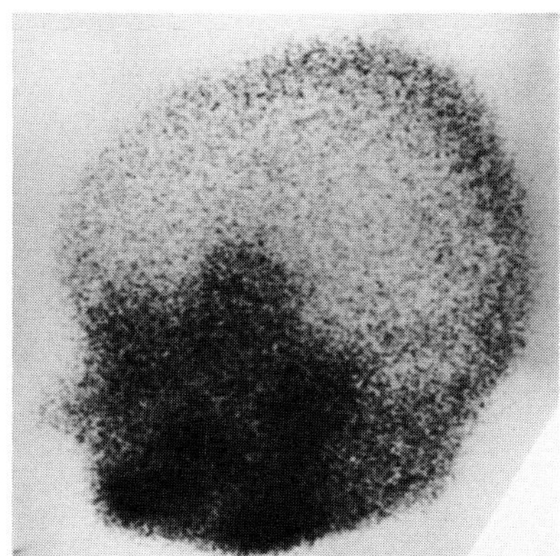

Fig. 56.10 Suprasellar tumour with high uptake—lateral view.

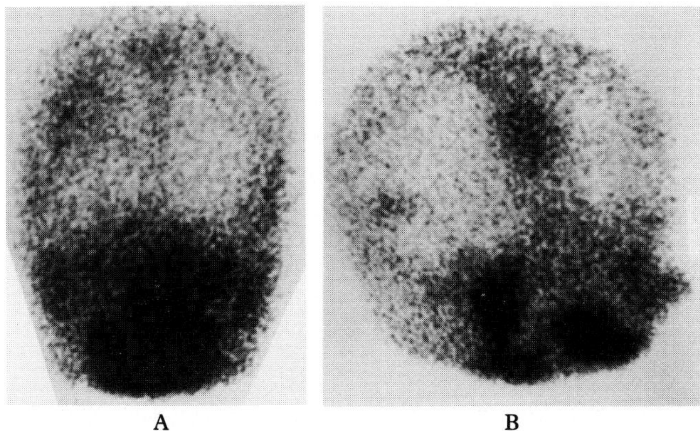

Fig. 56.11 Increased uptake in middle cerebral territory due to infarct. A repeat scan six weeks later showed no evidence of increased uptake. (A) Anteroposterior. (B) Right lateral view.

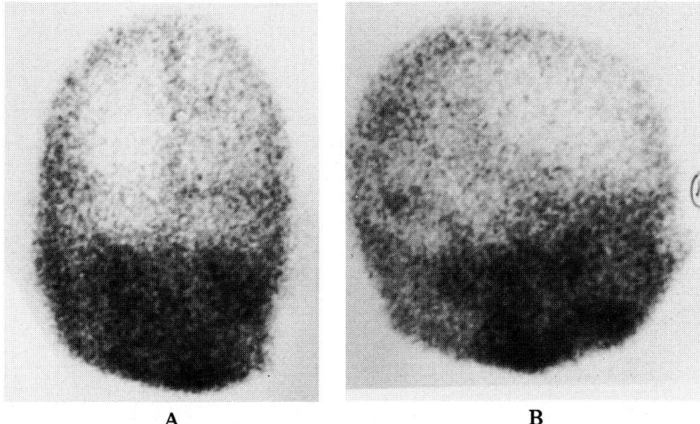

Fig. 56.12 Posterior cerebral infarction showing increased uptake in occipital region. A repeat scan a month later showed no increased uptake as is typical with established infarcts. (A) Postero-anterior. (B) Right lateral view.

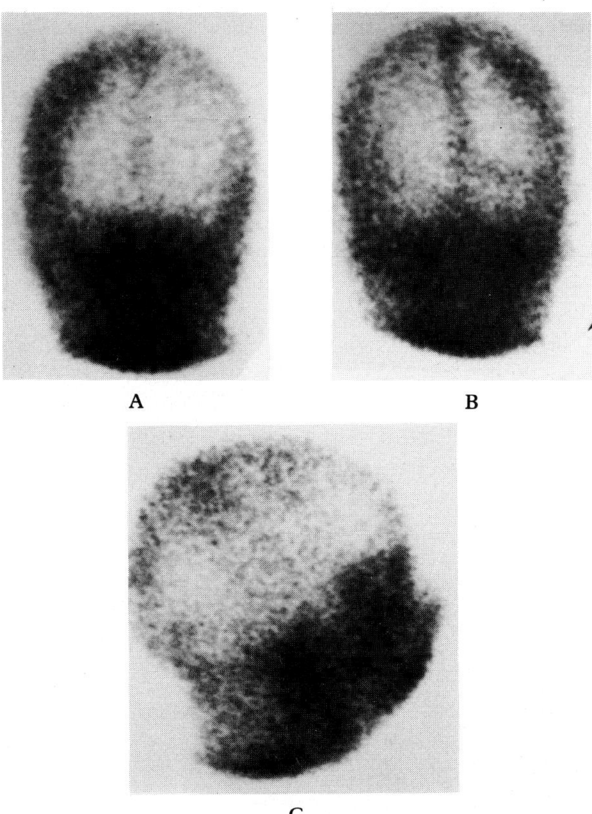

Fig. 56.13 Subdural haematoma showing superficial increased uptake in the right parietal region. (A) Anterior. (B) Posterior. (C) Right lateral view.

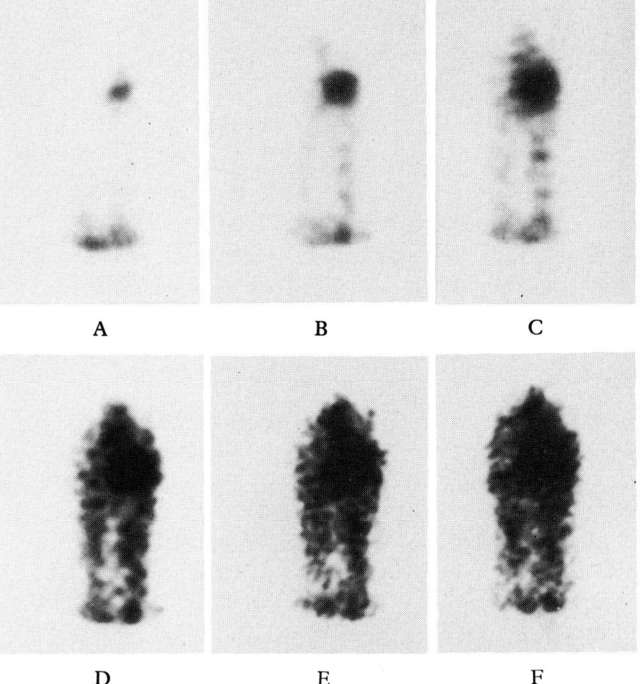

Fig. 56.14 Nuclear angiogram showing increased uptake in the left hemisphere with a large angioma, as the bolus passes up the neck vessels and through the brain. Films A to F at 1 second intervals.

Isotope encephalography

For this procedure the isotope was injected into the subarachnoid space by lumbar puncture. It then diffused up into the basal cisterns and cortical air channels and in some cases into the lateral ventricles.

In the normal patient the basal cisterns and cortical air channels are well outlined at 24 hours. There is no ventricular filling and radioactivity fades rapidly after 48 hours.

In patients with communicating hydrocephalus the isotope does not pass over the cortex but enters the dilated ventricles by 24 hours (Fig. 56.15) and it stays in the ventricles for several days. This characteristic behaviour has proved a useful feature in differentiating cerebral atrophy from low-pressure communicating hydrocephalus.

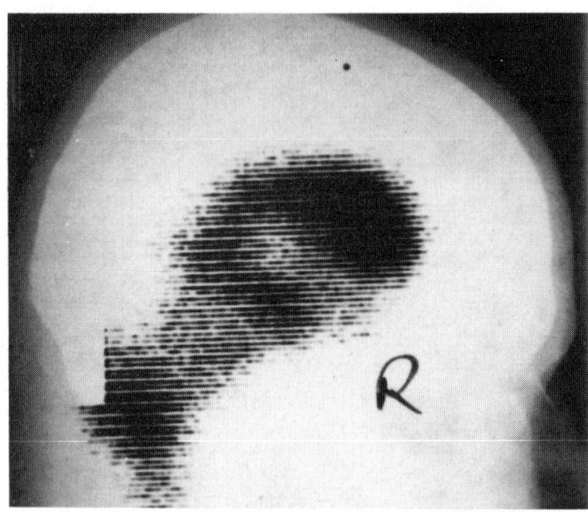

Fig. 56.15 Concentration of isotope in the ventricles following intrathecal injection in a patient with communicating hydrocephalus. Lateral view.

ULTRASONIC ENCEPHALOGRAPHY

The principles of echo-encephalography are similar to those developed for localization of submarines; they are also similar to the sound radar used by bats.

The use of sound for diagnosis in the basic forms of percussion and ausculation is of course well known and long established. Ultrasonic diagnosis, however, employs sound waves whose frequency is far higher than can be registered by the human ear. These ultrasonic waves are produced from a transducer and travel through human tissues at a velocity of some 1500 metres per second. When the wave reaches an object or surface with a different texture, or acoustic nature, a wave is reflected back from the surface of the object. These echoes are received back by the apparatus and changed into electric current. This can be amplified and shown on a cathode ray tube.

The use of echo-encephalography to measure the position of the midline structure in the brain was first described by Leksell (1956). He showed that by passing a beam of pulsed ultrasound through the skull vault and recording the echoes produced he was able to detect the presence of displacement of the midline structure. This was later confirmed by many other workers.

In skilled hands the method can predict a shift of the midline structures with a very high degree of accuracy. This is obviously important in deciding the correct side for cerebral angiography to be performed in patients with doubtful or equivocal lateralizing signs.

Leksell also suggested that echo-encephalography might be useful in the diagnosis of hydrocephalus. This was because echoes could be obtained from the ventricular walls in cases where the ventricles were dilated. This suggestion was later confirmed by other workers.

Echo-encephalography became established as a useful aid to the neurologist and neurosurgeon. It proved to be a very satisfactory method of indicating the position of the diencephalic midline, and had several advantages in the screening of patients for further and more complex in-

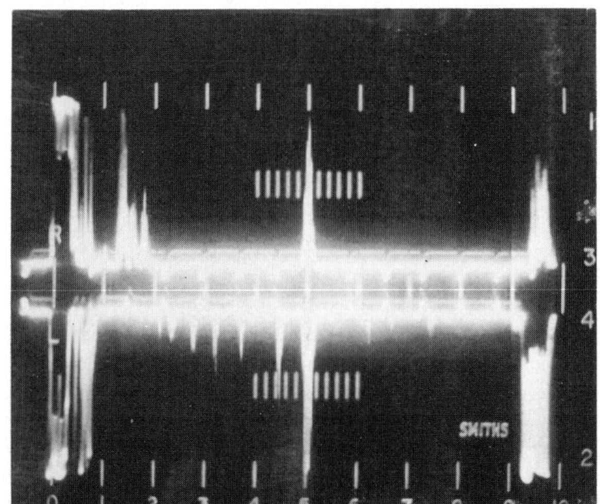

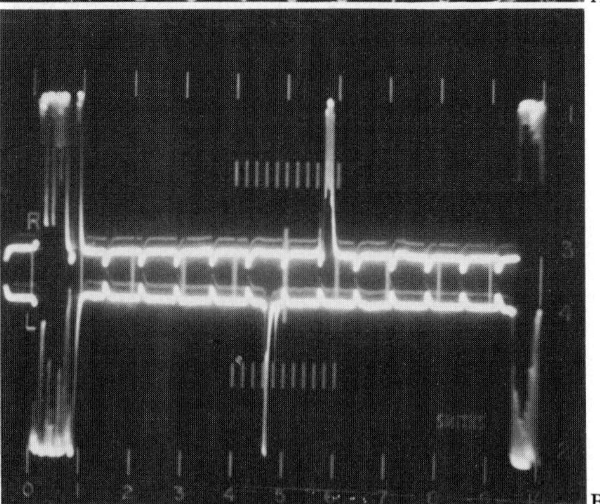

Fig. 56.16 (A) Echo-encephalogram. Diagrams showing central midline structures. (B) Echo-encephalogram. Diagram showing displacement of midline structures to the left.

vestigations by neuroradiology. The apparatus is very simple to use and causes no pain or discomfort to the patient. The procedure can be performed on seriously ill or comatose patients and can also be performed at the bedside or elsewhere in the hospital. Thus it was of routine use in patients with head injury where intracerebral, subdural or extradural haematomas were suspected. A shift of the midline structures as shown by the echo-encephalogram will indicate the presence of such a lesion and lateralize it prior to further investigation and treatment (Fig. 56.16A and B). It was also of use in patients with intracranial masses which were only vaguely or poorly localized by clinical methods. In these cases the echo-encephalogram will again demonstrate whether or not there is a shift of the midline structures. In some cases this indicated the correct side for carotid angiography, and saved the patient an unnecessary investigation on the contralateral side.

Despite the usefulness of ultrasound as just described, there is no doubt that the procedure is now obsolescent wherever there is free access to C.A.T. The latter can now provide so much more information in a non-invasive way that it is likely to be used whether the ultrasound findings are positive or negative. For this reason the preliminary ultrasound is now largely dispensed with except with infant skulls where both midline and ventricles can be easily shown.

STEREOTAXIS

Stereotaxic surgery was widely used in the treatment of Parkinsonism and other forms of involuntary movements. Since the introduction of successful drug control by Levodopa, the use of stereotaxic surgery in Parkinsonism has declined markedly though it is still used in selected cases.

Many different techniques have been described, all of which aim at destroying specific areas in the region of the basal ganglia. By using stereotaxic methods it is possible to obtain a very high degree of precision in the location of the tip of the brain probe.

The main agents used to produce the brain lesion are either alcohol or electrical coagulation. A cryogenic probe has also been used to kill the cells by freezing. The best target area in the basal ganglia is still a matter of some controversy, but it has been shown by post-mortem studies that good results can be achieved with different lesions, both large and small, in widely scattered areas.

A technique widely used in Britain is that elaborated by Bennett. The Bennett apparatus is firmly attached to the patient's skull with the patient in the sitting position.

The 3rd ventricle is opacified by the introduction of Myodil (Figs 56.17 and 56.18) and the X-ray tube is set

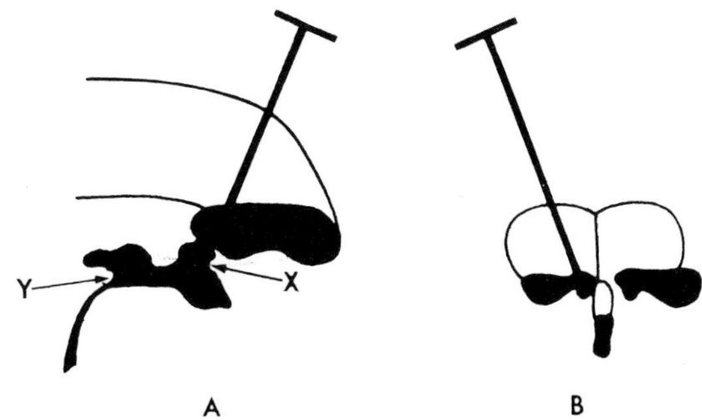

Fig. 56.17 Diagram to illustrate Figs 56.17A and B: X—anterior commissure; Y—posterior commissure. The pallidal target in one method is 3 mm below the intercommissural line, 5 mm behind the anterior commissure and 17 mm from the midline.

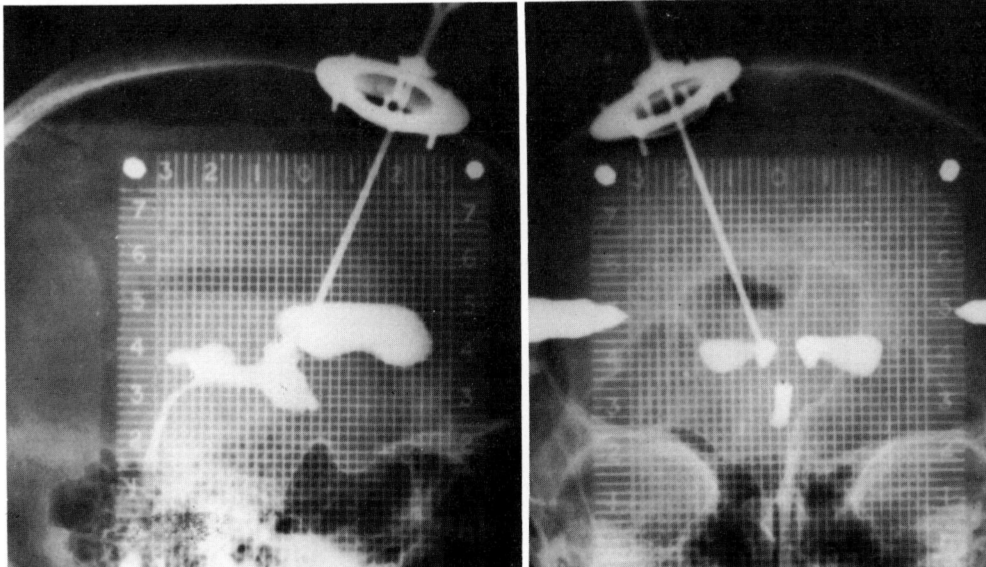

Fig. 56.18 Control films for siting the tip of a probe for stereotaxic surgery using the Bennett apparatus. (A) Lateral view. (B) A.P. view.

up at a distance of about 3·5 m from the film adjacent to the patient's head. The electrode is introduced through a burr-hole, made usually in a frontal site. This electrode is guided in all three planes by a steel ball with a hole in one of its diameters. The steel ball is anchored in the skull where it can safely remain for a few weeks if necessary. With the 3rd ventricle opacified and with films taken at the distance indicated, the tip of the electrode can be sited with great accuracy, using a superimposed wire mesh grid for checking measurements.

The coagulation is usually performed with the patient conscious and there is often a dramatic cessation of tremor when the electrode is inserted. If the result is unsatisfactory or there is a return of tremor within the first few days a further coagulation can be done.

Where it is necessary for both sides to be treated there is usually an interval of a few weeks or months before each operation. The operative mortality is about 2 to 3 per cent. Early deaths are usually due to intracerebral haemorrhage, though some other deaths are due to hypothalamic damage and bronchopneumonia.

Stereotaxic methods have also been used for trigeminal injections in the treatment of trigeminal neuralgia. However, this is being less frequently practised since the introduction of successful drug therapy by Tegretol.

C.T. has also been used for the control of stereotaxic procedures and may become the method of choice.

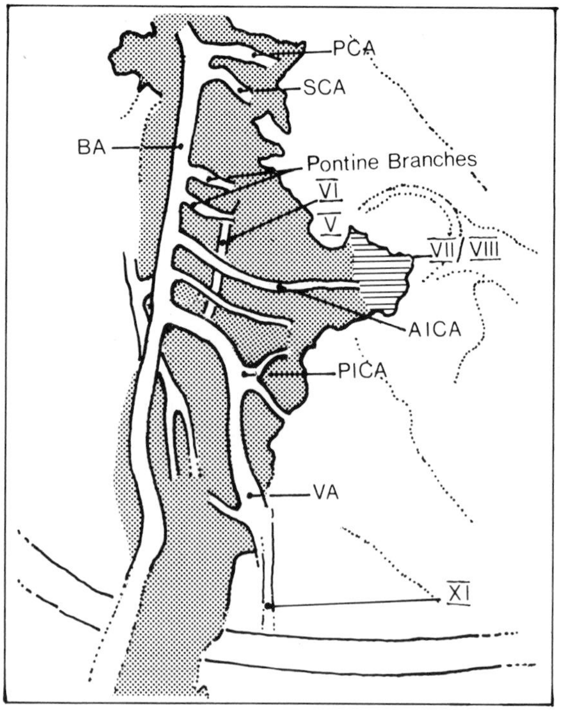

Fig. 56.19 Diagram to illustrate structures which may be identified in a normal cisternogram (courtesy of Dr E. H. Burrows, *British Journal of Radiology*, **42**, 904).

CISTERNOGRAPHY

The use of a positive contrast medium for outlining lesions in the basal cisterns has been fairly widely used for the demonstration of acoustic neuromas and other cerebello-pontine angle masses.

Myodil (ethyl iodophenylundecilate) was the medium most widely used. This was injected in the usual way by lumbar puncture and was then screened up the base of the skull and on to the clivus with the patient in the prone position and chin extended. The chin remains extended whilst the head is turned first to one side and then the other to fill the cerebellopontine angles. Films are obtained both in frontal view, and also in lateral view with a horizontal X-ray beam.

Some workers use fairly large amounts of contrast medium (6 ml) and fill the cerebellopontine angles. Acoustic and other tumours show as filling defects and in the normal angle Myodil will usually enter the internal auditory meatus. Other workers use only a small amount of Myodil (2 ml) and regard failure to fill the meatus as evidence of a tumour or other lesion obstructing it. The method is particularly valuable with small intracanalicular tumours which fail to show by any other technique. Fig. 56.19 shows the normal features seen in the cerebellopontine angle with this technique and Fig. 56.20 illustrates the appearances with a large acoustic neurinoma.

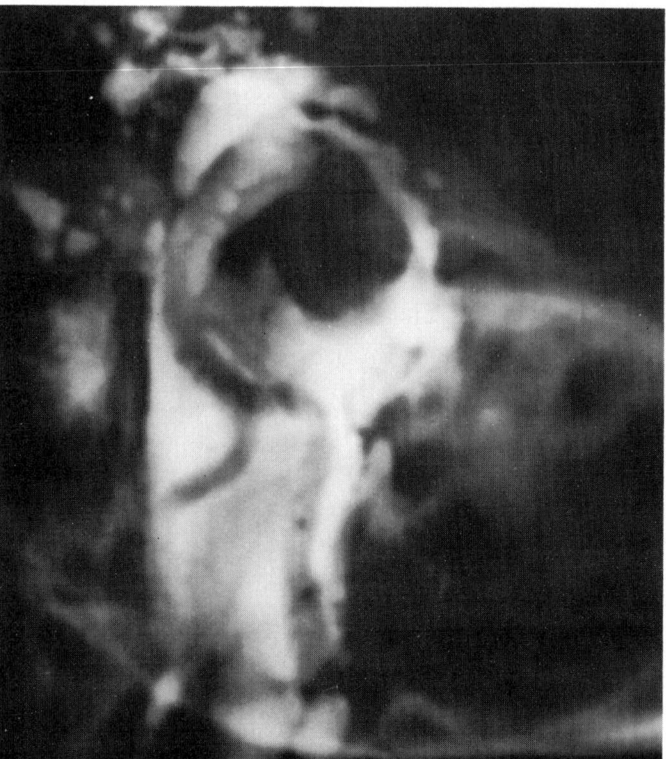

Fig. 56.20 Myodil cisternogram showing defect produced by a large acoustic tumour in the C.P. angle seen in the oblique view. Note the defects produced by the basilar and vertebral arteries.

Amipaque is a water-soluble contrast medium which is now being widely used for radiculography and myelography. It is also being used by some workers for cisternography using a similar technique to that just described for Myodil cisternography.

THERMOGRAPHY

Radiant heat is constantly emitted by the human skin and a thermograph is a graphic record of the infra-red radiation from the skin obtained by scanning its surface. The method is a simple and quite harmless technique for recording skin temperature. Indirectly it reflects cutaneous blood supply.

Clinical uses of thermography have been concerned with the detection of altered skin temperature. Thus increased skin temperature and abnormal radiant emissions are found with superficial neoplasms, with some deep tumours, and over the site of placental implantation. Reduced heat emissions, on the other hand, occur with impaired blood flow in the extremities.

In neuroradiology the practical use of the technique has been to record alterations in the heat of the skin of the forehead. This can be co-related with changes in cerebral circulation since the skin over and above the medial part of each eye is supplied almost exclusively by branches of the ophthalmic artery which is itself supplied by the internal carotid. Thus the frontal and supraorbital arteries can be regarded as terminal extensions of the internal carotid circulation. As a result patients with internal carotid occlusion or insufficiency show reduced blood flow and heat emission over the appropriate skin area (Fig. 56.21).

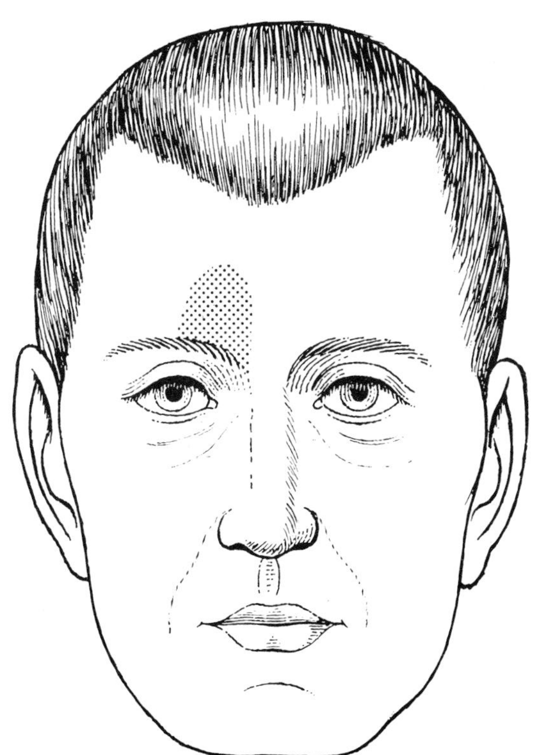

Fig. 56.21 Diagram to illustrate the area above the orbit supplied by the internal carotid and which shows up as a cool area in a patient with unilateral carotid insufficiency.

Apart from helping in the diagnosis of internal carotid insufficiency the thermogram has also been used after surgery as an index of the success of treatment.

The method is fairly reliable in showing reduced blood flow in one carotid, but it should be noted that changes have also been demonstrated where a large angioma in one hemisphere shunted blood from the contralateral carotid and its branches.

CYSTOGRAPHY AND PYOGRAPHY

When ventriculography was widely practiced the needle occasionally entered a tumorous cyst, usually gliomatous, and air was injected to outline the cyst and show any tumour nodule projecting into it (cystography).

Cerebral abscesses are becoming less frequent but are still encountered in fair numbers. They arise most commonly by direct extension of infection from an infected sinus or mastoid. Infected frontal sinuses give rise to frontal abscesses and infected mastoids to temporal lobe or cerebellar abscesses. In either case extradural abscesses may be seen. Some abscesses are haematogenous in origin and they may be encountered as a complication of bronchiectasis or of congenital heart disease with a right to left shunt. These haematogenous abscesses can be sited anywhere in the brain.

The treatment of cerebral abscesses is by antibiotics and repeated aspiration, with total excision in some cases. After the abscess was located and tapped it was usual until recent years to inject a radiopaque substance. Originally this was Thorotrast, later it was replaced by the sterile barium compound Steripaque. The resultant pyogram showed the cavity of the abscess well and films taken in different projections outlined the whole cavity and showed its size and shape. Serial aspiration and films demonstrated the progress and shrinkage of the abscess. If the abscess was biloculated the contrast could enter both cavities or if it only entered one the presence of a second cavity might be suggested by peaking or pointing of the primary cavity towards the second cavity. This was due to contrast entering the narrow neck between the two cavities.

Both cystography and pyography have become obsolete with the advent of C.A.T. A tumorous cyst is usually evident on a C.T. scan and abscesses are also well shown. Serial C.A.T. scans will show the effect of therapy on abscesses and can be used to control progress (see Chapter 64).

REFERENCES AND SUGGESTIONS FOR FURTHER READING

AMBROSE, J. (1973) Computerized transverse axial scanning. *British Journal of Radiology*, **46,** 1023–1047.

DELAND, F. H. & WAGNER, H. N. (1969) Brain, *Atlas of Nuclear Medicine*, vol. 1, Philadelphia: Saunders.

DOYLE, F. H. (1979) Radiology of the Pituitary. In *Recent Advances in Radiology—6*, ed. Lodge, T. & Steiner, R. E. Edinburgh: Churchill Livingstone.

GREENFIELD, J. G. (1958) *Neuropathology.* Baltimore: Williams and Wilkins.

HOUNSFIELD, G. N. (1973) Computerized axial scanning. *British Journal of Radiology*, **46,** 1016–1022.

PENMAN, J. & SMITH, M. C. (1954) Intracranial gliomata. *Medical Research Council, Special Report Series*, no. 284. London: H.M.S.O.

RUSSELL, D. S. (1966) Observations on the pathology of hydrocephalus. *Medical Research Council, Special Report Series*, no. 265. London: H.M.S.O.

RUSSELL, D. S. & RUBINSTEIN, L. J. (1977) *Pathology of Tumours of the Nervous System*, 4th edn. London: Arnold.

WHITE, D. N. & HANNA, L. F. (1974) Automatic midline echo-encephalography. *Neurology*, **24,** 80–93.

WOOD, E. H. (1965) Thermography in the diagnosis of cerebrovascular disease. *Radiology*, **85,** 270–283.

ZIMMERMAN, H. M. (1971) The ten most common types of brain tumor. *Seminars in Roentgenology*, **6,** 48.

CHAPTER 57

THE NORMAL SKULL

The skull is a complex structure composed of more than 20 different bones. A thorough radiological survey of the skull to demonstrate all possible anatomical points is impossible as a routine since it would require too large a number of X-ray films and be prohibitive in time and cost. For the routine survey of the skull it is customary in most departments of neuroradiology to rely on four standard projections.

1. The lateral view.
2. The postero-anterior (P.A.) view.
3. The Towne's view.
4. The basal view.

These are described below. They are not of course necessary in all cases, and a simple lateral view is the most useful single film where there is no clinical evidence of a localized lesion.

1. The lateral view is taken as shown in Figure 57.1A and the side of the suspected lesion is usually placed close to the film since this side will be shown most clearly on the X-ray (Figs 57.2A and B).

2. The so called 'postero-anterior' film is taken with the central ray tilted downwards 20° towards the feet and centred on the inion in order to project the dense petrous bones clear of the orbits (Fig. 57.1B). The resultant appearances are illustrated in Figures 57.3A and B.

3. The Towne's view or 30° fronto-occipital projection is obtained by tilting the central ray some 30° downwards towards the feet and centring as shown in Figure 57.1C. The resultant X-ray is illustrated in Figures 57.4A and B.

4. The basal view can be obtained by placing the patient's head in the 'hanging head' position and centring the X-ray beam vertical to the anatomical base-line and between the angles of the mandible. The film is placed beneath the patient's hanging head (Fig. 57.1D). Other techniques for achieving the basal view are described in standard textbooks of radiography. The resulting X-ray film and its anatomical features are illustrated in Figures 57.5A and B.

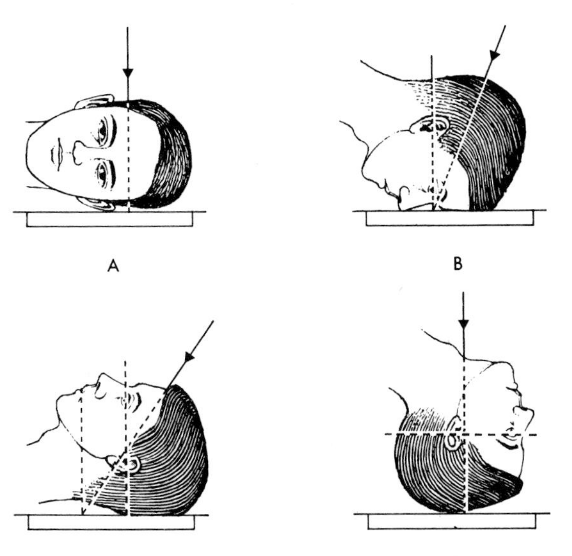

Fig. 57.1 The four standard skull projections. (A) lateral. (B) P.A. (C) Towne's. (D) Basal.

Whilst good-quality films can be achieved on general radiological apparatus it is now accepted practice to use specialized skull tables for neuroradiology. The original Swedish Lysholm-Schonander table was developed in the 1930s and has since been considerably improved. Special apparatus for neuroradiology is now available from several of the principal manufacturers of X-ray apparatus.

The advantage of specialized apparatus is that it enables routine views at fixed focus-film distances to be obtained on every patient and the radiologist can be certain that standard easily comparable films will result at each examination.

The student should be familiar with the normal appearances in the four standard projections described and should be able to recognize all the bony points in the diagrams.

Many cases will require further views to demonstrate specific points or specific anatomical landmarks. The special projections in most common use include:

1. Optic foramen views.
2. Sinus views.
3. Mastoid views.
4. Petrous bone views.
5. Coned views of the pituitary fossa.
6. Stereoscopic views.

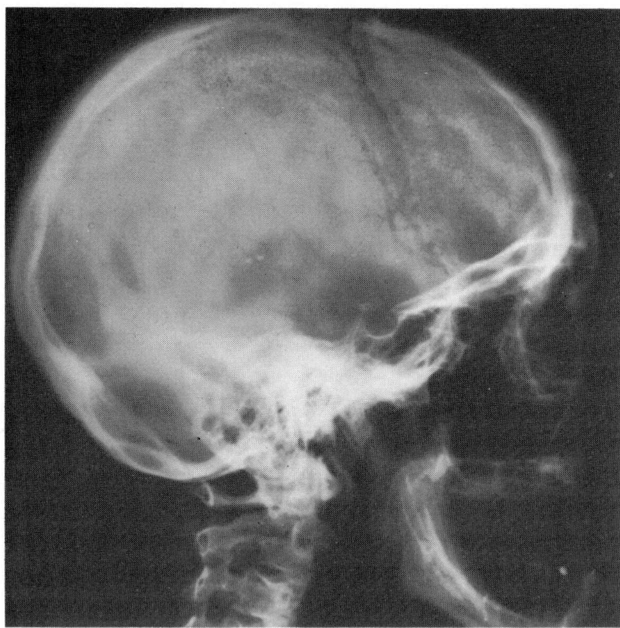

Fig. 57.2 (A) X-ray film of skull taken in standard lateral projection.

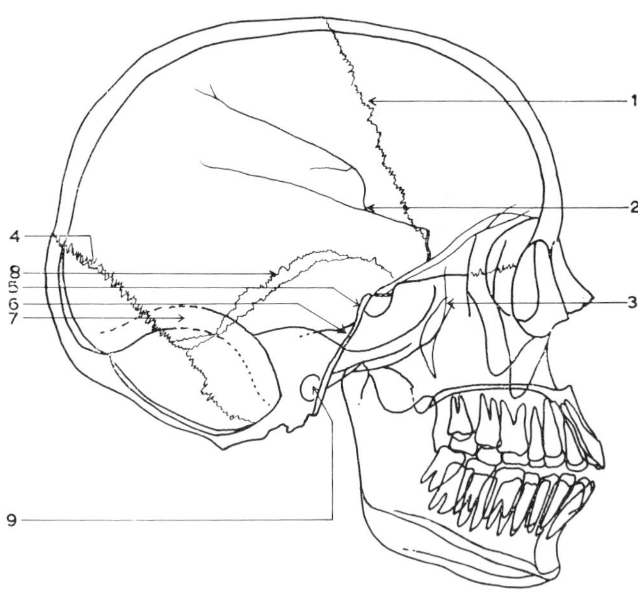

Fig. 57.2 (B) Diagram to illustrate the standard lateral view:

1. Coronal suture.
2. Meningeal vascular marking, anterior branch.
3. Anterior border of middle fossa.
4. Lambdoid suture.
5. Dorsum sellae.
6. Clivus.
7. Lateral sinus.
8. Squamo-parietal suture.
9. External auditory meatus.

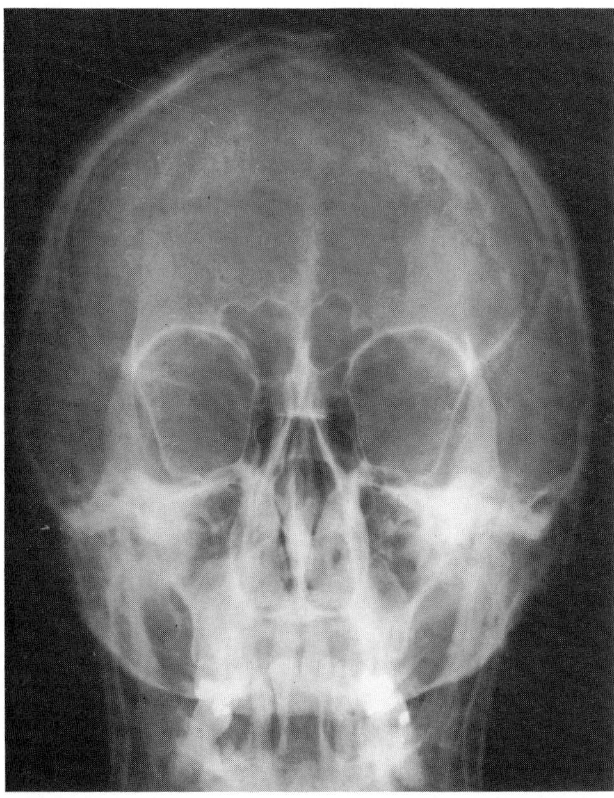

A

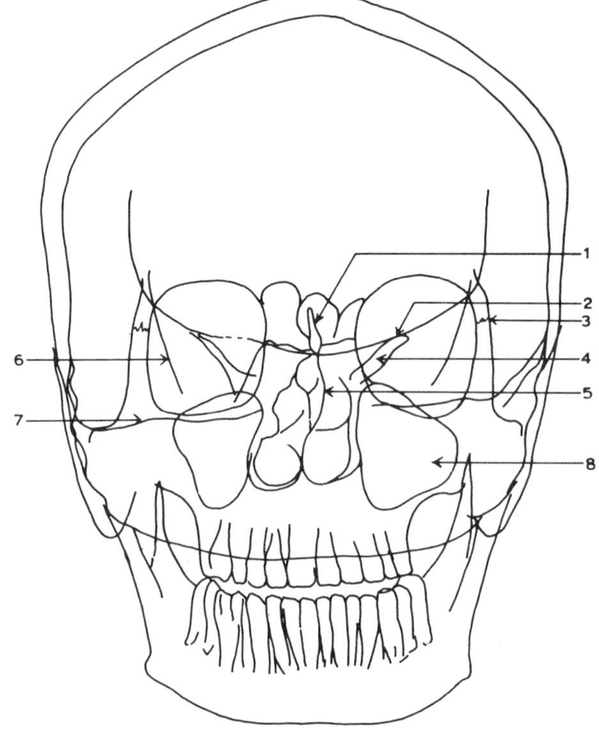

B

Fig. 57.3 (A) X-ray film taken in standard A.P. projection. (B) Diagram to illustrate Figure 57.3A:

1. Crista galli.
2. Lesser sphenoidal wing.
3. Zygomatic-frontal suture.
4. Superior orbital fissure.
5. Nasal septum.
6. Innominate line forming antero-lateral margin of middle fossa.
7. Superior margin of petrous ridge.
8. Maxillary antrum.

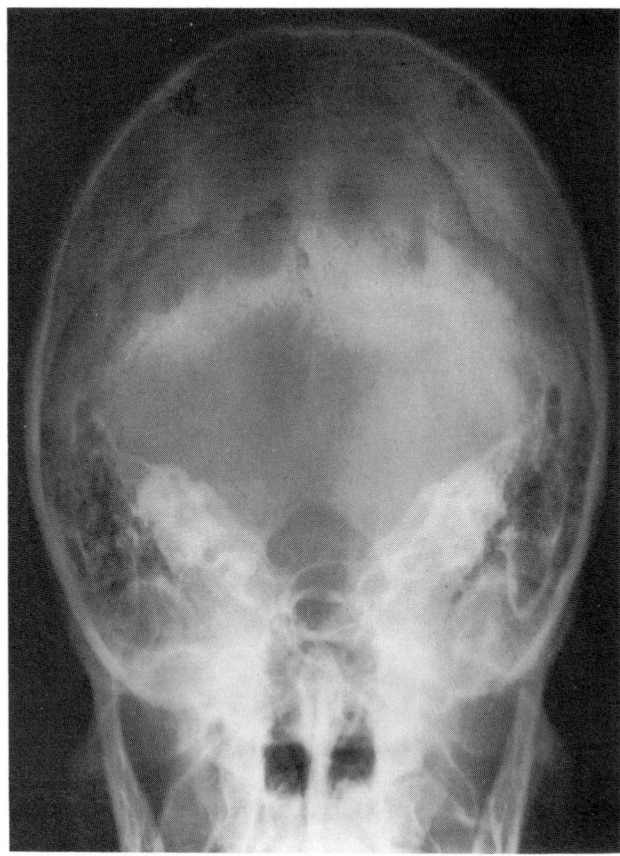

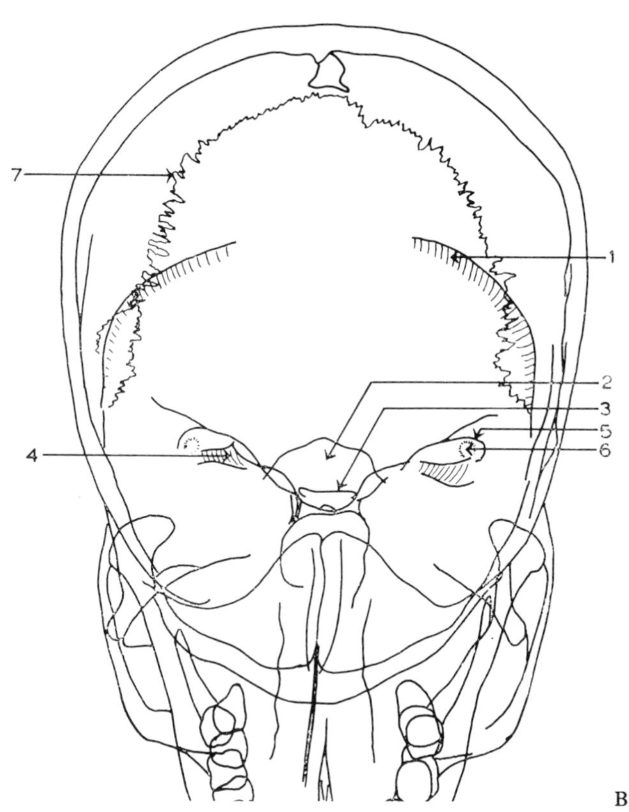

Fig. 57.4 (A) X-ray film taken in standard Towne's projection. (B) Diagram to illustrate Figure 57.4A.

1. Lateral sinus.
2. Foramen magnum.
3. Dorsum sellae.
4. Internal auditory meatus.
5. Arcuate eminence.
6. Superior semi-circular canal.
7. Lambdoid suture.

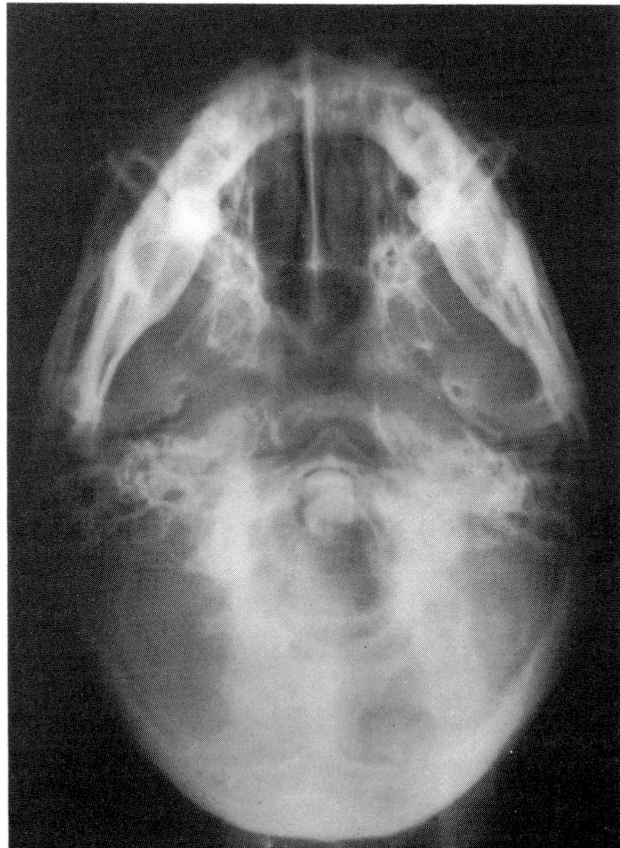

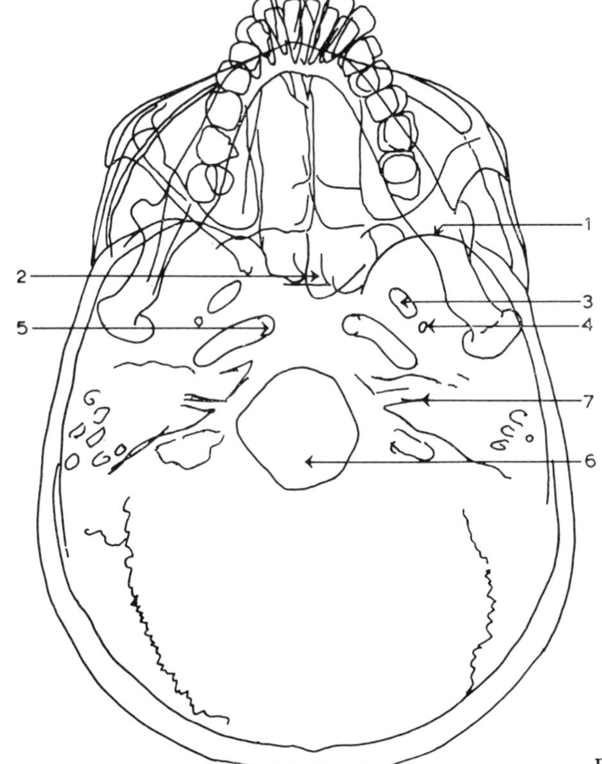

Fig. 57.5 (A) X-ray film taken in standard basal view. (B) Diagram to illustrate Figure 57.5A.

1. Greater sphenoidal wing.
2. Sphenoidal sinuses.
3. Foramen ovale.
4. Foramen spinosum.
5. Foramen lacerum medium.
6. Foramen magnum.
7. Internal auditory meatus.

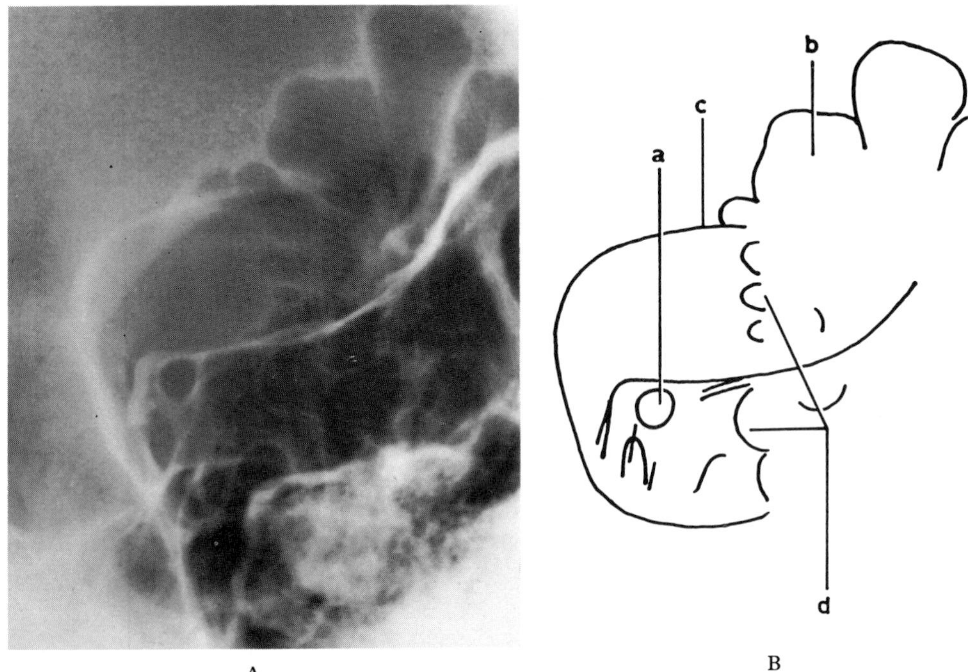

Fig. 57.6 (A) Special view of optic foramen. (B) Diagram to illustrate Figure 57.6A:

(a) optic formane
(b) frontal sinuses
(c) roof of orbit
(d) ethmoid sinuses.

Tomography is also frequently used to clarify detail in difficult cases.

Most of the special views listed above are described in standard textbooks of radiography, and the technical manuals describe how these can be obtained with the individual skull tables. The actual results achieved and the anatomical landmarks recognizable in a few of these Schonander projections are illustrated in Figures 57.6 to 57.10. Sinus and mastoid views are further discussed in Chapters 50 and 51.

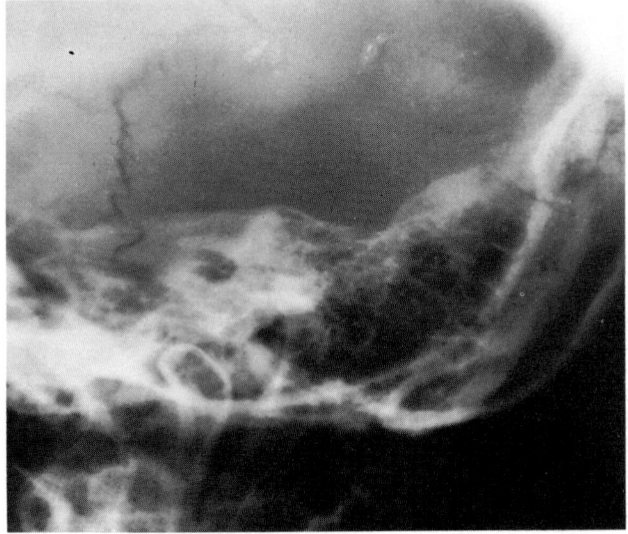

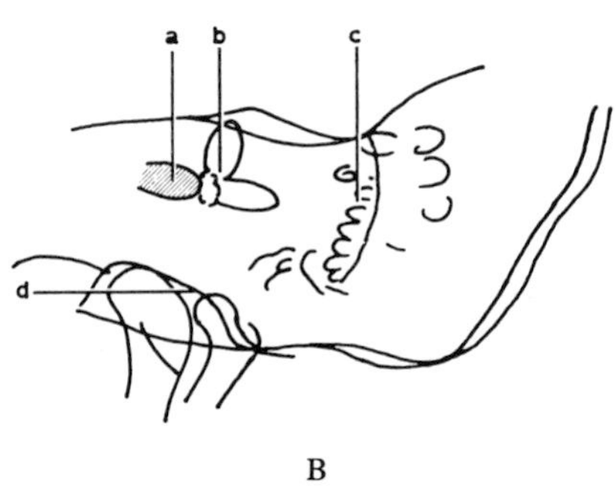

Fig. 57.7 (A) Petrous bones shown in Stockholm 'C' projection. (B) Diagram to illustrate Figure 57.7A.

(a) internal auditory meatus
(b) internal ear with semicircular canals
(c) mastoid air cells
(d) temporomandibular joint

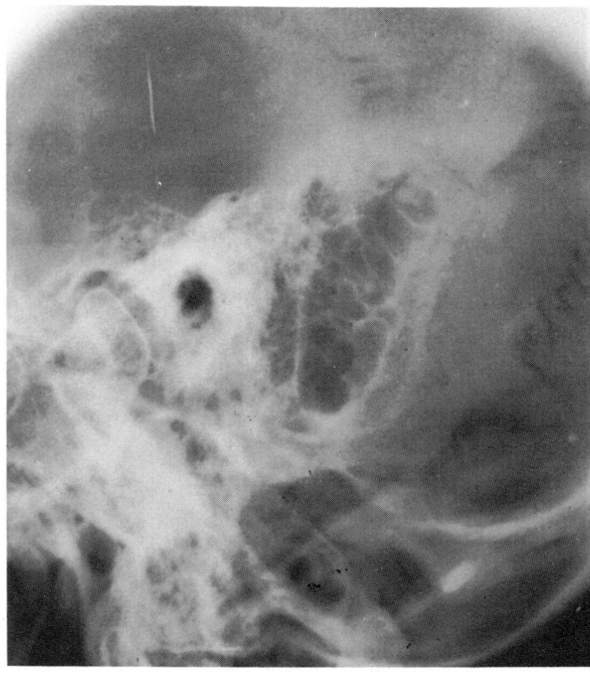

A

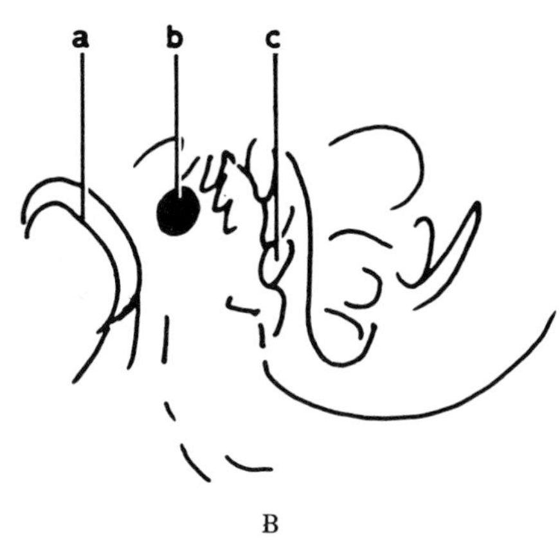

B

Fig. 57.8 (A) Cellular mastoids shown in Stockholm 'A' projection. (B) Diagram to illustrate Figure 57.8A:

(a) temporomandibular joint
(b) internal auditory meatus
(c) mastoid air cells.

The clinical usefulness and applications of particular projections will be referred to as pathological conditions are discussed in later chapters.

The optic canal. This often appears piriform in infants and children becoming more circular in adults. It passes from the middle fossa (sulcus chiasmaticus) to the back of the orbit and carries the optic nerve and ophthalmic artery, it is 4 to 9 mm in length and its size as seen on a standard view (Fig. 57.6) measures 4 to 6·5 mm in maximum diameter. The minimum diameter is usually 1 to 3 mm less. In about 4 per cent of normal people this canal has a 'keyhole' appearance, and this should be recognized as a congenital anomaly particularly when unilateral. Rarely the keyhole may be separated into two separate foramina divided by a fine strut ('figure of eight' optic canal); the optic nerve lies in the larger upper foramen and the ophthalmic artery in the smaller lower one.

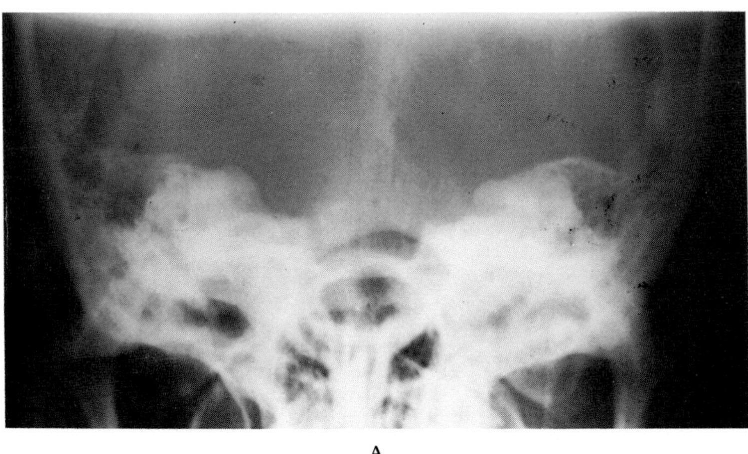

A

Fig. 57.9 (A) Both internal auditory meatus shown in Towne's projection.

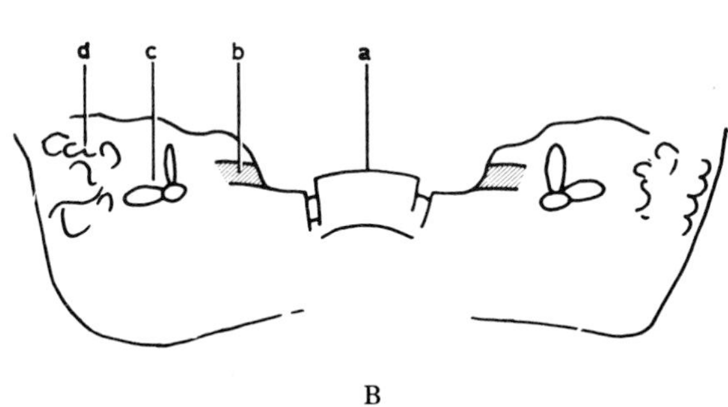

B

(B) Diagram to illustrate Figure 57.9A:

(a) dorsum sellae
(b) internal auditory meatus
(c) middle ear
(d) mastoid air cells.

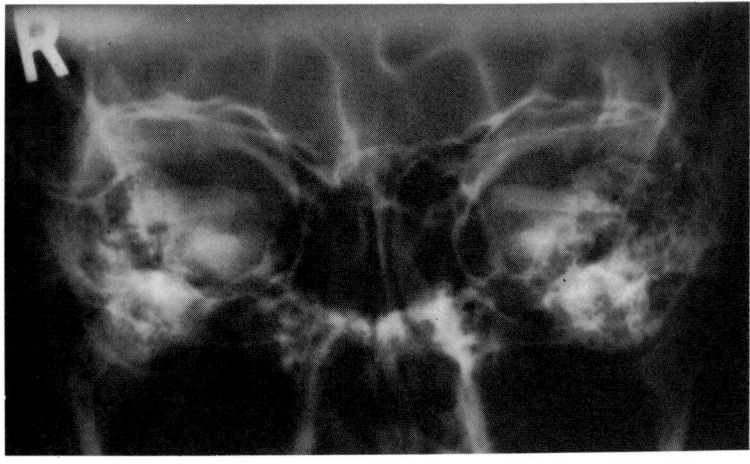

A

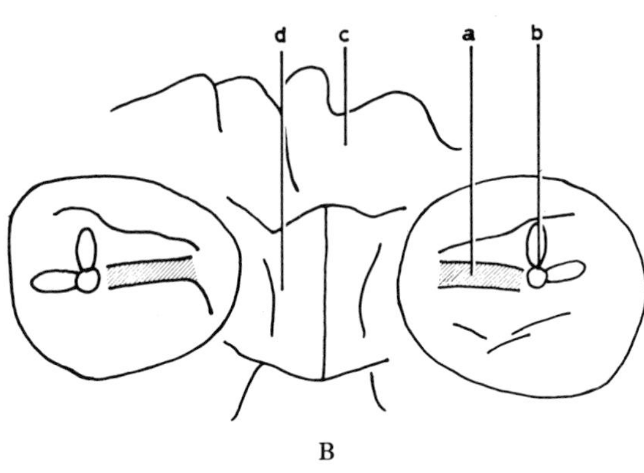

B

Fig. 57.10 (A) Internal auditory meatus in transorbital view. (B) Diagram to illustrate Figure 57.10A.

(a) internal auditory meatus
(b) semi-circular canals
(c) frontal sinus
(d) ethmoid sinuses.

The inferolateral border of the optic canal is known as the optic strut and separates it from the upper end of the sphenoidal fissure. Both the optic strut and the anterior clinoid process may be pneumatized, complicating the appearances seen. The caroticoclinoid canal if present may also cause confusion but should be projected inferior to the optic canal.

The sinuses

These are discussed in detail in Chapter 50.

It is important to realize that there is a wide variation in size and extent of the sinuses. Thus the frontal sinuses in an adult may be rudimentary or absent, or they may extend laterally to the lateral aspect of the skull. The paranasal sinuses are often unusually large in *acromegaly*. The extent of the frontal sinuses are of some importance when neurosurgical procedures involving the frontal areas are to be undertaken. It has been recorded that abnormally large frontal sinuses have been accidentally perforated during craniotomy operations in which a prior skull X-ray had not been taken.

The sinuses are rudimentary at birth and tend to increase in size with age, reaching their full development in the adult skull.

The mastoids

These are considered in detail in Chapter 51.

Like the paranasal sinuses the mastoid air cells are absent or rudimentary at birth and increase in size with age, reaching their full development in the adult. In some patients the mastoid air cells remain rudimentary or absent and the mastoid processes remain diploetic. The mastoid air cells, when present, also vary greatly in size and extent. Occasionally they may extend well forward into the squamous temporal bone, occupying a very large area and obscuring the sella in the lateral view of the skull.

Petrous bones

The petrous bones are of considerable importance in neuroradiological diagnosis. The *internal auditory meatus* is well shown in the Towne's view and in the Stockholm C projection (Figs 57.9 and 57.7). It is also well seen in the transorbital view (Fig. 57.10). In good-quality films the semicircular canals and cochlea are readily recognized. They can be demonstrated with even greater precision by tomography of the petrous bones.

Vascular markings

There is a very wide range in the appearance of the vascular markings in the normal skull. Two types of vascular markings can be readily identified, the *meningeal* and the *diploic*.

The *meningeal* vascular markings are constant in position; they follow the distribution of the anterior and posterior branches of the middle meningeal artery as these pass from the foramen spinosum to the periphery of the skull vault. They are thus quite easy to recognize, not only because of their constant position but because of their resemblance to the outline of a river on a map. They increase in size as they pass from the periphery downwards to the foramen spinosum and they form prominent grooves on the internal surface of the skull, easily recognizable in the dried specimen.

The groove associated with the anterior branch of the middle meningeal vessels is continuous in its lower part with the sphenoparietal sinus groove. The latter can be very large and extend up to the vertex.

The *diploic* vascular markings, in contrast, are extremely variable in size, shape and number. Charac-

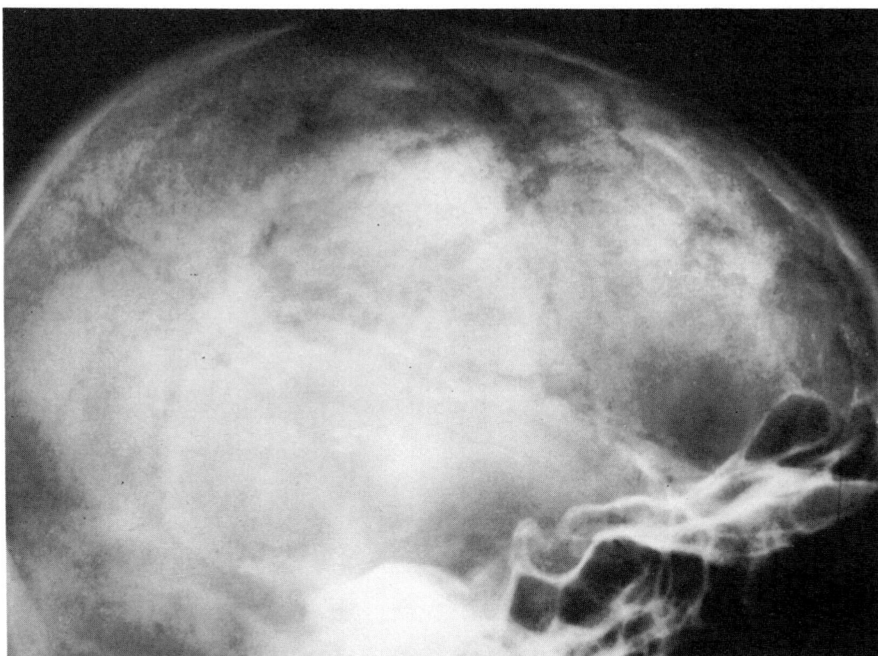

Fig. 57.11 Lateral film of skull showing prominent diploic vascular markings.

teristically their course appears quite purposeless; they may commence as a small channel, widen into a large one, and then peter out completely, or they may be stellate in pattern. In some skulls diploic vascular markings may be entirely absent. In others they may be extremely numerous and large. They are most numerous in the parietal region (Fig. 57.11). As they lie between the inner and outer tables of the skull vault, they cannot be identified in the dry skull.

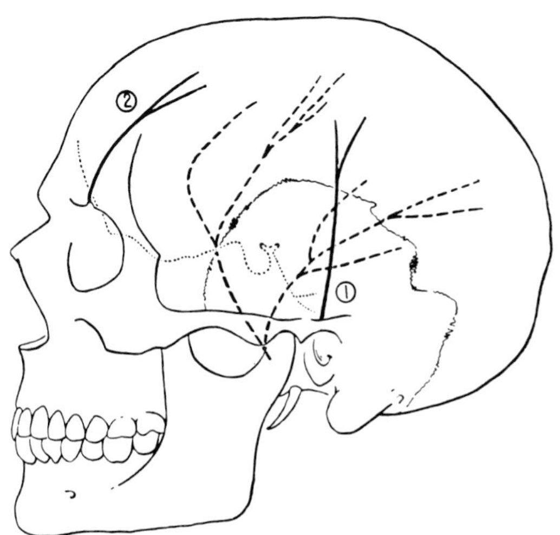

Fig. 57.12 Two vascular markings on the outer surface of the skull which may resemble fractures and are due to (1) the middle temporal artery (2) the supra-orbital artery. The meningeal vascular markings shown by dotted lines. (After Schunk, H. and Marayama, Y., 1960. *Acta radiologica Stockholm*, **54**, 186.)

The normal meningeal and diploic vascular markings should be distinguished from pathological vascular markings (described below) which are encountered with *meningiomas* or with cerebral *angiomas*.

The normal *foramen spinosum* has been referred to above and is readily recognized in the basal view of the skull.

Two linear vascular grooves on the outer table of the skull are sometimes unusually prominent on X-rays and because of their linear nature have been mistaken for fractures (Fig. 57.12). They are due to the supra-orbital and middle temporal arteries.

The pituitary fossa

The normal pituitary fossa can vary considerably in size. Several workers have attempted to define the normal limits of size of the pituitary fossa on an X-ray. This is said to vary between 11 and 16 mm in length and 8 to 12 mm in depth in the routine lateral film.

It is doubtful whether a very small pituitary fossa shown in a lateral skull film has any significance. In any case this only shows the pituitary fossa in one plane, and does not allow for the fact that the sella may be wider in the transverse plane. Certainly people who are X-rayed for suspected fractures or other non-pituitary lesions are occasionally found to have a very small pituitary fossa without clinical evidence of a pituitary lesion. A small sella is, however, frequently seen in patients with *myotonia congenita*.

The question of the upper limit of normal in size must remain largely subjective and few experienced workers

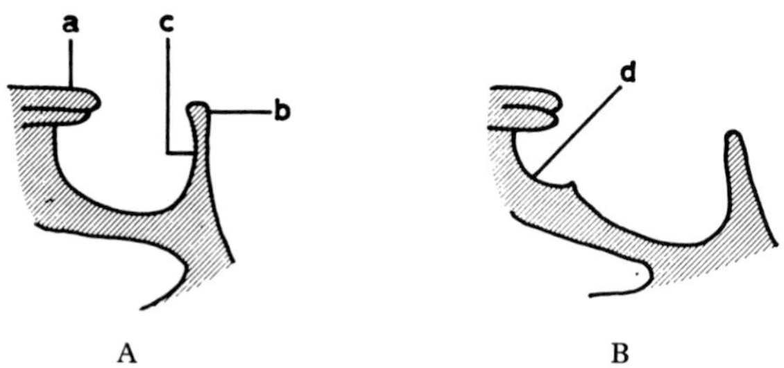

Fig. 57.13 (A) Diagram of normal sella:
(a) anterior clinoids
(b) posterior clinoids
(c) anterior cortex or 'lamina dura' of dorsum and floor of sella.
(B) J shaped sella:
(d) sulcus chiasmaticus.

rely on arbitrary figures such as those quoted above. Like all human measurements the upper limit of the normal overlaps the pathological.

The appearance of the normal dorsum sellae is of considerable importance in neuroradiology. Here again there is a wide range of normal. In a healthy adult a lateral view of the skull shows a dorsum with a well-defined cortex outlining its anterior and posterior margins (Fig. 57.13A). The medulla in between varies in thickness and has a spongy texture. Occasionally a large sphenoid sinus may extend into the dorsum sellae (pneumatisation of the dorsum). In the Towne's view the dorsum sellae is usually well defined and easily recognized as it is silhouetted within the foramen magnum.

The range of normal appearances is of considerable importance since changes in the dorsum sellae are of great value in diagnosing raised intracranial pressure (see below). Loss of definition of the dorsum may be pathological, but it can also occur in the normal. Osteoporosis may occur as a normal phenomenon in the elderly. Osteoporosis and loss of definition of the dorsum may also be seen in prolonged hypertension. In both cases the appearances have to be distinguished from the effects of raised intracranial pressure (Chapter 58). It has been claimed that the senile sella can be distinguished by the fact that the anterior cortex of the dorsum remains intact despite the porosis. The sellar changes due to prolonged arterial hypertension cannot, however, be differentiated from those of chronic raised intracranial pressure.

The J-shaped sella

The inaccurate term 'J-shaped sella' has been used by some authors to describe the appearance of a certain type of pituitary fossa. This has also been misnamed the 'omega shaped', 'shoe shaped' or 'hour glass' sella. The description refers to an elongated sella with a shallow anterior convexity (Fig. 57.13B). This can be regarded as an exaggeration of the normal slight impression of the sulcus chiasmaticus.

This impression is only rarely evident in a skull X-ray of an adult but it may be quite well shown in a small proportion of children.

A very prominent sulcus chiasmaticus was at one time thought to be diagnostic of glioma of the optic chiasm. However, apart from being a normal finding in a minority of children (about 5 per cent), a prominent sulcus chiasmaticus giving rise to a J-shaped sella is also seen in certain other pathological conditions. These include *gargoylism* in infancy and childhood, and *chronic low-grade hydrocephalus* in children.

The sutures

In the adult skull the sutures are readily recognized and their appearance in the various projections is illustrated in Figures 57.2 and 57.5.

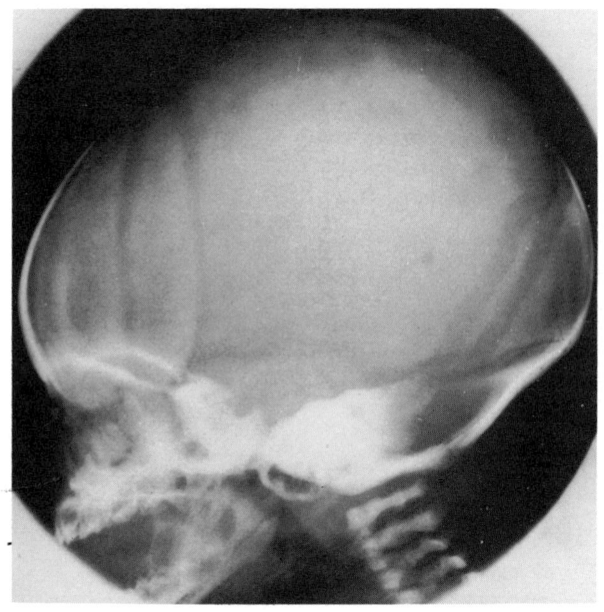

Fig. 57.14 Neonate skull. Note the wide fontanelles and sutures.

In infants the sutures are different in appearance, presenting as radiolucent linear bands, but are still readily recognized, as are the wide-open fontanelles (Figs 57.14 and 57.18). The adult suture is serrated at the outer table but linear on the internal surface of the skull.

Skull vault

In the adult skull the inner and outer tables of the vault are visible in most projections as is the diploe between. There is some variation in the normal appearances and in the thickness of both inner and outer tables, and the diploe. In certain pathological conditions (e.g. Paget's disease) the appearances and relationships will be much altered.

Pacchionian impressions are produced on the inner table by the Pacchionian bodies and appear as relative translucencies or small bone defects. Tangential views show that they are due to depressions of the inner table. They occur most frequently along the sagittal sinus but may be seen in other positions, particularly the region round the torcula, where they may simulate pathological bone defects due to deposits.

NORMAL INTRACRANIAL CALCIFICATION

Intracranial calcification which may be regarded as normal or physiological can occur in various situations. These are listed below:

1. Pineal.
2. Habenula.
3. Choroid plexuses.
4. Dura (falx, tentorium, vault).
5. Ligaments (petroclinoid and interclinoid).
6. Pacchionian bodies.
7. Basal ganglia and dentate nucleus.
8. Pituitary.
9. Lens.

The *pineal* is calcified in an increasing proportion of patients as they grow older. Thus it is rare to see calcification in the skull X-ray of children, but the majority of elderly patients have calcified pineals. In a general population a little over half the skulls X-rayed will show a calcified pineal. In most cases the calcification first appears in late adolescence or early adult life.

Pineal calcification varies considerably in size. It is usually concentrated in an area 3 to 5 mm in size but occasionally occupies a larger area (Fig. 57.15A). The calcification appears as amorphous deposit which may be nodular or ring-like. It is important to note that in routine skull X-rays, taken on a skull table and with correct centring and technique, the pineal always lies in the midline in both the postero-anterior and Towne's views. A displacement of more than 3 mm to one side of the midline can be regarded as pathological (Chapter 58). Where the pineal is faintly calcified it may be better seen in a postero-anterior view with a lesser degree of tilt than usual (5 to 10° instead of 20°). Stereo slit films are also helpful in localizing the pineal when using skull table techniques.

In the lateral position the pineal usually lies above the petrous block and slightly behind it. Displacement of the calcified pineal by intracerebral masses is discussed in the next chapter.

The habenular commissure lies directly anterior to the pineal and is directly related to the back end of the 3rd ventricle. Calcification is very common in this commissure and is often mistaken for pineal calcification. Typically the calcification is 'C' shaped, with the open part of the letter facing backwards (Fig. 57.15B).

Displacement of the habenula occurs in exactly the same way as displacement of the pineal by intracranial masses. These two different types of calcification can therefore be considered together from this point of view.

The choroid plexuses of the lateral ventricles also calcify frequently. The calcification varies in type from a few faint punctate dots to denser calcification occupying a circular area a centimetre or more in diameter. Calcification in the choroids is readily identified by its typical position in lateral view. It lies in the parietal region about one inch above and behind the pineal. In the Towne's

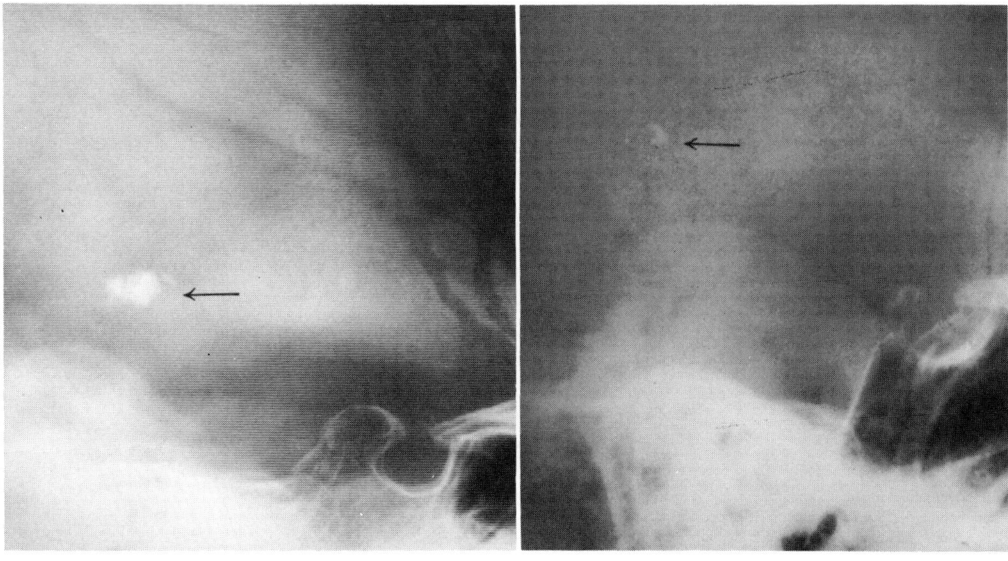

Fig. 57.15 (A) Heavily calcified but normal pineal. (B) Calcification in the habenular commissure.

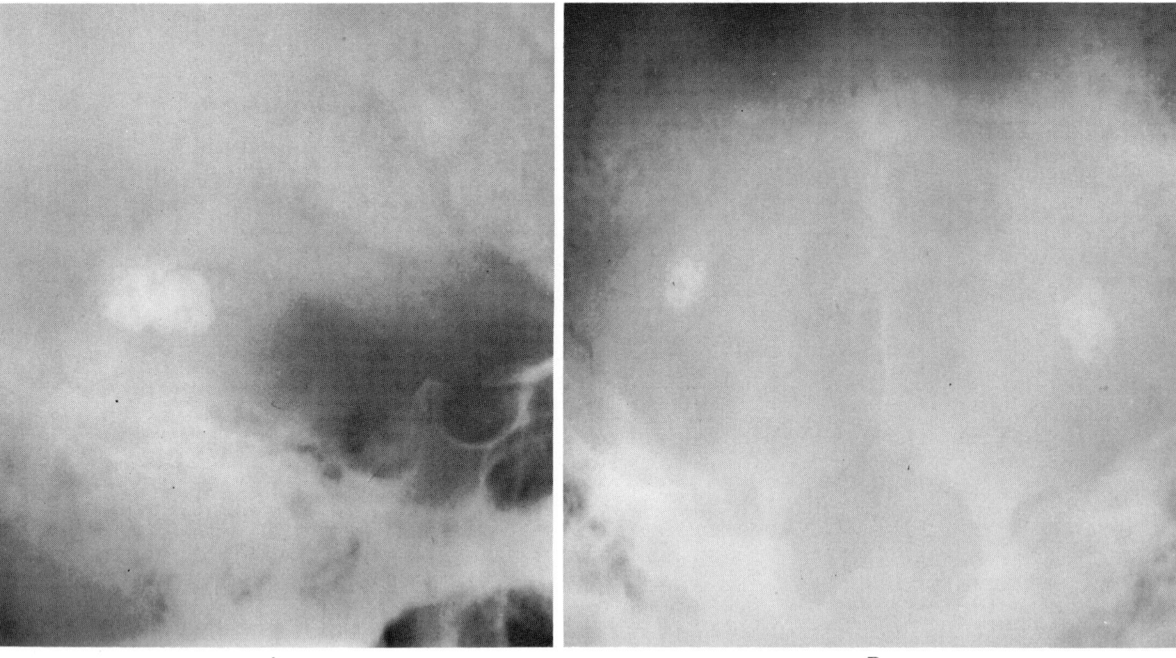

Fig. 57.16 Calcified choroid plexus. (A) lateral view. (B) Towne's view.

view or in the postero-anterior view, it lies lateral to and above the pineal in the region of the ventricular trigone. The calcification is nearly always symmetrical and bilateral in these projections; this is an important diagnostic feature which is helpful in distinguishing from other abnormal calcification (Fig. 57.16).

Dural calcification is common in the middle aged and elderly. It may occur anywhere over the vault. In this case, being close to the bone it may be difficult to identify except in tangential projection. Dural calcification is also quite common in the *falx* and is readily identified in the Towne's or postero-anterior views where it is seen end on Fig. 57.17). Calcification can also occur in the *tentorium* usually near its margin.

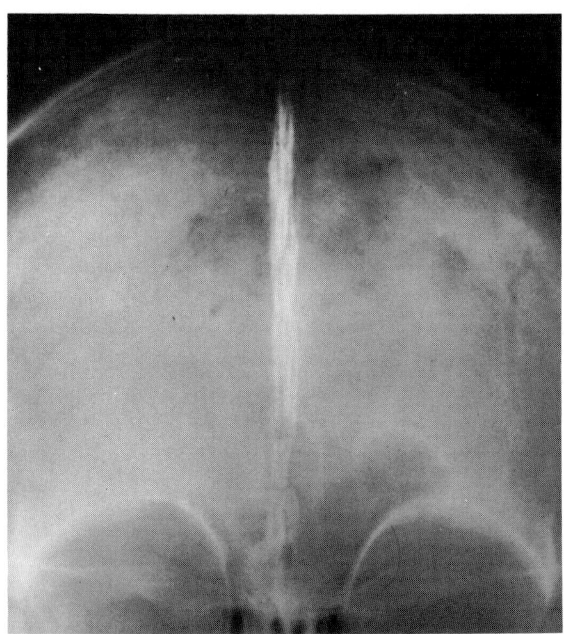

Fig. 57.17 Heavily calcified falx.

The *petroclinoid ligaments* may calcify and this is most common in the elderly. In the lateral view such calcification lies just behind the sella between the tip of the dorsum sellae and the apex of the petrous bone. The Towne's view will confirm the localization.

The *interclinoid* ligaments may also calcify and give rise to so called 'bridging' of the sella.

Calcification in *atheromatous carotid vessels* is commonly encountered in the internal carotid artery as it passes through the cavernous sinus. This will be further discussed in Chapter 58 under 'pathological calcification'.

Pacchionian bodies (Syn. arachnoid villi). Calcium deposition may occur in Pacchionian bodies. It will then lie close to the skull vault, usually near the superior longitudinal sinus. It may be readily recognized if it is in relation to a Pacchionian impression.

Calcification in the *basal ganglia* is usually pathological and is described below (Chapter 58). Occasionally, however, it has been described in patients with no demonstrable cause. In these rare cases it has been considered 'idiopathic'. Typically this calcification is bilateral and symmetrical and it commences in the region of the head of the caudate nucleus. It has been shown histologically that this calcification lies in and around the media of tiny arteries.

Calcification in the *dentate nucleus* has been described

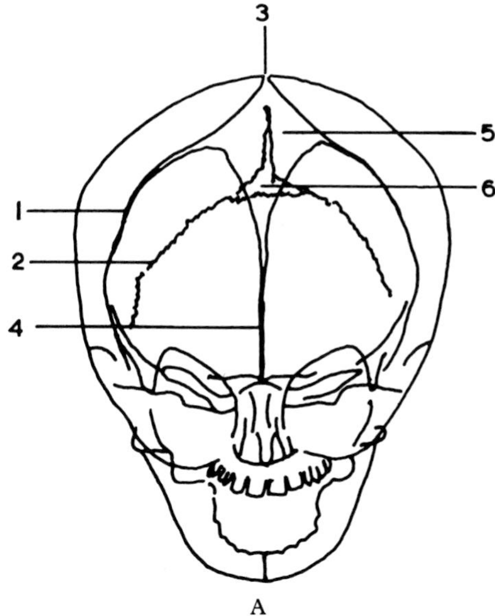

A

(A) Frontal view
1. Coronal suture.
2. Lambdoid suture.
3. Sagittal suture.
4. Metopic suture.
5. Anterior fontanelle.
6. Posterior fontanelle.

as a chance finding. It may also occur with calcification of the basal ganglia in the pathological conditions described below.

Pituitary calcification can be shown by histology but is rarely recognizable by radiology. Such cases as have been recorded have usually been in pituitary adenomas, though it has been noted in apparently normal patients with no evidence of pituitary adenoma.

Calcification in the *lens* may occur in elderly patients. It is recognized as a ring shadow in the characteristic situation of the lens in the orbit. In lateral view it is seen end on and appears as a linear shadow. Calcification can also occur in the choroid of the eye. The situation of the calcification is of course characteristic. It should not be confused with the opacity caused by the presence of an artificial eye.

THE SKULL IN INFANCY AND CHILDHOOD

The skull of the newborn child is affected by the moulding undergone during birth. Thus the skull may appear elongated, and sometimes overlapping of the cranial bones is seen. These appearances change within a week or two to

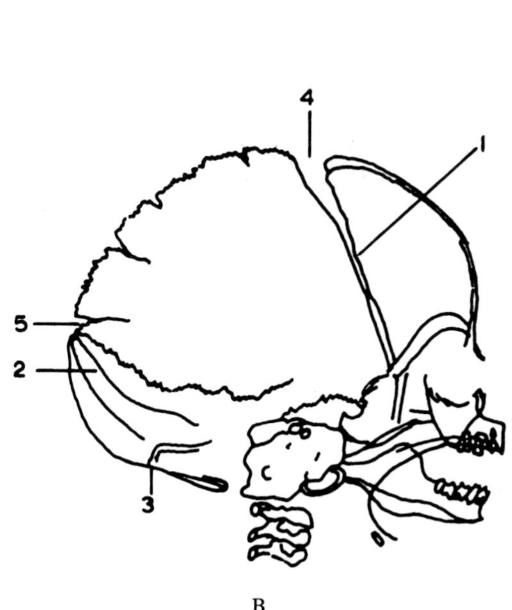

B

(B) Lateral view.
1. Coronal suture.
2. Lambdoid suture.
3. Mendosal suture.
4. Anterior fontanelle.
5. Posterior fontanelle.

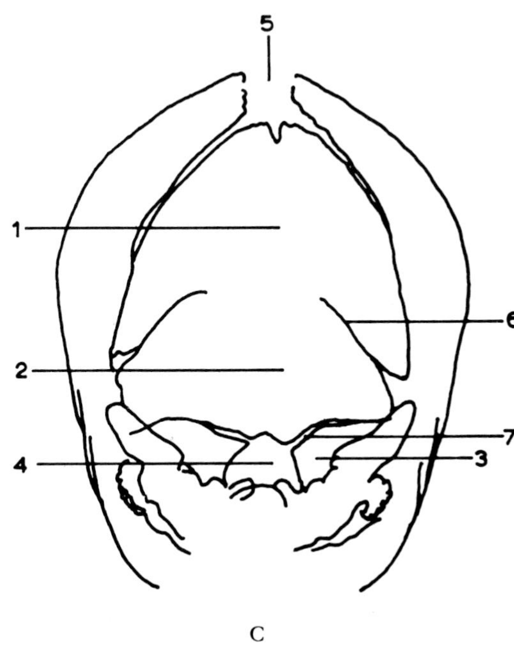

C

(C) Towne's view.
1. Interparietal bone.
2. Supra-occipital bone.
3. Exoccipital bone.
4. Foramen magnum.
5. Posterior fontanelle.
6. Mendosal suture.
7. Synchondrosis between supra-occipital and exoccipital.

Fig. 57.18 (A, B and C) Diagrams of neonatal skull showing features of note.

a more normal contour. In the lateral view of the newborn skull the vault appears thin, there is no differentiation into inner and outer tables, and there are no vascular markings to be seen. There are also no convolutional impressions. The sutures are shown as wide straight lines and the fontanelles are widely open. Within the suture lines Wormian bones may occasionally be seen though these unite with the vault as growth proceeds. The anterior fossa appears short and slopes downwards more than in the adult, and the middle fossa shows a similar appearance. The features of the neonatal skull are illustrated in Figures 57.14 and 57.18.

The sinuses and mastoids are rudimentary at this stage and it is only occasionally that small airspaces can be recognized in the region of the antra. The spheno-occipital suture is readily visible and a synchondrosis crosses the occipital bone, dividing it into upper and lower portions. The latter are termed the supra-occipital and lateral occipital regions. The occipital bone at this stage also shows an oblique suture (the *mendosal* suture) passing upwards and inwards from its lower part on both sides. There is also in the midline near the apex a vertical fissure best seen in the Towne's view. These normal occipital appearances should not be confused with fractures.

In premature infants the skin may be very lax and form folds which produce linear shadows on the skull X-ray. These again should not be mistaken for fractures.

The metopic suture of the frontal bone is evident at birth and begins to disappear from about the ninth month onwards. It is usually fused by the end of the second year, though occasionally it persists into adult life.

The facial bones are relatively small in the newborn skull and the mandible is divided into two lateral halves by a midline bar of cartilage.

The sella has dense walls as the sphenoid is not yet pneumatized and the anterior clinoids are relatively large and rounded. Closure of the posterior fontanelle usually occurs at 6 to 8 months and of the anterior fontanelle at 15 to 18 months. The smaller lateral fontanelles (sphenoid and mastoid) disappear after 6 months. In children with raised intracranial pressure the fontanelles may of course remain open for longer periods.

The width of the sutures at birth varies tremendously and the coronal and lambdoid sutures in lateral view may be between 1·5 and 10 mm in diameter. The wider normal sutures narrow rapidly and most are below 3 mm in width in a few months. By the end of the second year the appearance of the skull has begun to resemble that of an adult skull. The vault has increased in thickness and differentiated into inner and outer tables and a diploe. The sutures are assuming the serrated adult configuration.

At the sutures the inner tables usually meet in a straight line whereas the outer tables are serrated. On the X-ray this may show as a straight line apparently running through the middle of the serrated one. This appearance, which may also be recognized in the adult, should not be mistaken for a fracture.

As already noted the metopic suture is usually obliterated by 2 years of age, though it sometimes persists in adult skulls. Its slight interdigitations help to distinguish it from a fracture. The mendosal sutures disappear by the end of the first year, whilst the synchondrosis between the supra-occipital and exoccipital region vanishes by the end of the second or third year. The spheno-occipital synchondrosis begins to close during puberty, but may be still evident until the age of 20 or longer.

The so-called convolutional impressions have been mentioned above. They are rarely present before 2 years of age but rapidly increase in number and prominence until 4 or 5, when they can be very well marked. They remain prominent until the child is over 10 and then begin to slowly diminish until about 14 years. It is alleged that there is a relationship between brain growth and these impressions, and the term brain markings has also been used for them. However, their true mode of production has not yet been satisfactorily explained. They regress in prominence after the age of 10, though occasionally they may still be quite evident in adult skulls. It is rare however to find them in an adult skull after middle age.

The middle meningeal vascular markings first appear between the second and third years. The diploic vascular channels, however, appear rather later. The latter, as already noted, are much more variable than the meningeal markings both in extent and size.

The sinuses develop during childhood, the antra and ethmoids rather earlier than the frontal and sphenoidal sinuses.

REFERENCES AND SUGGESTIONS FOR FURTHER READING—See Chapter 58

CHAPTER 58

THE ABNORMAL SKULL

Abnormalities seen on plain X-ray of the skull will be discussed under the following headings:

1. Congenital lesions.
2. Raised intracranial pressure.
3. Localizing evidence of cerebral tumours.
4. Pathological intracranial calcification.
5. Abnormal vascular markings.
6. Erosions of the skull and osteoporosis.
7. Hyperostosis.
8. Skull trauma.

CONGENITAL LESIONS

There are many descriptive terms for variations in the shape of the skull. These variations in shape are not necessarily pathological and in any case there is a wide variation in the normal dimensions of the skull.

Skulls which appear excessively long in relation to their transverse diameter are termed *dolichocephalic*, whilst skulls which are excessively wide in relation to their length are termed *brachycephalic*. In *trigonocephaly* the frontal bone is rather sharply pointed anteriorly giving the head

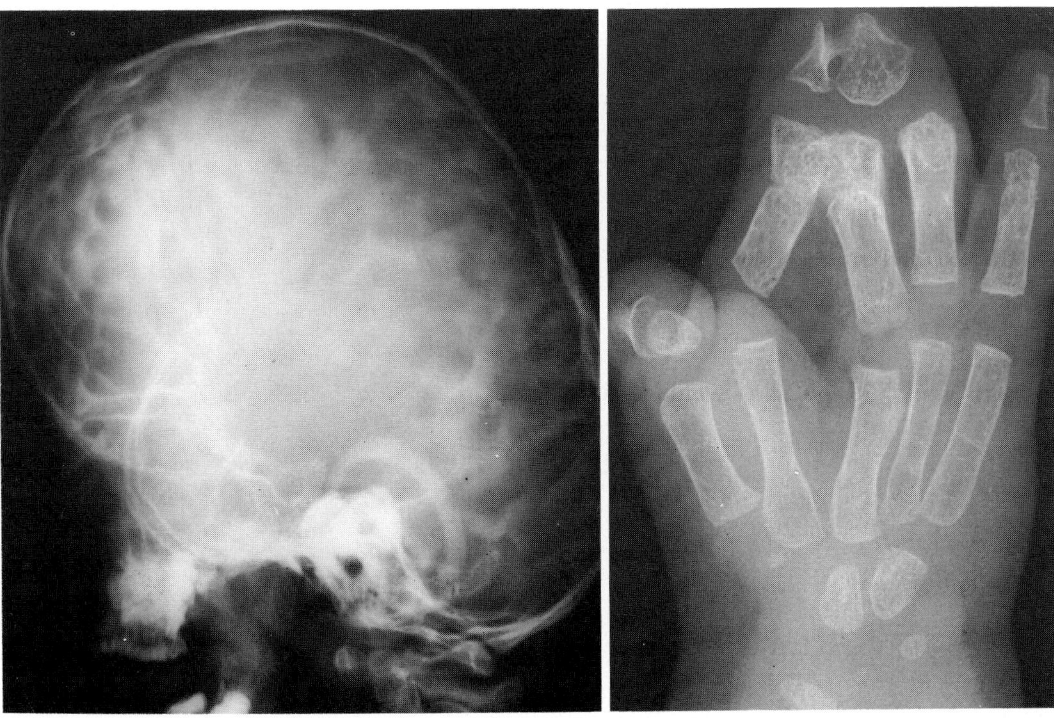

Fig. 58.1 *Fig. 58.2*

Fig. 58.1 Oxycephaly due to premature fusion of the coronal sutures.
Fig. 58.2 Hand of the same patient showing syndactyly. The combination of oxycephaly and syndactyly comprises Apert's syndrome.

a triangular appearance. This is due to premature *in utero* fusion of the metopic suture. In some patients a step-like deformity is seen at the back of the skull because the squamous occipital bone overlaps the parietal bones at the lambdoid suture. This is termed *bathrocephaly* and should not be confused with a traumatic lesion.

Craniosynostosis. Premature fusion of skull sutures is not uncommon and gives rise to various deformities. The type due to fusion of the coronal and lambdoid sutures is termed *oxycephaly*, *acrocephaly* or *turricephaly* because of the supposed tower-like or peaked appearance of the skull.

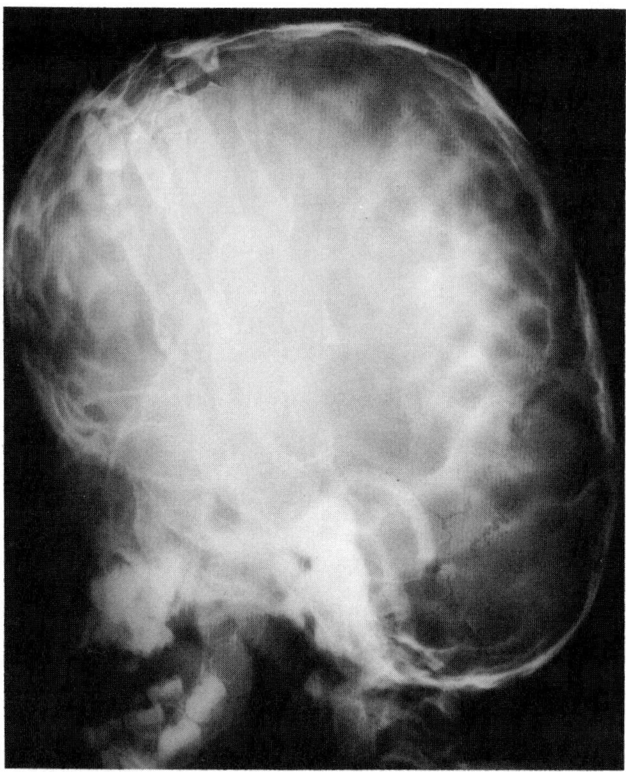

Fig. 58.3 Post-operative film of same patient as in Figure 58.1. The coronal suture has been excised and tantalum foil inserted between the bone and margins.

Whilst many of the cases result merely in a bizarre appearance, some may be associated with compression of the optic nerves. Eighth nerve lesions have also been described as has mental deficiency and other neurological disabilities. Patients with oxycephaly usually show prominent convolutional markings in the skull vault. Very rarely oxycephaly may be associated with syndactyly, a condition known as *acrocephalosyndactyly* or *Apert's syndrome* (Figs 58.1 and 58.2). *Acrocephalopolysyndactyly* or *Carpenter's syndrome* is characterized by polydactyly with mild soft tissue syndactyly and also less severe skull changes together with obesity and mental retardation.

Scaphocephaly with a narrow elongated skull results from premature fusion of the sagittal suture. It is the commonest form of craniosynostosis and is more frequent in boys than in girls. Apart from the shape of skull the condition is symptom-less. In *microcephaly* there is premature fusion of all the skull sutures and the skull vault is abnormally small. The condition is usually associated with mental defect. *Plagiocephaly* is a condition in which the skull is markedly asymmetrical, presumably as a result of premature closure of the coronal and lambdoid sutures on one side. *Trigonocephaly* (triangular head) is due to premature closure of the metopic suture.

Crouzon's disease (hereditary craniofacial dysostosis) is a form of generalized craniosynostosis associated with hypoplasia of the facial bones, hypertelorism, and exophthalmos.

Many operations have been used for the treatment of craniosynostosis, and it has been postulated that preventing premature fusion of the sutures will also prevent the development of mental retardation and neurological defects. However, it is probable that maldevelopment of the brain in microcephaly is associated with, rather than secondary to, the premature fusion of the sutures. It seems unlikely, therefore, that such operations can have any but cosmetic value in microcephaly, though they may prevent nerve compression in oxycephaly. Mere excision of the sutures is insufficient to prevent fusion. This rapidly recurs unless the bone surfaces can be kept separate by the interposition of such substances as tantalum (Fig. 58.3).

In their survey of craniostenosis Tod and Yelland (1971) made a plea that the traditional Greek terminology be abandoned and replaced by a classification based solely on the sutures affected, e.g. coronal fusion, sagittal fusion, or multiple suture fusion.

Lacunar skull (Luckenschadel). This condition is found in infantile skulls and is characterized by groups

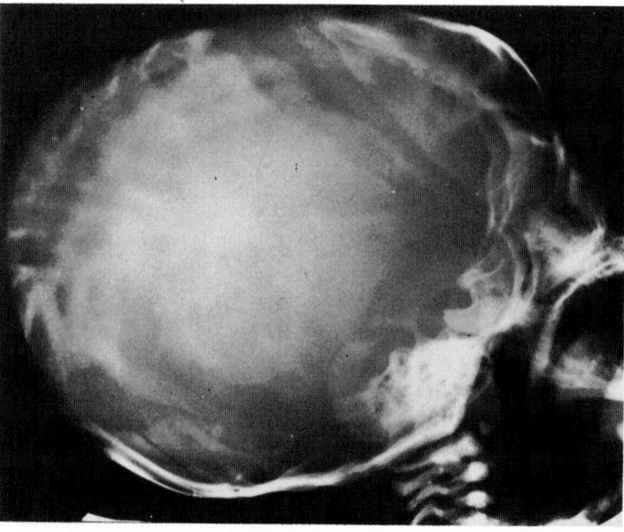

Fig. 58.4 Lacunar skull in an infant. Note the wide sutures.

of round, oval or finger-shaped pits on the inner surface of the cranial vault and separated by ridges of bone (Fig. 58.4). These lacunar markings in the skull appear in fetal life in the membranous part of the cranial vault. They lie in the thickest parts of the frontal, parietal and upper occipital bones. The markings begin to fade round the time of birth and they generally disappear by the age of 4 or 6 months. There are usually associated anomalies of the central nervous system, the commonest being myelomeningocele and encephalocele. Less often there is a simple meningocele. There may also be associated stenosis of the aqueduct or an Arnold Chiari malformation and either of these may lead to hydrocephalus. However, craniolacuna can occur without raised intracranial pressure. Children with this anomaly have a high mortality because of the associated multiple lesions of the central nervous system.

Cranial **meningoceles** and **encephaloceles** are commonest in the occipital region and in the frontal region. They can occur, however, elsewhere over the vault and have also been described as presenting in the skull base. Diagnosis is usually obvious clinically, but small lateral and basal meningoceles and encephaloceles can present diagnostic problems. If there is a bone defect beneath a swelling of the scalp then the possibility of encephalocele should always be borne in mind. An encephalocele in the nasofrontal region will give rise to one form of hypertelorism, and when minor in degree is often misdiagnosed as a dermoid or lacrimal sac cyst. The basal encephalocele can be even more difficult to diagnose and presents in infancy and childhood with nasal obstruction, though sometimes the lesions are not diagnosed until adult life. It is vital that the nasopharyngeal mass should be correctly diagnosed as surgical intervention could be disastrous. Again hypertelorism may be present and should suggest this diagnosis. A basal view of the skull will show a central defect in the sphenoid or spheno-ethmoid region. A lateral view of the skull will show the soft tissue mass in the nasopharynx. Air studies or C.A.T. may show the third ventricle extending down through the pituitary fossa into the sphenoid, giving rise to one form of 'empty sella'.

Platybasia is the term used for the condition in which the base of the skull appears relatively flattened. The 'basal angle' is the angle between the plane of the clivus and the plane of the midline of the anterior fossa. It is a measurement widely used by anthropologists particularly in comparative anatomy. Man has a basal angle of between 120° and 140° whilst primates have basal angles greater than 150°. In platybasia the basal angle is greater than 142°. The condition may be symptomless and of no pathological significance. However, the term is also used rather loosely to include *basilar impression* and *basilar invagination*, conditions with which it is usually, though not invariably, associated.

Basilar invagination results from diseases producing softening of bone. The commonest aetiological factor in this country is Paget's disease. The condition is also seen with rickets, osteomalacia, scurvy, fragilitas ossium, cleidocranial dysostosis, and occasionally with hyperparathyroidism.

Basilar impression indicates an elevation of the floor of the posterior fossa commonly associated with congenital anomalies of the cervical spine such as atlanto-occipital fusion or Klippel-Feil syndrome. The foramen magnum may also be abnormal in shape and size.

Platybasia is usually symptomless but, particularly when associated with basilar impression, symptoms from tonsillar herniation and obstruction of c.s.f. circulation may result.

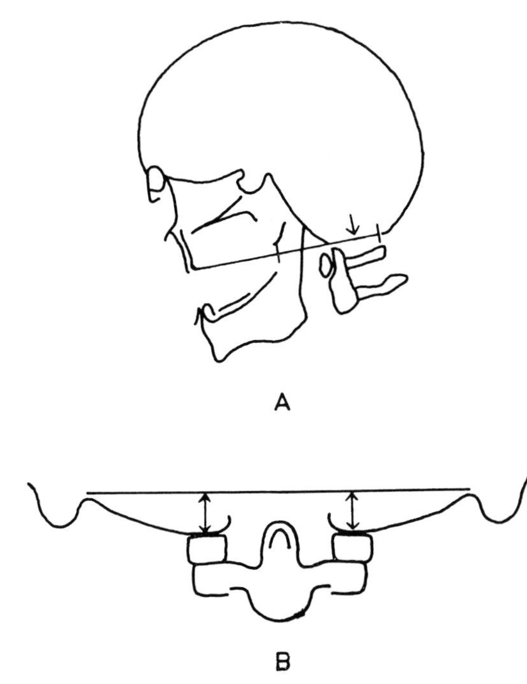

Fig. 58.5 (A) Diagram to show Chamberlain's line (↓). (B) Diagram to show normal relationship of digastric grooves and atlanto-occipital joint. The distance arrowed (↕) normally measures 1·1 cm (±0·4 cm).

A number of lines and measurements have been used in the past for assessing platybasia and basilar impression on plain X-ray of the skull.

The '*basal angle*' is defined as the angle subtended by a line drawn from the nasion to the tuberculum sellae in a lateral X-ray film of the skull, and a second line drawn from the tuberculum to the anterior margin of the foramen magnum. Normally this measures between 125° and 142°, and greater values are thought to indicate platybasia.

Chamberlain's line is drawn on a lateral film of the skull from the back of the hard palate to the posterior lip of the foramen magnum. Normally less than one-third of the odontoid peg lies above this line but more than half does so in platybasia.

Bull's angle is formed by a line drawn through the hard palate and another drawn through the plane of the atlas in a lateral skull film taken with the patient prone and his head turned laterally. In platybasia this angle is increased above the normal limit of 13°.

However, the most reliable method of assessing platybasia is by anterio-posterior tomography of the skull in the plane of the petrous bones and occipital condyles. The atlanto-occipital joints normally lie below the level of the digastric grooves (Fig. 58.5) but are elevated in basilar impression.

Cleidocranial dysostosis is a skeletal dystrophy in which there is complete or partial absence of the clavicles, persistence of the metopic suture and anterior fontanalle, and also failure of fusion of the lower lambdoid sutures. Multiple Wormian bones are usually visible at the open fontanelles and suture lines, and platybasia is frequently seen (see Fig. 1.28 p. 13).

Fragilitas ossium (osteogenesis imperfecta). This is fully described in the bone section (p. 14). The skull is of considerable interest. It is poorly mineralized with irregular thinning in the neonate, and multiple Wormian bones are present along the sutures.

Hypertelorism is a descriptive term for a condition in which the orbits seem widely separated. It may occur as an isolated congenital lesion (Grieg's disease). Apart from the wide separation of the orbits the only other radiological abnormality is the usual presence of a metopic suture and of well-developed ethmoid cells occupying the gap between the orbits. Other cases are associated with bone dysplasias such as osteogenesis imperfecta, cleidocranial dysostosis, and fibrous dysplasia; or with craniostenosis. Finally some cases are secondary to frontal encephalocele, and rarely acquired cases can occur from mucocele of the ethmoids (see above).

Hypophosphatasia is due to an inborn error of metabolism (see p. 31 and p. 180). This results in defective ossification. The skull of an affected child shows a very characteristic appearance. The vault is under-mineralized and the growing edges of the bone are particularly affected. As a result the sutures at birth appear abnormally wide and their margins irregular. Later there may be early suture fusion and craniostenosis.

Sinus pericranii. In this condition an emissary vein causes a small defect in the frontal bone. The vein is subcutaneous and can be distended by posture, i.e. by placing the forehead in the dependent position or by raising the venous pressure.

Congenital parietal foramina. In some patients a large parasagittal defect may be found in the posterior parietal region. The lesion is usually bilateral and symmetrical. In other patients a small emissary vein may produce a tiny defect in the bone here. Congenital posterior parietal foramina may be familial.

RAISED INTRACRANIAL PRESSURE

The radiological signs of raised intracranial pressure are generally listed under the following four headings:

1. Suture diastasis.
2. Erosion of the dorsum sellae.
3. Increased convolutional markings.
4. Pineal displacement.

It is most important to realize that the radiological signs are quite different in children and in adults. The difference depends on the fact that the sutures are firmly united in the adult and are not therefore affected by the chronic raised intracranial pressure.

CHILDREN

In children, and the younger the child the more marked the sign may be, **suture diastasis** or splaying apart of the sutures is the first and most prominent result of a rise in intracranial pressure (Fig. 58.6). It is most obvious and prominent at the coronal suture, though the sagittal suture may also be markedly affected (Fig. 58.7). It is usually least prominent at the lambdoid suture. Lesser degrees of diastasis of the coronal and sagittal sutures may be more obvious in the basal view of the skull. Neonates and young infants with raised intracranial pressure may show, in addition to large heads with suture diastasis, unusually *thin skull vaults*. They may also show *craniolacuna* particularly when the raised pressure is associated with such congenital anomalies as meningocele (Fig. 58.4).

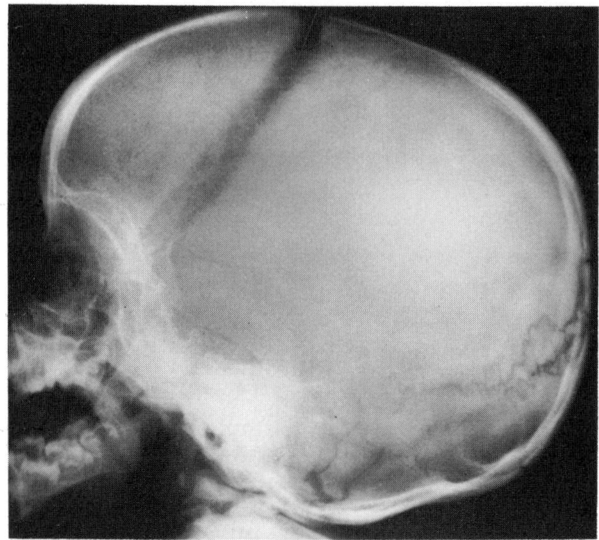

Fig. 58.6 Suture diastasis in a child with raised intracranial pressure. The coronal suture is mainly involved. The sella appears relatively normal.

Older children and adolescents with chronic raised intracranial pressure (Fig. 58.8) may show sutures which,

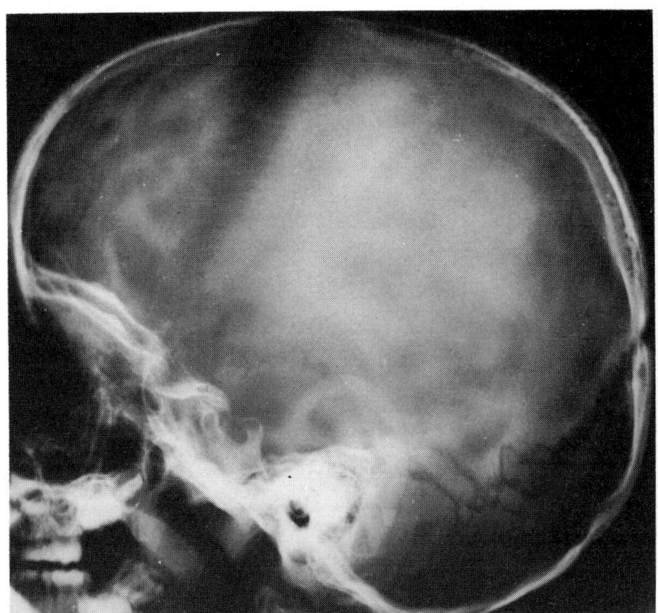

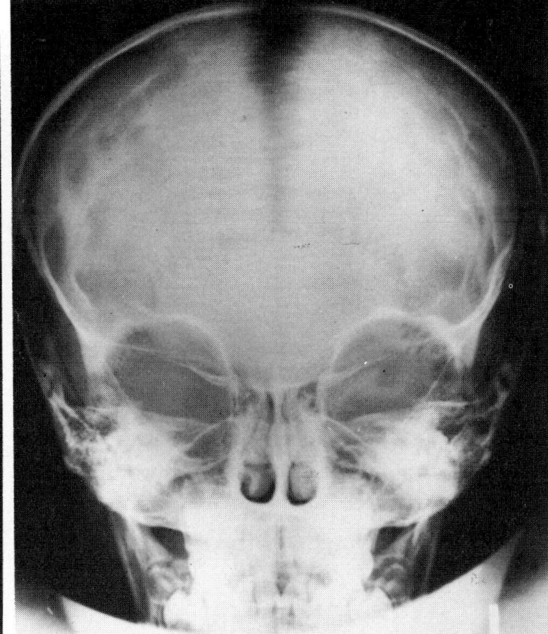

Fig. 58.7 Lateral and P.A. films of child with raised intracranial pressure and marked suture diastasis involving the coronal and sagittal sutures.

though not obviously splayed, are abnormal in that they are uniting with excessive interdigitations. The skull may be relatively large and there may be an abnormal depth of the central part of the anterior fossa (cribriform plate) as seen in lateral view.

It is important to realize that suture diastasis may be the only radiological sign of raised intracranial pressure in a child and it may be very well marked with no other apparent changes. However, in cases of long-standing raised intracranial pressure there is generally some loss of definition of the dorsum sellae with erosion of its tip, even in children.

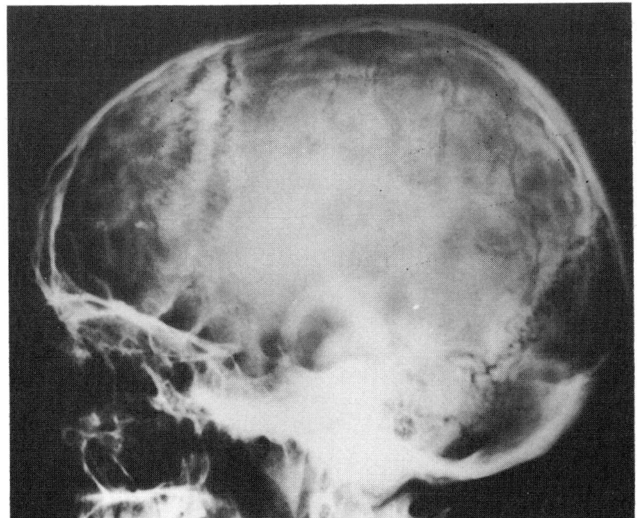

Fig. 58.8 Slight suture diastasis in an adolescent from chronic raised intracranial pressure. The dorsum sellae is also thinned.

Sellar erosion in children under 10, if it occurs without any suture diastasis is generally the result of a local lesion in the region of the sella.

Suture diastasis may occur very rapidly in small children and may be present within a few weeks of the onset of symptoms. Over the age of 10, however, it generally implies chronic raised intracranial pressure and sellar changes are proportionately more frequent as the child increases in age.

Increased convolutional markings have often been attributed to raised intracranial pressure in the past. However, the copper beaten or silver beaten appearance of the skull is commonly seen in normal children, being most marked between the ages of 4 and 10. Conversely severe raised intracranial pressure may exist with no visible changes in the skull vault. The sign therefore is of very little diagnostic significance. Convolutional markings may also be seen in certain congenital lesions which are not necessarily associated with raised pressure. It is quite common for instance in patients with craniostenosis.

ADULTS

In adults the evidence of raised intracranial pressure is very different from that seen in the child. Suture diastasis is not seen and increased convolutional marking is of no significance. *Erosion of the dorsum sellae* is the characteristic change (Figs 58.9 and 58.10). This commences first as slight porosis of the anterior cortex of the dorsum and of the cortex of the sellar floor which is best seen in the lateral film. Eventually there is marked loss of definition

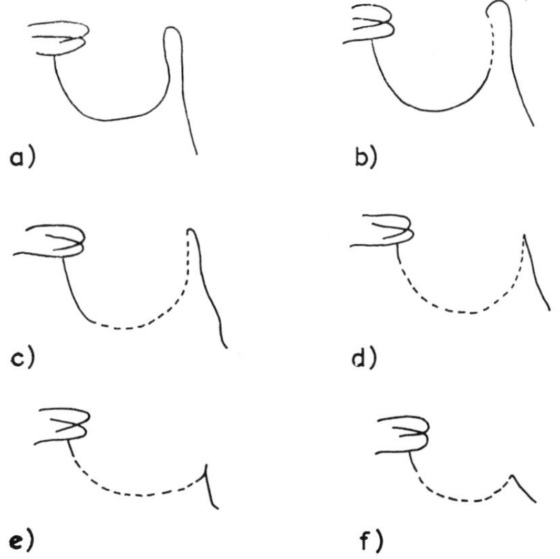

Fig. 58.9 Diagram of the sellar changes in raised intracranial pressure in the adult. (a) to (f) show progressive changes from slight in (b) to gross in (f).

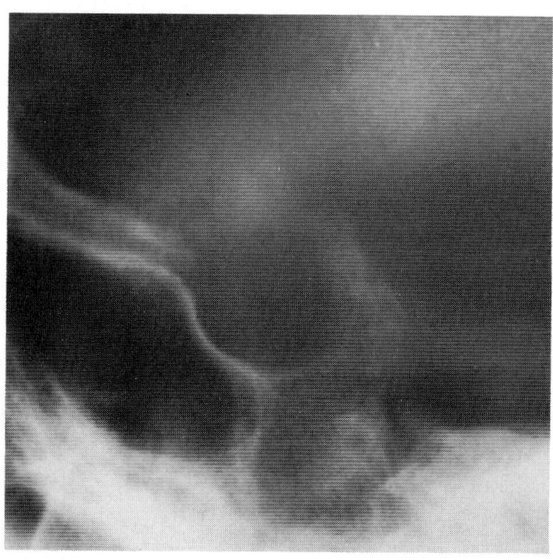

Fig. 58.10 Advanced changes due to chronic raised pressure. The dorsum sellae has become ill-defined. The anterior clinoids are also affected and the floor of the sella is indistinct.

of this cortex or 'lamina dura', and frank erosion of the dorsum may follow. The actual erosion commences at the top and progresses downwards. In a patient with long-standing raised intracranial pressure the whole of the dorsum sellae may completely disappear. However, at this stage the diagnosis is nearly always clinically obvious. Radiology is of most value in indicating that the early changes of raised pressure are present rather than by confirming the late case with gross evidence of raised intracranial pressure.

Frank erosion of the posterior clinoids and dorsum of the sella due to raised pressure is claimed to be largely due to pressure from a dilated third ventricle and therefore more common in patients with posterior fossa tumours and symmetrical hydrocephalus.

The sellar erosion of raised pressure must be distinguished from that due to local destructive lesions. Apart from pituitary adenoma, these include meningioma, chordoma, craniopharyngioma and aneurysm.

Pineal displacement. In good-quality films of the

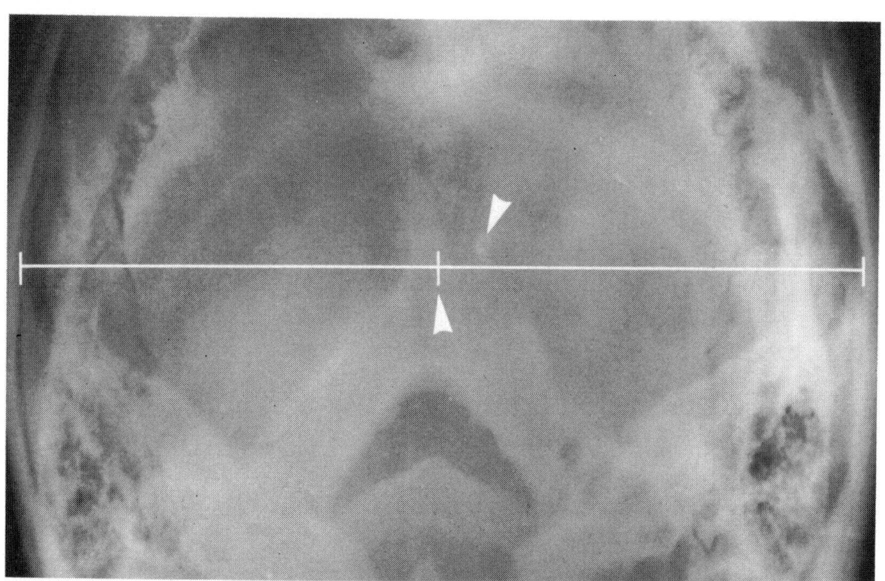

Fig. 58.11 Displacement of the calcified pineal by a right hemisphere tumour. The displacement measures 5 mm on the original film. ↑ = mid point ↓ = pineal.

skull the pineal lies in the midline in the Towne's projection. If the pineal is poorly calcified it may be better demonstrated in frontal projections by special coned views with a lesser degree of tilt than for the Towne's projection. With the Schonander apparatus such coned views are best obtained with the slit diaphragm, and stereo-slit films can be helpful in localizing faint calcification. With well positioned good quality films displacement of the calcified pineal more than 3 mm to one side of the midline can be regarded as good evidence of the presence of an intracranial mass displacing the pineal away from the side of the lesion (Fig. 58.11). The commonest cause of such a displacement is an intracranial tumour but such lesions as subdural haematoma or other non-neoplastic masses may produce the same effect.

The pineal may also be observed to be displaced in the lateral projection. With the presence of a large supratentorial tumour, the displacement in this view is backwards and downwards. There are several special charts or diagrams, such as those of Vastine and Kinney, aimed at assessing such displacement. These are little used in practice, and are poor substitutes for practical experience of skull film interpretation.

Occasionally forward and downward displacement of the pineal may be seen in a lateral film. This usually indicates the presence of an extra cerebral mass, such as a meningioma of the tentorial apex, lying behind the pineal.

LOCALIZING EVIDENCE OF CEREBRAL TUMOURS

Apart from the *general* signs of raised intracranial pressure just described, the presence of an intracerebral tumour may also be deduced from the presence of certain other signs which have in addition *localizing* value. In some cases not only the site of the tumour may be indicated but also its pathological nature. This radiological evidence can be classified under the following headings:

1. Intracranial calcification.
2. Abnormal vascular markings.
3. Skull erosion.
4. Hyperostosis.
5. Lateral displacement of pineal.

Lateral displacement of the calcified pineal, a sign which usually indicates the presence of a mass in one hemisphere, has already been discussed. The other radiological signs listed above are discussed in detail and with reference to differential diagnosis in the following pages.

PATHOLOGICAL INTRACRANIAL CALCIFICATION

The accompanying table (Table 58.1) lists most of the known causes of pathological intracranial calcification.

Table 58.1 Pathological intracranial calcification

1. *Tumours*
   (*a*) Glioma
   (*b*) Craniopharyngioma
   (*c*) Meningioma
   (*d*) Ependymoma
   (*e*) Pinealoma
   (*f*) Papilloma of choroid plexus
   (*g*) Chordoma
   (*h*) Dermoid and cholesteatoma
   (*i*) Hamartoma
   (*j*) Lipoma
   (*k*) Pituitary adenoma

2. *Vascular*
   (*a*) Atheroma
   (*b*) Aneurysm
   (*c*) Angioma
   (*d*) Subdural haematoma
   (*e*) Intracranial haematoma

3. *Infections and infestations*
   (*a*) Tuberculosis
   (*b*) Toxoplasmosis
   (*c*) Cytomegalic inclusion body disease
   (*d*) Cysticercosis
   (*e*) Pyogenic abscess
   (*f*) Hydatid
   (*g*) Paragonimas Westermani

4. *Metabolic and miscellaneous*
   (*a*) Idiopathic basal ganglia calcification
   (*b*) Hypoparathyroidism
   (*c*) Pseudohypoparathyroidism
   (*d*) Tuberous sclerosis
   (*e*) Sturge-Weber syndrome
   (*f*) Lissencephaly
   (*g*) Fahr's syndrome
   (*h*) Neurofibromatosis

TUMOURS

Calcification occurs in many cerebral tumours. The commonest tumour seen in clinical practice is the **glioma** which forms about half of the neoplasms encountered in most large centres. Calcification is estimated to occur in a radiologically visible form in between 5 per cent and 10 per cent of these cases. It is the slow growing and less malignant types of glioma which are most likely to develop such calcification and in the relatively rare oligodendroglioma the percentage is nearly 50 per cent. Posterior fossa gliomas show calcification in about 20 per cent of cases, but medulloblastomas and highly malignant astrocystomas (grades I and II) rarely show calcification. It has been alleged that specific types of gliomas may show a specific type of calcification. Thus oligodendroglioma has been said to have characteristic serpiginous calcification. However, little reliance can be placed on the appearance of the calcification. In any type of glioma this may consist of a few ill-defined punctate dots, a dense calcified nodule, hazy amorphous calcification or irregular linear streaks (Figs 58.12, 58.13 and 58.14).

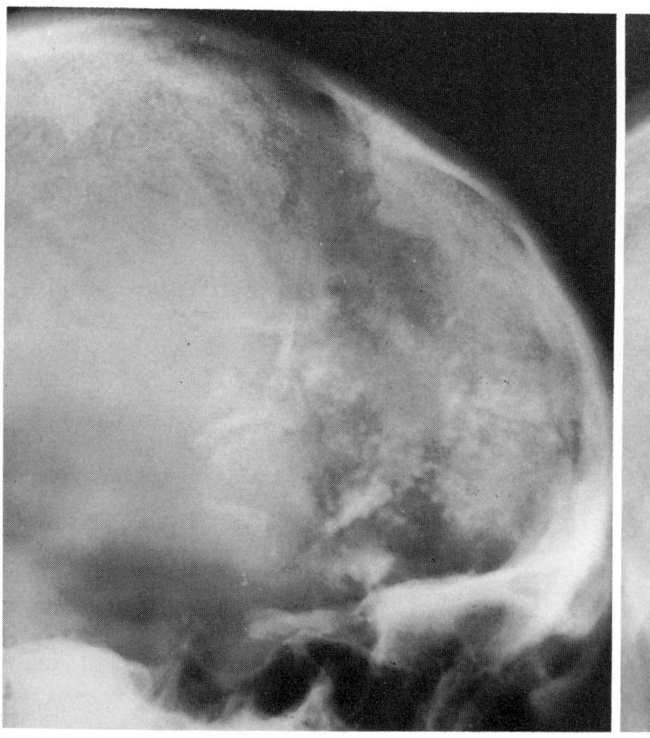

A

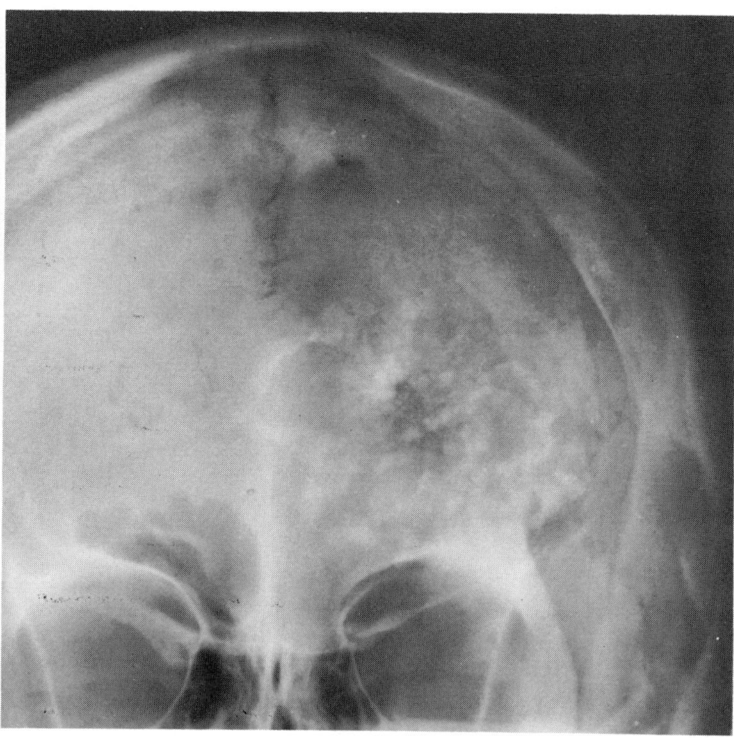

B

Fig. 58.12 Calcification in a slow growing frontal glioma. (A) Lateral view. (B) P.A. view.

Calcification is common in **craniopharyngiomas** and occurs in more than three-quarters of the cases. The majority of these tumours present in children. Calcification again varies in type from a few punctate dots to a large densely calcified mass (Figs 58.15 and 58.16).

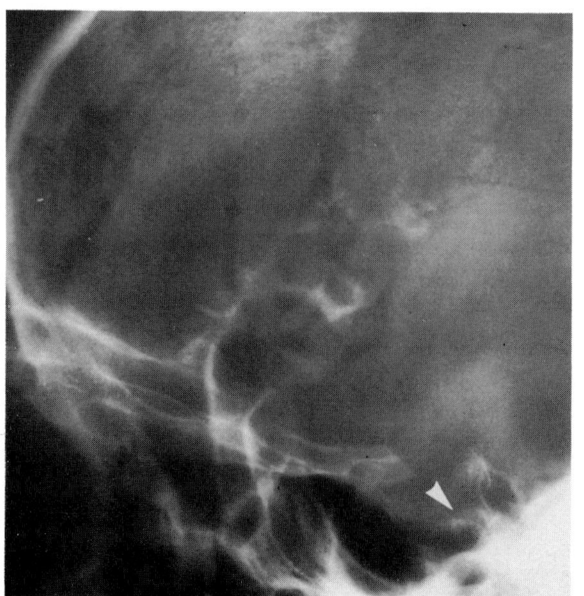

Fig. 58.13 Sinuous calcification in a frontal glioma. Note the evidence of raised pressure in the sella which shows loss of definition of its surrounding cortex (↘).

Occasionally, when cystic, curvilinear calcification may be seen in the cyst wall (Fig. 58.16). The characteristic feature is the position of the calcification, which is usually in the midline and just above the sella. Although the patient is nearly always a child, the tumours are occasionally encountered in adults. If they do present in adult life, differential diagnosis may be difficult, since calcification is less common than it is with children. A helpful point is the shape of the dorsum sellae, which often appears bent forward as if flattened from above. Occasionally these tumours with their calcification are actually intrasellar or partially so (Figs 58.16 and 58.17).

Meningiomas calcify in about 15 per cent of cases. Since they are benign tumours correct radiological diagnosis is of considerable importance. Apart from calcification there may be other features to suggest meningioma, e.g. an enlarged foramen spinosum and increased meningeal vascular markings leading up to the lesion, or associated hyperostosis of the skull vault (see below). Meningioma calcification is frequently very characteristic. In such typical cases it is usually circular in shape and amorphous in type, resembling a fairly well-defined ball of calcium (Fig. 58.18). Such calcification, if seen in a characteristic meningeal site (e.g. the parasagittal region or directly related to the skull base), should always suggest meningioma. Even when calcification is less characteristic, meningioma can be diagnosed with confidence if the other radiological signs mentioned above are also present, or if the site seems characteristic (Fig. 58.19).

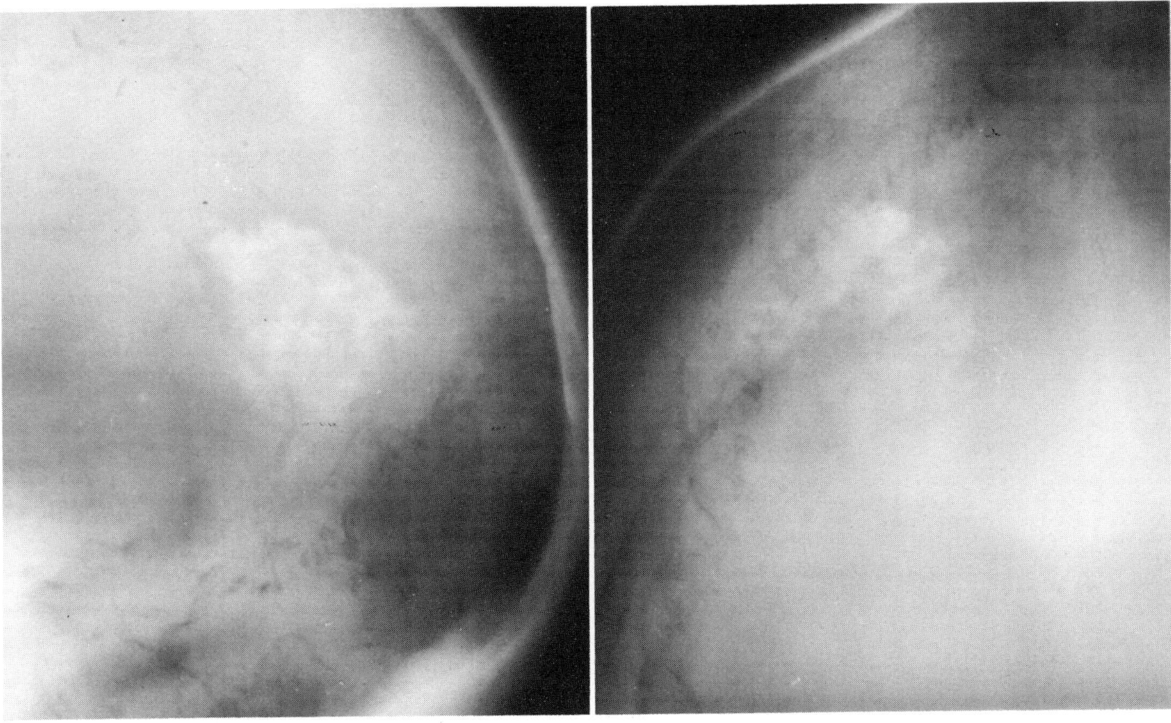

A B

Fig. 58.14 Hazy amorphous calcification in a glioma of the occipital lobe. (A) Lateral view. (B) Towne's view.

Ependymomas are rare tumours. They usually arise from the ventricular wall but occasionally appear to lie outside the ventricle and in the cerebral hemisphere. It is thought that these latter cases arise from cell rests. Calcification is unusual but can occur and can be quite dense.

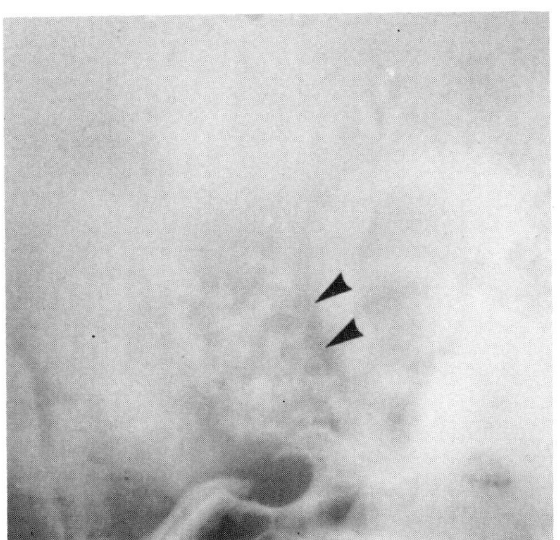

Fig. 58.15 Irregular calcification in a craniopharyngioma arrowed. Note the bowed shape of the dorsum sellae.

Dermoids and teratomas are found either in the posterior fossa or near the base of the skull. In the case of the rare teratomas, abnormal structures such as teeth may be identified and give a clue to the correct diagnosis. Posterior fossa dermoids may be associated with a characteristic small central defect in the occipital bone. They may show curvilinear or arc-like calcification similar to that seen in aneurysm (Fig. 58.20).

Cholesteatomas may also show arc-like calcifications which can be multiple.

Hamartomas may occur in the temporal lobe (Fig. 58.21) and be associated with temporal lobe epilepsy. Calcification in these lesions has no typical features and is usually diagnosed as calcification in a glioma.

Lipomas are rare benign tumours which may occur in relation to the *corpus callosum*. The author has described a highly characteristic calcification in these tumours. This is best identified in the postero-anterior or Towne's projection. It consists of two curvilinear streaks of calcium with the concavity facing the midline and symmetrically disposed around it in the region of the corpus callosum (Fig. 58.22). It is important to recognize this typical appearance since the lesion is benign. Surgical intervention is contraindicated and has resulted in tragedy since the anterior cerebral arteries are involved in the tumour.

Pineal tumours can also calcify. If calcification in the pineal area is abnormal in extent or type it should raise suspicion of neoplasm, particularly when occurring in a child.

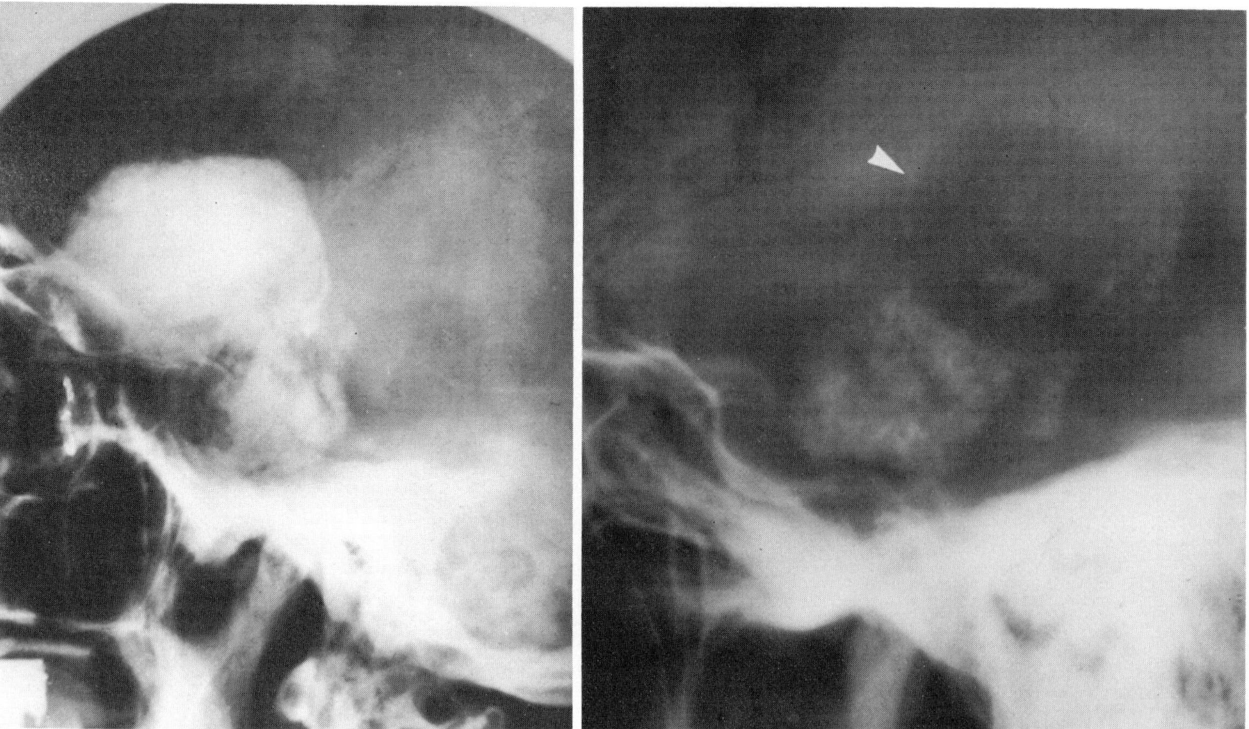

Fig. 58.16 Heavily calcified craniopharyngioma growing upwards and forwards from the sella.

Fig. 58.17 Calcified craniopharyngioma. The calcification in the upper part appears to be outlining a cyst (→) and the tumour is actually encroaching on the sella.

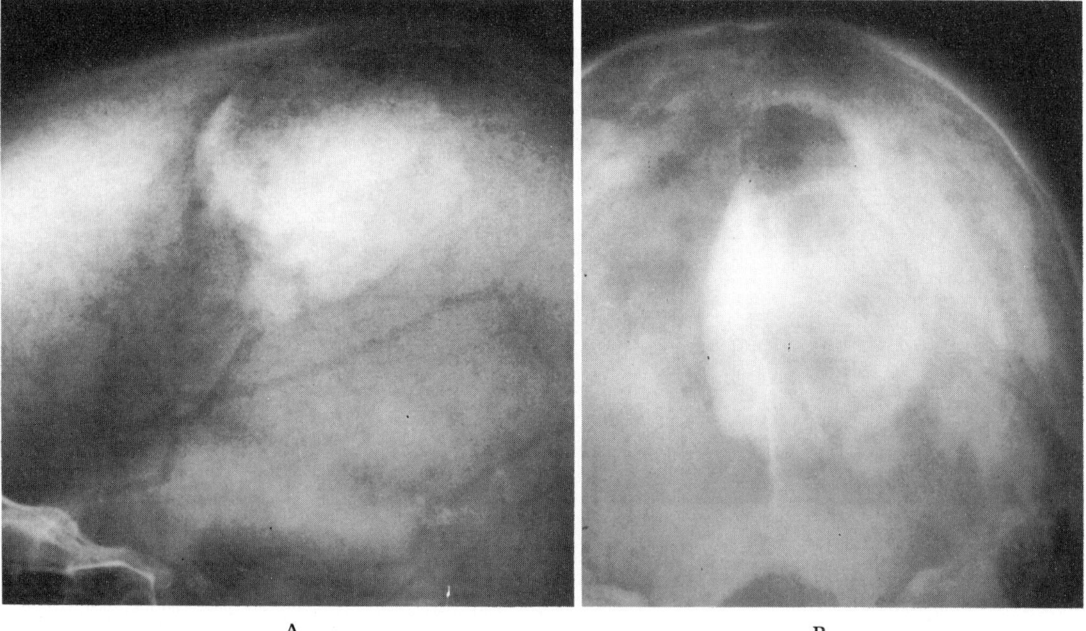

Fig. 58.18 Heavily calcified parasagittal meningioma. The site and type of calcification which outlines the whole tumour are characteristic.

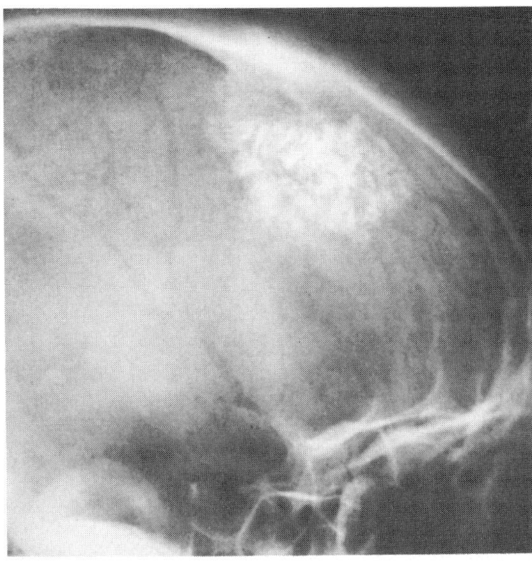

Fig. 58.19 Calcified meningioma. Calcification is less typical but again the site with the base of the tumour against the vault in the parasagittal region is characteristic. The presence of a local hyperostosis also helps to confirm the diagnosis.

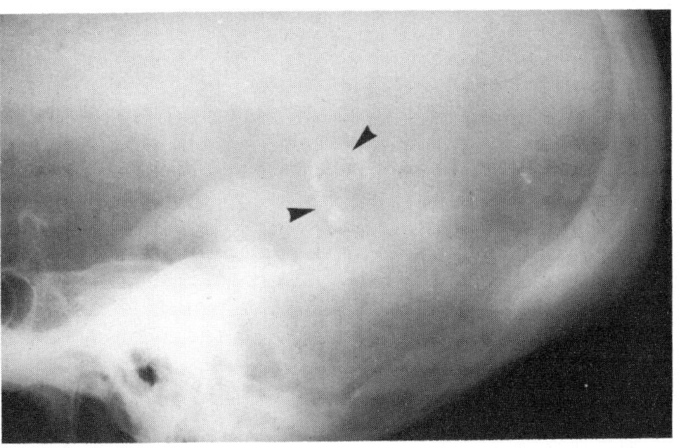

Fig. 58.20 Calcified dermoid in the posterior fossa.

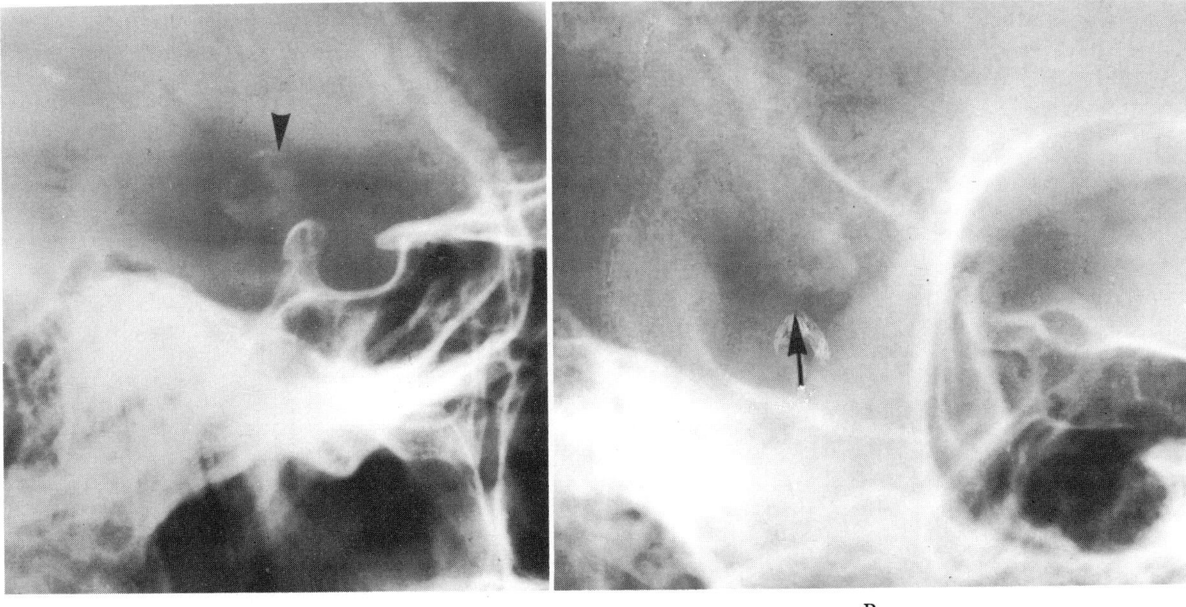

Fig. 58.21 Unusual calcified lesion in the anterior part of the temporal lobe. Histology: hamartoma. (A) Lateral view (↓). (B) Oblique view (↑).

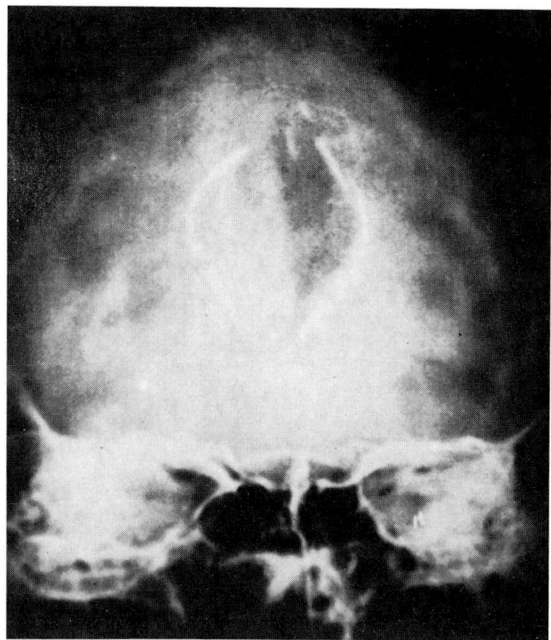

Fig. 58.22 Lipoma of corpus callosum.

Chordomas in a minority of cases may show irregular calcification (Fig. 58.23). They usually grow near the clivus and other radiological features such as erosion of the base or the presence of a soft-tissue mass in the pharynx may help in suggesting the diagnosis.

Secondary deposits in the brain have been described with radiologically demonstrable calcification, but this is so rare as to be a curiosity. It occurred in only two patients out of one series of 136 cases.

Pituitary tumours sometimes contain small areas of calcification, but again it is only in very rare cases that this can be recognized radiologically.

2. VASCULAR LESIONS

Aneurysms which have been present over a long period may show calcification in their wall. Most intracranial aneurysms occur in the region of the Circle of Willis and a ring shadow or an arc-like shadow in this region should always suggest the diagnosis of aneurysm. It must be emphasized however that the vast majority of aneurysms seen in clinical practice present by subarachnoid haemorrhage, and calcification is hardly ever seen in these cases. Thus, radiologically demonstrable calcification is seen in less than 1 per cent of the aneurysms diagnosed by angiography.

It is also important to realize that intracranial aneurysms can occasionally reach a very large size. Where a calcified ring shadow is more than an inch in diameter or where such a large shadow appears ovoid or lobulated in contour there has been a tendency to diagnose the lesion as a 'calcified cyst'. It is the author's experience, however, that even very large calcified ring shadows are almost always due to aneurysm and the marginal nature of the calcification is virtually pathognomonic (Fig. 58.24).

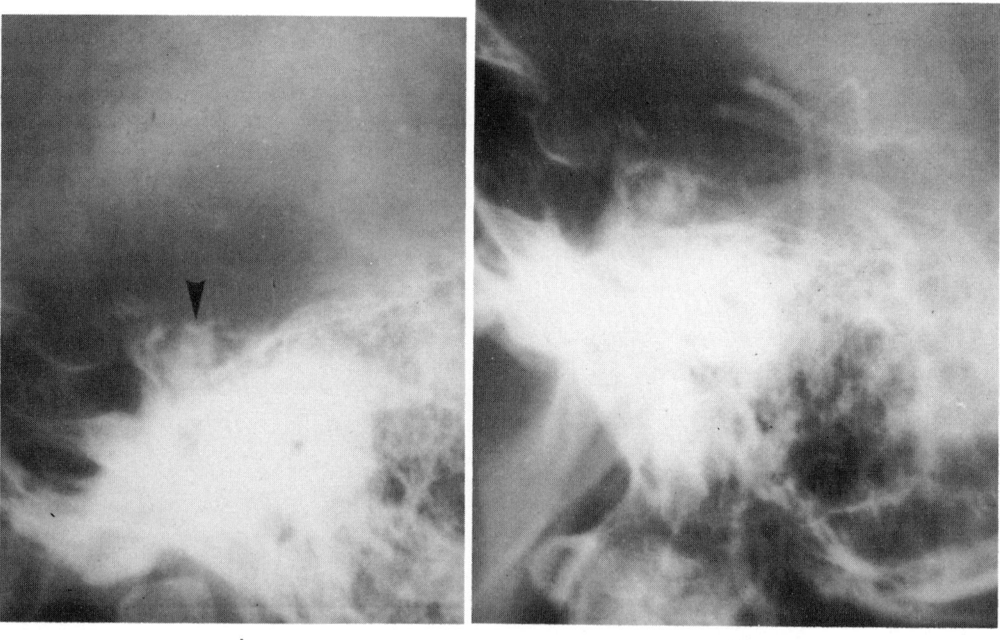

Fig. 58.23 (A) Calcification behind the clivus (↓) in a chordoma growing from the clivus. (B) Vertebral arteriogram showing backward displacement of the basilar artery by the tumour which is thus proved to be extra-cerebral and much larger than the calcification suggests.

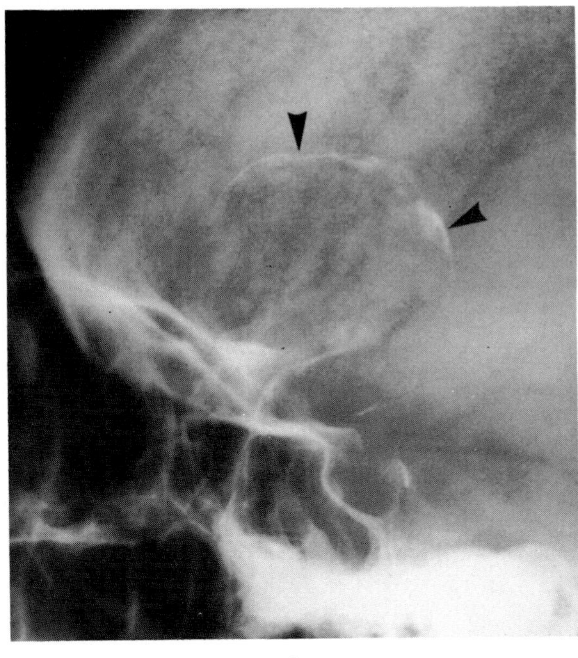

A

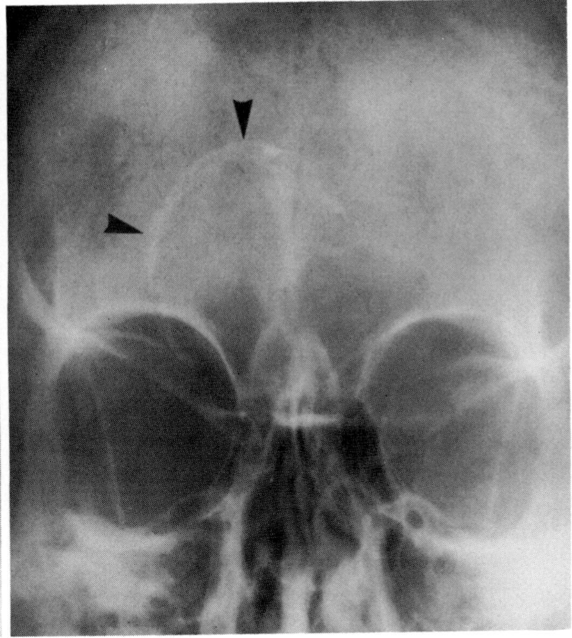

B

Fig. 58.24 Large calcified aneurysm of the anterior communicating artery. The lesion is unusually large but the calcification is typically marginal. Most calcified aneurysms are under 1 cm in diameter. (A) Lateral view (←). (B) P.A. view (→).

Angioma. Intracranial angiomas are relatively common intracranial lesions. In a small proportion of cases calcification may occur and this can be diagnostic. The calcification usually appears as a few irregular flecks of calcium and this may be associated with the presence of one or more small calcified ring shadows. The ring shadows are due to aneurysmal dilatation, usually on the venous side of the malformation. The flecks of calcium resemble those seen in atheromatous vessels. These characteristic features are illustrated in Figures 58.25 and 58.26.

Chronic subdural haematomas sometimes calcify, but only after a long period. The calcification can be recognized as outlining the subdural membrane (Fig. 58.27).

Intracranial haemorrhage with long survival of the patient may permit calcification in an **intracranial haematoma**. Calcification has also been demonstrated as developing in the course of the needle track following ventricular puncture for pneumography. The calcification

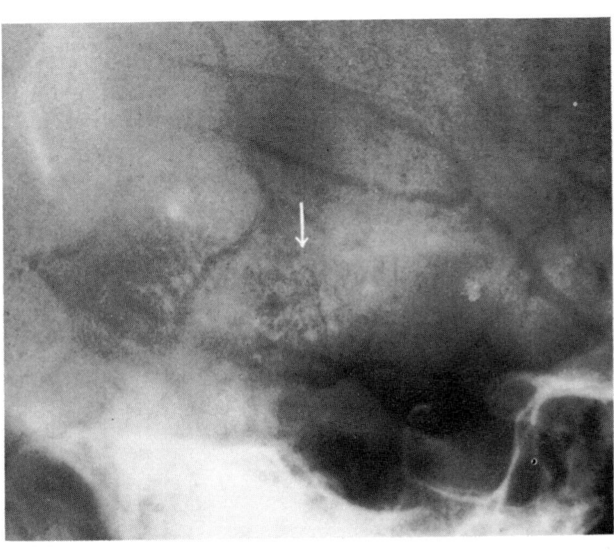

Fig. 58.25 Multiple flecks and specks of calcification in an angiomatous malformation (↓).

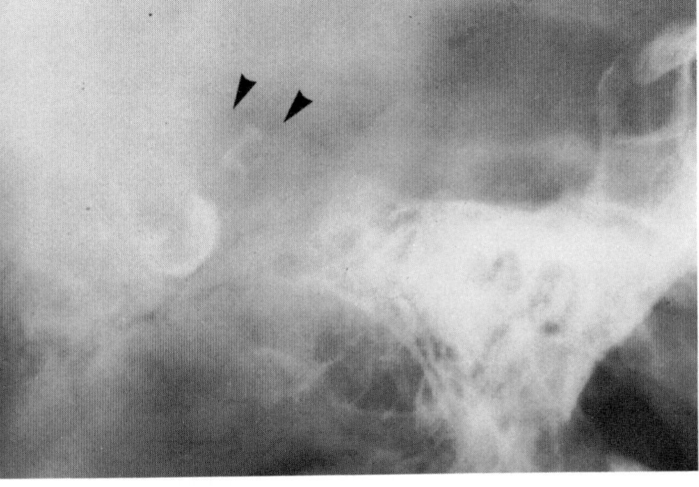

Fig. 58.26 Flecks of calcification associated with a calcified ring shadow in an angioma (arrowed).

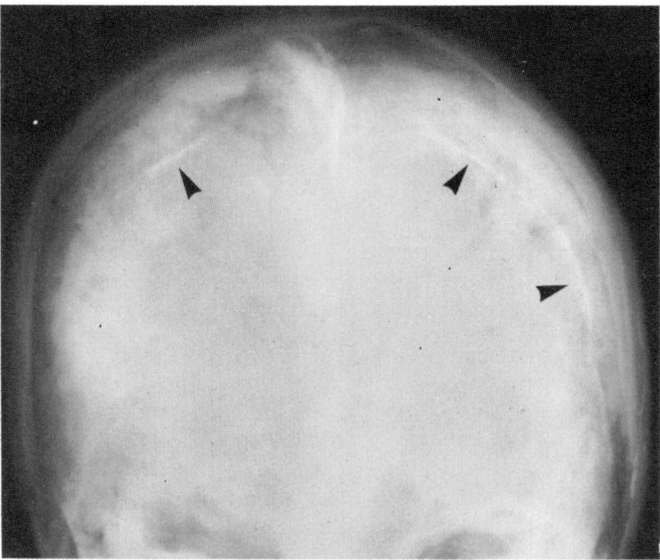

Fig. 58.27 Calcification in the margins of chronic bilateral subdural haematomas (arrowed).

is probably in small haematomas. The presence of a burr hole behind the line of calcification will usually point to the correct diagnosis.

Atheroma. Calcification may occur in atheromatous carotid arteries. Usually this type of calcification is seen in the cavernous sinus as a small fleck or flake of calcium superimposed on the sella. Occasionally it may be quite extensive (Fig. 58.28). It is unusual for calcification to occur in the more distal intracranial vessels though it is occasionally noted. Calcification may also be noted in atheromatous lesions near the common carotid bifurcation in the neck.

3. INFECTION AND INFESTATIONS

Tuberculoma. In the older textbooks tuberculoma is listed as a common cause of intracranial calcification. However, the evidence for the general belief that intracranial tuberculomas readily calcify is poor. Many of the reported cases are based merely on the association of pulmonary tuberculosis with a chronic non-progressive lesion in the brain which shows calcification. Radiologically detectable calcification in intracranial tuberculoma is very rare and has been said to occur in only 1 per cent of cases (Lorber). The diagnosis therefore is unjustified on a plain X-ray film. An exception to this rule is the patient with known healed tuberculous meningitis. Tuberculous meningitis was formerly a fatal disease, but since the introduction of antibiotics most cases can now be cured. A follow-up of cases of tuberculous meningitis cured by antibiotics has shown that they may develop intracranial calcification. This usually occurs in the healed exudate at the base of the brain though it can occur intracerebrally. The appearance of such calcification is characteristic (Fig. 58.29) and confirmation will always be provided by the history.

Toxoplasmosis is due to a protozoon which has been known for many years to infect animals and birds. Since 1942 it has also been known to infect humans. Infection of adult humans usually produces no symptoms, though the patient may become a carrier. Unfortunately, a pregnant woman who is a carrier can infect the fetus *in utero*. Such foetal infection produces serious results by involving the central nervous system. In the classical cases the infant is born with bilateral choroidoretinitis. Toxoplasmic granulomata are widespread throughout the brain and often show marked calcification. The calcification is characteristic and the diagnosis may be made on simple

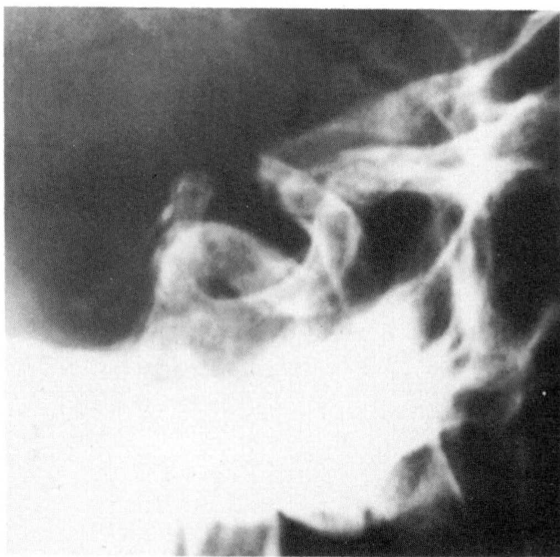

Fig. 58.28

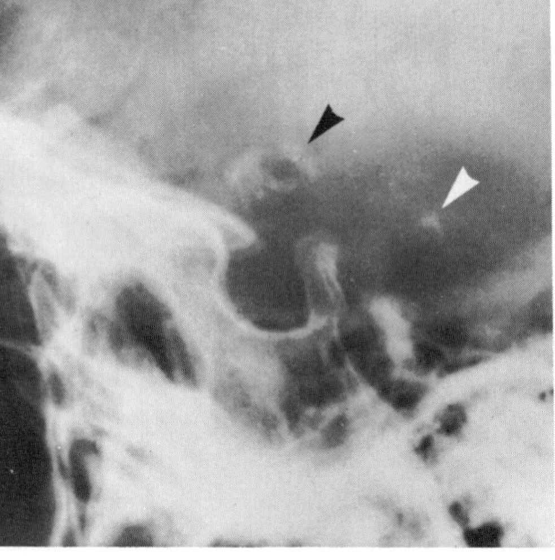

Fig. 58.29

Fig. 58.28 Unusually heavy calcification outlining the whole of the carotid syphon and shown to be bilateral in the frontal projection.

Fig. 58.29 Calcified basal exudate above the sella in a patient with healed tuberculous meningitis (arrowed).

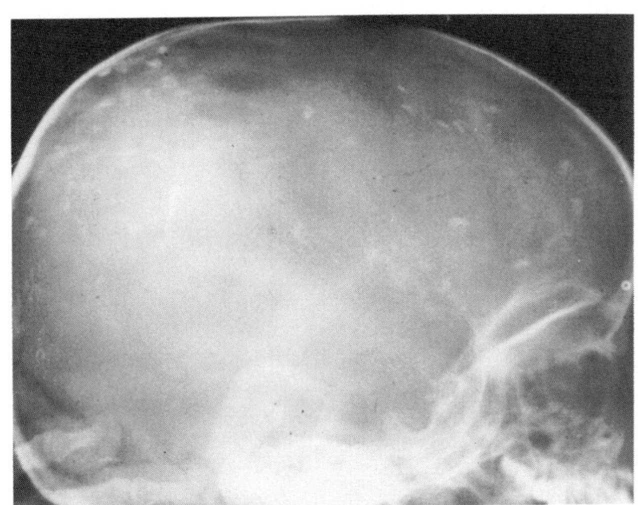

Fig. 58.30 Toxoplasmosis. Note characteristic multiple flecks of calcification.

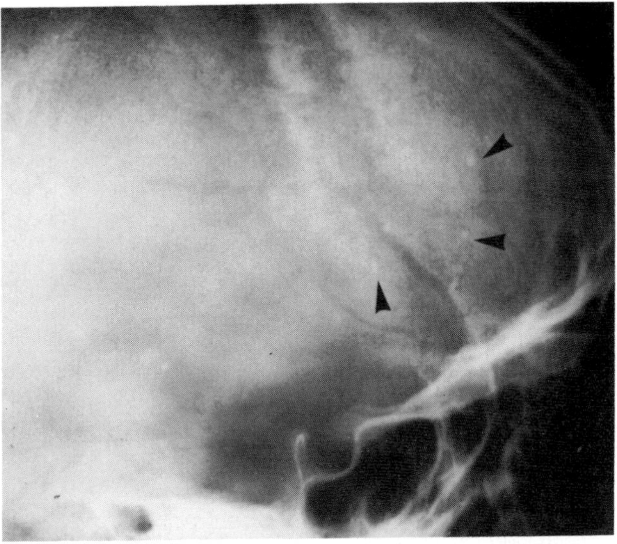

Fig. 58.31 Cysticercosis. There are multiple small calcified lesions 2 to 3 mm in diameter (arrowed).

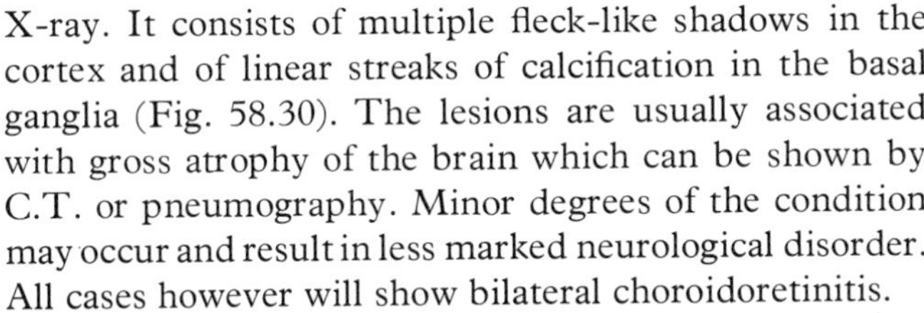

X-ray. It consists of multiple fleck-like shadows in the cortex and of linear streaks of calcification in the basal ganglia (Fig. 58.30). The lesions are usually associated with gross atrophy of the brain which can be shown by C.T. or pneumography. Minor degrees of the condition may occur and result in less marked neurological disorder. All cases however will show bilateral choroidoretinitis.

Cytomegalic inclusion body disease is caused by the widespread salivary gland virus. Intra-uterine infection produces serious effects on the fetus though the mother is symptomless. The brain infection results in widespread periventricular calcification which may 'outline' almost the whole of the dilated ventricles. The calcification is described as stippled in nature and since it outlines the walls of dilated ventricles it is bilateral and symmetrical. Microcephaly is usually present. Diagnosis may be confirmed by the finding of typical cells in the urine.

Cysticercosis. Human infestation is usually derived from eating infected pork. Most of the cases described in this country were in patients who had lived in India. The infestation is heaviest in the muscle masses where the calcified cysts show a very characteristic appearance (see Chapter 54). Infection of the central nervous system is relatively uncommon and intracranial calcification is seen in only about 10 per cent of the cases which show muscle calcification. The intracranial calcification differs in shape and size from that in the muscles. In the muscles the whole of the cyst calcifies giving rise to an oat-shaped shadow. In the skull only the scolex calcifies and the resultant shadow is pin point or nodular measuring 1 to 3 mm in diameter. Characteristically such calcified shadows are multiple and scattered over a wide area of the brain (Fig. 58.31).

Paragonimas Westermani is a trematode or fluke. Infection is acquired by the ingestion of cysts in the intermediate host, a crab or crayfish. Humans as final or definitive hosts develop pulmonary lesions, and in heavy infections, liver, mesentery, skeletal muscle and brain may become involved. The intracranial infection may give rise to focal neurological signs or epilepsy, and calcification may be shown radiologically. The disease is endemic in the Far East. Most of the recorded cases with intracranial calcification were reported from Korea and China. The lesions are usually in the parietal region and there may be extensive 'soap-bubble' calcification in cysts measuring up to 3 or 4 cm in diameter.

METABOLIC AND MISCELLANEOUS DISORDERS

Calcification of the basal ganglia may be observed as a chance finding in the X-ray film of an adult skull. Typically this calcification is amorphous or punctate. It is also bilateral and symmetrical and the region of the head of the caudate nucleus is first involved (Fig. 58.32). Calcification may also occur at the same time in the posterior fossa in the dentate nuclei (Fig. 58.33). Dentate nuclei calcification can also occur as an isolated phenomenon. In over half the cases of basal ganglia calcification no cause for the calcification is discovered. Where a cause is discovered *hypoparathyroidism* of spontaneous origin is the most frequent factor. Hypoparathyroidism may also occur following thyroidectomy and similar intracranial calcification may ensue.

Pseudo-hypoparathyroidism (Albright's syndrome) has also been cited as a cause of basal ganglia

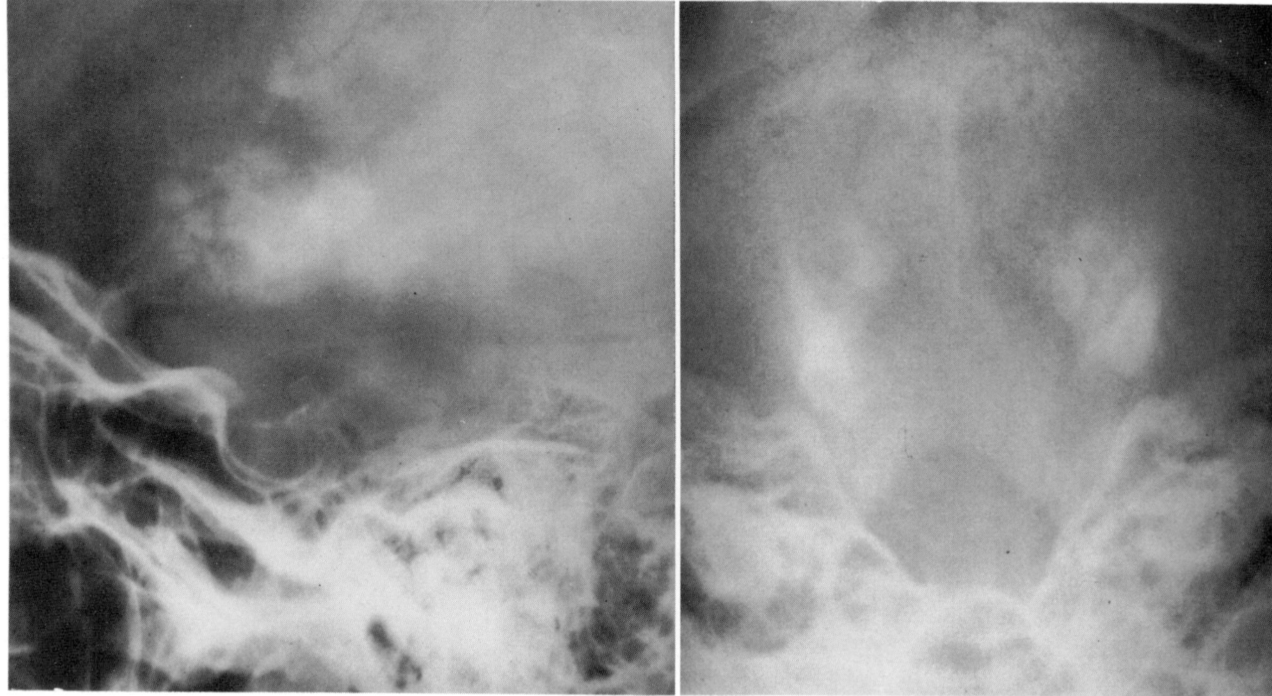

A B

Fig. 58.32 Calcified basal ganglia. (A) Lateral view. (B) Towne's view.

calcification. The other features of this syndrome are described on page 177.

Familial calcification of the basal ganglia is a very rare condition in which calcification has been demonstrated in several members of the same family. In none of these cases was an aetiology such as hypoparathyroidism demonstrated.

In *Fahr's syndrome* there is deposition of iron and calcium in the basal ganglia and dentate nuclei, and to a lesser extent in the cerebellum and cortical areas. The disease starts in childhood and presents with spasticity and choreo-athetoid movement proceeding to progressive mental deterioration.

In *Cockayne's syndrome* progeria is the most conspicuous clinical feature. There is also microcephaly and thickening of the skull vault. Calcification occurs in the basal ganglia and dentate nuclei, and also in the cortex.

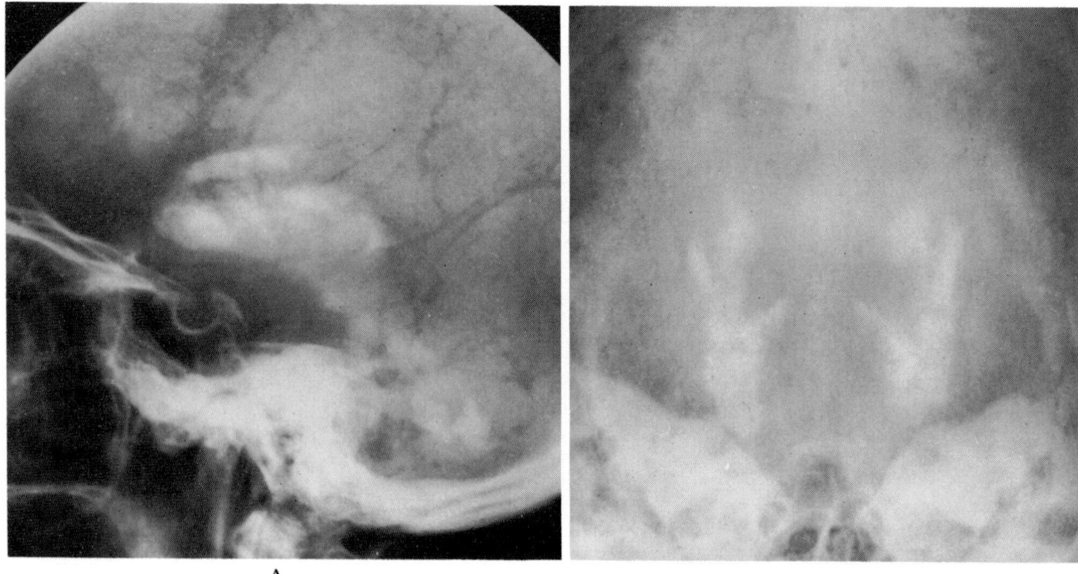

A B

Fig. 58.33 Heavy calcification in the basal ganglia and dentate nuclei. (A) Lateral view. (B) Towne's view.

Hyperparathyroidism with metastatic calcification in the brain has been described but it excessively rare.

Tuberous sclerosis (syn. Epiloia). Typical cases are characterized by such cutaneous lesions as adenoma sebaceum, subungual fibromata and the Shagreen patch in the loin. There are multiple areas of dysplasia in the brain containing abnormal and giant glial cells. These cerebral lesions often contain calcification (Fig. 58.34). Radiologically the calcification may appear as rounded or irregular shadows which are discrete and multiple. Calcification may also take less typical forms and appear as sinuous lines or dense nodules.

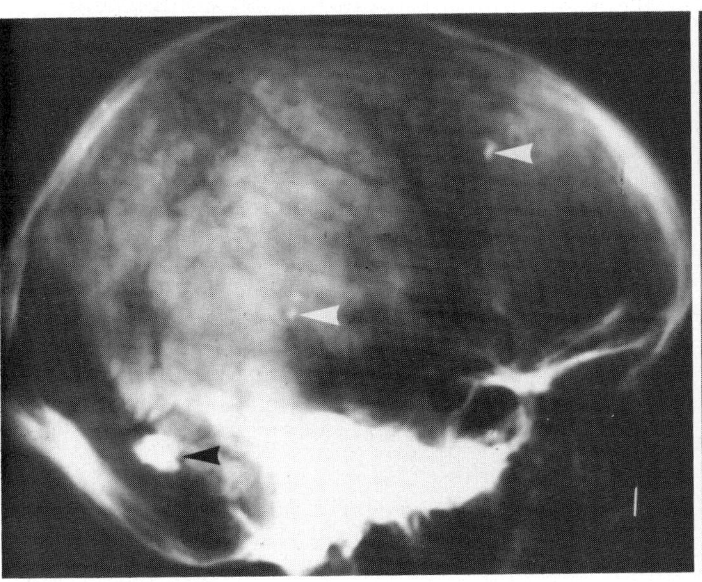

Fig. 58.34

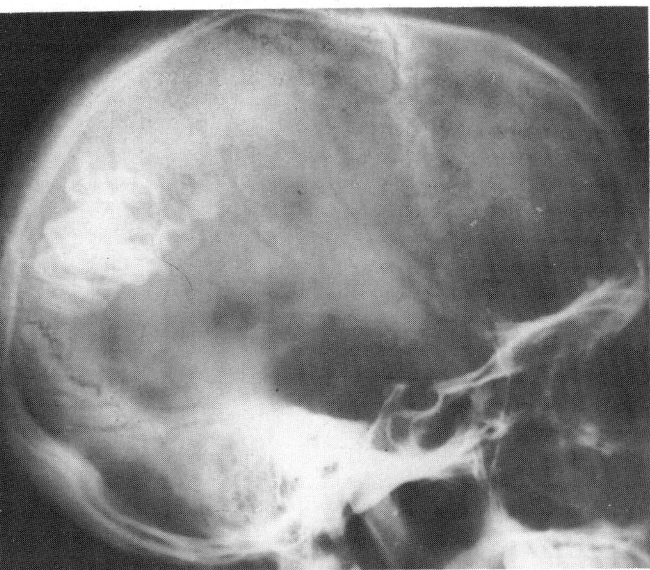

Fig. 58.35

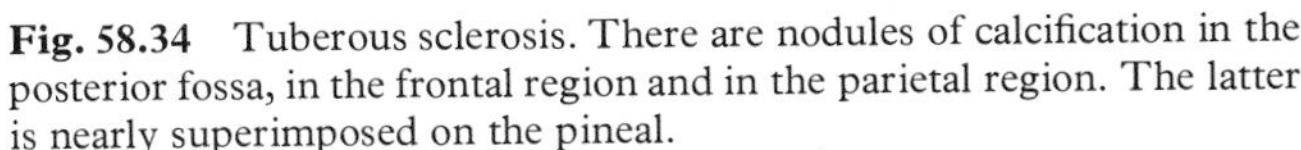

Fig. 58.34 Tuberous sclerosis. There are nodules of calcification in the posterior fossa, in the frontal region and in the parietal region. The latter is nearly superimposed on the pineal.

Fig. 58.35 Calcified cortex in Sturge-Weber syndrome.

In most cases the diagnosis is clinically obvious but there are 'formes frustes' where the cutaneous manifestations are minimal and the patient is not mentally defective or epileptic. In these cases radiology of the skull can be helpful in suggesting the true diagnosis. Other radiological manifestations of tuberous sclerosis are discussed under Pneumography, and in the sections on bones, lung and kidney.

Sturge-Weber syndrome (Syn. Trigeminal Angiomatosis). Clinically these patients are characterized by the 'port wine' naevus on the face or scalp. This represents a capillary haemangioma in the sensory distribution of one or more branches of the fifth nerve. Intracranial calcification in this condition normally lies in the occipital lobe and is unilateral (Fig. 58.35). It takes the form of parallel sinuous lines. These have been erroneously described in the past as calcification in an angioma; the calcification in fact lies in the surface of atrophic brain tissue, the parallel lines representing sulci of the brain seen end on. The atrophic brain is usually overlain by thickened meninges. Angiography in these cases may or may not show evidence of excessive vascularity or of macroscopic angiomatosis of the meninges.

Cases in which the calcification is more extensive and extends to the parieteal and frontal lobes are rare and bilateral calcification is even more uncommon.

Neurofibromatosis. Extensive calcification in the choroid plexus of the third and lateral ventricles has been described as a rare accompaniment of neurofibromatosis.

Lissencephaly is a rare condition in which there is congenital absence of gyri and sulci. This is normal before the 4th intrauterine month, but its persistence is associated with severe mental retardation, fits and decerebrate rigidity in the neonate. In these infants a characteristic 3 mm calcified nodule has been described in the septum pellucidum just behind the foramen of Monro.

ABNORMAL VASCULAR MARKINGS

Meningioma is the commonest cause of pathological vascular markings in the skull vault (Fig. 58.36). These tumours derive part of their blood supply from the middle meningeal artery. In addition they are, when large, supplied by the internal carotid artery and also when they invade the skull vault, by branches of the external carotid artery. The middle meningeal vascular markings leading up to the site of the tumour may be obviously enlarged

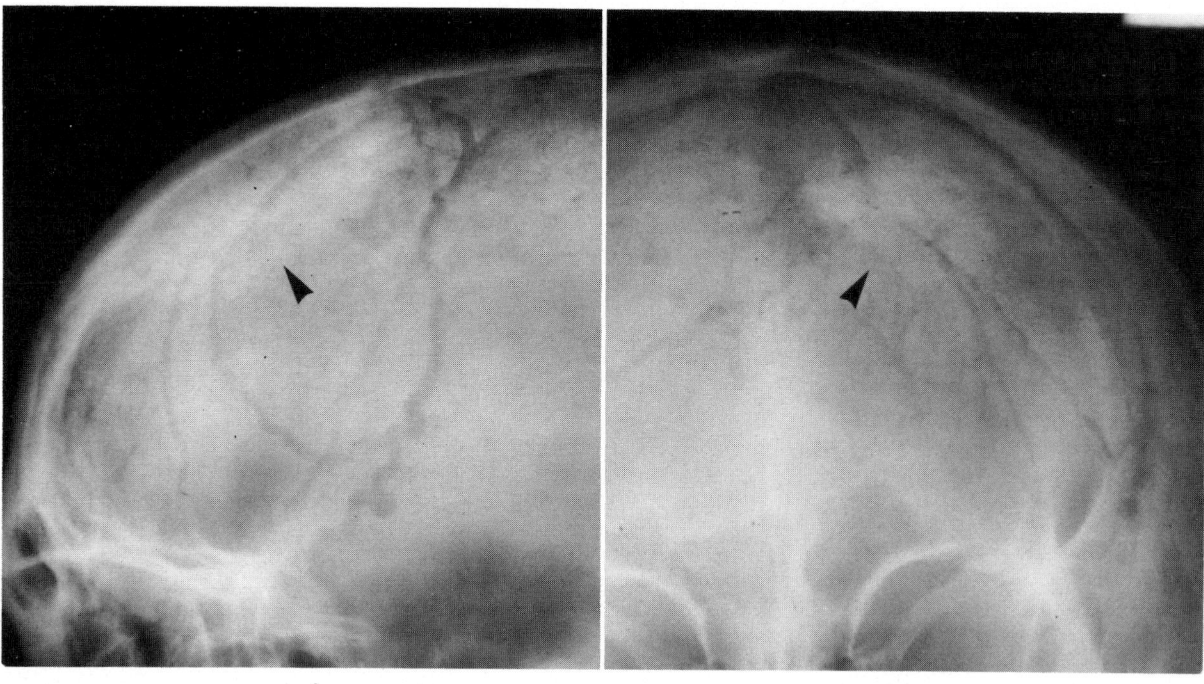

Fig. 58.36 Enlarged meningeal and diploic vascular markings associated with a parasagittal meningioma. There is also a localized hyperostosis (↑). (A) Lateral view. (B) P.A. view.

as compared with the normal side. In addition, they may be more tortuous than normal, particularly in their proximal segment just above the pterion.

The basal view of the skull will also show the appropriate *foramen spinosum* to be enlarged as a result of hypertrophy of the affected middle meningeal artery. It should be remembered, however, that the foramen spinosum can be larger on one side in the normal skull, and this sign has little significance except as a confirmatory sign.

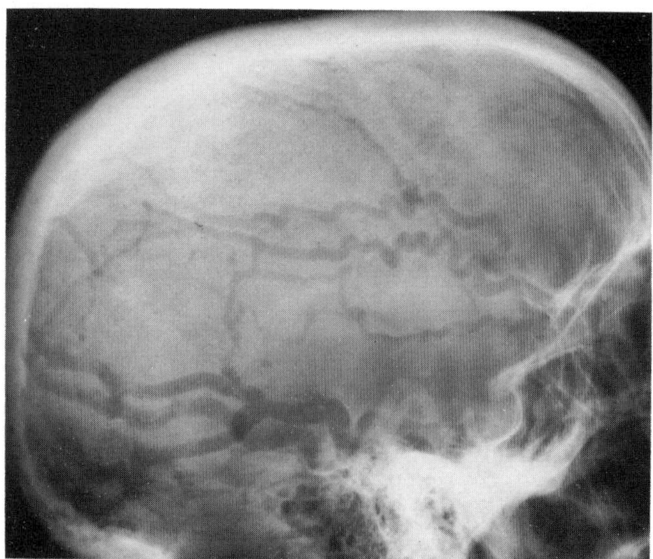

Fig. 58.37 Bilateral hypertrophy of the middle meningeal vascular markings in a patient with a large angiomatous malformation.

In addition to hypertrophied meningeal vascular markings there may also be locally increased diploic vascular markings and emissary venous markings in the region of the lesion. There may be further radiological evidence of the presence of a meningioma such as a local bony hyperostosis or erosion or intracranial calcification. Finally radiological evidence of generally raised intracranial pressure may also be present.

Angiomatous malformations are sometimes supplied by the meningeal arteries as well as by intracranial vessels. In these cases the hypertrophied middle meningeal vessels are also evidenced by increased meningeal vascular markings in the skull vault. These tend to be more generalized than those seen with meningioma and are often bilateral (Fig. 58.37). Prominent emissary vascular markings may also be seen with angiomatous malformations.

EROSIONS OF THE SKULL AND OSTEOPOROSIS

SKULL EROSIONS DUE TO TUMOURS

Skull erosions due to tumours may arise from:

1. Extracranial tumours.
2. Tumours of bone.
3. Intracranial tumours.

EXTRACRANIAL TUMOURS

Erosion of the skull vault or base from extracranial tumours is relatively rare but does occasionally occur.

Extracranial **dermoid cysts** can produce pressure erosion of the underlying bone. **Rodent ulcers** and **epitheliomas** can also invade and erode the bone of the vault. The rare **carcinoma of the sphenoid** may invade and erode the base of the skull in the region of the pituitary fossa.

Naso-pharyngeal carcinoma can also affect the base of the skull and produce bony erosion usually in the middle fossa (Fig. 58.38). However, frank bony erosion is relatively uncommon with these tumours as they tend to infiltrate through the bony foramina rather than produce bone destruction.

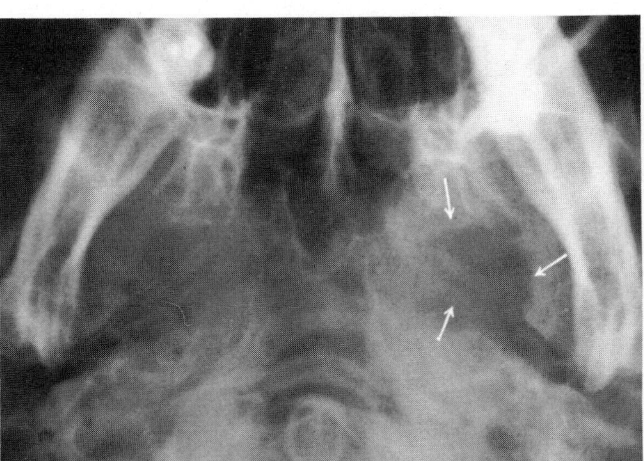

Fig. 58.38

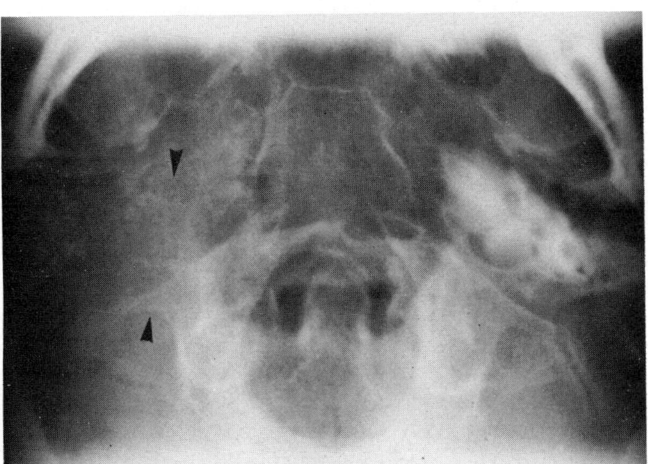

Fig. 58.39

Fig. 58.38 Nasopharyngeal carcinoma producing erosion of the floor of the middle fossa on the left (arrowed).

Fig. 58.39 Glomus jugulare tumour. This has completely destroyed most of the right petrous bone (arrowed).

Glomus jugulare tumours. These tumours may invade the base of the skull in the region of the jugular foramen and undersurface of the petrous bone (Fig. 58.39). They can also grow through into the posterior fossa. In its early stages the erosion around the jugular foramen and on the under surface of the petrous bone is best seen with a half-axial view of the base of the skull.

TUMOURS OF BONE

These may be primary or secondary. *Primary tumours* with skull erosion are relatively uncommon.

Dermoid tumours occur most commonly just above the outer angle of the orbit. They are associated with soft-tissue swelling and a bony defect may be apparent on X-ray which has a slightly sclerotic margin (Fig. 52.23, p. 1003).

Epidermoid tumours or cholesteatomas can also occur in the skull vault. They may expand the bone slightly and in classical cases have a scalloped corticated margin.

Haemangioma of the skull vault is rare but shows a fairly characteristic appearance of radiating spicules within a circular translucency which slightly expands the bone (Fig. 6.13, p. 118).

Chordoma is thought to arise from remnants of the primitive notochord in the basi-sphenoid. It can produce erosion in the clivus or at the petrous apex. Sometimes erosion is seen more anteriorly in the floor of the sella and at its lateral wall. A point which is helpful in differential diagnosis is the presence of a soft-tissue mass protruding into the nasopharynx, and occasionally of calcification within the tumour or its intracerebral extension.

Secondary tumours of the skull vault producing bone erosion are very common.

Secondary carcinoma usually produces irregular and ill-defined erosions. These may have a characteristic 'moth-eaten' appearance (Fig. 58.40) or present as large clear-cut defects (Fig. 58.41).

Myelomatosis with widespread deposits usually in volves the skull vault. The deposits in myeloma are very characteristic, appearing as multiple small rounded clear-cut holes in the bone (Fig. 7.32). Very rarely myelomatosis may present at first as *solitary myeloma* or *plasmacytoma* in the skull vault. These originally solitary lesions may produce large defects with a characteristic appearance (p. 141). Eventually, however, generalized bone lesions will develop. Such large solitary plasmacytomas usually present with a palpable swelling. Radiology shows a large irregular bone defect usually in the occipital or occipito-parietal region. The lesion commences in the diploe and expands the bone. Tangential views may show apparent spiculation extending into the superficial soft tissues and this, together with intracranial bulging has led to erroneous diagnoses of sarcoma or meningioma.

Neuroblastoma in children frequently metastasizes

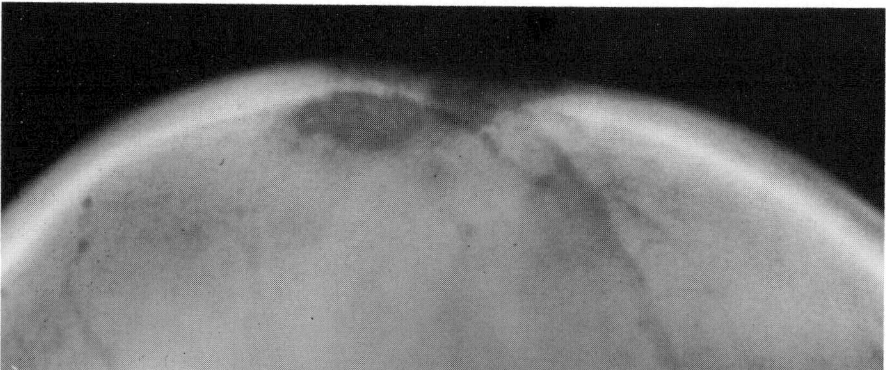

Fig. 58.40 Irregular erosion of the skull vault by secondary deposit.

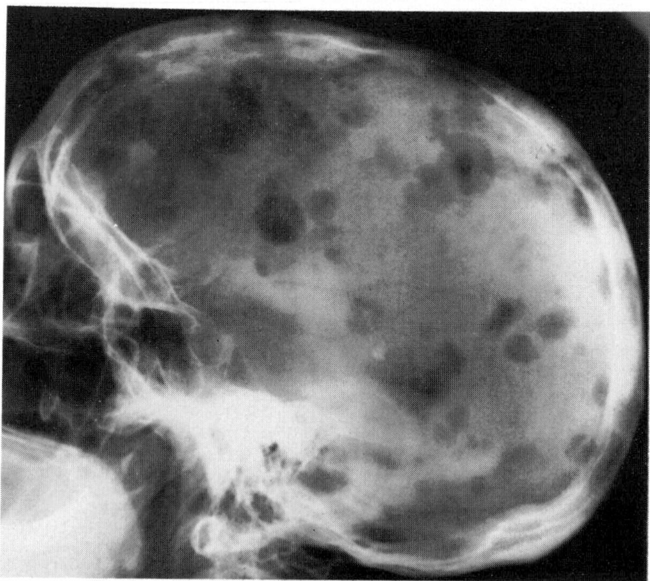

Fig. 58.41 Multiple lytic deposits in the skull vault in a patient with carcinoma of the breast.

to the skull. Metastases may involve the suture margins, particularly of the coronal suture, and produce a characteristic widening with irregular margins of the affected bone. The appearance may be accentuated by the presence of true suture diastasis from intracranial masses which are often extradural and continuous with the bony lesions. Orbital deposits with proptosis are also common in neuroblastoma.

Leukaemia of the meninges and central nervous system can also cause raised pressure and sutural widening in children.

Reticulosis and **lymphosarcoma** rarely affect the skull vault but can occasionally do so. The lesions are usually small multiple erosions which can become confluent and widespread.

Histiocytosis frequently involves the skull, particularly in **Letterer-Siwe** disease and in **Hand-Schüller Christian** disease (see Chapter 7). In these conditions the typical 'geographical' skull defects may be seen (Fig. 7.36).

Eosinophil granuloma may also affect the skull vault and produce similar lesions. It may also occur as an isolated lesion. This can expand the bone, and unlike the more malignant histiocytosis may have a sclerotic margin. An isolated eosinophil granuloma may be difficult to distinguish from similar lesions such as epidermoid or fibrous dysplasia.

PRIMARY INTRACRANIAL TUMOURS PRODUCING SKULL EROSIONS

Pituitary tumours as they increase in size erode and enlarge the pituitary fossa. In the classical case this gives rise to the so-called 'ballooned' sella with undercutting of the anterior clinoid processes, backward bowing of the dorsum and downward enlargement of the floor of the sella into the sphenoid bone or sphenoidal sinus (Fig. 58.42). In most cases the appearances are characteristic but occasionally if the dorsum sellae is completely eroded there may be a difficult radiological differential diagnosis from the effects of raised intracranial pressure. In most of these cases the clinical features will point to the correct diagnosis.

The *empty sella syndrome* is a condition in which a subarachnoid recess extends into the sella and compresses the pituitary. There is usually enlargement of the fossa, which can simulate expansion by a tumour. Diagnosis is by air encephalography or C.T. and is discussed further in Chapter 60.

Pituitary tumours have been classified into the following groups:

1. Chromophobe adenoma.
2. Eosinophil adenoma.
3. Basophil adenoma.
4. Prolactin secreting microadenoma.
5. Pituitary carcinoma.
6. Craniopharyngioma.

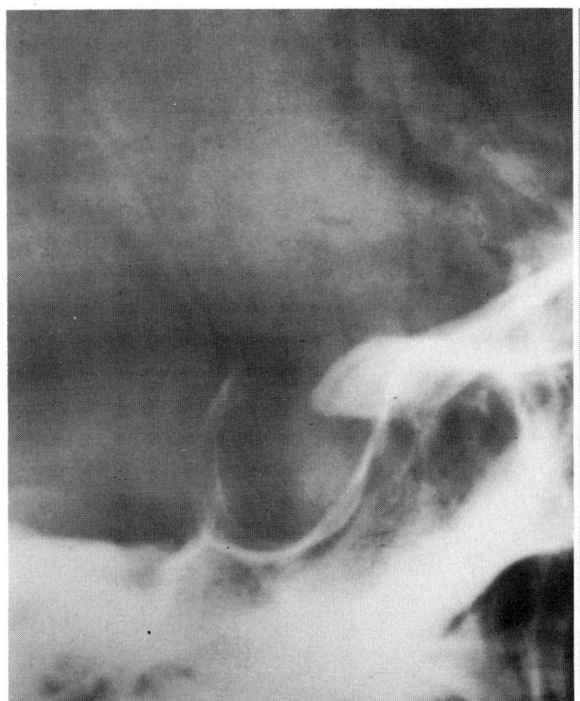

A

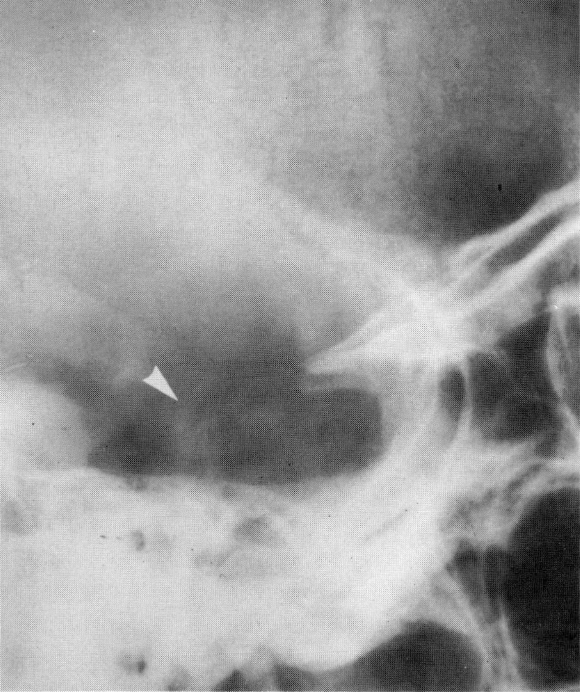

B

Fig. 58.42 (A) Chromophobe adenoma showing ballooning of the sella and backward bulging of the dorsum. (B) Chromophobe adenoma showing ballooning of the sella with undercutting of the anterior clinoids, backward bowing and thinning of the dorsum (arrowed).

Chromophobe adenomas nearly always produce enlargement of the pituitary fossa at the time of clinical presentation, since the majority of cases present with visual failure resulting from pressure of the enlarging tumour upon the optic chiasm. This results in the classical bitemporal hemianopia. On careful clinical examination some evidence of panhypopituitarism is usually found and a significant proportion are found to have hyperprolactinaemia.

Eosinophil adenomas are less common and give rise to acromegaly in the mature, and to gigantism in the adolescent. The pituitary fossa is usually, though not always, enlarged and shows the characteristic features already described. Even more characteristic however is the appearance of the skull vault which is thickened and enlarged. The thickening is mainly of the inner and outer tables with encroachment on the diploe, and the latter may be difficult to distinguish. At the same time the sinuses are unduly large; the frontal sinus is particularly involved giving rise to 'bossing'. The enlarged prognathous jaw is another classical feature of the acromegalic skull.

Basophil adenomas are said to give rise to Cushing's syndrome. In the majority of cases the tumours are microscopic and it is very unusual for the pituitary fossa to be enlarged. However, it has been shown that in cases of Cushing's disease treated by adrenalectomy enlargement of an adenoma may result with secondary enlargement of the sella (Nelson's syndrome).

As noted in Chapter 56 the long accepted classification of pituitary adenomas into basophil, acidophil and chromophobe according to function is no longer regarded as precise and it is now thought better to classify as 'functioning' and 'non-secretory'. Purely chromophobe adenomas have in fact been found in some patients with acromegaly and with Cushing's syndrome, and prolactin secreting adenoma is now well recognized.

Prolactin secreting microadenomas generally present with amenorrhoea and galactorrhoea. The tumours are small and in most cases the sella is not enlarged. Careful tomography may, however, demonstrate a unilateral depression or indent in the bony wall. In women with microadenomas the serum prolactin radioimmunoassay can be 10 to 1000 times the normal.

Craniopharyngioma is most commonly encountered in children and usually lies above the sella. In these cases there may be a typical deformity of the sella which is elongated and shows a short curved dorsum (Fig. 58.43). Very rarely a craniopharyngioma lies actually within the sella and produces rounded expansion of the pituitary fossa. Calcification is frequently present as described above.

Carcinoma of the pituitary is excessively rare. It appears to be only locally malignant and produces erosion of the bony walls of the sella.

Acoustic neuroma is a very common intracranial tumour. It is usually seen in middle-aged or elderly patients. The classical physical signs are of nerve deafness on the affected side, associated with 7th nerve weakness

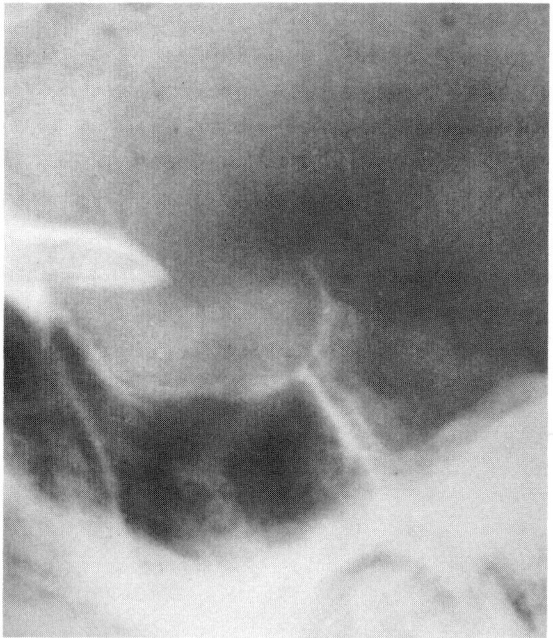

Fig. 58.43 Craniopharyngioma or suprasellar cyst without calcification. The shape of the sella which is elongated and the dorsum which is slightly bowed forwards is suggestive of the cause.

and evidence of involvement of the first division of the 5th nerve. The latter results in a depressed corneal reflex. Eventually the tumour may give rise to hydrocephalus and raised intracranial pressure. Radiological changes are present in a high proportion of cases at the time of clinical presentation. These consist of erosion and expansion of the internal auditory meatus. Where this is well marked it will be obvious on the routine Towne's view (Fig. 58.44). With minor degrees of bone involvement careful radiographic studies with special reference to the internal auditory meatus are necessary. The routine procedure with a Schonander skull table is to take stereo-slit views of the petrous bones in the Towne's and basal projections, and Stockholm C or Stenvers views of the petrous bone in addition.

With good-quality films of this type minor degrees of enlargement or asymmetry can readily be recognized. Another very useful projection is the transorbital view of the petrous bones and internal auditory meatus (Fig. 57.10). In doubtful cases tomography of the petrous bone may be helpful.

In addition to erosion and expansion of the internal auditory meatus there may be erosion of the petrous apex. If the lesion has produced hydrocephalus then the general radiological signs of raised intracranial pressure in an adult, as described above, may also be noted.

Glioma of the optic nerve is a rare tumour which usually occurs in children. It produces a pathognomonic radiological sign consisting of a localized expansion of the optic foramen on the affected side (Fig. 58.45). **Glioma of the optic chiasm** is one cause of so called 'J'-shaped sella, since it enlarges the sulcus chiasmaticus.

With an optic nerve glioma the enlargement of the optic canal is usually concentric and the cortical margin remains distinct. Chiasmatic glioma may extend into both orbits and enlarge both optic canals. Occasionally, but very rarely, such bilateral enlargement is seen with generally raised intracranial pressure since the subarachnoid space extends into the canal. Unilateral optic canal enlargement may also be seen with *meningioma* involving the optic nerve sheath. This also can rarely be bilateral. *Retinoblastoma* may also extend back into and enlarge an optic canal but this is relatively rare. *Neurofibromatosis* may be associated with optic nerve glioma and optic canal enlargement, and there may be other associated orbital

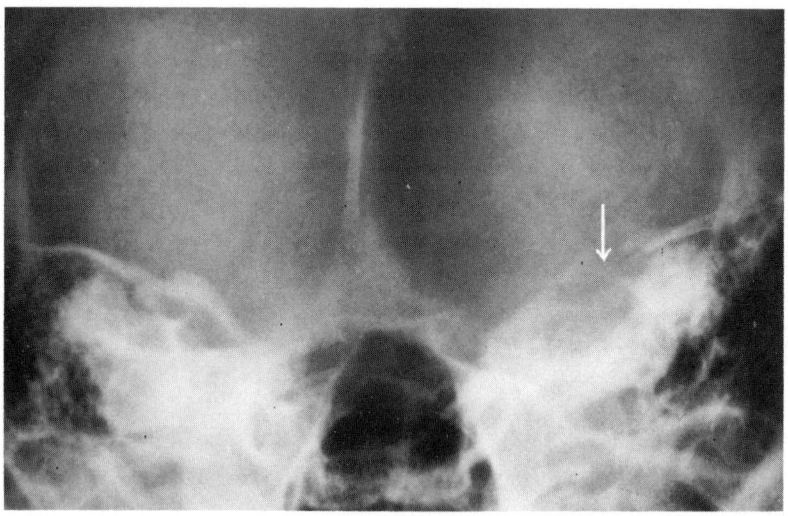

Fig. 58.44 Left acoustic neuroma producing erosion around the left internal auditory meatus (↓).

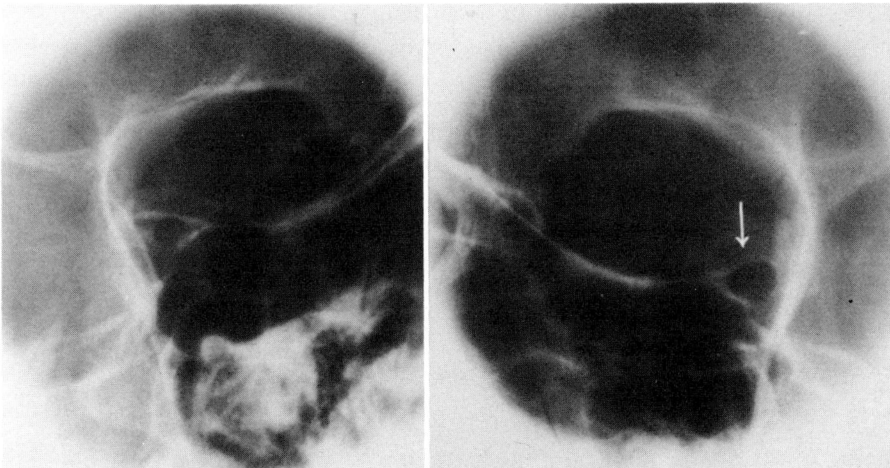

Fig. 58.45 Glioma of the left optic nerve. The left optic foramen (↓) is markedly expanded compared with the normal right.

anomalies such as generalized enlargement of the orbit. Defects in the sphenoid can also arise in neurofibromatosis.

Inflammatory lesions such as *sarcoid* have been cited as rare causes of optic canal enlargement both unilateral and bilateral, as has *chiasmatic arachnoiditis* with arachnoid cyst.

Meningiomas are intracranial tumours which can also grow outwards from the meninges and invade the skull vault. In most cases this results in a hyperostotic reaction of the bone to the tumour (see below). Sometimes there is a mixed osteoblastic and osteolytic response. In these cases the appearance may simulate such lesions as fibrous dysplasia or eosinophilic granuloma of the vault. Very occasionally meningioma produces a purely osteolytic reaction. In these cases evidence as to the true cause of the bone lesion may be provided by other features. Thus in the skull vault enlarged meningeal vascular channels may be seen extending to the lesion and the foramen spinosum may be enlarged on the affected side. Again, the characteristic meningioma site, i.e. parasagittal or along the sphenoidal ridge (Fig. 58.46) may suggest the true cause.

Gliomas have also been recorded as growing through the dura and producing bone erosion, but this sequence of events is excessively rare.

LOCAL BULGING OF THE SKULL

This is occasionally seen over superficial **gliomas**, particularly in children in the region where the expanding lesion impinges on the skull.

Chronic juvenile subdural haematomas may also expand the skull of children, particularly when they lie around the temporal lobe. There is a characteristic bulging of the temporal fossa and in the basal view the

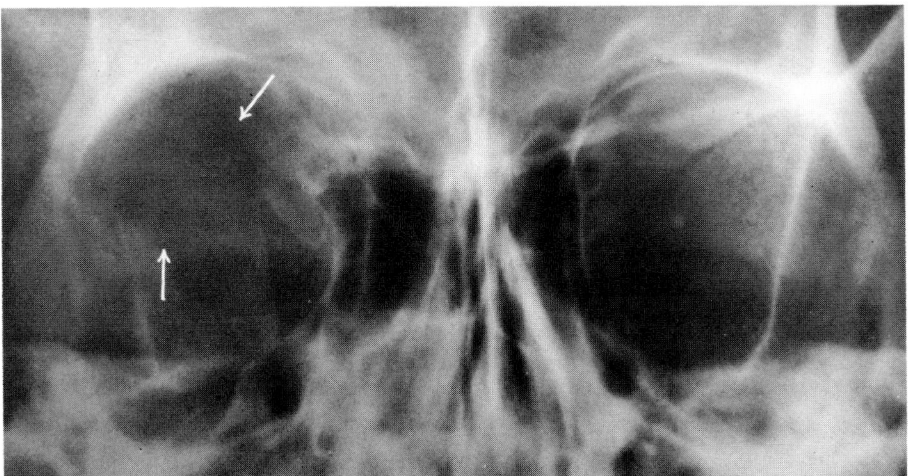

Fig. 58.46 Meningioma of the right sphenoidal ridge producing localized bone erosion (arrows). This is very unusual. Most meningiomas in this region produce hyperostosis.

middle fossa is seen to be expanded. The postero-anterior film also shows absence of the linear shadow representing the junction of anterior and lateral walls of the middle fossa which is normally superimposed on the lateral aspect of the orbit (the innominate line—see Fig. 57.3). The sphenoidal ridge may also be elevated.

Arachnoid cysts are extracerebral lesions of obscure and possibly developmental origin which can occur anywhere over the brain. When they lie over the vault they can produce local displacement and thinning of the bone which may be bulged outwards over the cyst. In the temporal region the bone changes just described for juvenile subdural haematoma are seen.

NON-TUMOUROUS SKULL EROSIONS

Erosion of the skull due to tumour has to be differentiated from defects and erosion due to other causes. The causes of normal or physiological defects have been discussed in Chapter 57. Erosion of the skull may also occur from other non-tumourous lesions. Thus it may be seen with inflammatory lesions, as a result of trauma, with fibrous dysplasia, and with congenital anomalies. The latter have been discussed above.

Acute and subacute osteomyelitis involving the skull vault is most commonly seen as a result of spread of infection from the frontal sinus or following compound fracture or other trauma. It results in patchy erosion of the affected bone.

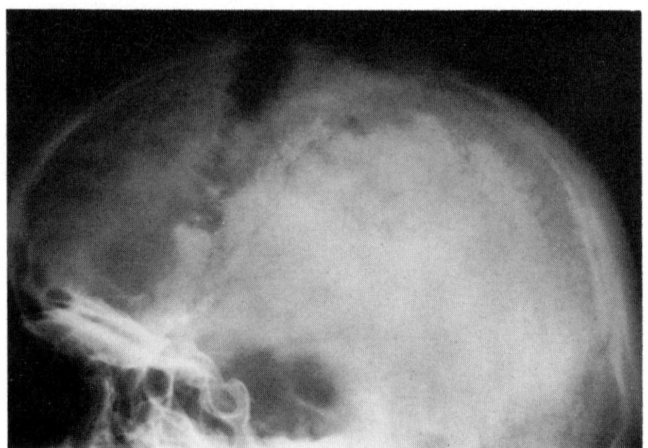

Fig. 58.47 Extensive erosion of the skull vault along the sagittal and coronal sutures. This was due to unrecognized chronic osteomyelitis following a minor scalp wound which was sutured.

With acute osteomyelitis the diagnosis is usually clinically obvious. Occasionally, however, skull infection may follow a relatively minor trauma which has been forgotten by the patient (Fig. 58.47). Infection may also occur in bone flaps after craniotomy. Radiologically this is manifest by erosions of the bone margin and the development of radiolucent areas in the bone flap.

Radiation necrosis may occur in bone flaps after radiotherapy and results in small marginal and central bony erosions. The appearances are similar to those of infection of a bone flap. Very rarely such radiation necrosis may be seen in the intact skull vault.

Chronic infections of the skull vault are now very rare. **Tuberculosis** was occasionally seen in the past and tended to produce a localized rounded and purely destructive lesion. A soft-tissue abscess was often associated. Bone tuberculosis has now virtually disappeared in this country; the occasional cases still seen are usually in Asian immigrants.

Syphilis of the skull vault has now become extremely rare. Involvement of the skull by tertiary syphilis gives rise to an extensive 'moth-eaten' appearance (Fig. 2.38). Clinical features usually enable a ready differentiation from acute osteomyelitis or extensive deposits.

Hydatid cysts may occasionally involve the skull vault when they give rise to a multilocular cystic mass expanding the bone and bulging in outwards. This is, however, very rare since less than 2 per cent of patients with hydatid disease have bone involvement and in only a small proportion of these has the skull been involved.

Neurofibromatosis can give rise to congenital bone defects, the commonest site being in the occipital bone adjacent to the lower part of the lambdoid suture. Defects have also been described adjacent to the squamous temporal suture and at the back of the orbit in the greater wing of sphenoid. In the latter case proptosis may result.

Trauma to the skull vault occasionally gives rise to **post-traumatic defects** which develop slowly after the initial injury. In these cases the story is usually of a skull fracture in childhood. Follow-up films sometime later show a bony defect to have developed at the old fracture site. It is thought that these are the result of a meningeal tear allowing c.s.f. to pulsate into the region of the fracture and form a leptomeningeal cyst.

Aneurysm. Large retro-orbital aneurysms in the cavernous sinus can erode the bony structures at the back of the orbit. Characteristically this type of aneurysm produces erosion of the inferolateral margin of the optic foramen and of the anterior clinoid process. There may also be slight expansion of the sphenoidal fissure at its upper end.

Erosion of the sphenoidal fissure may also occur with atypical meningiomas, and it can also be seen with secondary deposits in this region.

Large aneurysms in the region of the sella occasionally erode the lateral aspect of the sella or of the dorsum sellae. In rare instances uniform enlargement of the sella simulating a pituitary tumour has been produced by an intrasellar aneurysm.

OSTEOPOROSIS

Osteoporosis of the skull vault may occur in several different conditions. It may be seen as a normal physiological change in the elderly in parallel with the general osteoporosis of the skeleton. It may also be seen with the various metabolic disroders giving rise to osteomalacia and osteoporosis (see Chapter 8).

Hyperparathyroidism (see Chapter 8) will give rise to osteoporosis of the skull vault, usually with a characteristic pattern. This has been described as 'miliary osteoporosis' or 'pepper-pot' porosis (Fig. 8.22). Another typical appearance in the skull in hyperparathyroidism is loss of definition of the lamina dura around the teeth. In primary hyperparathyroidism large bone cysts may occur which can give rise to diagnostic difficulty and are often mistaken for areas of simple fibrous dysplasia.

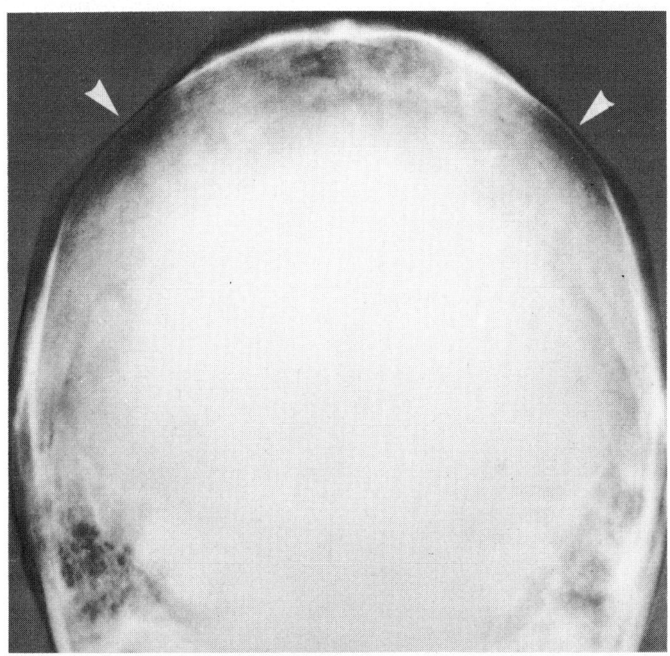

Fig. 58.48 Parietal thinning. The Towne's or P.A. projections show clearly that the external table and diploe are affected whilst the internal table remains (arrows).

Localized porosis or thinning of the skull vault is seen in **parietal thinning**. This unusual condition occurs mainly in elderly males and is characterized by symmetrical thinning of the parietal bone involving the outer table of the skull. In the affected area this may almost disappear as may the diploe giving rise to a peculiar 'scalloped' appearance of the bone. The appearance in both lateral and postero-anterior projections are characteristic (Fig. 58.48). In the Towne's view there is absence of the outer table and diploe over the affected parietal area. In the lateral view there is an apparent band of porosis over the same area. The aetiology remains obscure.

Osteoporosis circumscripta is the name given to a type of Paget's disease involving the skull vault. This is characterized by large areas of osteoporosis with clear-cut, well-defined margins between normal and affected bone (Fig. 3.31). The changes are often bilateral and symmetrical and there may be evidence of Paget's disease in other bones, a feature which helps in differential diagnosis. The osteoporosis spreads upwards from the base of the skull and characteristically spreads over a wide area without being limited by sutures.

HYPEROSTOSIS

Hyperostosis or thickening of the skull vault may occur as a generalized or local phenomenon.

Generalized hyperostosis is seen with **acromegaly** and has been described above. It is also seen with such bone dystrophies as **marble bones** and **Engelmann's disease** (Chapter 1). Increase in thickness of the skull vault may also occur in epileptic patients treated for prolonged periods with the drug **phenytoin**. The increase consists mainly of widening of the diploic space.

Dystrophia myotonica is usually accompanied by a rather thick skull. The small pituitary fossa in this condition has already been noted.

Gross increase in the thickness of the skull vault may also be seen in one form of **Paget's disease**. However, at the same time as the bone becomes widened and thickened there are also osteomalacic changes and the bone becomes softer and more pliable frequently giving rise to platybasia with basilar invagination. The radiological appearances are characteristic (Fig. 3.30). In addition to the softening of the bone the texture of the thickened bone in Paget's disease is quite abnormal. Usually it shows an irregular mottled appearance sometimes described as the 'woolly' form of Paget's disease.

Another condition in which there may be gross generalized thickening of the skull vault is **Cooley's anemia**. This is described in detail in Chapter 7. The skull appearances in this condition can be quite characteristic. The main abnormality is a widening of the diploe. Its texture is also abnormal showing radiating linear spicules of the sun-ray or hairbrush type (Fig. 7.2). Sometimes the bone changes in this form of anaemia may be more localized, particularly to the frontal region.

Localized hyperostosis of the skull is seen in a wide variety of conditions.

Fibrous dysplasia is a common cause of localized areas of bone thickening in the skull vault, facial bones and the skull base (Fig. 1.42). It may occur as an isolated phenomenon or, less commonly, in association with lesions in other bones (polyostotic fibrous dysplasia and Albright's syndrome—see Chapter 1).

Leontiasis ossia is the term used for a form of hyperostosis seen in the facial bone and frontal region. The term is a descriptive one relating to the peculiar facies. The condition is now rare and the aetiology is thought

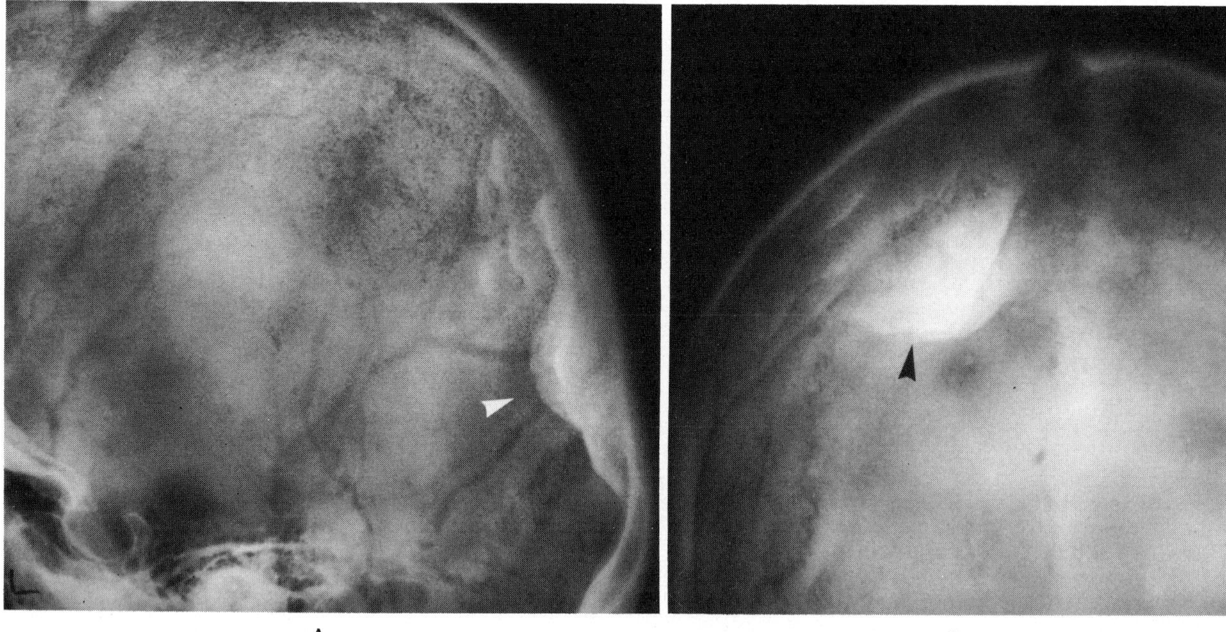

Fig. 58.49 Large internal hyperostosis associated with an occipital meningioma. Note also the increased vascular markings extending to the lesion. (A) Lateral view. (B) Towne's view.

to be either a creeping chronic periostitis or a widespread involvement by fibrous dysplasia.

Localized hyperostosis is quite common with **meningiomas** that invade the skull vault. Typically this occurs in the classical meningioma sites of the parasagittal region (Fig. 58.49) or the sphenoidal ridge. It may however occur elsewhere over the vault and present clinically with a palpable bony lump or with proptosis. Eventually the hyperostosis involves the whole thickness of the bone though in the early stages it may be confined to the inner table (Fig. 58.50). When protruding externally on the skull vault sun-ray spicules are sometimes shown on the radiograph (Fig. 58.51). In addition there may be other evidence of meningioma such as increased vascular markings, an enlarged foramen spinosum, and general radiological evidence of the presence of an intracranial tumour.

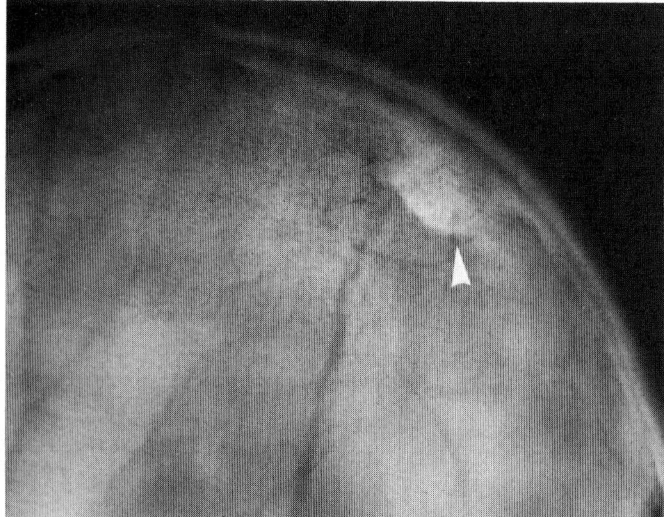

Fig. 58.50 Small parasagittal hyperostosis in the parietal region associated with a meningioma (↑). Note the prominent vascular channels leading to the lesion.

Primary osteogenic sarcoma is very rare in the skull vault but has been described as giving rise to localized hyperostosis. Sun-ray spicules may also be seen in this rare type of tumour. Osteogenic sarcoma of the vault is most commonly seen as a complication of Paget's disease.

Hyperostosis frontalis interna. This mysterious condition is frequently seen in middle-aged and elderly females. Its cause is quite unknown though there may be a hormonal element in its production, since the majority of the patients are post-menopausal. The lesions consist of irregular thickening of the inner tables of the skull vault mainly in the frontal regions. The lesions are characteristically bilateral and symmetrical and spare the midline.

Occasionally such hyperostotic lesions can be very extensive and involve the parietal region. It is very unusual, though not unknown, for such changes to be present in male patients.

Hemiatrophy. In infantile hemiplegia associated with porencephalic cysts or other conditions in which one half of the brain is maldeveloped or atrophied, the skull vault overlying the hemiatrophy is usually quite different from the vault on the normal side. As well as being smaller, the vault on the abnormal side is thicker, a feature which is obvious in the postero-anterior or Towne's view. There is no ready explanation for this curious phenomenon,

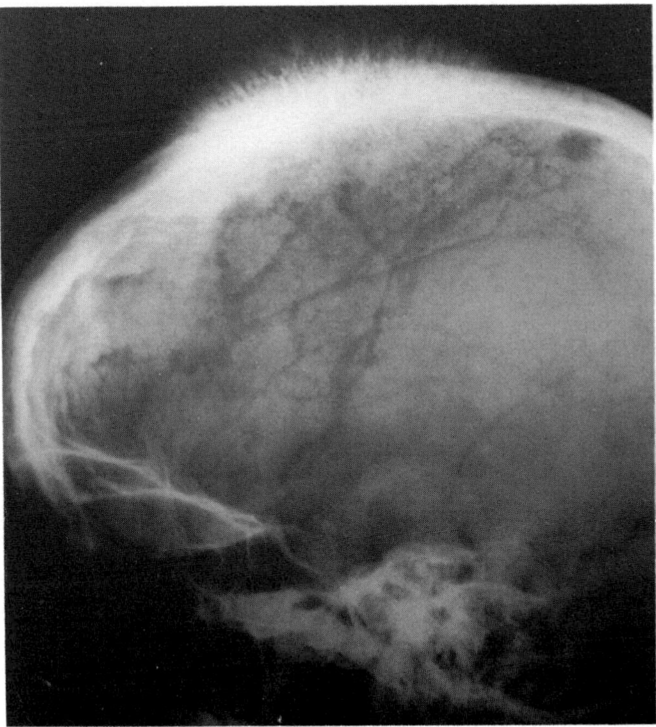

A

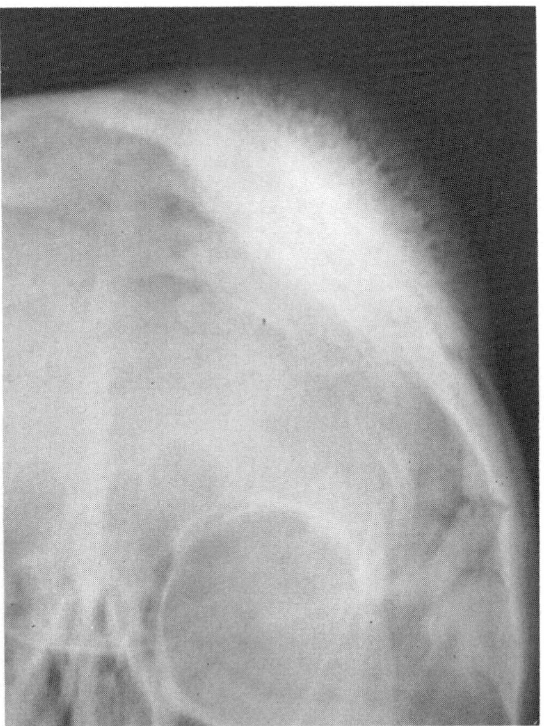

B

Fig. 58.51 Meningioma growing through the skull vault. Note the sunray spiculation and the enlarged vascular channels of the skull vault. (A) Lateral view. (B) P.A. view.

though it suggests that normal growth of the underlying brain is necessary for normal growth and moulding of the overlying skull vault.

Osteomas may occur in the skull vault. Small flat ivory osteomas are occasionally encountered as dense nodules on the surface of the vault. More commonly osteomas are encountered in a frontal sinus as a chance finding. Occasionally these lesions can be very large and perforate through the sinus into the skull. They have even been encountered as a cause of pneumocephalus.

Ossifying fibromas are rare cranial lesions which have been most commonly described as commencing in the paranasal sinuses, the antrum being the most frequently involved. These lesions which may be densely calcified are particularly common in East Africa. Occasionally they grow from other sinuses and in a case encountered by us a lesion in the sphenoid sinus grew through the base of the skull.

SKULL-TRAUMA

Cephalhaematoma is due to birth injury and the infant presents clinically with a swelling in the parietal region either on one or both sides. The haematoma which lies under the pericranium rapidly becomes hard and its margins become calcified. As growth proceeds the lesion becomes less prominent and finally merges with the underlying skull.

Fractures of the skull following head injury have been classified as *linear*, *stellate* and *depressed*.

There is a tendency in many casualty departments to X-ray head injuries immediately on admission of comatose or confused patients with temporary head-dressings. This usually results in poor-quality films and difficulty in confirming or excluding a fracture. Unless a depressed fracture is suspected, or it is desired to confirm suspicion of extradural haemorrhage by demonstrating a fracture involving the middle meningeal vascular markings, such emergency skull radiology is to be deprecated.

In most cases the demonstration or exclusion of a fracture is largely of medicolegal or academic importance. Severe brain injury may occur in the absence of any visible fracture and severe fractures may occur with relatively little brain damage. The treatment of the patient will depend entirely on the clinical features and not on the radiological demonstration of a fracture, except in the circumstances mentioned above.

In most cases, therefore, radiology of the skull should be deferred until it is possible to obtain first-class radiographs in non-emergency circumstances. After a severe head injury, particularly one associated with fractures of the frontal or ethmoid sinuses, the possibility of a complicating **aerocele** should always be borne in mind. In these cases it is particularly important that follow-up films should be obtained within a few days. These should be taken in the lateral brow-up position with a horizontal

X-ray beam so that small air collections can be identified by their air fluid level (Fig. 58.52).

Linear fractures of the skull are in most cases easy to identify particularly when the X-ray beam passes vertically through the fracture. Difficulty, however, may be experienced where the margins overlap in relation to the X-ray beam. In these cases the fracture may be seen not as a translucent shadow but as an apparent dense line (Fig. 58.53). Fractures may also be confused with normal vascular markings and occasionally with the internal suture line. The latter is linear and not serrated like the external suture line. It can usually be differentiated by its characteristic position being superimposed on a normal suture line. If a fracture is superimposed on a suture line it will usually deviate from it at some point. Linear fractures of the skull vault are slow in healing and may be visible for periods up to four years or longer.

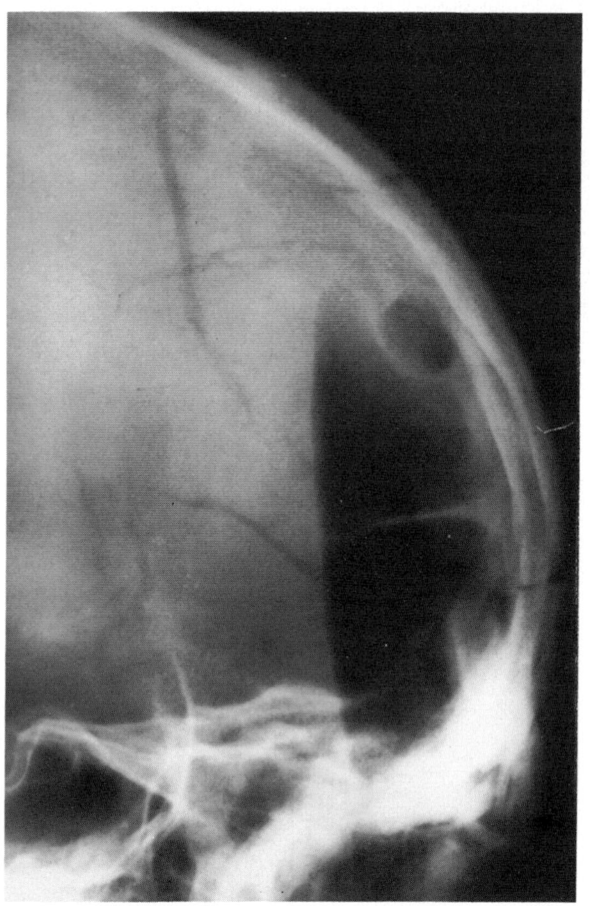

Fig. 58.52 Brow-up film showing pneumocephalus following frontal fractures. Note the air-fluid level best seen in brow-up lateral films.

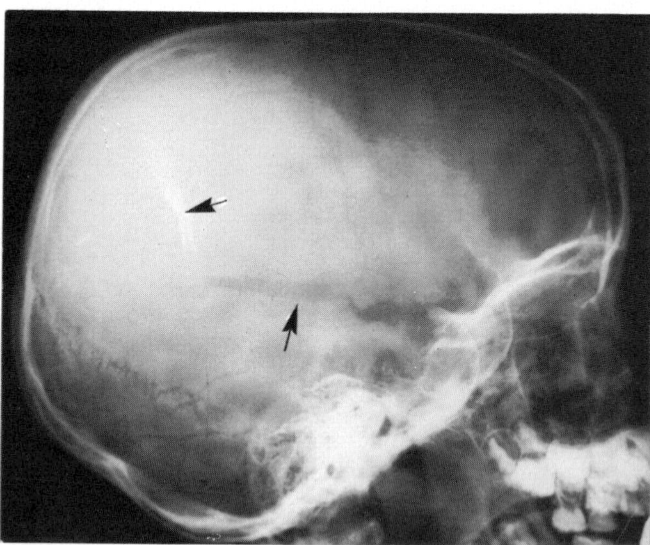

Fig. 58.53 Transverse linear fracture of the skull vault showing as a translucency (↑). There is also a vertical fracture showing as an increased density (↙).

Depressed fractures will usually require tangential views to show their exact relationship to the skull margins. They are also well shown by C.T.

Post-traumatic cysts (Leptomeningeal cyst). Where a fracture involves the meninges there may be an escape of cerebrospinal fluid from the subarachnoid space. This will give rise to local cyst formation under the fracture. As a result atrophy of the overlying bone may occur and quite large skull defects may result. In some of these cases the original fracture may be difficult to identify. Thus a difficult diagnostic problem may arise where the original trauma was minor or has been forgotten.

Juvenile subdural haematoma. In subdural haematoma resulting from trauma in childhood local expansion of the skull can occur from the pressure of the haematoma. The lesions are usually localized around the temporal lobe and the middle fossa is therefore expanded in a characteristic manner as described above.

Juvenile subdural haematomas may also occur near the skull vault and result in local bulging of the skull. In old cases the diagnosis may become obvious from linear calcification at the internal margin of the haematoma.

Pneumocephalus. Demonstration of air within the cranial cavity following head injury was first described as long ago as 1913. Pneumocephalus most commonly results from a fracture involving the frontal or ethmoid sinuses. There is usually a dural tear and c.s.f. rhinorrhoea may be present. The importance of follow-up films (including brow-up lateral films with a horizontal ray) in the case of patients with fractures of the frontal and ethmoid region has already been emphasized. Cerebrospinal fluid rhinorrhoea is always an indication for such follow-up. Gas may be demonstrated either in the subdural or the subarachnoid space in the early stages. In more severe cases gas will be shown in the brain itself (aerocele), or even in the ventricles. Surgery with closure of the dural tear is indicated in these cases.

REFERENCES AND SUGGESTIONS FOR FURTHER READING

General

Du Boulay, G. H. (1964) *The Skull*. London: Butterworth.

Newton, T. H. & Potts, D. G. (1971) *The Skull*. St Louis: Mosby.

Shapiro, R. & Janzen, A. M. (1960) *The Normal Skull—A Roentgen Study*. New York: Paul B. Moeber.

Taveras, J. M. & Wood, E. H. (1976) *Diagnostic Neuroradiology*, 2nd ed. Baltimore: Williams & Wilkins.

Specific

Alexander, G. L. & Norman, R. M. (1960) *The Sturge Weber Syndrome*. Bristol: John Wright & Sons Ltd.

Babbitt, D. P., Tang, T., Dobbs, J. & Berk, R. (1969) Idiopathic familial cerebrovascular ferrocalcinosis (Fahr's disease) and review of differential diagnosis of intracranial calcification in children. *American Journal of Roentgenology*, **105**, 352–358.

Banna, M. (1976) Craniopharyngioma—based on 160 cases. *British Journal of Radiology*, **49**, 206–223.

Bennett, J. C., Maffly, R. H. & Steinbach, H. L. (1959) The significance of bilateral basal ganglia calcification. *Radiology*, **72**, 368–378.

Bull, J. W. D. (1953) The radiological diagnosis of intracranial tumours in children. *Journal of the Faculty of Radiologists*, **4**, 149–170.

Burrows, E. H. (1963) Bone changes in orbital neurofibromatosis. *British Journal of Radiology*, **36**, 549–561.

Castro, M. & Lepe, A. (1963) Cerebral tuberculoma. *Acta radiologica (diagn.)*, **1**, 821–827.

Dixon, H. B. F. & Hargreaves, W. H. (1944) Cysticercosis (Taenia-solium) further ten years clinical study covering 284 cases. *Quarterly Journal of Medicine*, **13**, 107–121.

Dorfsman, J. (1963) The radiologic aspects of cerebral cysticerosis. *Acta radiologica (diagn.)*, **1**, 836–842.

Duggan, C. A., Keever, E. B. & Gay, B. B. (1970) Secondary craniosynostosis. *American Journal of Roentgenology*, **109**, 277–293.

Falconer, M. A., Pond, D. A., Meyer, A. & Woolf, A. L. (1953) Temporal lobe epilepsy with personality behaviour disorders caused by an unusual calcifying lesion; report of two cases in children relieved by temporal lobectomy. *Journal of Neurology, Neurosurgery and Psychiatry*, **16**, 234–244.

Falk, B. (1951) Calcifications in the track of the needle following ventricular puncture. *Acta radiologica*, **35**, 304–308.

Fieldman, H. A. (1968) Toxoplasmosis. *New England Journal of Medicine*, **279**, 1370–1375, 1431–1437.

Galatius-Jensen, F. & Uhm, I. K. (1965) Radiological aspects of cerebral paragonimiasis. *British Journal of Radiology*, **38**, 494–502.

Gautier-Smith, P. C. (1970) *Parasagittal and Falx Meningiomas*. London: Butterworth.

Gold, L. H. A., Kieffer, S. A. & Peterson, H. O. (1969) Intracranial meningiomas; a retrospective analysis of the diagnostic value of plain skull films. *Neurology*, **19**, 873–878.

Hastrup, J. & Reske-Nielsen, E. (1965) Symmetrical brain calcification in infants. *Acta neurologica, Scandinavica*, supp. **13**, 637.

Kalan, C., Burrows, E. H. (1962) Calcification in intracranial gliomata. *British Journal of Radiology*, **35**, 589–602.

Lagos, J. C., Holman, C. B. & Gomez, M. R. (1968) Tuberous sclerosis neuroroentgenologic observations. *American Journal of Roentgenology*, **104**, 171–176.

Lorber, J. (1958) Intracranial calcifications following tuberculous meningitis in children. *Acta radiologica*, **50**, 204–210.

McRae, D. L. (1965) Habenular calcification as an aid in the diagnosis of intracranial lesions, *American Journal of Roentgenology*, **94**, 541–546.

Mascherpa, F. & Valentino, V. (1959) *Intracranial Calcification*, Springfield Ill.: Charles C. Thomas. Publisher.

Mussbichler, H. (1968) Radiologic study of intracranial calcifications in congenital toxoplasmosis. *Acta radiologica (diagn.)*, **7**, 369–379.

Oh, S. J. (1968) Roentgen findings in cerebral paragonimiasis. *Radiology*, **90**, 292–299.

Palacios, E. & Schimke, N. (1969) Craniosynostosis—syndactilism. *American Journal of Roentgenology*, **106**, 144–155.

Potts, G. & Svare, G. T. (1964) Calcification in intracranial metastases. *American Journal of Roentgenology*, **92**, 1249–1251.

Ross, R. J. & Greitz, T. V. B. (1966) Changes in the sella turcica in chromophobe adenomas and eosinophilic adenomas. *Radiology*, **86**, 892–899.

Rumbaugh, C. L. & Potts, D. G. (1966) Skull changes associated with intracranial arteriovenous malformations. *American Journal of Roentgenology*, **98**, 525–534.

Samiy, E. & Zadeh, F. A. (1965) Cranial and intracranial hydatidosis with special reference to roentgen-ray diagnosis. *Journal of Neurosurgery*, **22**, 425–433.

Santin, G. & Vargas, J. (1966) Roentgen study of cysticerosis of central nervous system. *Radiology*, **86**, 520–528.

Stauffer, H. M., Snow, L. B. & Adams, A. B. (1953) Roentgenologic recognition of habenular calcification as distinct from calcification in pineal body, its application in cerebral localisation. *American Journal of Roentgenology*, **70**, 83–89.

Sutton, D. (1951) The radiological diagnosis of lipoma of the corpus collosum. *British Journal of Radiology*, **22**, 534.

Sutton, D. (1951) Intracranial calcification in toxoplasmosis. *British Journal of Radiology*, **24**, 31–37.

Sutton, D. (1958) Radiology of cerebral angiomas with special reference to neuro-ophthalmology. *Journal of the Faculty of Radiologists*, **9**, 90–96.

Tod, P. A. & Yelland, J. D. N. (1971) Craniostenosis. *Clinical Radiology*, **22**, 472–486.

Tytus, J. S. & Pennybacker, J. (1956) Pearly tumours in relation to the central nervous system. *Journal of Neurology, Neurosurgery and Psychiatry*, **19**, 241–259.

Vezina, J. L. & Sutton, T. J. (1974) Prolactin-secreting pituitary micro-adenomas. *American Journal of Roentgenology*, **120**, 46–54.

Wesenberg, R. L., Juhl, J. H. & Daube, J. R. (1966) Radiological findings in lissencephaly (congenital agyria). *Radiology*, **87**, 436–444.

Wilson, C. B. & Roy, M. (1964) Calcification within congenital aneurysm of the vein of Galen. *American Journal of Roentgenology*, **91**, 1319–1326.

Zatz, L. M. (1968) Atypical choroid plexus calcification associated with neurofibromatosis. *Radiology*, **91**, 1135–1139.

CHAPTER 59

THE SPINE AND MYELOGRAPHY

In addition to lesions of the spinal cord itself, this chapter is concerned with bony abnormalities of the spinal canal which produce neurological disorders. The site of lesions of the spinal cord and nerve roots may usually be defined with a fair degree of accuracy by clinical examination, although their nature frequently remains obscure. By showing associated bone and soft-tissue changes, plain radiography can confirm the anatomical level and help to establish the true cause of the symptoms.

Well-penetrated films are essential to show as much bone detail as possible, particularly of the pedicles and laminae which form most of the boundary of the spinal canal. Localized coned views, sometimes supplemented by appropriate tomographic cuts, may be required. Oblique projections are essential to show the intervertebral foramina in the cervical region although in the lower thoracic and lumbar areas these foramina are readily seen in lateral films. It is extremely difficult to obtain lateral views of the upper thoracic vertebrae owing to the overlying shoulders and a high-voltage technique, tomographic cuts, or carefully positioned oblique views are necessary.

ANATOMY

Several bony prominences serve as useful landmarks for localization. The first large vertebral spine at the base of the neck is that of C.7. The angle of the scapula is usually at the level of T.7. The last rib defines T.12. The iliac crest is at the level of the L.4–5 interspace.

In assessing films of the spine, the vertebrae and all their appendages should be examined systematically. This should include general alignment, the intervertebral bodies and disc spaces, the pedicles, laminae and spinous processes, the posterior intervertebral joints, the intervertebral foramina, and the transverse processes. Finally, the adjoining ribs and paravertebral soft-tissue shadows should also be carefully noted.

The vertebral canal is bounded anteriorly by the vertebral bodies, intervertebral discs and posterior longitudinal ligament. Posterolaterally, it is enclosed by the pedicles and laminae, forming the neural arches, which are roofed in by the tough ligamentum flavum.

Spinal cord. The vertebral column, particularly *in utero*, grows more rapidly in length than the spinal cord. Because of this, the adult spinal cord terminates at its lower end at the level of the upper border of L.2. From the conus medullaris, the thin threadlike filum terminale formed of glial tissue covered by meninges runs caudally to be attached to the coccyx.

Because the spinal cord is shorter than the bony spine, the spinal nerve roots gradually take an increasingly vertical course within the vertebral canal from the cervical to the sacral areas, as they pass to their exit foramina. Thus, the upper cervical nerve roots pass horizontally to the intervertebral foramina. In the lower cervical spine, the segmental cord level is approximately one segment above the corresponding exit foramen, in the dorsal spine two segments, and in the upper lumbar area three segments, above the exit foramina. Finally the cauda equina is formed of bundles of nerve roots surrounding the filum terminale and passing almost vertically downwards in the lumbar canal.

Local expansions of the cord are found in the lower cervical and lower thoracic areas, where the limb plexuses originate. This is reflected in the increased width of the spinal canal as shown by the interpedicular distance in anteroposterior films. The cervical enlargement extends from C.3 to T.5 vertebrae, with the maximum interpedicular width at C.5 and 6. The smaller lumbar enlargement starts at T.10 vertebra, is maximal at T.12, and tapers into the conus medullaris. Comprehensive figures of the normal range of measurements of the interpedicular distance have been published by Elsberg and Dyke (1934).

Spinal arteries. The spinal cord carries a long indentation, the anterior spinal sulcus on its anterior aspect in the midline which contains the anterior spinal artery and vein. The anterior spinal artery is formed by anastomosing radicles from the subclavian, aorta and internal iliac arteries, of which the most important are the vertebral, intercostal and lumbar arteries. It supplies the anterior three-quarters of the spinal cord. The posterior columns are supplied separately by small posterior arterial branches. More detail is given in the section on spinal angiography in Chapter 61.

Meninges. The subarachnoid space, filled with cerebrospinal fluid, is divided incompletely into anterior and posterior compartments by the thin, serrated dentate ligaments. These extend from the pia mater on either side, laterally to the dura, and from the foramen magnum above to L.1 below. These help to suspend the cord centrally in the spinal canal.

The arachnoid usually extends as far down as the second segment of the sacrum, although its termination varies slightly. Small, sleeve-like projections of arachnoid usually accompany the spinal nerve roots towards their exit from the spinal canal through the intervertebral foramina.

The subdural space is potential rather than actual. Not infrequently after lumbar puncture, cerebrospinal fluid leaks through the puncture in the arachnoid, and accumulates in the subdural space, where it is sometimes described as a subdural hygroma. Such a collection of subdural fluid occasionally impairs the satisfactory injection of contrast medium for subsequent myelography.

The main contents of the extradural space are a large venous plexus and a variable amount of fat. The dura itself is attached by connective tissue strands to the bony walls and longitudinal ligaments of the spinal canal.

MYELOGRAPHY

History. Pasteur's observation that 'change favours the prepared mind' is well illustrated in the development of myelography. The use of *air* to outline the spinal cord within its bony canal was forecast by Dandy, who in 1919 exploited the chance finding of a traumatic aerocele to develop the technique of cerebral pneumography. Dandy forecast that air could also be used to outline the spinal cord, and the first air myelograms were reported by Jacobeaus in 1921. In France, the following year, Sicard and Forestier, in treating sciatica by extradural injections of *Lipiodol*, on one occasion accidentally injected some into the subarachnoid space. Observing its lack of toxic reaction, mobility and radiopacity, they at once realized its application in the demonstration of spinal tumours. Lipiodol, however, in addition to being viscous and forming large globules, causes some meningeal irritation with danger of subsequent adhesive arachnoiditis and its use has been discontinued.

In 1944, Ramsey, French and Strain introduced *Pantopaque* (*iodophenylundecylic acid*) an oily organic iodine compound, marketed in Britain as *Myodil.* This substance is less viscous and less irritant than Lipiodol, and is currently in general use.

Gas (air or oxygen) has the chief merit of utilizing the least irritant contrast media. It is difficult to manipulate and keep in the areas under examination, and fluoroscopy is not possible. Because of the low contrast produced, tomographic cuts rather than plain X-ray films are desirable. Relatively large amounts of air, at least 50 ml, and withdrawal of the same volume of cerebrospinal fluid, are necessary for adequate demonstration of the relevant parts of the spinal cord and canal. Because of these practical difficulties, gas myelography has not been widely employed. It has, however, a specific application in the diagnosis of syringomyelia (see later).

Water-soluble contrast media were first introduced in 1931, when Arnell and Lidström described the use of *Abrodil*, an organic iodide. This compound is water miscible and shows excellent detail of the intrathecal structures. Owing, however, to its high neurotoxicity, its use is now only of historic interest. In the present decade, major pharmacological developments have taken place in water-soluble contrast media. Initially, *meglumine iothalamate* (*Conray*) and later *meglumine iocarmate* (*Dimer X*) were employed for lumbar radiculography. These salts greatly reduced meningeal and neurotoxic side effects, but these were still too great to permit examination of the cervical and thoracic cord. In 1969, however, Almen formulated the non-ionic compound *metrizamide (Amipaque).*

Because it does not dissociate in solution, metrizamide had a much lower osmolality than all previous water soluble contrast media. Since neurotoxicity is principally related to hyperosmolality, Almen's innovation represents a major advance in myelographic contrast media.

At the time of writing, extensive clinical trials of metrizamide have been completed in many countries and it is gradually being introduced into general use, throughout the spinal canal and ventricular system.

In these circumstances, separate descriptions will be given of the techniques of myelography using Myodil (Pantopaque) and metrizamide (Amipaque).

Indications. As most contrast substances may be slightly irritant to the meninges, myelography should not be employed without clear indications. In general there are two:

1. To confirm or exclude the presence of a tumour or other operable lesion in cases where the clinical diagnosis is in doubt. This usually involves the distinction between compression by a tumour or prolapsed disc, and the different forms of degeneration of the cord.

2. The precise localization of a compressing lesion, usually as a pre-operative measure. This is because neurological localization is not always accurate and can be very misleading. In some cases occlusion of small spinal arteries may give false localizing signs. In addition, the vertebral spines may not be easily palpable to help the surgeon place his incision.

MYODIL MYELOGRAPHY

The slight inflammation of the meninges sometimes seen following the use of positive contrast media is due to the liberation of free iodine in the cerebrospinal fluid. This often produces a small increase of cells in the fluid for one or two days, accompanied by a transient rise of temperature. The oily medium usually remains mobile in decreasing amounts in the theca for a few weeks or months. It finally becomes fixed in small pockets by arachnoid adhesions, mainly in the sacral cul-de-sac. Occasionally a few drops become fixed in the intra-cranial subarachnoid cisterns. These pockets give quite spectacular appearances in subsequent radiographs, but very rarely cause any symptoms. Nevertheless, it is wise to shake Myodil from the basal cisterns back into the spinal canal after myelography.

Sometimes, however, neurological symptoms can be aggravated by myelography. Thus, in disseminated sclerosis, the slight irritation of the contrast medium may exacerbate symptoms. The escape of some cerebrospinal fluid at lumbar puncture tends to reduce pressure below an obstruction caused by a spinal tumour, resulting in increased pressure of the mass on the cord. Myelography of spinal tumours is thus best performed as a pre-operative examination.

Myodil, a slightly viscous oily solution, contains 30 per cent iodine. It is usually injected in a dose of 5 to 6 ml by lumbar or cisternal puncture. At the end of the examination, an attempt should be made to aspirate the contrast medium under fluoroscopic control. It is permissible in some cases, particularly with dorsal lesions, to inject volumes up to 20 ml, but if this is done the Myodil must always be aspirated when the examination is completed.

Technique

Injection of contrast. Myodil is injected into the subarachnoid space by lumbar puncture; a 20 s.w.g. needle is suitable. Cisternal or lateral cervical puncture is employed when necessary to define the upper border of an obstruction causing complete spinal block, or when lumbar puncture is technically not practicable.

A meticulous puncture technique is essential. If Myodil is carelessly injected, with leak into the subdural or extradural spaces, it may obscure the diagnostic field for weeks or even months. This is liable to happen with a long-bevelled needle, when only part of the bevel is in the subarachnoid space. It is a helpful precaution when this space has been tapped, to rotate the hub of the needle through 180°. If this rotation causes reduction of the back-flow of c.s.f., the whole of the bevel is not cleanly in the space, and the needle position should be slightly readjusted.

A further helpful precaution to avoid incorrect contrast injection, particularly in inexperienced hands, is to perform this under fluoroscopic control. This is best carried out with the patient in lateral decubitus position for lumbar injections, with slight downward tilt of the table. The syringe is connected to the needle by a fine polythene tube. After the lumbar puncture there is a tendency for c.s.f. to leak through the needle hole in the arachnoid, forming a small pool in the subdural or extradural spaces. This pool may be accidentally tapped instead of the subarachnoid space and Myodil injection should therefore not be made within a week of a previous lumbar puncture.

Lumbar puncture is safe through any intervertebral space below L.2. It is obviously desirable to avoid making the puncture at the level of the suspected lesion. Thus the injection should be made through the L.2–3 inter-space in suspected herniation of a lower lumbar disc.

Myodil should be removed at the end of the examination. This is done under fluoroscopic control through the original injection needle left *in situ* where prone screening only has been performed, as in lumbar disc lesions. However as supine screening is frequently necessary and often essential removal of the injection needle and a second lumbar puncture may be needed.

Subdural injection. It is important that extrathecal injections should be clearly recognized, for they may simulate the appearance of tumours within the canal, spinal block, or arachnoiditis. The Myodil may remain in a solid column as it dissects the subdural space, but it usually has an irregular shape and it does not descend completely into the sacrum when the patient is erect. It moves abnormally slowly on tilting the patient's head downwards, and usually does not pass above the upper dorsal area in this position.

With the patient prone, a lateral film shows Myodil disposed around the cord with some dorsal to it. Myodil in the subarachnoid space would descend by gravity through the cerebrospinal fluid to the anterior part of the spinal canal (Fig. 59.1). Sometimes the injection is made into both the subarachnoid and subdural spaces. In this case, the subarachnoid Myodil flows freely on tilting the patient, whilst the subdural Myodil moves very sluggishly.

Extradural injection. The characteristic feature of an extradural injection is the gradual tracking of globules of Myodil along the course of the spinal nerves outside the spinal canal (Fig. 59.2). When in doubt, a delayed film taken one or two days later will confirm this. The remaining Myodil is usually dispersed in globules throughout the extradural space. Some will be shown dorsal to the cord on lateral films with the patient prone.

Needle defects. Following lumbar puncture, the escape of cerebrospinal fluid along the needle track has been mentioned. The small pool of fluid which collects in the subdural or extradural space can constrict the Myodil column, simulating a prolapsed disc or extradural tumour (Fig. 59.3). In the same way, a traumatic puncture may

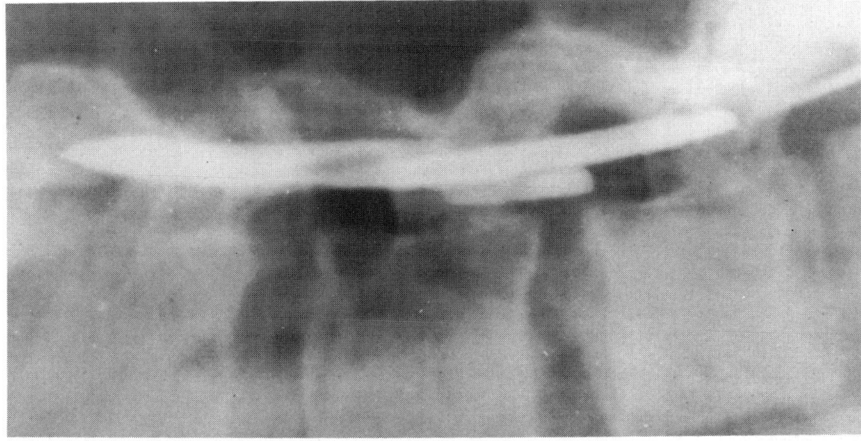

A

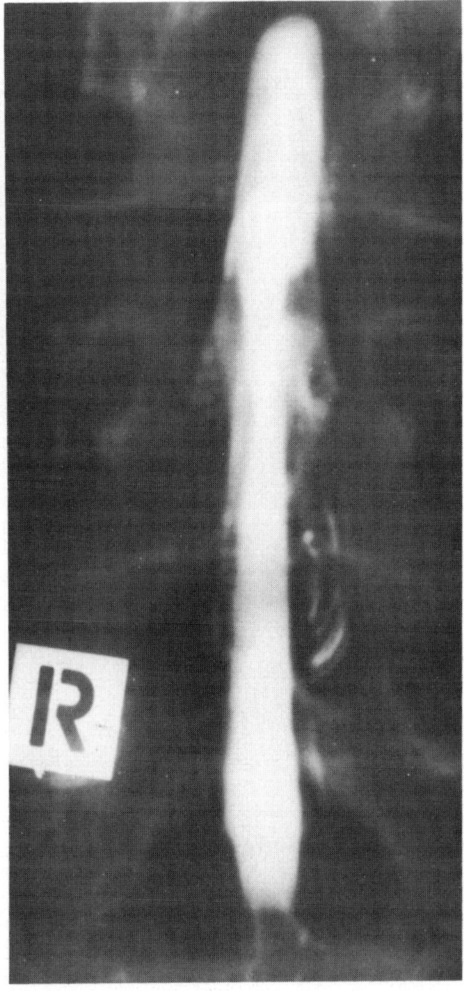

B

Fig. 59.1 Subdural injection. (A) Horizontal ray, lateral film with patient prone; Myodil should lie in the anterior part of the spinal canal in this position. (B) Antero-posterior film.

tear one of the extradural veins, causing a small haematoma which can also cause a false picture by displacing or constricting the Myodil column.

Fortunately, such needle artefacts are rare, although they may perhaps be more readily recognized when the injection needle remains *in situ* during subsequent fluoroscopy.

Fluoroscopy. The patient should be prone and accommodated securely and comfortably in a supporting harness on a tilting table. A large, soft pad beneath the chin maintains extension of the head to prevent Myodil entering the basal cisterns when the table tilts the patient head downwards. One learns by experience to check harness adjustments, screen traverse, position of markers and the like before commencing fluoroscopy. To have to attend to such matters with the patient in a diving position rapidly induces a state of near-hysteria in all concerned.

An over-couch tube is necessary to take lateral films with a horizontal beam across the table, to correspond with the anteroposterior films taken with the undercouch tube.

The table is slowly tilted, the head moving downwards, and the cephalad flow of the Myodil column is followed on the television monitor. Anteroposterior and lateral films are taken of the areas to which the clinical symptoms point, and also of any other abnormalities observed on the screen. With the patient prone, the normal lumbar and cervical curves lie with the convexity downwards, and the Myodil will readily pool in these areas. The thoracic spine, however, forms a curve with the convexity upwards, and as the Myodil runs over this arch, the column breaks up into droplets which reform when the cervical lordosis is reached. To obtain prone lateral films, the table should be tilted until the upper border of the Myodil column lies at about the level of T.10. The cross table tube and lateral film are then centred over the mid-thoracic area. The table is then tilted a further 15° head downward, and after a few seconds delay, the exposure made. This is a matter of careful judgement, and it may be necessary to repeat the manoeuvre to obtain a satisfactory film. It is, however, of importance, particularly in cases of suspected prolapsed thoracic disc.

When all the Myodil has been collected in the cervical theca, the table may be returned to the horizontal position. Minor degrees of table tilt, or flexion or extension of the head, may then be applied to outline the areas between the foramen magnum and T.3. For lateral films of the cervicodorsal area, the shoulders should be depressed as much as possible, or alternatively a swimming position with one arm extended above the head may be adopted.

When examination of the cervical canal is complete, the patient may be turned on to his back, the head being flexed at the same time. The dorsal curve is now convex downwards, and the Myodil will pool in the mid-dorsal area. The resulting picture differs from the previous ones

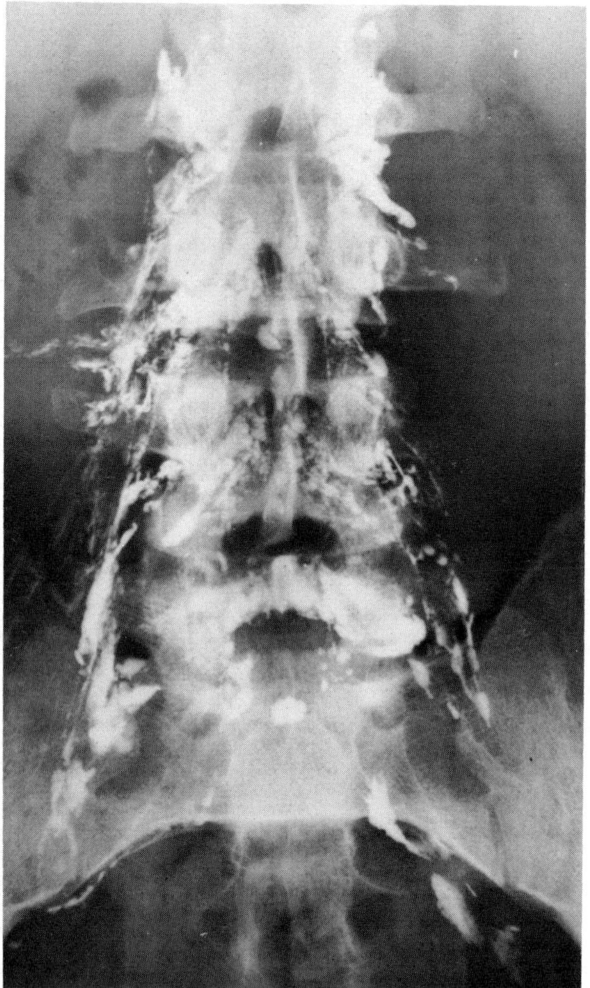

Fig. 59.2 Extradural injection. Myodil has tracked outside the bony canal along the course of the spinal nerves.

in that the Myodil is now lying dorsal to the cord on the neural arches and ligamenta flava. With the patient prone, on the other hand, the Myodil surrounds the anterior part of the cord and lies against the vertebral bodies.

In patients with a pronounced dorsal kyphos, there may be difficulty in manipulating the Myodil over the kyphos in the prone position. To spare the patient an uncomfortable degree of tilt, the Myodil can be run past this curve with only a little tilt if the lateral decubitus position is utilized. The prone position is then resumed.

It is important that any obstructions or filling defects observed should be proved constant, and to resolve any doubts on this point the fluoroscopic tilting should be repeated, with any appropriate variations.

In the prone position, Myodil passing through the foramen magnum runs up the clivus in the pontine cistern. From here it readily returns to the cervical theca. Myodil droplets passing laterally round the cerebellar hemispheres will remain within the skull, however, and this particularly applies if any pass upwards through the tentorial hiatus. Although this causes no symptoms, it should be avoided if possible.

Small, slow-growing tumours can cause symptoms, but no obstruction at myelography. The dense Myodil may surround the obscure these small masses, so that the examination may be considered normal. In such cases, re-screening, or a repeat examination at a later date should always be considered if symptoms persist.

When there is a complete block to the cephalad flow of Myodil, the upper border of the obstruction can be outlined by Myodil injected by cisternal puncture, and run caudally down the canal to the obstruction.

If operation is planned, a transverse scratch should be made on the skin to mark the level of the lesion. This mark should be about 5 cm from the midline to avoid the line of the proposed incision.

It is essential that any films taken should be large enough to include unequivocal anatomical landmarks to localize the lesion. The first or last ribs are usually most helpful in this respect.

NORMAL APPEARANCES

The aim of fluoroscopy is to maintain a solid Myodil column, which will outline both the thecal sac and the spinal cord within it. The theca normally extends laterally to lie against the medial border of the pedicles. The cord itself appears with varying clarity in different areas as a solid filling defect, occupying the central half of the theca, except at the level of the cervical and lumbar enlargements, where it occupies two-thirds of the theca.

Root sleeves. Small triangular outpouchings of the theca are seen at each segmental level in the cervical and lumbar areas. These are due to small outpouchings of arachnoid which enclose the origins of the nerve roots, and are referred to as root sheaths or sleeves. It is sometimes possible to trace the linear filling defect of a nerve root through the Myodil to its origin from the cord. The anterior and posterior nerve roots unite immediately distal to the posterior root ganglion. The spinal nerve so formed runs down the medial border of the pedicle to the foramen below. Here it lies above the intervertebral space. Thus the L.5 root emerges above the lumbosacral disc space, and prolapse of a lumbosacral disc will compress the S.1 root. In the prone position, owing to the anatomical ventral curve, the Myodil does not distend the theca sufficiently to reach the root sheaths and fully outline them. The root sheaths lie in the acute angle below the origin of the spinal nerves.

Spinal arteries. In the prone position, a thin vertical linear midline filling defect due to the anterior spinal artery is frequently seen. It usually takes a fairly straight course, unlike the tortuous dilated vessels supplying a spinal angioma. Small radicular tributaries from the aortic intercostals may sometimes be seen. They usually run

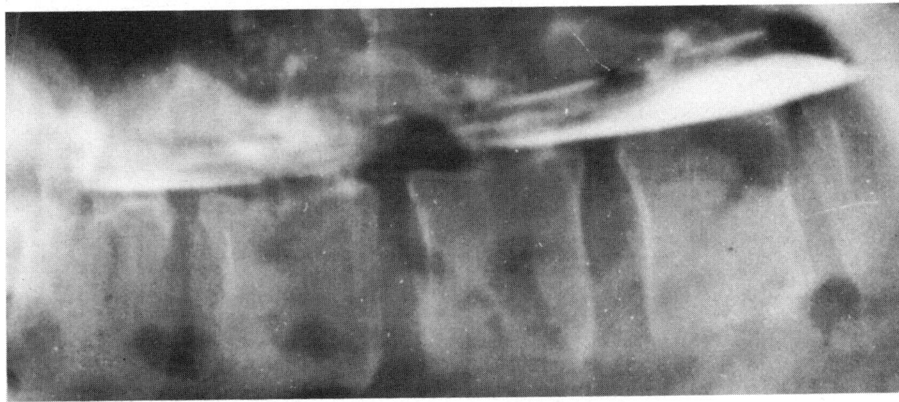

A

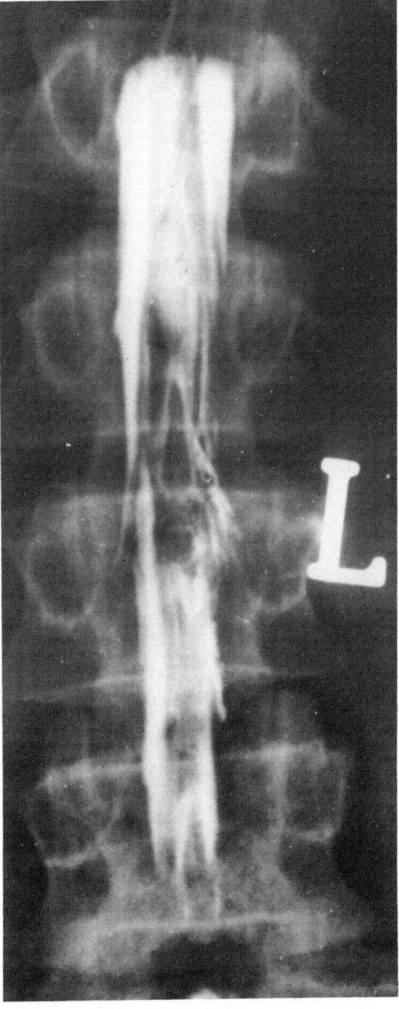

B

Fig. 59.3 Needle defect. (A) Filling defect in the Myodil column simulating prolapsed disc. Myodil fragments shown posteriorly in the soft tissues at the puncture site. (B) Anteroposterior films of patient in erect position; Myodil in the subdural plane has not descended freely to the sacrum.

obliquely upward towards the anterior spinal artery, their course being roughly parallel to the spinal nerve roots. Tortuous linear filling defects are sometimes seen at the level of C.1 and 2. These are due to the vertebral arteries and their posterior inferior cerebellar branches, and should not be misinterpreted as an angioma. Similarly, the basilar artery may be outlined in the pontine cistern (Fig. 59.4).

In the prone position, the bulge of the odontoid may form an oval filling defect in the midline in the anterior view. In lateral projections, the odontoid causes a slight posterior displacement of the Myodil column. Also, in the prone lateral cervical view, a thin, linear filling defect may be seen in the centre of the Myodil column, running parallel to the spine. This is due to the dentate ligament.

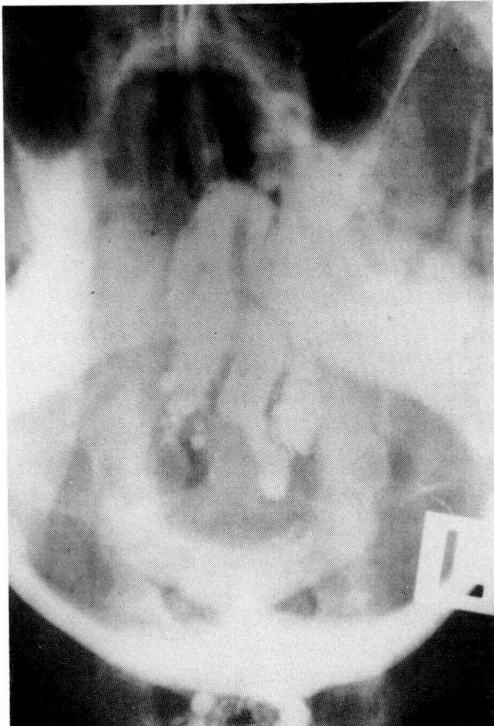

Fig. 59.4 Vertebral and basilar arteries outlined in the pontine cistern.

The theca normally ends at S.2, and this is best seen in an erect lateral film. The end point may not be clearly identified on anteroposterior films, owing to foreshortening due to the curve of the sacrum. Occasionally, the theca ends at L.5. In this event, prolapse of a lumbosacral disc cannot be recognized.

In the prone position, the Myodil usually lies very closely against the back of the vertebral bodies, the intervertebral discs and the posteriorly longitudinal ligament, due to the narrowness of the anterior extradural space. In the lumbosacral area, however, the extradural space is much wider, so that there will be a slight gap between the Myodil and the vertebral bodies and discs. When such a gap is observed, it must be remembered that a small disc herniation will not be demonstrable.

WATER-SOLUBLE (METRIZAMIDE) MYELOGRAPHY

Water-soluble compounds have major advantages over oily contrast media for myelography. Water-soluble compounds are freely permeable throughout the subarachnoid and ventricular spaces without the surface tension effects and droplet formation which are disadvantages of oily media. This property renders the cerebrospinal fluid radio-opaque, through which can be seen the detailed structure of the spinal cord and nerve roots (Fig. 59.5A). Because of this reduced surface tension, water-soluble media will often traverse an apparent complete block to oil or air contrast.

The *radiographic contrast* produced is optimal, being less than that of Myodil and greater than that of air. The contrast may also be varied for particular examinations, according to the concentration and volume of metrizamide injected. A low kilovoltage (preferably under 75) radiographic technique results in the best contrast.

The medium is excreted rapidly (24–48 hours) and completely in the urine, eliminating the need for subsequent aspiration.

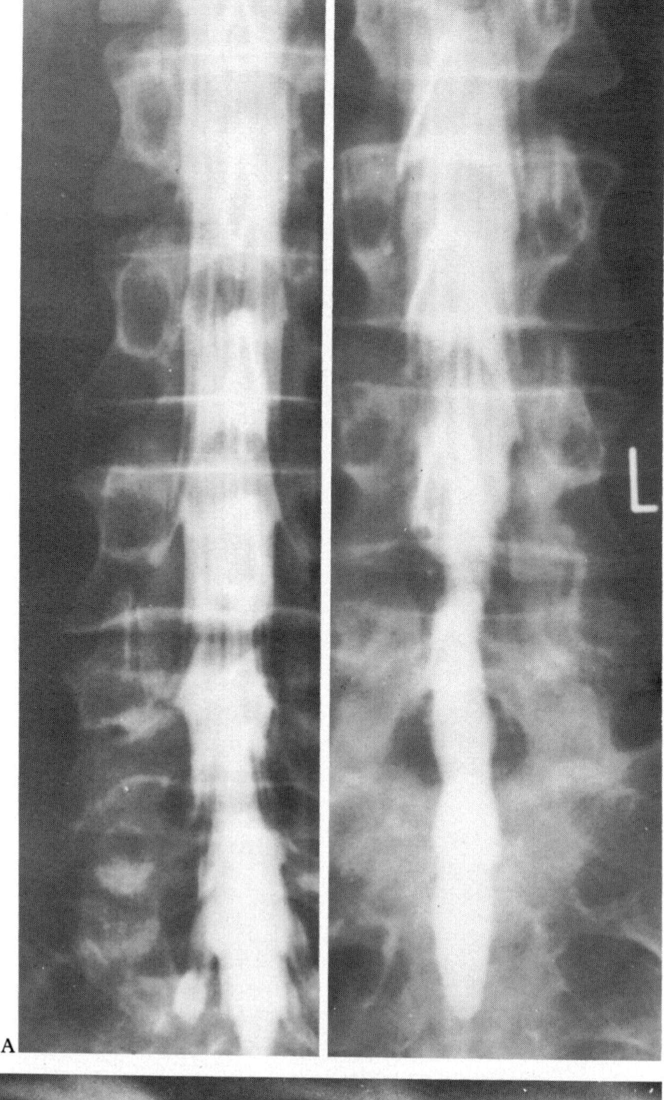

Fig. 59.5A Water soluble myelogram. The roots of the cauda equina and root pockets are shown through the opacified cerebrospinal fluid.

Fig. 59.5B Arachnoiditis following previous myelograms with Myodil and Dimer X. Below the level of L.4 the whole of the thecal sac is narrowed and the root pockets obliterated.

Fig. 59.5C Oblique view of lumbar theca showing root pouches.

Fig. 59.5D Thoracic myelogram (metrizamide). Horizontal beam with patient supine. Both cord and theca are clearly outlined.

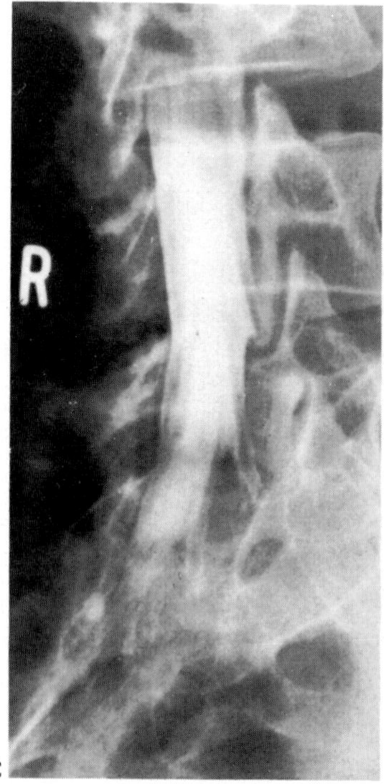

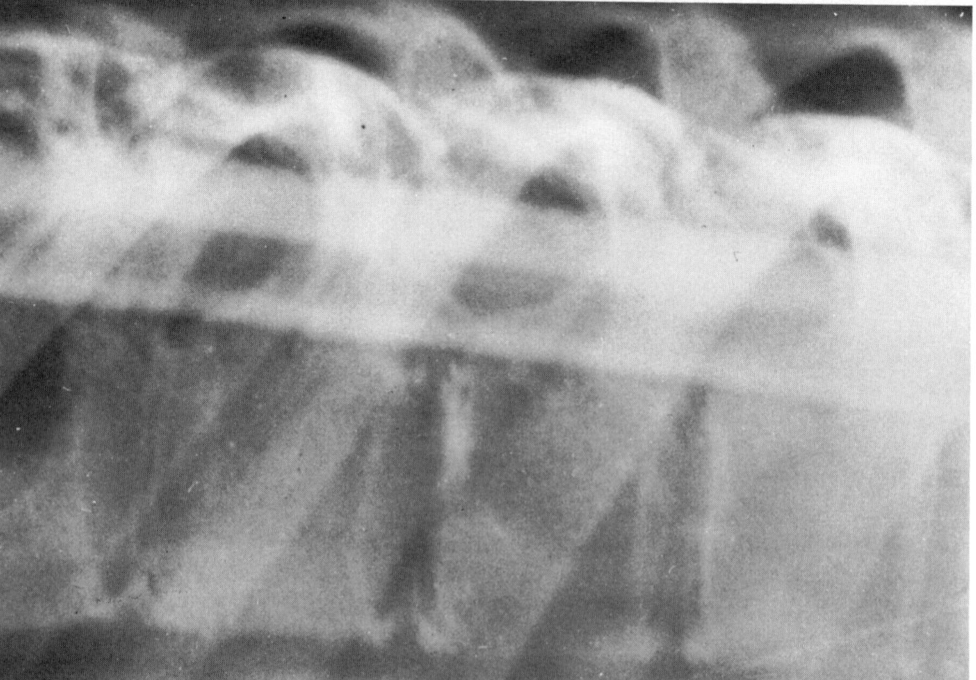

Neurotoxicity of metrizamide is low, although it can be very weakly epileptogenic, particularly if, through faulty technique, it comes into contact with the meninges over the cerebral cortex. For this reason, it is usually contraindicated if there is a history of previous epilepsy. It is also contraindicated if there is a previous history of significant allergy. Rarely, fits or muscle spasms may follow the use of metrizamide. These can readily be controlled by the immediate administration of diazepam intravenously.

There is evidence to suggest that this epileptogenic tendency is increased in patients being treated by neuroleptic drugs such as chlorpromazine. Such drugs should be withheld for 48 hours before myelography with metrizamide. If fits do occur, then diazepam should be supplemented by the longer acting phenobarbitone.

In about half the patients, headache lasting about 24 hours is experienced, but the incidence of this is only slightly greater than that following simple lumbar puncture. The headache is worse after cervical injection of contrast and is reduced by recumbency for 24 hours, with the head raised 10–15° for the first six hours. The headache is not affected by the use of diazepam.

Adhesive arachnoiditis. There appears to be little or no tendency for metrizamide to produce thecal scarring as a sequel to myelography. This often follows myelography with Myodil, Dimer X or Conray (Fig. 59.5B). It is also more pronounced after laminectomy and the irritant effect of blood in the subarachnoid space. The relation between such contraction of the theca and root pockets to symptoms is problematical. It is obvious, however, that a symptomatic disc prolapse will no longer be demonstrable when the theca and root pockets are contracted in this way. Thecal scarring may follow oil myelography even when the contrast medium is aspirated at the end of the examination.

Technique

Premedication with diazepam is usually satisfactory. The low viscosity of metrizamide permits a fine (22 s.w.g.) needle to be used. The small bevel of such a needle helps to ensure complete subarachnoid injection of contrast, without artefacts. Details of technique vary with the area to be examined, and will be described in turn.

Lumbar myelogram. Lumbar puncture is made in either the sitting position, or in lateral decubitus with the head end of the table raised 10°. An average dose of metrizamide is 14 ml, 200 mg I_2 per ml. The patient is then placed in the prone position, and the following films taken:

Vertical beam—anteroposterior, right and left obliques (Fig. 59.5A and C).

Horizontal beam—lateral, right and left lateral decubitus.

Thoracic myelogram. The object is to introduce the metrizamide into the thoracic area as directly as possible, without dilution in the lumbosacral canal. Accordingly, lumbar puncture is made in lateral decubitus with the head end of the table lowered 10–15°. A pillow is placed below the head to prevent intracranial passage of contrast. The average dose is 12–14 ml, 200 mg I_2 per ml, but 5–10 ml with spinal block. Following injection of contrast, an anteroposterior film may be taken with horizontal beam. The table is returned to horizontal and the patient placed supine, when the contrast medium will be collected in the thoracic canal. Anteroposterior and lateral films are taken with vertical and horizontal beams respectively (Fig. 59.5D). These may be supplemented with oblique views as required. Finally, the patient is placed in the opposite lateral decubitus position and an anteroposterior film with horizontal beam taken.

After the examination, the patient should sit upright for a few minutes, and then return to bed for 24 hours, with the head slightly elevated as described earlier.

Cervical myelogram. (a) *Cervical injection.* Direct injection of metrizamide into the cervical canal will give the best contrast, and with less chance of intracranial passage of the medium. It should not be used, however, if there is clinical suspicion of either a high cervical tumour, or a caudal block.

Either lateral cervical (between C.1 and 2), or sub-occipital puncture may be used. The patient is in the prone position, with the head slightly extended by a soft pad under the chin. Television/film control of the puncture in both vertical and horizontal planes is desirable. As with other punctures it is often helpful to use a short polythene connecting tube between syringe and needle for contrast injection. The average dose is 10 ml metrizamide, 200 mg I_2 per ml, though some workers use higher concentrations. In the prone position, the contrast pools in the cervical canal and the usual anteroposterior and lateral films are taken (Fig. 59.6A and B) supplemented by oblique views as required.

(b) *Lumbar injection.* Water-soluble contrast media have insufficient density to permit screening up the spinal canal in the anteroposterior plane of the patient. With lumbar injection of metrizamide, when the patient is tilted head downwards, the arrival of contrast in the cervical canal can only be monitored and controlled by lateral screening of the cervical spine. When the equipment possesses this capability, there is no problem in screening the patient in the necessary prone position with the head extended. When only single plane screening is available, however, the patient must be tilted head downwards in lateral decubitus position. There must also be a pillow under the head during this manoeuvre to produce sharp lateral flexion and prevent intracranial passage of contrast. It is important that the contrast medium should not ascend above the lower part of the clivus, else some will pass irretrievably into the middle fossa, with increased

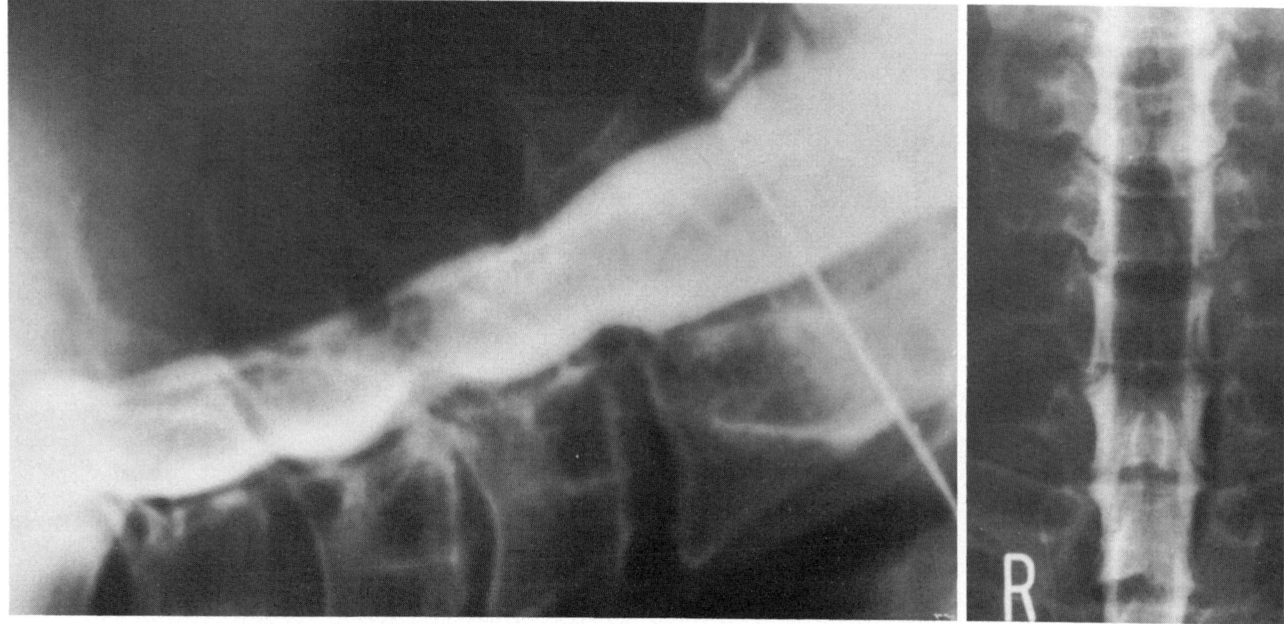

A B

Fig. 59.6A Cervical myelogram (metrizamide). Contrast injection by lateral cervical puncture between C.1 and 2—lateral view. B A. P. view. Minor spondylitis indents anteriorly and on l.h. side.

risk of neurotoxic manifestations. These manoeuvres are assisted by the use of a smaller volume of metrizamide in higher concentration, which gives increased viscosity. This also allows for some dilution in the cephalad passage of the medium. An average dose is 7 ml, 300 mg I_2 per ml. When the metrizamide is collected in the cervical canal, the patient is placed in the prone position, and the usual series of films taken.

At the end of cervical myelography, the patient should sit upright for a short time before returning to bed as described above.

DEVELOPMENTAL ABNORMALITIES

MENINGOCELE AND SPINA BIFIDA

Incomplete fusion of the developing neural arches may result in the formation of a meningocele, which is herniation of a sac covered by leptomeninges through an associated defect in the vertebral laminae. The most common sites are the lumbosacral and suboccipital regions (Fig. 59.7). All grades of this anomaly may be encountered. The least significant is a simple bony defect, spina bifida occulta, in the first cervical or first sacral vertebrae, which may be considered almost a normal anatomical variant. In the most severe degrees, a meningomyelocele may be found, in which the neural arch is widely open over several segments, and the sac containing elements of spinal cord or cauda equina. This latter condition is incompatible with life.

The sac of a meningocoele usually contains cerebrospinal fluid, and transmitted pulsation may cause still further erosion of adjacent bones. Anteroposterior films of the spine show the bone defect in the neural arch and also enlargement of the spinal canal as evidenced by widening of the interpedicular distance. The bone defects may be difficult to identify in lateral films, although the projecting soft-tissue mass is outlined. Other developmental vertebral abnormalities are often seen in association with meningocele and spina bifida, in particular an Arnold-Chiari malformation. Two variants merit separate description.

Lateral thoracic meningocele. Occasionally a meningeal sac herniates through an enlarged thoracic intervertebral foramen into the posterior mediastinum. This produces a well-defined, round, soft-tissue paravertebral shadow. This condition is often associated with neurofibromatosis, and should always be suspected when this lesion coexists. Differential diagnosis may be difficult, as the condition can closely simulate neurofibroma, ganglioneuroma, bronchial and secondary neoplasm, and the various forms of intrathoracic cyst. The diagnosis of thoracic meningocoele may be confirmed by myelography, when Myodil will be seen to enter the sac of the meningocele (Fig. 59.8). This may occasionally necessitate screening in the lateral decubitus position.

Anterior sacral meningocele. Well-defined bone defects are occasionally found in the anterior part of the sacrum (Fig. 59.9A). A meningocele may prolapse through this defect, presenting as a soft-tissue mass in the pelvis both clinically and radiologically. Barium enema may show displacement of the recto-sigmoid (Fig. 59.9B). Diagnosis can be confirmed by myelography (Fig. 59.9C)

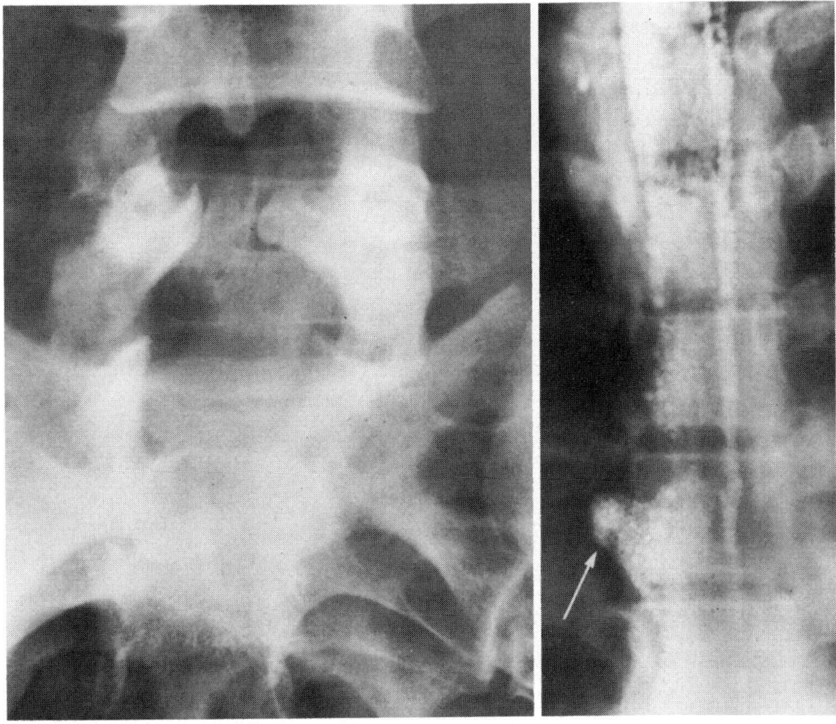

Fig. 59.7 *Fig. 59.8*

Fig. 59.7 Spina bifida. Wide defects in the neural arches of L.5 and S.1.

Fig. 59.8 Lateral thoracic meningocele. Myodil has entered a small sac to the right of the spinal canal (↗). Patient with neurofibromatosis.

which will exclude the alternative possibility of a malignant pelvic tumour eroding the sacrum. This is also of surgical importance, as an anterior approach to the mass carries the obvious risk of infection and meningitis. Several fatalities have been recorded from such intervention in the past.

Sacral cysts. Arachnoid cysts arising within the sacrum are frequently large, usually contain cerebrospinal fluid, and communicate freely with the subarachnoid space. Being pulsatile, they often cause erosion and expansion of the sacral canal. This is best shown on lateral films, and particularly on lateral tomograms.

As the majority of sacral cysts communicate freely with the subarachnoid space, myelography makes the diagnosis obvious (Fig. 59.10A and B). Occasionally, however, delayed erect films may be necessary to outline the cyst, if there is only a narrow opening between it and the thecal sac.

Other variants of these large single cysts are small perineural cysts associated with nerve roots. These are small arachnoid cysts associated with nerve roots, most commonly found in the S.2 and 3 segments. They may or may not communicate with the subarachnoid space. When they do, Myodil will be seen at myelography to enter the small lateral outpouchings overlying the sacral foramina (Fig. 59.11). If the neck of communication is narrow, it will take some time for the contrast to enter the sac. Thus a delayed film taken with the patient erect one or two days after injection of contrast may show them to be more extensive than was originally supposed. They are found in about 8 per cent of patients when films are taken some time after a myelogram.

These cysts may or may not cause symptoms. They are a rare cause of sciatica when the sacral nerve roots are compressed. Sometimes they erode bone and cause enlargement of the sacral exit foramina.

Corresponding small arachnoid diverticula may very occasionally be seen in relation to the root sleeves in the cervical and thoracic areas, but they rarely cause symptoms.

ARNOLD-CHIARI MALFORMATION

In this condition there is downward displacement of the lower brain stem and tonsils and occasionally the lower part of the cerebellum through the foramen magnum into the upper part of the cervical canal. The lower part of the cerebellum is itself often malformed, and the fourth ventricle may be present in the upper cervical canal. There may be enlargement of the foramen magnum, and spina bifida of the upper cervical vertebrae. Sometimes there is an associated meningomyelocele. Plain

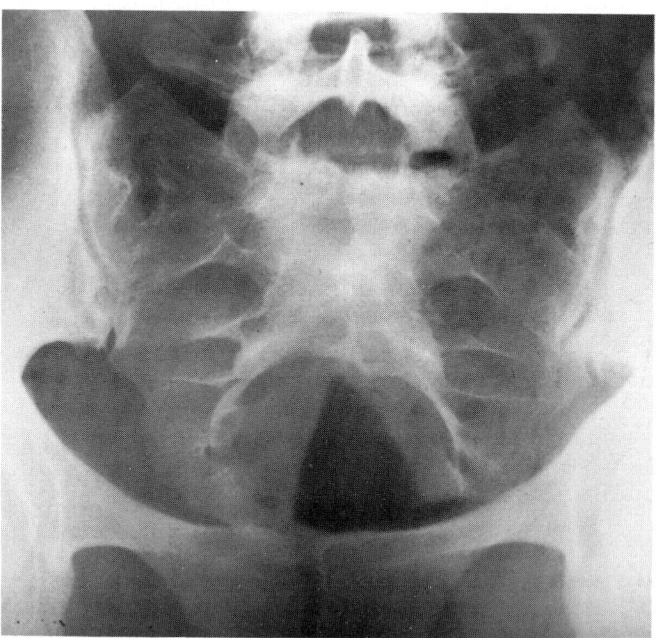

A

films may be normal, or may show spina bifida if present. The posterior fossa can appear rather shallow and flat on a lateral skull film.

Unlike the tonsillar herniation resulting from obstructive hydrocephalus due to a posterior fossa tumour, the herniated brain stem is not usually compressed in an Arnold-Chiari malformation except as a late event. An obstructive hydrocephalus does, however, develop if the exit foramina of the fourth ventricle become obstructed in the upper cervical canal.

Not unexpectedly, other developmental anomalies such as platybasia and a Klippel-Feil deformity may be found in association with an Arnold-Chiari malformation.

Myelography, if not contra-indicated by raised intracranial pressure, will usually show an obstruction in the upper cervical canal, normally at C.1 or 2, or sometimes lower. The herniated cerebellar tonsils usually produce a symmetrical filling defect in the Myodil column on each side of the cord at the point of obstruction. The tonsils lie postero-lateral to the cord which may be

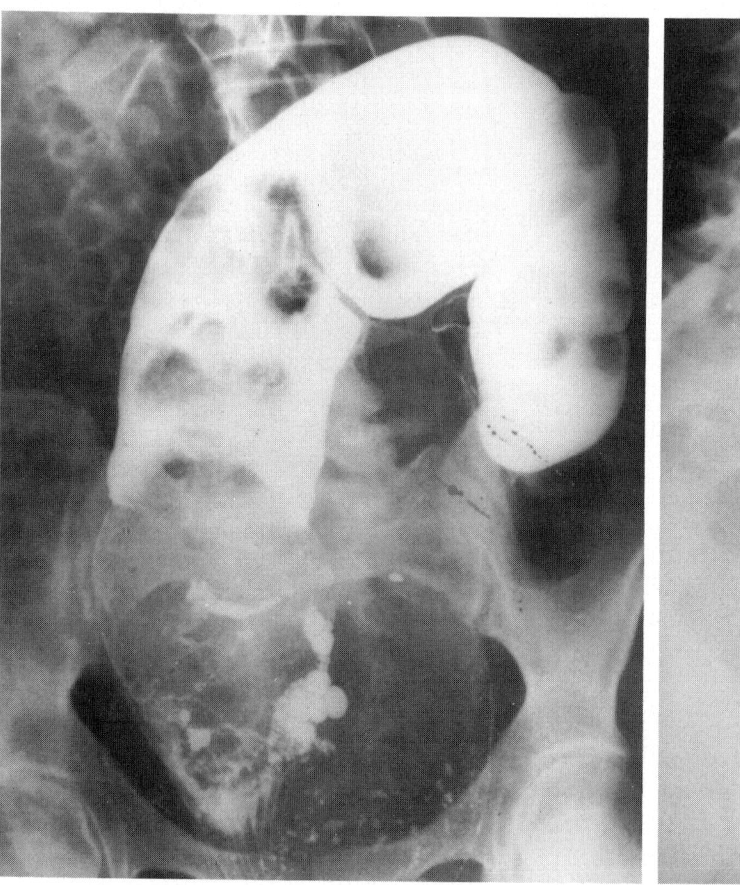

B

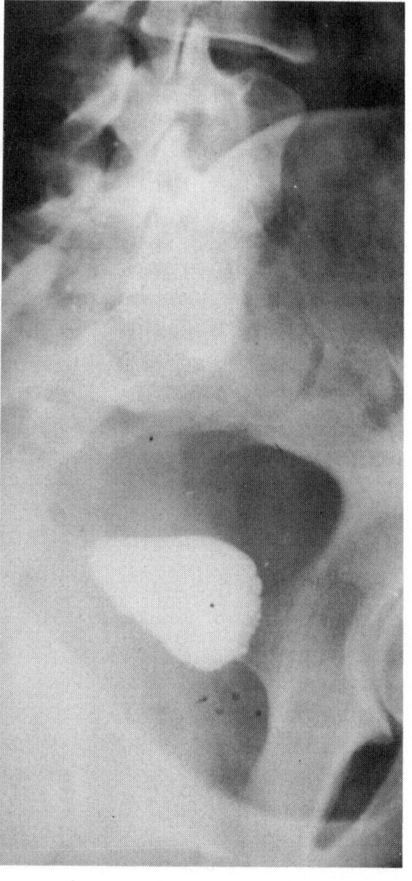

C

Fig. 59.9 (A) Anterior sacral meningocele. Large defect in the lower half of the sacrum. There is also spina bifida occulta, shown by a small defect in the posterior arch of S.1. (B) Anterior sacral meningocele. Myodil remnants outline the large sac of the meningocele, which is compressing and displacing the rectum. (C) Anterior sacral meningocele. Myodil has left the spinal canal to enter the large pelvic sac.

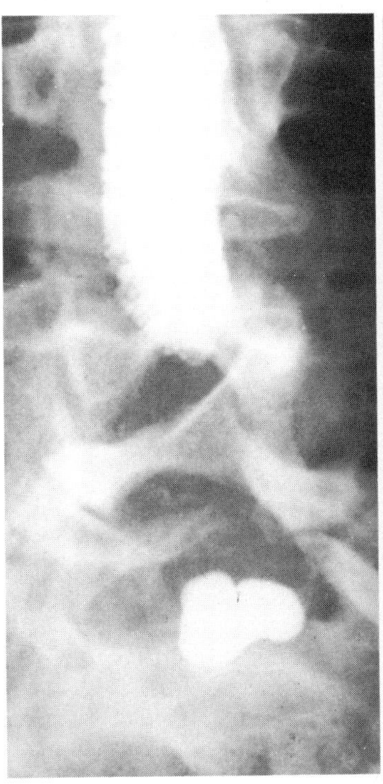

Fig. 59.10A

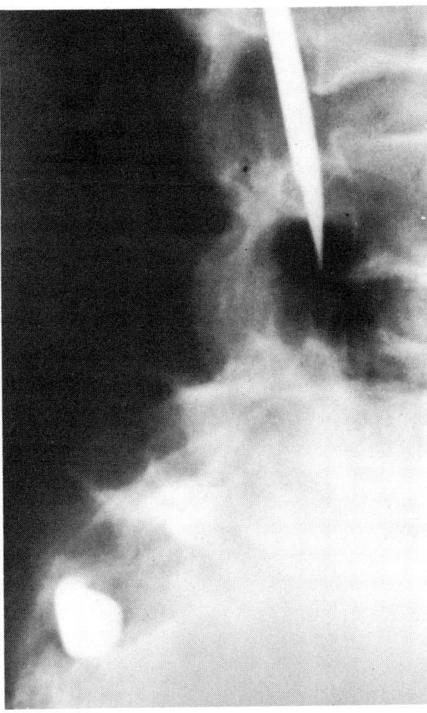

Fig. 59.10B

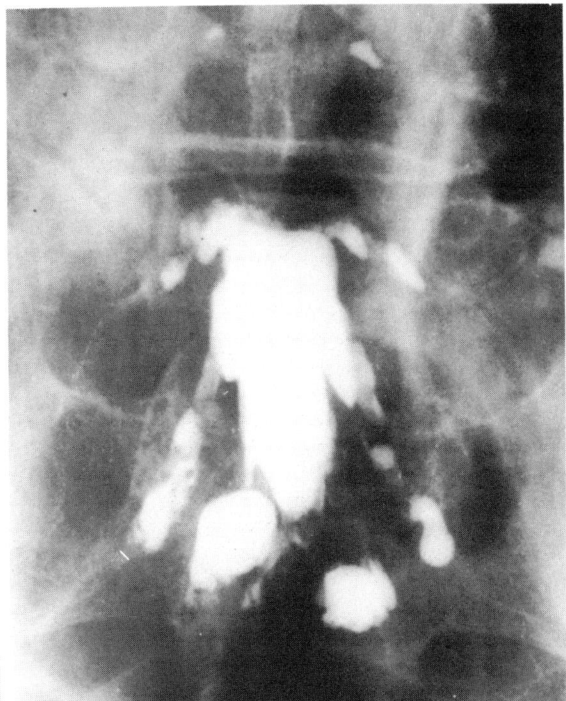

Fig. 59.11

Fig. 59.10 (A and B) Sacral cyst. The sacral canal is deepened and enlarged. There is also associated spina bifida.

Fig. 59.11 Sacral arachnoid diverticula.

displaced forwards, and are best shown by screening the patient supine.

Minor degrees of the Arnold-Chiari malformation (cerebellar ectopia) can only in fact be shown by such supine screening. Sometimes these appearances simulate an intradural tumour. Absolute confirmation of the diagnosis may be given by air encephalography or Myodil ventriculography, when the caudal part of the fourth ventricle will be shown in the upper cervical canal (Figs 60.21 and 60.22).

With recent technical developments in computed tomography, it has become possible to scan the craniovertebral junction with head machines. The whole of the spinal canal may, of course, be examined by body machines.

Detail of the upper cervical cord and herniation of cerebellar tonsils through the foramen magnum can however only be reliably demonstrated after injection of metrizamide into the cerebrospinal fluid. The subarachnoid space is then demonstrated as a zone of increased density. Herniated tonsils are demonstrated as filling defects in this zone posteriorly, of the same density as the cord itself. In some cases, metrizamide may occasionally be demonstrated in the central cavity within the cord. Any associated hydrocephalus is, of course, shown by the cranial scan.

KLIPPEL-FEIL ABNORMALITY

This developmental malformation results from defective segmentation of the vertebrae. It is usually seen in the cervical spine, but may rarely be observed in the thoracic or lumbar areas. Two or more vertebral bodies are fused, forming a 'block vertebra' (Fig. 59.12A). This fusion may also involve the neural arches (Fig. 59.12B). The condition may need to be distinguished from post-inflammatory fusion of the vertebral bodies. In the Klippel-Feil abnormality, the antero-posterior diameter of the vertebral bodies is often reduced (Fig. 59.12A), there is no angulation in the block vertebra due to previous inflammatory destruction, and there may be some fusion of the posterior arches.

Other developmental anomalies are associated with a Klippel-Feil malformation, particularly spina bifida, meningocele, hemivertebra, Arnold-Chiari malformation and cervical ribs.

Clinically the Klippel-Feil anomaly is manifest by a short neck with restricted movements. Owing to the absence of movement in the fused segments, compensatory increased movement takes place above and below the block vertebra. This often results in the premature development of spondylosis at the intervertebral spaces adjoining the block vertebra.

ATLANTO-OCCIPITAL FUSION

Developmental occipitalization of the atlas may result in compression of the spinal cord at the medullospinal junction. When the atlas is fused with the occiput, the

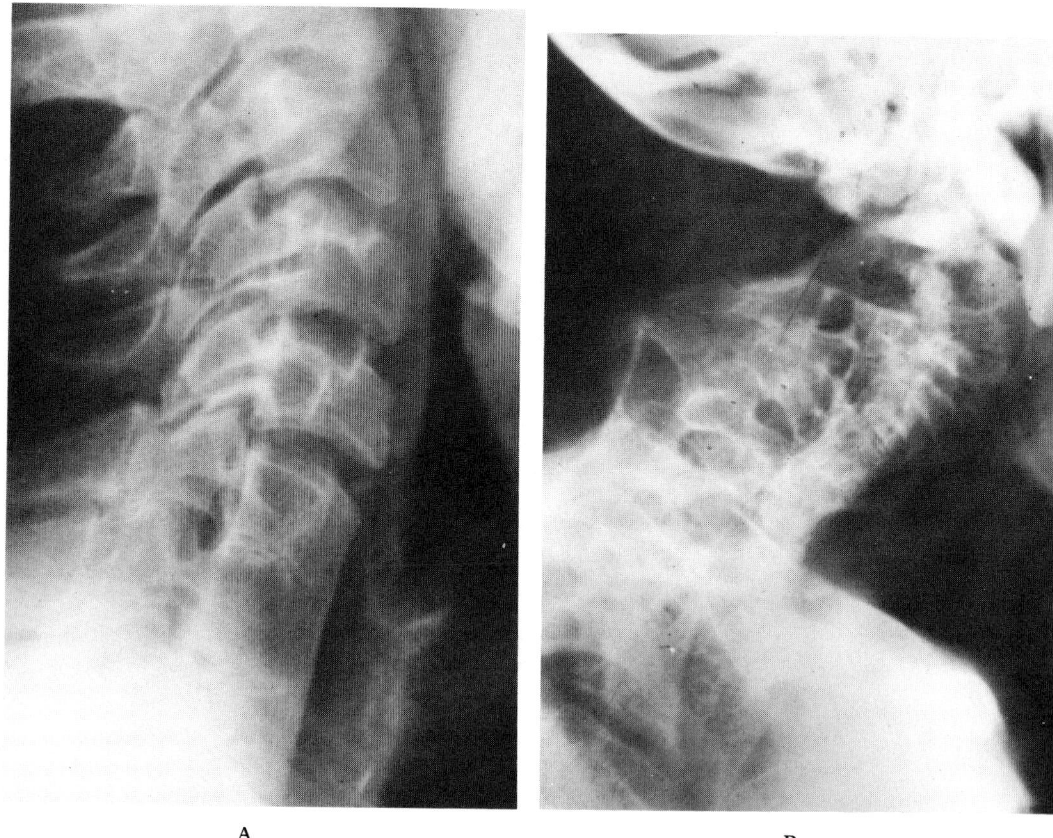

A

Fig. 59.12A Klippel-Feil abnormality. Block vertebra due to fusion of the bodies of C.5, 6 and 7.

B

Fig. 59.12B Klippel-Feil abnormality. More severe degree with fusion also involving the posterior arches.

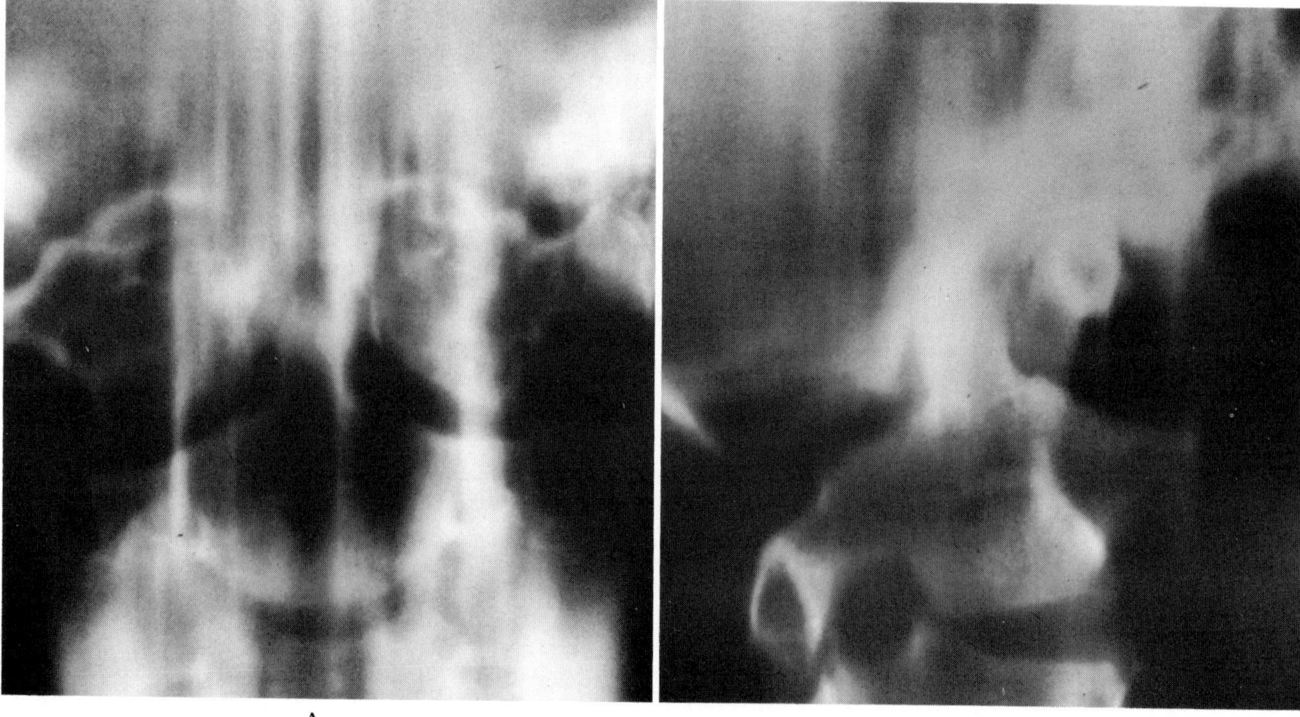

A

Fig. 59.13A Atlanto-occipital fusion. Anteroposterior tomograms.

B

Fig. 59.13B Atlanto-occipital fusion. Lateral tomogram shows forward subluxation of the atlas on the axis, with posterior displacement of the odontoid.

odontoid process extends in effect into the foramen magnum. When the head is flexed, partial forward subluxation of the fused atlas takes place on the axis, and the medullospinal junction may be compressed by the odontoid (Fig. 59.13). This may be best shown by lateral tomographic cuts with head in flexion, extension and neutral positions.

This compression is recognized clinically by varying degrees of spastic quadriparesis, with sensory disturbance, fifth and twelfth nerve palsies, and possibly nystagmus and ataxia.

DETACHED ODONTOID PROCESS AND ATLANTO-AXIAL DISLOCATION

Detachment of the odontoid process may be *traumatic* or *congenital* and it may or may not be associated with atlanto-axial dislocation. Such a dislocation is also seen rarely as a complication of *inflammatory* disease, such as tuberculous caries or retropharyngeal abscess. It is also seen occasionally as a late manifestation in severe cases of *rheumatoid arthritis*, and has also been recorded as a complication of *ankylosing spondylitis*.

When subluxation or dislocation occurs, the atlas moves forwards and downwards on the axis. For this to happen, there must be defects or abnormal laxity in the ligamentum flavum and transverse ligament of the atlas. The onset of symptoms in chronic cases may be delayed for many years, and the symptomatology is similar to that described under atlanto-occipital fusion.

The condition is best demonstrated by lateral films, preferably tomograms, with the head in full flexion and full extension.

SPONDYLOLISTHESIS

Bony fusion of the interarticular part of the neural arch is sometimes incomplete, with fibrous rather than bony union occurring between the separate ossific centres. This developmental weakness predisposes to forward subluxation of the vertebral body, pedicles and superior articular processes. The spinous process, laminae and inferior articular processes remain in normal position. When present, such spondylolisthesis nearly always occurs at the lumbo-sacral junction with forward subluxation of L.5 on S.1, but is occasionally seen at higher levels. The defect in the pars interarticularis is often bilateral, and is readily shown by oblique views. When large, it can sometimes be seen on a lateral film.

The forward subluxation causes narrowing of the intervertebral foramen, and compression of the nerve roots. Thus the clinical features may be indistinguishable from prolapse of an intervertebral disc. Indeed, there is frequently an associated disc lesion, as the forward subluxation results in rupture of the annulus fibrosus. When a defect is present in the pars interarticularis, but without any subluxation, the condition is known as *spondylolysis*. The condition is discussed in detail in Chapter 9 (p. 203).

DIASTEMATOMYELIA

This is a linear vertical division or reduplication of the spinal cord in the midline. The lower thoracic and upper lumbar areas are the most common sites. This part of the cord is often transfixed by a bony or fibrous ridge or spicule extending from the vertebral body in front to the dura behind the cord. In anteroposterior films the spinal canal is widened over several segments. The interpedicular distance is increased, although the pedicles are not eroded. When the midline septum is ossified (Fig. 59.14), it may be shown as a short linear shadow and can be better demonstrated by tomography in either the anteroposterior or lateral plane.

In some cases, however, the spur transfixing the cord may be fibrocartilaginous and therefore radiolucent, and the condition can only be diagnosed by myelography. At the site of the lesion, the contrast column will be split into two halves by the septum. This filling defect is constant and either linear or round, as the spur is in the form of either a ridge or a spike (Fig. 59.15).

DYSRAPHISM

This term relates to the presence in the lumbar area of spina bifida occulta associated with abnormally low fixation of the cord. It results from abnormal fusion of the posterior midline structures. In normal foetal development, after the third month, the spinal column elongates at a faster rate than the cord. As a result, the cord normally ends at the level of L.2. In dysraphism, the conus medullaris is attached more firmly than normal to the coccyx by the filum terminale, which may also be thickened. The cord may thus extend to the lower lumbar area, as far as L.5.

The resultant symptoms include pain, weakness, wasting and sensory loss in the legs. There may be trophic ulceration. These children are slow in learning to walk, and there may be progressive deformities of the feet, leading to pes cavus. There is often bladder dysfunction, with incontinence or enuresis.

Abnormal hair patches may be found on the skin in the lumbosacral area. Alternatively, at this site there may be skin dimpling, or a lipoma or a pilonidal sinus. Within the spinal canal, in addition to thickening of the filum terminale, there may be a lipoma or epidermoid, or intrathecal bands. It is important that the diagnosis should be made in the first five years for the best surgical results.

Plain films show spina bifida occulta, and possibly other developmental anomalies due to abnormal segmentation.

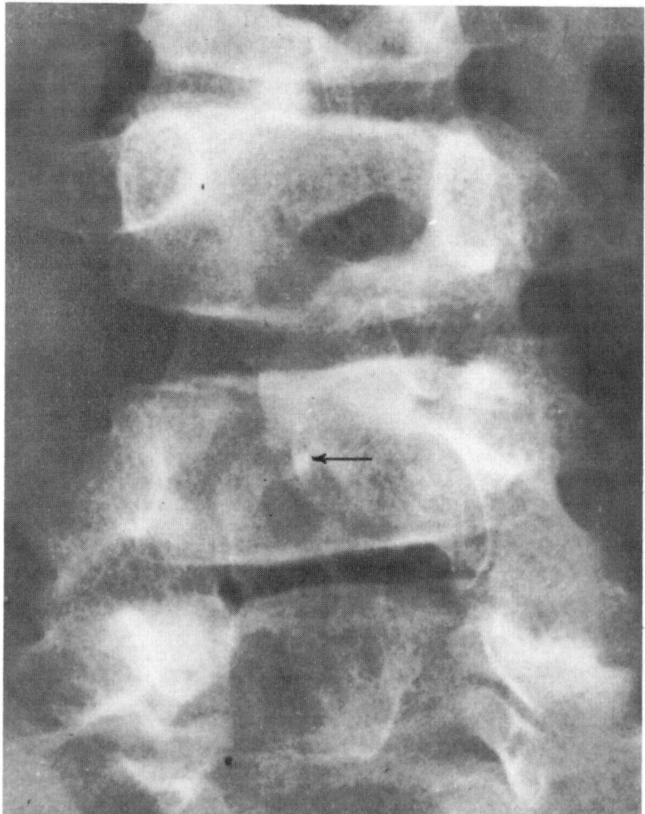

Fig. 59.14 Diastematomyelia. Midline bony spicule (←). There are also developmental defects in the posterior arches.

Fig. 59.15 Diastematomyelia. Filling defect in Myodil column caused by central bony spur.

The spinal canal is often widened, and there may be a bony spur due to associated diastematomyelia. There may also be a scoliosis.

Definitive diagnosis depends on myelography, and for this metrizamide is preferable to Myodil (Fig. 59.16A and B). The high density of the latter in addition to its tendency to break up into droplets are disadvantages. The injection is preferably made by careful low lumbar puncture, as there is too much dilution and loss of contrast when the injection is made cisternally. The injection should always be made under fluoroscopic control, and the volume adjusted according to the age of the patient and the volume of the lumbar canal. A concentration of 200 mg I_2 per ml is appropriate.

Screening and radiography should be carried out with the patient supine. The cord is usually tethered posteriorly, and metrizamide being denser than cerebrospinal fluid will tend to layer posteriorly in the supine position. The thickened filum may not be demonstrated by prone screening. The filum may be shown to exceed its normal width of 2 to 3 mm.

Metrizamide will also show clearly any intrathecal masses such as lipoma or dermoid, and also diastematomyelia, regardless of whether a midline septum is present.

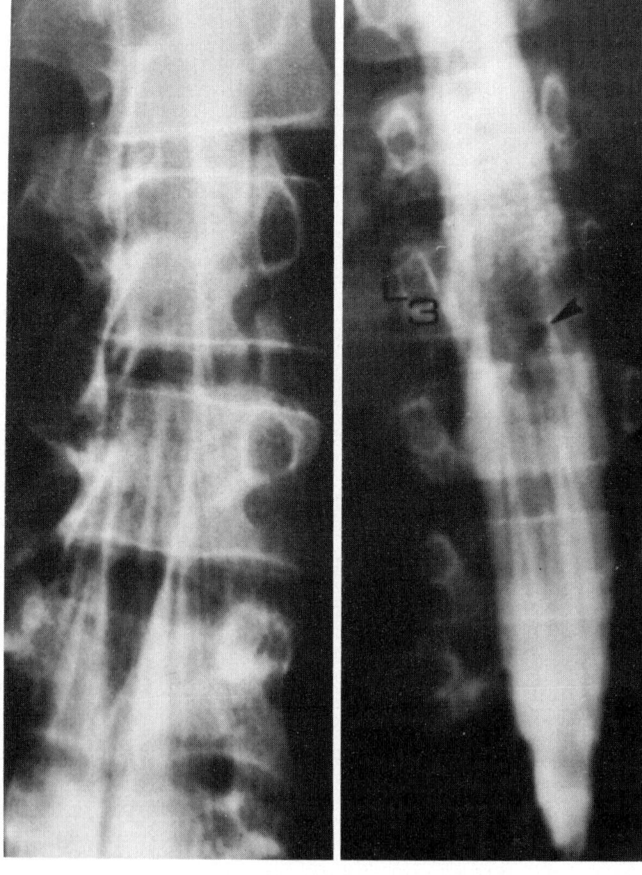

Fig. 59.16 (A) Metrizamide study in a patient with scoliotic spine clearly showing details of the cord and a low conus extending to L.4. (Dr V. L. McAllister.) (B) Low conus with a typical rounded radiolucent shadow (arrow) due to a tethering band. (Dr V. L. McAllister.)

INFLAMMATORY DISEASE

EXTRADURAL ABSCESS

Inflammatory disease of the spinal cord may arise either as direct extension of a local infective focus, such as vertebral osteomyelitis, or as a haematogenous infection from a distant lesion, such as a boil on the skin. The epidural space is vulnerable to involvement, either inflammatory or neoplastic, by virtue of its large venous plexus. In inflammatory disease the organisms concerned may be either tuberculous or pyogenic, the latter being more common. Tuberculous infection usually occurs by direct extension from an infected vertebra. Staphylococcal infection is usually of metastatic origin.

All grades of infection may occur, from diffuse suppuration or a localized abscess, to a chronic low-grade granuloma. An acute abscess constitutes one of the major neurosurgical emergencies. In addition to mechanical compression of the cord, the inflammatory changes involve its blood vessels, leading to thrombosis and infarction. Unless the compression is treated as an acute emergency and relieved rapidly, the paralysis may become irreversible. In contrast, a chronic granuloma may develop so slowly as to simulate compression by a tumour.

Radiographic film changes will obviously depend on the type and source of the infection. Thus an acute metastatic abscess will produce cord compression before any infective bone destruction has time to develop, and plain X-rays will be normal. In tuberculous cases, however, the onset is more gradual, the primary source is in the bone, and characteristic vertebral changes are seen on plain radiographs. The corresponding disc space is narrowed, with varying destruction and collapse of the adjacent bone of the vertebral bodies (Fig. 59.17A). A paravertebral soft-tissue mass may be evident in antero-posterior films. This is most easily seen in the thoracic area, as the abscess displaces outwards the mediastinal pleura and a silhouette is formed by air in the overlying lung (Fig. 59.17B).

Extradural abscesses are most frequently found in the thoracolumbar spine, and usually on the back of the cord, as the epidural space, occupied by fat and a rich network of veins, is largest in these areas. The epidural space is much narrower anteriorly and above the level of T.4.

Diagnosis is usually obvious in tuberculous cases, but myelography is necessary to show an extradural abscess in acute cases, owing to the absence of plain film changes.

DEGENERATIVE LESIONS

SPONDYLOSIS AND PROLAPSE OF THE INTERVERTEBRAL DISC

The clinical syndromes of sciatica and brachial neuralgia were the subject of much confused thinking until the

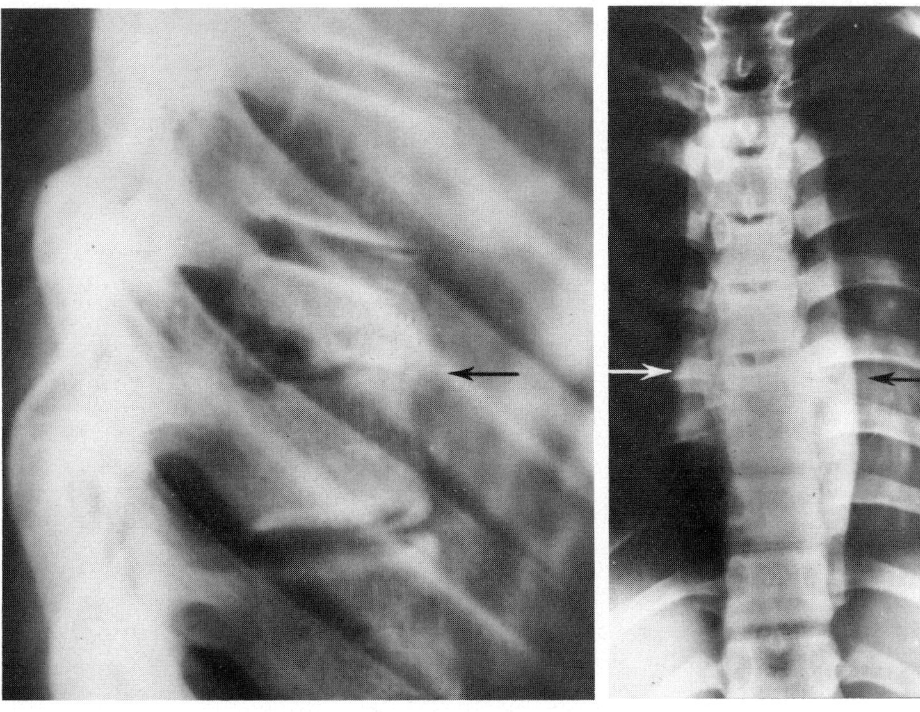

A B

Fig. 59.17 (A) Spinal tuberculosis. Lateral film showing destruction of the vertebral body and adjoining disc (←). (B) Spinal tuberculosis. Same case. Paravertebral soft tissue abscess shown in A.P. view (→ ←).

classic paper of Mixter and Barr in 1934, which drew attention to the fact that the commonest cause of these complaints is degeneration and herniation of the intervertebral disc into the spinal canal. Here it may compress the spinal cord or nerve roots, producing the characteristic neurological disturbances.

Two main types of syndrome are encountered. Firstly an acute disc prolapse, which is related to minor strain or injury, and usually occurs in an otherwise normal spine. The second type is part of the degenerative ageing process, is often widespread and is known as *spondylosis*.

Anatomy

Each intervertebral disc has three components.

1. *The articular plate*. This is a disc of hyaline cartilage attached to the upper and lower surface of the vertebral body.

2. *The annulus fibrosus*, a ring of fibrous tissue attached to the edge of the articular plate and containing in its central part.

3. *The nucleus pulposus*. This is a semigelatinous remnant of the notochord, composed of fibrous strands, connective tissue and cartilage cells.

The intervertebral discs are connected to the anterior and posterior longitudinal ligaments. In the thoracic area, they are also connected to the vertebral ends of the ribs, and in the cervical spine they have small prolongations into the neurocentral joints (of Luschka), which are of some clinical importance in the production of symptoms.

The intervertebral discs are thickest in the lumbar spine, and in the cervical and lumbar areas are wider anteriorly, maintaining the anatomical lordosis in these areas. They form a quarter of the height of the vertebral column.

With increasing age, there is loss of water from the nucleus pulposus, which becomes thinner and flatter.

Acute disc prolapse

Symptoms are generally only produced by posterior and postero-lateral disc herniations, when the extruded fragment causes compression of the spinal cord or nerve roots. Anterior and anterolateral disc protrusions usually cause few symptoms. Posterior disc herniation occurs more commonly where the annulus is thinner and attached to the weaker posterior longitudinal ligament. Some previous degeneration of the nucleus may also have occurred, as loss of fluid makes it more rigid and inelastic. A minor injury or strain, as in lifting or twisting, often precipitates the occurrence.

Following rupture of the annulus, there is escape of nuclear material into the vertebral canal. Rarely this fragment passes slightly upwards or downwards from the level of the intervertebral space and can simulate an extradural tumour. All degrees of compression of the

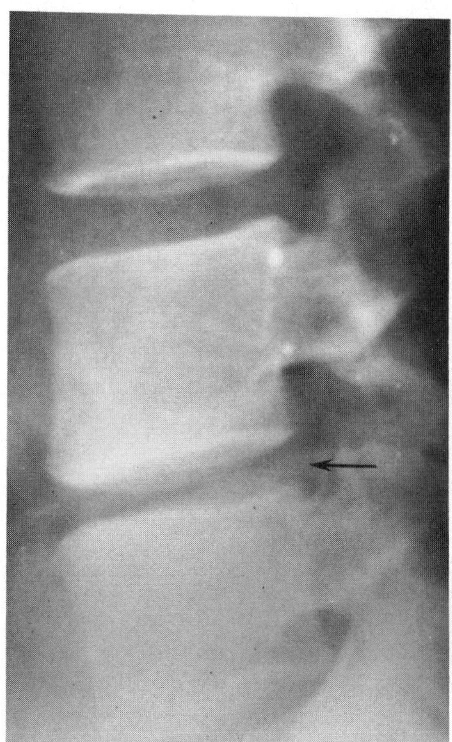

Fig. 59.18

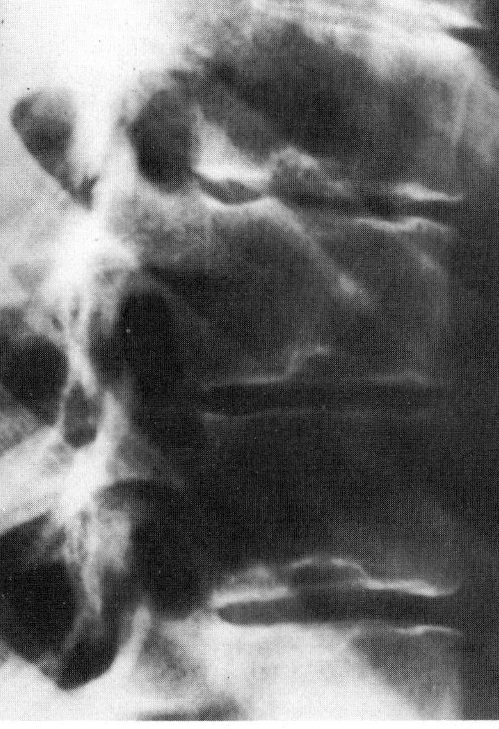

Fig. 59.19

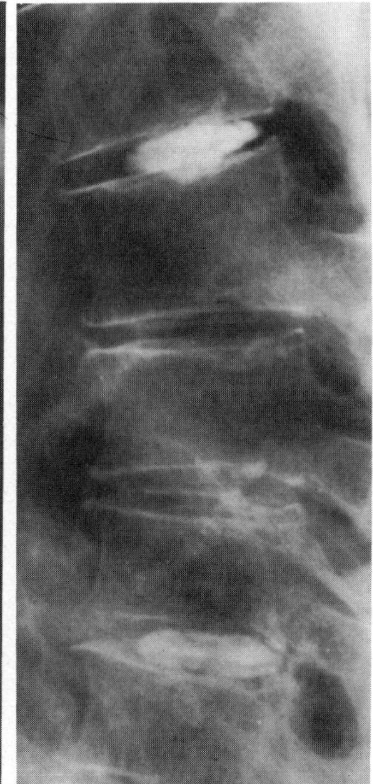

Fig. 59.20

Fig. 59.18 Acute disc prolapse (←). The intervertebral space between L.4 and 5 is narrowed. (The corresponding space at the lumbosacral junction is often anatomically narrow.)

Fig. 59.19 Schmorl's nodes.

Fig. 59.20 Calcification in intervertebral discs.

spinal cord or cauda equina may occur, up to complete spinal block; nerve roots may be affected alone or in combination.

Disc prolapse tends to occur in the most mobile parts of the spine such as the lower cervical and lower lumbar regions. Disc lesions are often found adjacent to developmentally or pathologically fused vertebrae. In the cervical spine, the discs between C.5, 6 and 7 are particularly vulnerable; prolapse of the C.5–6 disc will compress the C.6 nerve root. In the lumbar area, the discs between L.4 and 5 and S.1 are most frequently affected; prolapse of the lumbosacral disc compresses the S.1 root. Disc prolapse in the thoracic spine is relatively uncommon.

Radiological appearances. It is important to realize that plain X-rays may be entirely normal following an acute disc prolapse. More often, however, the affected disc space is narrowed (Fig. 59.18). This may appear as symmetrical narrowing of the intervertebral space, or on one side only, as following a lateral disc prolapse. The affected intervertebral space should be carefully compared with the adjoining disc spaces above and below, in both anteroposterior and lateral radiographs.

Narrowing of a disc space is also observed in early tuberculous infection, although in this condition the clinical presentation is different, and there tends to be associated bone destruction in the adjoining vertebral bodies.

In addition to narrowing of the disc space, some alteration of spinal alignment is frequently seen, either flattening of an anatomical lordosis, or scoliosis. This is due to reflex muscle spasm, which attempts to reduce tension in the nerve root which is stretched over the protruded disc.

Spondylosis

Long-standing herniation or degeneration of an intervertebral disc usually gives rise to some bony overgrowth in the adjoining vertebral margins, a condition known as spondylosis. Small tears in the annulus and posterior longitudinal ligament elevate the periosteum from the edge of the vertebral body and osteoblasts lay down new bone in the bulge so formed. Thus a fibrous or bony ridge may develop on the anterior aspect of the spinal canal at the level of the intervertebral space. This can compress either the spinal cord, or nerve roots, giving rise to the characteristic symptoms. Sometimes several discs are affected. As with acute disc herniation, these changes most commonly occur in the lower

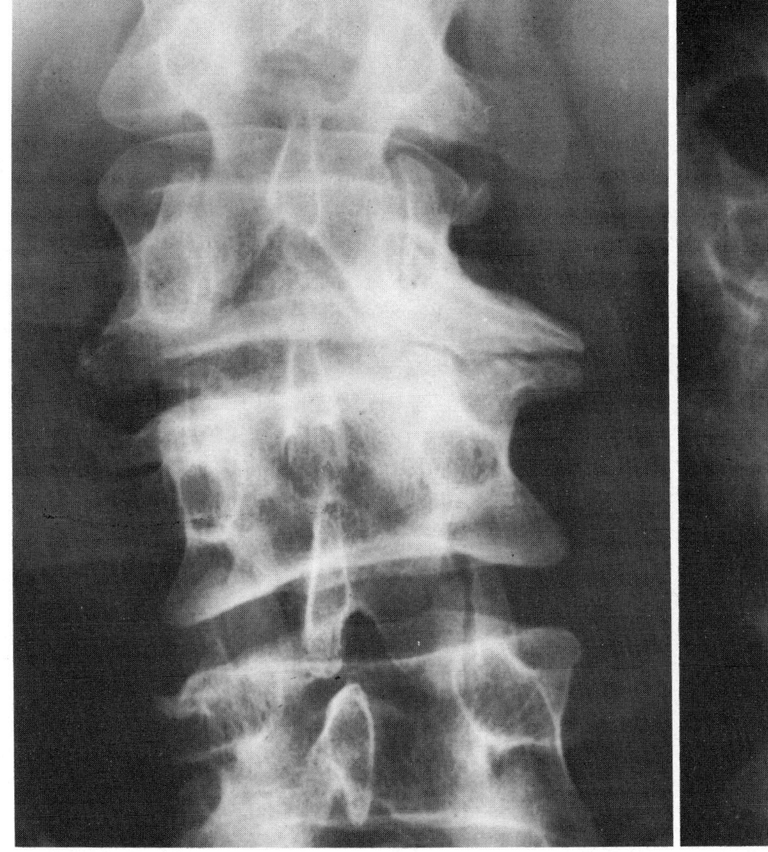

A

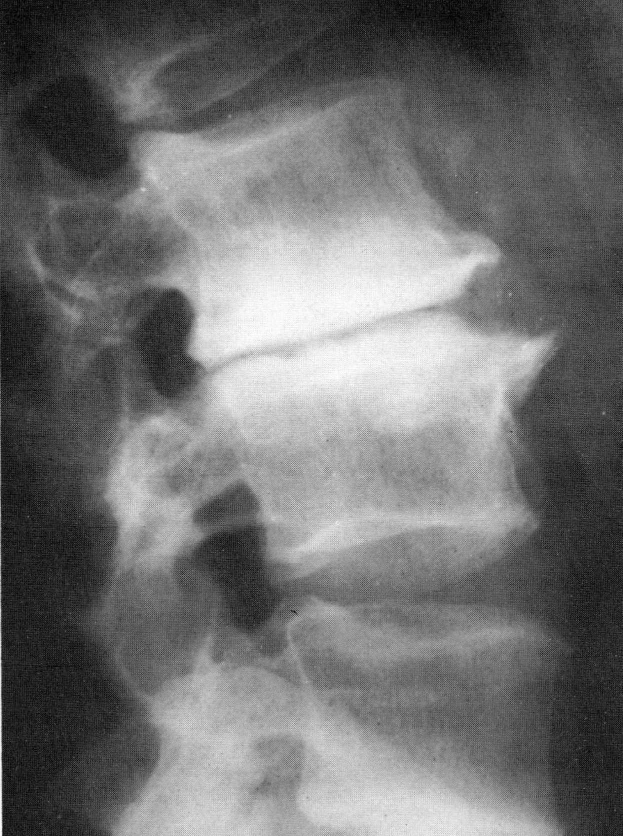

B

Fig. 59.21 (A and B) Spondylosis. Narrowing of the disc space, sclerosis of adjoining vertebral surfaces and osteophytic outgrowth.

cervical and lower lumbar segments. Long-standing abnormality of curvature, as in scoliosis, also predispose to the condition.

Occasionally, vertical prolapse of the nucleus pulposus into the adjoining vertebral body may take place. This occurs through a small traumatic or developmental defect in the cartilaginous end plate of the vertebral body, and is known as a *Schmorl's node*. It is most easily seen in lateral films and results in a small rounded defect in the cancellous bone of the vertebral body adjoining the disc space usually in the thoracic area (Fig. 59.19). This is sometimes bounded by a sclerotic margin of condensed bone. No nerve compression results, the condition is asymptomatic, and is of no clinical significance.

Calcification in the nucleus or annulus is seen only occasionally, and then most commonly in the thoracic spine (Fig. 59.20). Diffuse degeneration of the disc usually leads to a posterior bulging of the annulus rather than extrusion of disc material into the spinal canal.

Spondylolisthesis normally leads to an adjacent disc degeneration or prolapse, as vertebral subluxation inevitably results in a tear of the annulus fibrosus.

Radiological appearances. In addition to narrowing of the intervertebral space, an osteophytic rim may be seen on the posterior margin of the vertebral body at the level of the cartilage plate in lateral radiographs. This rim can extend laterally to the intervertebral foramen and cause compression of a nerve root at its exit from the spinal canal. Particularly in the cervical spine this may be clearly seen in oblique views. Sometimes some subchondral sclerosis and irregularity is seen in the surface of the vertebral body adjoining the disc space. Lateral films taken in flexion and extension may occasionally show some slight subluxation and abnormal mobility. It should be remembered that the intervertebral space at the lumbosacral junction is anatomically narrow when a transitional vertebra is present—either sacralization of L.5, or lumbarization of S.1, as with this condition the disc is often rudimentary. Such an anatomically narrow lumbosacral intervertebral space may be present, even if there is no transitional vertebra, and one should always be wary of making a diagnosis of disc prolapse at this site without the additional evidence of osteophytic lipping or bony sclerosis.

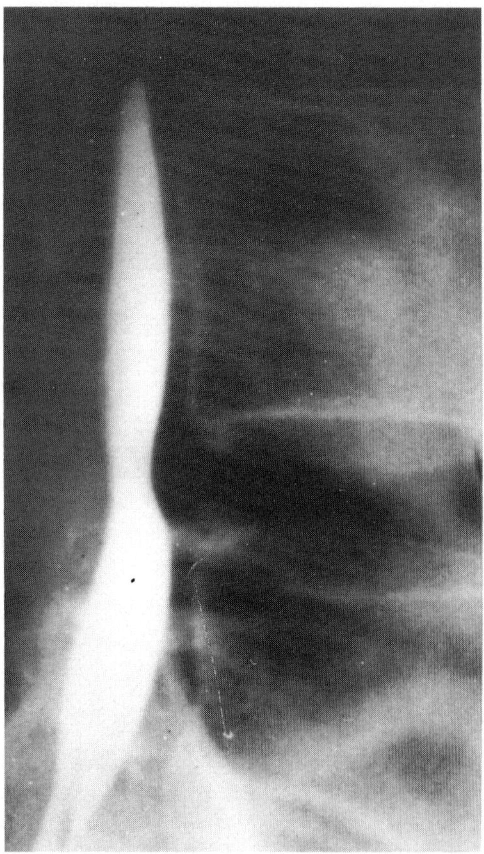

Fig. 59.22

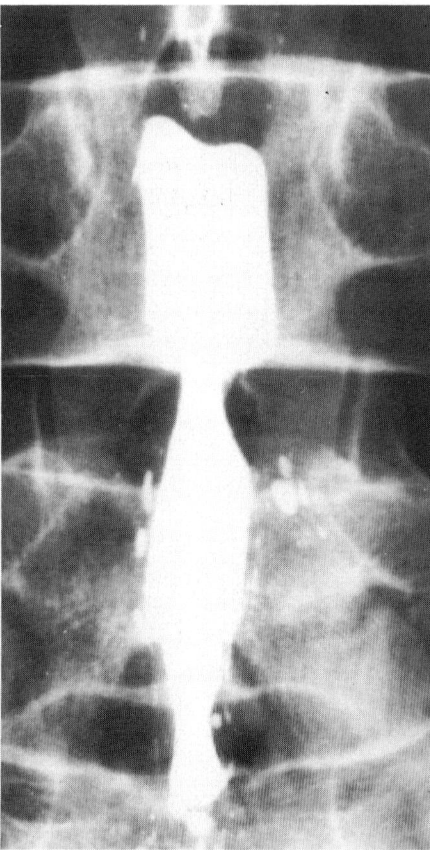

Fig. 59.23

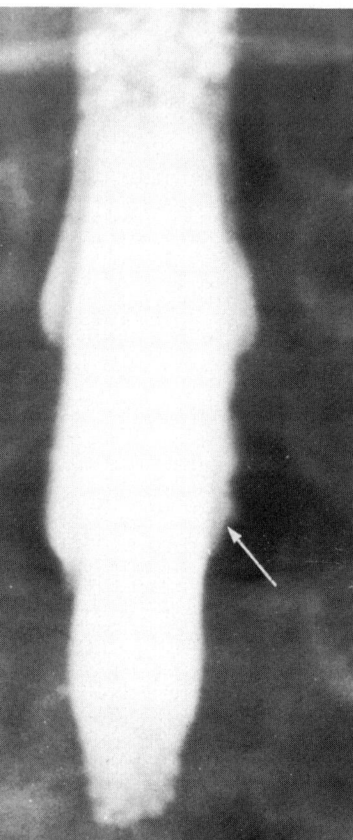

Fig. 59.24

Fig. 59.22 Posterior disc protrusion in lateral view. The contrast column is indented at the level of the intervertebral space.

Fig. 59.23 Disc prolapse in A.P. view in same patient. The contrast column is constricted at the level of the intervertebral space.

Fig. 59.24 Posterolateral lumbar disc prolapse (↖). The root sheath is obliterated. Lateral film normal.

Myodil myelography

Plain X-rays only provide indirect evidence of disc prolapse. Myelography provides more precise confirmation of this condition, and shows the extent to which the spinal cord and nerve roots are compressed. Anterior or anterolateral indentations are shown in the theca when the subarachnoid space is outlined by positive contrast.

Myelography is frequently performed as a preoperative measure, both to confirm a clinical diagnosis and to give accurate localization of the lesion. Sometimes an additional unsuspected lesion may be shown, and the myelogram must then be interpreted in conjunction with the clinical presentation.

The osteophytic overgrowth round the disc margins found in spondylosis produces the same myelographic abnormalities as a herniated disc, and is essentially a chronic form of the same lesion.

There are four principal myelographic signs of disc prolapse, any one of which is alone sufficient for the diagnosis, provided it is constantly present:

1. In lateral films an indentation is seen on the anterior border of the Myodil column at the level of the affected disc. This sign is seen with posterior rather than lateral disc prolapse (Fig. 59.22).
2. In the anterior view, an hour-glass constriction or horizontal defect is seen with posterior disc prolapse (Fig. 59.23). Lateral disc prolapse produces a lateral indentation in the Myodil column.
3. In the anterior view there may be obliteration, or deformity, of the affected nerve root sheath (Fig. 59.24).
4. In severe cases, complete spinal block can occur.

There are certain special features in different regions of the spine.

Lumbar disc lesions

With posterolateral disc protrusions, the prone lateral film may show no abnormality. This is because overlying Myodil on the normal side obscures the filling defect round the compressed nerve root. Oblique views are of value in confirming root sheath deformities and thecal indentations which appear doubtful on anteroposterior films.

The extradural space becomes wider at the lower end of the spinal canal as the subarachnoid space tapers to its caudal cul de sac. Thus there may be an increased gap in lateral films between the Myodil column and the posterior surfaces of L.4 and 5 and S.1. Hence, a small symptomatic disc protrusion causes little deformity of the theca.

In the same way, it would be impossible to show prolapse of a lumbosacral disc if the subarachnoid space ends at L.5, which is an occasional anatomical variant.

A large disc prolapse may produce a complete spinal block. This is normally readily distinguished from an extradural tumour, since it is shown to be lying anteriorly at the level of the intervertebral space. When, however, an extruded fragment of disc migrates upwards or downwards, it causes an obstruction above or below an intervertebral space and is indistinguishable from an extradural tumour.

Cervical disc lesions. The cervical cord occupies most of the space in its spinal canal. The subarachnoid space is relatively narrow and small disc protrusions or osteophytes thus give rise to relatively severe symptoms. Central disc protrusions or the bony bars of spondylosis cause an indentation of the anterior margin of the Myodil column and are usually best shown in lateral films (Fig. 59.25).

Occasionally the posterior margin of the Myodil column may show multiple indentations particularly when the head is extended. This is due to thickening and buckling inwards of the ligamentum flavum due to the reduced height between the bodies of the vertebrae (Fig. 59.26). This posterior compression often produces a spurious spinal block at myelography when the table is tilted head-downwards with the head extended. If the head is then flexed, this obstruction is usually relieved. This is readily seen at fluoroscopy.

Symptomatic disc protrusion is more likely with a congenitally small spinal canal. In this respect a sagittal diameter of 14 mm or less should be regarded with suspicion.

Lateral disc protrusions or osteophytes are usually well shown in anteroposterior films and oblique views contribute very little. Indentations or complete breaks in the Myodil column may be seen on one or both sides, usually without spinal block.

Thoracic disc lesions. Prolapse of a thoracic intervertebral disc is relatively uncommon. When present, it usually occurs in the lower thoracic spine, the area of greatest mobility. It is frequently associated with some calcification of the disc at the corresponding intervertebral space. Scheuermann's disease or a dorsal kyphosis predispose to its occurrence.

Demonstration of the anterior part of the thoracic spinal canal with the patient prone is difficult owing to the upward convexity of the thoracic curve. The technique of obtaining lateral myelographic films has been described earlier. It is to be anticipated that diagnosis will become easier with the introduction of the newer water-soluble contrast media.

A precise anatomical diagnosis of site is of considerable importance to the surgeon, who may otherwise employ a posterior approach when a lateral approach is necessary. The diagnosis is greatly facilitated when there is a partial or complete spinal block. In the latter case, it may not be possible to distinguish the lesion from an extradural or on occasions intramedullary tumour. Filling defects are frequently seen in the thoracic Myodil column, and these

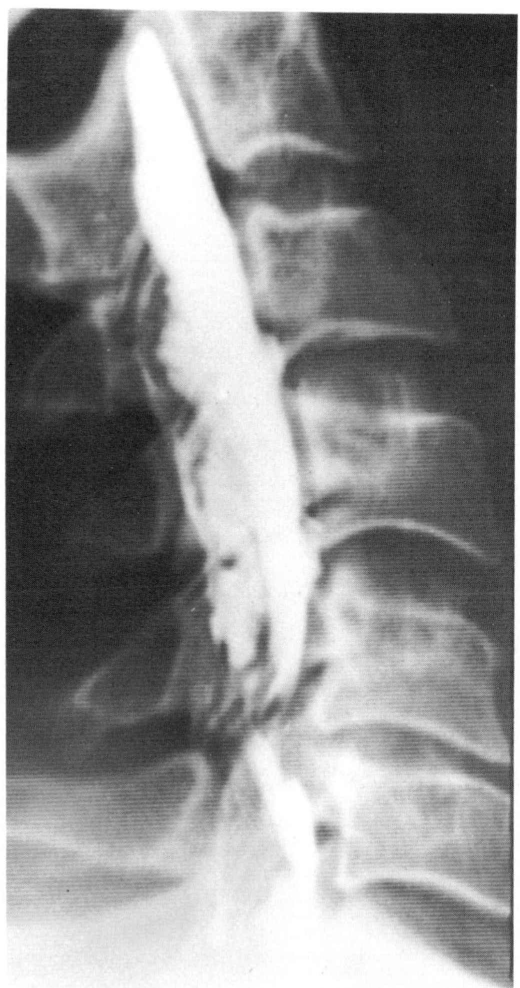

Fig. 59.25

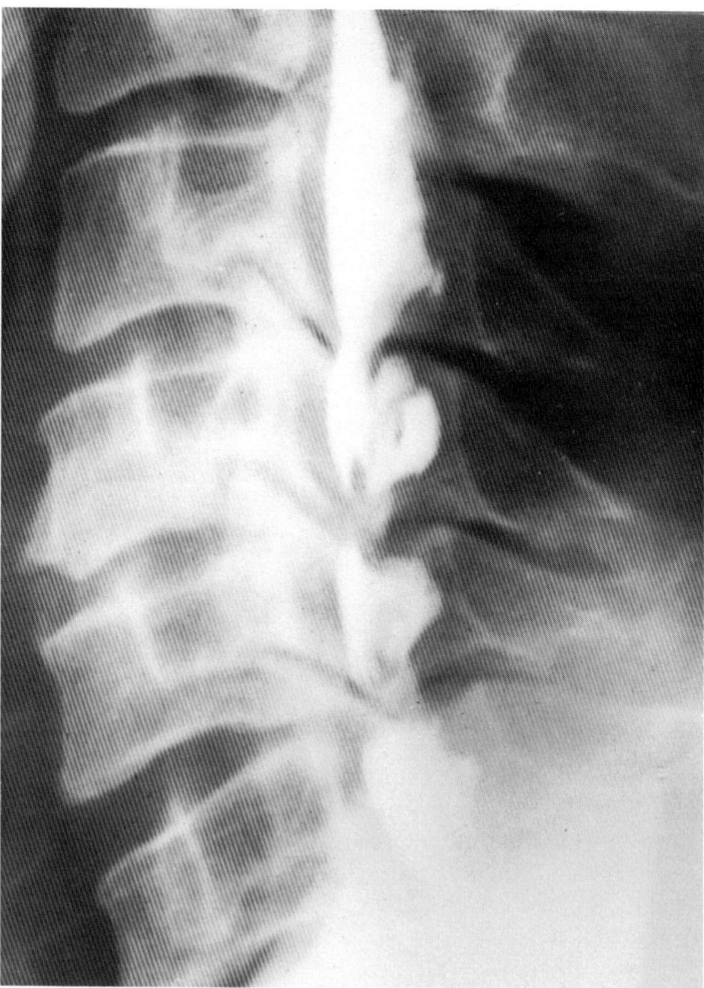

Fig. 59.26

Fig. 59.25 Cervical spondylosis. Compression of theca by bony bar.

Fig. 59.26 Cervical spondylosis. Indentation of the contrast column posteriorly by thickened ligamentum flavum.

must be constant and reproducible before a confident diagnosis of a lesion can be made. Otherwise, some negative explorations will result.

Water soluble myelography

Because of its permeability and the fact that it opacifies the c.s.f., metrizamide completely outlines the root sheathes, and shows in great detail the shape and course of the nerve roots of the cauda equina. For this reason it is now replacing Myodil as contrast medium. Normal appearances are shown in Figure 59.5A and C. Antero-posterior films with the patient in lateral decubitus using a horizontal beam give a particularly good demonstration of the dependent root pockets.

Prolapse or symptomatic degeneration of an intravertebral disc may cause compression with medial displacement, elevation or complete obliteration of the root sheath (Figs 59.27 and 59.28). The nerve root is often displaced medially.

It should be remembered that a nerve root will be compressed by a disc one space above its emergence from the spinal canal. Thus prolapse of the L.4–5 disc will compress the L.5 root, and the S.1 root will be compressed by the lumbosacral disc.

Most published series report a diagnostic accuracy of 90 to 95 per cent acuracy in lumbar disc disease, using water-soluble contrast media. This is appreciably better than the results obtained with oily compounds.

SPINAL STENOSIS

In this condition, the spinal canal is developmentally narrow (Fig. 59.29). Its capacity is reduced, and any further intrusion on the canal, even though small, produces disproportionally severe symptoms. The lumbar area is commonly affected, and symptoms result from compression of the cauda equina. The cervical area is also frequently affected, as noted above.

The lumbar canal is abnormally narrow if lateral

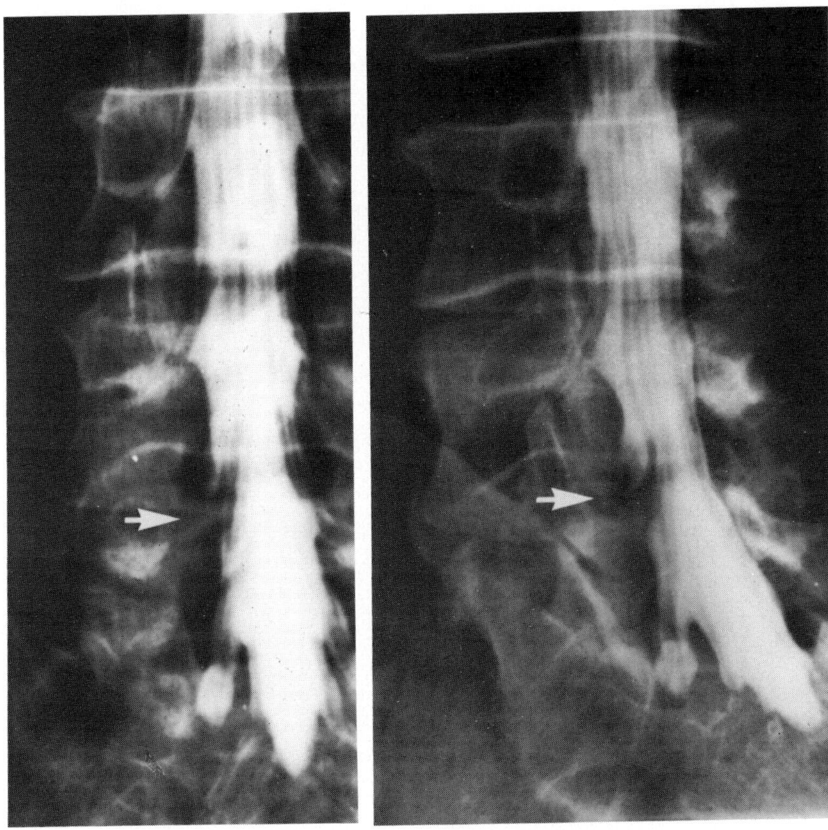

Fig. 59.27 *Fig. 59.28*

Fig. 59.27 Water-soluble radiculogram. The first sacral root and sheath are compressed by a lateral disc protrusion in the lumbosacral junction (→). A.P. view.

Fig. 59.28 Oblique view of same case.

films show its diameter, in the anteroposterior plane, to be less than 15 mm. In anterior views the sagittal plane of the apophysial joints may lie close to the midline, although the interpedicular distance may be normal.

Symptoms are precipitated by relatively minor aggravating factors—small disc protrusions, spondylotic bars or osteophytic overgrowth of the articular facets. The latter produce narrowing of the lateral recesses, and nerve root compression. There is often inward protrusion of the ligamentum flavum and thickened laminae.

In spondylolisthesis, either with or without laminar defects, subluxation will produce stenosis without concomitant disc herniation.

Symptoms. These are unusual and may be characteristic. They consist of pain in the back, with or without signs of cord or root compression, and the so-called *intermittent claudication of the cauda equina.* In spinal stenosis, the dural sac is under pressure. This compression prevents hyperaemia of the cauda equina which normally follows exercise. Pain, numbness and weakness of the legs is precipitated by walking and relieved by rest. Later pain may occur at rest, but is not affected by coughing or sneezing. There are usually no signs of peripheral vascular disease, but arteriography may be requested in error. The diagnosis is dependent on myelography.

Back pain is more severe than with a simple disc protrusion. It is unremitting and progressive, often bilateral, with femoral and sciatic distribution. Progressive paraparesis and sphincter disturbance may lead to a tumour of the cauda equina being suspected.

Diagnosis. The condition may be frequently suspected on examination of the plain films (v.s.). In addition to narrowing of the anteroposterior diameter of the canal, the plane of the intervertebral joints may lie close to the midline. This narrowing is accentuated if these joints are arthritic, with sclerosis and osteophytic overgrowth. More recently it has been shown that such narrowing of the spinal canal can be shown in clear cross-sectional detail by computed tomography when a body scanner is available.

Myelography is of obvious importance in diagnosis, often showing a spinal block of extrathecal type. Two punctures may be needed to show the upper and lower

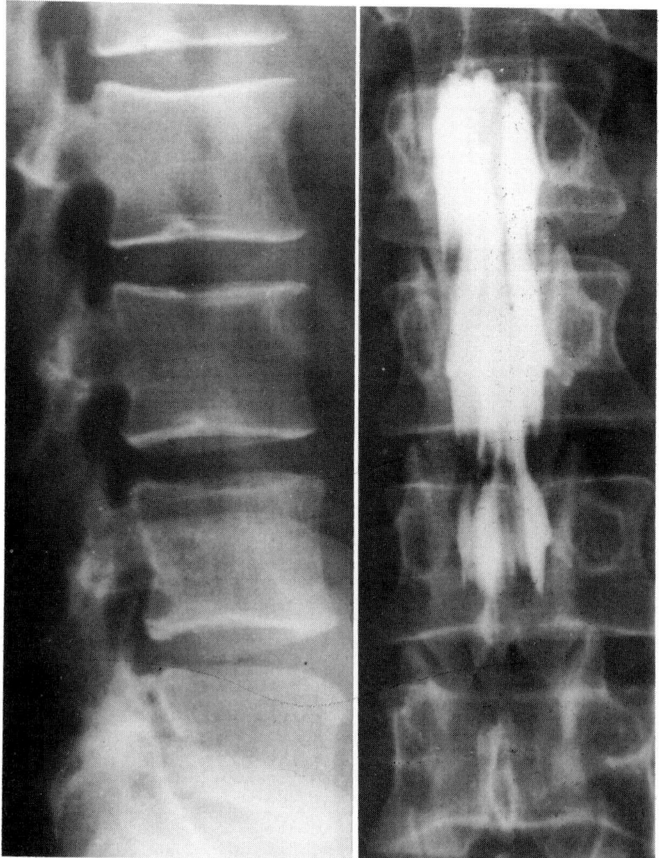

Fig. 59.29 *Fig. 59.30*

Fig. 59.29 Spinal stenosis. Narrowing of anteroposterior diameter of lower lumbar canal.

Fig. 59.30 Same case as Figure 59.29. Complete block to caudal flow at level of L.3 with partial obstruction between L.2 and L.3. Symptoms precipitated by sequestrated disc L.3–4.

borders of the obstruction. Lumbar puncture may be difficult because the interlaminar space is narrowed, and the subarachnoid space tight due to external compression. These difficulties may result in subdural injection of contrast, and it may be necessary to make a further injection by cisternal puncture.

Myelography often shows flattening of the column, with posterolateral and posterior indentations. Complete block usually occurs at or near a disc space. Sometimes partial obstruction occurs at several levels, usually upper and mid-lumbar (Fig. 59.30). Shallow lateral recesses may indicate nerve root compression. Narrowing of the antero-posterior diameter of the canal results in compression of the medial roots.

Treatment by laminectomy and decompression usually relieves symptoms. At operation, the dura is tight, and the narrowed canal is seen. Adequate decompression is necessary, both longitudinally and laterally, including removal of superior articular facets to unroof the whole of the lateral recess.

DISCOGRAPHY

This technique outlines the anatomy of the intervertebral disc by direct injection of contrast medium into it. It is most commonly used in the lumbar area, but in some centres is also employed in the cervical spine, using a posterolateral approach.

Its use occasionally provides additional diagnostic information, particularly when the clinical presentation does not correlate with the myelographic findings. In problem cases, it may assist a surgical decision on the need for exploration.

Under X-ray control, needles of 21 gauge are positioned against the appropriate intervertebral spaces. Through these needles, further needles of 26 gauge are advanced directly into the disc substance, and approximately 1 ml of water soluble contrast is injected under fluoroscopic control.

The normal disc is outlined as an oval or biconvex shadow occupying the central third of the intervertebral space. Following rupture of the annulus, or disc degeneration, the contrast outlines an irregular narrowed area occupying the whole of the intervertebral space (Fig. 59.31) which may or may not project into the spinal canal.

TUMOURS

Tumours in the spinal canal are divided into three main groups—*extradural, intradural extramedullary*, and *intramedullary*. Myelography is frequently necessary to distinguish between these three groups, and the combination of the plain film and myelographic appearances frequently enables a precise pathological diagnosis to be made.

A wide variety of tumours, both benign and malignant, occur in the spinal canal. Neurological symptoms are produced by compression of the cord or spinal nerves.

The largest single group of spinal tumours are secondary deposits involving the extradural compartment and among these the site of the primary lesion is most commonly the breast or bronchus.

In only a minority of spinal tumours—less than 20 per cent—are changes seen in plain radiographs, when there is evidence of bone erosion or destruction by the expansive process. With intraspinal tumours the medial border of the pedicle may appear concave in antero-posterior films, instead of having a normal convex or flat profile. With a malignant tumour, the pedicle may be destroyed completely. The expansion of the vertebral canal may be shown by widening of the interpedicular distance in anteroposterior views, and occasionally by concavity of the posterior border of the vertebral body in lateral radiographs. In so-called dumb-bell tumours

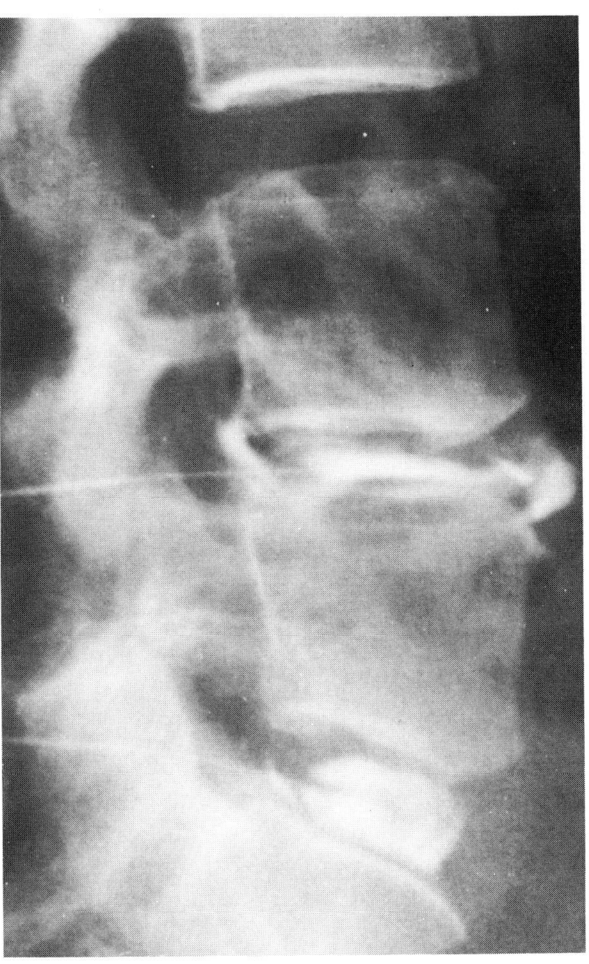
A

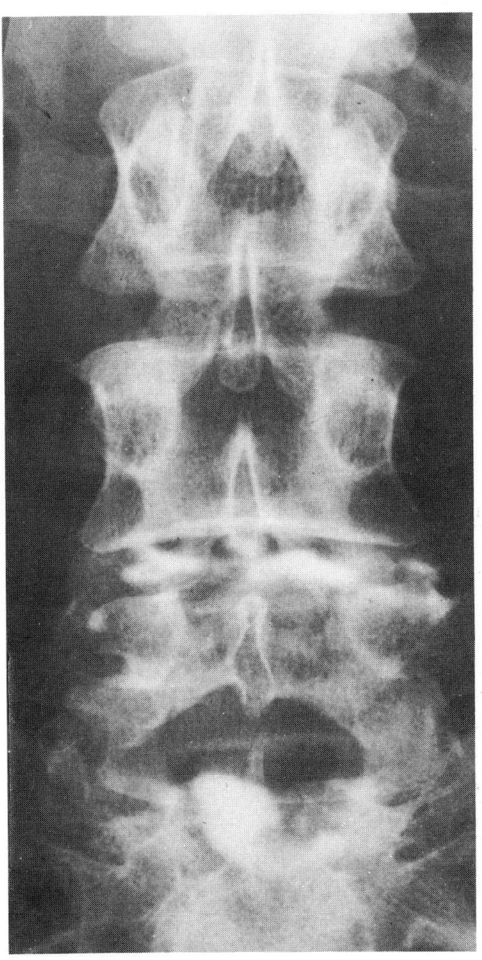
B

Fig. 59.31 Discogram. Ruptured annulus L4/5. Normal disc at lumbosacral junction. (A) Lateral view. (B) A.P. view.

the erosion may be confined to the intervertebral foramen—these tumours are usually neurofibromas.

In addition to local expansion of the spinal canal, changes should be sought in the surrounding structures. There may be abnormal sclerosis or destruction in the corresponding vertebral body or appendages. There may be destruction of the vertebral disc, and there may be a paravertebral soft-tissue mass.

Myelography contributes much to the precise diagnosis of tumours occurring in the spinal canal. Not only may the degree of spinal cord or nerve root compression be shown directly, but the size, shape and limits of the mass may be defined accurately. Myelography usually shows whether the mass is extradural, intradural extramedullary, or intramedullary. In conjunction with plain film changes it may permit an accurate pathological diagnosis to be made. Finally, when the clinical diagnosis is in doubt, myelography is of value in distinguishing between a tumour and degenerative or ischaemic spinal cord disease as the cause of symptoms.

EXTRADURAL TUMOURS

These may be either benign or malignant; the latter group is by far the most common. In addition to these, which are mainly secondary deposits, several non-neoplastic conditions may give rise to a mass in the extradural space and cause cord compression. These include fractures, prolapsed intervertebral disc (Fig. 59.32A, B and C) and spondylosis, extradural abscess, dural cysts and Paget's disease.

Benign tumours. Primary extradural tumours are rare, and benign neoplasms in the extradural space usually result from extension of a tumour originating in the intradural compartment. This group includes *meningiomas*, *neurofibromas*, *dermoids* and *lipomas*. A meningioma is normally intradural, and does not erode bone, but when extradural extension occurs, bone erosion may take place and the tumour may resemble a neurofibroma. An extradural haematoma is a relatively rare cause of cord compression. It is almost invariably due either to injury, or to haemorrhage from a spinal

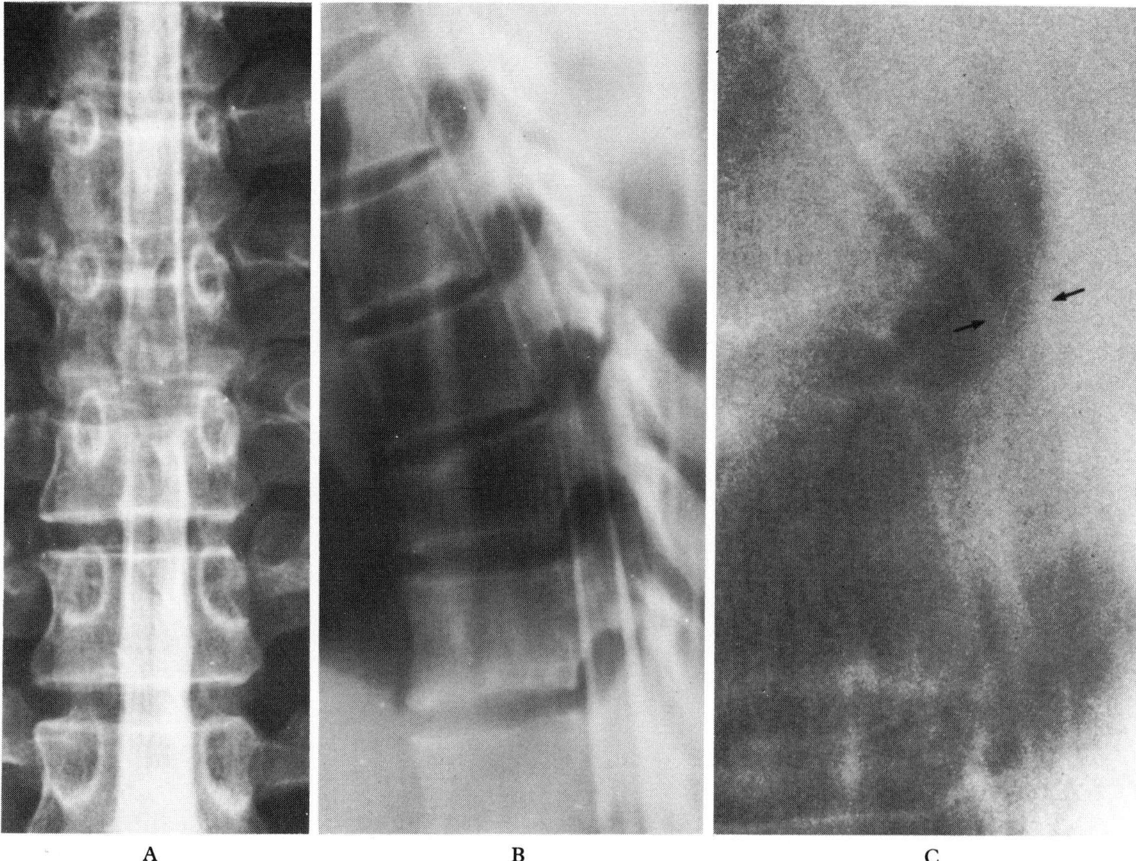

Fig. 59.32A and B Fracture of thoracic vertebral body and lamina. Compression of theca and cord outlined by metrizamide. (A) Antero-posterior view. (B) Lateral view. (C) Prolapsed thoracic disc. Theca displaced posteriorly and cord compressed (arrows).

angioma. Benign bone tumours such as chondroma or osteoma arising from a vertebra may implicate the vertebral canal or foramina. Perhaps more common is cord compression due to Paget's disease or other bone malacia. In these conditions, there may be some vertical compression of the abnormal softened bone, causing flattening of the vertebral body and sometimes constriction of the vertebral canal. This may be shown by a convex bulging of the posterior margin of the vertebral body in lateral films.

Extradural cyst. An arachnoid cyst or hygroma containing cerebrospinal fluid is a rare cause of spinal cord compression. This is essentially a pulsion diverticulum, with prolapse of a fluid-containing meningeal cyst into the extradural space. The condition is most likely to be found in the thoracic area, with symptoms of gradual cord compression usually appearing in the second decade. Transmitted pulsatile pressure may cause expansion of the spinal canal over several segments, with thinning and flattening of pedicles and widening of the interpedicular distance in anteroposterior films, and scalloping of the posterior vertebral margins in lateral views.

Its true nature is shown at myelography. Contrast may enter and remain within the cyst cavity, whilst the remaining subarachnoid contrast traverses the spinal canal on tilting the table. To demonstrate this phenomenon, it may be necessary to screen the patient in prone, supine and oblique positions, depending on the position of the ostium of the cyst.

Malignant tumours. The majority of lesions in this group are due to metastatic deposits, usually carcinoma or less commonly, reticulosis. As mentioned earlier, the primary neoplasm is most commonly found in the breast or bronchus. The extradural space is implicated either by extension from a vertebral metastasis or directly from the blood stream. Cord compression may occur with or without radiological evidence of vertebral metastasis. This particularly applies when the secondary deposit originates in the vertebral arch, as minor degrees of bone destruction are difficult to recognize in this situation. Evidence of vertebral involvement is usually shown by erosion and destruction of pedicles (Fig. 59.33A), areas of abnormal sclerosis, or more commonly destruction, in the vertebral bodies and appendages. These should be carefully sought for in both antero-posterior and lateral films. In cases of doubt, coned localized views or tomographic cuts are frequently helpful. Pathological compression fractures are often seen. With metastatic malignant disease, the disc space is usually normal, a point of the greatest importance

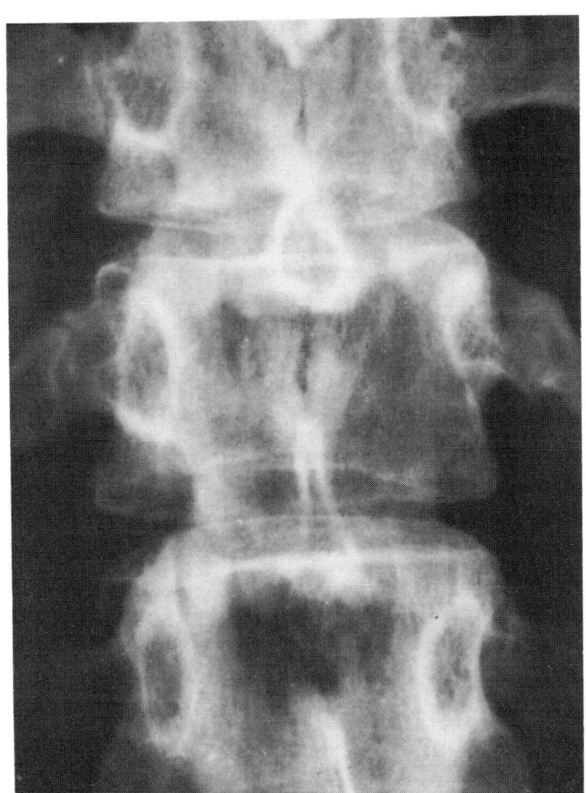

A

in the differentiation from tuberculous infection (Fig. 59.33B and C).

The extradural space may be the initial site of metastasis, owing to its large venous plexus and lymphatic connections. In Hodgkin's disease, lymphosarcoma, or other reticuloses, direct infiltration along lymphatics occurs from paravertebral glands in the thorax or abdomen. Sometimes a malignant extradural mass may extend beyond the confines of the spinal canal, causing a paravertebral soft-tissue shadow. Conversely, a malignant paravertebral tumour, such as a bronchial carcinoma, can erode adjacent bone and invade the extradural space.

Primary vertebral tumours, although rare, usually cause compression of the cord or nerve roots. Of this group, two of the most important are so-called 'solitary' myeloma, and chordoma.

Myeloma causes vertebral destruction and collapse. It may also extend laterally, produce a paravertebral soft-

Fig. 59.33A Secondary carcinoma. Destruction of left pedicle of T.12. Compare normal pedicle on right side.

Fig. 59.33(B and C) Hodgkin's disease. Sclerotic bony involvement with pathological compression fracture. Note preservation of disc spaces.

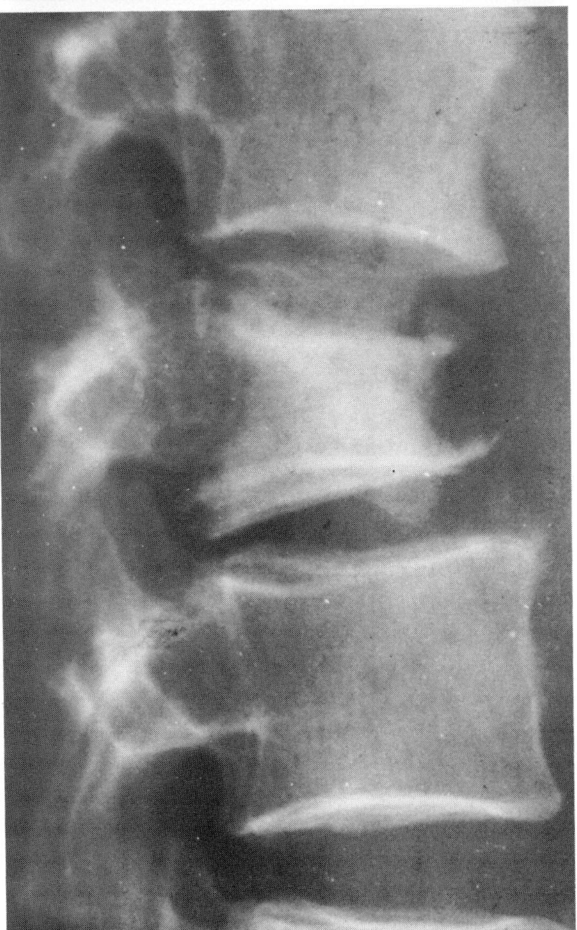

B

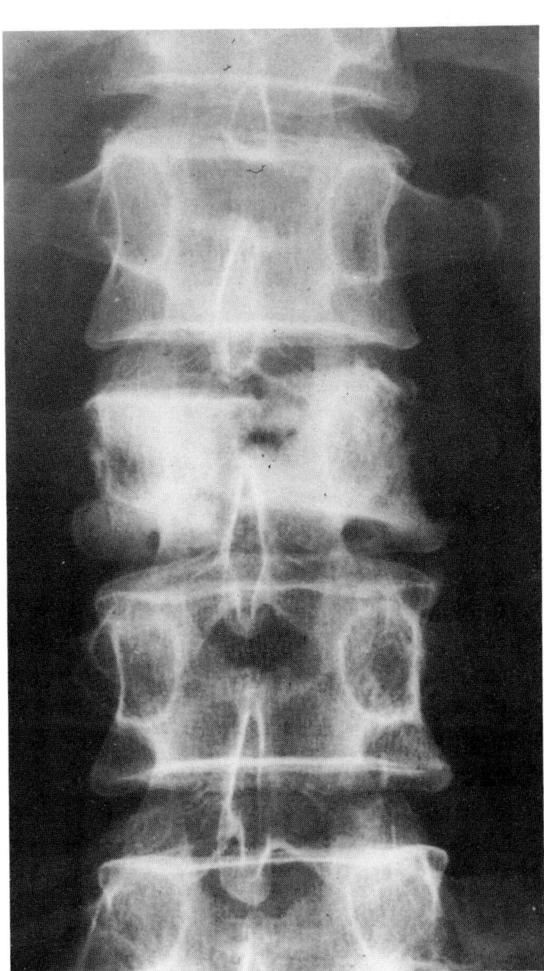

C

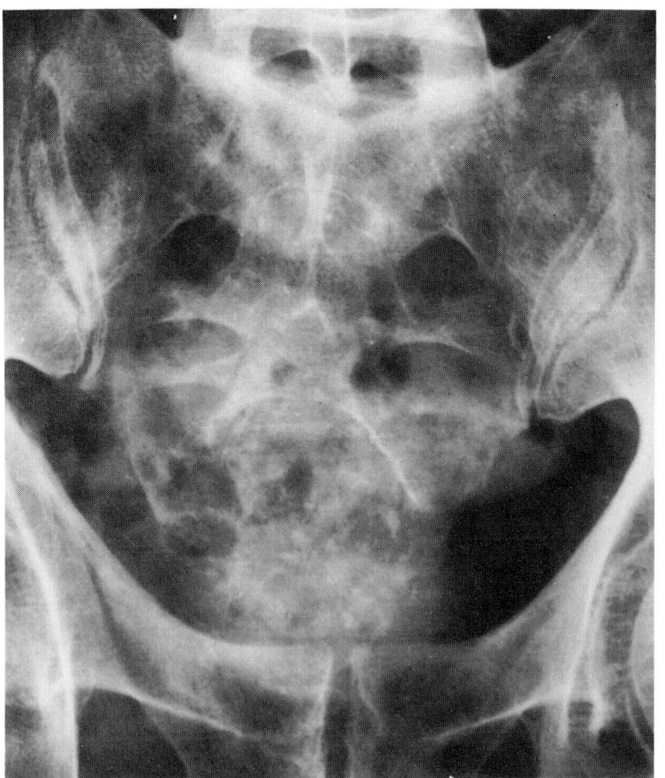

tissue shadow on anteroposterior films. These appearances can be indistinguishable from tuberculous osteomyelitis. In myeloma, however, the changes progress much more rapidly, and the tumour is unlikely to penetrate the intervertebral discs and invade adjoining vertebrae.

A *chordoma* is a locally malignant tumour arising from embryonic remnants of the notochord. Although it may occur anywhere in the spinal column, it is commonest in the sacrum or in the region of the clivus. Growth is slow, and the tumour does not metastasize, although it invades local structures. The radiological signs are a well-defined area of bone destruction, with an associated soft-tissue mass which enlarges both anteriorly and posteriorly from the vertebral body displacing nearby structures including the spinal cord (Fig. 59.34). Calcification is sometimes seen in the tumour.

At *myelography*, extradural masses displace the theca away from the bony wall of the spinal canal. In anteroposterior films, the contrast column normally extends to the medial border of the pedicles. An extradural tumour will produce a gap between contrast and the pedicles

Fig. 59.34 Chordoma. Well-defined area of destruction in the sacrum with patchy calcification in the associated soft-tissue tumour mass.

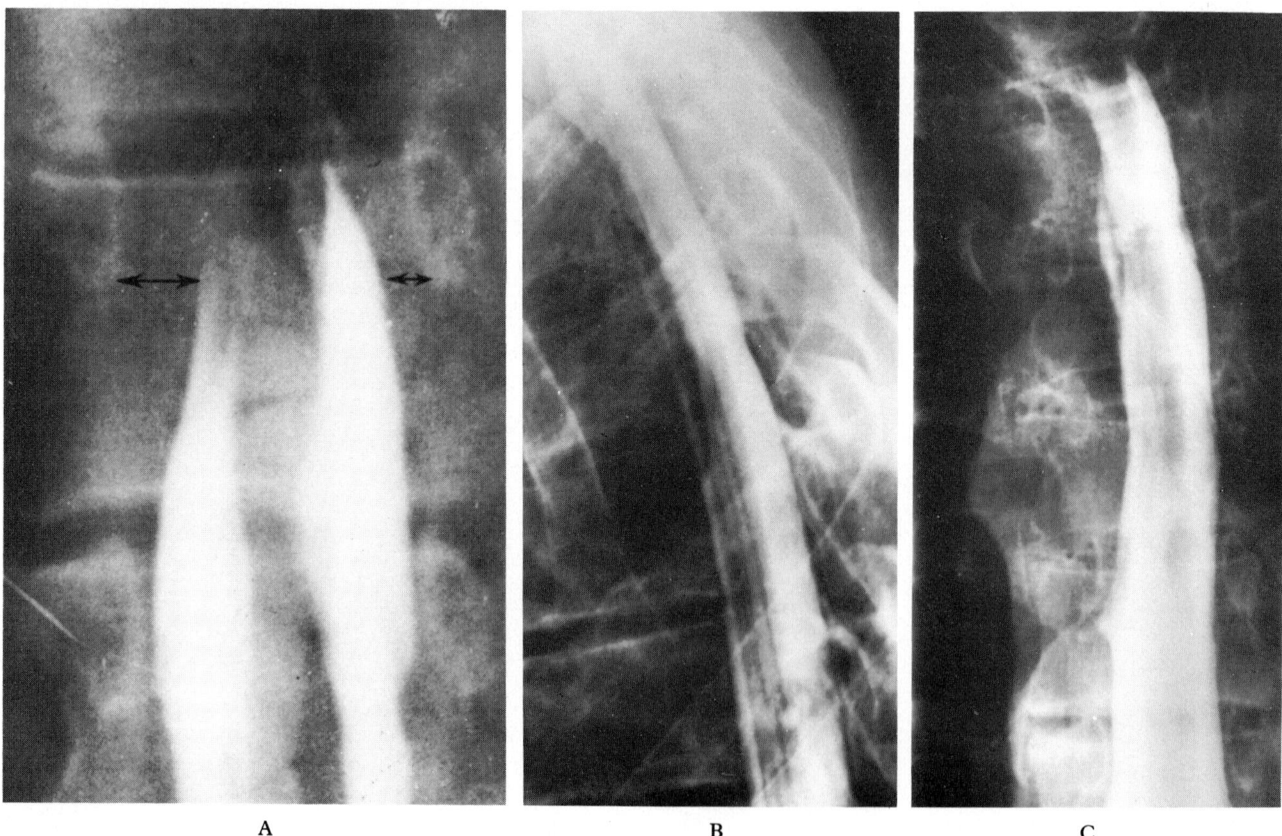

Fig. 59.35A Extradural tumour causing spinal block. Note displacement of theca away from pedicles by tumour mass (↔) and central cord impression.

Fig. 59.35(B and C) Metrizamide column displaced from pedicles over several segments by lymphoma deposit.

(Fig. 59.35). In lateral films, the column may be displaced away from the vertebral body or disc.

Small masses may cause no obstruction, but show varying displacements of contrast from the pedicles, vertebral bodies or neural arches. When obstruction is complete a horizontal cut-off of contrast is shown at the level of the lesion. In lateral films, its edge is often serrated by compressed nerve roots, and had been likened to a bundle of sticks.

INTRADURAL EXTRAMEDULLARY TUMOURS

In contrast to extradural neoplasms, intradural tumours are usually benign. By far the commonest are meningiomas and neurofibromas. Other rare causes are dermoids, lipomas and metastatic gliomas and secondary carcinomas which have seeded through the cerebrospinal fluid.

Meningiomas. These are well-defined, slow-growing tumours which compress and indent the cord. Because of this, there is often a long history of symptoms, as with intracranial meningiomas. Plain radiographs are usually normal, bone erosion being rare unless, as already mentioned, there is extradural spread of the tumour. If pedicle flattening is seen, only one pedicle is usually involved. Meningiomas are usually found in the thoracic spine. They are rare in the lumbar or cervical region except near the foramen magnum. For some unknown reason there is a strong female sex incidence—over 80 per cent.

Spinal meningiomas are firm, and they frequently contain small grains of calcification. Very rarely this calcification is dense, and may be demonstrable on plain X-rays. In cases of doubt, such intraspinal calcification can be confirmed by tomography (Fig. 59.36). The differential diagnosis will then be between a meningioma or calcified prolapsed disc. The latter will usually be seen opposite an intervertebral space, which may be narrowed, with osteophytic lipping of the vertebral margins.

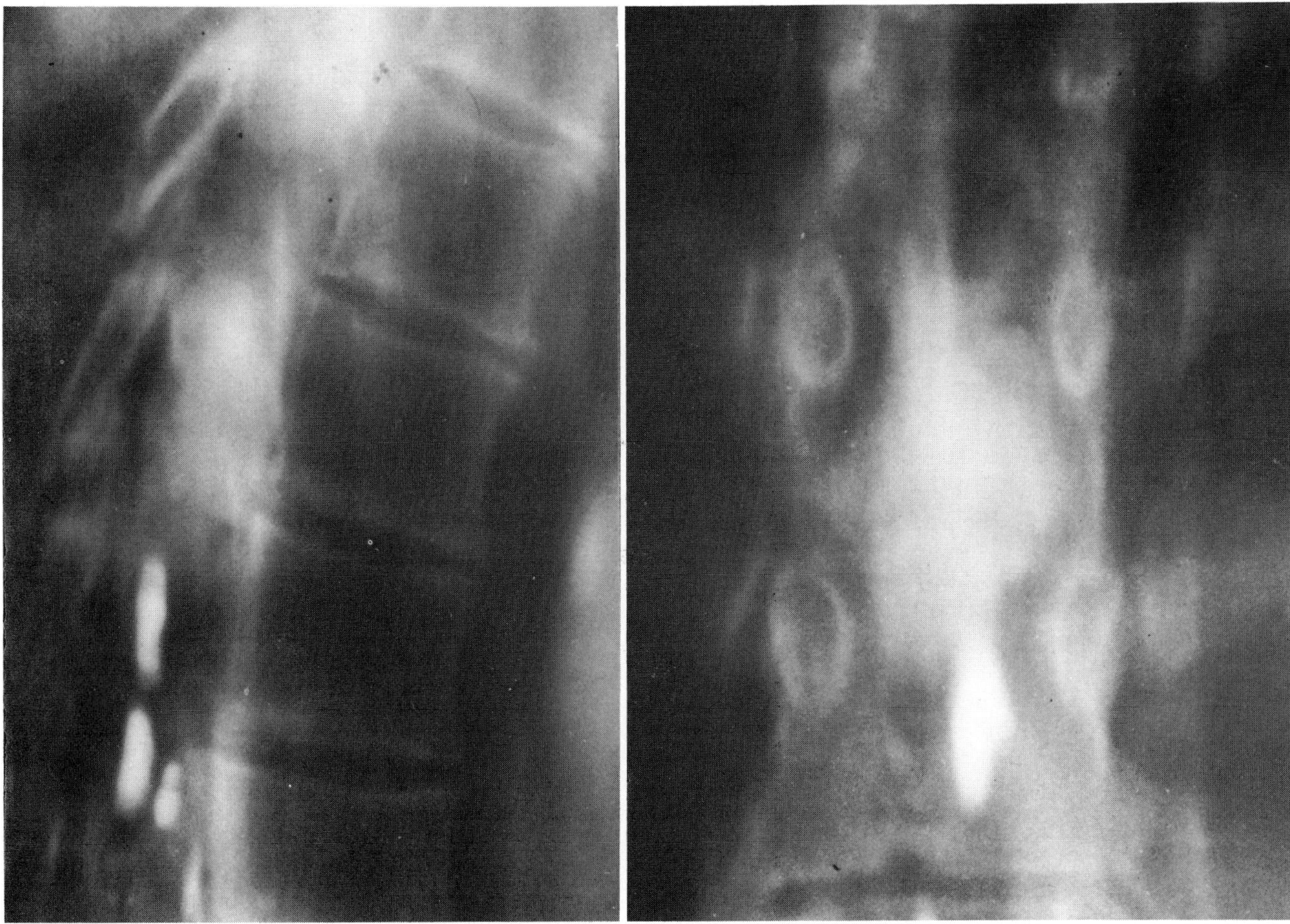

Fig. 59.36 (A and B) Meningioma. Tomograms show calcification within the spinal canal. This is a rare phenomenon, and meningiomas usually produce no changes on plain films. (Myodil fragments are shown caudal to the calcified tumour.)

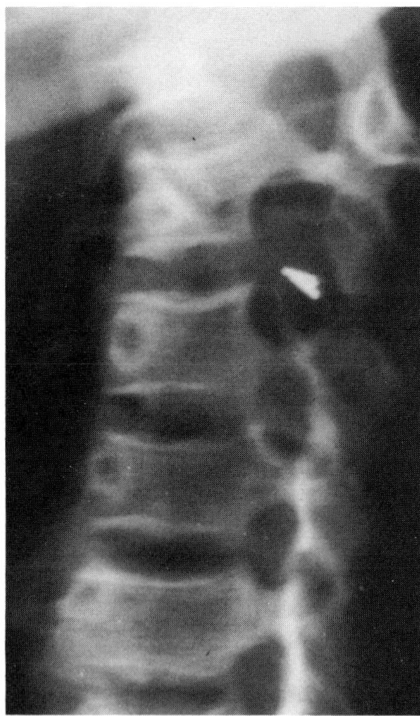

Fig. 59.37 Neurofibroma in cervical region. Typical bone erosion, expanding intervertebral foramen marked by postoperative clips.

Neurofibromas. These tumours arise from cells in the sheath of Schwann, and their characteristics are very different from meningiomas. Thus, they erode bone, do not calcify, occur at any level in the spine, and are found equally in men or women. They can be solitary or associated with generalized neurofibromatosis. Rarely they undergo sarcomatous degeneration. They are soft tumours, usually attached to posterior nerve roots. From this situation, they may grow through the dura and out through an intervertebral foramen and expand into a paraspinal mass. Thus they form a so-called *hour-glass* or *dumb-bell* tumour. When this happens, the intervertebral foramen is expanded, and this is well shown by oblique or lateral views. This sign is best seen in the cervical region (Fig. 59.37). The paravertebral mass may cause erosion or splaying apart of the vertebral ends of the ribs in the thoracic region. This characteristic appearance strongly favours a diagnosis of neurofibroma in preference to other causes of a paravertebral shadow. Soft neurofibromas sometimes cause expansion of the spinal canal, evidenced by thinning of the pedicles, widening of the interpedicular distance, and scalloping of the posterior border of the vertebral body.

Neurofibromas arising from the cauda equina can become very big, producing much expansion of the lower lumbar spinal canal or forming a so-called 'giant tumour of the cauda equina'. An ependymoma of the caudal end of the spinal cord can produce a similar 'giant tumour'.

Dermoid. These are uncommon tumours of developmental origin. They are usually intradural, but may be extradural. They are often associated with spina bifida, and a tuft of hair or a naevus on the overlying skin. The conus and cauda equina are the most common sites of origin. There are usually no plain film changes, although occasionally pressure erosion of adjacent bone may be seen.

Myelography shows the cord to be displaced within the theca. The cord is normally outlined occupying the central half of the contrast column. With an intradural tumour, the cord is seen to be displaced within the Myodil column to the opposite side of the spinal canal away from the tumour. There is usually a sharp cut-off of contrast on the side of the tumour. This cut-off is usually concave as the contrast caps the pole of the tumour (Fig. 59.38). There can be complete obstruction to the flow of Myodil, but if not, the oil may flow round and outline the whole of the tumour. The lower surface tension of water soluble contrast facilitates this. Both neurofibromas and meningiomas produce the same myelographic appearances. Important points in their differentiation, however, are that meningiomas are usually

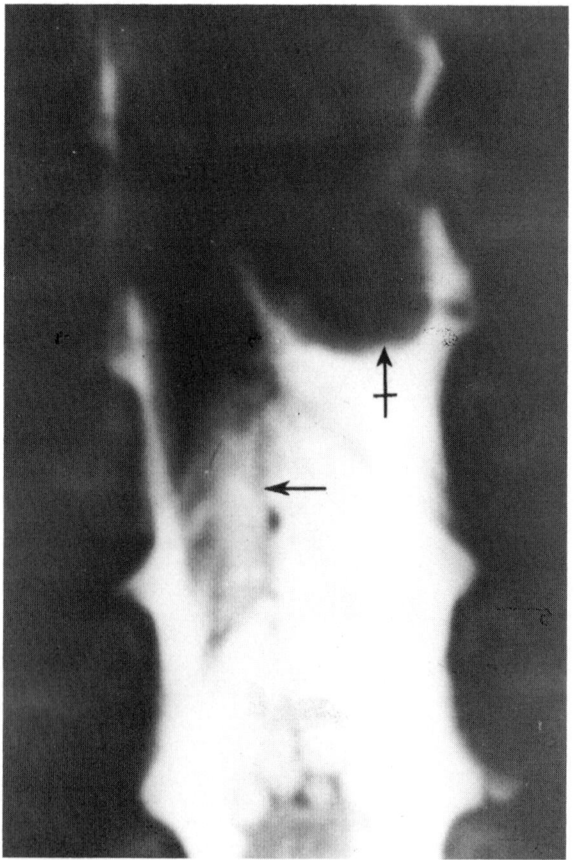

Fig. 59.38 Intradural extramedullary tumour causing almost complete spinal block. Cord displaced within theca (←). Pole of tumour outlined by contrast (↑).

found in women, in the thoracic area, and usually do not erode bone though local flattening or erosion of a single pedicle may be seen. Neurofibromas occur at any level in the spine, in either sex, and usually cause local bone erosion.

INTRAMEDULLARY TUMOURS

This group of tumours is uncommon. It consists mainly of ependymomas, gliomas and haemangioblastomas, but syringomyelia, a non-tumorous condition, may also be considered with this group. These lesions cause fusiform enlargement of the spinal cord and sometimes of the vertebral canal. Distinction between intramedullary and intradural extramedullary tumours is usually made by myelography.

Ependymomas. These are the commonest intramedullary spinal tumours. They originate from the ependymal lining of the central canal of the cord, and are most frequently found in the lumbar segments and conus. From the latter area they may extend along the filum terminale to the sacrum. They sometimes become massive both in length and diameter, causing great erosion and expansion of the lumbosacral canal, and together with neurofibroma are referred to as the 'giant tumour of the cauda equina'. This gross expansion of the vertebral canal is evident in both antero-posterior and lateral films (Fig. 59.39).

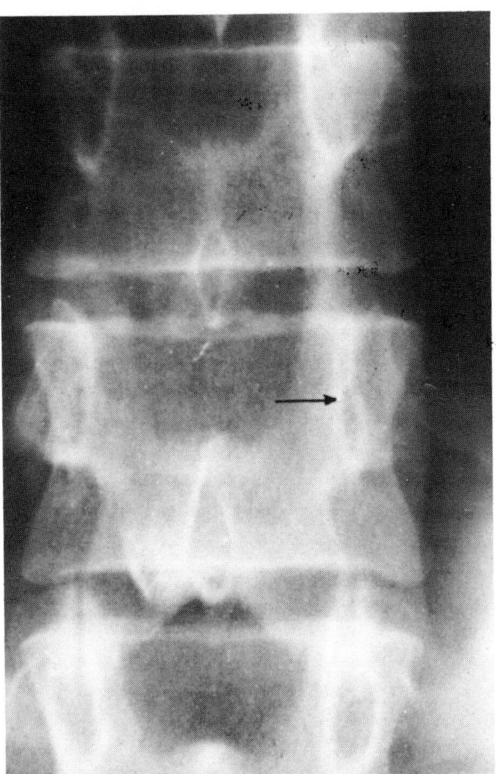

Fig. 59.39 Ependymoma. Expansion of spinal canal with pronounced local thinning of one pedicle (→). In the dorsal region such localized change is usually due to meningioma.

Glioma is a very similar tumour to ependymoma, but may occur anywhere in the cord. It does not produce massive erosion and expansion of the vertebral canal, perhaps because of the shorter history and more rapid onset of neurological disability than ependymoma. The most common type is an astrocytoma.

With all these lesions myelography shows the cord to be expanded within the Myodil column, which is not displaced from the bony walls of the canal. There is fusiform expansion of the cord within the theca usually extending over several segments. The cord lies centrally in the Myodil column, and the margins of the column are in their normal apposition to the pedicles, arches and vertebral bodies (Fig. 59.40). Obstruction to the flow of Myodil may be partial or complete. In the lower cervical and lower thoracic areas, the anatomical cervical and lumbar enlargements must not be confused with intramedullary tumour. Ependymomas may also be found in the cauda equina region, presumably arising from the filum terminale.

Syringomyelia and the Arnold-Chiari malformation. The pathogenesis of syringomyelia has been elegantly explained by the hydrodynamic theory of Gardner. This postulates a partial mechanical obstruction to the outflow of cerebrospinal fluid from the fourth ventricle through the foramen of Magendie. The degree of obstruction is delicately balanced, permitting the flow of ventricular fluid at the rate at which it is being formed, but precluding the sudden displacements of ventricular fluid which occur during each cardiac systole. Instead of fluid being ejected into the cisterna magna with each systolic pulse wave, it is funnelled into the upper part of the central canal of the spinal cord. This results in the cystic cavitation found in the cord in syringomyelia.

The cause of this foraminal obstruction in 90 per cent of cases is a Chiari malformation with downward prolapse of the cerebellar tonsils through the foramen magnum. Rarer causes include basal adhesive arachnoiditis and the Dandy-Walker syndrome. Hydrocephalus is unusual.

The resulting neurological syndromes are variable, depending on whether central cord cavitation or medullospinal compression by the herniated tonsils predominates. Thus bulbar palsies and cerebellar signs may be seen with or without limb neuropathies and dissociated anaesthesia.

Positive contrast myelography. Conventional myelography with the patient prone shows an expanded cord, often with free flow of Myodil through the foramen magnum (Fig. 59.41). The vital examination in this condition, however, is supine myelography. In the presence of a Chiari malformation, previously unsuspected obstruction may be shown at the foramen magnum. The herniated cerebellar tonsils causing the

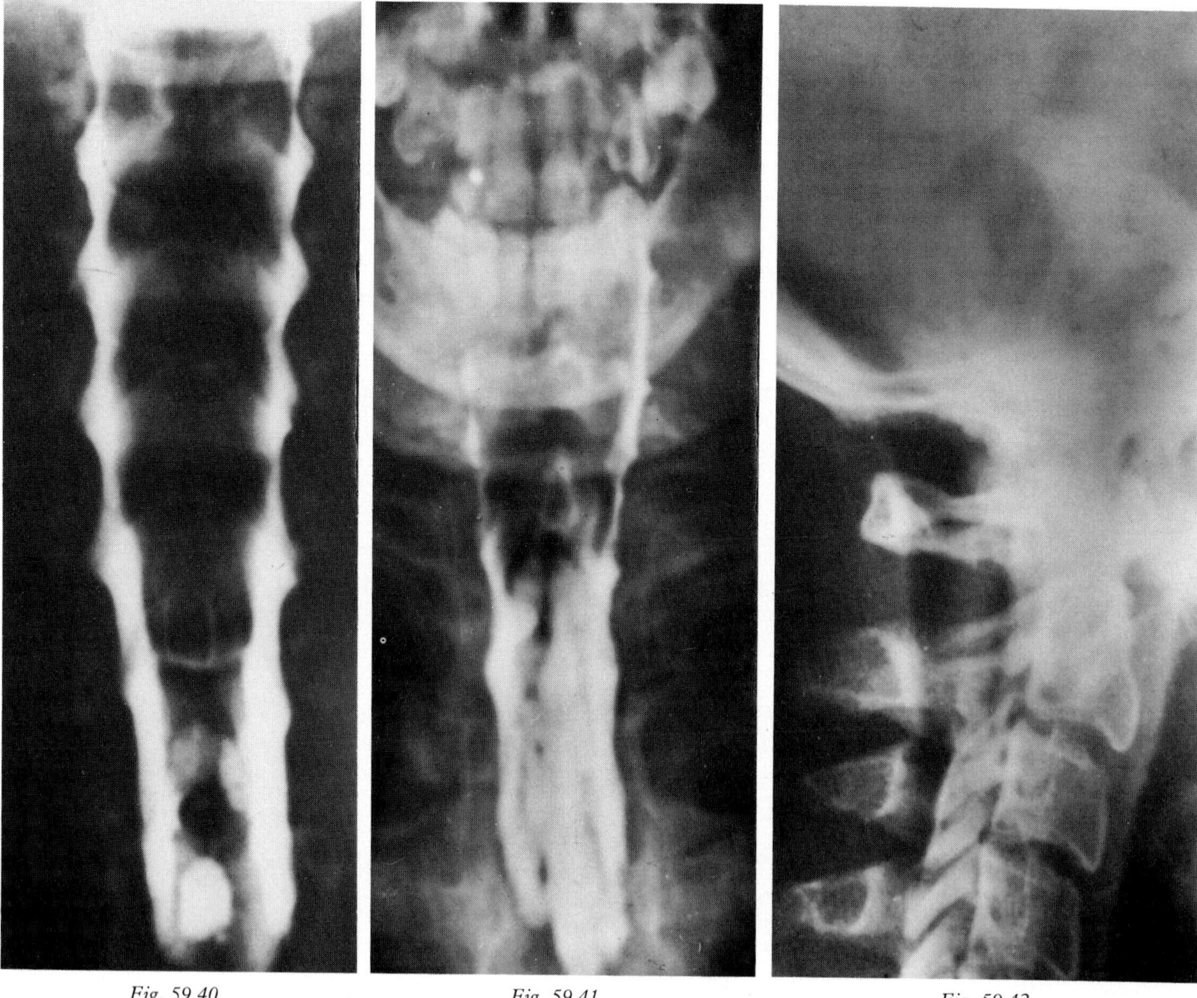

Fig. 59.40 Fig. 59.41 Fig. 59.42

Fig. 59.40 Intramedullary tumour. The cord is expanded and occupies almost all the spinal canal in the upper cervical area.

Fig. 59.41 Syringomyelia, prone myelogram. Expanded cervical cord. In this case there was complete obstruction to the cephalad flow in the upper cervical canal.

Fig. 59.42 Same case as Figure 59.41. Lumbar air myelogram with patient sitting shows collapsed atrophic upper cervical cord. Chiari malformation at operation.

obstruction may be outlined in both lateral and antero-posterior projections (Fig. 60.22, p. 1162).

Air myelography. A sign pathognomonic of syringomyelia may be shown by air myelography. This is the phenomenon of the collapsing cord. When the cord is outlined by air, its width varies with the position of the patient. In the head-down position, the cyst fluid fills the upper cervical part of the cavity in the cord, which thus appears swollen. With downward tilting of the feet, the cyst fluid gravitates to the lower part of the cavity. The upper cervical cord then appears collapsed, thin and atrophic. These appearances are diagnostic of cord cavitation (Fig. 59.42).

For this technique, air is injected by lumbar puncture with the patient either sitting or in lateral decubitus with caudal tilt, the head positioned to retain the air in the cervical canal. Lateral films will then confirm a collapsed and atrophic cord. Gardner's hypothesis and these techniques have encouraged a more positive surgical approach to the management of syringomyelia. The inevitable progression of the disease may often be arrested following high cervical laminectomy and posterior fossa decompression.

MISCELLANEOUS CONDITIONS

Angioma

Arteriovenous malformations of the spinal cord are much less common than those occurring in the brain. Symptoms are usually those of progressive cord malacia, although in a third of cases presentation may be by subarachnoid haemorrhage.

Plain radiographs of the spine are almost always normal. Diagnosis is made by myelography, which shows

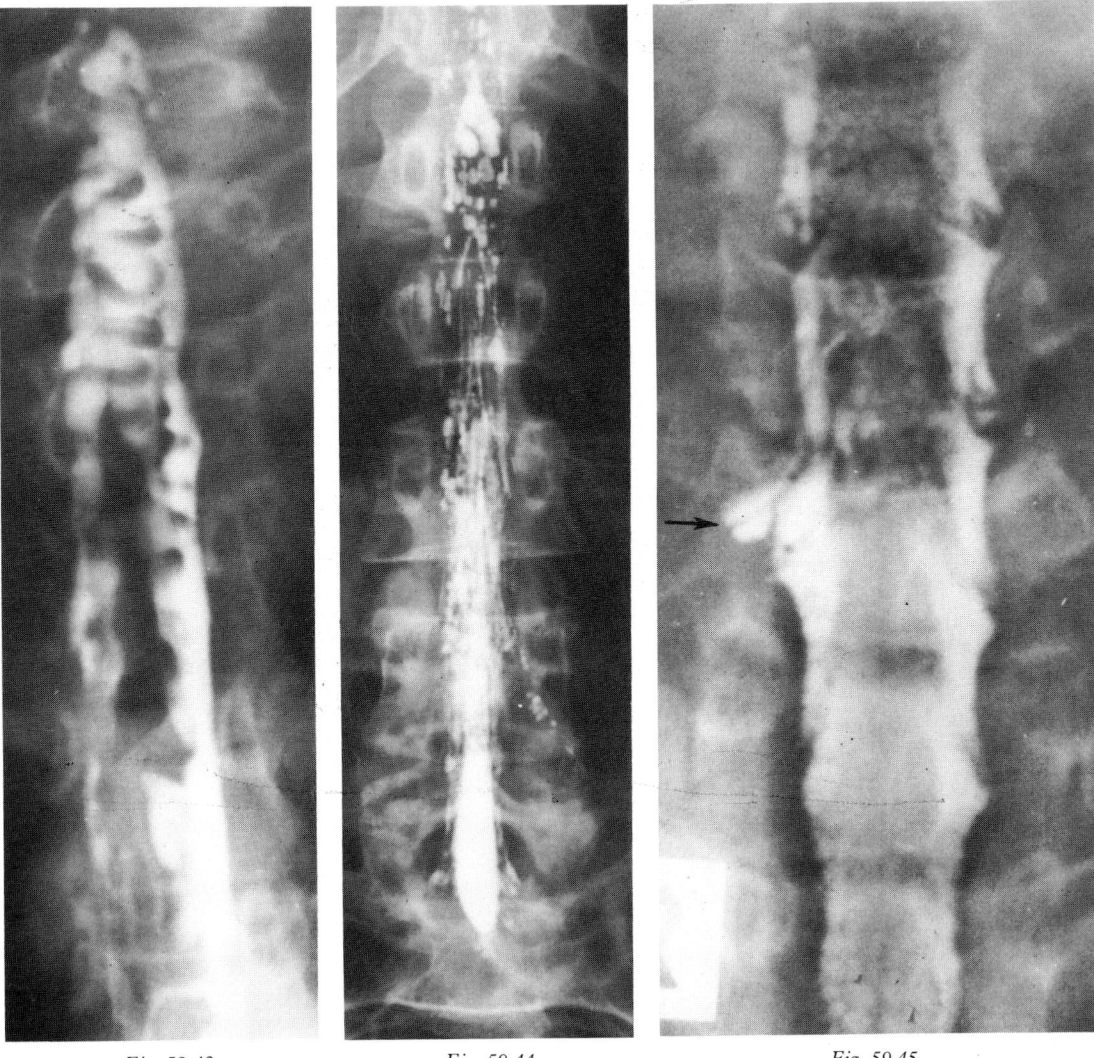

Fig. 59.43 *Fig. 59.44* *Fig. 59.45*

Fig. 59.43 Angioma. Tortuous filling defects in contrast due to dilated vessels on the surface of the cord.

Fig. 59.44 Arachnoiditis. Multiple and widespread pockets of Myodil due to the irregularly thickened meninges.

Fig. 59.45 Post-traumatic meningocele (→). Small, irregular, extradural diverticulum following shoulder dislocation.

tortuous serpiginous linear filling defects in the opaque column (Fig. 59.43). There is normally little or no obstruction to the flow of Myodil, unless haemorrhage or thrombosis with cord softening have occurred. The filling defects extend over several segments and are largely due to dilated feeding arteries and draining veins, the actual malformation being relatively small. It should be remembered that much smaller varicosities are sometimes shown at the site of tumours producing spinal block. This is due to distended veins, obstructed by pressure from the tumour.

Screening should always be carried out in the supine as well as the prone position, since the majority of angiomas occur on the dorsal aspect of the cord. The majority are also on the surface of the cord rather than being intramedullary.

The demonstration of the precise anatomy, which is of the greatest importance to surgical attack, is dependent on selective spinal angiography. This is described in Chapters 61 and 62.

Arachnoiditis

Fibrous adhesions between pia, arachnoid and dura follow infection, haemorrhage, injury or operation. Symptoms may result from traction and distortion of nerve roots or cord. The diagnosis is almost entirely dependent on myelography. Small cysts and loculi are formed between the adhesions, which usually extend over several segments. At myelography, there is slow flow of Myodil through this area, although obstruction is usually incomplete. There are irregular filling defects in the column, and once droplets of Myodil have entered the small arachnoid pockets they usually remain within them, despite repeated tilting (Fig. 59.44). These features are reminiscent of artefacts due to subdural injection of Myodil, although an early lateral prone film confirms the latter condition.

Traumatic meningocele

Injuries causing tears or avulsion of spinal nerve roots sometimes also tear the meningeal root sheath. This leads to the formation of small irregular arachnoid diverticula extending outside the bony spinal canal along the affected nerve root. These post-traumatic meningoceles may be outlined by myelography (Fig. 59.45). They are most common in the cervical area following injuries to the brachial plexus nerve roots.

REFERENCES AND SUGGESTIONS FOR FURTHER READING

Acta Radiologica (1973) Metrizamide. Suppl. 335.

Acta Radiologica (1977) Metrizamide-Amipaque. Suppl. 355.

DiChiro, G. & Wener, L. (1973). Angiography of the spinal cord; a review of contemporary techniques and applications. *Journal of Neurosurgery*, **39**, 1–29.

Djindjian, R. (1970) *Angiography of the Spinal Cord*. Paris: Masson.

Elsberg, C. A. & Dyke, C. G. (1934) *Bull. Neurol. Inst. New York*, **3**, 359–394.

Epstein, B. S. (1976) *The Spine : A radiological text and atlas*, 4th edn. Philadelphia: Lea & Febiger.

Gardner, W. J. (1965) Hydrodynamic mechanism of syringomyelia; its relationship to myelocele. *Journal of Neurology, Neurosurgery and Psychiatry*, **28**, 247–259.

Grainger, R. G. (1979) In *Recent Advances in Radiology*, 6th edn., pp. 177–194, eds. Sir Thomas Lodge & R. E. Steiner. London: Churchill Livingstone.

Heinz, E. R. & Goldman, R. L. (1972) The role of gas myelography in neuroradiologic diagnosis. *Radiology*, **102**, 629–634.

Lindblom, K. (1950) Technique and results in myelography and disc puncture. *Acta Radiologica*, **34**, 321–330.

Logue, V. (1971) 14th Crookshank Lecture. Syringomyelia: a radiodiagnostic and radiotherapeutic saga. *Clinical Radiology*, **22**, 2–16.

Mixter, W. J. & Barr, J. S. (1934) Rupture of the intervertebral disc with involvement of the spinal canal. *New England Journal of Medicine*, **211**, 210–215.

Roberson, G. H., Llewllyn, H. J. & Taveras, J. M. (1973) The narrow lumbar spinal canal syndrome. *Radiology*, **107**, 89–97.

Schatzker, J. & Pennal, G. F. (1968) Spinal stenosis, a cause of cauda equina compression. *Journal of Bone and Joint Surgery*, **50B**, 606–618.

Shapiro, R. (1975) *Myelography*, 3rd edn. Chicago: Year Book Publishers.

Skalpe, I. O. & Amundsen, P. (1975) Thoracic and cervical myelography with metrizamide. *Radiology*, **116**, 101–106.

Skalpe, I. O. & Sortland, O. (1978) *Myelography—Textbook and Atlas*. Oslo: Tanum-Notli.

Sutton, D. (1963) Sacral cysts. *Acta Radiologica*, **1**, 787–795.

Taveras, J. M. & Wood, E. H. (1976) *Diagnostic Neuroradiology*, 2nd edn. Baltimore: Williams and Wilkins.

CHAPTER 60

ENCEPHALOGRAPHY AND VENTRICULOGRAPHY

The diagnosis of intracranial disease was revolutionized by Dandy in 1918. Dandy, an American neurosurgeon, was the first to perceive that the introduction of a contrast medium into the ventricles followed by radiography of the skull would reveal ventricular deformities. This enabled exact topographical localization of brain tumours to be made. In preliminary experiments, solutions used in pyelography were injected into the ventricles of dogs. These injections were fatal, however, due to toxic brain injury. Dandy then realized that air would be non-toxic and would be readily absorbed. It would also be radiolucent, from analogy with radiographs of the chest and abdomen and a reported case of accidental air pictures of the ventricles following a traumatic aerocele (Luckett, 1913). This reasoning led him to perform the first air ventriculogram by replacing ventricular cerebrospinal fluid with air injected directly through a needle introduced through a burr-hole.

In the ventriculograms so obtained, Dandy observed that some air escaped from the ventricles and passed over the surface of the brain, outlining the sulci between the convolutions. Since many brain lesions affect the subarachnoid space, Dandy appreciated that the outlining of these spaces by air would give additional diagnostic information. He effected this in 1919 by injecting air directly into the subarachnoid space by lumbar puncture. The air passed into the ventricles, into the subarachnoid cisterns and over the surface of the brain. This procedure is known as **air encephalography**. The injection of air or a positive contrast medium directly into a ventricle through a burr-hole is known as **ventriculography**.

By appropriate positioning of the head, the air introduced may be manipulated into the different parts of the ventricular system. From radiographs taken with the head in different positions, a complete 'cast' of the ventricular system may be built up. Intracranial masses cause displacements and deformities of the ventricles. From these deformities, the position of tumours, blood clots and abscesses may be accurately determined. In cases of obstructive hydrocephalus, the point of obstruction to the cerebrospinal fluid pathway is usually made plain. Tumours in or near the base of the skull deform the basal subarachnoid cisterns. The shrunken convolutions of the hemispheres in cerebral atrophy are outlined by air in the widened sulci. The overall diagnostic accuracy of the examination in the diagnosis of tumours is of the order of 95 per cent. The choice of diagnostic method and the hazards involved will be discussed later.

Air encephalography is, however, a very unpleasant examination for the patient, which may cause severe and persistent headache, with nausea and vomiting. It may also carry considerable risk if the intracranial pressure is raised as may ventriculography (see below). For these reasons both investigations have since 1973 been largely replaced by the non-invasive computed tomography and other supplementary neuroradiological investigations. The account which follows has accordingly been curtailed and for more detailed description reference should be made to the monographs listed at the end of this chapter.

ANATOMY

CEREBROSPINAL FLUID CIRCULATION

Fluid is secreted by the choroid plexuses in the lateral ventricles. It flows through the foramina of Monro to the third ventricle, and thence down the aqueduct of Sylvius (iter) in the midbrain to the fourth ventricle. It leaves the fourth ventricle via the midline foramen of Magendie, and the lateral foramina of Luschka, and enters the cisterna magna. From here some diffusion occurs with the fluid in the spinal canal. The fluid then passes upwards through the basal subarachnoid cisterns to the tentorial hiatus. Flow continues through the tentorial opening surrounding the midbrain, and once above the tentorium diffuses over the cerebral hemispheres, being finally absorbed into the dural sinuses through the arachnoid villi (Pacchionian granulations). The total volume of the cerebrospinal fluid is about 150 ml.

This circulatory pathway is of obvious importance in encephalographic diagnosis. Ventricular dilation proximal to the point of the obstruction usually indicates the site of the lesion. Thus a cerebellar tumour obstructing the aqueduct causes symmetrical dilatation of the lateral and third ventricles. Arachnoiditis blocking the exit foramina of the fourth ventricle causes symmetrical dilatation of all four ventricles. In their later stages, cerebral tumours frequently cause obstructions to the c.s.f. circulation at the tentorial opening and at the foramen magnum. This is due to the formation of pressure cones by the mass of the tumour, or the dilated ventricles. The uncus, the anterior part of the hippocampal gyrus on the medial surface of the temporal lobe may be forced into the tentorial opening, compressing vital structures in the midbrain. Similarly, the cerebellar tonsils may herniate down through the foramen magnum causing medullary compression. These events may be manifest clinically by a progressively deepening coma, and are of the gravest significance.

LATERAL VENTRICLES

The lateral ventricles lie in the central part of the cerebral hemispheres (Figs 60.1 and 60.2). They have a thin endothelial lining, the ependyma, and lie directly beneath the corpus callosum. The latter is the great transverse commissure of the hemispheres, from which fibres radiate into the different lobes. Its anterior and posterior ends are broader and curve downwards, and are known as the genu and splenium respectively.

Each lateral ventricle consists of:

(a) *Frontal* (*anterior*) *horn*, which lies anterior to the foramen of Monro, and within the frontal lobe.

(b) *Body*, from the foramen of Monro to the splenium.

(c) *Trigone* (*atrium*). This is a small, local expansion at the junction of body and temporal horn, and occipital horn if the latter is present.

(d) *Temporal*, or *descending*, or *inferior horn* which runs

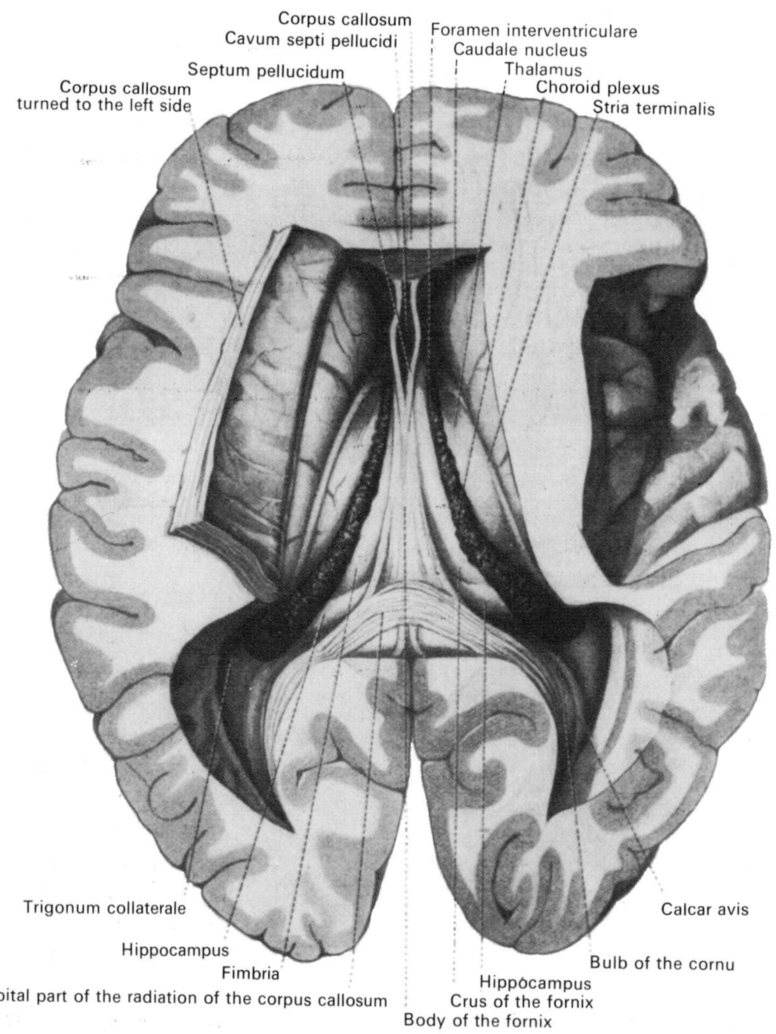

Fig. 60.1 Horizontal section to show the lateral ventricles from above. (Reproduced from Cunningham's *Anatomy*.)

forwards, downwards and outwards and lies within the temporal lobe.

(e) *Occipital (posterior) horn.* This is inconstantly present, and runs posteriorly within the occipital lobe.

Frontal (anterior) horn

This lies within the frontal lobe, running forwards and slightly outwards from the foramen of Monro. Thus, in anteroposterior radiographs taken with the brow up and with full air filling of the frontal horns, the latter are projected lateral to the bodies of the lateral ventricles.

The boundaries of the anterior horn are:

Roof—corpus callosum

Anterior wall—posterior surface of genu of corpus callosum

Medial wall—septum pellucidum

Floor—anterior end of the caudate nucleus.

Body

This part of the lateral ventricle extends from the foramen of Monro to the trigone and splenium. In section it is triangular, and its boundaries are:

Roof—corpus callosum

Medial wall—septum pellucidum

Floor and lateral wall—basal ganglia—i.e. caudate nucleus anteriorly and thalamus posteriorly. The body of the fornix and the choroid plexus also lie in the floor.

Trigone (atrium)

This is a small dilatation of the posterior part of the body of the lateral ventricle at its junction with the origin of the temporal horn. It contains a large tuft of choroid plexus (*glomus*) which appears as a rounded, irregular filling defect on encephalograms, and which must not be mistaken for an intraventricular tumour.

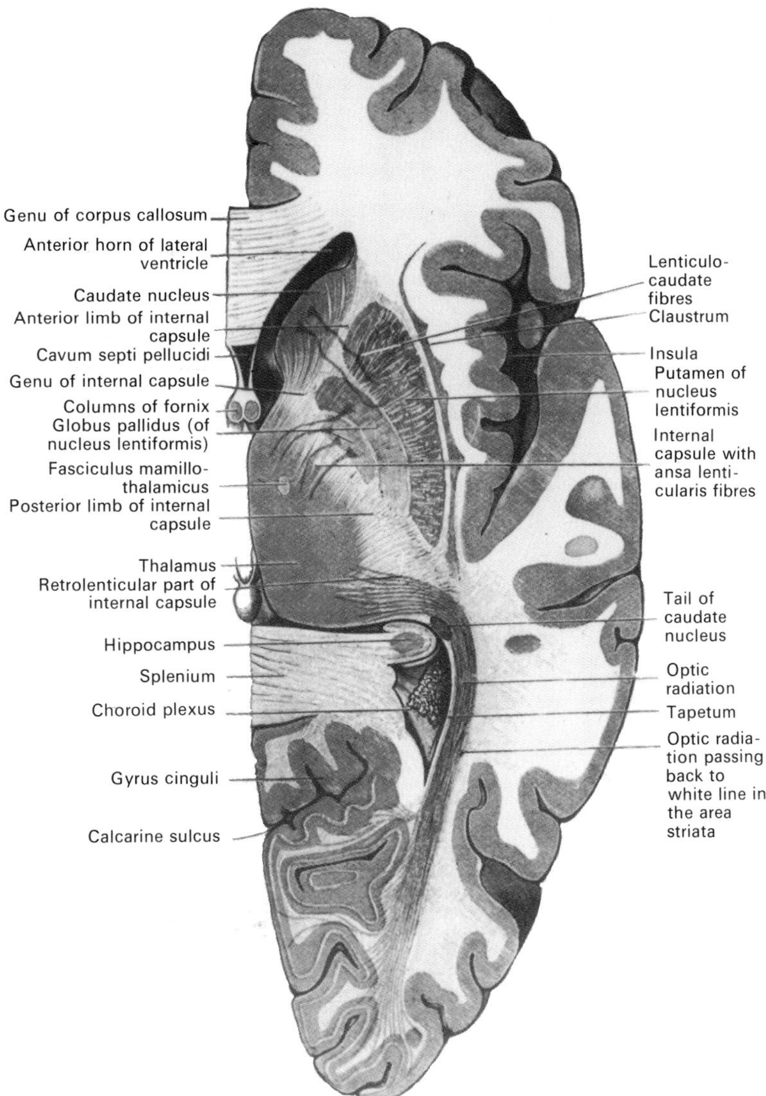

Fig. 60.2 Horizontal section to show basal ganglia, corpus callosum and lateral ventricles. (Reproduced from Cunningham's *Anatomy*.)

Temporal (descending or inferior) horn

This runs forwards, downwards and outwards from the trigone, lying within the temporal lobe. Anteriorly, it ends 4 cm from the tip of the temporal lobe. The choroid plexus lies in its roof. Other than the temporal lobe, its boundaries are:

Roof—outer parts of caudate nucleus and corpus callosum

Floor—Hippocampus. This forms the inferomedial gyrus of the temporal lobe. Anteriorly, its uncus lies close to the side of the midbrain above the tentorial opening, and its significance in the phenomenon of tentorial herniation has already been mentioned.

Occipital (posterior) horn

This runs posteriorly from the trigone into the occipital lobe. In 90 per cent of cases it is either vestigial or absent, and is subject to very great anatomical variation. Occasionally, it may be present on one side only, and this is usually the left side.

THIRD VENTRICLE (Figs 60.3 and 60.4)

The third ventricle is the narrow cleft in the midline between the two thalami. It extends from the foramina of Monro anteriorly to the opening of the aqueduct (iter) posteriorly. Its anterior end dips down from the foramen of Monro into the suprasellar area. Two separate projections from its antero-inferior end are usually clearly outlined at encephalography. The anterior one lies above the optic chiasm, and is known as the *chasmatic* or *supraoptic recess*. The posterior projection lies above the pituitary stalk and is known as the *infundibular recess*.

Two comparable projections are outlined at the posterior end of the third ventricle. The short lower one extends up to 4 mm into the pineal gland and is known as the *pineal recess*. The upper projection is larger and lies between the pineal and splenium; it is termed the *suprapineal recess*. Both these recesses are seen clearly on lateral encephalograms in relation to the calcified shadow of the pineal. The suprapineal recess varies in size, and is usually from 2 to 10 mm in length. It is occasionally still further

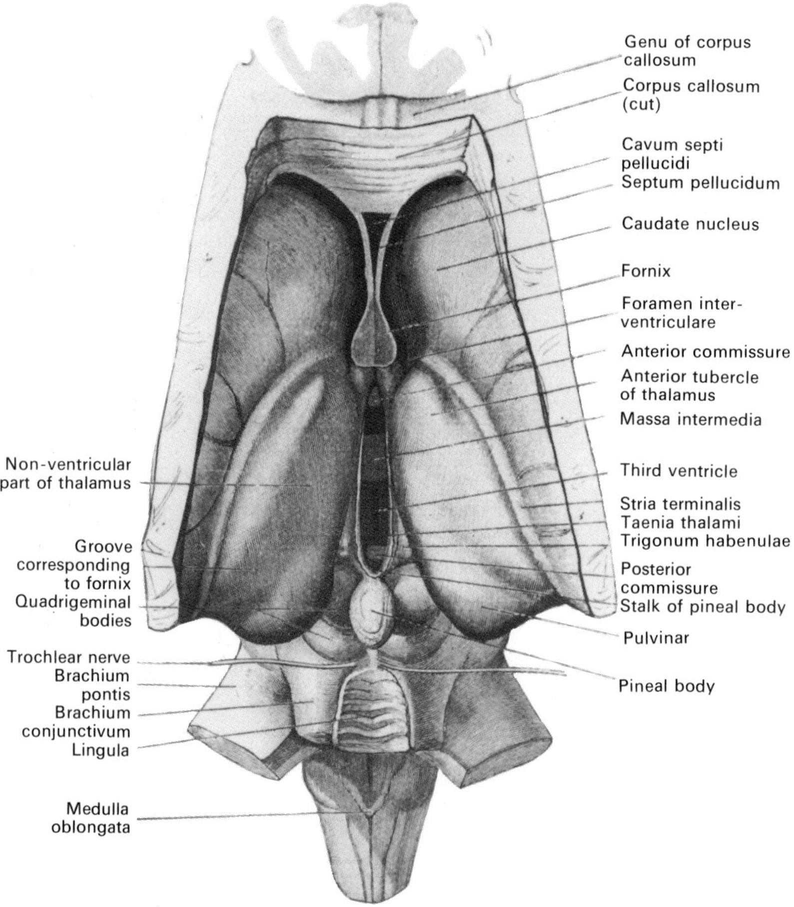

Fig. 60.3 Horizontal section showing relationships of third ventricle. (Reproduced from Cunningham's *Anatomy*.)

expanded or 'ballooned' in the presence of obstructive hydrocephalus, when it extends backwards beneath the corpus callosum into the quadrigeminal cistern.

It should be appreciated that the axis of the body of the third ventricle lies horizontally, but its anterior portion is inclined steeply downwards from the foramen of Monro towards the suprasellar area. This downward inclination lies immediately behind the anterior commissure. The three commissures are bands of white matter connecting the two hemispheres. The *anterior commissure* connects the temporal lobes of the two hemispheres. The *middle commissure* or *massa intermedia* connects the two thalami in the middle of the third ventricle, when it appears as a filling defect in lateral encephalograms. The *posterior commissure* (or habenular commissure) lies immediately below the pineal and thus marks the posterior end of the third ventricle.

The anterior wall of the third ventricle is formed by the anterior commissure and the lamina terminalis. The *lamina terminalis* is a thin layer of grey matter passing downwards from the genu of the corpus callosum to the optic chiasm.

The roof of the third ventricle is formed by a layer of pia mater, the *velum interpositum* (*tela choroidea*), which is invaginated by the choroid plexus of the third ventricle. Above the velum interpositum lies the fornix and corpus callosum. The *fornix* consists of two white longitudinal bands beneath the corpus callosum, separated in front and behind forming the columns, but joined in the middle forming the body. The body is attached anteriorly to the septum lucidum and it forms the floor of the lateral ventricle and roof of the third ventricle. The anterior columns pass downwards in front of the foramen of Monro to reach the mammillary bodies in the suprasellar area. The posterior columns curve laterally and downwards round the thalami into the floor of the temporal horn where they pass to the hippocampal uncus.

The choroid plexus of the body of the lateral ventricle emerges from beneath the lateral margin of the body of the fornix and extends into the floor of the lateral ventricle. The floor of the third ventricle is formed by those structures which lie between the pituitary fossa and the cerebral peduncles. From before backwards, these are the lamina terminalis, optic chiasm, tuber cinereum, mammillary bodies and posterior perforated substance.

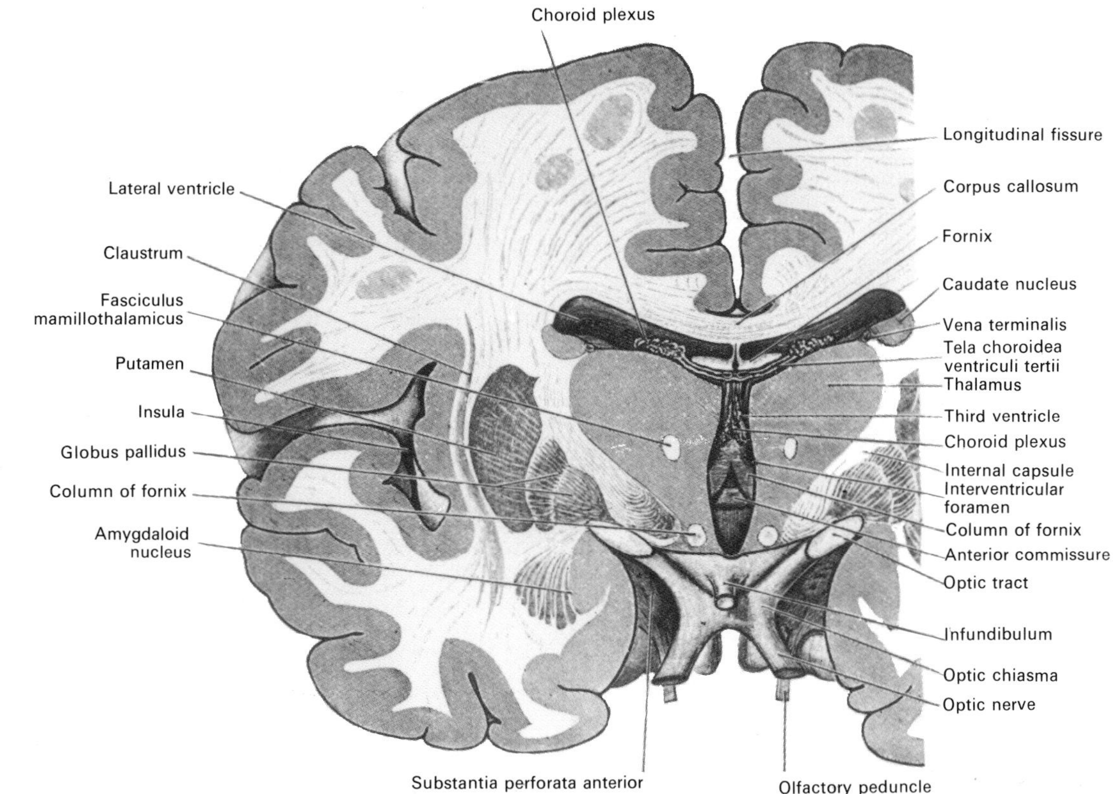

Fig. 60.4 Coronal section showing third ventricle, basal ganglia and corpus callosum. (Reproduced from Cunningham's *Anatomy*.)

AQUEDUCT OF SYLVIUS (ITER)

This narrow canal runs through the midbrain from the postero-inferior angle of the third ventricle (Fig. 60.5).

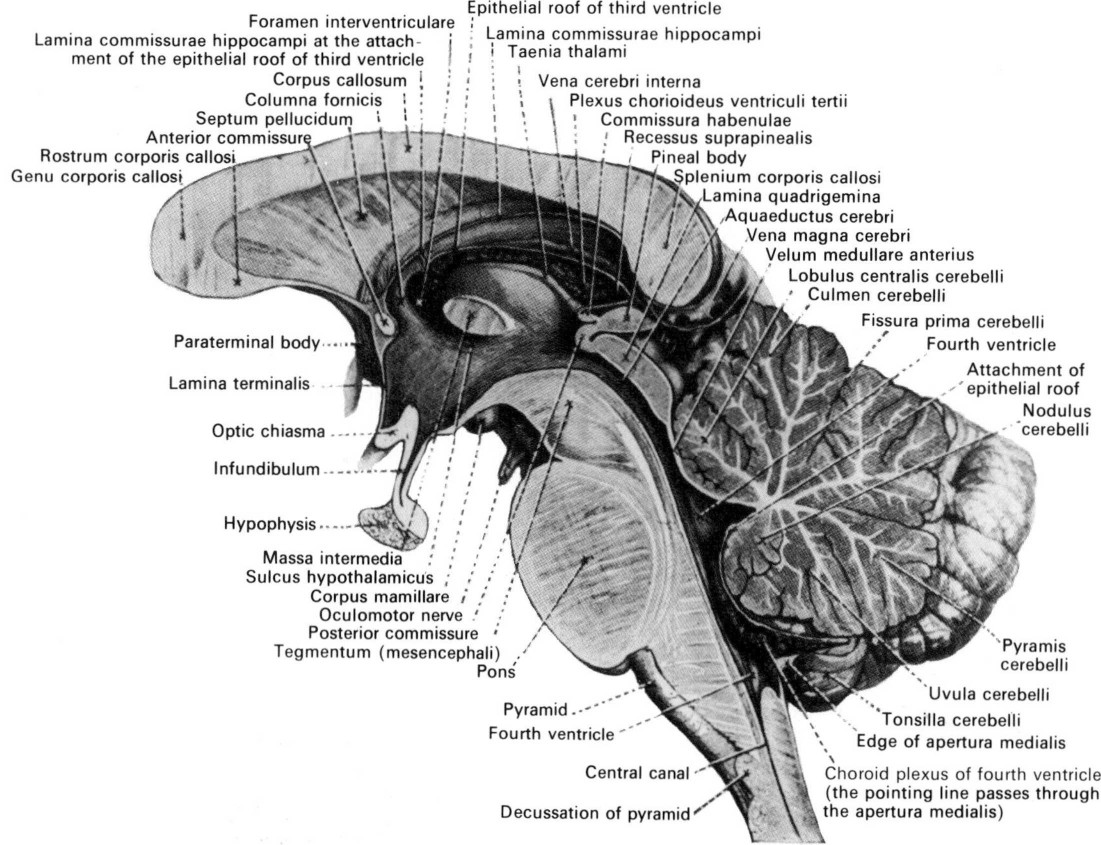

Fig. 60.5 Midline section showing relationships of third ventricle, aqueduct, and fourth ventricles. (Reproduced from Cunningham's *Anatomy*.)

It is about 1·5 cm long and ends at the lower border of the quadrigeminal plate, wherein it opens into the cavity of the fourth ventricle. In the midbrain, the quadrigeminal plate lies on its posterior wall, and the tegmentum of the cerebral peduncles forms its anterior wall.

Its diameter is only 1 to 2 mm and since it passes through the fixed and rigid tentorial opening it is very easily obstructed by lateral brain displacement due to tumours. This applies particularly to tumours in the posterior fossa displacing the fourth ventricle. The resulting kink in the aqueduct at the tentorial opening leads to the development of obstructive hydrocephalus.

FOURTH VENTRICLE

The fourth ventricle lies between the anterior surface of the cerebellum and the posterior surface of the pons and upper part of the medulla (Fig. 60.5). The uppermost point of the cavity lies at the level of the inferior quadrigeminal body (inferior colliculus). This point is known as the *fastigium,* which is the summit of the posterior extension of the roof. The posterior wall of the cavity is known as the roof, and is formed by the vermis and superior cerebellar peduncles which form lateral connections from the pons to the cerebellum. The floor, or anterior wall, is formed by the pons and medulla. In lateral projection the fourth ventricle is triangular. In anteroposterior projection it is rhomboidal, with a short easily recognizable flat roof. This is quite unlike the thin oval appearance of the third ventricle in anteroposterior projection.

There is a small choroid plexus in the lower part of the roof of the fourth ventricle. There are also three exit foramina for the circulation of cerebrospinal fluid into the subarachnoid space. The *foramen of Magendie* lies in the midline at the lower end of the fourth ventricle and opens between the cerebellar tonsils into the cisterna magna. The lateral recess of the ventricle contain the two *foramina of Luschka* which open into the cisterns of the cerebellopontine angles. On the lateral side of the fourth ventricle lie the middle and inferior cerebellar peduncles.

THE SUBARACHNOID CISTERNS

The subarachnoid spaces at the base of the skull and over the surface of the brain contain more cerebrospinal fluid then the ventricles themselves (Fig. 60.6). The largest spaces or cisterns lie in the base of the skull and round the tentorial opening. A knowledge of their anatomy is of importance, as deformities of the cisterns may enable a diagnosis to be made at encephalography even if ventricular filling is not obtained. In general, the cisterns may be compressed or deformed by tumours, and are enlarged in the presence of atrophy. The main cisterns of diagnostic significance are:

1. Cisterna magna
2. Cisterna pontis
3. Cisterna interpeduncularis (crural cistern)
4. Suprasellar cisterns
5. Pericallosal cistern
6. Quadrigeminal cistern (cisterna venae magnae)
7. Ambient cisterns.

Cisterna magna. This is continuous through the foramen magnum with the spinal subarachnoid space. It is an irregular space with a capacity of about 10 ml. It lies behind the medulla and below the cerebellar hemispheres. Its lateral borders are formed by the cerebellar hemispheres and tonsils. Posteriorly, it extends for a variable distance upwards round the occiput behind the cerebellum.

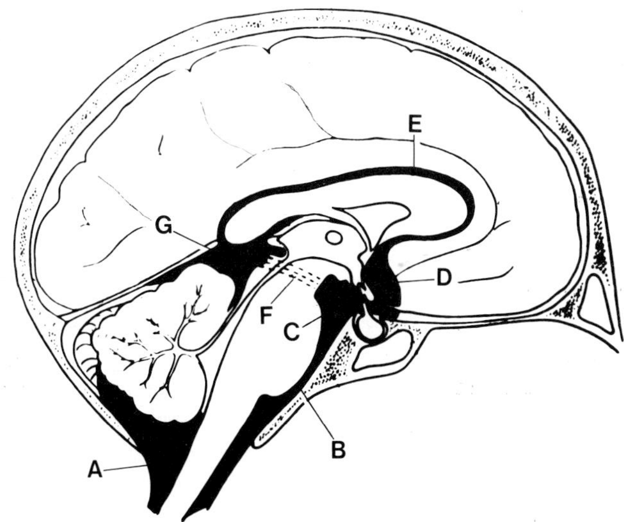

Fig. 60.6 The subarachnoid cisterns.
(A) Cisterna magna
(B) C. points
(C) C. interpeduncularis
(D) C. chiasmatis
(E) C. corporis callosum
(F) C. ambiens
(G) C. venae magnae (quadrigeminal cistern)

Cisterna pontis. This lies between the pons and clivus and communicates below with the cisterna magna and above with the cisterna interpeduncularis. It contains the basilar artery, which is frequently outlined by air in lateral encephalograms. Lateral recesses of the cisterna pontis extend out into the cerebellopontine angles, and tumours in this situation may be outlined by air in the cistern.

Cisterna interpeduncularis. This cistern lies anterior to, and between, the cerebral peduncles. The bifurcation of the basilar artery and first parts of the posterior cerebral arteries may be seen within the cistern in lateral encephalograms. It communicates inferiorly with the pontine cistern and anterosuperiorly with the suprasellar cisterns. In lateral encephalograms, it is projected above and behind the dorsum sellae and posterior clinoids. Above the interpeduncular cistern lie the mammillary bodies and posterior perforated substance which form the posterior part of the floor of the third ventricle.

Suprasellar cisterns. The suprasellar subarachnoid spaces are sometimes referred to as the cisternae infundibularis and chiasmatis. These cisterns extend forwards from the cisterna interpeduncularis above and to the side of the pituitary fossa. They are bounded above by the anterior part of the floor of the third ventricle, and below by the diaphragma sellae. They are traversed by the optic nerves passing to the chiasm, and these nerves may be outlined by air. Laterally, these cisterns extend round the carotid arteries into the parasellar area, and thence still further laterally into the lower end of the Sylvian fissure.

Pericallosal cistern. The cistern above the optic chiasm extends upwards along the anterior wall of the third ventricle as the cisterna lamina terminalis. This narrow subarachnoid channel is continued in the midline over the upper surface of the corpus callosum as the pericallosal cistern. This cistern runs backwards over the corpus callosum where, behind the splenium, it enters the large and important quadrigeminal cistern (cisterna venae magnae).

Quadrigeminal cistern. This cistern is so named since it invests the quadrigeminal plate and quadrigeminal bodies (colliculi). Its older name, cisterna venae magnae, derives from the fact that it also contains a large venous confluence. Thus, the cistern contains the junction of the inferior sagittal and straight sinuses, and the vein of Galen which is joined within the cistern by the basal vein of Rosenthal. The quadrigeminal cistern is an irregular space which is usually well outlined in both lateral and antero-posterior encephalograms. Its boundaries are:

Anterior—quadrigeminal plate, pineal and third ventricle

Superior—splenium and vein of Galen

Posterior—tentorium and falx

Inferior—upper part of vermis between the two cerebellar hemispheres.

It has been mentioned earlier that patency of the subarachnoid space round the brain stem in the tentorial opening is essential for the free circulation of subarachnoid fluid. Fluid must pass upward through this opening to be absorbed by the arachnoid villi near the vertex. The dural margin of the tentorial opening is rigid and fibrous, and deformities and compression of the quadrigeminal cistern by tumours promote the occurrence of obstructive hydrocephalus, in addition to compressing the aqueduct.

Ambient cisterns. The ambient cisterns extend from the interpeduncular cistern round each side of the brain stem to meet behind it in the quadrigeminal cistern. They thus complete the chair of subarachnoid cisterns from the base of the skull to the supratentorial area.

Lying within the anterior part of the ambient cistern are the posterior cerebral artery and basal vein. Lateral extensions of the upper part of the ambient cistern pass round the posterior part of the thalamus, and are referred to as the wings of the ambient cistern, or ambient wing cisterns. The ambient and ambient wing cisterns outline the midbrain at encephalography. In half axial postero-anterior films they define the lateral margins of the midbrain and outline the quadrigeminal plate on the posterior aspect of the brain stem behind the aqueduct. In lateral projection, the ambient wing cisterns cross the quadrigeminal plate at right angles as they run upwards and backwards from the interpeduncular cistern to the quadrigeminal cistern.

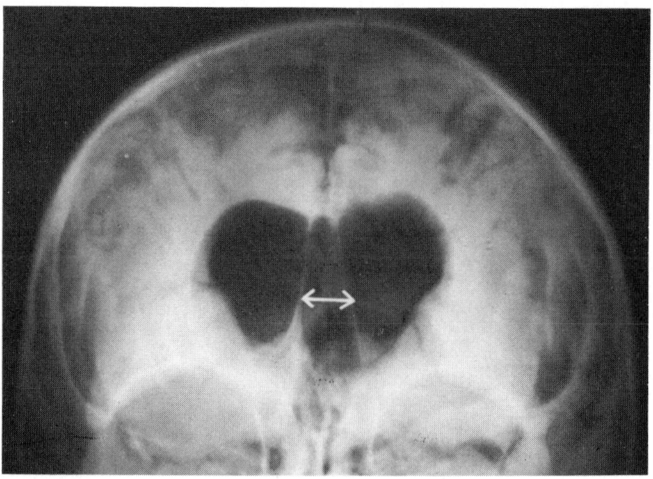

Fig. 60.7 Cavum septum pellucidum (↔).

Cavum septum pellucidum (fifth ventricle) (Fig. 60.7). This is an anatomical variant of the septum pellucidum which is occasionally seen. The septum is a double membrane, and occasionally a narrow cavity containing cerebrospinal fluid is present between these membranes. This is sometimes referred to as the *fifth ventricle* and when present may be outlined with air, lying between the two lateral ventricles, in anteroposterior encephalograms. The roof of the cavum septum pellucidum is formed by the corpus callosum and its floor by the anterior pillars of the fornix.

Occasionally, posterior extensions of the cavum septum pellucidum towards the splenium are seen. This latter cavity is known as the *cavum vergae*, or *sixth ventricle*.

AIR ENCEPHALOGRAPHY

Lumbar encephalography is the method of choice in performing air studies. The injection of air by lumbar puncture is safer and allows easier positioning of the head during injection than does the alternative method of cisternal puncture. Ventriculography is a more formidable procedure and is usually reserved for those cases with raised intracranial pressure in which lumbar puncture carries the risk of precipitating tentorial or foraminal herniation. Ventriculography is a procedure for the neuro-

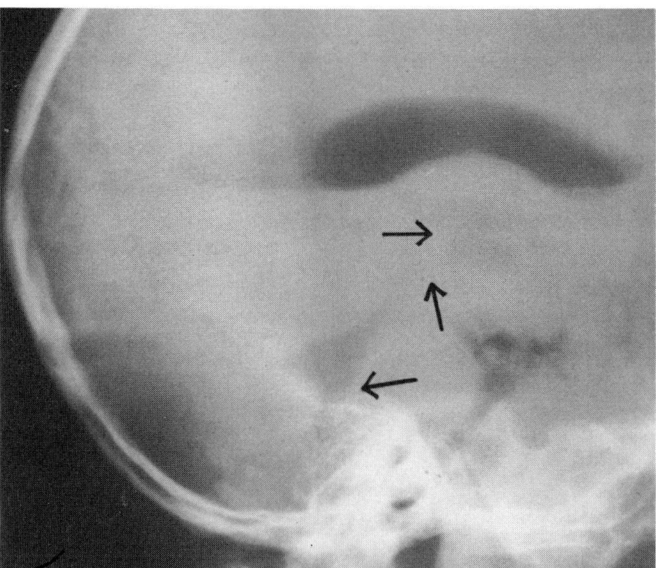

Fig. 60.8 Erect film taken during air injection. The fourth ventricle (←), aqueduct (↑) and posterior end of the third ventricle with its recesses (→) are outlined. The roofs and bodies of the lateral ventricles are also shown, as are the pontine and interpeduncular cisterns.

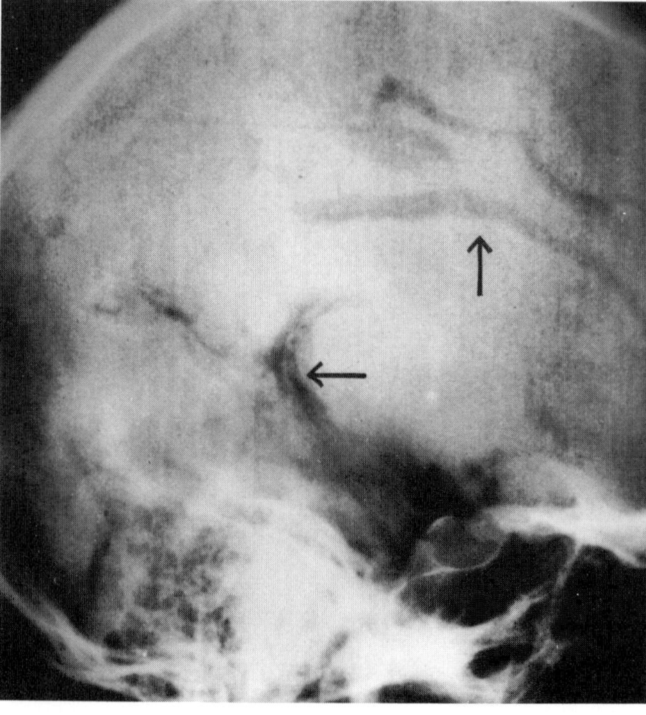

Fig. 60.9 No air has entered the ventricles. The pontine, interpeduncular, ambient (←) and pericallosal cisterns (↑) are outlined.

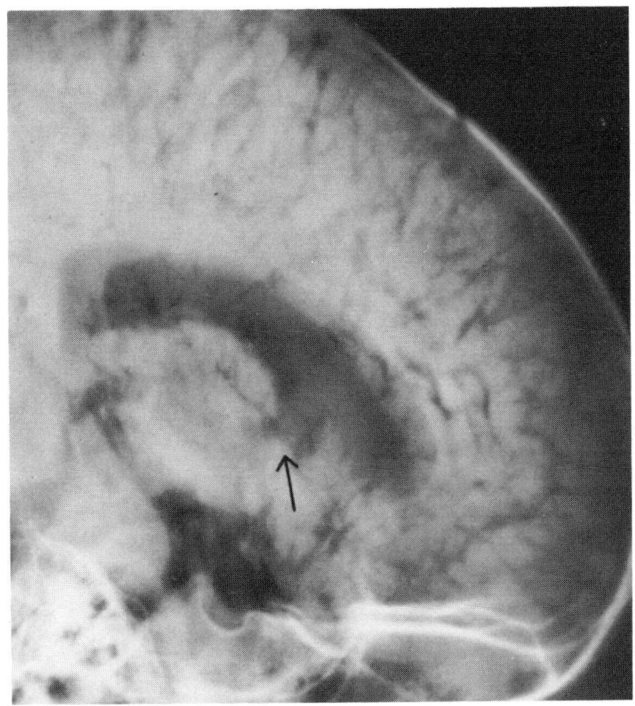

Fig. 60.10 Brow-up. The position is shown by the fluid levels in the bodies of the lateral ventricles. The third ventricle and the foramen of Monro (↑) can be identified.

surgical theatre. The head must be shaved, burr-holes made, and either air or positive contrast injected directly into the ventricle.

Technique. The introduction of neuroleptanalgesia, using *droperidol* and *phenoperidine* have greatly increased patients' comfort during the examination. These drugs should preferably be given in large doses, under skilled anaesthetic supervision.

Air injection is made by lumbar puncture with the patient in the sitting position, with the head flexed 20°. Air is very slowly injected and c.s.f. withdrawn in 5 ml fractions. Lateral and reversed Towne (half axial) films are taken at intervals during this period (Fig. 60.8). At this stage, the 4th ventricle, aqueduct, 3rd ventricle and roofs of the lateral ventricles should be demonstrated in both lateral and postero-anterior planes. In addition, the pontine, interpenduncular and ambient cisterns may be outlined (Fig. 60.9). The positions of the needle and head may be adjusted if necessary to promote ventricular filling.

When adequate ventricular filling has been obtained (usually by injection of 20 to 30 ml air), the needle is withdrawn and the patient placed in the horizontal position. With repositioning, the different parts of the ventricular system are progressively shown as in Figures 60.12, 60.13, 60.14, 60.15 and 60.16.

Tomography. Greatly enhanced detail of the anatomy of the third and fourth ventricles may be shown by tomography (Figs 60.15, 60.16 and 60.17). For this purpose, specialized equipment permitting cuts to be made in both horizontal and vertical planes is of the greatest assistance. This is of particular value in lesions in the area of the third ventricle, midbrain, fourth ventricle and cerebellopontine angle. When such equipment is not available, *autotomography* improves detail of the third and fourth ventricles and aqueduct.

Hazard and contraindications. When the intracranial pressure is raised, lumbar puncture is dangerous because it may precipitate tentorial or tonsillar herniation. The selection of patients for air encephalography must therefore be made after careful clinical assessment. Nowadays, any obstructive hydrocephalus is usually demonstrated previously by computed tomography.

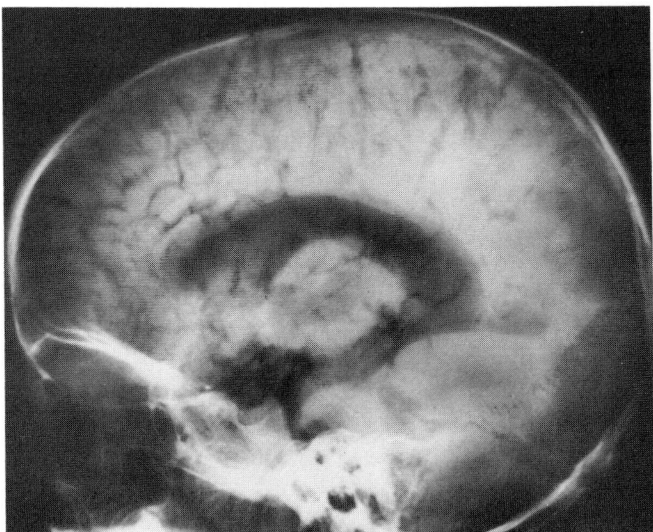

Fig. 60.11 Recumbent lateral film showing the temporal horn. The third ventricle is partly outlined, and the fourth ventricle is also seen.

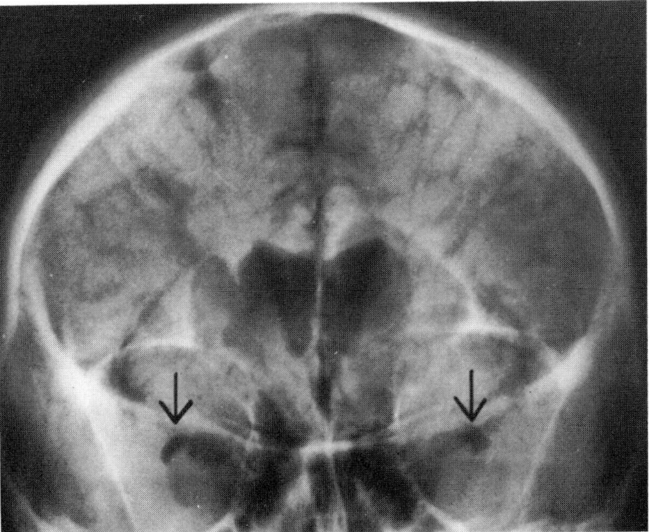

Fig. 60.12 Air in the tips of the temporal horns is shown by the small crescentic shadows in the centre of the orbits (↓).

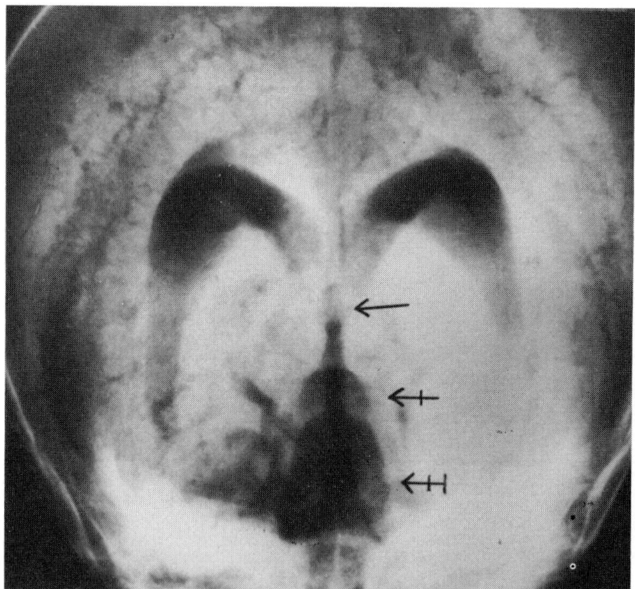

Fig. 60.13 Brow-down. The trigonal area and temporal horns are outlined. The third (←) and fourth ⇸) ventricles and cisterna magna (⇹) are outlined from above downwards in the midline. More laterally, air has passed into the cerebello-pontine angles.

Fig. 60.14 Brow-down. The trigone (→) and adjoining parts of the lateral ventricle are shown. The third (⊥) and fourth ventricles (⇻) and aqueduct may also be identified.

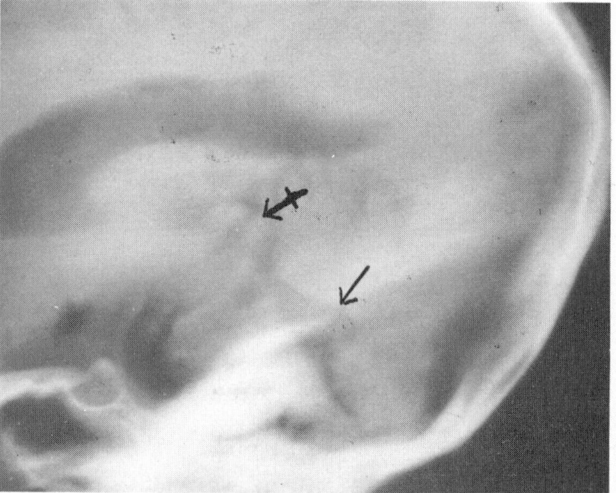

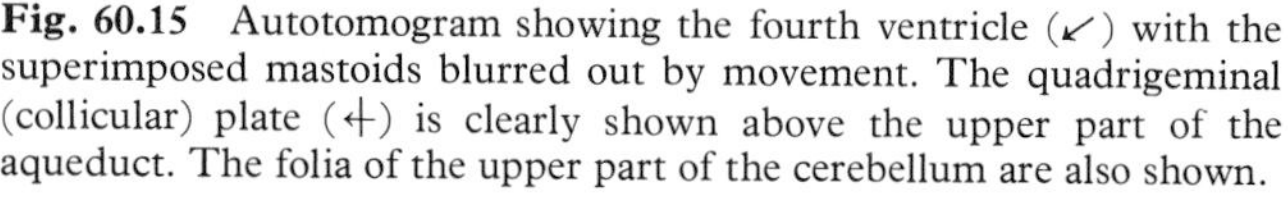

Fig. 60.15 Autotomogram showing the fourth ventricle (↙) with the superimposed mastoids blurred out by movement. The quadrigeminal (collicular) plate (⇸) is clearly shown above the upper part of the aqueduct. The folia of the upper part of the cerebellum are also shown.

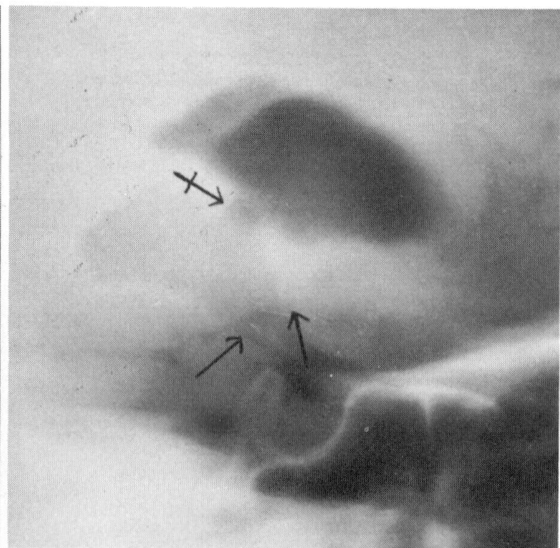

Fig. 60.16 Autotomogram showing the antero-inferior recesses of the third ventricle (→ ←) and the foramen of Monro (⇸).

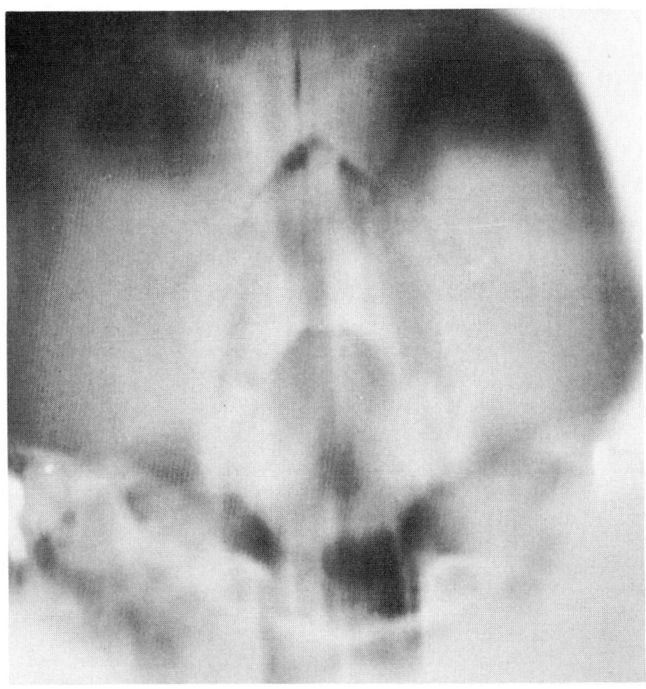

Fig. 60.17 Anterior tomogram of brain stem obtained with a Mimer III. The brain stem and fourth ventricle are well shown, as are the c.p. angles and cranial nerves.

Ventriculography. This is usually the final investigation when all other methods have failed to establish a precise diagnosis. It is usually employed for lesions in the region of the midbrain or posterior fossa, which frequently produce obstructive hydrocephalus with raised intracranial pressure. In this surgical procedure, burr holes are made in the skull, and contrast injected directly into a ventricle. The contrast substances used may be Metrizamide, Myodil (Pantopaque) or air. Following this injection, appropriate anteroposterior and lateral films are taken (Fig. 60.18A and B). The advantage of positive contrast is that a smaller volume (2 to 5 ml) is injected. This causes less disturbance to patients, many of whom are in a precarious clinical condition.

PATHOLOGICAL CONDITIONS

Encephalography and ventriculography give remarkably detailed information about the intracranial anatomy. The presence of a *tumour* is shown in more than 95 per cent of cases, and in the majority of these, accurate localization is usually possible. Obstruction to the cerebrospinal fluid pathway may be shown by ventricular dilatation proximal to the obstruction. Extrinsic tumours in the base of the skull may be outlined by air in the basal subarachnoid cisterns, confirming their extracerebral location.

Cerebral atrophy may be shown indirectly by *ex-vacuo* dilation of the ventricles, and more directly by the outlining of surface cortical scars and widening of the sulci by air.

Air studies may, however, reveal no abnormality in two main groups of conditions:

1. Multiple small tumours, as in metastatic deposits or meningeal carcinomas. In some cases there may be no deformity of the ventricular system or basal cisterns, and no ventricular dilatation.

2. Ischaemic disease and some diffuse inflammatory lesions, e.g. encephalitis. Air studies are frequently

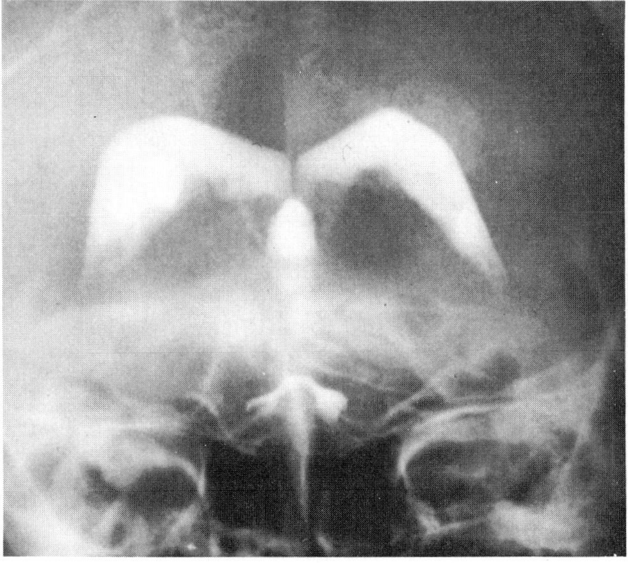

A

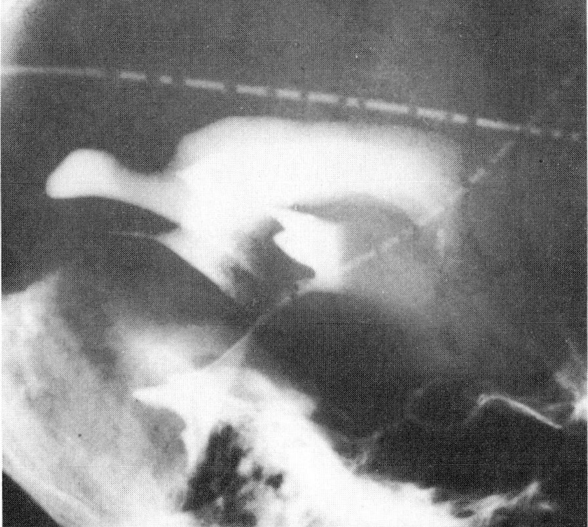

B

Fig. 60.18A and B Water soluble ventriculogram. The whole of the posterior half of the ventricular system is outlined.

normal in such cases, unless vascular occlusion leads to areas of infarction and oedema which cause ventricular narrowing and displacement. Cortical atrophy, however, may be shown by encephalography as a late sequel to these conditions, together with *ex-vacuo* dilatation of the ventricles.

Tumours and other mass lesions such as *blood clot*, *oedema* and *abscess* produce displacement and deformity of the ventricular system. Masses lying near the surface of the brain tend to produce *en-bloc* displacement of the ventricles, which retain their normal contour. Deeply placed masses produce more local deformity of the ventricular outline and may extend into the cavity of the ventricle, appearing as filling defects outlined by air. The cavity of a ventricle may be compressed, or even obliterated, by a tumour lying near it. The greatest displacements most commonly affect the anterior horns of the lateral ventricles, and the fourth ventricle. Lateral displacements are less marked in the central and posterior part of the intracranial cavity, as they are restrained by the relatively rigid attachments of the falx and tentorium in these areas.

With some tumours causing much swelling of a cerebral hemisphere, little or no air may be seen in the sulci over the surface of the affected hemisphere, in comparison with the unaffected side. This sign is somewhat variable, and little reliance may be placed on it. Lastly, much diagnostic information may be given by compression and deformity of the subarachnoid cisterns, enabling some tumours to be recognized, even when no air can be introduced into the ventricles.

HYDROCEPHALUS

Ventricular dilatation occurs in two contrasting circumstances:

1. *Obstructive hydrocephalus*, when the ventricles are dilated by increased pressure of cerebrospinal fluid due to an obstruction in its circulatory pathway.

2. *Non-obstructive hydrocephalus*, or *ex-vacuo* ventricular dilatation is found when the brain substance is reduced in volume as in cerebral atrophy, degeneration, destruction, or hypoplasia. This is accompanied by enlargement of the subarachnoid cisterns and the sulci on the surface of the hemispheres.

The size of the ventricles is somewhat variable, so that precise measurements are not practicable. It increases gradually, with age, when the superolateral angles as seen in brow-up anteroposterior films become slightly rounded. In general, the width of one lateral ventricle as measured on an anteroposterior brow-up X-ray film is usually less than 2 cm and the distance from the septum to the upper outer margin of the anterior horn is not more than one-third of the distance from the septum to the inner table of the skull in its widest part.

OBSTRUCTIVE HYDROCEPHALUS

Ventricular dilatation is found proximal to the site of the obstruction of the c.s.f. pathway. *Communicating hydrocephalus* refers to an obstruction lying outside the ventricles. The commonest site of such an obstruction is the tentorial hiatus due to such factors as the formation of a *pressure cone* or a *chronic arachnoiditis* after meningitis. A rarer cause of communicating hydrocephalus is *sinus thrombosis*, when the absorption of cerebrospinal fluid through the arachnoid villi into the venous sinuses is impaired.

Tumours are the most common cause of obstruction to the cerebrospinal fluid circulation within the ventricular system. The most vulnerable sites are the exit foramina of the lateral, third and fourth ventricles, and the narrow aqueduct in the midbrain. Adjacent tumour masses readily block these foramina or cause kinking or occlusion of the aqueduct. When this occurs, cerebrospinal fluid secreted by choroid plexus proximal to the obstruction cannot escape, and ventricular dilatation occurs. The same mechanism is operative in *non-neoplastic obstructions*, such as congenital stenosis of the aqueduct, and occlusion of the exit foramina of the fourth ventricle by arachnoid adhesions.

Dilatation of one lateral ventricle indicates some obstruction of the foramen of Monro. Symmetrical dilatation of the lateral ventricles with incomplete filling of the third ventricle may indicate a tumour within the third ventricle. Symmetrical hydrocephalus of the lateral and third ventricles without dilatation of the fourth ventricle signals a tumour in the region of the pineal, midbrain or posterior fossa, or congenital stenosis of the aqueduct. Dilatation of all four ventricles, if not due to communicating hydrocephalus, indicates obstruction to the exit foramina of the fourth ventricle by tumour, arachnoid adhesions or developmental atresia (the Dandy-Walker syndrome).

Hydrocephalus of the lateral and third ventricles due to aqueduct obstruction is not uncommon. Three different groups of lesions may produce this phenomenon:

1. Strictures of the aqueduct.

2. Local tumours in the brain stem and pineal region. (These may be in the posterior fossa.)

3. Tumours in the posterior fossa, particularly in the cerebellum. These latter cause lateral displacement of the fourth ventricle, which produce angulation or 'kinking' of the aqueduct which is anchored in the tentorial opening. This kinking frequently obstructs the cerebrospinal fluid circulation.

It is of considerable importance in management that these three groups of causes of aqueduct obstruction should be differentiated, as different operative approaches are employed. Direct operation is not usually feasible on lesions in the brain stem and pineal region, and a bypass operation (ventriculo-atrial or ventriculo-peritoneal shunt) has to be performed. For infratentorial lesions, a posterior fossa exploration with direct attack on a tumour may be practicable. Contrast ventriculography is usually safer and more informative than air ventriculography or encephalography in such cases, as the intracranial pressure may be very high. This often results in considerable local expansion or 'ballooning' of the suprapineal recess, which usually extends posteriorly, with possible rupture of the ependymal wall into the quadrigeminal cistern (Fig. 60.19).

In the present section, the non-neoplastic causes of obstructive hydrocephalus will be briefly described. Tumours causing such obstruction will be considered in the systematic regional account which follows later.

usually has a smooth or tapering margin, and the aqueduct is not displaced (Fig. 60.20). It is commonly found in the upper third of the midbrain. In aqueduct obstruction due to a *local tumour*, the margin of the stenosis is often irregular, and the aqueduct may be slightly displaced. Kinking of the aqueduct due to a *posterior fossa tumour* rarely produces a complete obstruction, and the fourth ventricle is usually outlined and shown to be displaced.

Acquired stenoses of the aqueduct are rare. They may be seen as a late sequel to diffuse inflammatory disease—*meningo-encephalitis*. The commoner infections producing this are *tuberculous meningitis*, *toxoplasmosis*, and *cytomegalic inclusion disease*. The aqueduct may be similarly obstructed by *seeding* through the cerebrospinal fluid of

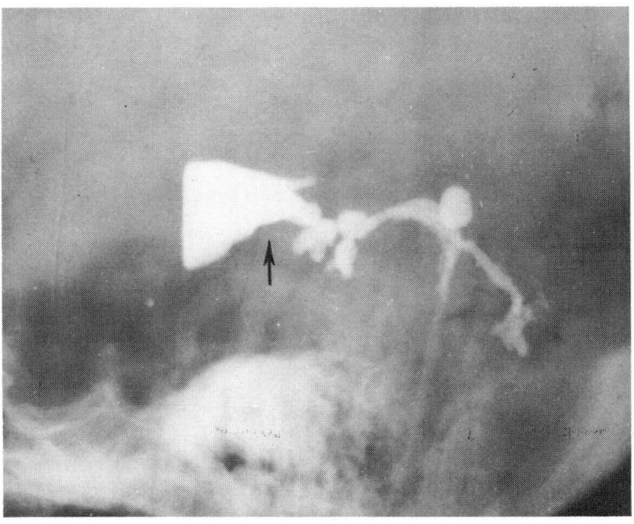

Fig. 60.19 Ruptured suprapineal recess. Aqueduct obstructed by midbrain tumour. Myodil has entered the quadrigeminal cistern and passed over the upper surface of the cerebellar hemispheres. Irregular indentation by tumour of floor of third ventricle posteriorly (↑).

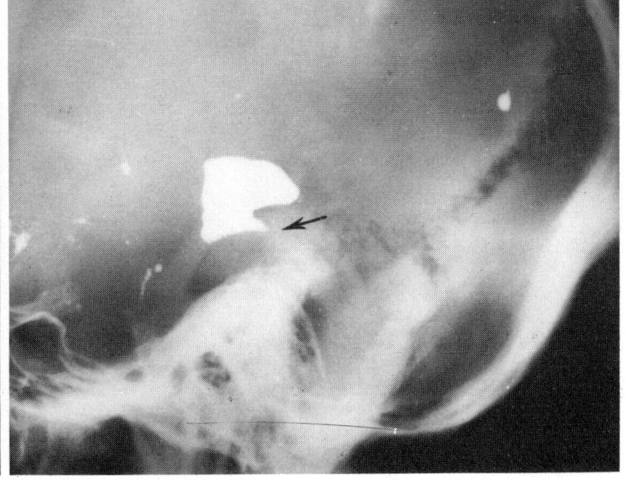

Fig. 60.20 Aqueduct stenosis (↙). Patient supine. Myodil obstructed in upper aqueduct. The third ventricle lay in the midline.

Aqueduct stenosis

Developmental strictures in the aqueduct are not uncommon. Symptoms may be present from birth, with rapid and progressive enlargement of the head. It is none the less remarkable that patients with pin-hole narrowing of the aqueduct may experience no symptoms until adult life. Presumably some minor traumatic or inflammatory episode then upsets the precarious hydrodynamic balance, so that the minute channel is no longer adequate and the obstruction becomes relatively complete.

Air and Myodil ventriculography tend to show a greater degree of obstruction than actually prevails. Both these contrast media have a greater surface tension than cerebrospinal fluid, which may be able to traverse a very tight stricture. This does not apply to water-soluble media.

In differential diagnosis, a *benign aqueduct stenosis*

ependymomas and *gliomas* invading the ventricle. Subependymal metaplastic nodules of *tuberose sclerosis* may also obstruct the aqueduct though more commonly they obstruct the foramen of Monro. In the inflammatory lesions, ependymitis or gliosis occurring at the site of old inflammatory foci causes the obstruction. In all these conditions the previous history and other stigmata of the disease may suggest the diagnosis. Nodules elsewhere in the walls of the ventricles may be seen in tuberose sclerosis and cytomegalic inclusion disease (the latter is a viral prenatal meningo-encephalitis). Widespread intracerebral calcifications are often present in tuberose sclerosis, in addition to the facial adenoma sebaceum and history of mental retardation with epilepsy. Toxoplasmosis, also a prenatal focal encephalomyelitis, is characterized by calcifications in the basal ganglia and cortex (Fig. 59.30).

Fourth ventricle obstruction

Obstruction to the cerebrospinal fluid circulation at the exit foramina of the fourth ventricle are encountered in two groups of non-neoplastic conditions: (1) adhesive arachnoiditis and the Dandy-Walker syndrome and (2) the Arnold-Chiari malformation.

Arachnoid adhesions and the Dandy-Walker syndrome. After meningitis, the meninges are often thickened, fibrosed and adherent, particularly round the base of the brain. Such adhesive arachnoiditis may implicate the foramina of Magendie and Luschka and obstruct the exit of cerebrospinal fluid from the fourth ventricle. A purulent meningitis or any of the specific infections referred to under aqueduct stenosis can be the primary cause. In post-tuberculous cases, punctate meningeal calcifications may be seen elsewhere in the basal subarachnoid cisterns. Ventriculography is the examination of choice to show such foraminal obstruction. The intracranial pressure is often raised, and the adhesions would in any event prevent air entering the fourth ventricle at air encephalography.

The same phenomena are found in the *Dandy-Walker syndrome*, when there is developmental atresia of the foramina of Magendie and Luschka.

Diagnosis is really made by exclusion, as there is symmetrical hydrocephalus affecting all four ventricles, with no displacement to suggest a tumour. In the Dandy-Walker syndrome, the fourth ventricle may balloon out to a huge size, occupying most of the posterior fossa.

Arnold-Chiari syndrome. In a major degree of this condition there is downward prolapse of medulla, pons and cerebellar tonsils through the foramen magnum into the upper cervical spinal canal. Minor degrees with prolapse of tonsils only are more frequently seen. Various associated developmental bony anomalies may be found, including defects in the foramen magnum, spina bifida and a shallow posterior fossa. The caudal part of the fourth ventricle may be displaced downwards to the level of C.2 or even lower (Fig. 60.21). The ensuing compression in the narrow cervical spinal canal may occlude its outlet and lead to obstructive hydrocephalus. The demonstration of this abnormality is obviously best undertaken by ventriculography, for reasons similar to those given in the preceding section. However, the displaced tonsils may be outlined by air at encephalography. They can also be shown by myelography (Fig. 60.22), which will also reveal any associated hydromyelia or syringomyelia.

More recently, herniated cerebellar tonsils have been demonstrated by computed tomography of the craniovertebral junction following intrathecal injection of metrizamide (see Ch. 65, p. 1292).

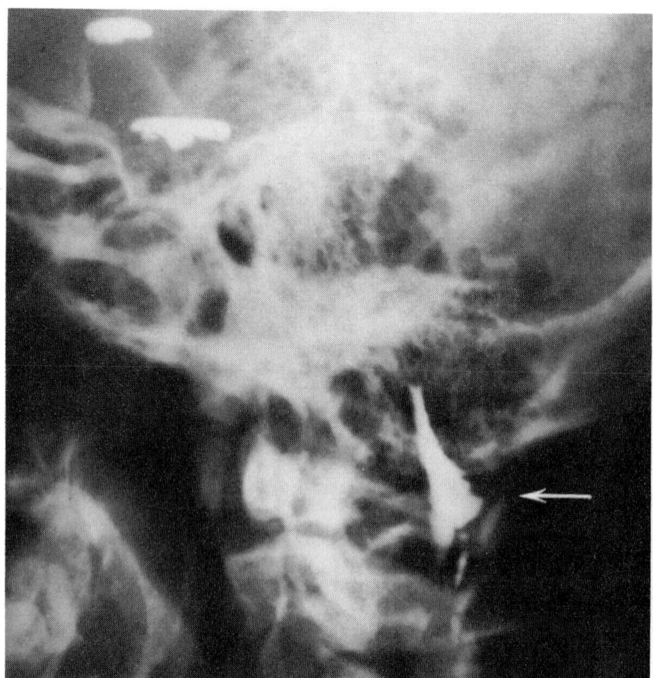

Fig. 60.21 Arnold-Chiari malformation. Fourth ventricle at level of C.1 (←).

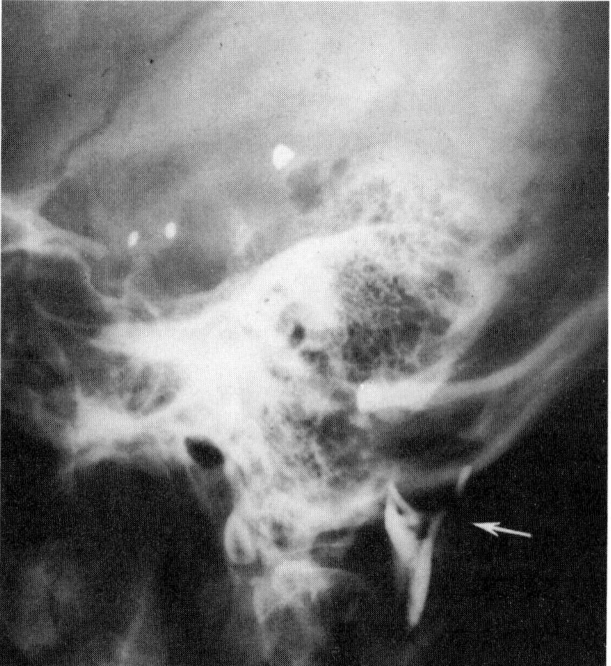

Fig. 60.22 Supine myelogram with patient tilted head downwards. Myodil outlines cerebellar tonsils displaced below posterior margin of foramen magnum (←).

Normal pressure hydrocephalus

In recent years, a group of patients has been recognized

in which communicating hydrocephalus is present, with ventricular dilatation, but with normal intracranial pressure. The obstruction to c.s.f. flow lies outside the ventricular system and is usually due to arachnoid adhesions in the basal cisterns or tentorial opening. In many patients, this follows subarachnoid haemorrhage or head injury, with irritant blood in the c.s.f. In others, there may be a previous history of meningitis. In other patients still, there may be no history of such illnesses, and the adhesions appear to have arisen spontaneously.

The resulting symptoms consist of progressive dementia, ataxia, incontinence and spastic paraparesis. Their recognition is of great importance, since these symptoms are reversible and may be relieved by ventriculo-atrial shunt in carefully selected cases (Adams *et al.*, 1965). The diagnosis may be established by air encephalography or by metrizamide or isotope cisternography.

At air encephalography, the ventricles and sometimes the basal cisterns are enlarged. Little or no air passes over the brain surface, however, due to the adhesions, and the sulci are not enlarged.

At isotope cisternography, the isotope injected by lumbar puncture passes into the ventricles, where it remains, instead of circulating over the surface of the hemispheres to the vertex, and being absorbed in 24 to 48 hours. This method is now being replaced by a combination of intrathecal metrizamide and computed tomography (see Ch. 63, p. 1234).

NON-OBSTRUCTIVE HYDROCEPHALUS

Atrophy and hypoplasia

In these conditions, the brain volume is reduced. This results in *ex-vacuo* dilatation of the ventricles, and both the subarachnoid cisterns and sulci over the hemispheres are enlarged. The condition may be general or local, is usually acquired, but may be congenital, and affects mainly the hemispheres of the cerebrum or cerebellum.

The ventricular dilatation due to atrophy may be distinguished from that due to obstructive hydrocephalus both by the clinical features and by the enlargement of the sulci and basal cisterns. When atrophy is unilateral, there may be some ventricular displacement towards the affected side. This mechanism should be remembered and not misinterpreted as being due to a tumour in the contralateral hemisphere.

Atrophy or hypoplasia results from several main groups of lesions:

1. **Congenital and neonatal.** Developmental hypoplasia and atrophy following birth injuries.
2. **Vascular.** Generalized arteriosclerosis, and arteriosclerosis with thrombo-embolism producing infarction.
3. **Traumatic.** Local scars, and general ventricular dilatation following major head injuries.
4. **Degenerative.** Presenile (Pick-Alzheimer's disease) and senile dementia. Heredofamilial cerebellar atrophies.
5. **Inflammatory.** Following encephalitis and general paresis.

INTRACRANIAL TUMOURS

In the following pages, the word 'tumour' will be used in its wider neurosurgical sense to refer to any intracranial mass, including oedema, blood clot, abscess and cyst as well as neoplasm. Air studies do not usually permit distinction between the different pathological types of mass lesion.

The presence of obstructive hydrocephalus is usually an indirect sign of the presence of an intracranial tumour. More direct evidence is given by displacement and deformity of the ventricles, which enable precise anatomical localization of the mass to be made.

Three-quarters of brain tumours are found in the cerebral hemispheres, and of these, half occur in the frontal lobes, perhaps because of the greater relative size of these structures.

Displacement of the lateral ventricles is a sign that the mass lies above the tentorium, and not in the posterior fossa. Local deformity of a lateral ventricle indicates a tumour placed near the ventricle, usually lying deeply. Superficial masses situated on or near the convexity produce *en-bloc* displacement of the ventricular system.

Filling defects within the ventricle are another sign of a deeply placed tumour, arising in, or which has invaded, the ventricular cavity.

Unequal air-filling of the ventricles should be interpreted with caution, as it may be due to technique during air injection. Dilatation of one lateral ventricle should also be interpreted with caution. This may result from distortion of the foramen of Monro by a tumour in the contralateral hemisphere—or to direct obstruction of this foramen by an ipsilateral tumour. The possibility of dilatation of one lateral ventricle due to ipsilateral cortical atrophy must also be remembered.

Lateral brain displacement is clearly shown in anteroposterior encephalograms. The alignment of the septum pellucidum and third ventricle frequently indicates whether the mass lies in the upper or lower half of the hemispheres. Displacements affect mainly the septum lucidum and upper half of the third ventricle. The lower part of the third ventricle is relatively anchored by the pituitary stalk.

Tumours situated high on the convexity of the hemisphere exert thrust and consequently cause most displacement of the upper part of the septum lucidum. Displacement of the lower half of the septum and upper half of the third ventricle is correspondingly less. In this type of displacement, the septum and third ventricle maintain their normal alignment—i.e. a straight line (Fig. 60.23).

Low hemisphere tumours, lying in the temporal lobe or basal ganglia, produce a different configuration. Here the maximum thrust occurs at the junction between the septum and third ventricle. The greatest lateral displacement is, therefore, seen in the lower part of the septum and upper part of the third ventricle. This produces angulation between the lines of the septum and third ventricle (Fig. 60.24).

Such lateral brain displacements produce secondary changes in the roofs of the lateral ventricles in anteroposterior films. In the frontal area there may be herniation of the lateral ventricle beneath the falx. This results in depression of the roof of the herniated ventricle. Such an appearance may be difficult to distinguish from depression of the roof by a parasagittal tumour. The appearance of the upper and outer angle of the body of the lateral ventricle may help to distinguish between these two causes. In herniation beneath the falx, this angle is sharper and at a higher level than the medial part of the roof (Fig. 60.24). In the presence of a parasagittal tumour, this angle is at the same level or lower than the medial part of the roof, and may also be slightly rounded.

It is, however, in the diagnosis and exclusion of tumours, that air encephalography has been so greatly replaced by computed tomography and angiography. This is especially so in tumours of the cerebral hemispheres. For this reason, such lesions will not be described in detail. The encephalographic changes they produce are included in the diagrammatic summary shown in Figures 60.37 to 60.41.

Tumours which will be described in more detail are those near the skull base, especially near the midline and those arising in the posterior fossa. At the time of writing, these areas are the most diagnostically difficult by the newer methods, and it is here that further information may be sought by encephalography or ventriculography, for either diagnosis or management.

Third ventricle. Whilst the third ventricle may be invaded by infiltrating tumours arising in adjacent structures, the two characteristic masses found within the ventricle are the colloid cyst and the pinealoma.

Colloid or *paraphysial cysts* are derived from cells of the anterior part of the choroid plexus in the roof of the third ventricle. They are usually small, 1 to 2 cm in diameter, with a smooth border, and produce symptoms when they obstruct the foramina of Monro. Such obstruction may be related to the position of the head, as the cyst is often pedunculated, and may impact in the foramen. This intermittent foraminal obstruction causes the characteristic postural paroxysmal headache. Colloid cysts are best demonstrated in anteroposterior projections with the brow-up, when they appear as rounded defects at the base of the septum. The round, soft-tissue mass may also be outlined in lateral view behind the foramen of Monro (Fig. 60.25). With foraminal obstruction, a considerable degree of symmetrical hydrocephalus is often seen. In the differential diagnosis of a colloid cyst, large *suprasellar cysts*, *tuberose sclerotic nodules* near the foramen of Monro, and *basilar aneurysms* must be remembered. Large

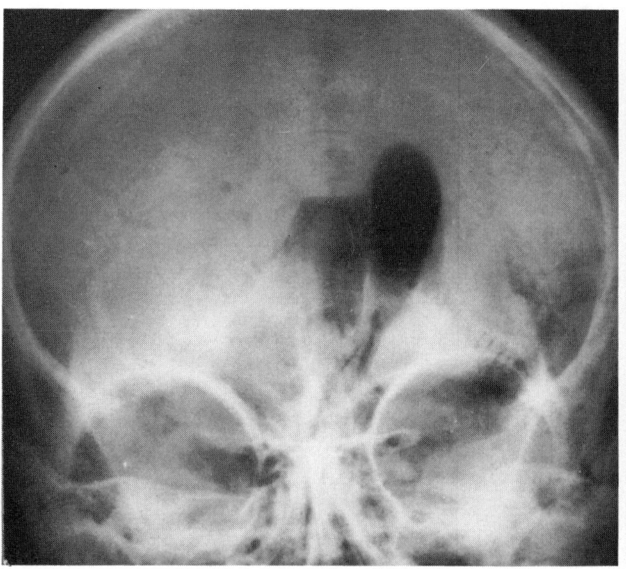

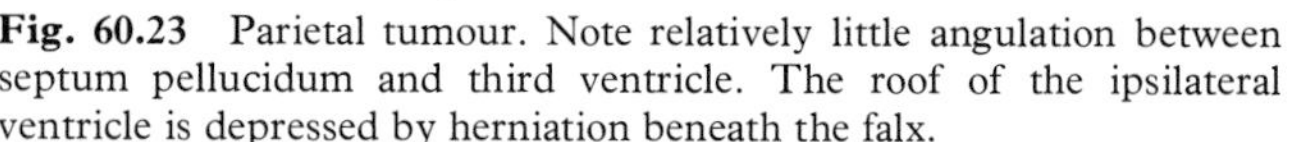

Fig. 60.23 Parietal tumour. Note relatively little angulation between septum pellucidum and third ventricle. The roof of the ipsilateral ventricle is depressed by herniation beneath the falx.

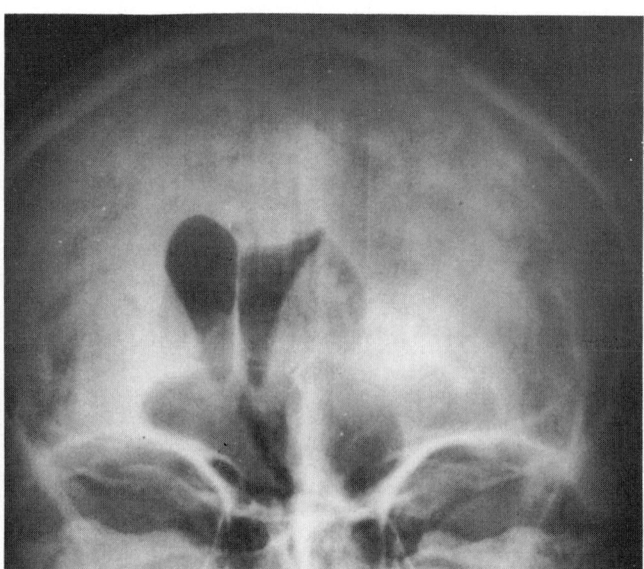

Fig. 60.24 Low hemisphere tumour, showing angulation between septum pellucidum and third ventricle. The roof of the ipsilateral ventricle is slightly depressed owing to lateral herniation beneath the falx.

aneurysms arising from the bifurcation of the basilar artery may very rarely extend up through the floor of the third ventricle as high as the foramina of Monro. If the diagnosis is in any doubt, vertebral angiography may be performed, and the prudent surgeon will always insert a fine needle into the sac before attempting excision.

Pinealoma. Although not a true intraventricular tumour, a pinealoma enlarges into the posterior end of the third ventricle, and in so doing may obstruct the aqueduct. Other tumours occur in this area and may produce similar appearances. They include third ventricle *ependymomas* and brain stem and posterior thalamic *gliomas*. The latter produce some lateral displacement of the third ventricle, whereas with tumours of the pineal and brain stem the third ventricle remains in the midline. Pinealomas obliterate the suprapineal recess and produce a smooth convex indentation of the posterior half of the third ventricle. There is often an unusually large, irregular area of calcification in the pineal on plain films (Fig. 60.26). In differential diagnosis, a congenital stricture obstructing the upper aqueduct leads to a dilated pineal recess in the posterior end of the third ventricle. Gliomas encroaching on the posterior end of the third ventricle produce an irregular indentation in contradistinction to the smooth curve of a pinealoma. As mentioned earlier, pinealomas may metastasize by seeding through the cerebrospinal fluid.

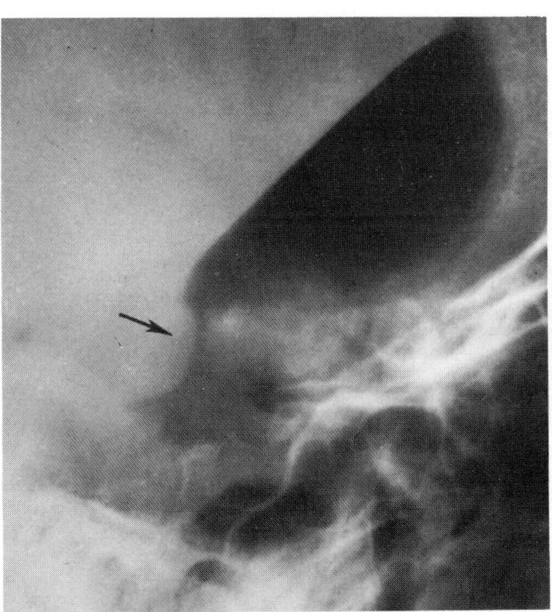

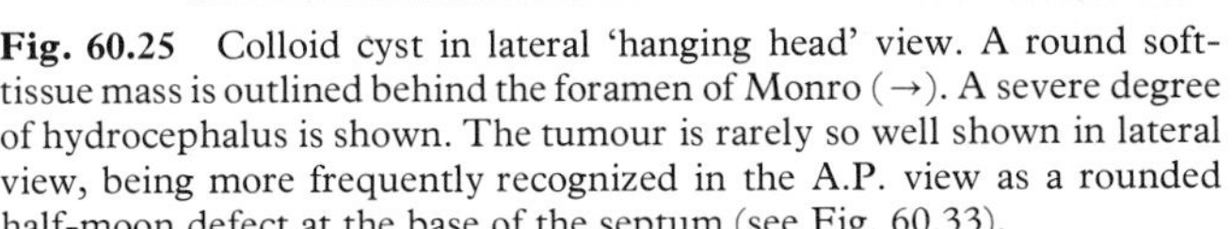

Fig. 60.25 Colloid cyst in lateral 'hanging head' view. A round soft-tissue mass is outlined behind the foramen of Monro (→). A severe degree of hydrocephalus is shown. The tumour is rarely so well shown in lateral view, being more frequently recognized in the A.P. view as a rounded half-moon defect at the base of the septum (see Fig. 60.33).

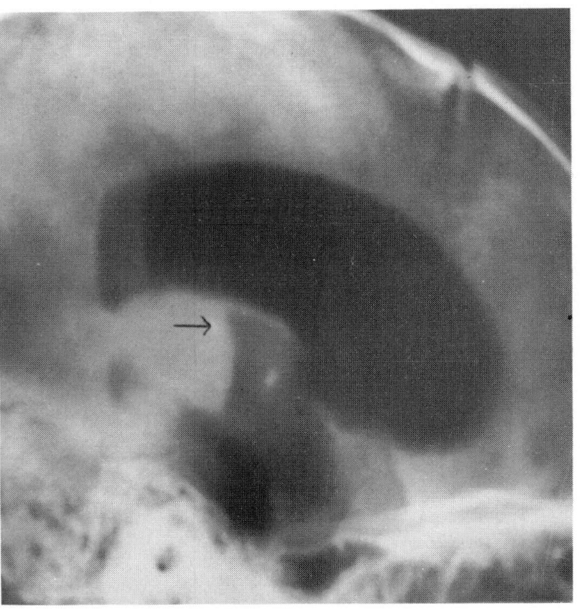

Fig. 60.26 Pinealoma. Typical smooth indentation of the posterior end of the third ventricle. Punctate calcification within tumour (→). Obstruction of the aqueduct has caused hydrocephalus.

Suprasellar tumours

A well-defined group of tumours occurs in the suprasellar area. Typical syndromes are produced, enabling precise clinical localization. These tumours are usually encapsulated, rather than invasive, and the symptomatology results from local pressure. Hypopituitarism follows pressure atrophy of the pituitary gland. Pressure on the optic nerve chiasm or optic nerves produces bitemporal hemianopia and blindness. Sometimes these tumours are sufficiently large to extend upwards and obstruct the foramina of Monro, producing obstructive hydrocephalus of the lateral ventricles.

The tumours most commonly occurring in this group are:

1. *Pituitary tumours*, usually chromophobe adenoma.
2. *Craniopharyngiomas* (Rathke pouch or suprasellar cysts).
3. *Aneurysms*—arising from the supraclinoid portion of the carotid artery.
4. *Meningiomas*—arising from the diaphragma sellae, and dural convexity of the medial part of the sphenoid bone.
5. *Optic nerve gliomas*—arising from the optic nerve or chiasm.

Other tumours less commonly found in this area include *glioma of the hypothalamus*, *secondary deposit*, and supra and parasellar extensions of *chordomas* and *nasopharyngeal carcinomas*.

Valuable information regarding the nature of the lesion is given by plain films. Air encephalography is necessary to show the precise extent of the suprasellar mass, which cannot be assessed clinically.

Chromophobe pituitary tumours cause erosion of the dorsum sellae and floor of the pituitary fossa. This is often asymmetrical, giving a double contour in lateral films. Soft-tissue calcification is frequently seen in craniopharyngiomas and in the walls of aneurysms. Meningiomas often invade the underlying bone, producing thickening and sclerosis, seen in the clinoid processes and adjoining medial parts of the sphenoid bone. Calcification is also sometimes seen in meningiomas. Optic nerve gliomas may cause erosion and enlargement of the optic foramen. These tumours, with craniopharyngiomas, are most commonly encountered in childhood.

In the clinical management of this group of conditions, it is important to know the exact size of the suprasellar mass in order to decide whether treatment shall be surgical, or by radiotherapy, or by both methods. Tumours extending to the foramen of Monro are usually considered too large for surgical attack. This extent of the suprasellar mass may only be shown by encephalography (or ventriculography if the intracranial pressure is raised (Fig. 60.27A and B)). Suprasellar tumours compress and obliterate the basal subarachnoid cisterns, the cisternae chiasmatis and interpeduncularis. The upward extension of such tumours causes elevation and indentation of the anterior end of the third ventricle (Fig. 60.27A). Large masses extending up to the foramina of Monro obliterate the anterior third of the third ventricle and elevate and project into the floor of the anterior horn of the lateral ventricles (Fig. 60.20B). Such changes are readily seen in both anteroposterior and lateral encephalograms. Smaller masses may only be recognizable in lateral projections.

The diagnostic radiographs are those taken with the brow-up, particularly the lateral films with a horizontal beam. The head should be over-extended to enable good air filling of the dependent antero-inferior recesses of the front of the third ventricle. These recesses may not be completely outlined in the supine brow-up position, as the antero-inferior part of the third ventricle is directed downwards towards the skull base.

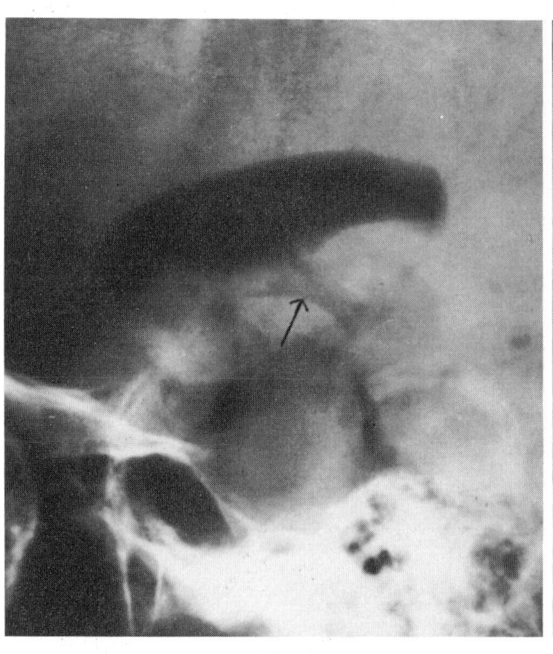

A

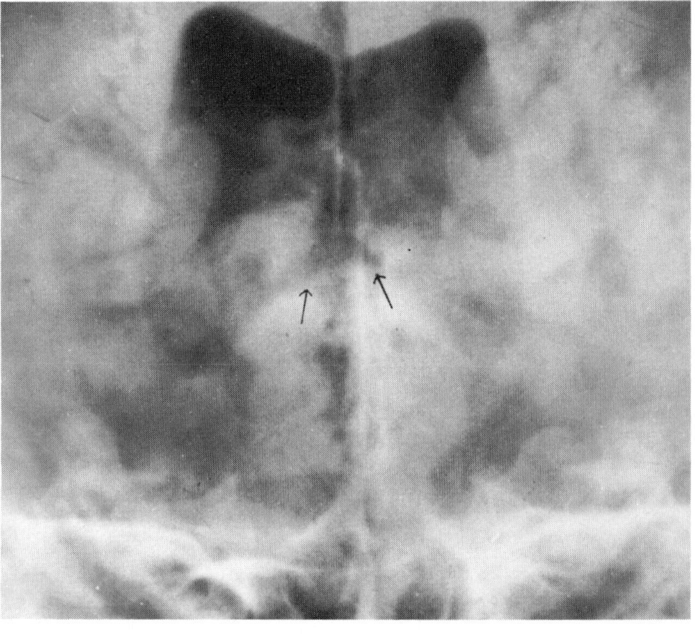

B

Fig. 60.27 (A) Indentation and elevation of the anterior end of the third ventricle (↗) by suprasellar extension of chromophobe adenoma. (B) The midline tumour mass (↖↗) encroaches on the floor of both the third and lateral ventricles.

Suprasellar tumours compress and may obliterate the basal subarachnoid cisterns situated above the pituitary fossa. Anterior masses occlude the cisterna chiasmatis, and posterior masses extend into the cisterna interpeduncularis. Occasionally the tumour mass may be outlined by air in these cisterns. More commonly, however, air in these cisterns depict a suprasellar mass smaller than is actually found at operation or autopsy. The reason for this is that large subarachnoid spaces extend laterally from the cisterna chiasmatis into the parasellar area around the carotid arteries. Air in this space will obscure midline suprasellar masses in lateral projections. In such projections, subarachnoid air lying laterally in the lower part of the Sylvian fissure will also obscure the suprasellar structures. The crux of the examination is the demonstration of the antero-inferior end of the third ventricle. When this area is not clearly shown on plain lateral films with the head overextended, tomography or autotomography will usually give very satisfactory detail. Suprasellar tumours usually obliterate the recesses in the anterior end of the third ventricle and cause a smooth convex indentation of its anterior end. This indentation is very similar to that produced in the posterior end of the third ventricle by a pinealoma.

Metrizamide cisternography

At the time of writing, metrizamide cisternography is replacing air encephalography in the demonstration of suprasellar anatomy. This method of examination is equally precise, but is far less unpleasant for the patient, causing only a minor degree of side reaction, such as headache, nausea and vomiting. It can also be supplemented effectively by computed tomography (Sheldon and Molyneux, 1979).

For this examination, metrizamide (250 mg 1 per ml) is injected by lumbar or lateral cervical puncture. Appropriate doses would be 5–7 ml by lumbar puncture, and 1–2 ml less than this by cervical injection. The prone patient is then tilted head downward under lateral fluoroscopic control. The contrast medium flows up the clivus, and through the suprasellar cisterns. When appropriate contrast distribution is obtained, the patient is returned to the prone horizontal position. Lateral films and tomograms are then taken (Fig. 60.36). Following this, the supine patient is transferred for C.T. scanning, when axial basal views and also coronal scans are made of the suprasellar cisterns (see Ch. 63).

The 'empty' sella

Enlargement of the pituitary fossa on lateral radiographs is usually due to either an intrasellar tumour or to raised intracranial pressure. In recent years, interest has been aroused by a third cause, the syndrome of the 'empty' sella. In this condition, a subarachnoid recess extends into the pituitary fossa. The pituitary gland itself is often compressed into a thin rim of tissue lying in the postero-inferior part of the floor of the pituitary fossa.

The aetiology of this condition has not yet been finally established. The most probable cause is a developmental defect in the diaphragma sellae, a finding not uncommonly seen at routine post-mortem examinations. This allows prolapse of a small fluid-containing pocket of arachnoid into the pituitary fossa. The fluid-transmitted pulsation then results in enlargement of the sella. Other mechanisms have been postulated, including primary pituitary shrinkage, either following necrosis in a tumour or after surgery or radiotherapy.

Although the gland is compressed, pituitary function is often normal, although occasionally diminished. An intrasellar subarachnoid cistern is also occasionally observed in relation to raised intracranial pressure.

The normal maximum length of the sella in the sagittal plane is 17 mm and the depth 13 to 14 mm. An intrasellar subarachnoid recess results in an enlarged, deepened and globular sella on lateral radiographs.

There is no erosion of the lamina dura, and no posterior displacement of the dorsum sellae. These changes are not invariable, and the sella may have a normal outline, despite the presence of an intrasellar recess.

Diagnosis is obviously dependent on air encephalography. It may also be suggested by computed tomography. It is important that the condition should be recognized when present, lest the enlarged sella be mistakenly attributed to a pituitary tumour, with the potential hazard of unnecessary surgery or radiotherapy. Tomography is necessary for the air studies to differentiate between air within the pituitary fossa and in the adjoining suprasellar and parasellar subarachnoid spaces. Tomographic cuts should be taken in lateral and preferably also the anteroposterior planes.

Air will enter the intrasellar cistern in the sitting position with the head extended, and also in the brow-up positions. This air can be shown to leave, and re-enter the pituitary fossa with repositioning of the head. Sometimes a fluid level may be demonstrable within the pituitary fossa.

Tumours of the midbrain and tentorium

The narrow aqueduct of Sylvius, or iter, is particularly vulnerable to obstruction as it passes downwards through the tentorial opening in the midbrain. Tumours in this area are thus often accompanied by raised intracranial pressure and symmetrical obstructive hydrocephalus of the lateral and third ventricles.

When the intracranial pressure is high, ventriculography is the examination of choice, and positive contrast, using Myodil or metrizamide, is particularly valuable in outlining the aqueduct clearly. In the absence of obstructive hydrocephalus, air encephalography is preferable, for in addition to outlining the third and fourth ventricles and aqueduct, it will also show detail of the quadrigeminal, pontine and interpeduncular cisterns.

Local deformities produced by tumours in the tentorial hiatus affect the aqueduct, posterior end of third ventricle and quadrigeminal and interpeduncular cisterns. The most common tumour in this area is a *midbrain glioma.* Less common masses include *tentorial meningioma*, *aneurysm of the basilar artery* or *vein of Galen*, *glioma of the quadrigeminal plate*, posterior extension of *pinealoma*, *midbrain angioma*, and *meningioma* and *chordoma* arising from the upper part of the clivus and dorsum sellae. Because of the frequency of vascular lesions in this area, vertebral angiography may be advisable as a complementary investigation.

Midbrain. Tumours in the midbrain usually obstruct the aqueduct early. An irregular occlusion of the aqueduct is in favour of a glioma rather than a simple stricture.

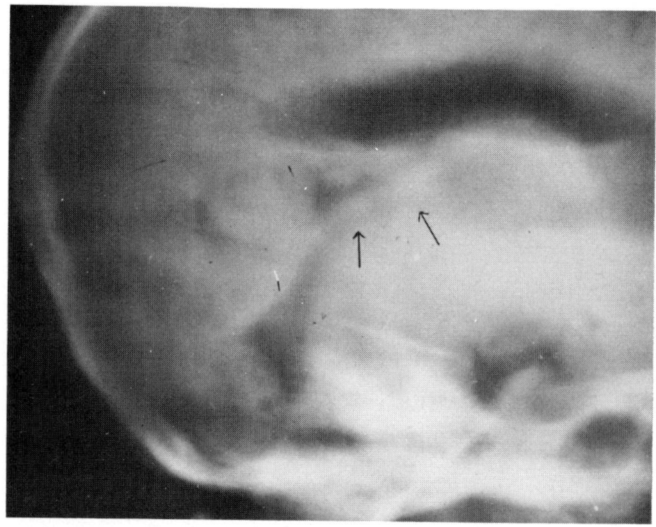

Fig. 60.28 Midbrain tumour. Autotomogram shows the upper part of the aqueduct displaced upwards and posteriorly (↖).

The aqueduct may be displaced posteriorly (Fig. 60.28). The posterior end of the third ventricle is not deformed, although it is frequently dilated. When a midbrain tumour extends forward into the cerebral peduncles, it may compress the interpeduncular cistern and elevate the floor of the posterior end of the third ventricle. Tumours of the quadrigeminal plate deform and may obliterate the quadrigeminal cistern. Their forward extension may deform the posterior end of the third ventricle. Pinealomas and pineal cysts tend to produce rounded defects, whilst the defects due to quadrigeminal plate tumours are more irregular.

Tentorium. *Meningiomas* are the most common tentorial tumours. They are often related to the tentorial opening and may lie on its anterior, lateral or posterior aspect. Meningiomas of the clivus and cerebellopontine angle may also extend into the anterior and lateral portions of the tentorial hiatus. Of the vascular masses, *aneurysm of the basillar artery* may occur anteriorly in the tentorial opening, and *aneurysm of the vein of Galen* posteriorly.

Extrinsic masses are less liable to occlude the aqueduct than intrinsic tumours. Thus the aqueduct may be displaced but patent throughout its length, whilst the third and fourth ventricles show little displacement. This is an important diagnostic feature. The aqueduct is displaced posteriorly by tumours in the anterior half of the tentorial opening, laterally by lateral tumours, and anteriorly by posterior tumours. Anterior tumours may elevate the floor of the posterior end of the third ventricle. Posterior tumours compress and deform the quadrigeminal cistern.

Posterior fossa tumours

Tumours arising beneath the tentorium in the posterior cranial fossa form an important and well-defined group of lesions both clinically and radiologically. They are common in both childhood and adult life, and frequently obstruct the aqueduct or fourth ventricle. The ensuing hydrocephalus often results in high intracranial pressure with false localizing signs clinically. A precise radiological diagnosis may be crucial, because of the special operative approach, or alternatively, the decision in inoperable cases of referring the patient direct for radiotherapy.

It is necessary to confirm whether a tumour lies in the posterior fossa, and if possible whether it is *intrinsic* in the brain stem or cerebellum, or *extrinsic*. Extrinsic and cerebellar tumours are usually operable. Tumours of the *brain stem*—medulla, pons and midbrain—are not, and are referred for radiotherapy, if applicable. Tumours of the brain stem usually show a clear difference, both clinically and radiologically from cerebellar and extrinsic tumours.

Plain films of the skull often show signs of raised intracranial pressure—spreading of sutures in children and pressure erosion of the dorsum sellae in adults. Extrinsic tumours in the cerebellopontine angles may cause erosion of a petrous apex, or expansion of an internal auditory meatus. Nasopharyngeal tumours may show a soft-tissue mass in the nasopharyngeal area in lateral films, and bony erosion of the skull base above in basal views and tomograms. Chordomas may produce bony destruction in the area of the clivus. They may also produce a soft-tissue mass in the pharynx, and may show calcification in their substance. Calcification within the brain substance is occasionally seen in gliomas.

It has been mentioned earlier that displacements of the fourth ventricle and lower aqueduct cause local angulation, usually referred to as kinking, of the upper part of the aqueduct where it is relatively fixed in the tentorial opening. Such a kink may block the circulation of cerebrospinal fluid and produce obstructive hydrocephalus. The resulting symmetrical dilatation of the lateral and third ventricles without displacement usually points to a lesion in the midbrain or posterior fossa.

In the distinction between intrinsic and extrinsic masses in the posterior fossa, examination of the basal subarachnoid cisterns, and also vertebral angiography, may be of considerable help.

Radiological technique. In the investigation of patients with posterior fossa tumours the tendency of these lesions to produce obstructive hydrocephalus must always be remembered. In such cases the intracranial cerebrospinal fluid is in precarious hydrodynamic balance. Injudicious lumbar puncture, even without air injection, may result in the formation of dangerous and even fatal pressure cones, due to impaction of the midbrain in the tentorial opening by the herniated hippocampal uncus or of the medulla in the foramen magnum, by the herniated cerebellar tonsils.

For patients with raised intracranial pressure, the diagnostic examination was ventriculography. Positive contrast is preferable to air for this purpose, as this gives outstandingly clear detail, and only a small volume needs to be injected. Vertebral angiography does not affect the intracranial pressure, and should be employed when any vascular lesion is suspected such as aneurysm, angioma, subdural haematoma, and haemangioendothelioma (haemangioblastoma). When there is clinical doubt as to the intracranial pressure, a preliminary carotid angiogram is often helpful if C.T. is not available. This will show whether any hydrocephalus is present, as evidenced by stretching and increased sweep of the pericallosal artery and by the disposition of the deep veins. If no ventricular dilatation is shown on the carotid angiogram, it is usually safe to proceed to air encephalography. As noted, however, C.T. is now the primary investigation of choice and may be diagnostic.

Air encephalography is normally employed when it is known that there is no obstructive hydrocephalus and by some workers is even used in the presence of raised intracranial pressure. This examination gives the most information about the anatomy of the posterior fossa. In addition to outlining the third and fourth ventricles and aqueduct, it also outlines the basal subarachnoid cisterns. This assists in the distinction between extrinsic and intrinsic masses. It is unnecessary to inject large amounts of air at lumbar encephalography to show the anatomy of the posterior fossa. Ten to fifteen millilitres are sufficient to outline the third and fourth ventricles and pontine, interpeduncular and quadrigeminal cisterns. Erect films, with the patient sitting during air injection, are the most important. Improved detail of the fourth ventricle in lateral projection is given by tomography or autotomography. In the coronal plane, the most informative films are the half-axial postero-anterior view (reverse Towne's projection). The technique of positive contrast ventriculography has already been described.

Pathology. One-third of all intrinsic brain tumours occur in the posterior fossa. The cerebellum is the second most common site for such tumours, after the frontal lobe. There is also a striking predilection for tumours to occur in the posterior fossa in childhood. Three-quarters of brain tumours in children are found in the cerebellum.

There is a strong tendency for particular tumours to occur at specific sites in different age-groups. From the site of a tumour, and the age of the patient, it may often be possible to predict the type of tumour.

In children, the most common tumour is the *medulloblastoma.* This is found in the medial part of the cerebellum, vermis and roof of the fourth ventricle. The other tumours of childhood are *gliomas*. These are astrocytomas, and occur in the pons and cerebellum. In the latter site, these tumours are cystic and often slow-growing.

A variety of tumours is found in the posterior fossa in adults. These include *glioma* (usually astrocytoma) *metastasis*, *acoustic neuroma* and *meningioma*. *Haemangioendothelioma* (haemangioblastoma) is a common primary tumour of the cerebellum in adults. A very rare variant of this condition is *Lindau's disease*, which has a hereditary predisposition, and in which multiple angiomatous tumours may occur, often in other systems, and particularly in the retina. Intraventricular tumours, *ependymoma* and less commonly, *choroid plexus papilloma*, are also found in the fourth ventricle.

Non-neoplastic masses are fairly common in the posterior fossa. A middle-ear infection is prone to extend posteriorly through the petrous bone, and result in a *cerebellar abscess*. *Tuberculomas* and *cholesteatomas* are also found in the cerebellum.

Extrinsic tumours, particularly *acoustic neuromas* and *meningiomas*, are common in adults. They are usually found in the cerebellopontine angle, where they may erode the petrous apex. Acoustic neuromas are of the same nature as the multiple neurofibromata of von Recklinghausen's disease, and may occasionally be associated with multiple peripheral nerve tumours, and patchy skin pigmentation.

Radiological anatomy. In anteroposterior projection, the third and fourth ventricles and aqueduct lie in the midline. Any lateral displacement of these structures is readily recognizable. In lateral projection, the aqueduct runs downwards and backwards in a gentle curve from the postero-inferior angle of the third ventricle to the apex of the fourth ventricle. Its position may be checked by reference to the Lysholm (Stockholm) line. This defines its position as lying below the junction of the anterior and middle thirds of a line drawn from the posterior clinoid processes to the inner table of the skull vault. The pons and cerebral peduncles lie ventral to the fourth ventricle and aqueduct, whilst dorsally they are bounded, from below upwards, by the superior cerebellar peduncles, vermis and quadrigeminal plate. The normal calibre of the aqueduct is 2 mm. Between the pons and the clivus lies the cisterna pontis, with lateral recesses extending out into the cerebello-pontine angles. These are bounded anteriorly by the petrous apex and internal auditory meatus. The normal width of the pontine cistern is 5 mm.

Twining's line joins the tuberculum sellae to the internal occipital protuberance. Its midpoint normally lies in the fourth ventricle (Fig. 60.41).

Cerebellar tumours. Tumours in the cerebellar hemispheres displace the fourth ventricle and lower half of the aqueduct laterally. This results in kinking of the aqueduct at the tentorial opening, which commonly produces obstructive hydrocephalus, with symmetrical dilatation of the lateral and third ventricles (Fig. 60.29A and B). The lateral displacement of the fourth ventricle is readily recognized in postero-anterior or reverse Towne's films (Fig. 60.29A). In lateral projection the kinking produces a characteristic angulation, in the upper part of the aqueduct (Fig. 60.29B).

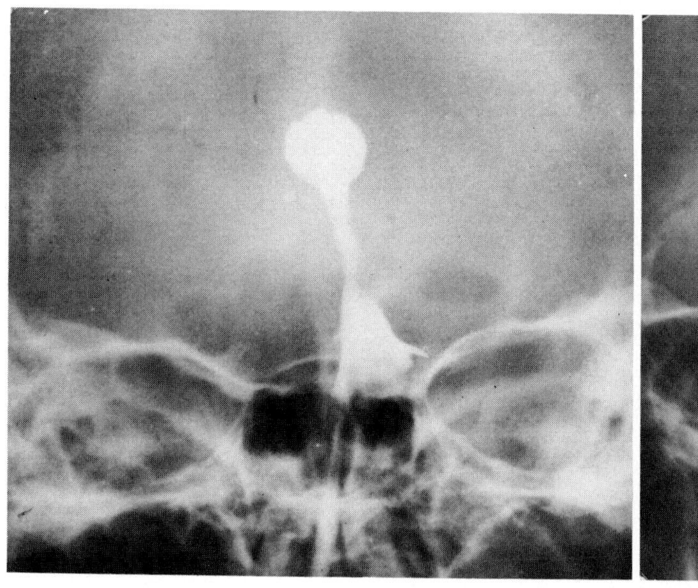

A

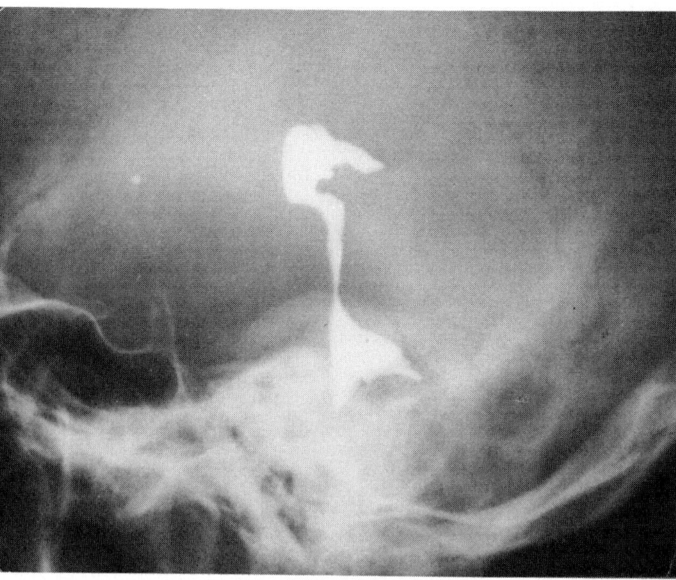

B

Fig. 60.29 (A) Right cerebellar tumour. Lateral displacement of fourth ventricle to the left. (B) Right cerebellar tumour. Typical Twining's kink in the aqueduct.

Similar displacements are also produced by laterally placed extrinsic masses—*meningioma* or posterior fossa *subdural haematoma*. The outline of the fourth ventricle in lateral films is usually normal, unless the ventricle has been invaded by a deeply placed invasive tumour. Cerebellar tumours also result in narrowing of the pontine cistern in lateral projection.

Vermis tumours. The vermis lies in the midline between the cerebellar hemispheres and immediately behind the aqueduct and fourth ventricle. Tumours often occur in this situation, particularly *medulloblastomas* in children, and *astrocytomas* in adults. They result in forward displacement of the aqueduct or fourth ventricle (Fig. 60.30). High vermis tumours displace mainly the aqueduct, and low vermis tumours the fourth ventricle, which is often compressed from behind. High vermis tumours may cause upward herniation through the tentorium, with elevation of the posterior part of the third ventricle. Vermis tumours usually cause kinking of the aqueduct. There is usually no lateral displacement of the aqueduct and fourth ventricle.

Pontine tumours. *Glioma of the pons* occurs most fre-

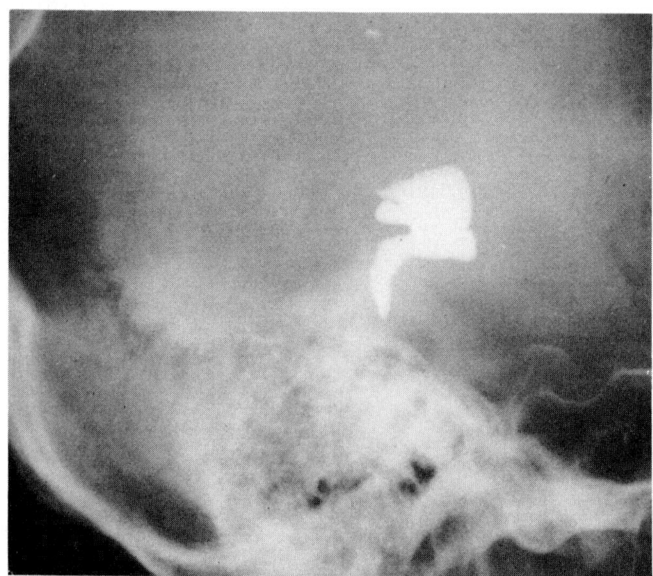

Fig. 60.30 Vermis tumour. The aqueduct is kinked forwards and obstructed.

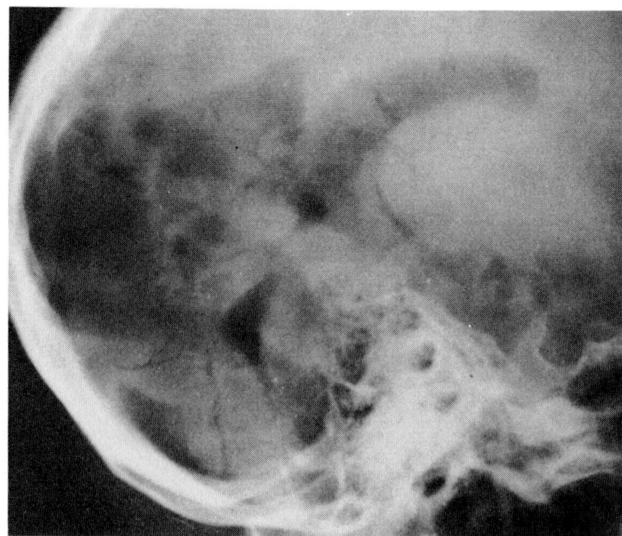

Fig. 60.31 Pontine tumour. The fourth ventricle is displaced posteriorly.

quently in children and is occasionally seen in adults. Neurological symptoms—multiple cranial nerve palsies with long tract and cerebellar signs—are experienced early, before obstructive hydrocephalus develops. For this reason, the third and fourth ventricles usually outline clearly at encephalography. The fourth ventricle is displaced posteriorly in lateral projections (Fig. 60.31). As these tumours are often not completely in the midline, there may be slight lateral displacement of the aqueduct and fourth ventricle in postero-anterior views.

Pontine tumours also cause narrowing of the pontine cistern. Air in the pontine cistern can be often of value in distinguishing between intrinsic and extrinsic tumours in this area. Vertebral angiography is also helpful. Intrinsic tumours compress the basilar artery against the clivus, whilst extrinsic tumours displace the basilar artery backwards from the clivus. Since pontine gliomas are inoperable and are usually referred direct for radiotherapy, it is of great importance in management to make the distinction between intrinsic and extrinsic tumours in this area.

Extrinsic tumours. These tumours are not uncommon. The majority arise anteriorly between the pons and clivus, or in the cerebellopontine angles. Lateral and posterior extrinsic tumours are very rare, and when they occur, are usually due to *meningiomas*. This latter group cannot be distinguished from cerebellar tumours by pneumography.

Anterior masses. *Meningiomas* arising from the clivus, and *chordomas* are the most common tumours. More rarely, *aneurysms* of the basilar artery or *angiomatous malformations* may be found. On plain films, chordomas may cause destruction of the clivus, best shown by tomography, and may also produce a soft-tissue mass in the nasopharyngeal area in lateral projection. Meningiomas may produce bony sclerosis in the clivus, or soft-tissue calcification with the tumour. At encephalography, these tumours cause similar displacements to pontine masses; the aqueduct and fourth ventricle are displaced posteriorly, although remaining in the midline. The ventricular system usually fills readily, and there is no hydrocephalus. Vertebral angiography is of considerable help in the distinction between extrinsic and pontine tumours. Meningiomas and chordomas usually displace the basilar artery posteriorly from the clivus (Fig. 62.35). Intrinsic pontine masses compress the basilar artery against the bone in lateral films. Both groups tend to obliterate the pontine cistern in encephalograms. Vertebral angiography will, of course, outline any aneurysm or angioma.

Cerebellopontine angle tumours. *Acoustic neuromas* and *meningiomas* are the frequent lesions, being amongst the more common of posterior fossa tumours. They are also of great clinical importance, since they are not invasive, and are operable. Air encephalography is usually a safe procedure, unless the tumours are sufficiently large to have produced obstructive hydrocephalus, when positive contrast ventriculography should be employed. These tumours displace the fourth ventricle and lower aqueduct laterally and posteriorly. This postero-lateral displacement also causes some rotation of the fourth ventricle. The special manoeuvres for filling the pontine angle cistern with air at encephalography have already been described. By this means, the tumour mass may be directly outlined with air in half-axial views (Fig. 60.32).

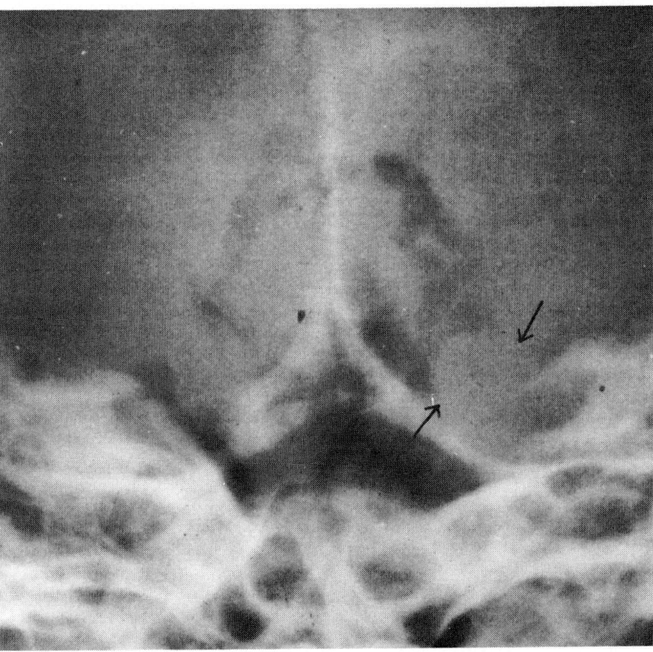

Fig. 60.32 Left acoustic neuroma (→ ←). Air filling of pontine angle cisterns shows left side is occluded by soft-tissue mass (compare right side which is filling well). There is also some bone erosion of the affected petrous apex.

CEREBELLOPONTINE CISTERNOGRAPHY

This is a most useful auxillary technique for demonstrating tumours in the cerebellopontine angle. It is much less disturbing for the patient than the traditional methods of air encephalography, vertebral angiography or positive contrast ventriculography. Its use, however, must be restricted to those patients with normal intracranial pressure.

The examination is best performed using small amounts of positive contrast (1 to 1·5 ml Myodil). Larger amounts tend to obscure detail round the internal auditory meatus, particularly when acoustic neuromas are under investigation.

The Myodil is injected by lumbar puncture, and the patient placed in lateral decubitus on a tilting table, with the affected side downwards. The table is then tilted 45° with the head downwards, and rotated slightly forwards,

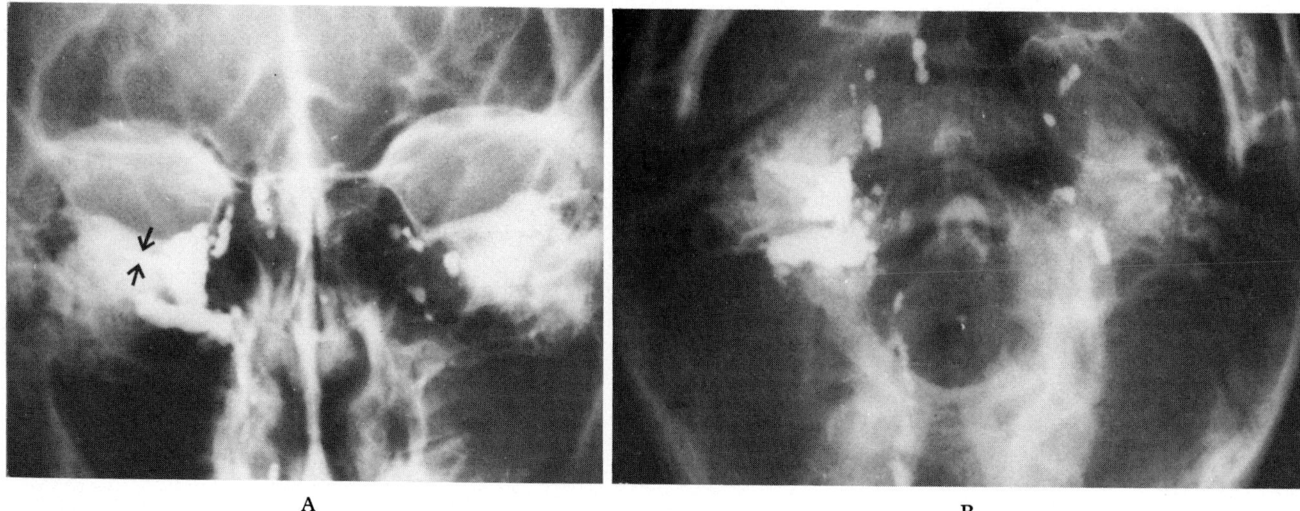

Fig. 60.33A and B Normal cisternogram. Contrast has entered the internal auditory canal.

for two minutes. During this time, the head must be kept extended to prevent Myodil running over the clivus into the middle fossa, from where it cannot be returned. With this manoeuvre, the Myodil will surround the internal auditory meatus and, in normal cases, enter the canal. Fluoroscopy is usually unnecessary. The table is then returned to the horizontal position, the patient remaining in lateral decubitus. Two films are then taken with the overcouch tube and a horizontal beam. The most useful projections are straight anteroposterior (per-orbital) and submentovertical. These show the cerebellopontine angles and internal auditory canals outlined by Myodil in two planes at right angles.

When satisfactory films have been obtained, the Myodil may be returned to the spinal theca by elevating and extending the head. The procedure may then be repeated to obtain comparative views of the opposite side.

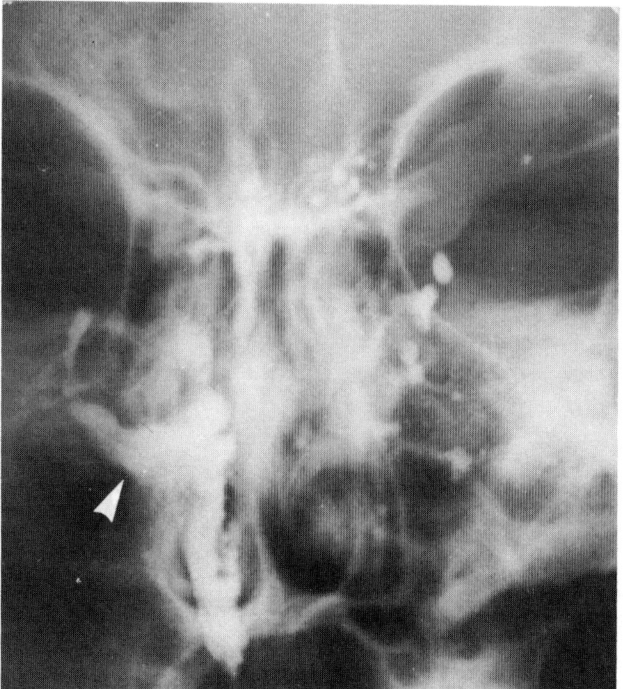

Fig. 60.34 Acoustic neuroma. Lower pole of tumour outlined by contrast.

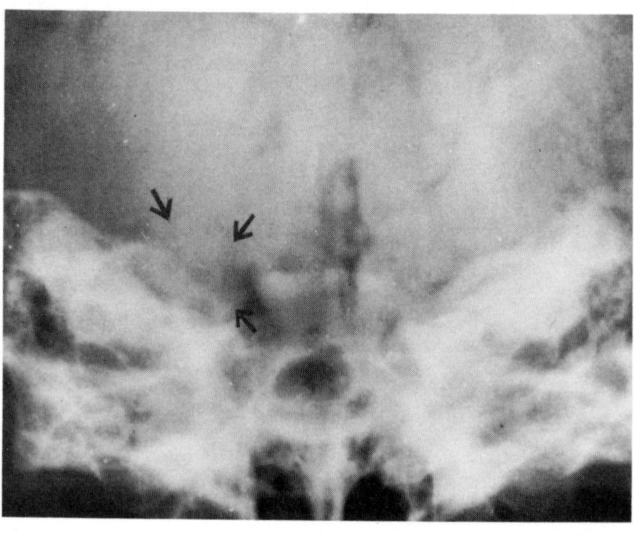

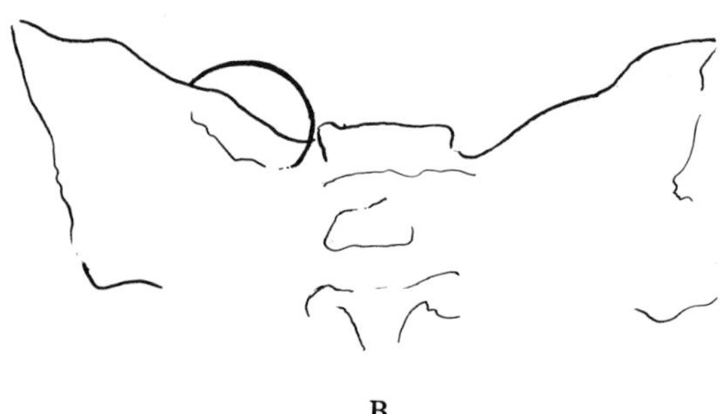

Fig. 60.35 (A) Same case as Figure 60.34. Tumour outlined by air at encephalography. (B) Diagrammatic representation.

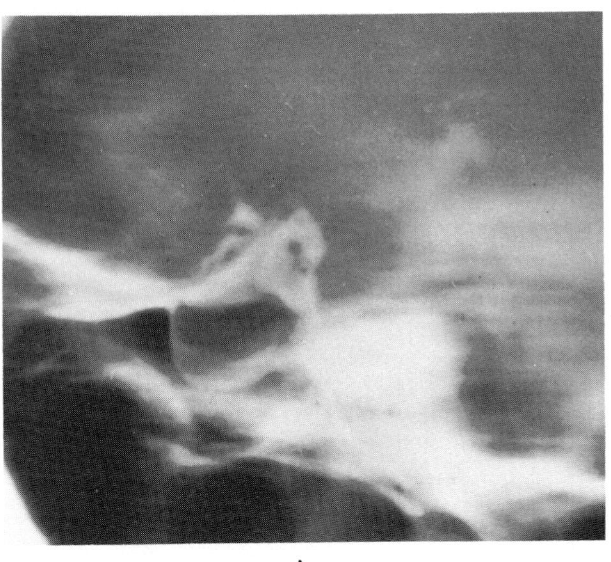

A

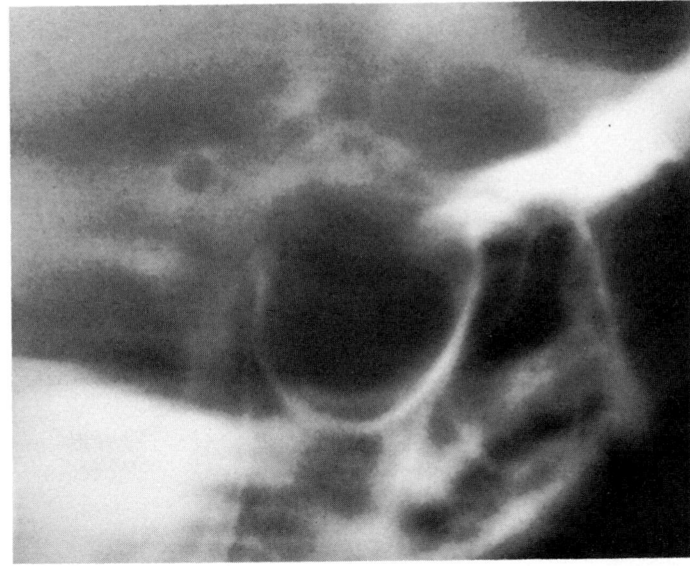

B

Fig. 60.36 (A) Suprasellar cisternogram with metrizamide showing normal appearances. (B) Suprasellar cisternogram with metrizamide showing small suprasellar extension of a pituitary tumour (Prolactinoma).

Using this method, a normal internal auditory canal is almost invariably outlined with Myodil (Fig. 60.33A and B). Non-filling may be due to a tumour, arachnoid adhesions, or obstruction by a brain stem displaced by a contralateral tumour. When a tumour is present in the cerebellopontine angle, its medial border is outlined by the Myodil (Fig. 60.34 and Fig. 60.35A and B). With this technique, tumours down to 1 cm in size may be demonstrated.

Recently metrizamide has been increasingly used for cerebellopontine cisternography with excellent results. This water soluble contrast medium has also been used for suprasellar cisternography where it will demonstrate small suprasellar masses (Fig. 60.36) or will enter an empty sella.

TUMOURS AND VENTRICULAR DEFORMITIES

A diagrammatic summary of the ventricular deformities produced by tumours is shown in Figures 60.37 to 60.41.

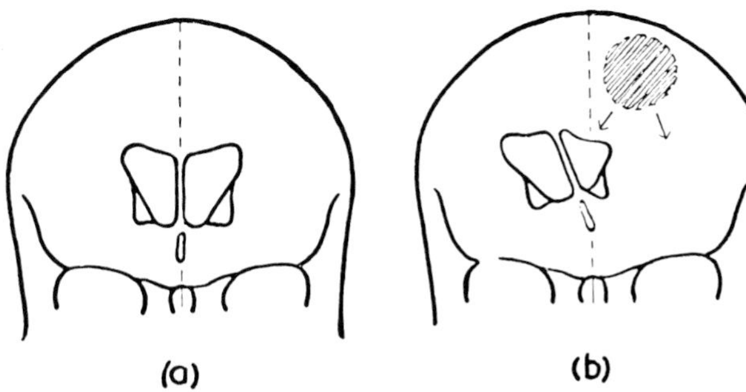

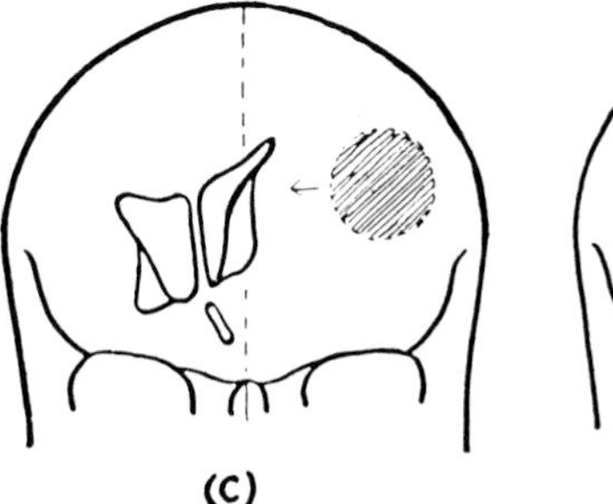

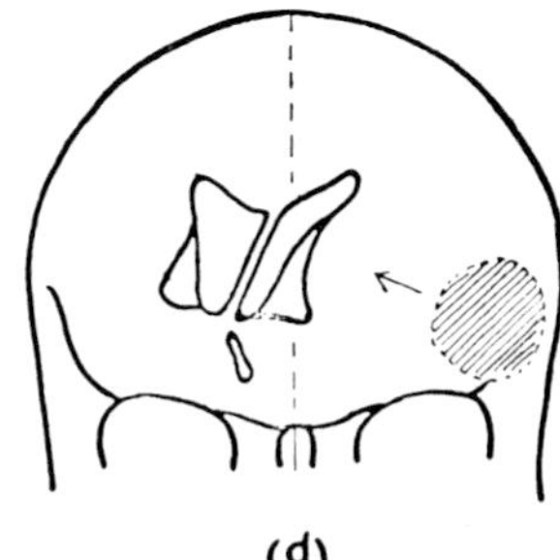

Fig. 60.37 Supratentorial tumours. Diagram to illustrate tumour localization in the frontal plane.

(*a*) Normal.

(*b*) High parasagittal tumour.
Note: (i) the septum and 3rd ventricle lie in the same plane,
(ii) the supero-lateral angle of the lateral ventricle is blunted on the side of the tumour.

(*c*) Laterally placed tumour.
Note: (i) Displaced septum and 3rd ventricle are slightly angled to each other.
(ii) Supero-lateral angle of the adjacent ventricle is slightly narrowed.

(*d*) Low lying (temporal) tumour.
Note: (i) Septum and 3rd ventricle are sharply angled.
(ii) Supero-lateral angle of lateral ventricle is squeezed and narrowed.

(From Sutton, in Brain's *Recent Advances in Neurology*, 6th edition, 1955.)

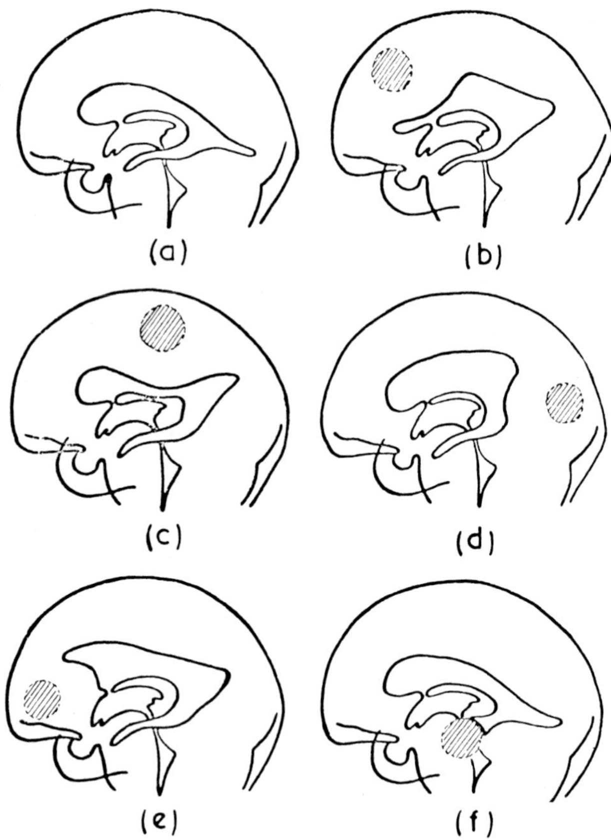

Fig. 60.38 Supratentorial tumours; tumour localization in the lateral view.

(*a*) Normal appearances
(*b*) High frontal tumour.
(*c*) Parasagittal parietal tumour.
(*d*) Occipital tumour.
(*e*) Subfrontal tumour.
(*f*) Temporal tumour.

(From Sutton, in Brain's *Recent Advances in Neurology*, 6th edition, 1955.)

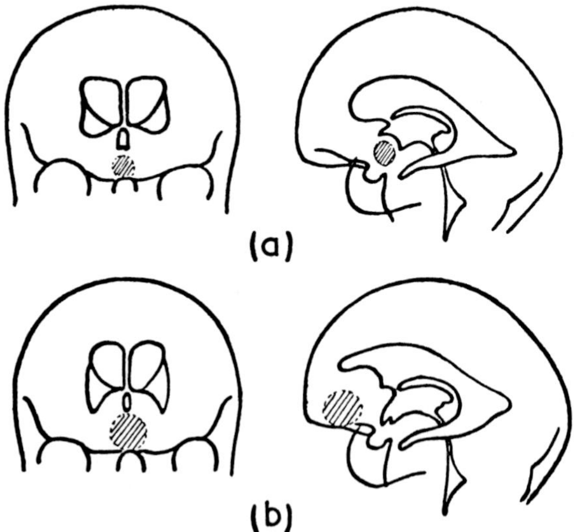

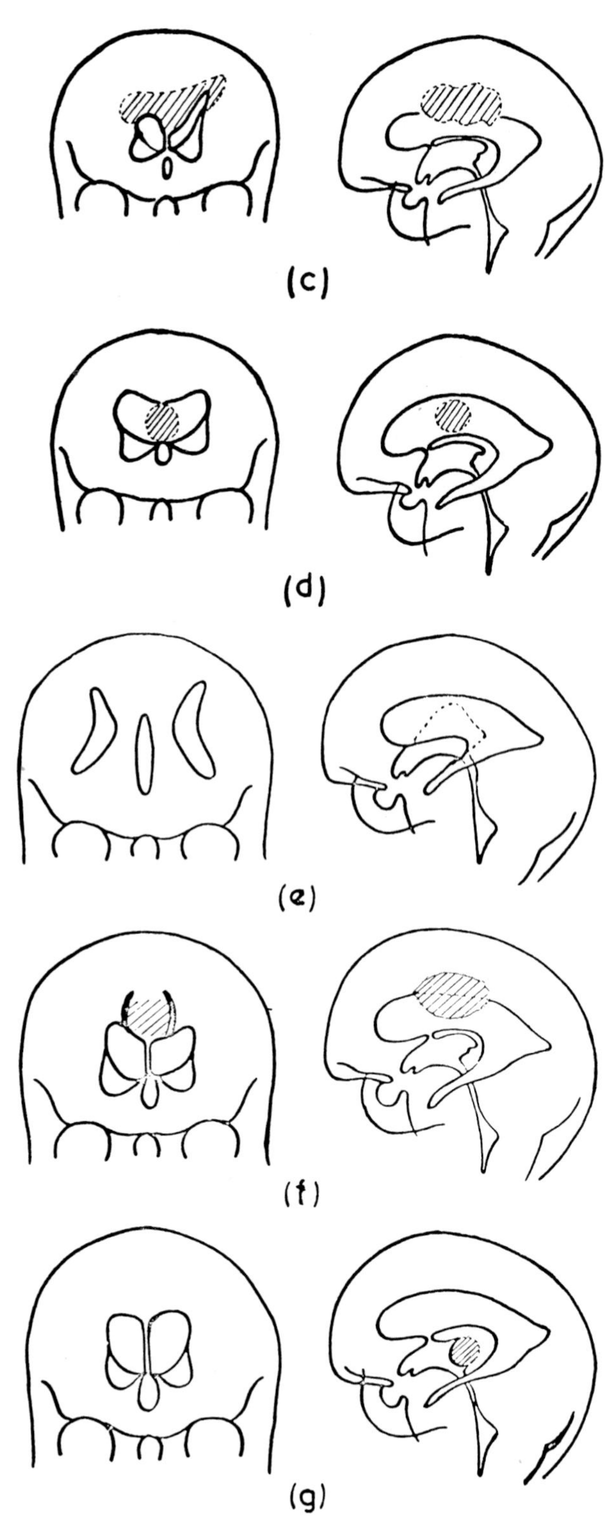

Fig. 60.39 Midline supratentorial tumours and other conditions.

(*a*) Suprasellar tumour.
(*b*) Subfrontal tumour.
(*c*) Tumour of the corpus callosum.
(*d*) Tumour of septum pellucidum (cysts of the septum are biconvex rather than rounded). The above two conditions should be differentiated from *e* and *f*.
(*e*) Agenesis of the corpus callosum.
(*f*) Lipoma of the corpus callosum. (Note pathognomonic, crescentic calcifications facing the midline in anteroposterior view.)
(*g*) Pineal tumour or cyst.

(From Sutton, in Brain's *Recent Advances in Neurology*, 6th edition, 1955.)

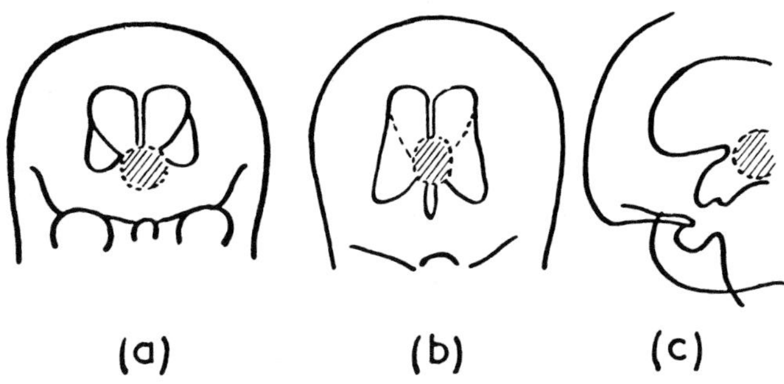

Fig. 60.40 Colloid cyst of the 3rd ventricle.
(From Sutton, in Brain's *Recent Advances in Neurology*, 6th edition, 1955.)

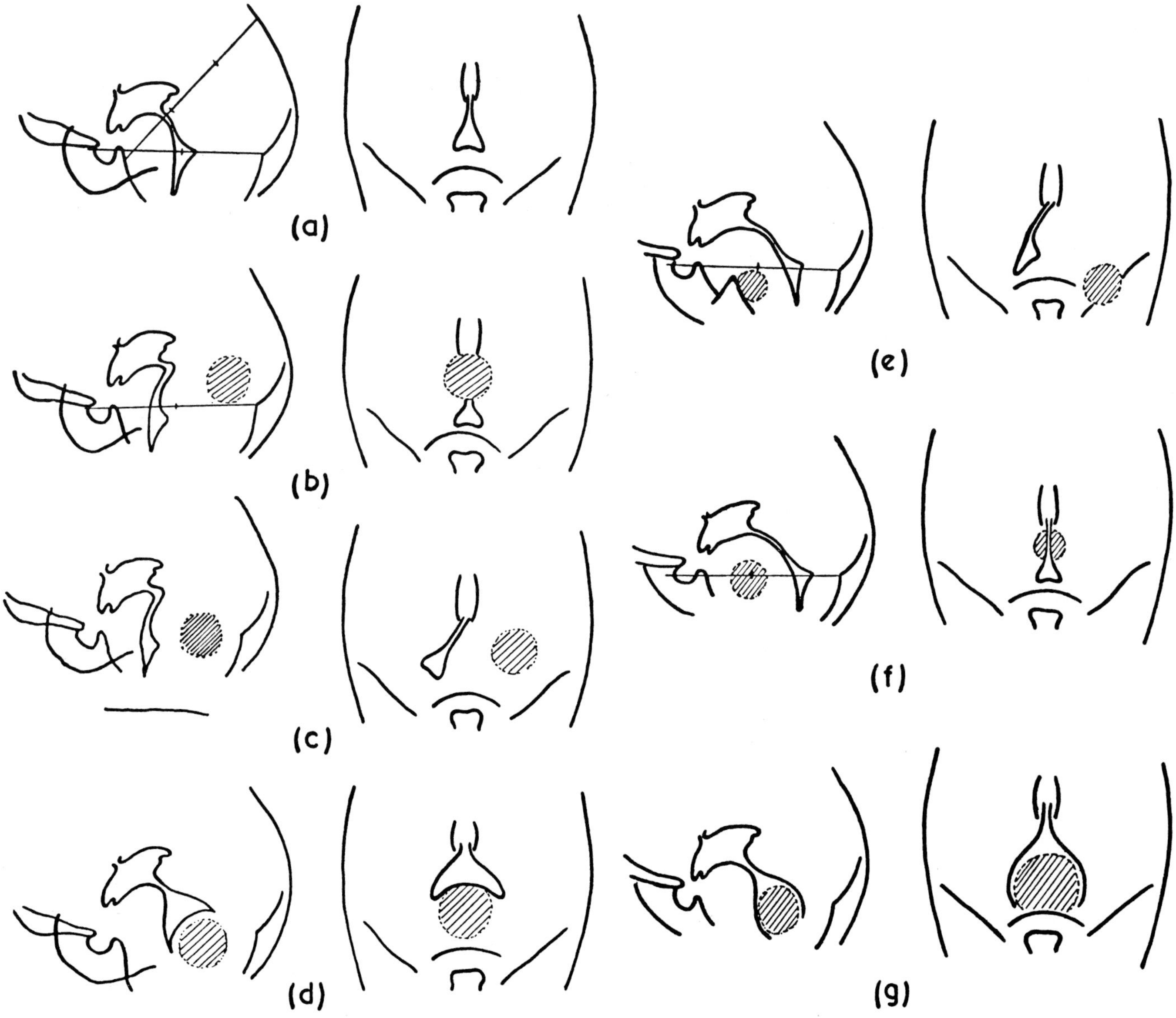

Fig. 60.41 Tumours of the posterior fossa.
(*a*) Normal relationships with Twining's line, and Lysholm's line. (See text.)
(*b*) Vermis tumour. (Note 'Twining's kink'.)
(*c*) Cerebellar hemisphere tumour.
(*d*) Midline infra-fastigial tumour.
(*e*) Cerebello-pontine angle tumour.
(*f*) Pontine tumour.
(*g*) Fourth Ventricle tumour.
(From Sutton, in Brain's *Recent Advances in Neurology*, 6th edition, 1955.)

REFERENCES AND SUGGESTIONS FOR FURTHER READING

Acta Radiologica (1973) Metrizamide. Suppl. 335.

Acta Radiologica (1977) Metrizamide-Amipaque. Suppl. 355.

ADAMS, R. D., FISHER, C. M., HAKIM, S., OJEMANN, R. G. & SWEET, W. H. (1965) Symptomatic occult hydrocephalus with 'normal' cerebrospinal fluid pressure; a treatable syndrome. *New England Journal of Medicine*, **273**, 117.

BRITTON, B. H., HITSELBERGER, W. E. & HURLEY, B. J. (1968) Iophendylate examination of posterior fossa in diagnosis of cerebello-pontine angle tumours. *Archives of Otolaryngology*, **88**, 608–617.

DANDY, W. E. (1918) Ventriculography following the injection of air into the cerebral ventricles. *Annals of Surgery*, **68**, 5.

DANDY, W. E. (1919) Röntgenography of the brain after the injection of air into the spinal canal. *Annals of Surgery*, **70**, 397.

DI CHIRO, G. (1967) *An Atlas of Pathologic Pneumoencephalographic Anatomy*. Springfield, Illinois: Thomas.

DI CHIRO, G. (1971) *An Atlas of Detailed Pneumoencephalographic Anatomy*, 2nd edn. Springfield, Illinois: Thomas.

GRIETZ, T. & HINDMARSH, T. (1974) Computer assisted tomography of intracranial c.s.f. circulation using a water-soluble contrast medium. *Acta Radiologica (Diag.)*, **15**, 497–507.

KAUFMAN, B. (1968) The 'empty' sella turcica—a manifestation of the intrasellar subarachnoid space. *Radiology*, **90**, 931–941.

LILIEQUIST, B. (1959) The subarachnoid cisterns, an anatomic and roentgenologic study. *Acta Radiologica*, Suppl. 185.

LINDGREN, E. (1949) Some aspects of the techniques of encephalography. *Acta Radiologica*, **31**, 161.

LUCKETT, W. H. (1913) In *Surgery, Gynecology and Obstetrics*, **17**, 237.

ROBERTSON, E. G. (1957) *Pneumoencephalography*. Oxford: Blackwell.

SCHECHTER, M. M. & GUITIERREZ-MAHONEY, C. G. (1962) Autotomography. Showing the normal and abnormal mid-line ventricular structures and basal cisterns. *British Journal of Radiology*, **35**, 438–461.

SHELDON, P. & MOLYNEUX, A. (1979) Metrizamide cisternography and C.T. for the investigation of pituitary lesions. *Neuroradiology*, **17**, 83–87.

TAVERAS, J. M. & WOOD, E. H. (1976) *Diagnostic Neuroradiology*, 2nd edn. Baltimore: Williams and Wilkins.

CHAPTER 61

ANGIOGRAPHY IN NEURORADIOLOGY (1)

TECHNIQUES

Angiography is widely used in the diagnosis of neurological and neurosurgical conditions. The investigations practised are:

1. Carotid angiography
2. Vertebral angiography
3. Arch aortography
4. Spinal angiography
5. Orbital phlebography.

Magnification arteriography is widely practised in cerebral angiography. With modern high powered fine focus (0·1 mm) X-ray tubes true magnifications can be readily obtained. The technique is particularly useful in showing pathological vessels in tumour circulations and in demonstrating small aneurysms.

Subtraction films are also extremely valuable and are widely used in cerebral angiography to show tumour circulations and vessels clear of overlying bone. The combination of subtraction techniques and magnification angiography often provides much information not evident on conventional standard films.

1. **Carotid angiography** was originally performed by percutaneous puncture of the common carotid artery in the neck. In most centres needles of 18 s.w.g. were used. The technique of needle arteriography is described in Chapter 29. Carotid angiography is also practised by the introduction of catheters or cannulae into the lumen of the common carotid artery. The latter techniques permit selective catheterizations or cannulation of the internal and external carotid arteries. However, caution should be observed in passing cannulae or catheters into the internal carotid artery in middle-aged and elderly patients, particularly if there is any suspicion of atheromatous internal carotid artery stenosis.

In recent years needle puncture of the carotid artery has been largely replaced by transfemoral catheter techniques. Specially designed 'head hunter' catheters are widely used for this purpose. In most patients these can be fairly easily passed into the common carotid arteries on both sides, and then into the internal or external carotid arteries so that selective injections can be achieved. In a few older or hypertensive patients the technique can prove more difficult or impossible.

For direct injections into the carotid arteries only the lower concentrations of contrast medium are used. There is evidence that the meglumine salts are preferable to sodium salts and are less toxic in cerebral tissue. Urografin 310 is a satisfactory contrast medium for cerebral work, as is Conray 280.

About 10 ml of contrast medium are usually injected within 1 to 2 seconds into the common carotid artery. A slightly smaller quantity, about 8 ml, is adequate for selective injection of the internal carotid artery. Selective injection of the external carotid artery can be accomplished with a similar amount of contrast media (8 ml). In the case of the external carotid artery the injection can be made more slowly, taking 2 to 4 seconds.

Carotid angiography can be carried out either under local anaesthesia or under general anaesthesia. In cases where more than one artery is to be injected at one session, or if the patient is likely to be very unco-operative or nervous, general anaesthesia is more commonly used.

As with other forms of arteriography, it is important to obtain rapid serial films as the contrast medium passes through the circulation. Many types of apparatus are available for achieving this. In routine practice we use Puck film changers. These enable different 'programmes' to be used tailored to the individual case. A standard series would consist of seven films taken at 1 per second for 7 seconds and timed so that arterial, capillary and venous phases of the angiogram are all covered. With angiomas and arteriovenous fistulas the early films would be taken at two or three films per second to allow for the rapid arteriovenous shunting.

2. **Vertebral arteriography.** Direct needle puncture was widely performed for many years but has now been largely superseded by catheter techniques.

Needle puncture of the vertebral artery was usually done from an anterior percutaneous approach. Different workers preferred to puncture at different levels, some high, some low. As the vertebral artery is small it is difficult to obtain a clean puncture with a long bevelled

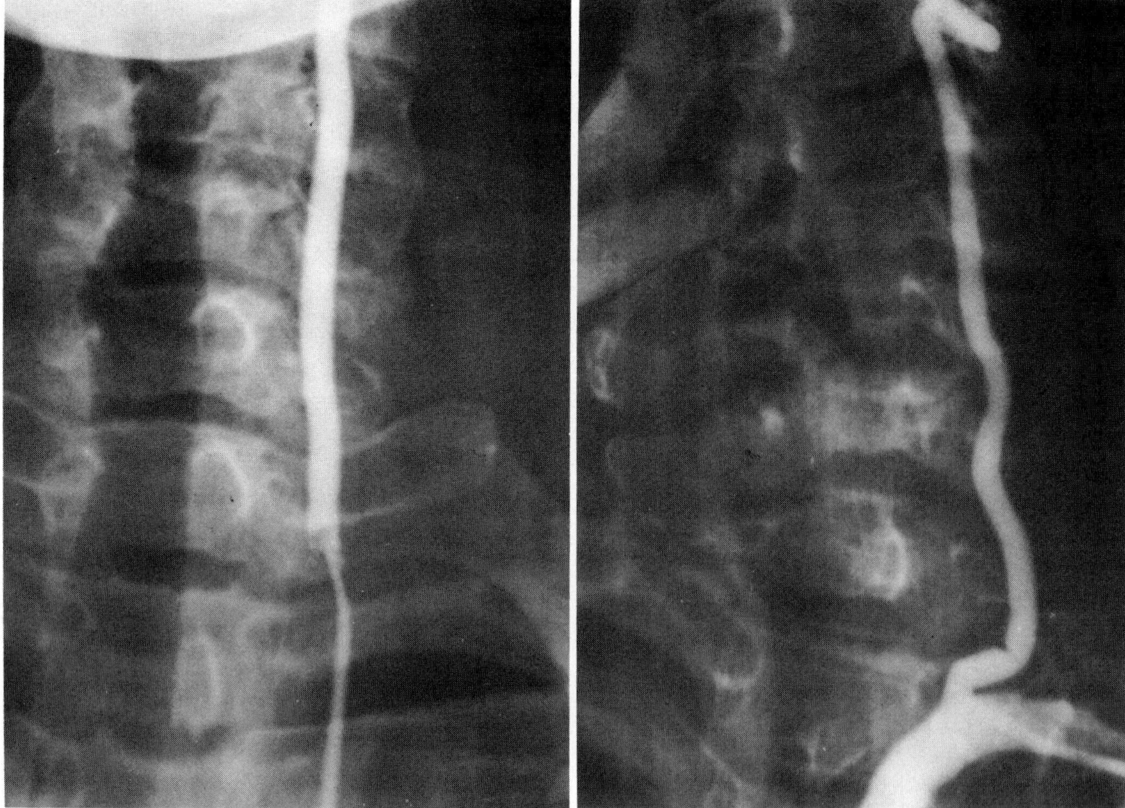

Fig. 61.1 *Fig. 61.2*

Fig. 61.1 Vertebral artery catheterized from the femoral artery.

Fig. 61.2 Vertebral artery catheterized from the axillary artery.

needle and there is always a danger of peri-arterial injection. This led to the development of different types of side-hole needle with the object of ensuring that the contrast was injected into the lumen.

The needles used for vertebral arteriography may be of 18 s.w.g. or the smaller 19 s.w.g.

The vertebral artery has also been outlined by needle puncture and injection of the first part of the subclavian artery, or by retrograde brachial injection.

For **catheter** demonstration of the carotid or vertebral artery several alternative catheters are available, and different workers have preference for different types of catheter. The main ones used in the early seventies were the Judkins type (7F) 'headhunter' catheters. Other workers achieved good results with preshaped Hannafee (5F) catheters. We prefer the Mani (5F) headhunter catheters. The smaller catheters have the added advantage of being less liable to form clot or to damage arterial walls.

Normally the left vertebral is easier to catheterize than the right (Fig. 61.1) but if one side proves difficult the other can usually be entered. It is normally only necessary to catheterize one vertebral artery as a forced injection will fill the contralateral vertebral artery by reflux as well as filling the basilar artery.

Sometimes the catheter can be passed into the subclavian artery but will not enter the vertebral artery. In these cases an injection can be made into the subclavian artery and an indirect vertebral arteriogram obtained. In patients whose vessels are too tortuous for the subclavian arteries to be catheterized from below, or in whom diseased iliacs prevent passage of a catheter, success can still be obtained by transaxillary catheterization (Fig. 61.2). In about 5 per cent of cases the left vertebral artery arises direct from the aortic arch. If no vertebral artery can be found arising from the left subclavian this condition should be suspected, the catheter withdrawn into the arch, and an attempt made to manipulate it into the anomalous vertebral. If this fails the right vertebral should be attempted.

For direct injection into the vertebral artery either by needle or by catheter we use only 6 to 8 ml of contrast medium. We regard Urografin 310 as the contrast medium of choice. As with carotid angiography improved detail can be obtained by the use of magnification with a fine focus tube and by the use of subtraction films.

Where the first part of the subclavian artery is injected about 15 ml of contrast medium are injected in about 2 seconds. It may help to obtain better filling of the vertebral artery in these cases if the appropriate brachial artery is occluded at the time of injection.

3. **Arch aortography.** It has been shown that cerebral symptoms frequently arise from stenosis or thrombosis of the origins of the internal carotid arteries or of the vertebral arteries. It has also been shown that intra-thoracic lesions of the innominate, left common carotid and left subclavian arteries can be a cause of cerebral symptoms.

Injections of contrast medium into the aortic arch enables all the great vessels in the thorax and the vertebral arteries in the neck, together with the carotid bifurcations, to be demonstrated.

The technique most widely used is percutaneous trans-femoral catheterization and the passage of a catheter into the ascending aorta. The ascending aorta may also be catheterized by percutaneous right transaxillary catheterization.

The right transaxillary approach can also be used to inject:

(*a*) the first part of the right subclavian artery and the right vertebral artery;

(*b*) the innominate artery, thus showing the right carotid and right subclavian and vertebral arteries.

In North America direct pressure injection into the right brachial artery was at one time widely used with retrograde filling of the aortic arch and great vessels. This method has been little used by European workers, who on the whole prefer to use selective catheter techniques, as more easily controllable.

The important features of arch aortograms are illustrated in Figure 61.3. It is usual to take rapid serial films with the supine patient rotated about 45° to the right and the head turned to the right lateral position. This normally avoids super-imposition of the carotid and vertebral arteries and shows the carotid bifurcations clearly.

4. **Spinal angiography.** In recent years this procedure has been increasingly practised. It involves selective angiography and a careful radiographic subtraction technique. The arterial supply to the spinal cord is illustrated in Figure 61.4A and B. The main blood supply to the cord is from the longitudinal midline anterior spinal artery, which is in effect an anastomotic chain between the feeding arteries (Fig. 61.4C). This receives feed vessels from the vertebral, deep cervical, intercostal and lumbar arteries. There is a smaller posterior longitudinal system supplied by posterior radicular branches of the vessels indicated. These consist of a network of anastomosing channels on the back of the cord which communicates

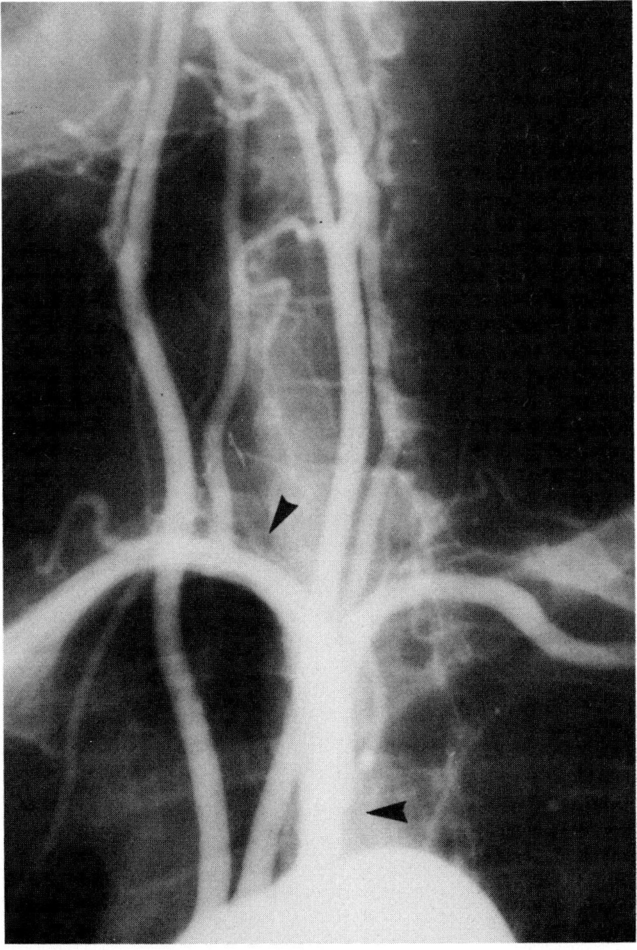

Fig. 61.3 Arch aortogram in right posterior oblique position. There is a congenital anomaly in that the right subclavian artery arises distally from the aortic arch (arrows). Its origin is superimposed on the left subclavian origin.

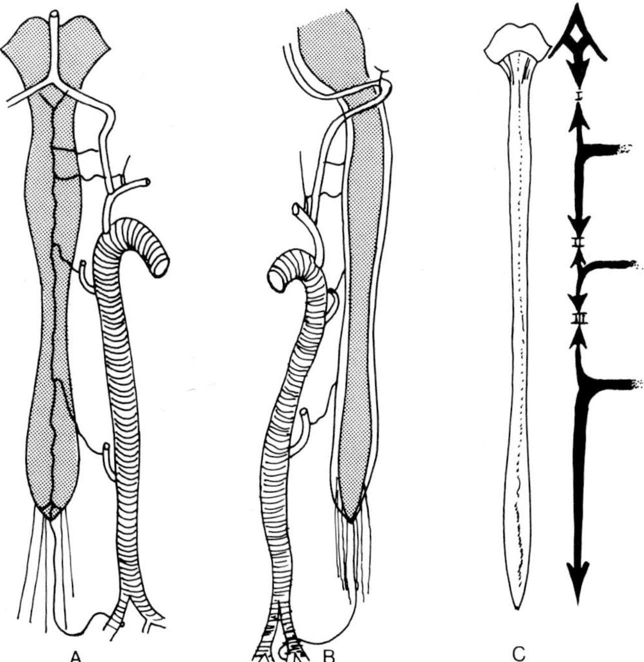

Fig. 61.4A, B and C Normal blood supply to the spinal cord as seen (A) in anterior view and (B) in lateral view. (C) Blood flow currents in the longitudinal spinal arteries. (After Di Chiro.)

freely with the anterior system. Since the anterior spinal artery is not one continuous vessel but an anastomotic chain supplied from multiple radicular feeding arteries, no single injection will opacify its whole extent. It must therefore be opacified in segments, i.e. cervical, dorsal, and dorsilumbar. Usually there are four or five feeding radicles in the cervical segment, two or three in the dorsal segment and a single large radicle in the dorsilumbar region. This is known as the artery of Adamkiewicz, or *arteria radiculomedullaris magna.*

Spinal angiography has so far proved most valuable in the diagnosis and elucidation for surgery of spinal *angiomas.* It has only a limited use in the diagnosis of spinal tumours. In this context its most valuable use is to differentiate a spinal *haemangioblastoma* from other forms of spinal tumour. The haemangioblastoma shows a characteristic tumour stain as it does in the posterior fossa.

With angiomas, the main feeding vessel may arise at quite a distance from the site of the lesion so spinal angiography may involve injection of many arteries before an angioma is excluded or its main feeding vessel identified.

Spinal angiography is performed by transfemoral catheterization. For lesions in the cervical region both vertebrals and both costocervical trunks need to be injected. For the upper dorsal region the upper intercostals must be injected, and for the lower dorsal and lumbar region the lower intercostal and lumbar arteries. Selective bilateral intercostal and lumbar arteriography from T.8 to L.3 may be required before the artery of Adamkiewicz is identified. The lower left intercostals are usually the most rewarding. As each intercostal is entered a test dose of 1 ml of contrast medium is injected and observed on the intensifier screen. Serial films are then obtained using very small doses of low concentration contrast medium; 3 to 4 ml of Urografin 310 are adequate unless an obvious angioma with arteriovenous shunting is observed at the test dose. A preliminary film for subtraction studies is always taken with each injection. If an angioma or tumour is identified a lateral series of films should be obtained to establish whether the lesion is anterior or posterior to the cord. An anterior angioma is unusual but important as it cannot be dealt with by direct surgery.

Most angiomas have in the past been treated by surgical ligation of the main feeding vessels. Recently however, successful results have been claimed for treatment by embolism with metallic pellets or Gelfoam after percutaneous catheterization of the vessel supplying the main feeder.

5. **Orbital phlebography.** This procedure aims at outlining the veins of the orbit. It is now performed by percutaneous puncture of the frontal vein. The vein can be distended and made more prominent by compressing

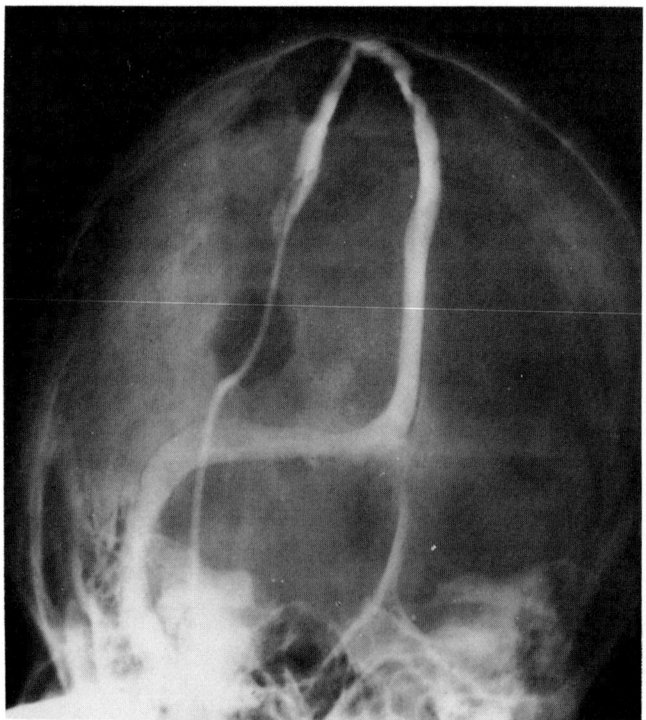

Fig. 61.5A Normal dural sinus phlebogram, oblique projection. The sagittal sinus is clearly shown together with its drainage into the right lateral sinus.

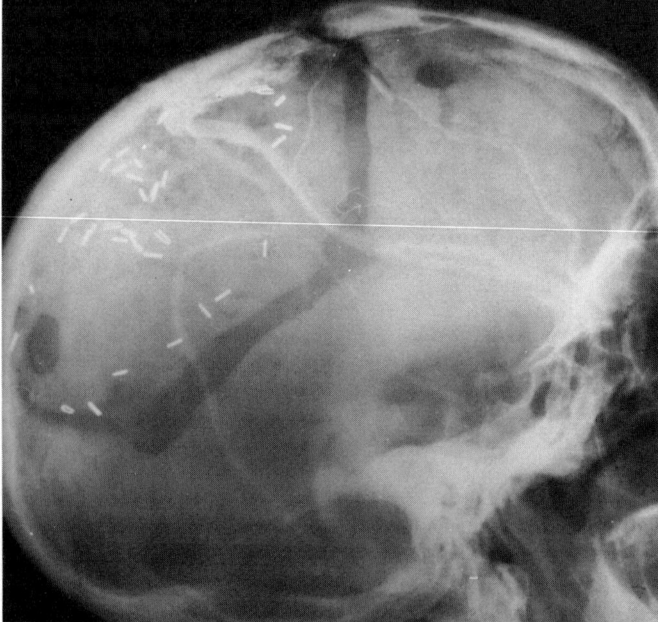

Fig. 61.5B Sagittal sinogram in a patient who has previously had a craniotomy for parietal parasagittal meningioma. Lateral view. The sinogram shows the sagittal sinus to be occluded by recurrence in the parietal region. There is a collateral circulation over the hemisphere.

the venous return at the forehead with a compression band and by partial compression of the veins in the neck with a tourniquet. If the procedure is performed under local anaesthesia, the patient is asked to co-operate by distending the head and neck veins with a Valsalva manoeuvre (see Ch. 52).

Dural sinus phlebography. This is undertaken to demonstrate more clearly the superior sagittal sinus and its drainage into the lateral sinuses. The investigation is indicated in cases where obstruction of the superior sagittal sinus by tumour or thrombosis is suspected. During normal carotid angiography, the superior sagittal sinus may be shown, but the contrast is diluted by blood from the opposite hemisphere and detail may, therefore, be poor. Better detail can be obtained by injection of one carotid artery, whilst compressing the opposite carotid in the neck. This permits cross-flow of contrast through the anterior communicating artery with contrast filling of both hemispheres, and improved visualization of the sinuses.

The sagittal sinus can also be shown by operative insertion of a catheter into its anterior end. A small parasagittal burr hole is made in the frontal region and a fine polythene catheter inserted through it into the sinus by the neurosurgeon. Contrast is then injected directly into the sinus and appropriate X-ray films taken. This technique was once used to assess involvement of the sagittal sinus by meningioma, but with modern contrast media the sinus is usually adequately shown by carotid angiography as just described.

For dural sinus phlebography films are usually taken in both the lateral and in the A.P. oblique projections (Fig. 61.5).

COMPLICATIONS OF CEREBRAL AND SPINAL ANGIOGRAPHY

The general complications of angiography have been discussed in Chapter 29. Cerebral angiography carries particular local hazards, since the brain is such a vital organ. As has already been explained, the major causes of accidents in the past have been either excessive doses of contrast medium or local trauma to a carotid or vertebral artery resulting in local dissection or thrombosis. With the increasing use of catheters clot embolus has also increased in incidence. Such accidents at carotid angiography have given rise to hemiplegia, temporary or permanent, or to acute cerebral infarction and death. Vertebral angiography has given rise to death from brainstem lesions, to spinal-cord damage, and to cortical blindness. Arch aortography has also resulted in severe brain damage, or death from acute cerebral infarction. Particular caution is needed in patients with atheroma and stenotic lesions in major vessels, since hypotension may precipitate thrombosis in such cases.

The possibility of these grave accidents makes it obvious that cerebral angiography should only be practised by experienced workers who are fully aware of the hazards and how best to avoid them.

Selective spinal angiography carries the special hazard of damage to the cord and must be practised with due caution. As mentioned above, only small doses of a low concentration contrast medium should be injected into intercostals, lumbar arteries or other small arteries which may be providing direct spinal feeding arteries. Irritation of the cord may result in muscle spasms. Should these occur they may need to be controlled by anaesthesia. Excessive doses of contrast can result in quadriplegia or paraplegia depending on the level of damage to the cord. In this context arteriographers should be aware that a bronchial artery may arise in common with an intercostal feeding the spinal cord, and that the thyroid axis can supply the costocervical trunk. Cord damage has resulted both from bronchial angiography and thyroid angiography. It has also been reported as a complication of lumbar and abdominal aortography with the older types of contrast medium. Presumably this was due to excessive doses entering the artery of Adamkiewicz.

THE NORMAL INTERNAL CAROTID ANGIOGRAM

The features of the normal internal carotid arteriogram are illustrated in Figures 61.6 and 61.7.

The normal circulation time from injection of the contrast into the internal carotid artery to its disappearance from the veins of the brain varies with the individual and averages from 5 to 7 seconds. In certain pathological conditions it may of course be appreciably slower. With angiomatous malformations or arteriovenous fistula it may be extremely rapid.

It is customary to divide the angiogram into four phases. The first phase lasts 1 to 2·5 seconds and is referred to as the *arterial* phase. A film taken during this period shows the arterial tree. The second or *capillary* phase lasts about 1 second or less but is rarely clearly defined on the X-ray film since there is usually some late arterial or early venous filling superimposed. The third and fourth phases are characterized by *venous* filling and lasts 4 or 5 seconds. They include the early and late phlebograms respectively. The early phlebogram outlines the superficial veins of the hemisphere, and the late phlebogram shows the deep veins.

The blood flow through the internal carotid artery is considerably more than through the external carotid artery. Thus, following injection of the common carotid artery the intracranial vessels are usually visible in the lateral films a second or so before the branches of the external carotid become superimposed. The experienced worker has no difficulty in differentiating branches of the

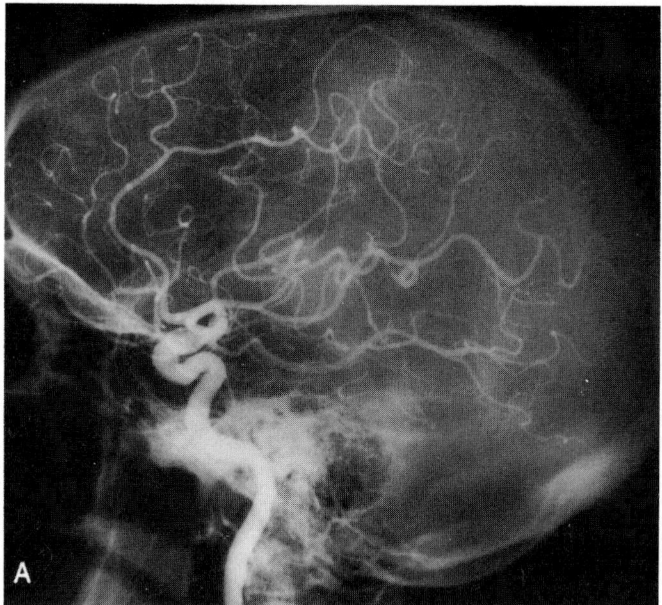

Fig. 61.6A Normal internal carotid arteriogram lateral view.

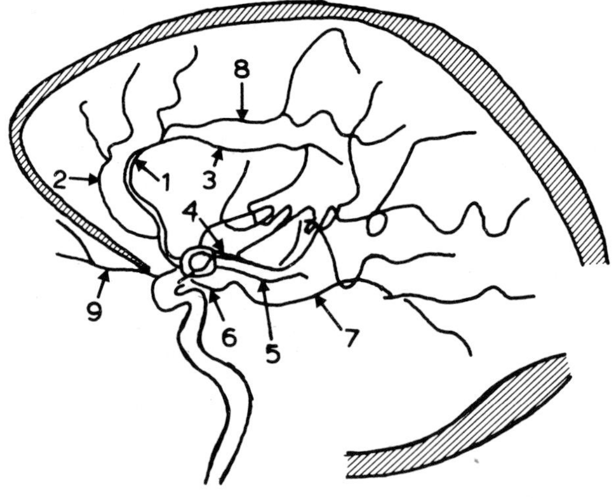

Fig. 61.6B Diagram to illustrate Fig. 61.6A.
1. Anterior cerebral artery
2. Frontopolar artery
3. Pericallosal artery
4. Middle cerebral artery and its branches
5. Anterior choroidal artery
6. Posterior communicating artery
7. Posterior cerebral artery
8. Callosomarginal artery
9. Ophthalmic artery.

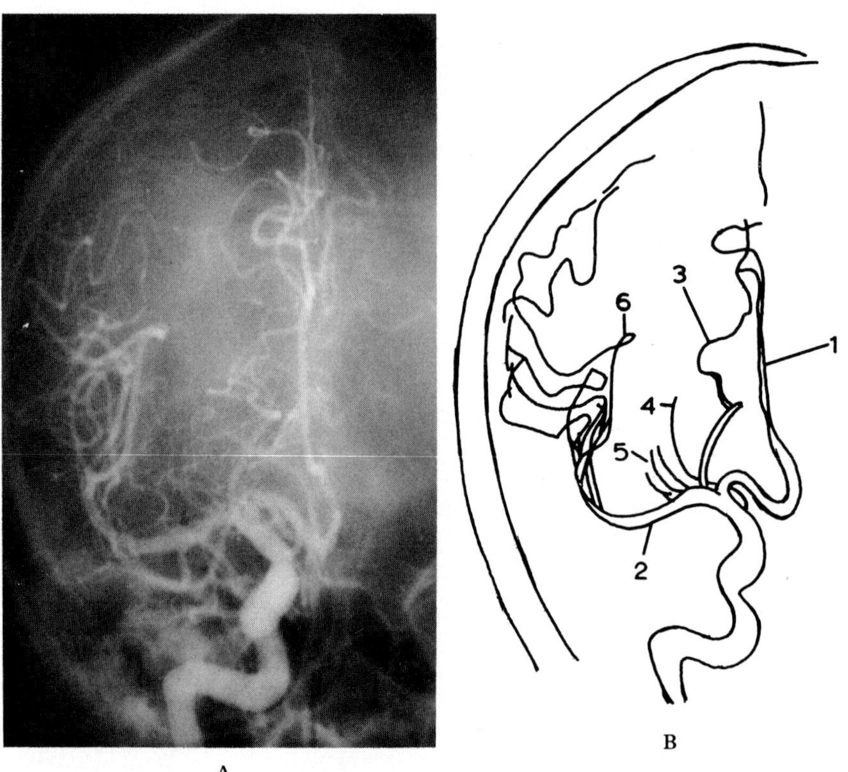

Fig. 61.7A Normal internal carotid arteriogram A.P. film. B Diagram to illustrate Figure 61.7A.
1. Anterior cerebral artery
2. Middle cerebral artery and its branches
3. Posterior cerebral artery
4. Anterior choroidal artery
5. Lenticulostriate arteries
6. Sylvian point.

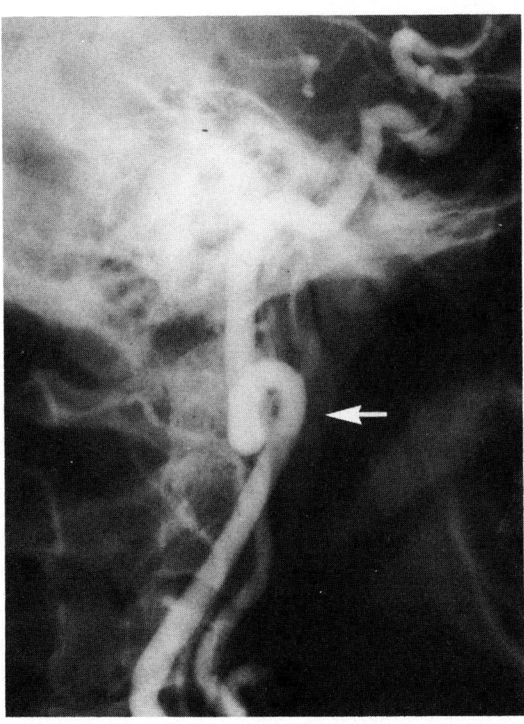

Fig. 61.8 Carotid arteriogram showing 'tonsillar loop' (←) in the neck.

external from branches of the internal carotid as the distribution of these vessels follows a standard pattern. The middle meningeal artery and its branches which stem from the internal maxillary branch of the external carotid also fill slightly later than the internal carotid branches. Early filling of the middle meningeal artery together with internal carotid branches can occur if the vessel is hypertrophied to supply a meningioma or angioma. This point is further commented on below.

Sometimes the internal carotid artery shows a prominent loop as it lies lateral to the oropharynx, and this is known as the 'tonsillar loop' (Fig. 61.8). It can be regarded as a normal variant.

The normal internal carotid artery also forms a loop as it lies in the lateral wall of the cavernous sinus which is usually referred to as the 'carotid syphon'. The suprasellar portion of the internal carotid artery just before its bifurcation is normally inclined laterally (from below upwards) as seen in the antero-posterior view. In this view the major branches of the anterior and middle cerebral arteries pass respectively medially and laterally. These two vessels together with the termination of the internal carotid resemble the letter T when seen in this projection (Fig. 61.7).

The major branches of the internal carotid artery all arise above the cavernous sinus, but there are some minor branches arising in its *intrapetrosal* and *intracavernous* segments. The former include the coroticotympanic and pterygoid (Vidian) arteries which are rarely recognizable at angiography. The intracavernous branches include:

1. The important *meningohypophyseal trunk* (see Fig. 62.15) which gives rise to
   (a) the tentorial artery
   (b) the dorsal meningeal artery
   (c) the inferior hypophyseal artery.

The tentorial artery may be enlarged and easily recognizable with tentorial meningiomas.

2. The *inferior cavernous artery* which supplies the wall of the cavernous sinus and its contents and anastomoses with the middle meningeal artery.

3. The capsular artery.

Under normal circumstances these arteries are only recognizable in high quality subtraction films with magnification as are the tiny *superior hypophyseal arteries* which arise above the sella.

The **ophthalmic artery** arises from the internal carotid just above the sella and medial to the anterior clinoid process. It passes forward to the optic canal beneath the optic nerve and then into the orbit. A good quality films will show its terminal branches outlining the posterior aspect of the globe (Fig. 61.9). Displacements of the ophthalmic artery have occasionally been helpful in the diagnosis of orbital tumours. Its terminal supraorbital branch supplies a small cutaneous area above the medial aspect of the orbit.

The *artery of the falx* arises from the anterior ethmoidal branch of the ophthalmic artery and passes through the cribriform plate to supply the anterior part of the falx. It

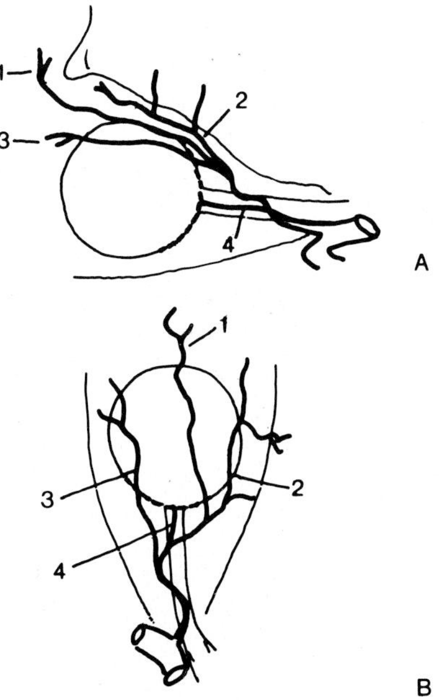

Fig. 61.9 Diagram of Rt. ophthalmic artery, (A) in lateral view; (B) in axial view (Cp. Fig. 52.17).
1. Supra orbital branch
2. Main artery with ethmoidal branches
3. Lachrymal branch
4. Central retinal branch.

may be markedly hypertrophied to supply meningiomas or arteriovenous malformations.

The **posterior communicating** and **posterior cerebral** arteries fill in only about a third of common carotid arteriograms. However, they fill in a higher proportion of cases following selective injection of the internal carotid artery. In other cases the dominant blood supply to the posterior cerebral artery is through the vertebrobasilar circulation. Sometimes the origin of the posterior communicating artery as seen in lateral view is slightly expanded. This appearance, known as the 'infundibulum' of the posterior communicating artery, has been regarded as a normal variant. On the other hand, there is some pathological evidence that it may be associated with a defect in the vessel wall and predispose to aneurysm formation.

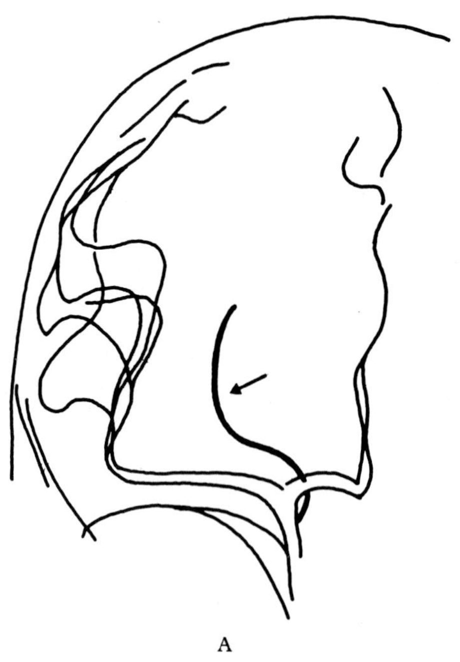

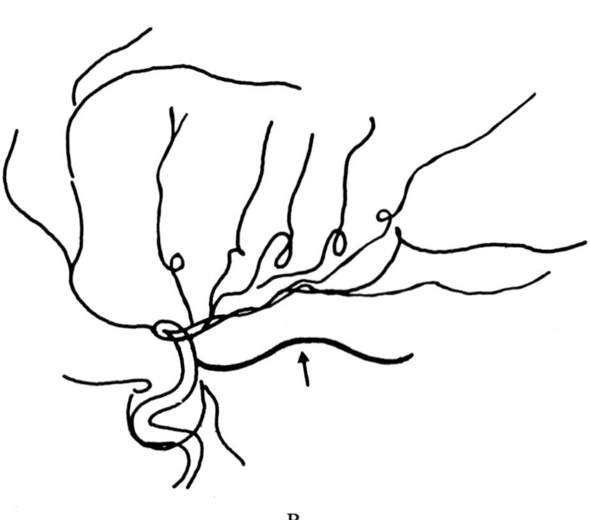

Fig. 61.10 Diagram of the anterior choroidal artery in (A) A.P. and (B) lateral projections.

The **anterior choroidal** artery is small but is readily identifiable. Its normal position in both lateral and antero-posterior views is illustrated in Figure 61.10. Displacement of this vessel can be of considerable help in identifying and localizing mass lesions, and is discussed in Chapter 62.

The normal anterior choroidal artery arises from the posterior aspect of the internal carotid just distal to the origin of the posterior communicating artery, but rarely it arises from the middle cerebral or posterior cerebral artery. The artery is directed backwards and medially to the medial aspect of the anterior part of the temporal lobe. It then passes round the uncus and turns laterally and backwards into the choroidal fissure to enter the temporal horn. There it supplies the choroid plexus which is sometimes seen as an ill-defined blush of contrast.

As with the posterior communicating artery an infundibulum is occasionally seen at the origin of the artery from the internal carotid artery.

The **lenticulostriate** arteries arise in two groups of two to four tiny arteries, the *medial* and the *lateral*. Normally they stem from the upper surface of the middle cerebral artery trunk and pass directly up through the anterior perforated substance into the basal ganglia and internal capsule. Some of them may arise from the internal carotid bifurcation or the origin of the anterior cerebral. They are readily recognized in good quality antero-posterior films, but are usually obscured by larger overlying vessels in the lateral view. The normal disposition of these vessels is illustrated in Figure 61.11. They pass upwards and medially for a short distance and then laterally in an arc that is concave inwards.

The **anterior cerebral** artery passes medially from the bifurcation of the internal carotid to reach the midline. This small segment of the artery lies above the optic chiasm or optic nerve and is usually convex upwards. It is best seen in the antero-posterior projection. Near the midline it is joined by the anterior communicating artery to its fellow on the opposite side. Beyond the anterior communicating artery the anterior cerebral turns forwards and upwards in the interhemispheric fissure. It passes around the anterior aspect of the corpus callosum and turns backwards along its upper surface. It continues as the pericallosal artery to the back end of the corpus callosum.

In lateral view the segments between the anterior communicating artery and the genu of the corpus callosum usually has a gentle concavity downwards. This is variable

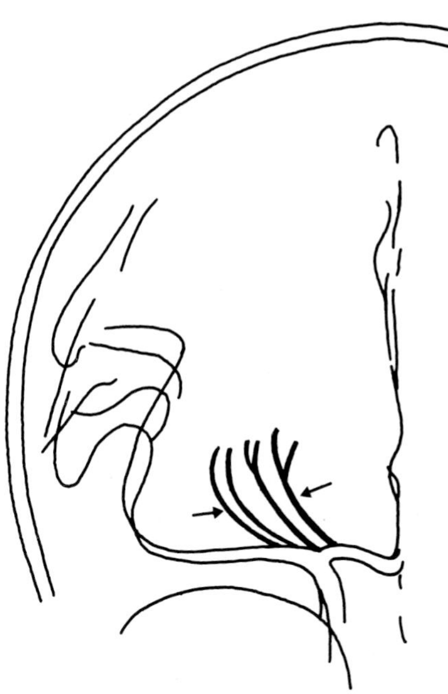

Fig. 61.11 Diagram of the lenticulostriate arteries in A.P. projection. They are difficult to identify in lateral projection because of the superimposed middle cerebral vessels.

in degree and should not be mistaken for displacement by a mass. There are a few tiny perforating branches given off from the proximal horizontal segment of the anterior cerebral artery, but these are variable and difficult to identify on angiograms.

The *frontopolar* branch is generally the first major branch of the anterior cerebral and arises proximal to the knee or bend of the vessel around the corpus callosum. This vessel passes forwards and upwards towards the anterior pole of the frontal lobe and is best seen in lateral view. It divides into two or three branches which pass to the superomedial margin of the hemisphere and over on to the convexity.

The next major branch of the anterior cerebral is the *callosomarginal*. This usually arises near the genu and passes backwards and upwards giving off anterior, middle and posterior internal frontal branches. It terminates in the paracentral branch around the paracentral lobule. The branches just described are variable and may arise directly from the anterior cerebral. The callosomarginal artery lies in the callosomarginal sulcus for part of its course and whilst in the sulcus may be lateral to the midline. This should not be mistaken for a true displacement by a mass. The terminal branches of the artery, like those of the frontopolar artery, reach the superomedial border of the hemisphere and pass over it to the convexity. Here they anastomose with terminal ascending branches of the middle cerebral artery.

The *pericallosal* artery represents the continuation of the anterior cerebral after it has given off the major branches just described. Normally it is fairly closely applied to the upper surface of the corpus callosum and terminates in a precuneal or posterior callosal branch.

The proximal segment of the anterior cerebral artery is occasionally hypoplastic forming one of the many variations of the circle of Willis. In these cases the major part of the vessel fills from the opposite side through the anterior communicating artery. Such congenital hypoplasia should be distinguished from spasm associated with subarachnoid haemorrhage. This is described in Chapter 62.

The **middle cerebral** artery passes laterally and slightly forward from the bifurcation of the internal carotid artery. This segment is best seen in the A.P. view and is horizontal or convex upwards. It gives rise to the *lenticulostriate* arteries which have just been described. About 2 cm from its origin it reaches the insula (or island of Reil) where is usually bifurcates. The main branches pass backwards over the surface of the insula and are hidden by the opercula. These branches lie deep in the Sylvian fissure and deep to the external surface of the brain. The branches loop downwards on the under surface of the inferior parietal operculum and then pass out through the Sylvian fissure to reach the surface of the hemisphere. These downward loops can be identified in the lateral angiograms and the margins of the triangular insula can thus be defined. The surface of the insula is also identified in the same way on the A.P. film (Fig. 61.12).

The appearance of these vessels and their relationship to the skull vault in the frontal projection are of considerable importance in detecting displacement by tumours and other masses. Taveras refers to the posterior

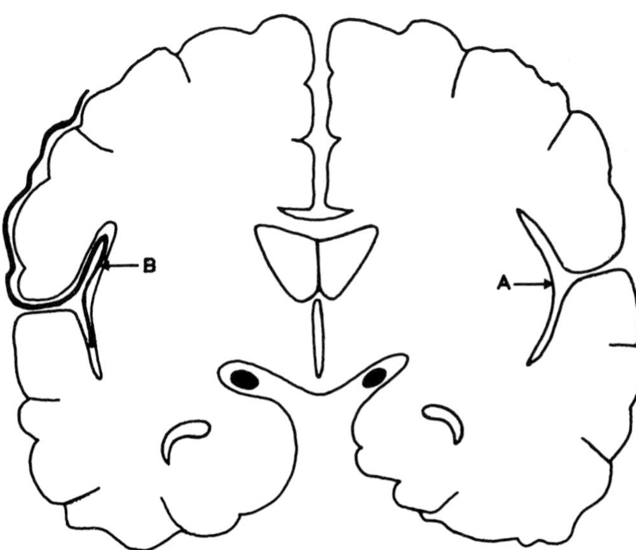

Fig. 61.12 Diagram to show the relationship of the middle cerebral artery and its branches to the insula in a sagittal brain section. (A) Insula. (B) Middle cerebral artery.

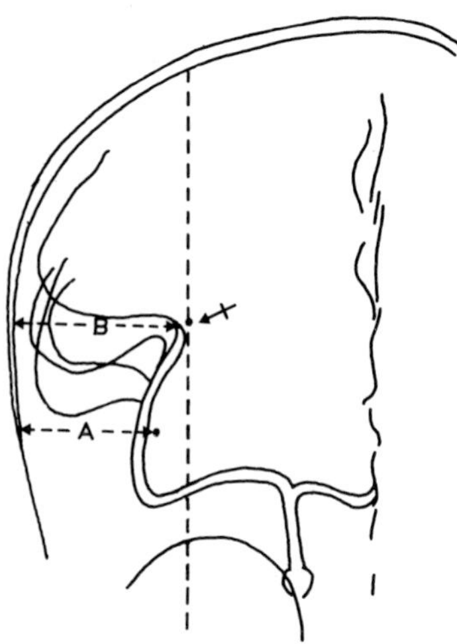

Fig. 61.13 Diagram showing relationship of middle cerebral vessels to skull vault in the A.P. projection. Arrow points to the angiographic Sylvian point (+) which represents the posterior limit of the insula. Distance A, from the skull vault to the lateral aspect of the insula, varies from 20 to 30 mm. Distance B, from the Sylvian point to the skull vault measures 30 to 40 mm. (After Taveras.)

limit of the Sylvian triangle as the 'angiographic Sylvian point' and shows how this can be identified in the frontal projection. The last artery to emerge from the insula occupies at its medial bend the position of the angiographic Sylvian point.

The Sylvian vessels and Sylvian points should appear symmetrical on the two sides. Taveras also gives measurements for the distances of the angiographic Sylvian point from the skull vault under standard conditions (40-inch target film distance). With the head 1 to $1\frac{1}{2}$ inches from the film this distance measures 30 to 43 mm. Under the same conditions the lateral surface of the insula lies 20 to 30 mm from the skull vault (Fig. 61.13).

As the branches of the middle cerebral artery emerge from the Sylvian fissure they turn, in the case of the anterior branches, upwards, and in the case of the posterior branch, backwards. The anterior or ascending branches pass upwards in the pre-rolandic areas to supply the lateral surface of the hemisphere in the frontal and parietal regions. These arteries are rather variable and tortuous. The posterior branches are more regular and three major arteries can usually be identified. From above downwards these are the *posterior parietal*, *angular* and *posterior temporal* arteries.

THE CEREBRAL VEINS

The superficial cerebral veins are very variable in position and distribution. Most of the veins of the hemisphere run upwards and backwards to end in the superior longitudinal sinus (Fig. 61.14). They usually enter the sinus against the direction of the blood flow which is from before backwards. Two large veins are named by the anatomists. The first, the *vein of Trolard*, is a large vein which passes upwards and backwards over the hemisphere to enter the superior sagittal sinus in the parietal region. The second is the *vein of Labbé*. This large vein passes horizontally across the temporal region to enter the lateral sinus. In most angiograms one or other of these veins can be recognized but it is unusual for both veins to be present in the same angiogram. The smaller middle cerebral veins run forwards in the Sylvian fissure and then to the sphenoidal ridge to end in the sphenoparietal sinus.

The deep cerebral veins fill slightly later than the superficial veins just described. They are of considerable importance in angiographic diagnosis since their position is much more constant than that of the superficial veins.

The **internal cerebral veins** lie one on each side of

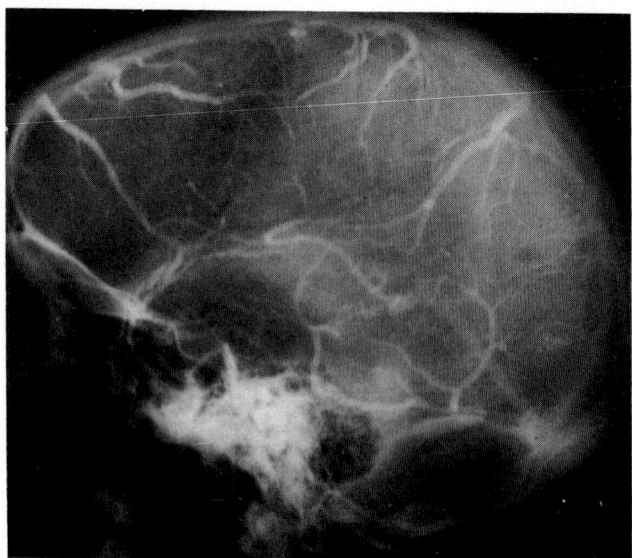

Fig. 61.14A Phlebogram showing superficial and deep veins.

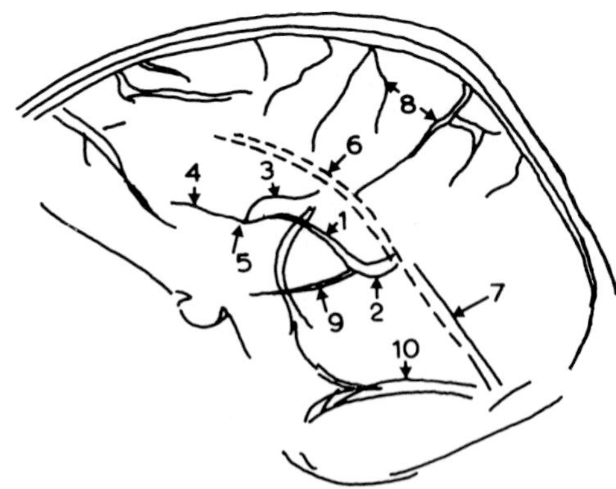

Fig. 61.14B Diagram to illustrate Figure 61.15A

1. Internal cerebral vein
2. Vein of Galen
3. Striothalamic vein
4. Septal vein
5. Venous angle
6. Inferior sagittal sinus
7. Straight sinus
8. Superficial cortical veins
9. Basal vein
10. Lateral sinus.

the midline. They commence just behind the foramen of Monro and pass backwards in the roof of the third ventricle lying in the Tela Choroidea. Two smaller veins drain into each internal cerebral vein at its commencement. These are the *septal vein* which runs on the medial surface of the frontal horn and the *striothalamic vein* which runs in the floor of the lateral ventricle to reach its lateral wall (Fig. 61.15). In the lateral view the junction of the striothalamic vein with the septal vein forms the origin of the internal cerebral vein and is known as the '*venous angle*'. This provides in most cases a recognizable landmark since it normally lies just behind the foramen of Monro. However, the anatomy is not constant and in some cases the strio-thalamic vein may enter the internal cerebral vein more posteriorly. At its posterior end the internal cerebral vein unites with its fellow on the opposite side and enters the vein of Galen. This is constant in position and is easily identified. Just proximal to the vein of Galen other small tributary veins may enter the internal cerebral veins. The *auricular vein* drains the area of the trigone. The *basal vein* arises anteriorly above the sella and passes round the midbrain to enter the back end of the internal cerebral vein. Less commonly, it drains directly into the vein of Galen.

The appearance of these deep veins in the A.P. projection is illustrated in Figure 61.16. Normally the internal cerebral vein lies just to one side of the midline. Thus displacement across the midline is good evidence of the presence of an intracranial mass. Sometimes as with deep-seated tumours of the basal ganglia the deep veins may be displaced across the midline whilst the anterior cerebral artery remains central. The striothalamic vein lies in the floor and lateral wall of the body of the lateral ventricle. Thus it indicates the size of the ventricle and ventricular dilatation can easily be recognized by its appearance in the antero-posterior view.

Ventricular size can also be assessed in the lateral view since the septal, striothalamic and auricular veins all commence in the walls of the ventricles. Thus the shape of the ventricle can be roughly outlined by drawing in a line around the origins of these vessels. These small veins drain the subependymal veins of the cerebral white matter. Normally the latter are very tiny and are rarely recognizable in a routine angiogram. In certain patho-

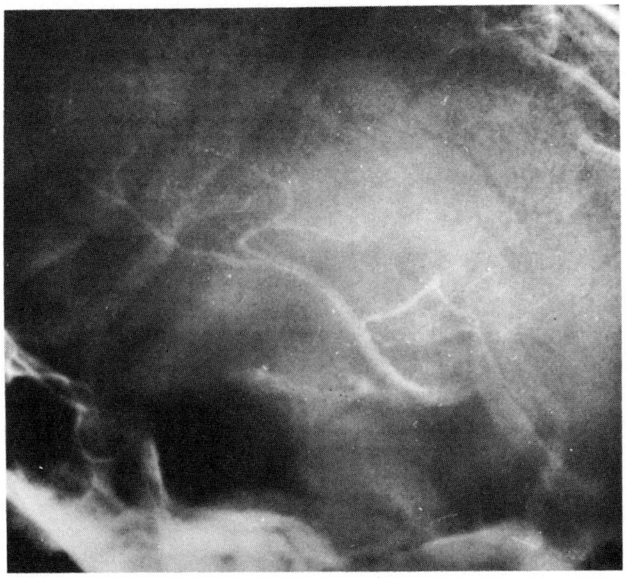

Fig. 61.15A Deep veins shown at late phlebography.

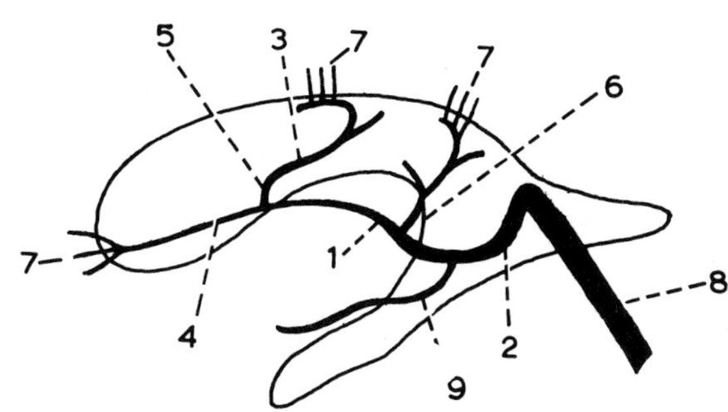

Fig. 61.15B Diagram of late phlebogram (lateral vein) showing relationship to the ventricle.
1. Internal cerebral vein
2. Vein of Galen
3. Striothalamic vein
4. Vein of the septum pellucidum
5. Venous angle
6. Atrial vein
7. Subependymal veins
8. Straight sinus
9. Basal vein

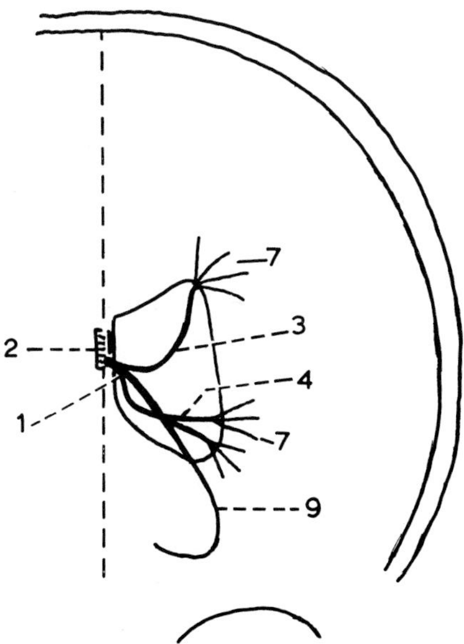

Fig. 61.16 Diagram of late phlebogram at carotid angiography (A.P. view) showing relationship to the ventricle.
1. Internal cerebral vein
2. Vein of Galen
3. Striothalamic vein
4. Vein of the septum pellucidum
7. Subependymal vein
9. Basal vein

logical conditions, however, these veins may become hypertrophied. Thus with highly malignant cerebral gliomas where there is rapid arteriovenous shunting through large tumour vessels and with angiomatous malformations, the subependymal veins may be quite large and readily visible (Fig. 62.32B).

The **vein of Galen** is a short thick vein which curves upwards and backwards behind the splenium of the corpus callosum. Here it joins the *inferior sagittal sinus* to form the *straight sinus* which passes downwards in the apex of the tentorium to the Torcular Herophili. The straight sinus usually drains into the *left lateral sinus*, whilst the *right lateral sinus* usually drains the superior sagittal sinus.

3. Facial artery
4. Ascending pharyngeal artery
5. Occipital artery
6. Posterior auricular artery
7. Internal maxillary artery
8. Superficial temporal artery.

The first three branches arise from the anteromedial aspect of the proximal segment of the artery. The upper or lower of these two, or occasionally all three arteries, may arise in common, as may the ascending pharyngeal and occipital arteries which arise from the postero lateral aspect of the external carotid.

The posterior auricular artery is a small branch which arise just before the main terminal branches, the super-

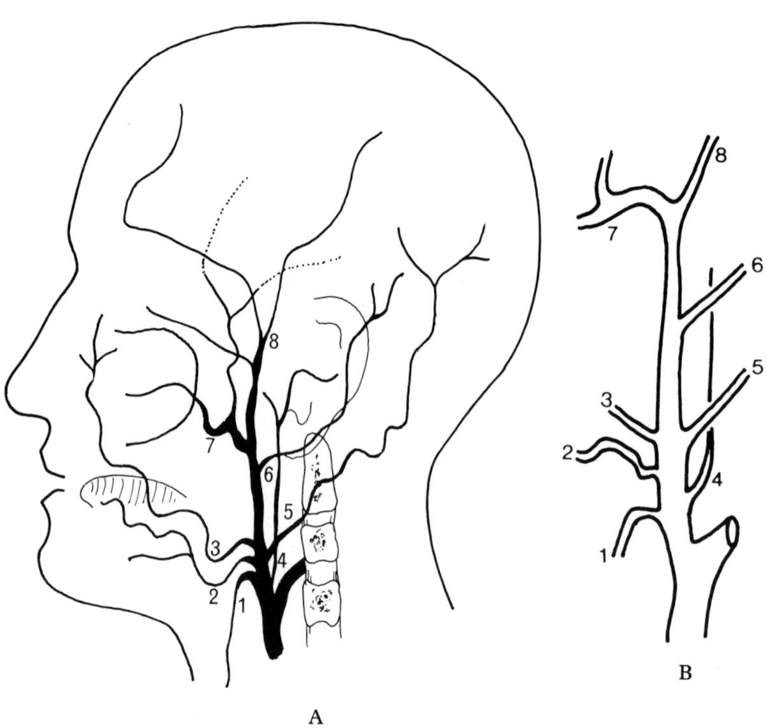

Fig. 61.17A and B Diagram of the external carotid artery branches.
1. Superior thyroid artery
2. Lingual artery
3. Facial artery
4. Ascending pharyngeal artery
5. Occipital artery
6. Posterior auricular artery
7. Internal maxillary artery
8. Superficial temporal artery.

THE NORMAL EXTERNAL CAROTID ANGIOGRAM

The detailed angiographic anatomy of the smaller branches of the external carotid artery is described in great detail in the excellent monograph of Djindjian and Merland (1978). The named major branches of the external carotid artery may be listed as follows (Fig. 61.17):

1. Superior thyroid artery
2. Lingual artery

ficial temporal and internal maxillary. The large internal maxillary artery gives rise to the important middle meningeal artery as well as supplying the nasal fossa, palate, mandible, and infra-orbital region.

The external carotid artery normally arises at the level of C.3 vertebra from the bifurcation of the internal carotid artery. Selective injection of the external carotid has been practised in the past for the better demonstration of intracranial tumours such as meningiomas deriving most of their blood supply from the middle meningeal artery. It is also useful for demonstrating the contribution of the external carotid artery to the blood supply of other intracranial tumours such as acoustic neurinomas and glomus jugulare tumours, and for the demonstration of dural arteriovenous fistulas supplied mainly or entirely by the external carotid artery.

With the increasing use of embolization techniques for the treatment of tumours and angiomatous malformations superselective angiography of the external carotid artery is being increasingly practised. The technique has been used for the demonstration and embolization of *angiomas* of the face, lips and tongue. It has also been used in the investigation and treatment of tumours. These include *meningiomas*, *glomus jugulare tumours*, and *nasopharyngeal angiofibromas*. Another indication is the demonstration and treatment of *dural arteriovenous fistula*.

THE NORMAL VERTEBRAL ANGIOGRAM

The vertebral artery arises from the subclavian artery at the root of the neck. It passes backwards to enter the transverse process of C.6.

In its cervical course the vertebral artery gives off muscular branches which supply the paraspinal muscles. It also gives rise to tiny spinal or radicular branches.

The muscular branches anastomose with branches of the occipital artery and with the ascending pharyngeal arteries. These anastomoses assume some importance in cases of carotid occlusion or stenosis of the vertebral origins.

The spinal branches are tiny and are rarely recognized on routine angiograms. They supply the meninges and may anastomose with the anterior and posterior spinal arteries which supply the cord.

The normal vertebro-basilar intracranial circulation is illustrated in Figures 61.18 and 61.19.

The termination of the vertebral artery in its intracranial portion gives rise to several important vessels. These are the *posterior inferior cerebellar artery*, the *anterior* and *posterior spinal arteries*, and a small *posterior meningeal artery*.

The anterior and posterior spinal arteries are tiny and difficult to identify, though the *anterior spinal artery* is frequently visible in a good quality vertebral arteriogram. It is seen passing downwards into the spinal canal as a very fine vessel directly anterior to the cord. Like most small vessels in the posterior fossa, it is best identified in good subtraction films.

The *posterior meningeal artery* when identified, is seen as a near midline vessel passing upwards and just anterior to the occipital bone in the lateral view.

The **posterior inferior cerebellar artery** usually arises from the terminal segment of the vertebral artery. With the more widespread use of catheter vertebral angiography it is usually possible to fill by reflux the termination of the contralateral vertebral artery. Thus both posterior inferior cerebellar arteries can be shown

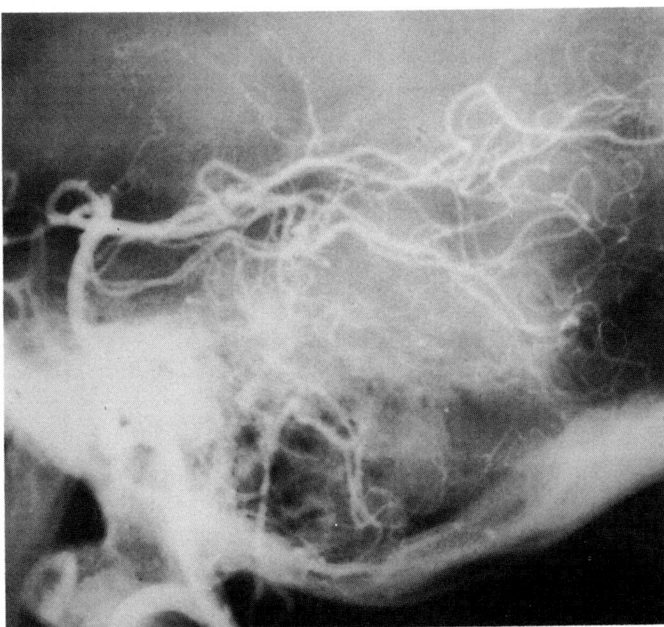

Fig. 61.18A Normal vertebral arteriogram lateral view.

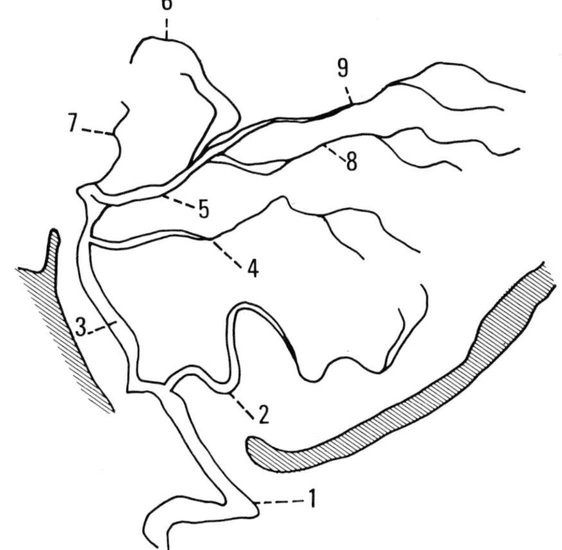

Fig. 61.18B Diagram to illustrate Figure 61.18A.
1. Vertebral artery
2. Posterior inferior cerebellar artery
3. Basilar artery
4. Superior cerebellar arteries
5. Posterior cerebral artery
6. Posterior choroidal arteries
7. Thalamoperforate arteries
8. Posterior temporal artery
9. Internal occipital artery.

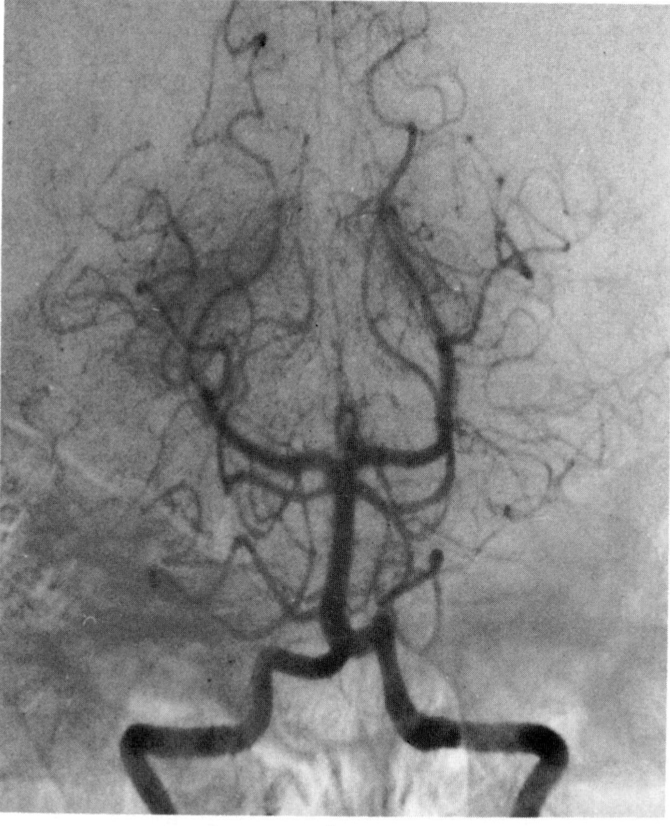

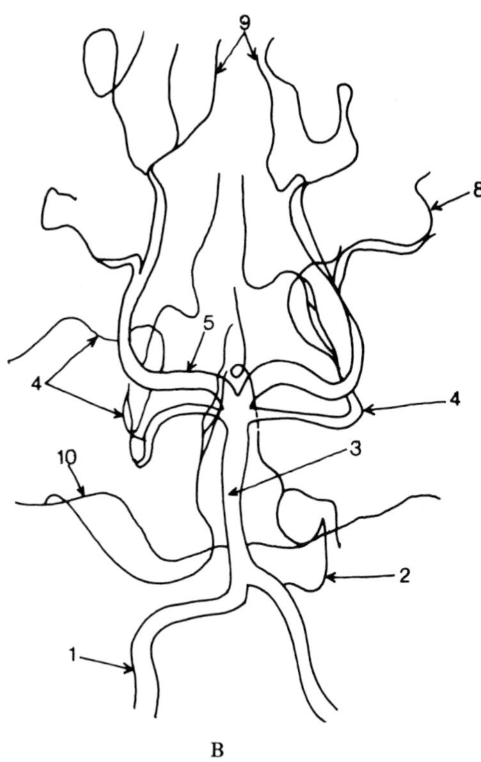

Fig. 61.19A Vertebral arteriogram A.P. view. (Subtraction print.)

Fig. 61.19B Diagram to illustrate Figure 61.19A.
1. Vertebral artery
2. Posterior inferior cerebellar artery
3. Basilar artery
4. Superior cerebellar artery
5. Posterior cerebral artery
8. Posterior temporal artery
9. Internal occipital artery
10. Anterior inferior cerebellar artery.

The right P.I.C.A. arises from the right A.I.C.A. in this case.

from the injection of a single vertebral artery (Fig. 61.19).

The normal anatomy of the posterior inferior cerebellar artery is illustrated in Figures 61.20 and 61.21. This vessel is of considerable importance in angiographic diagnosis in the posterior fossa. There is a wide variation in its course and distribution but a fairly typical pattern is followed in most cases. The point of origin of the artery may be from the vertebral artery below the foramen magnum or as high as the junction of vertebral and basilar arteries. Sometimes it arises from the basilar or in common with the anterior inferior cerebellar artery. Normally it arises from the vertebral artery just above the foramen magnum.

The first part of the artery as seen in lateral view loops round the medulla and then downwards to curve round the lower margin of the tonsil. It then passes up anterior and medial to the tonsil to reach the roof of the fourth

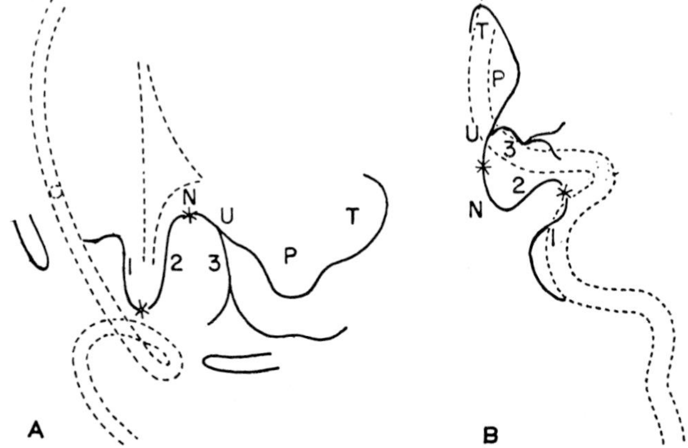

Fig. 61.20 Diagram of the posterior inferior cerebellar artery. (A) *Lateral view.* Asterisks mark the apices of the caudal and cranial loops. The apex of the cranial loop is closely related to the nodulus (N) and roof of the fourth ventricle (dotted). The upper or vermis branch runs near the midline around the inferior vermis (including uvula (U), pyramid (P) and tuber (T)). The lower or tonsillohemispheric branch runs near the posterior margin of the tonsil giving off anterior or tonsillar branches and posterior or hemispheric branches. The tonsil lies between 2 and 3.

(B) *Antero-posterior view,* in half axial projection. The segments marked in the lateral view are identified by the same numbers and letters. Segment 3 (the tonsillohemispheric branch) may be difficult to identify in this view. The apex of the cranial loop (*N) lies usually within 2 mm of the midline, and the terminal portion of the artery (T) returns to the midline.

(Reproduced from Wolf *et al.* (1962) *American Journal of Roentgenology,* 87, 323.)

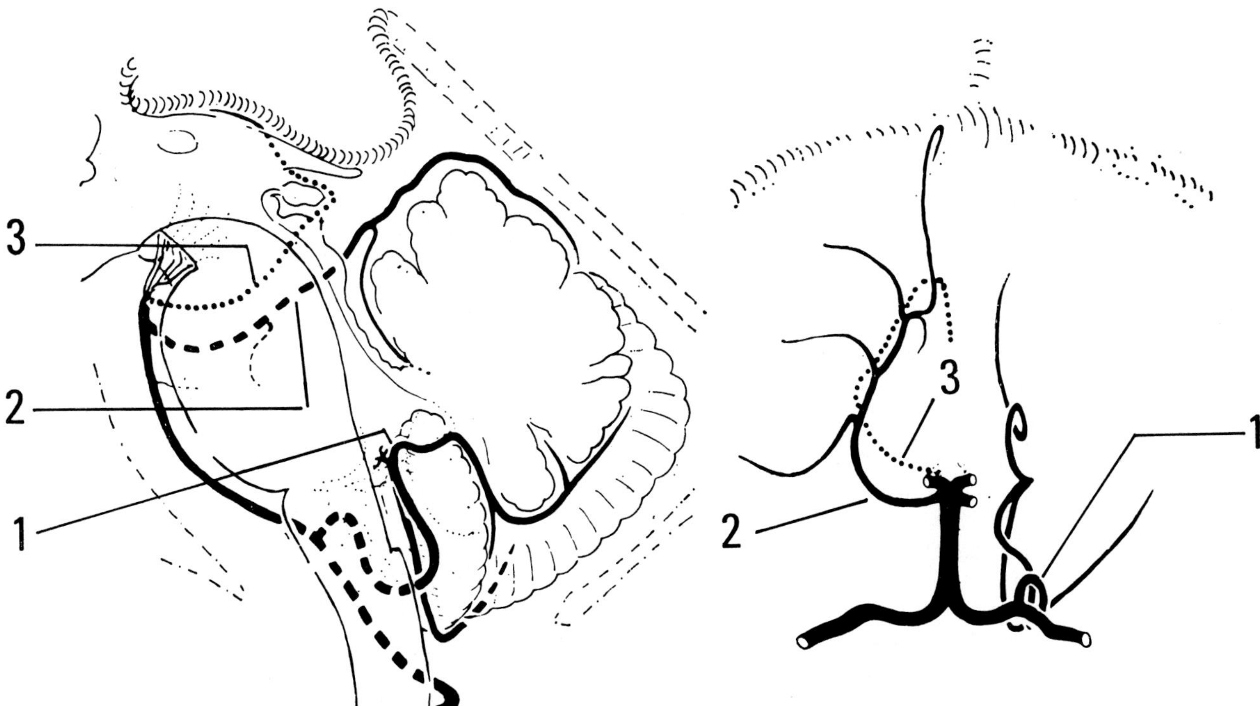

Fig. 61.21 Relationship of normal arteries in the posterior fossa to the brain stem.
1. Posterior inferior cerebellar artery
2. Superior cerebellar artery
3. Medial posterior choroidal artery
(After Huang & Wolf, 1970, *Neuroradiology*, **1**, 4.)

ventricle in the region of the inferior medullary velum. The downward loop just described usually marks the lower limit of the tonsil and has therefore been used as an index of tonsillar herniation. However, this sign should be treated with caution since the loop may reach below the foramen magnum in normal patients as an anomaly. In these latter cases the loop tends to be narrower with a 'hair-pin' appearance.

Just below the apex of the fourth ventricle the posterior inferior cerebellar artery as seen in lateral view loops slightly backwards again before dividing into its major branches. This important landmark is known as the 'choroidal loop', since it supplies choroidal branches to the 4th ventricle and marks out the inferior roof of the fourth ventricle.

The *vermis* branch which lies near the midline forms a flat loop convex downwards with a local exaggeration in the region of the pyramid. Its terminal portion curves round the tuber in the posterior cerebellar notch. Normally the vermis branch, as seen in the axial view, does not cross the midline and displacement across the midline can be regarded as evidence of a mass on the ipsilateral side of the posterior fossa.

The other major branch of the posterior inferior cerebellar artery is the *tonsillohemispheric*. This arises at the same point as the vermis branch but runs farther downwards in lateral view along the posterior margin of the tonsil. It gives off anterior or tonsillar branches and posterior or hemispheric branches which curve down and back around the under aspect of the cerebellar hemisphere.

This 'typical' distribution in lateral view is illustrated in Figure 61.20A. The typical distribution in the half axial view is shown in Figure 61.20B. The appearances in the latter view depend on the degree of obliquity with which the film is taken. Anteroposterior films of the vertebral arteriograms can be taken with varying degrees of tilt though the most usual projection is one corresponding to the Towne's projection.

It is possible, nevertheless, to recognize in most cases the first or caudal loop of the posterior interior cerebellar artery. This extends laterally as far as the lateral aspect of the medulla. The second or cranial loop can also be recognized and its apex is located within 2 mm of the midline in the roof of the fourth ventricle. The tonsillohemispheric branch is more difficult to identify in this projection than in the lateral projection, but the apex of the loop of the vermis branch can be recognized by its laterally convex outline. The terminal part of the vermis branch returns to the midline on the superior aspect of the vermis. The opposite curvature of the cranial and posterior loops given a characteristic 'S' appearance in this projection.

The appearance just described and illustrated can be regarded as the standard configuration of the posterior inferior cerebellar artery, but it should be appreciated that there are many variations from this standard pattern.

The **basilar artery** is formed by the junction of the two vertebral arteries just above the foramen magnum. It passes upwards directly behind the clivus in the lateral view and it terminates behind or just above the tip of the dorsum sellae. In the anterior or Towne's projection the basilar artery lies in the midline. However, displacement from the midline, or lateral kinking, is quite common in the middle aged and elderly, particularly in hypertensive patients, and such kinking does not necessarily imply displacement by a mass. In elderly and hypertensive patients the basilar artery may also be elongated and kinked as seen in lateral view. Sometimes it terminates well above the dorsum sellae and these cases of a high basilar termination may cause an indent in the floor of the third ventricle. Such an indent can be recognized at pneumography and should not be mistaken for displacement by a tumour. Lateral kinking of the basilar artery may also be seen in young patients. In these patients the kinking is always to the side away from a large dominant vertebral artery, and has no pathological significance.

The basilar artery has numerous small branches which supply the pons and are difficult or impossible to visualize in an angiogram. There are however larger branches which can be recognized in many cases. These include the paired **anterior inferior cerebellar arteries**. These two vessels arise within a centimetre of the origin of the basilar artery. In lateral view they are obscured by the mastoids and petrous bones, but they can often be identified in the Towne's view or in the direct antero-posterior view. Subtraction films will usually show them best and clear of overlying bone. They extend directly laterally and supply branches to the internal auditory meatus and also to the inferior surface of the cerebellum. Here they anastomose with branches of the posterior inferior cerebellar artery.

The **superior cerebellar arteries** arise just before the termination of the basilar artery. These paired arteries curve round the midbrain to reach the superior surface of the cerebellum where they divide into several branches. In a lateral film they lie below the posterior cerebral arteries and are seen to pass over the surface of the cerebellum. In this view they are partially superimposed on the posterior temporal branch of the posterior cerebral artery, as this lies on the other side of the slanting tentorium.

The **posterior cerebral arteries** are the terminal branches of the basilar artery. Both posterior cerebral arteries fill readily through the basilar in nearly 90 per cent of cases. In most of the remaining cases only one posterior cerebral artery fills well. Very rarely neither posterior cerebral artery is filled. In these latter cases there is probably a dominant supply from the carotid artery through large posterior communicating arteries. The posterior cerebral arteries curve around the cerebral peduncles to reach the dorsal aspect of midbrain. Here they pass through the tentorium to reach the under surface of the temporal lobes. Each posterior cerebral has two main branches, a **posterior temporal** which supplies the under surface of the posterior part of the temporal lobe, and an **internal occipital** branch which passes to the medial aspect of the occipital lobe. This divides into terminal branches named as the *calcarine* and *parieto-occipital* arteries.

The **thalamoperforating arteries** arise from the proximal segment of the posterior cerebral artery and lie close to the midline. They are easily seen in the lateral view, where they appear to be one to three in number and show as fine vertical vessels passing up into the thalamus. They are difficult or impossible to define in the A.P. view.

Posterior choroidal arteries. Each posterior cerebral artery gives off a *medial* posterior choroidal artery and also two or more *lateral* posterior choroidal arteries. The medial posterior choroidal artery arises first, just lateral to the bifurcation of the basilar artery. It passes round the midbrain together with and usually obscured by the posterior cerebral artery.

On the postero-lateral aspect of the midbrain it describes a figure 3 curve and passes lateral to the pineal to reach the midline. It then enters the tela choroidea in the roof of the third ventricle. The two or more lateral posterior choroidal arteries arise from the distal posterior cerebrals as these vessels pass round the brain-stem. They usually describe a curve which is concave forward as they ascend and this corresponds to the posterior aspect of the thalamus. Their marked forward curve differentiates them from the medial posterior choroidal artery which ascends more vertically with a double curve and arises more anteriorly. All these arteries are more difficult to identify in frontal angiograms. Thalamic tumours usually increase the depth of the curve and stretch the choroidal vessels on one side. Pineal tumours will cause stretching on both sides but usually involve the medial choroidal arteries only.

In the capillary phase the choroidal plexus is outlined as a well-defined blush of contrast. This is a normal appearance and should not be mistaken for a pathological circulation.

A small splenium branch of the posterior cerebral artery also supplies the pial plexus on and behind the splenium of the corpus callosum which may thus be outlined on the vertebral angiogram.

The **posterior communicating artery** is occasionally outlined, but it is unusual to see good ante-grade filling of the carotid system from the posterior communicating artery in a normal patient. However, the phenomenon can be demonstrated in certain pathological conditions. In one case we have demonstrated filling of the whole of the cerebral circulation from the vertebrobasilar system in a patient with bilateral internal carotid thromboses. Retrograde filling has also been demonstrated following compression of the carotids in the neck and simultaneous injection of the vertebral artery.

THE VEINS OF THE POSTERIOR FOSSA

At one time little attention was paid to the veins of the posterior fossa, but careful anatomical studies have shown that many are constant in position and can be consistently recognized. They are thus of considerable importance in demonstrating the presence of tumours in the posterior fossa (Figs 61.22 and 61.23).

A mass in the pineal region will press the precentral cerebellar vein downwards. The precentral cerebellar vein drains into the great vein of Galen at its posterior end where it joins the straight sinus. In the frontal view the vein is difficult to recognize because of the other larger overlying midline veins. Occasionally its origin can be seen in the A.P. view as an inverted 'Y' draining up from the fourth ventricle.

The **anterior pontomesencephalic vein** runs on the anterior surface of the pons where it forms an irregular concave curve. It marks out the posterior wall of the pontine cistern and the anterior surface of the pons. Below, it communicates with the right and left petrosal vein. Above, it drains into the **posterior mesencephalic vein**. The latter is superimposed on the basal vein in lateral view and may drain into it.

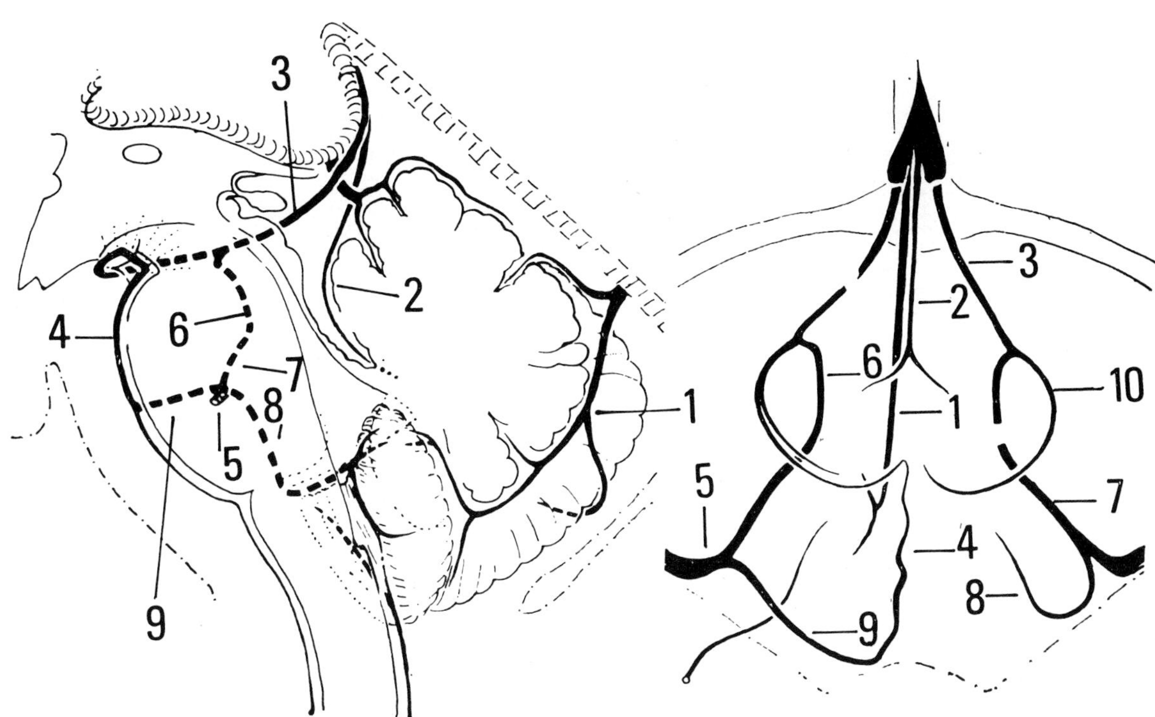

Fig. 61.22 Normal veins of the posterior fossa and their relationship to the normal structures.
1. Inferior vermian vein
2. Precentral cerebellar vein
3. Posterior mesencephalic vein
4. Anterior pontomesencephalic vein
5. Petrosal vein
6. Lateral mesencephalic vein
7. Brachial vein
8. Vein of the lateral recess of fourth ventricle
9. Transverse pontine vein
10. Peduncular vein.

(After Huang & Wolf, 1970, *Neuroradiology*, 1, 4.)

Precentral cerebellar vein. This small vein is easy to recognize in the lateral phlebogram. It passes in the midline over the superior surface of the cerebellum and lies dorsal to the midbrain. If the aqueduct and fourth ventricle are pressed backwards the precentral cerebellar vein will be pressed backwards with them. A mass in the upper vermis will displace the vein forwards and upwards.

The **lateral mesencephalic vein** also communicates with the posterior mesencephalic or basal vein. It passes downwards and forwards at an angle of about 80° in the lateral view and connects with the superior petrosal sinus, via the brachial and petrosal veins.

Superior vermian vein. This passes along the superior vermis to terminate in the great vein of Galen near the termination of the precentral cerebellar vein. It may join the precentral vein, or the basal vein, or be continuous with the inferior vermian vein. Again it is difficult to identify in the anterior view though easily seen in the lateral view.

Inferior vermian vein. The paired inferior vermian veins lie near the midline. Both commence with a superior

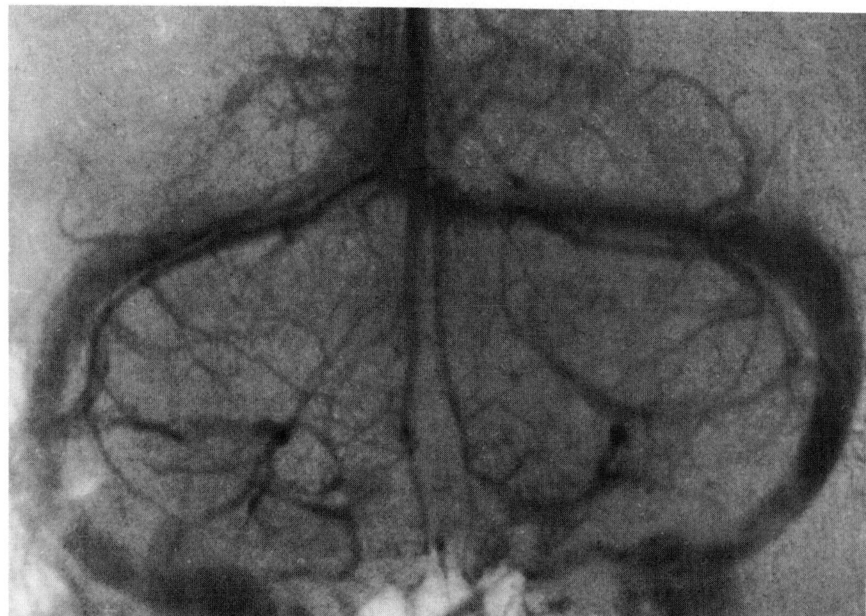

Fig. 61.23 Subtraction print of venous phase of vertebral angiogram in a normal patient. The reader should identify many of the veins marked in Figure 61.22.

and inferior retrotonsillar vein and drain up the inferior vermis. They usually end in the straight sinus but can join the superior vermian vein. In lateral view they are easily recognized as they lie as much as 1 cm from the occipital bone and mark the anterior margin of the cisterna magna.

The **petrosal vein** lies just above and lateral to the internal auditory meatus. It is fed by the brachial vein and drains into the superior petrosal sinus. It is best seen in the Towne's view and is of considerable importance in the assessment of angle tumours, since acoustic neurinomas or other angle tumours usually elevate or obliterate the petrosal vein.

The **brachial vein** drains into the petrosal vein and is best seen in the Towne's view where it lies at an angle of 45° to the midline. The lateral mesencephalic vein may connect it with the posterior mesencephalic vein.

THE NORMAL ARCH AORTOGRAM

This is illustrated in Figure 61.24. The majority of patients show the arrangements of great vessels shown in Figure 61.24A, but anomalies of the great vessels are present in at least a quarter of the cases (Sutton and Davies, 1966).

The variation which was seen most often was a common origin for the innominate and the left common carotid artery. Obvious cases are recognized readily but it is sometimes difficult, or even impossible, to distinguish minor degrees, even in the oblique position, because of overlapping of vessels. About one-fifth of our cases had this

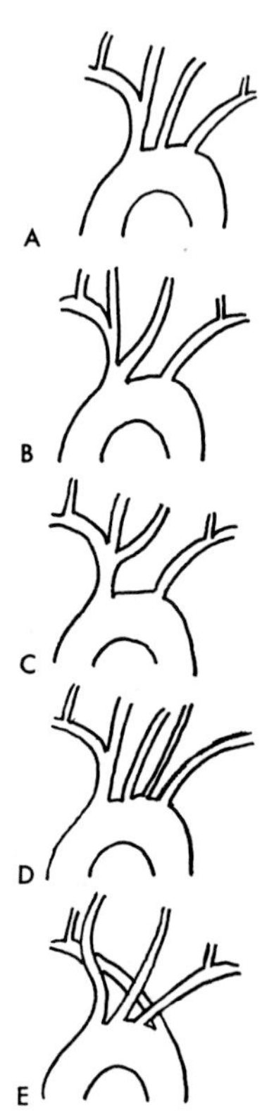

Fig. 61.24 Anomalies of the aortic arch branches. A = normal, B = joint origin of innominate and L. common carotid, C = L. common carotid arises from innominate, D = L. vertebral arises from arch, E = anomalous R. subclavian (Sutton, D. and Davies, E. R. (1966) *Clinical Radiology*, 17, 330).

anomaly, but it is commoner in Negroes, being present in 36 per cent of reported autopsies among coloured patients.

The remaining anomalies show a fairly constant incidence and are also of importance. Thus the left vertebral arises from the aortic arch in 5 per cent of patients so that its origin can only be seen in these cases by arch aortography and not by subclavian catheterization.

An aberrant right subclavian artery is present in 1 to 2 per cent of patients. This is also important because it may be a cause for right transaxillary catheterization failing to enter the ascending aorta.

The two carotid arteries are of similar calibre but the vertebral arteries can vary greatly in size as described in the following section.

CONGENITAL ANOMALIES

Congenital anomalies of the intracranial circulation are relatively uncommon, with the exception of anomalies of the circle of Willis (Fig. 61.25). The first part of the *anterior cerebral* artery may be small or hypoplastic on one side. In these cases both anterior cerebral arteries fill from the other side with the aid of the anterior communicating artery.

The *posterior communicating* artery may also be small or hypoplastic. Such anomalies of the circle of Willis can be very important when stenosis or obstruction of a major extracranial vessel occurs, since it normally provides a collateral circulation.

Congenital hypoplasia of the intracranial part of the *internal carotid* arteries has been described and in such cases a collateral circulation may develop from the primitive vascular 'rete' or network present in the embryo at the base of the skull.

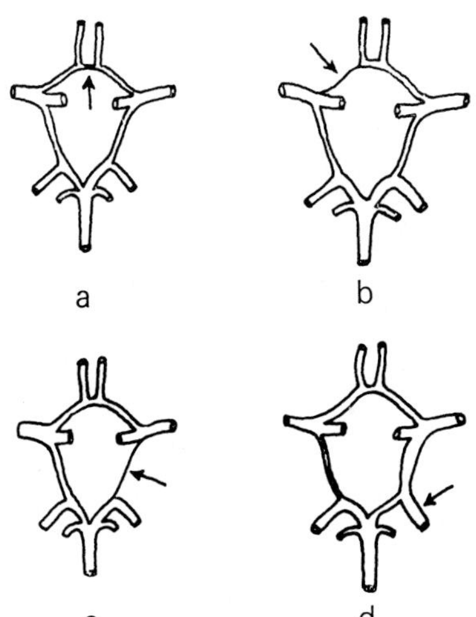

Fig. 61.25 Anomalies of the circle of Willis (after Alpers, Berry and Paddison, 1959). The posterior communicating artery is most frequently involved and combined lesions are common.
(a) Hypoplastic anterior communicating (3%)
(b) Hypoplastic proximal segment of anterior cerebral (2%)
(c) Hypoplastic posterior communicating (22%)
(d) Carotid origin of posterior cerebral (15%)

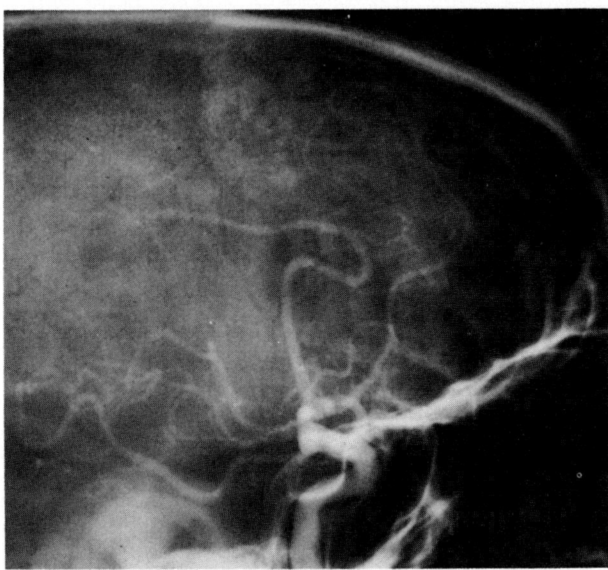

Fig. 61.26 Agenesis of the corpus callosum. Note the unusual vertical course of the anterior cerebral artery.

Congenital anomalies of the brain such as *agenesis of the corpus callosum* may also be associated with arterial anomalies. In this condition the anterior cerebral arteries may be represented by a large common trunk in the midline, or two arteries may be present. In either case the anterior cerebral artery pursues an abnormal course. It passes more vertically upwards, and since there is no corpus callosum the pericallosal branch is abnormal in course and situation (Fig. 61.26).

Some congenital anomalies of the extracranial circulation have been mentioned above. Thus the left common carotid artery arises in common with the innominate artery in some 20 per cent of cases.

The common carotid artery usually bifurcates at the level of C.3 just below the angle of the jaw. In some cases, however, it may bifurcate at a much lower level and occasionally at a higher level.

Occasionally a vertebral artery will arise normally but pass into the vertebral canal at a higher level than the normal C.6.

Size of arteries. The vertebral arteries vary markedly in size. On the one hand the vertebral artery may be almost as large as an internal carotid artery, on the other hand it may have a lumen as small as 1 mm and may appear on the arteriogram almost as a thread of cotton. Such a small vertebral (usually the right) may terminate in the posterior inferior cerebellar artery, and not join the basilar artery. The average vertebral artery lies somewhere between these extremes and on the X-ray film its lumen measures 3-4 mm in diameter. In the same individual the two vertebral arteries can be very different in

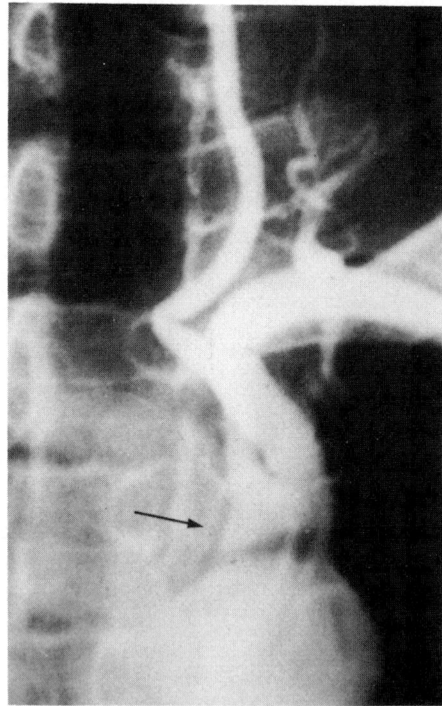

Fig. 61.27 Origin of the left vertebral artery from the aortic arch.

size, though in approximately 30 per cent of patients the two vertebral arteries are equal. In the remaining 70 per cent of patients, about 40 per cent have a larger left vertebral than the right and about 30 per cent have a larger right vertebral than the left. The basilar artery can also vary greatly in diameter, being quite small when both posterior cerebrals are supplied from the internal carotids.

Anomalous vertebral arteries. An important anomaly in the origin of the left vertebral artery direct from the aortic arch between the left common carotid and the left subclavian arteries. This happens with sufficient frequency (5 per cent of cases) to be of practical importance. Left vertebral catheterization from the femoral artery in these cases is more difficult, and from the axillary artery it is impossible. There are a number of other but much rarer anomalous origins for a vertebral artery. Thus it may arise from the innominate artery, from the inferior thyroid artery or even from the common carotid artery in

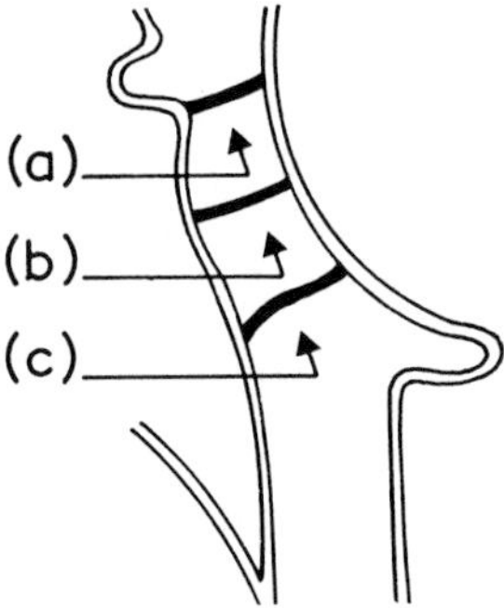

Fig. 61.29 Anomalous communications between the carotid and vertebrobasilar systems. (a) Trigeminal artery, (b) acoustic artery, (c) hypoglossal artery. (From Sutton, D., 1971, *Clinical Radiology*, **22**, 271.)

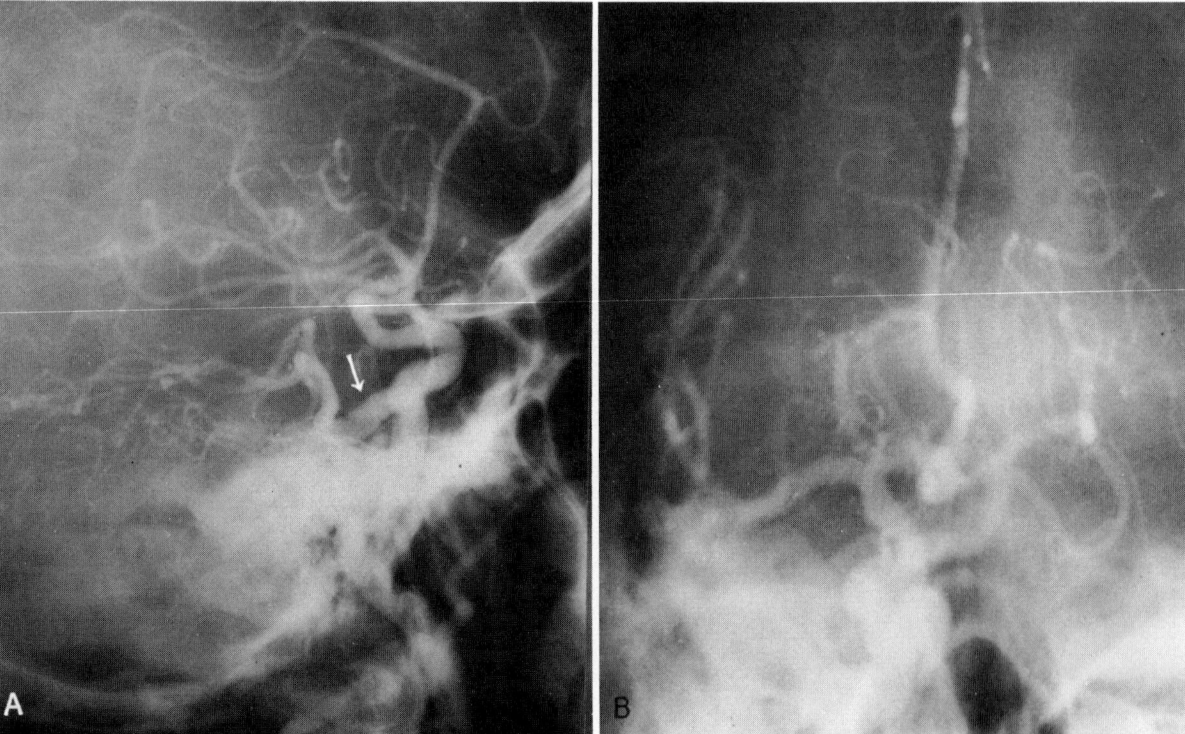

Fig. 61.28 Anomalous carotid basilar anastomosis (↘). This is an example of the trigeminal artery. A. Lateral view. B. A.P. view.

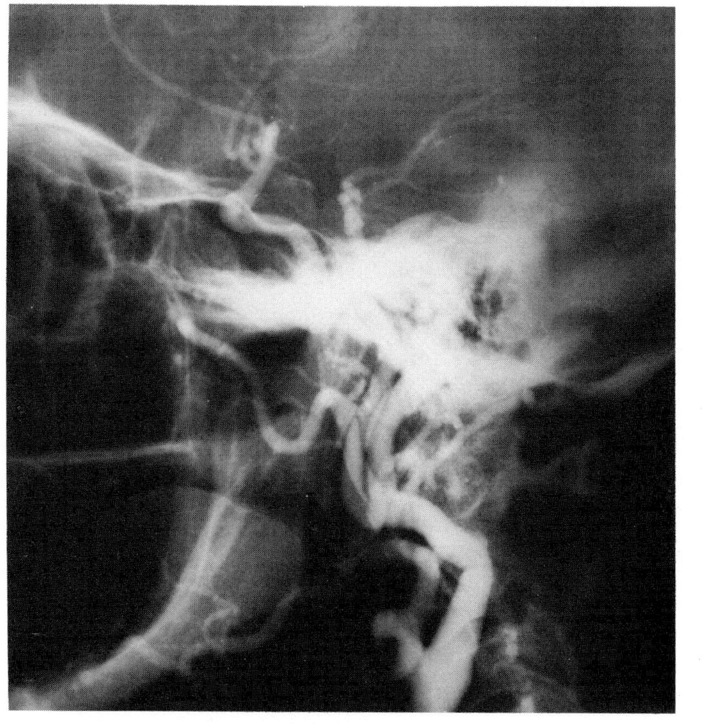

A

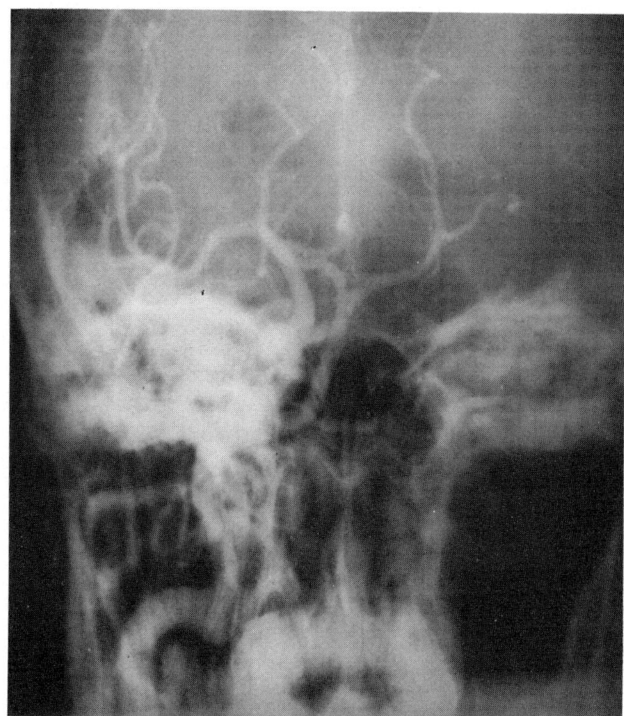

B

Fig. 61.30 Hypoglossal artery connecting carotid and basilar arteries. (A) Lateral view. (B) A.P. view.

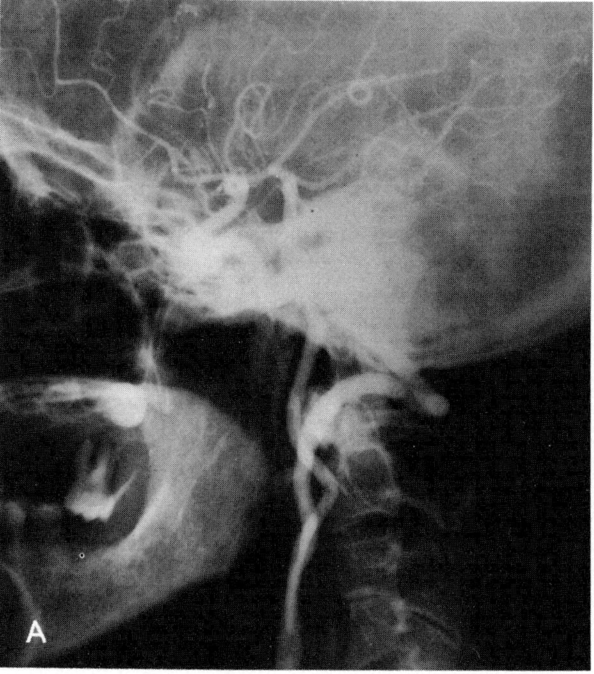

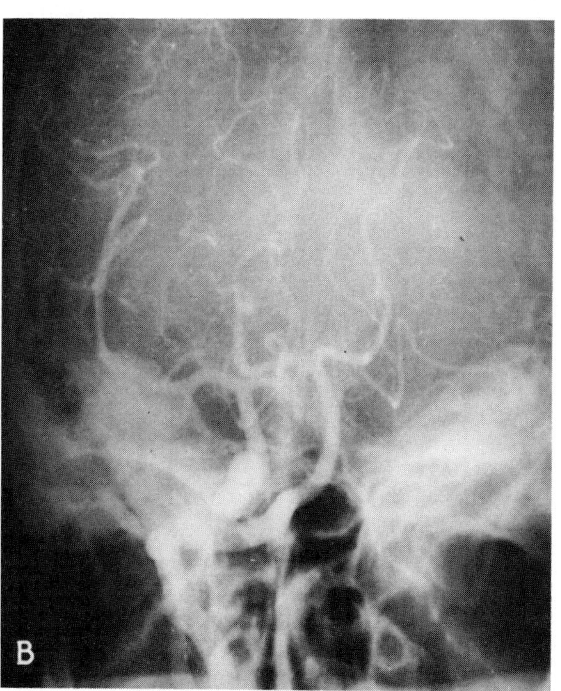

Fig. 61.31 Origin of the vertebral artery from the common carotid in the neck. This is an example of the pre-atlantal intersegmental artery. (A) Lateral view. (B) A.P. view.

the neck. Another very rare anomaly is the origin of the right vertebral from the distal part of the aortic arch. Such a vessel must pass behind the oesophagus like an anomalous subclavian artery in order to reach the right side of the neck.

Communications between the carotid and vertebrobasilar systems may also occur, the most frequent of these (about one in 500 cases) is between the internal carotid artery as it enters the cavernous sinus and the termination of the basilar artery. This artery passes round the base of the sella and is often termed the *trigeminal artery* because of its close relationship to the trigeminal nerve (Fig. 61.28). Anastomosis at a more proximal level is less frequent. Named communications are the *acoustic artery* and the *hypoglossal artery*, so called because they accompany the corresponding cranial nerves (Fig. 61.29).

The *acoustic artery* connects the internal carotid artery with the basilar by an artery accompanying the 7th and 8th nerves through the internal auditory meatus. It is excessively rare and special projections including a basal view are necessary before a case can be regarded as authenticated.

The *hypoglossal artery*, which passes through the anterior condyloid foramen at the base of the skull after arising from the carotid in the neck, is less rare, though still much less common than the trigeminal artery (Fig. 61.30).

The *pre-atlantal intersegmental artery*. This vessel is also very rare though we have personally encountered a case (Fig. 61.31). The essential feature is that the artery arises from the internal carotid and joins the horizontal part of the vertebral artery as it lies on the atlas. In our case the anomalous vessel arose opposite C.4 and there was no external carotid artery apparent.

Anomalous middle meningeal artery. The middle meningeal artery or its anterior branch may occasionally arise from the ophthalmic artery. The converse, an ophthalmic artery arising from the middle meningeal, can occur but is very rare.

REFERENCES AND
SUGGESTIONS FOR FURTHER READING

(See end of next chapter)

CHAPTER 62

ANGIOGRAPHY IN NEURORADIOLOGY (2)

VASCULAR LESIONS

The diagnosis of vascular lesions affecting the central nervous system was revolutionized by the widespread practice of arteriography. Many conditions which were previously only diagnosed at operation or autopsy were rapidly elucidated by the advent of the techniques described above.

In this chapter vascular lesions will be considered under the following headings:

1. Aneurysm
2. Angiomatous malformation
3. Arteriovenous fistula
4. Haematoma
    (*a*) extradural
    (*b*) subdural
    (*c*) intracerebral
5. Embolus
6. Vascular stenosis and thrombosis

1. ANEURYSM

Before the days of cerebral arteriography there was only one certain radiological sign to indicate the presence of an intracerebral aneurysm. This was ring calcification in the wall of the aneurysm. Unfortunately such a sign is extremely rare and it usually implies the presence of a clotted aneurysm of long standing.

Aneurysms may present clinically in three different ways. By far the commonest mode of presentation and that seen in over 90 per cent of the cases encountered is by *subarachnoid haemorrhage*. The second method of presentation is by pressure upon cranial nerves, particularly around the Circle of Willis and lateral to the cavernous sinus and giving rise to *oculomotor pareses*. The third cranial nerve is the one most commonly involved. Finally in a few cases the aneurysm may reach a very large size and simulate an *intracranial tumour*.

Before the advent of C.T. scanning a patient who had suffered a **subarachnoid haemorrhage** usually had the diagnosis confirmed by lumbar puncture. Once confirmation was obtained, angiography was proceeded with in order to define the cause of the haemorrhage and if possible to localize its site. This information is vital if neurosurgical treatment is to be undertaken. In large series of subarachnoid haemorrhages investigated by arteriography an aneurysm has been shown to be the cause in a majority of cases. Less commonly the haemorrhage may arise from rupture of an angiomatous malformation or from rupture of an atheromatous vessel. Extremely rare causes are haemorrhage from tumours, and haemorrhage in blood dyscrasias (Table 62.1).

Table 62.1 Causes of subarachnoid haemorrhage

A. Trauma
B. Spontaneous
    1. Aneurysm
    2. Angioma
    3. Atheroma
    4. Tumour
    5. Blood dyscrasia

Since the development of C.T. scanning the management of this serious condition has been radically changed. The non-invasive scan will, in many cases, confirm the diagnosis of subarachnoid haemorrhage without lumbar puncture by showing the presence of blood in the basal cisterns or over the cortex of the brain. In some cases an intracerebral haematoma or intraventricular haemorrhage may be demonstrated, and the source of the haemorrhage in many cases may be inferred from the localizing evidence of the scan (see Fig. 64.7). Whilst a lesion will be demonstrated in some two-thirds of the cases a significant proportion will have negative findings, and investigation will proceed as above by lumbar puncture and angiography. If the C.T. findings are positive the causative lesion may be successfully localized to one hemisphere or to the posterior fossa. Angiography may then be limited, if clinically advisable, to a single carotid angiogram or vertebral angiogram thus saving the patient from the more extensive four vessel studies. In non-localized subarachnoid haemorrhage a very high degree of accuracy in the diagnosis of subarachnoid haemorrhage can be achieved by careful and systematic angiography. First-class radiography is essential and it is usually necessary to take films in several projections before an aneurysm can be confidently excluded.

For the carotid angiogram *lateral*, *A.P.*, and *oblique* films are usually required; it may also be necessary to take an *oblique transorbital* view, and occasionally an *axial* view. The aim is to show the aneurysm clearly and the relationship of its neck to the vessel of origin.

In cases where there are no localizing signs and C.T. is negative it may be necessary to delineate the whole of the arterial supply to the brain before the lesion is discovered. Thus if bilateral carotid arteriography proves negative, vertebral arteriography is next undertaken. In a small proportion of cases it was also necessary to inject the second vertebral artery, if the previous injections had failed to show the posterior inferior cerebellar artery arising from this contralateral vertebral (see Fig. 62.5). However, with modern catheter techniques it is usually possible to show the contralateral vertebral artery by reflux. Follow-up of cases which had negative findings at four vessel angiography suggests that the prognosis in these patients is much better than in those patients where aneurysms were demonstrated.

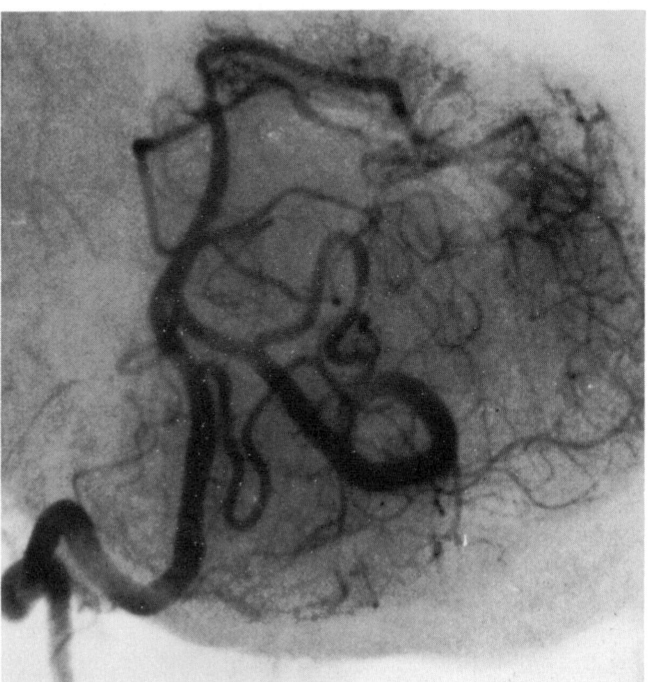

Fig. 62.1 Right vertebral arteriogram. Oblique view showing reflux down the left vertebral and clear definition of the origin of PICA on both sides (subtraction print).

For the vertebral angiogram, *lateral* and *Towne's* views are required with good subtraction films. A *lateral oblique* view, to show the origins of the posterior inferior cerebellar arteries clearly, may also be helpful (Fig. 62.1).

The following table shows the percentage of positive findings in large series of cases of subarachnoid haemorrhages investigated by cerebral angiography (Table 62.2). Bilateral carotid angiography provided a diagnosis in about 75 per cent of the cases. Subsequent vertebral angiography reduced the 25 per cent of negative cases by over a third.

Table 62.2 Findings after bilateral carotid angiography for subarachnoid haemorrhage

Findings	Walsh (1956) (461 cases)	Sutton and Trickey Group 1 (1962) (557 cases)
	Per cent	Per cent
Aneurysms	54	54
Angiomas	11·5	7·5
Haematomas	7·5	12·5
Tumour	0	1
Negative	27	25

Cerebral aneurysms were found to be multiple in between 5 and 15 per cent of cases in different series investigated. In some patients more than two aneurysms have been demonstrated (Fig. 62.2A). In such cases the clinical features or C.T. scan may help to decide the source of the haemorrhage, or local vascular *spasm* may point to the aneurysm responsible. Following a recent bleed the vessels in the region of the ruptured aneurysm often become spastic and narrowed. Sometimes the spasm is more widespread, involving most of the intracranial arteries. This spasm is readily identified on the arteriograms (Fig. 62.2B) and may be a contributory factor to the clinical symptoms. Other features which may help to identify the bleeding aneurysm when multiple aneurysms are present, are the size of the aneurysm and the presence of local haematoma. In the majority of cases it is the largest aneurysm which bleeds (Fig. 62.3).

Ruptured aneurysms may haemorrhage into the brain and produce large *intracerebral haematomas*. These may act as mass lesions and produce displacement of superficial vessels and even shift of the anterior cerebral artery across the midline. In these cases and in the absence of a C.T. scan the diagnosis of haematoma will be based on the history and the demonstration of a source for the haemorrhage, such as an aneurysm or angioma. C.T. scanning will of course show an intracerebral haematoma clearly prior to angiography. Such intracranial haematomas may themselves be the cause of symptoms and require surgical treatment by evacuation. Sometimes an anterior communicating aneurysm may fill from one carotid yet have ruptured into the contralateral frontal lobe.

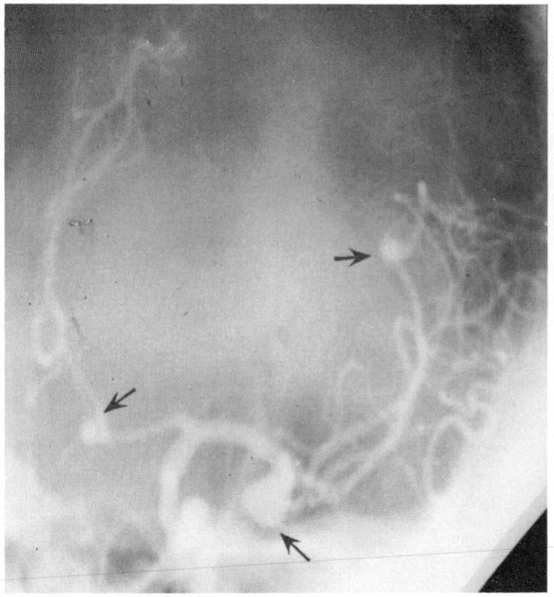

A

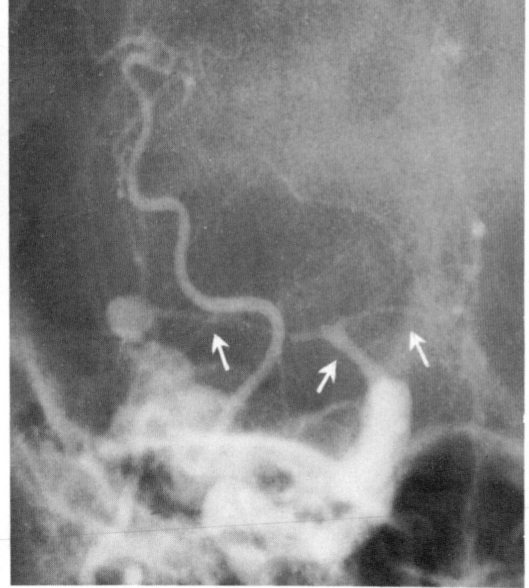

B

Fig. 62.2A Multiple aneurysms in a patient with subarachnoid haemorrhage. Three aneurysms are demonstrated (arrows).

Fig. 62.2B Middle cerebral aneurysm in a patient with subarachnoid haemorrhage showing local spasm of the adjacent vessels (arrows).

Subdural haematomas, usually shallow, may also result from ruptured aneurysms and should be carefully looked for when inspecting the angiograms or preliminary C.T. scan.

It is probable that a subarachnoid haemorrhage is a sudden incident lasting only a short time. It is followed by a drop in blood pressure with sealing off of the point of haemorrhage by clot. It is therefore extremely unlikely that haemorrhage will be shown at angiography by contrast extravasation. However, like other investigators, we have on isolated occasions seen evidence that the aneurysm was actually bleeding at the time of injection. It should be emphasized that this is excessively rare and we have only seen it 3 times in some 1000 cases of subarachnoid haemorrhage examined by angiography.

Many neurosurgeons when they consider intracranial surgery or carotid ligation feel that it is important to have *cross-compression* angiographic studies in order to determine whether there is free flow across the anterior communicating artery. Such cross-compression studies are

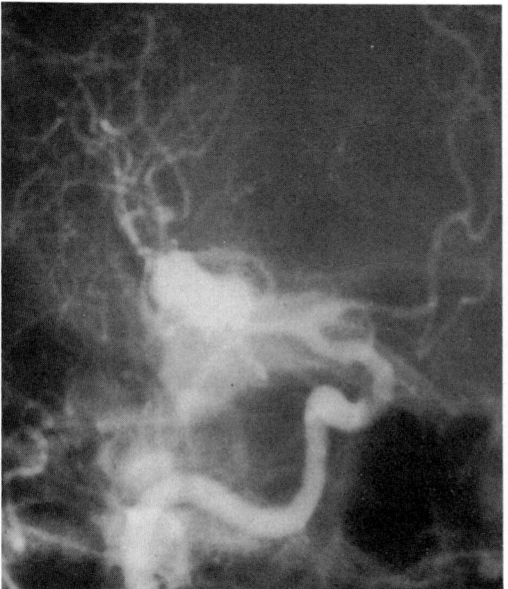

A

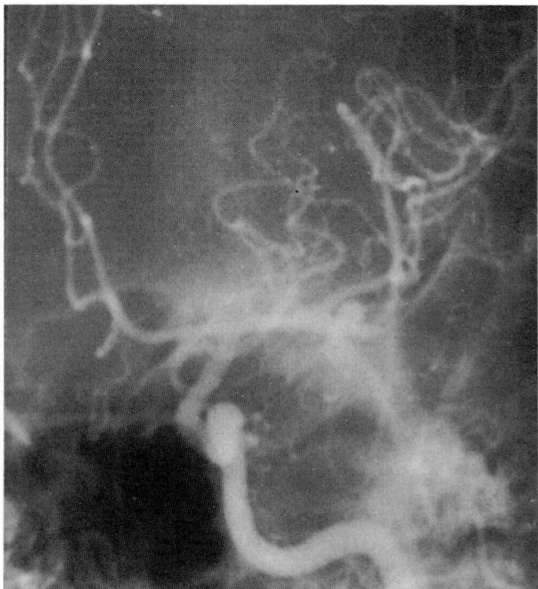

B

Fig. 62.3A and B Bilateral middle cerebral aneurysms.

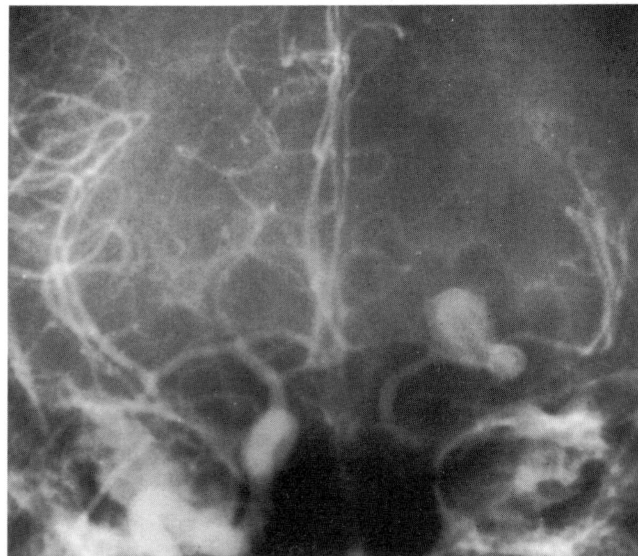

Fig. 62.4 Cross compression study of large biloculated left carotid bifurcation aneurysm. There is good cross-flow from right to left with filling of the aneurysm.

made by compressing one carotid artery whilst the other is injected with contrast. With a freely patent anterior communicating artery there will usually be good filling of the anterior and middle cerebral arteries on both sides (Fig. 62.4).

Aneurysms giving rise to subarachnoid haemorrhage may occur anywhere in the cerebral circulation but they are most frequent around the circle of Willis and in one or two other sites. Thus in one large series supratentorial aneurysms occurred most frequently at:

1. The origin of the posterior communicating artery (27 per cent).
2. The junction of anterior communicating and anterior cerebral artery (27 per cent).
3. The bifurcation or trifurcation of the main middle cerebral trunk (20 per cent).
4. The terminal segment of the internal carotid artery (6 per cent).

Aneurysms of the peripheral vessels are relatively uncommon, although occasionally encountered.

In the posterior fossa aneurysms causing subarachnoid haemorrhage and shown by vertebral arteriography have been found mainly:

1. At the basilar termination.
2. At the junction of posterior communicating and posterior cerebral arteries.
3. At the origin of the posterior inferior cerebellar artery from the vertebral artery (Fig. 62.5).

They have also been shown at the origin of other smaller vessels from the basilar artery and very rarely on more peripheral vessels.

Aneurysms, with the exception of the large atheromatous aneurysms, to be described later, usually arise at

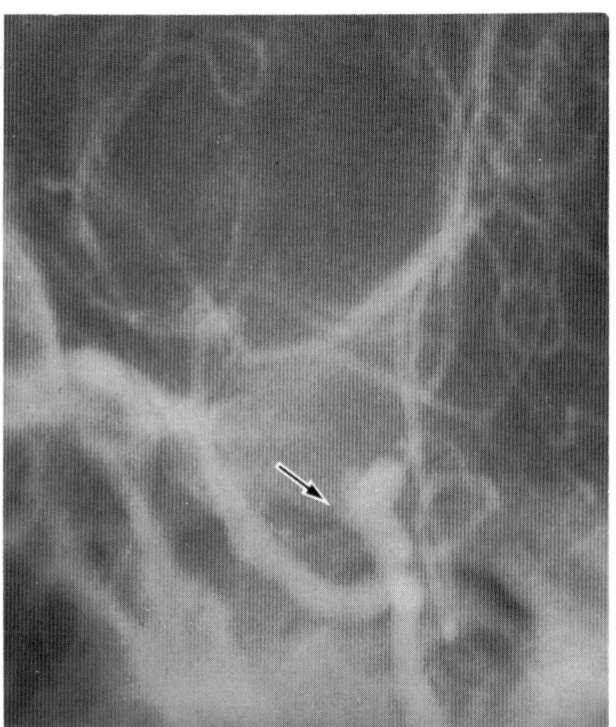

Fig. 62.5 Aneurysm of the origin of the posterior inferior cerebellar artery (↘). It is biloculated and was only demonstrated after both carotids and the other vertebral had previously been injected with negative results. Oblique projection.

points of bifurcation of cerebral arteries. There is evidence of a defect in the muscle coat at this point and this has given rise to the *congenital* theory of origin of these lesions. However, there is no doubt that other factors such as *age*, *atheroma* and *hypertension* are most important in their aetiology.

The vast majority of cases present in middle-aged or elderly patients and there is a higher incidence amongst hypertensives.

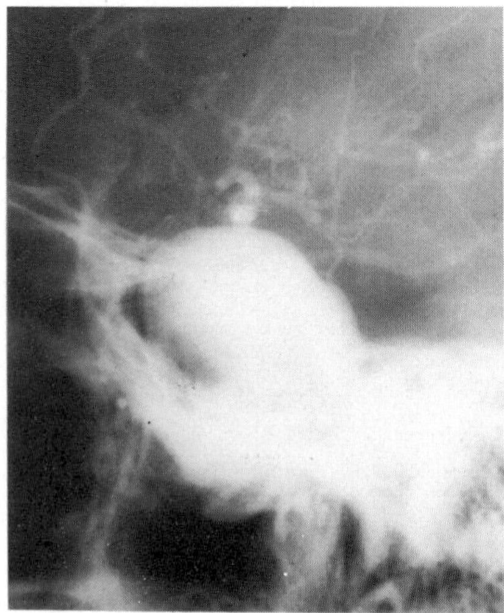

Fig. 62.6 Large parasellar aneurysm arising from the internal carotid artery in the cavernous sinus and producing oculomotor palsies.

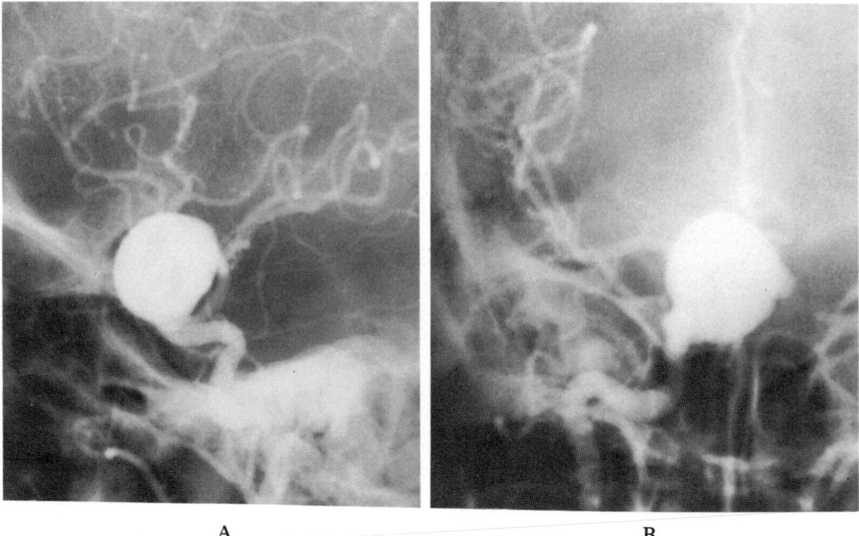

Fig. 62.7 Large aneurysm which presented as a suprasellar mass. (A) Lateral view. (B) A.P. view.

We have noted above that some cases of aneurysm may present by **pressure upon cranial nerves** leading to the orbit. The commonest nerve to be involved is the 3rd nerve, but the 4th, 5th and 6th nerves can also be affected. These lesions are usually produced by aneurysms lying in the cavernous sinus or affecting the posterior communicating artery (Fig. 62.6). Occasionally a suprasellar aneurysm may involve the optic chiasm or an optic nerve (Fig. 62.7).

Large supratentorial aneurysms presenting as **tumours** are relatively rare. The true diagnosis may not be suspected before C.T. or angiography unless marginal calcification is present. The author has seen several cases where large calcified ring shadows were shown on plain X-ray of the skull of patients with suspected tumours. Such a calcified ring or arc shadow should always raise suspicion of aneurysm even when it is much larger than one would normally expect an aneurysm to be (Fig. 58.24).

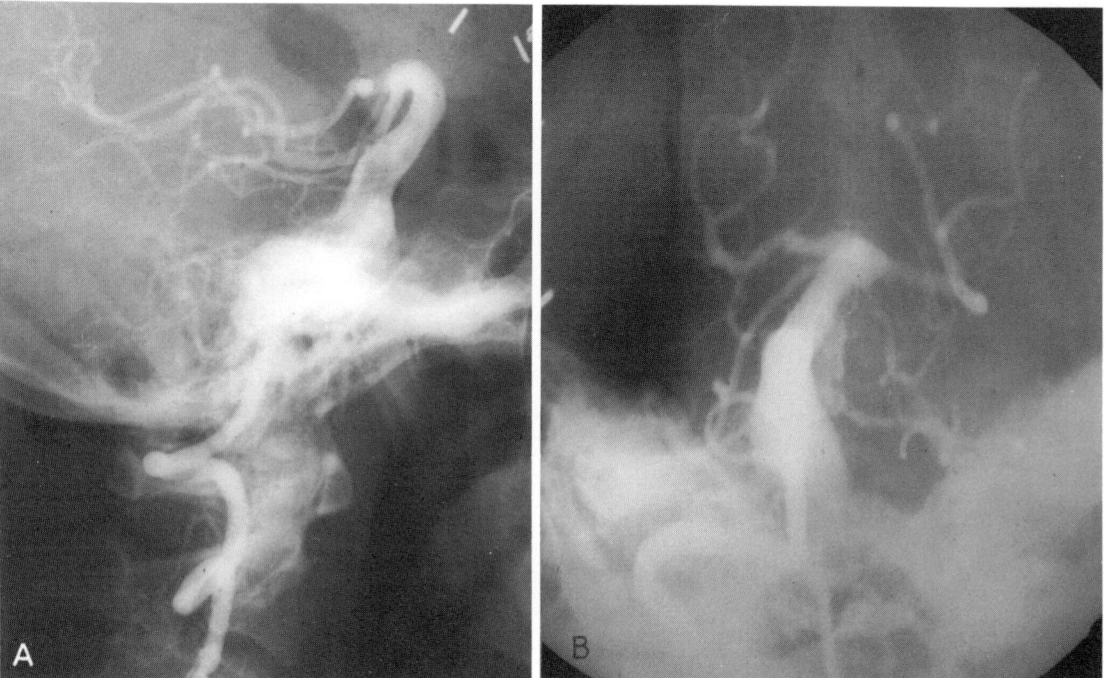

Fig. 62.8 Large basilar aneurysm presenting as a suspected pontine tumour. (A) Lateral view. (B) A.P. view.

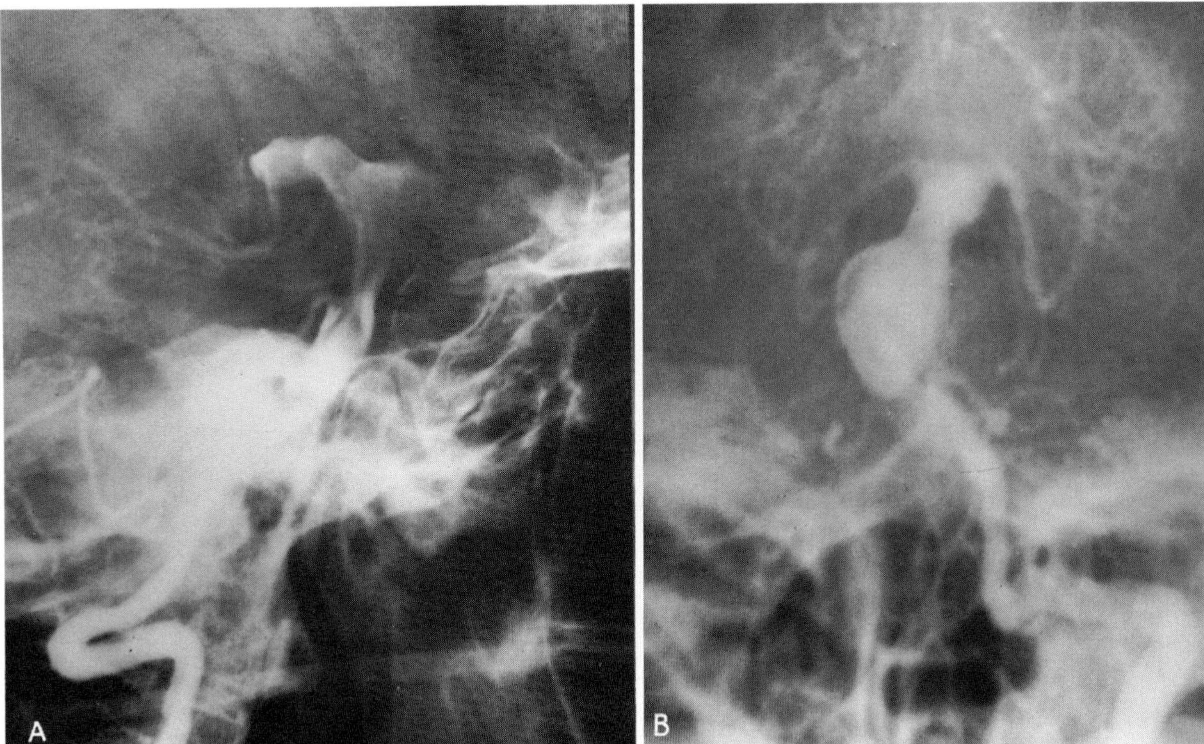

Fig. 62.9 Large basilar aneurysm with suprasellar extension. Unusual clinical presentation as chiasmal compression. (A) Lateral view. (B) A.P. view.

Clinically the patient illustrated was thought to have a frontal tumour. Angiography proved the presence of an aneurysm.

Large atheromatous aneurysms of the basilar artery are also rare, but when they do occur they may also simulate tumours. Vertebral angiography will demonstrate an aneurysm as a surprise finding in such cases unless a prior C.T. scan has suggested its presence (Figs. 62.8 and 62.9).

Occasionally large aneurysms of the internal carotid artery may bulge forwards into the orbit. Such aneurysms will erode the sphenoidal fissure and may even produce proptosis. In these cases differential diagnosis at simple X-ray is from a *secondary deposit* or the rare erosive type of *meningioma*. However, the erosion produced by an aneurysm is fairly characteristic, and usually involves the lateral margin of the optic foramen.

Aneurysm of the vein of Galen is a lesion usually seen in children. In most of these cases it is thought that the aneurysmal dilatation of the vein has been associated with an angiomatous malformation and an arteriovenous shunt. Occasionally such an aneurysm shows calcification in its wall.

2. ANGIOMATOUS MALFORMATION

(syn. angioma or congenital arteriovenous fistula)

These lesions are of congenital origin and are to be differentiated from the simple arteriovenous fistula which is usually due to trauma.

Although they are generally accepted as being of congenital origin the majority of cases present in early adult life. It is probable that they increase in size with age and that this increase proceeds more rapidly once adult blood pressure has been established. The communication between the arteries and veins lies over the surface of the brain, but if large in size they extend down into the brain substances in the manner of an inverted cone. In the silent areas of the brain they may be completely symptomless. Should they lie, however, in such sensitive areas as the motor cortex or the occipital cortex, they will produce appropriate symptoms and physical signs. In the former case Jacksonian epilepsy is likely to result; in the latter case cortical field defects may be demonstrated. Apart from the physical signs, these lesions may give rise to headaches, usually of a migrainous character. A small but significant proportion of cases present by rupture of the angioma and subarachnoid haemorrhage.

Simple X-ray of the skull in these cases has been discussed above (see p. 1099). Occasionally it may show the diagnostic appearances described, consisting of flecks of calcification with one or more characteristic ring shadows.

If an angioma is suspected clinically a dynamic radioisotope study or 'isotope angiogram' is a useful preliminary study (see Fig. 56.14). This is performed by taking rapid serial films on a gamma camera at one second

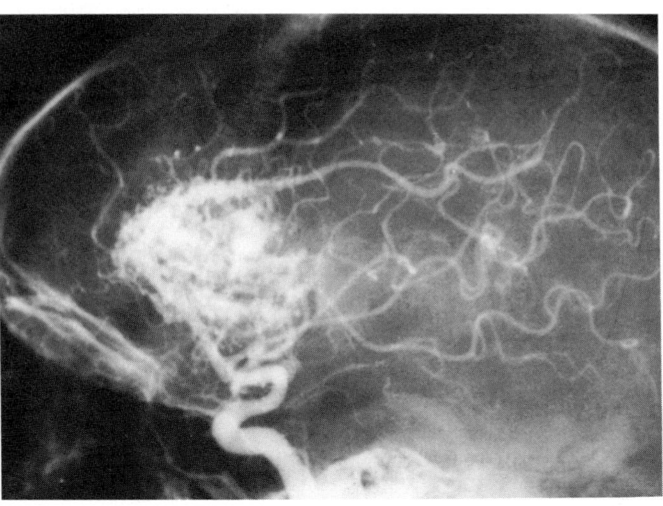

A

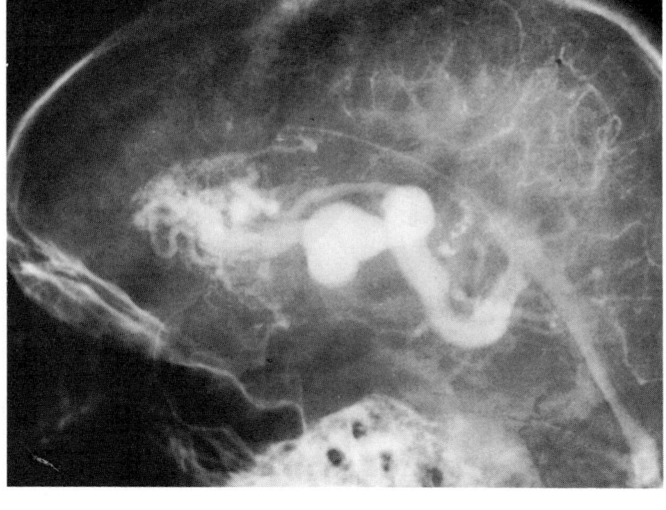

B

Fig. 62.10A Large angiomatous malformation in the region of the anterior end of the corpus collosum. B. Drainage is mainly by a hypertrophied internal cerebral vein to the vein of Galen and straight sinus.

intervals immediately after intravenous injection of a small dose of $^{99}Tc^{m}$. However, arteriography will still be required for accurate delineation of the lesion for neurosurgical purposes.

C.T. scanning will show the presence of a cerebral lesion and will suggest its angiomatous nature in a fair proportion of cases (see Ch. 64). Angiomatous malformations were once considered to be very rare but with the increasing use of angiography it has been shown that they are very common. They vary in size from small lesions difficult to demonstrate at angiography to large and spectacular vascular masses (see Figs 62.10 and 62.11).

It is a characteristic angiographic feature of angiomas that the drainage veins fill in the normal arterial phase. This is because the blood is passing direct from arteries to veins with no intervening capillary circulation. Depending on the size of the arteriovenous shunt, there will be compensatory hypertrophy of the afferent vessels supplying it, and also increase in size of the drainage veins. With large angiomas blood appears to be diverted away from the remaining normal cerebral vessels. Indeed, the lesion has been likened to a 'sponge' or parasite in this respect. This diversion of blood may possibly give rise to cerebral ischaemia and account for some of the symptoms.

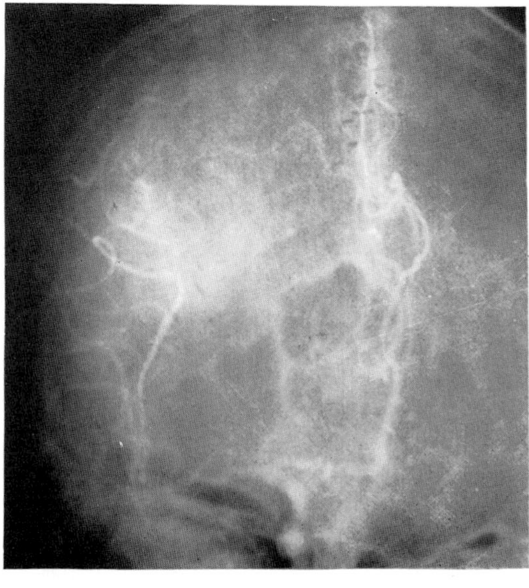

A

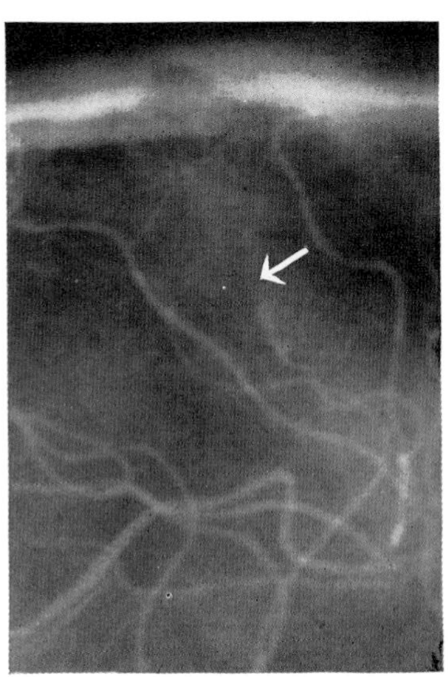

B

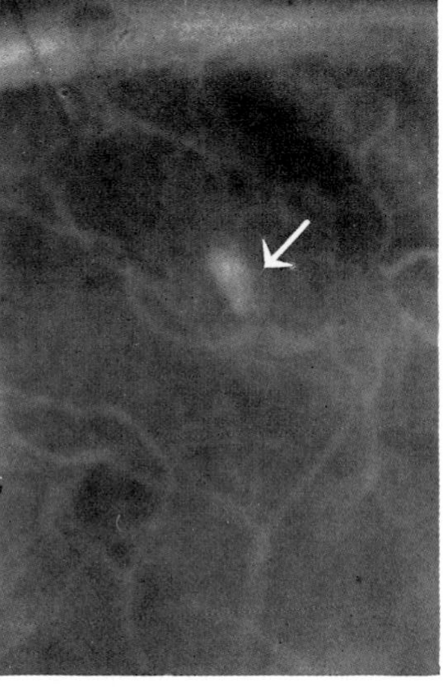

C

Fig. 62.11 Small angioma following haemorrhage and clotting. (A) Anterior view shows displacement of anterior cerebral artery by haematoma. (B and C) Lateral views. The evidence of the lesion is delayed filling of a partially clotted drainage vein (arrows).

In cases where an angioma has ruptured an intracerebral haematoma may result with displacement of vessels as by any other intracranial mass. Such intracranial haematomas are well shown by C.T.

With small angiomas which have ruptured there may be clotting of the angioma and it may be difficult or impossible to demonstrate the lesion at angiography. However, the clinical history of a subarachnoid haemorrhage with radiological evidence of an intracerebral haematoma at a peripheral site may cause suspicion. Sometimes some evidence of a lesion may remain—for example, delayed filling in a peripherally clotted vein (see Fig. 62.11).

Surgical treatment of angiomas requires full demonstration of all feeding arteries and drainage veins. In some cases this will require bilateral carotid angiography; in others vertebral angiography may also be required even though the lesion is supratentorial. Some angiomas are fed by meningeal vessels as well as by branches of the internal carotid so that the external carotid artery should be shown as well as the internal carotid. In one large series 80 per cent of supratentorial angiomas were supplied purely by pial vessels, 15 per cent by both pial and dural vessels, and 5 per cent were purely dural in blood supply (see Dural A.V. malformations, p. 1207). Infratentorial angiomas are not uncommon and constituted 20 per cent of the cases in the series just quoted; among these infratentorial angiomas dural lesions were relatively more frequent (33 per cent).

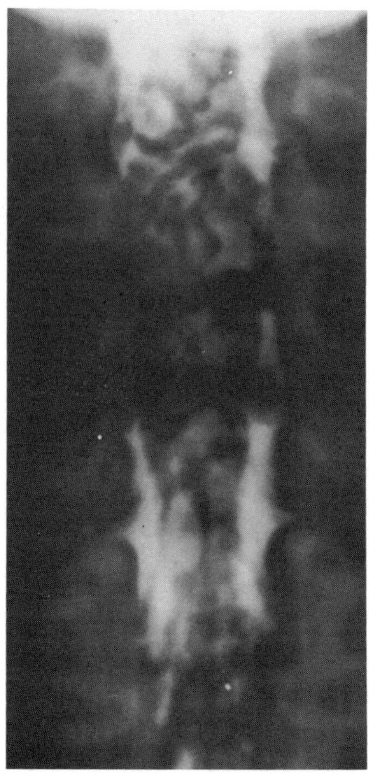

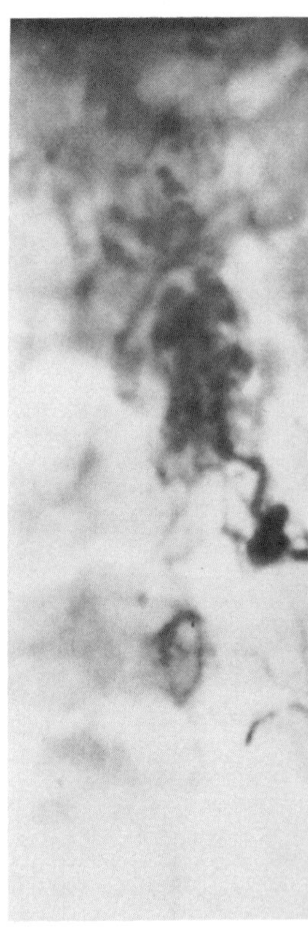

A B

Fig. 62.12 (A) Myelogram showing angiomatous vessels in the cervical region. (B) Angioma outlined by selective injection of the left costocervical trunk. It was not supplied by the vertebral arteries (subtraction print).

Spinal angiomas

With the increasing use of spinal angiography spinal angiomas are being demonstrated in increasing numbers and treated by surgery. The technique of selective spinal angiography has been described in Chapter 61. When the lesion is supplied by only one or two feeding vessels ligation of the arterial supply is usually performed, though embolization is advocated by some, and others practise complete ablation if feasible.

DiChiro describes three different types of spinal angioma.

Type 1 is characterized by one or two tightly coiled continuous vessels spread along a large longitudinal section of the cord. The fistulas are direct, and the recognition of the change from arterial to venous character is difficult, even by histological analysis of the specimen. Flow through this type of fistula is generally sluggish.

Type 2 presents as a localized plexus or congeries of vessels into which single or multiple arterial feeders converge and from which one or several venous drainers depart (Fig. 62.12). Circulation through the area of confluence of vessels, referred to as the glomus, nidus or core of the lesion, is generally fast, with slowing down in the discharging venous channels. The draining veins can be quite long and extend all the way to the endocranium or down to the pelvic vessels.

The third pattern (Type 3, or juvenile) is seen more frequently in children and some of its haemodynamic features are reminiscent of cerebral A.V. aneurysms. Multiple large feeding arteries supply voluminous malformations that often appear to fill the spinal canal. Flow through these lesions is rapid; markedly-dilated densely-opacified veins and early contrast filling of the azygos and caval systems are observed.

The important information to be derived from selective spinal angiography in angiomas is the number and localization of the feeding arteries, the extent of the angioma and its localization in front or behind the cord. The presence or absence of an associated aneurysm is also important since these are frequently associated with spinal subarachnoid haemorrhage. Such aneurysms are usually located on the main feeding vessel.

In about 15 per cent of cases a cutaneous angioma is present and can be helpful in localizing the cord lesion.

Spinal angiography is of little help in the diagnosis of spinal tumours except in the rare spinal haemangioblastoma where a characteristic appearance similar to that seen in the posterior fossa will be shown.

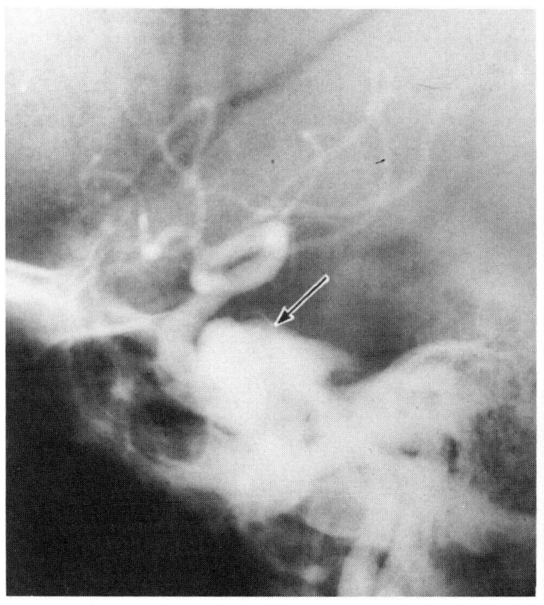

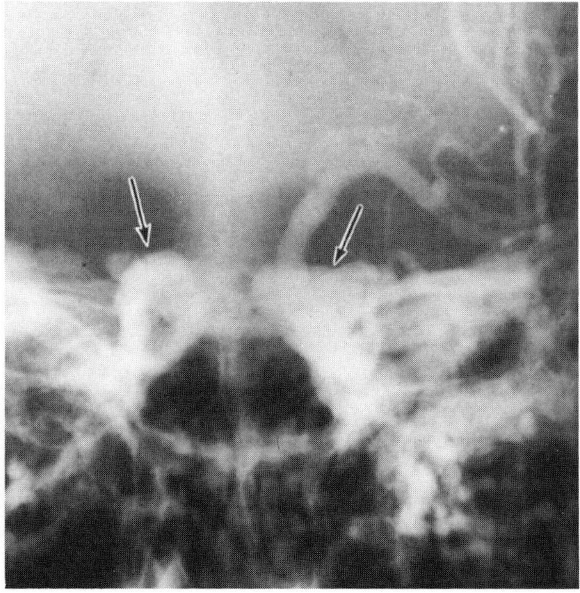

Fig. 62.13 A.V. fistula in the cavernous sinus (carotico-cavernous fistula). (A) Lateral view showing contrast entering cavernous and superior petrosal sinus (↙). (B) A.P. view showing contrast entering left cavernous sinus (↙ on right) and crossing over to fill the right cavernous sinus (↘ on left). The right carotid syphon appears as a defect in the opacified sinus

3. ARTERIOVENOUS FISTULA

This may be due to trauma causing a direct communication between an artery and a vein. It may also be due to rupture of the wall of an aneurysm or diseased artery into an adjacent or adherent vein.

Intracranial arteriovenous fistula is rare and is most frequently seen in the cavernous sinus. Most of the cavernous sinus cases encountered are due to trauma, but a significant proportion, particularly in female patients, are due to the second of the mechanisms mentioned, i.e. spontaneous rupture of a diseased arterial wall.

The condition may be very difficult to demonstrate by angiography. If there is a large shunt through the fistula it will best be shown by using larger doses of contrast and higher concentrations than usual. Figure 62.14 illustrates a case of spontaneous A.V. fistula. In this case there is a cross flow of contrast to the cavernous sinus on the opposite side. The contralateral internal carotid artery appears as a filling defect in the opacified sinus.

With cavernous sinus fistula several different venous outflow pathways may occur. These include:

1. The superior ophthalmic vein→the facial veins; or the inferior ophthalmic vein→pterygoid plexus→the facial veins.
2. The superior petrosal sinus→the sigmoid sinus.
3. The basal vein→the straight sinus.
4. The convexity veins→various sinuses.

As already noted, the venous outflow may pass to the contralateral as well as the ipsilateral veins.

Subtraction films are essential in elucidating the complex venous anatomy.

Vertebral A.V. fistula has been encountered in the past mainly as a complication of vertebral angiography by needle puncture. It has also been encountered following closed trauma. So called 'congenital' cases have also been described, though birth trauma cannot be excluded in these cases.

In recent years successful treatment of both carotico-cavernous and vertebral fistulae has been effected by detachable balloon catheters (Debrun *et al.*, 1979).

DURAL A.V. MALFORMATION

(*Syn. Dural A.V. fistula*)

It has been shown in recent years that many apparent spontaneous carotid cavernous fistulas are dural shunts between meningeal branches of the internal or external carotid artery and dural veins near the cavernous sinus. Differentiation of these dural shunts from direct internal carotid cavernous sinus fistula is important both for prognosis and treatment. Clinically the signs of an arteriovenous fistula are less marked with a dural shunt, but they include proptosis, chemosis, and elevated intraocular pressure. The shunt is one of low pressure and low flow and needs first class subtraction films for its demonstration. Selective angiography of both internal and external carotid artery will be required since the lesion may be fed by meningeal branches of the internal or external carotid artery, and can have multiple feeders. From the external carotid artery either the middle meningeal or the distal internal maxillary arteries may supply the fistula. From the internal carotid the meningohypophyseal trunk may be the source of supply (Fig.

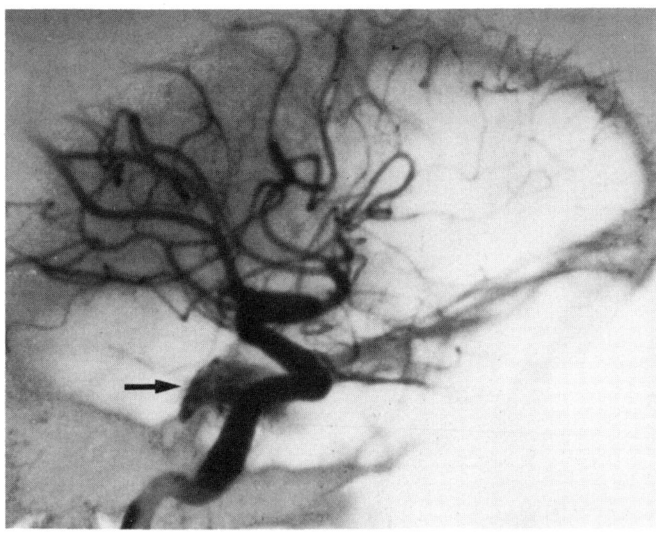

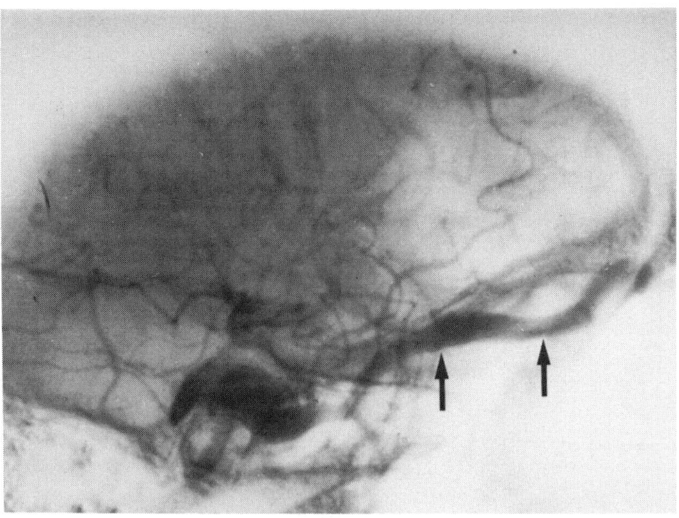

Fig. 62.14A and B Dural A.V. fistula supplied by meningio-hypophyseal trunk (arrow). The drainage is into the superior ophthalmic vein (arrows). Subtraction prints.

62.14). This small vessel arises from the internal carotid just before it enters the cavernous sinus. Bilateral injections will be necessary since once a fistula is established it can be fed from both meningohypophyseals.

Similar dural arteriovenous malformations can occur at other sites, but they are commonest at the base of the skull and in the occipitomastoid area. Figure 62.15 shows diagrammatically the meningeal vessels from which these lesions can arise.

In a review of 28 cases Houser *et al.* reported that 14 were basal mostly in the middle fossa and involving the cavernous sinus. Eleven were occipitomastoid, one was on the convexity, and one at the free edge of the tentorium. Lesions that are entirely fed by branches of the external carotid are eminently suitable for treatment by embolization (Fig. 62.16). This is a particularly valuable treatment of these lesions since direct surgery is difficult and carries a high complication and recurrence rate.

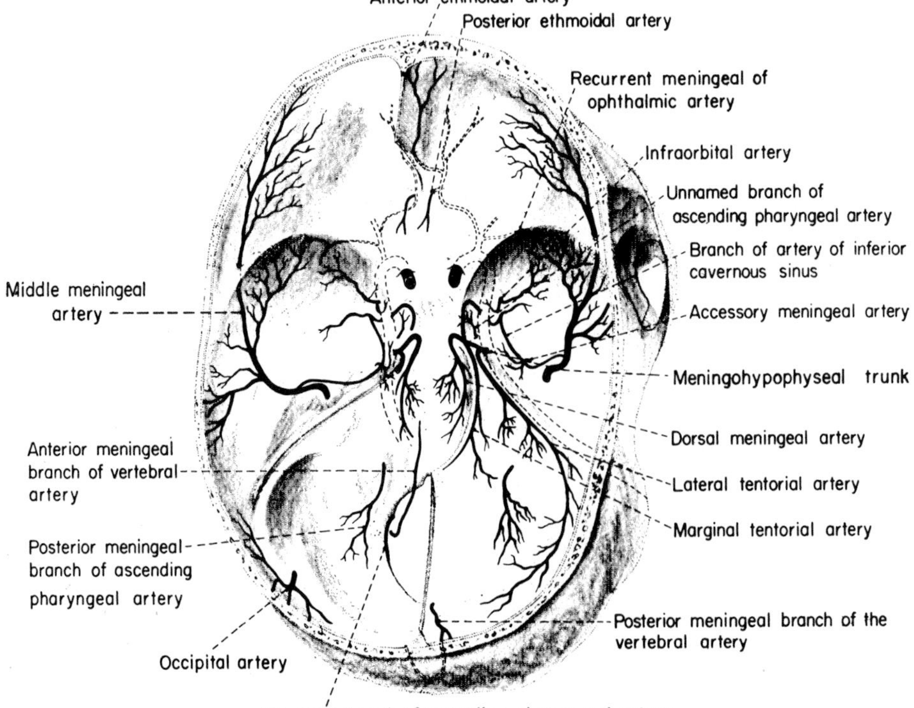

Fig. 62.15 Meningeal arterial supply to the cranial base. (From Houser, O. W. *et al.*, 1972, *Radiology*, **105**, 55.)

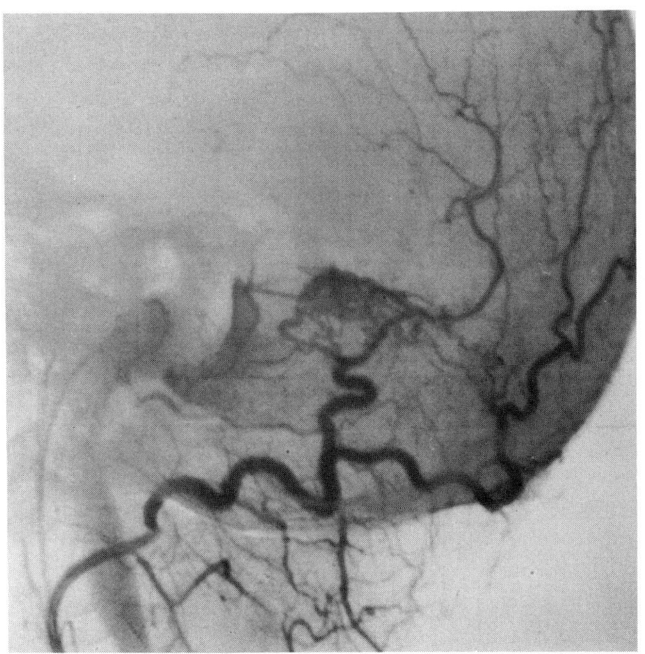

Fig. 62.16 Dural A.V. fistula supplied by the occipital artery and draining into the lateral sinus and internal jugular vein. Superselective occipital artery injection (subtraction print). This case was successfully treated by percutaneous embolization.

4. INTRACRANIAL HAEMATOMA

(*a*) **Extradural haematoma.** These usually result from severe head injury and are commonly associated with skull fractures. In most cases the diagnosis is suspected on clinical grounds. The diagnosis may be supported by the demonstration of a fracture at plain X-ray of the skull, particularly if the fracture involves the middle meningeal vascular marking.

An extradural haematoma can be demonstrated by arteriography as displacing the normal intracranial vessels away from the skull vault. Displacement of the sagittal sinus downwards has also been shown by angiography in cases of extradural haematomas. In most centres, however, the diagnosis was made on clinical grounds, possibly aided by the demonstration of a shift of the midline structures using the simple technique of echo sounding.

The development of C.T. scanning has resulted in a non-invasive method of assessing severe head injuries with suspected extradural haematomas. This has the added advantage of demonstrating the extent of direct cerebral trauma as well as the haematoma (see Ch. 64), and is now the primary investigation of choice.

(*b*) **Subdural haematoma.** Post-traumatic subdural haematoma may be very difficult to diagnose clinically and most neuroradiologists have seen cases where the diagnosis was not suspected clinically. In some cases the original trauma is so slight that the patient has difficulty in remembering the incident.

These lesions also occur relatively frequently in patients unable to give an adequate history. The possibility should therefore be borne in mind in the case of chronic alcoholics or in psychotic patients, two groups who are more liable to head injuries than the normal population. Subdural haematomas are also more liable to occur in patients in whom hydrocephalus has been relieved by ventricular shunting operations.

Angiography is no longer the method of choice for demonstrating subdural haematomas. C.A.T. will show an acute subdural haematoma as a high density peripheral lesion and a chronic subdural as a low density lesion (see Ch. 64). However, the diagnosis by C.T. can be difficult if, as sometimes happens, the lesion is isodense. Small isodense bilateral lesions can be missed completely at C.T. since there is no ventricular shift. Angiography may still be required in such cases, or where the C.T. scan is equivocal even after contrast enhancement.

The typical subdural haematoma in an adult patient occurs in the parietal region and displaces the cerebral structures away from the skull vault in a characteristic manner at angiography. This is best seen in the antero-posterior film (see Fig. 62.17). In an acute case the inner margin of the haematoma remains roughly parallel to the skull vault, but in the chronic case it bulges medially so that the haematoma appears biconvex.

It is important to realize that subdural haematomas may be frontal or occipital in situation and can then be missed in the direct anteroposterior view. If this is suspected, it is vital to obtain films tangential to the haematoma by appropriate rotation of the head. The same is true of subtemporal haematomas.

Some 10 to 20 per cent of subdural haematomas are bilateral. The possibility of a haematoma on the contralateral side should always be suspected if the anterior cerebral artery remains midline or is relatively little displaced in the presence of a subdural haematoma (Fig. 62.17).

In addition to the subdural haematoma of traumatic, or presumed traumatic, origin, subdural haematomas may also be seen in association with subarachnoid haemorrhage. Whatever the underlying cause these latter are usually shallower and smaller than the traumatic haematomas. They should always be carefully looked for when investigating patients with subarachnoid haemorrhage.

The treatment of subdural haematoma is by surgical evacuation of the clot. This is usually done through burr holes and in a recent case the brain expands fairly readily to occupy the area of the haematoma. In chronic cases, however, the inner membrane becomes thickened and the displaced brain does not readily come back to its normal position. Following aspiration the cavity of the haematoma becomes replaced by air. This is visible on X-ray, and serial films or C.T. scans can be taken to check on the re-expansion of the brain. In some cases craniotomy

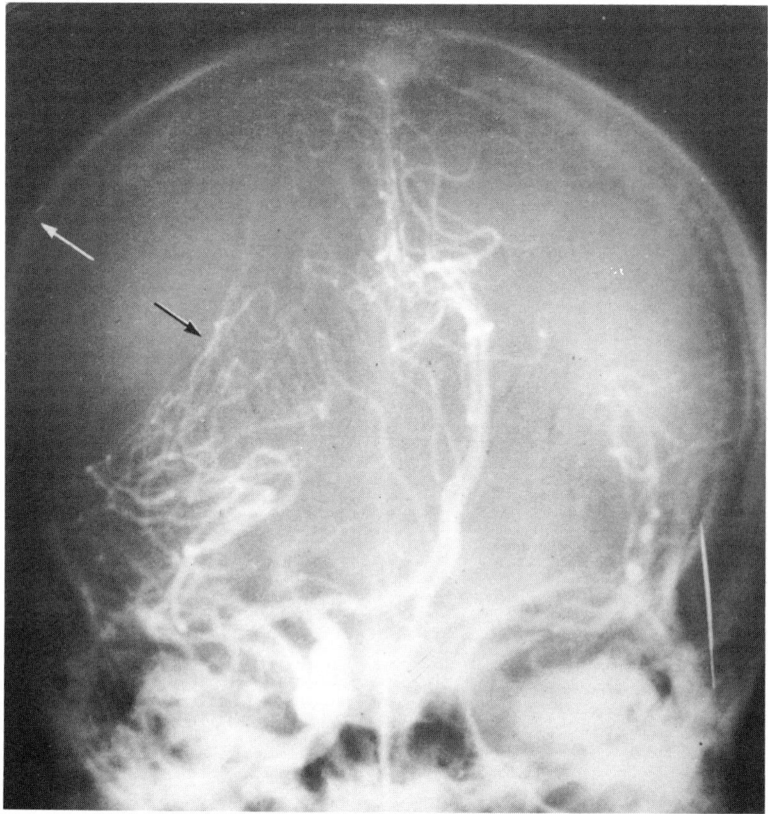
A

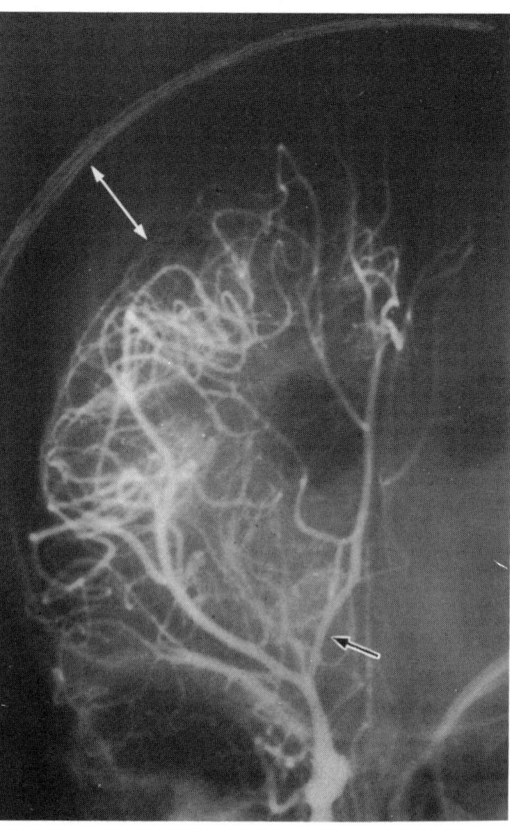
B

Fig. 62.17A Large chronic subdural haematoma seen in the A.P. projection (arrows).

Fig. 62.17B Large acute infantile subdural haematoma (↘). Despite the large haematoma the anterior cerebral is midline indicating a lesion on the other side also. The child also has a glioma of the chiasm displacing the anterior cerebral (↖).

and removal of the thickened membrane may eventually become necessary.

(*c*) **Intracerebral haematoma.** An intracerebral haematoma usually results from rupture of a diseased vessel into the brain substance.

Often no underlying cause can be demonstrated and the aetiology is thought, in most of these cases, to be atheromatous or hypertensive, or both. In other cases an aneurysm or an angioma may be demonstrated by angiography as the source of the haemorrhage.

Trauma with cerebral laceration is another cause of intracerebral haemorrhage.

C.A.T. is now the primary investigation of choice and will clearly demonstrate an intracerebral haematoma (see Ch. 64).

There are no specific angiographic features for an intracerebral haematoma, though the history of an acute vascular accident may suggest the diagnosis, and angiography may show an underlying lesion such as an aneurysm or angioma.

The angiographic diagnosis of basal ganglia or capsular haemorrhage is suggested by lateral displacement of the middle cerebral artery in the anterior projection, and by displacement of the lenticulostriate arteries medially or laterally. The anterior cerebral artery and internal cerebral vein will be displaced to the opposite side. Thalamic haematoma causes upward and medial bowing of the thalamostriate vein. A small haemorrhage deep in the hemisphere white matter may produce little angiographic evidence of its presence, though superficial extension may displace local blood vessels.

On the angiogram a large intracerebral haematoma appears as an intracerebral mass displacing normal vessels according to its situation. Thus such a haematoma will usually displace the anterior cerebral artery across the midline. If temporal in situation the middle cerebral vessels may be displaced upwards. If frontal in situation, it may show the characteristic displacement seen with any intracerebral frontal mass. A deep temporal lesion will also displace the deep veins in a characteristic manner. The displacement of cerebral vessels by intracerebral masses is discussed in detail below.

As already noted the new technique of computerized axial scanning, described in detail in Chapter 64, offers a non-traumatic method of diagnosing extradural, subdural and intracerebral haematomas, and localizes the lesions with great accuracy.

Juvenile subdural haematoma. Children with subdural haematoma react differently from adults and the haematoma is frequently localized around and under the temporal lobe rather than over the parietal region. In the case of chronic juvenile subdural haematoma local expansion of the skull may be demonstrable. This is best seen in the P.A. view, where the lateral orbital or innominate line, representing the junction of the anterior and lateral walls of the middle fossa, is seen to be displaced outwards or is no longer evident. This line is formed where the greater wing of the sphenoid turns backwards to form the lateral wall of the middle fossa. In the basal view of the skull the line formed by the greater wing of the sphenoid and representing the anterior floor of the middle fossa is also shown to be displaced forward and to bulge laterally.

Infantile subdural haematoma. Subdural haematomas in infants do not loculate as readily as those in children and adults, and the haematoma usually extends over the whole of the subdural space. Diagnosis is normally by aspiration of the subdural space from the fontanelles rather than by angiography. Following aspiration, air in the subdural space can be shown to move freely from the frontal to the occipital pole.

Both juvenile and infantile subdural haematomas are well shown by C.A.T.

5. EMBOLUS

Cerebral embolus most commonly arises from clot in a fibrillating auricle. It is therefore most frequently seen as a complication of mitral stenosis. Like embolus elsewhere, it is sometimes seen following coronary infarction and clot formation in the left ventricle. It may also result from paradoxical embolus, or from dislodgement of clot in an aortic aneurysm. Finally, it is thought that small emboli can result from clot forming on the surface of atheromatous plaques in the aorta and great vessels.

A cerebral vessel occluded by embolus is readily shown by arteriography, provided it is sufficiently large. In the writer's experience the middle cerebral artery is the commonest site for a major cerebral embolus. This is not surprising as the middle cerebral artery takes the major blood flow after bifurcation of the internal carotid artery. Embolus of smaller peripheral vessels may require careful study of rapid serial angiographic films before the lesion is recognized. A major embolus is now readily diagnosed by C.A.T. (see Ch. 64).

6. VASCULAR STENOSIS AND THROMBOSIS

Atheromatous stenosis and thrombosis of the arteries to the brain before they enter the cranium is a common cause of cerebral symptoms. Thus the internal carotid artery may be stenosed or thrombosed just distal to its origin from the common carotid artery (Figs 62.18 and 62.19). In the same way the vertebral artery may be stenosed or thrombosed by atheroma near its origin from the subclavian artery (Fig. 62.20).

It has also been claimed that the vertebral artery can be compressed in its cervical portion by pressure from

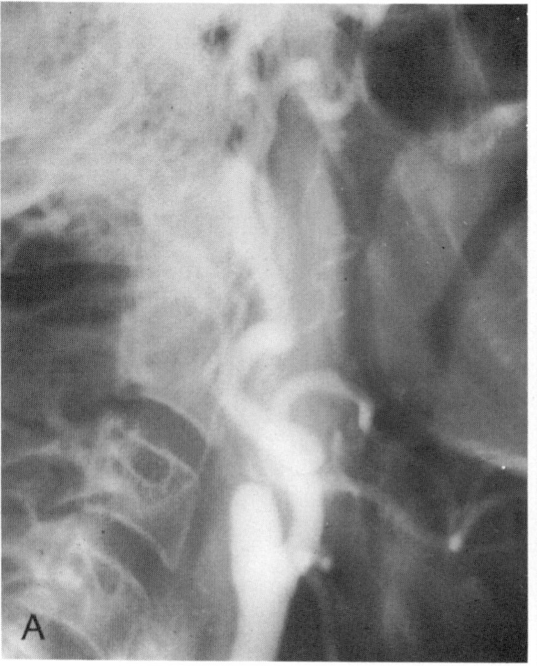

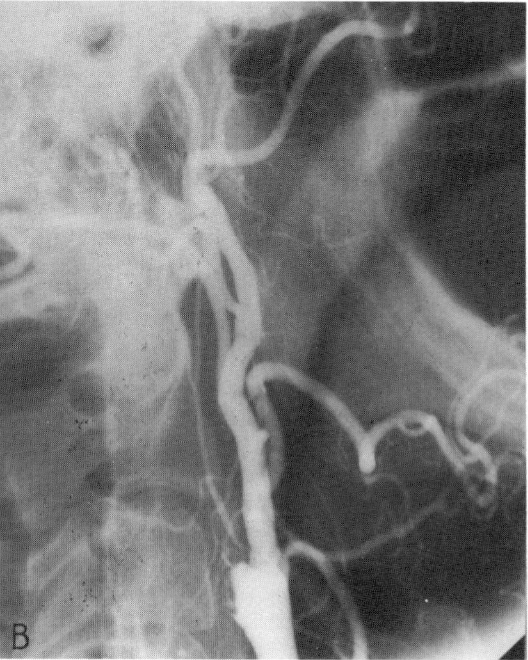

Fig. 62.18A and B Thrombosis of the internal carotid artery in the neck. Two different cases.

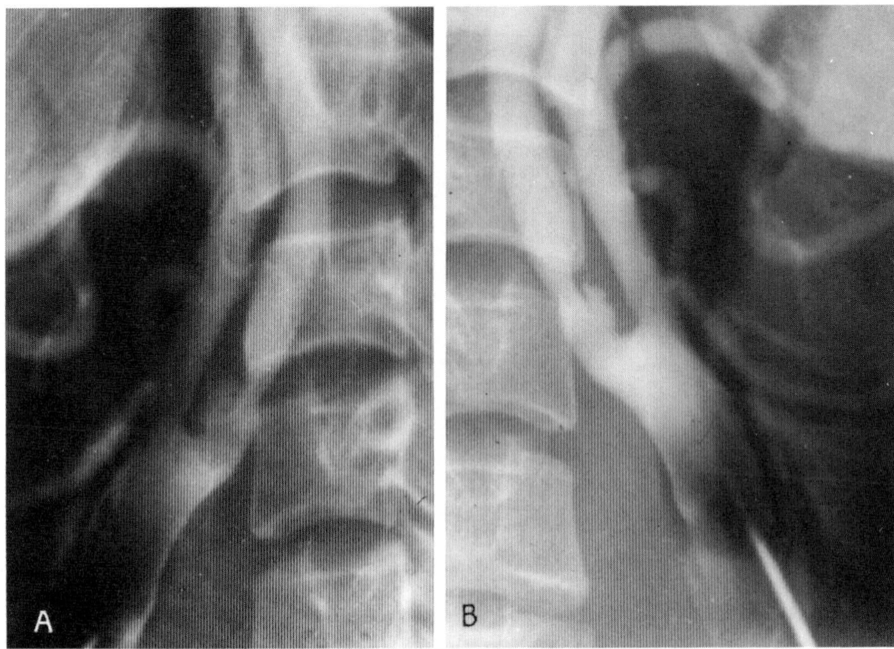

Fig. 62.19A and B Bilateral stenosis of the internal carotid arteries. Note the ulcerated plaque in B, a probable source of emboli.

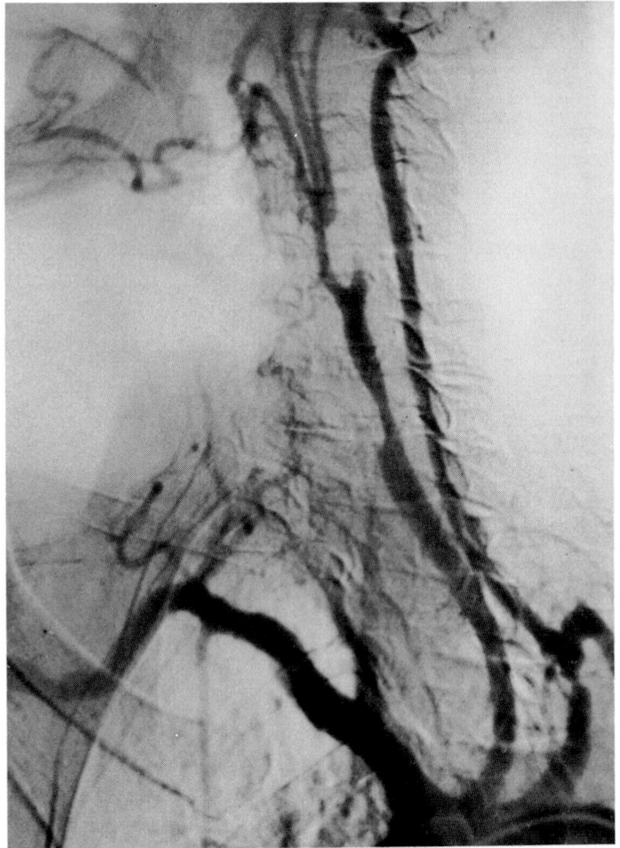

Fig. 62.20 Arch aortogram showing occlusion of right common carotid artery and left internal carotid artery and severe stenosis of the left subclavian artery. The right vertebral is also occluded. (Subtraction print.)

osteophytes, and further that rotation of the neck may compress the vertebral artery in some elderly patients.

Finally, stenosis or thrombosis of the innominate, common carotid and subclavian arteries may occur in the thorax, and affect the cerebral blood supply (Fig. 62.21). In the simple unilateral case of internal carotid *thrombosis* a collateral circulation may develop from several sources. Blood may reach the affected hemisphere through the circle of Willis, i.e. by flow across the anterior communicating artery from the opposite side, and by retrograde flow along the posterior communicating artery from the basilar to the internal carotid artery. In addition, an anastomosis usually opens up between the terminal branches of the maxillary artery and those of the ophthalmic artery. This permits blood from the external carotid artery to reach the ophthalmic artery and flow retrogradely into the cerebral circulation. Anastomoses may also develop between the muscular branches of the vertebral artery in the neck and branches of the external carotid artery such as the occipital artery (see Fig. 62.22).

Symptoms will vary greatly depending on:

1. whether there are large anterior and posterior communicating arteries,
2. whether there are associated lesions of the other internal carotid artery and of the vertebral arteries,
3. whether an adequate collateral circulation of the type described above develops, and
4. the blood pressure and general cardiovascular efficiency.

For these reasons it can be difficult to assess symptoms

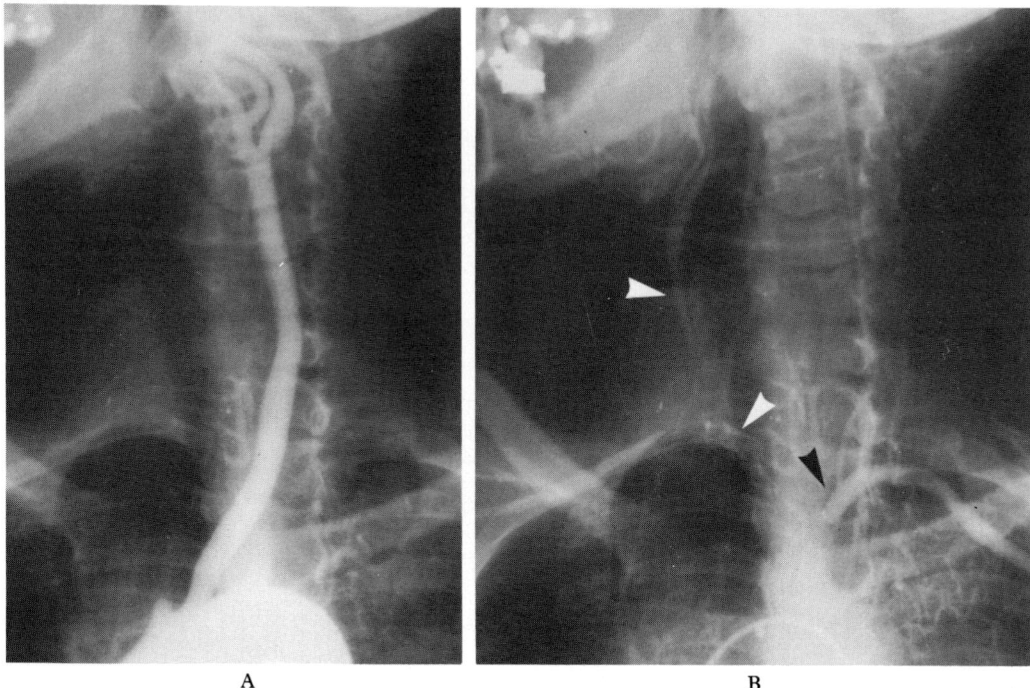

Fig. 62.21 Arch aortogram showing carotid and vertebral lesions. (A) The innominate and left subclavian arteries are occluded. The only major vessel still patent is the left common carotid. (B) Serial filmshows filling of the right carotid (top left arrow) and both vertebrals (arrowed) from collaterals with retrograde flow to the subclavians. This is an example of 'carotid steal' and bilateral 'subclavian steal' in the same patient.

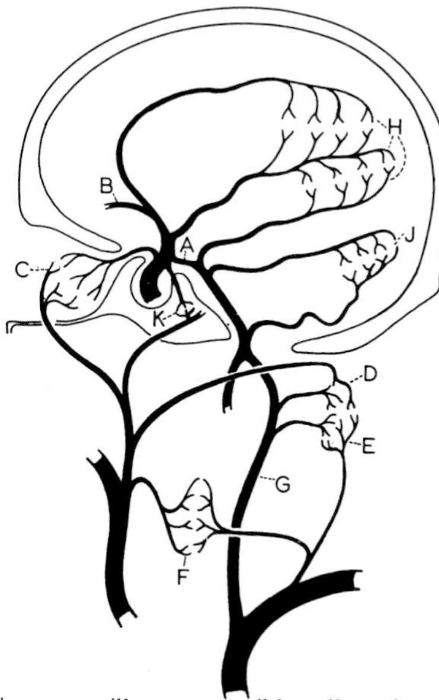

Fig. 62.22 Diagram to illustrate possible collateral pathways in cerebrovascular insufficiency. (A and B) Posterior communicating and anterior communicating arteries of the circle of Willis. (C) Communications between maxillary and ophthalmic artery. (D) Communication between muscular branches of the vertebral and the occipital artery. (E) Communication between the vertebral and ascending cervical arteries. (F) Communications between the inferior thyroid and superior thyroid arteries of the same and opposite sides. (G) The vertebral artery providing retrograde flow to the subclavian (subclavian steal). (H) Pial anastomoses between terminal branches of the anterior cerebral, middle cerebral, and posterior cerebral arteries. (J) Pial anastomoses in the posterior fossa. (K) Meningeal anastomoses and rete mirabile. (From Sutton and Davies, 1966.)

and prognosis in an individual case since so many variable factors are involved. This explains why one patient may have complete bilateral internal carotid artery occlusions and yet remain virtually symptomless, whereas another patient with a unilateral lesion develops major cerebral infarction with severe hemiplegia or even fatal complications.

In a suspected case of internal carotid artery stenosis or thrombosis it is necessary to consider the lesion not as an isolated phenomenon but in relation to the state of all the vessels to the brain. Thus it is desirable to perform at least bilateral carotid arteriograms as a routine even though only a unilateral lesion is suspected clinically. In the presence of a unilateral carotid thrombosis injection of the contralateral carotid, if it is normally patent, will usually show cross-flow through the anterior communicating artery and filling of both anterior and middle cerebral arteries from the one injection.

This phenomenon is occasionally seen as an unexpected finding at common carotid angiography. The radiologist should immediately suspect a compensated carotid thrombosis on the non-injected side.

It is now generally accepted that symptoms in cases of internal carotid *stenosis* are mainly due to small platelet emboli detached from the surface of ulcerating atheromatous plaques. These give rise to transient ischaemic attacks (T.I.As) with focal symptoms such as hemiparesis, hemiparaesthesia, or monocular amblyopia which recover fairly rapidly. If untreated, carotid thrombosis may eventually ensue. Rather surprisingly this can result in clinical improvement with spontaneous cure of the T.I.As. On the other hand thrombosis may result in the grave consequences described above. As there is no reliable method of predicting the outcome, surgery is now generally accepted as the treatment of choice and internal carotid endarterectomy, an operation pioneered at St Mary's Hospital, London (Eastcott, Pickering and Rob, 1954), is now widely practised.

Many workers feel that it is desirable to show the origins of both internal carotids and both vertebrals in all cases of suspected carotid or vertebrobasilar insufficiency.

The cervical course of the vertebral artery can be well shown either by arch aortography or by catheterization of the subclavian arteries.

Arch aortography has the advantage that it enables the intrathoracic great vessels to be studied as well as all four vessels to the brain. Atheromatous stenosis of the vertebral artery and compression by osteophytes have been mentioned above; so also has the claim that rotation of the head can produce vertebral artery compression in some patients and that this is a cause of *postural vertigo*.

Thrombosis of the common carotid artery may occur near its origin from the innominate on the right side, or from the aorta on the left side.

The vertebral circulation may be seriously affected by thrombosis of the left subclavian artery in its first part and proximal to the left vertebral origin. When this occurs, the left vertebral artery acts as a collateral to the left subclavian artery. Blood flows up the right vertebral artery and then retrogradely down the left vertebral artery to the left subclavian artery, where blood pressure has been lowered by the proximal subclavian block. This syphonage of blood from the vertebrobasilar system to the arm has been christened the '*subclavian steal*' phenomenon. It has been claimed that the diversion of blood from the brain may be considerable and result in cerebral symptoms. The lesion is well demonstrated by arch aortography (Fig. 62.23). Less commonly, syphonage of blood down the right vertebral artery may occur if there is an innominate or proximal right subclavian block.

In the same way 'carotid steal' may result from occlusion of a common carotid or innominate artery.

In addition to the vertebral artery acting as a collateral to the arm a further collateral circulation may be derived from the external carotid artery and its branches to the thyroid axis. Collaterals have also been demonstrated passing from the external carotid to the muscular branches of the vertebral and this provides a further contribution to the vertebral blood flow. Other sources of collateral supply are through the intercostals to the scapular and internal mammary arteries.

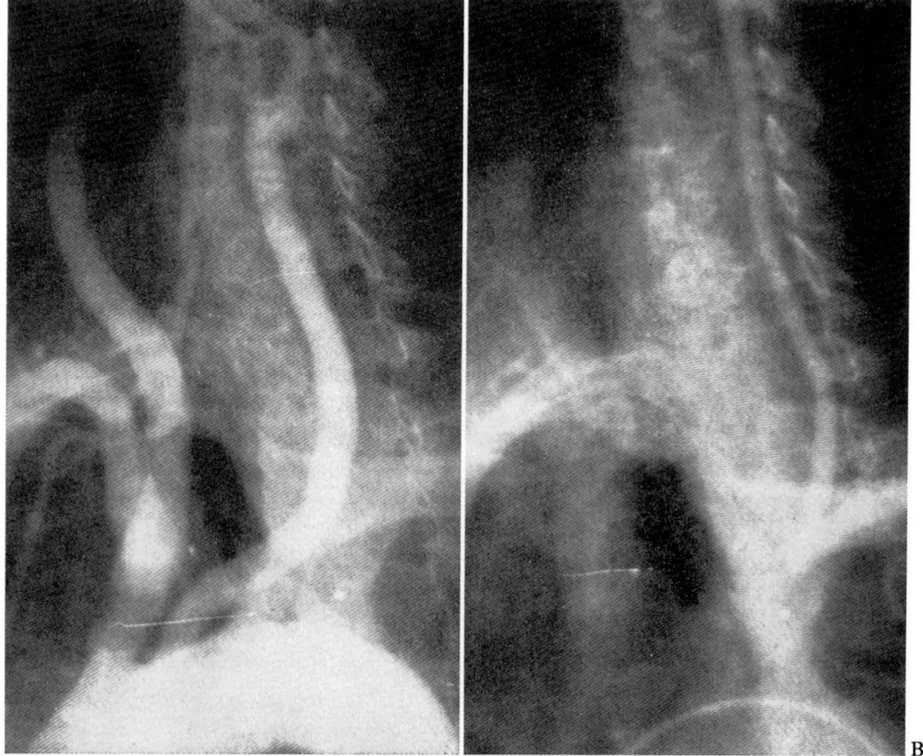

Fig. 62.23 Subclavian steal. (A) Early film shows no filling of L. subclavian and L. vertebral artery. (B) Late film shows L. vertebral filling from above and supplying L. subclavian artery.

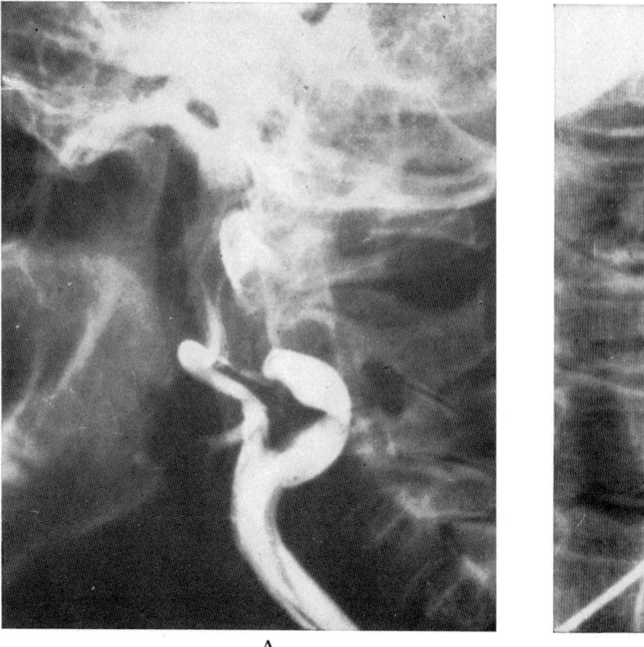

A

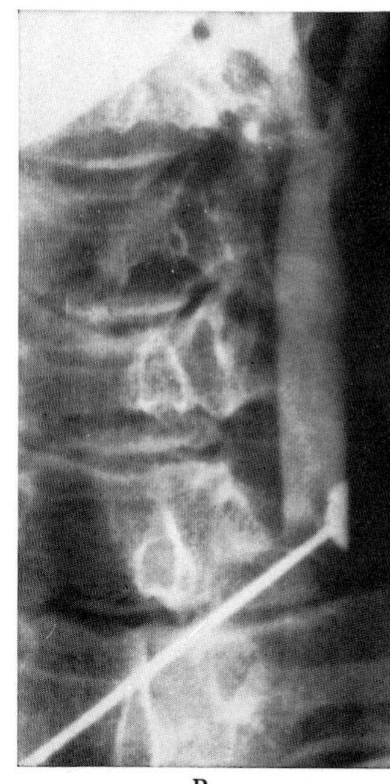

B

Fig. 62.24 Subintimal injections of contrast at carotid angiography. (A) Major degree. (B) Minor degree.

Pseudothrombosis of the internal carotid artery may result from several causes.

1. With needle injection of the common carotid artery the injection, particularly in the hands of an unskilled worker may be accidentally made into the arterial wall. If the injection is *subintimal* an appearance results superficially resembling thrombosis. This appearance is quite characteristic and should not give rise to any difficulty of interpretation (Fig. 62.24). Should this accident occur, the procedure should be abandoned and the patient carefully observed because there is a danger of initiating a true thrombosis of the artery by such iatrogenic trauma.

2. Thrombosis of the internal carotid artery has sometimes been wrongly diagnosed when the tip of the needle, cannula or catheter, has been at the bifurcation of the common carotid artery and the *main injection has entered the external carotid artery*. As a result the internal carotid artery, though patent, was not visualized (Fig. 62.25). In all cases where internal carotid thrombosis is suspected the needle point must be clearly shown on the X-ray film and it must be demonstrated to be below the point of bifurcation of the common carotid artery.

3. Another condition in which apparent thrombosis of the internal carotid artery may be seen is *grossly raised intracranial pressure in a comatose and moribund patient*. In these cases cerebral blood flow may be so reduced that even on delayed serial films the contrast passing through the internal carotid artery has still not progressed beyond the cavernous sinus (Fig. 62.26). We have seen several

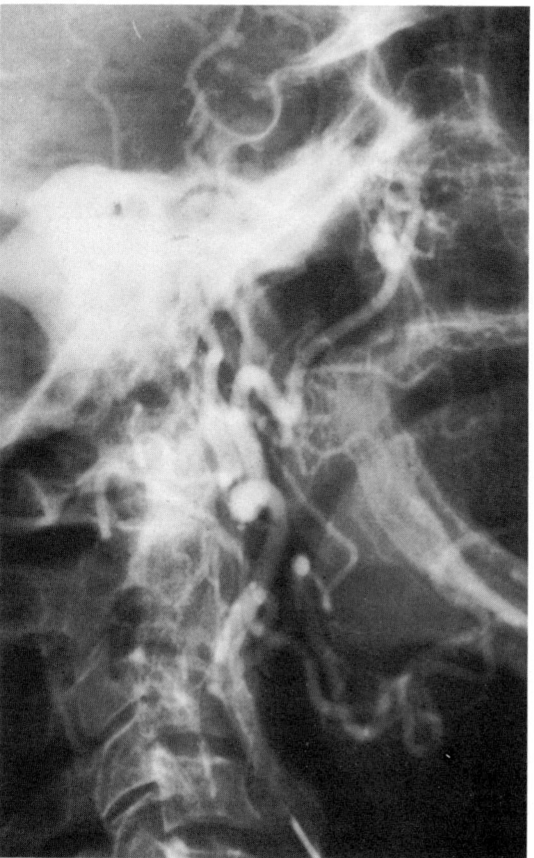

Fig. 62.25 Pseudothrombosis of the internal carotid artery due to injecting the external carotid artery.

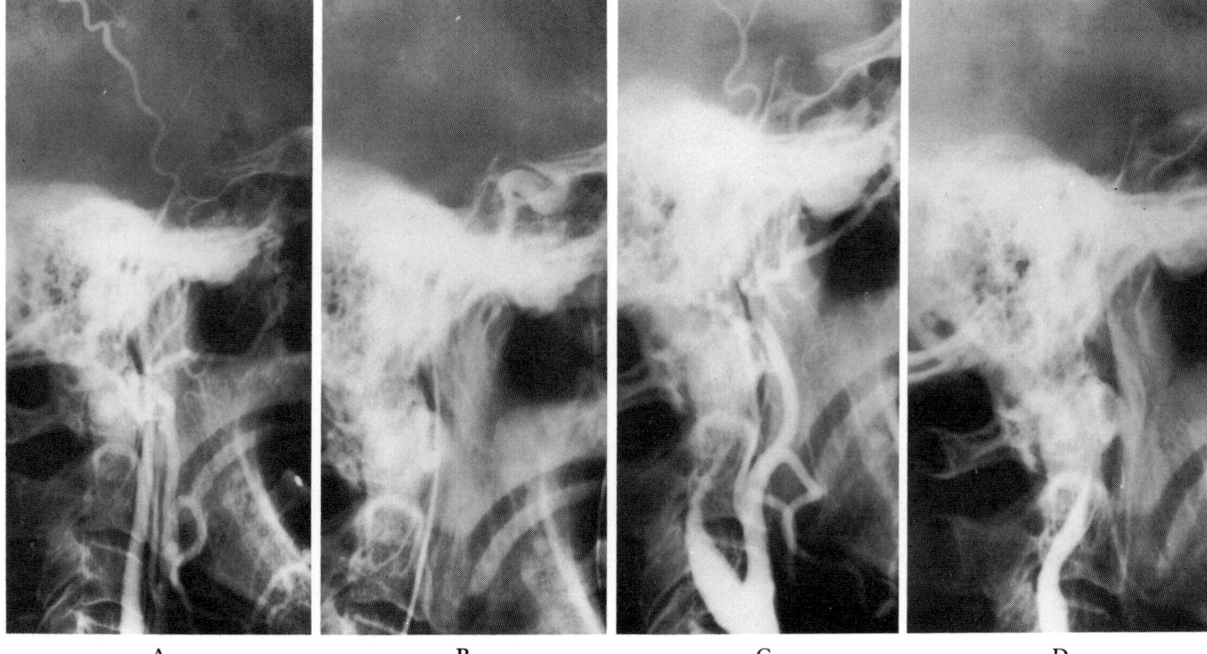

Fig. 62.26 Pseudo-thrombosis of the internal carotid artery. (A) and (B) Serial films of right side. (C) and (D) Serial films of left side.

such cases where autopsy has shown the vessels to be patent intracranially. When this phenomenon is seen it implies that cerebral perfusion is at an extremely slow rate and the prognosis is invariably bad.

An interesting feature is that the contrast as it passes slowly up the cervical carotid sinks to the posterior aspect of the vessel producing a 'layering' effect. This is better appreciated if the radiograph is viewed in the position in which it was taken.

It has been shown experimentally in animals that spontaneous respiration invariably ceases when intracranial pressure becomes equal to the diastolic blood pressure. The parallel between this observation and the clinical fact that most of the patients with pseudo-occlusion are in need of artificial respiration is clear.

Intracranial thromboses

Thromboses of intracranial vessels is less commonly diagnosed than before the days of angiography as it is now realized that many of these suspected cases were suffering from extracerebral thromboses. However, intracranial thromboses are encountered developing either from atheroma or, less commonly, from ruptured aneurysms. We have encountered atheromatous stenosis of the internal carotid artery intracranially either in or just above the cavernous sinus. Of the other major intracranial vessels, the middle cerebral artery is most frequently involved (Fig. 62.27).

Thrombosis of small peripheral vessels is easily missed and if it is suspected rapid serial films may be necessary to demonstrate the lesion clearly.

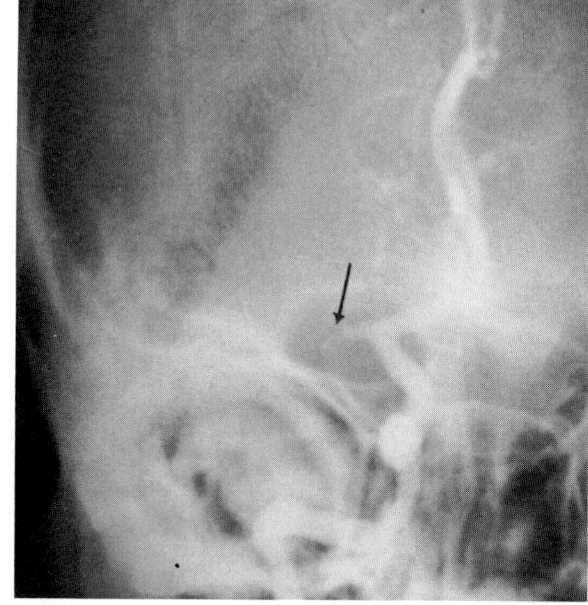

Fig. 62.27 Middle cerebral artery thrombosis (↓).

With intracerebral thrombosis a collateral circulation may be demonstrated filling the occluded vessel retrogradely (see Fig. 62.22).

Intracranial thrombosis of the internal carotid artery may also occur from atheroma in the cavernous sinus or just before the termination of the artery.

Basilar thrombosis is usually fatal but can occur with survival of the patient, and cases have been diagnosed by vertebral angiography.

A syndrome consisting of multiple progressive intracranial arterial occlusions in children originally thought to occur only in Japanese (moyamoya disease) has since been reported in American and British cases. The disease results in rapidly progressive stenoses of the major vessels of the circle of Willis leading to occlusion and multiple tiny basal collateral vessels. The process stops once occlusion occurs, so that survival is possible if collaterals are adequate. The distal arterial vessels are not involved and the aetiology is unknown.

The place of C.T. in the diagnosis of infarcts and T.I.A.s is discussed in Chapter 64.

DURAL SINUS AND CEREBRAL VEIN THROMBOSIS

Thrombosis of cerebral veins and dural sinuses is not uncommon. Clinically, the commonest cause is infection either local or distant. Meningitis or encephalitis may be complicated by venous thrombosis, often fatal and infection may spread from the paranasal sinuses or ear and mastoid. Thrombosis may also occur as a complication of pregnancy (about 1 case per 2500 births). Rarer causes include skull trauma and craniotomy, cardiac disease with right heart failure, oral contraception, dehydration and blood disorders. The symptoms and signs vary with the localization and extent of the lesion and with associated brain oedema, infarction, haemorrhage or infection. They include hemiplegia, papilloedema, and epilepsy, general or focal, and drowsiness or coma.

Superior sagittal sinus. Thrombosis of the anterior part is usually asymptomatic because of excellent pial collaterals. In any case absence of the anterior part of the sagittal sinus is a common congenital finding when the ascending frontal vein courses parallel to the midline to join the sagittal sinus more posteriorly. Thrombosis of the more posterior part of the sinus is more serious and produces symptoms of the type just described. The thrombosis may extend into the cortical veins and produce areas of infarction.

Transverse and sigmoid sinuses. Thrombosis is frequently septic arising from the middle ear or mastoid. Congenital absence of one transverse sinus may occur and should not be considered as thrombosis without supportive evidence.

Cavernous sinus. Involvement of the cavernous sinus is associated with exophthalmos, chemosis, oedema of the eyelids, and oculomotor palsies.

Radiological appearances. Oblique antero-posterior views give the best demonstration of the sagittal sinus. This can be well shown by serial angiography of the internal carotid with compression of the contralateral carotid. With thrombosis of the sagittal sinus there is usually slowing of the circulation, failure of a section of the sinus to outline, and dilated collateral venous channel bypassing the obstruction or draining to other areas. The bridging veins may be abnormal and 'corkscrew' in appearance. The lateral sinuses are best seen in the frontal projection and partial occlusions identified. Cortical venous thrombosis, apart from local absence of venous filling and presence of surrounding collaterals, may show evidence of a local mass due to infarction and oedema.

Obstruction of venous sinuses may also occur with tumours. Thus meningiomas frequently involve the sagittal and sometimes the lateral sinus, and glomus jugulare tumours may invade the internal jugular vein and sigmoid sinus.

ANGIOGRAPHY IN CEREBRAL TUMOURS

There are two common mechanisms by which angiography may demonstrate the presence of an intracranial tumour. These are:

1. the displacement of vessels from their normal position; and
2. the visualization of abnormal or pathological vessels in the tumour area due to the fact that many tumours have quite different vascular systems from that of the surrounding normal brain.

Occasionally a third feature is observed. The normal arteries supplying a tumour may be involved by the neoplasm resulting in localized narrowing of the artery by a tumour 'cuff'. This is commonest with a meningioma but can occur with other tumours.

DISPLACEMENT OF VESSELS

Small superficial lesions may manifest only by local stretching of one or more peripheral vessels. These may appear arc like and stretched instead of normally tortuous. Larger masses will produce displacement of the major vessels. The latter may also be locally displaced by smaller lesions closely related to them.

The **anterior cerebral artery** normally lies in the midline. With most tumours or other intracranial mass lesions lying superficially in a cerebral hemisphere the anterior cerebral artery will be displaced to the contralateral side. With A.P. films taken on standard skull tables a displacement of 3 to 4 mm or more can, with certain exceptions, be regarded as evidence of the presence

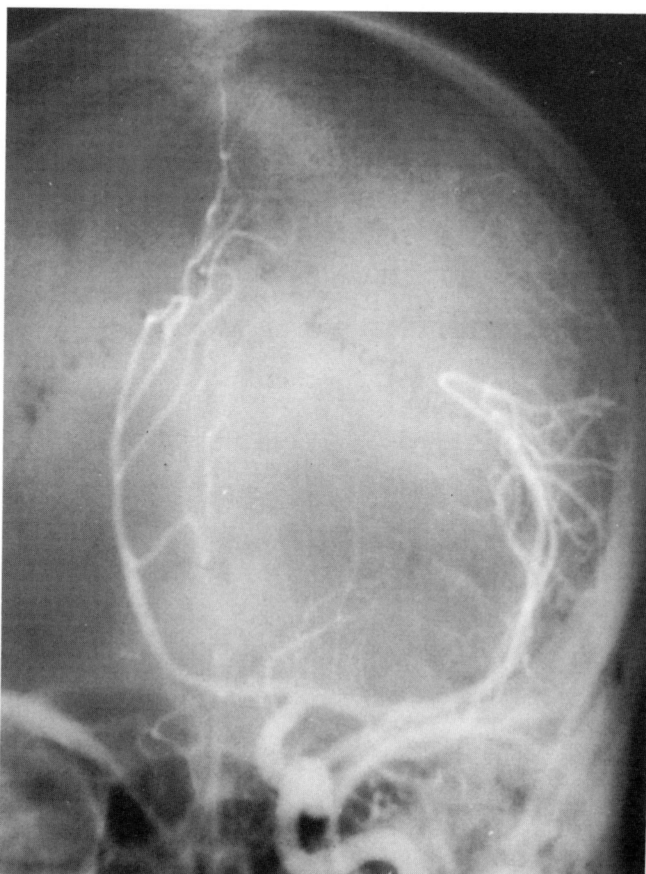

Fig. 62.28 Displacement of the anterior cerebral artery by a frontal tumour.

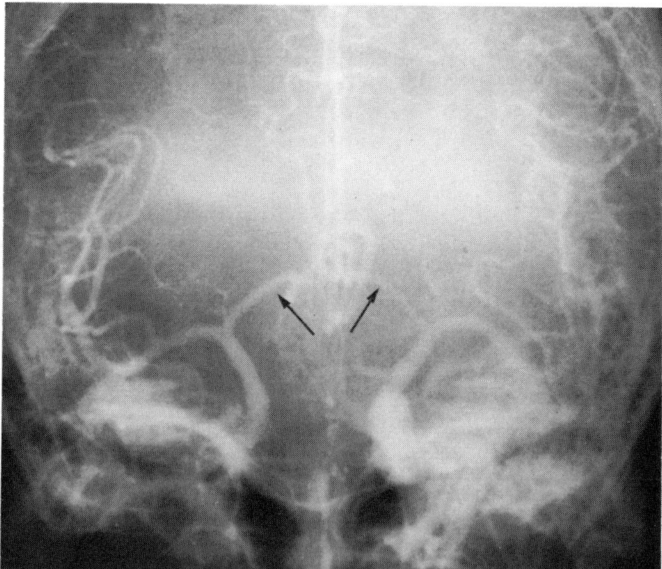

Fig. 62.29 Upward displacement of the proximal segment of the anterior cerebral artery by a suprasellar mass.

of a tumour. Marked tortuosity of the vessels, when the artery meanders from one side to the other, should of course be differentiated. This is particularly likely to occur in hypertensive patients with elongated and kinked arteries.

Lesions in different areas of the brain tend to produce different patterns of displacement. Thus a *frontal tumour* produces a rather wide separation of the anterior and middle cerebral groups of vessels in the P.A. film with a bow-like displacement of the anterior cerebral to the opposite side (Fig. 62.28). Posteriorly placed and *parietal* tumours produce relatively less displacement of the anterior cerebral artery unless they reach considerable size, and the displaced anterior cerebral artery appears vertical with a horizontal limb or 'step' as it passes back under the falx (Fig. 62.38A). High parietal tumours can produce remarkably little displacement of the anterior cerebral artery. Central tumours and deep-seated temporal masses may produce no displacement at all. In these latter cases however there is usually considerable displacement of the deep veins (see below). Superficial *temporal* masses displace mainly the lower or anterior part of the anterior cerebral artery across the midline. They also displace medially the terminal suprasellar segment of the internal carotid artery as seen in the antero-posterior projection. The latter normally tilts laterally in this view. The displacement will render it almost vertical, or even tilt it medially.

The proximal part of the anterior cerebral artery shows a characteristic displacement with suprasellar tumours. With a large midline suprasellar mass the proximal segments of both anterior cerebral arteries together with the anterior communicating artery are stretched upwards forming an arc over the tumour (Fig. 62.29).

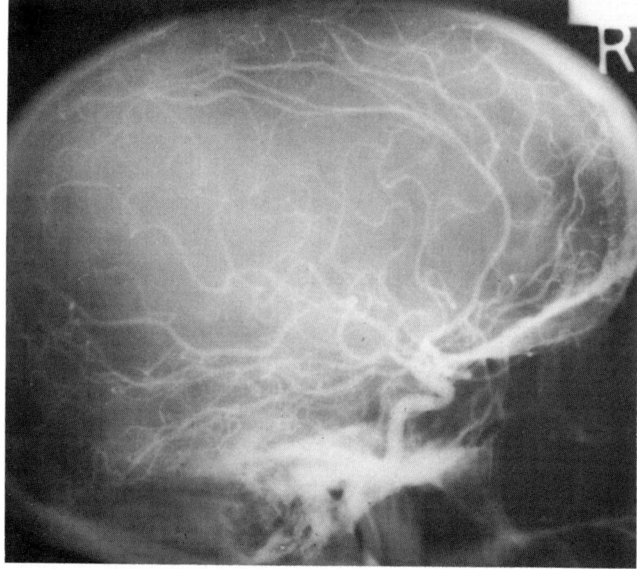

Fig. 62.30 Symmetrical hydrocephalus showing stretching of the anterior cerebral artery and downward displacement of the anterior choroidal and posterior communicating arteries. The anterior cerebral artery lay in the midline.

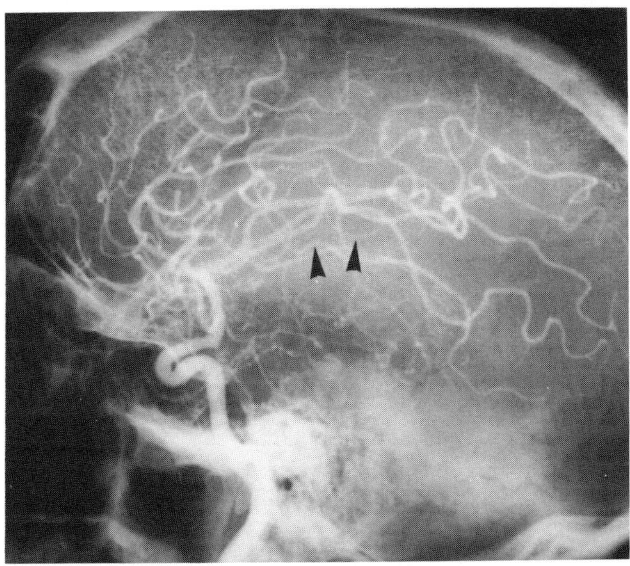

Fig. 62.31 Displacement of the middle cerebral vessels by a temporal tumour (↑ ↑).

Such displacements are most commonly seen with a suprasellar extension of a *pituitary tumour*; they will also occur with *suprasellar meningiomas* and with *glioma of the optic chiasm* (Fig. 62.17). Large pituitary tumours in addition to displacing the anterior cerebral artery may also displace and distort the carotid syphon in the cavernous sinus. In the lateral film the vessel appears stretched around the pituitary mass; in the A.P. films the syphon is displaced laterally.

Subfrontal tumours, such as *olfactory groove meningiomas*, will produce upward and backward displacement of the proximal midline portions of the anterior cerebral arteries.

Central and deep-seated lesions which produce no lateral displacement of the anterior cerebral artery, or upward displacement of the middle cerebral vessels, may, by obstructing the third ventricle or foramen of Munro, give rise to symmetrical hydrocephalus.

Symmetrical hydrocephalus, either from this type of lesion or from a posterior fossa tumour, produces stretching of the anterior cerebral artery as seen in the lateral film (Fig. 62.30). Instead of pursuing its normal tortuous course the artery appears wide swept and stretched. The dilatation of the ventricles can also be recognized by reference to the appearance of the deep veins (see below).

The middle cerebral vessels show most displacement with temporal lobe tumours (Fig. 62.31). These displace the middle cerebral vessels upwards, and a large temporal lobe mass may elevate the middle cerebral branches to such an extent that they appear superimposed on the anterior cerebral artery in the lateral films. Large temporal tumours may also displace the termination of the internal carotid artery medially as seen in the A.P. films. The anterior choroidal artery will also be displaced (see below). Smaller temporal lesions may produce local elevation of middle cerebral vessels either in the anterior middle, or posterior temporal region.

The *anterior choroidal artery* is of some importance in the assessment of cerebral tumours. Its normal position has been described above. With temporal lobe tumours it may be pressed medially and with deep-seated central tumours it may be pressed laterally.

With large intracranial masses there is downward herniation of the brain into the tentorial hiatus. Such *tentorial pressure cones* may be suspected at angiography by downward displacement of the *posterior communicating* and proximal part of the *posterior cerebral artery*. The

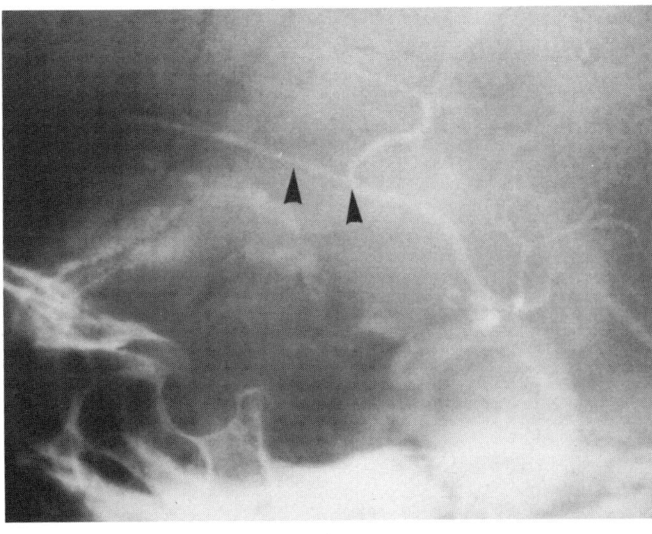

A

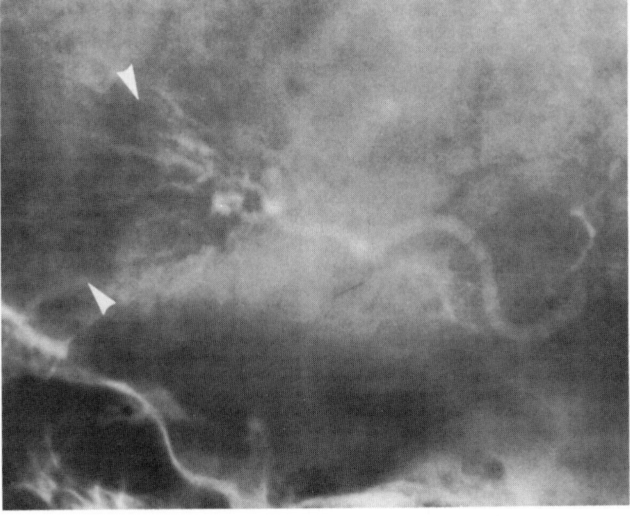

B

Fig. 62.32 Displacement of the deep veins. (A) Suprasellar meningioma displacing the septal veins and venous angle upwards and backwards (↖↖). Note the meningioma 'blush'. (B) Backward displacement of the venous angle and backward buckling of the internal cerebral vein with a large frontal glioma. Note the pathological veins draining into the septal vein (↖ ↙).

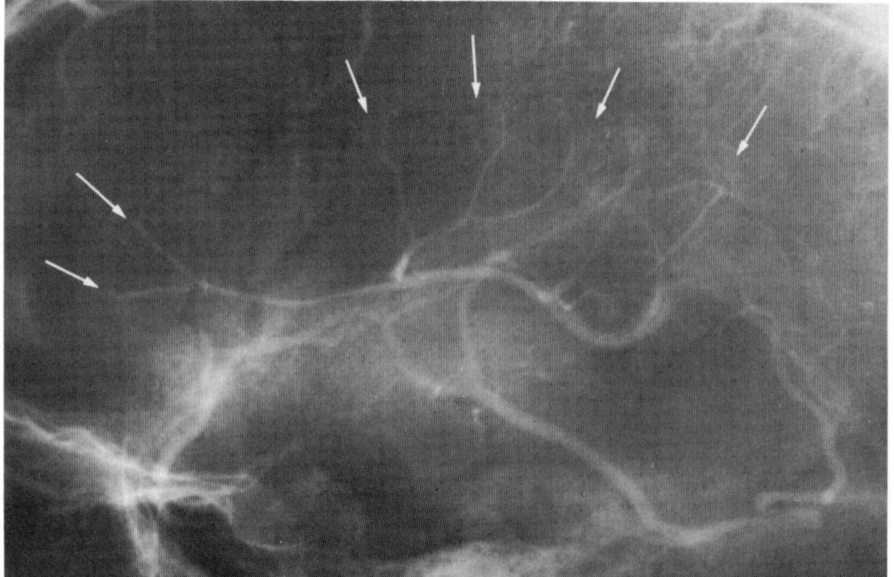

A

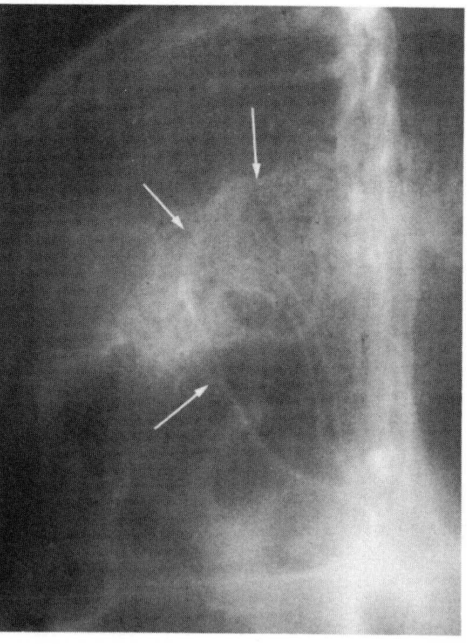

B

Fig. 62.33 Symmetrical hydrocephalus shown by the appearance of the deep veins. Arrows point to the ventricular margin. (A) In lateral projection. (B) In the A.P. projection.

anterior choroidal artery may also be seen to be pressed downwards in the lateral films.

The antero-posterior films may also suggest tentorial herniation by showing medial displacement of the posterior communicating and anterior choroidal arteries and of the proximal part of the posterior cerebral artery.

The **superficial veins** may be locally stretched or displaced by a large superficial tumour, and in some cases this may help considerably in localizing the tumours. Such stretched superficial veins are most frequently seen in the parasagittal region.

The deep veins. The normal position of the *internal cerebral vein* and its tributaries has been described above. These vessels may show considerable displacement by intracranial masses.

Thus a frontal tumour will displace the venous angle backwards (Fig. 62.32). Central masses will displace the internal cerebral vein across the midline even though there is no displacement of the anterior cerebral artery. Large non-central masses may also displace the internal cerebral vein to the opposite side. With a tumour of the basal ganglia the striothalamic vein may be elevated. Local distortion of the ventricles may be recognized in good-quality serial films where the subependymal veins are well shown.

With malignant gliomas and vascular deposits pathological vessels in the white matter may be seen draining into the deep veins. This is an important differential point between intracerebral tumours and extracerebral lesions, such as meningiomas (Fig. 62.32).

Hydrocephalus can be diagnosed from the appearance of the deep veins both in lateral and in A.P. projections. In lateral view the margins of the ventricles can be roughly assessed by linking in the points of origin of the deep veins from the subependymal veins (see Fig. 61.15 and Fig. 62.33A). The internal cerebral vein may be pressed downwards by the dilated ventricles and the septal and strio-thalamic veins appear elongated and stretched.

In A.P. view the striothalamic veins give a good impression of the size of the ventricle (see Figs 61.16 and 62.33B).

With unilateral hydrocephalus the internal cerebral vein may be displaced to the normal side and the appearance of the deep veins on the two sides will be quite different, suggesting a normal sized ventricle on the one side and a dilated one on the other.

Downward displacement of the *basal vein* may be seen in cases of tentorial herniation, and the vein may be displaced medially in the anteroposterior projection.

THE POSTERIOR FOSSA

For many years it was considered that vertebral arteriography was much less useful than carotid angiography in the localization of tumours and pneumography was the method of choice for localizing posterior fossa masses. However, as a result of painstaking anatomical studies it has been shown that many small arteries and veins can be consistently recognized at vertebral angiography and their displacement by tumours assessed. The normal anatomy of these vessels has already been described.

Pre-brainstem masses will displace the basilar artery backwards, a feature which is seen in lesions such as chordoma or meningiomas (Figs 62.34 and 62.35). Generally speaking, pontine or brain-stem gliomas from which these tumours have to be differentiated will press the

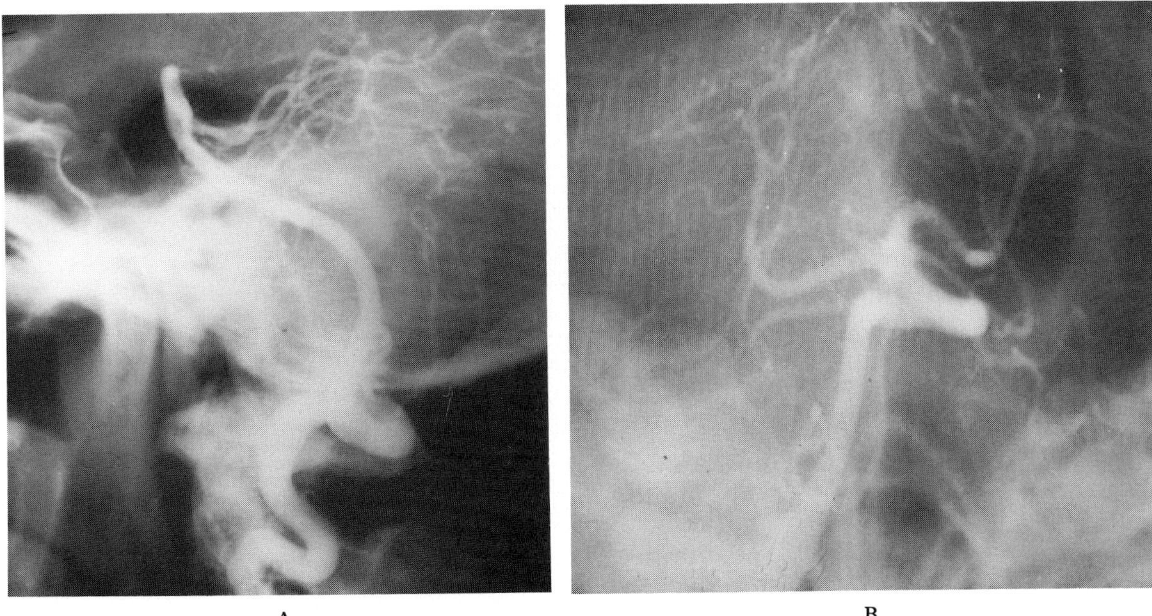

A B

Fig. 62.34A and B Vertebral arteriogram with a chordoma showing backward displacement of the vertebral and basilar arteries.

basilar artery forwards. It should be noted, however, that occasionally a *brainstem tumour* which is eccentric or enveloping the basilar artery will appear to displace the latter backwards. There are, however, other features which enable differentiation to be made. Usually a brainstem tumour displaces the basilar artery and the anterior pontomesencephalic vein forwards. At the same time the precentral cerebellar vein is pressed backwards and the choroidal loop is displaced backwards and downwards with the fourth ventricle. Downward displacement of the caudal loop of the posterior inferior cerebellar artery is seen with *tonsillar herniation*, whether this is primary (Arnold-Chiari malformation), or secondary to a mass in the posterior fossa. However, it should be remembered that this tonsillar loop can normally project down below the foramen magnum. When such a problem of differential diagnosis arises it is helpful to examine the hemispheric branch. In pathological cases this will be seen to be stretched in its proximal segment and its origin may be below the foramen magnum. This is best identified

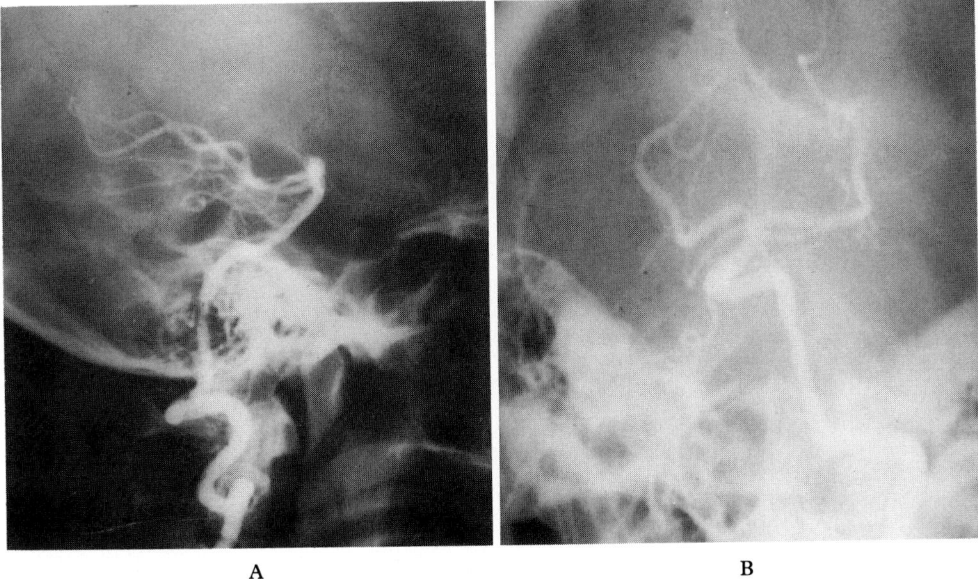

A B

Fig. 62.35A and B Clivus meningioma displacing vertebral and basilar arteries backwards.

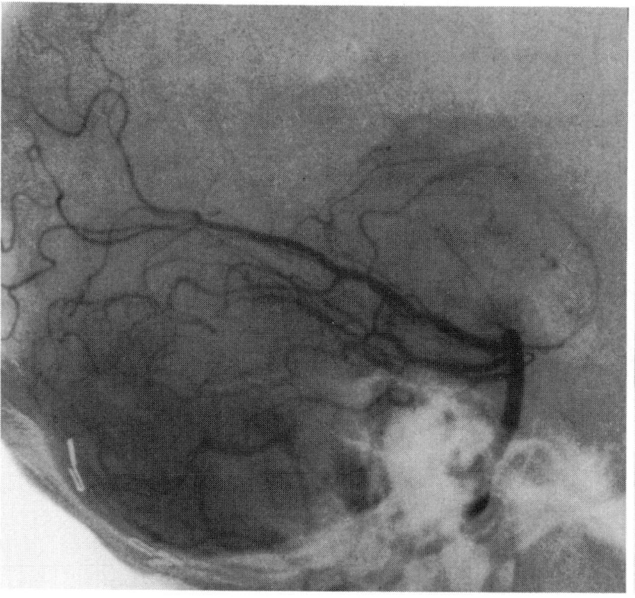

A

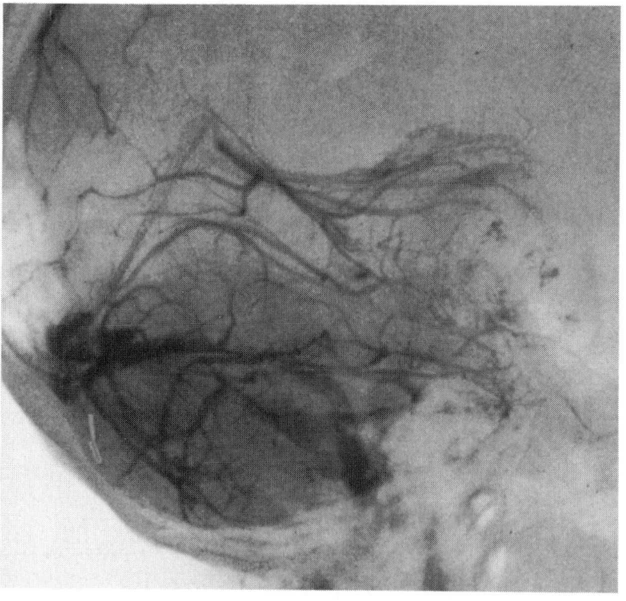

B

Fig. 62.36A and B Glioma involving thalamus, hypothalamus and upper brain stem shown by vertebral angiography. (Subtraction prints.) Note stretched vessels and abnormal circulation.

in an A.P. projection. This feature is not seen where the low vascular loop is an anatomical variation.

Tumours in the *cerebellar hemisphere* will tend to stretch the local cerebellar veins and to displace the inferior vermian vein across the midline. The fourth ventricle is also pressed forwards and this can be assessed from the position of the choroidal loop. It is also displaced to the contralateral side together with the vermis branch of the posterior inferior cerebellar artery.

Tumours in the *inferior vermis* will displace the inferior vermian vein backwards and the choroidal loop forwards. Tumours in the *superior vermis* will displace the precentral cerebellar vein forwards and also the choroidal loop. In both cases there will be no lateral displacement of the midline structures. With most large masses in the posterior fossa the basilar artery and the anterior pontomesencephalic vein will be pressed forwards.

Tumours in the *cerebellopontine angle* will displace the anterior inferior cerebellar artery upwards and medially. They will also displace upwards or occlude the petrosal vein. Large tumours will also displace the superior cerebellar artery upwards. The fourth ventricle and its choroidal loop may be displaced backwards, it may also be displaced to the contralateral side, though it can remain relatively normal in position.

Occasionally, a brain-stem tumour will produce a large nodule in the C.P. angle. Such a lesion can be differentiated from an extra-axial tumour by downward displacement of the anterior inferior cerebellar artery.

Tumours in the *fourth ventricle* are difficult to assess but if large they will displace both choroidal loops laterally in the A.P. or Towne's projection. Normally the distance between the choroidal loops is less than 5 mm. A distance of 5 to 10 mm is suggestive of neoplasm and distances greater than this are definitely pathological. Some fourth ventricle tumours may show a pathological circulation as noted below.

Tumours in the *pineal region* will show local displacement of the vein of Galen and precentral cerebellar vein. *Thalamic* tumours will show unilateral backward and upward displacement of the lateral posterior choroidal arteries and, if large enough, backward displacement of the precentral cerebellar vein. They may also show evidence of a gliomatous pathological circulation (Fig. 62.36). The thalamic veins will also be displaced.

THE DEMONSTRATION OF PATHOLOGICAL VESSELS

Malignant gliomas vary in vascularity. The more slow growing and benign tumours are relatively avascular, whilst the highly malignant and rapidly growing tumours may be excessively vascular. Over one-third of malignant tumours will show pathological vessels at arteriography. Clearly prognosis becomes worse the more numerous and obvious such pathological vessels are. Abnormal vessels are often small and tortuous. Little pin-points or irregular lacunae of contrast may also be seen (Fig. 62.37). These probably represent sinuses or venous lakes within the tumour. Direct arteriovenous communications may also be present and with vascular tumours there may be very early filling of the drainage veins. This is a feature normally seen in angiomatous malformations, and an excessively vascular tumour may superficially resemble such an angiomatous malformation. However, there is seldom

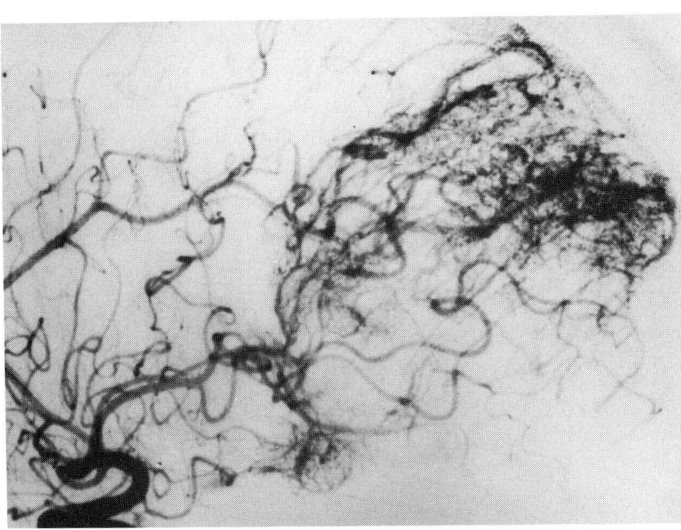

A

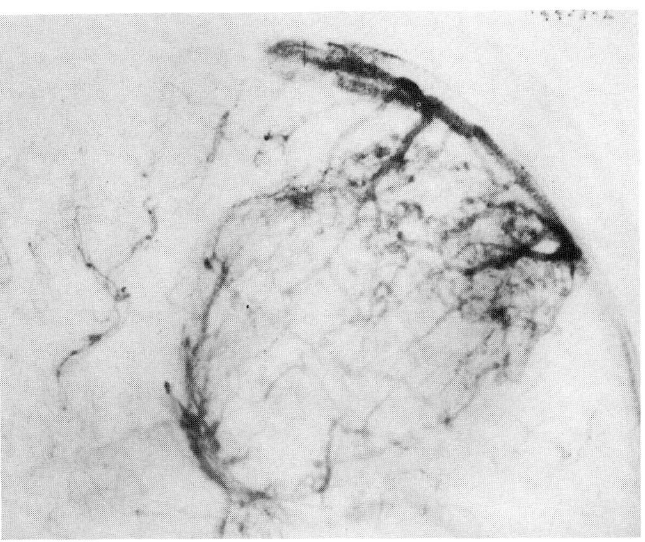

B

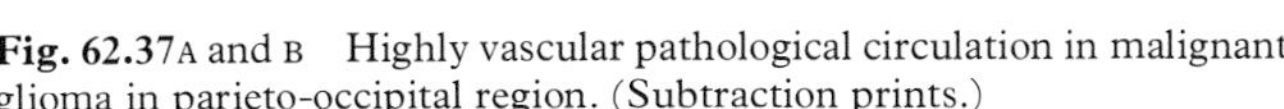

Fig. 62.37A and B Highly vascular pathological circulation in malignant glioma in parieto-occipital region. (Subtraction prints.)

real difficulty in differential diagnosis, since the drainage veins are rarely as large and tortuous as those seen in angiomas of similar size. In addition, the clinical history is usually quite different. The area of pathological vessels in a malignant glioma has no clear-cut margins and it merges imperceptibly into normal tissue.

Secondary deposits may show appearances very similar to those of malignant gliomas. Angiographic differentiation can therefore be quite difficult but is usually possible because deposits are on the whole small, rounded, well circumscribed tumours (Fig. 62.38). Gliomas on the other hand are often large, ill-defined and infiltrating. In addition secondary deposits may be multiple and two or more separate rounded areas of pathological vessels may be recognized in the brain.

Not all secondary deposits are vascular and the proportion showing pathological vessels is similar to the proportion of malignant gliomas showing such abnormal vessels (about 40 per cent).

Certain deposits are more vascular than others. The most vascular of all are usually those from renal carcinoma or thyroid carcinoma. Such excessively vascular deposits, like vascular gliomas, can closely resemble

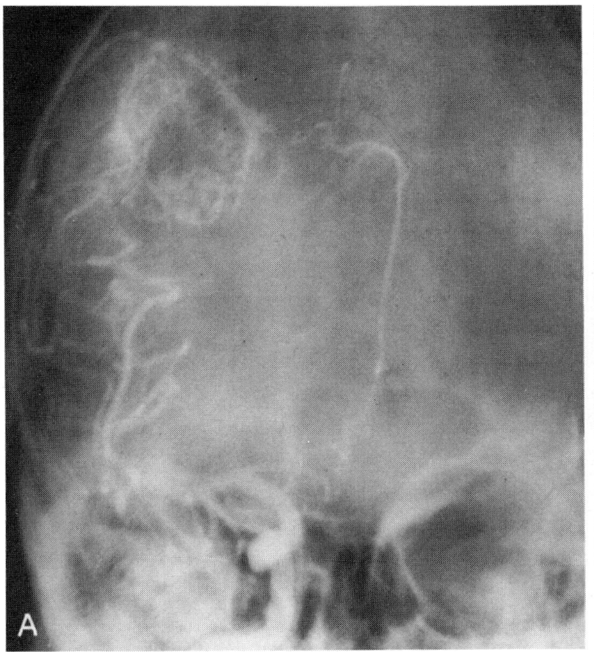

Fig. 62.38A and B Pathological vessels outlining secondary deposit in parietal region.

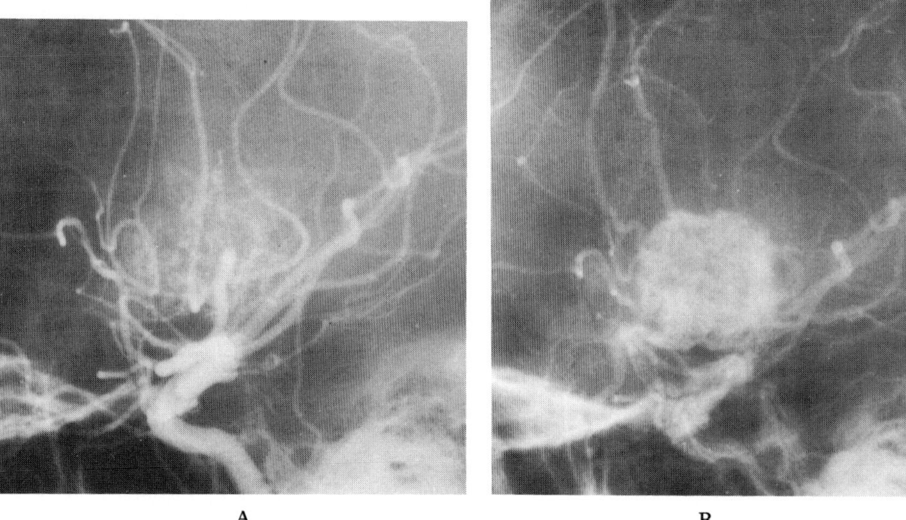

A B

Fig. 62.39 Pathological vessels. Very vascular deposit from hypernephroma. A and B. Serial films.

angiomatous malformation, but they do not show the typically large drainage veins of angiomatous malformation.

Figure 62.39 shows a case which presented as a cerebral tumour. Because of the angiographic appearance a post-arteriogram pyelogram film was taken which showed a clinically unsuspected primary in the kidney. Such pyelogram films should always be obtained immediately after the angiogram should a very vascular deposit be seen on the cerebral films.

Meningiomas. The pathological circulation at angiography can be characteristic of meningioma. As with the other tumours mentioned above, the characteristic appearance is only seen in the more vascular tumours representing some two-thirds of those examined by common or internal carotid angiography. In these cases selective external carotid angiography with good subtraction films will identify the tumour in a higher proportion of cases. The vascular nature of the tumour appears on the angiogram as a diffuse and fairly homogeneous smear of contrast best seen in the capillary or early venous phase. As a result the whole of the tumour may be outlined against the brain (Figs 62.32A, 62.40 and 62.41).

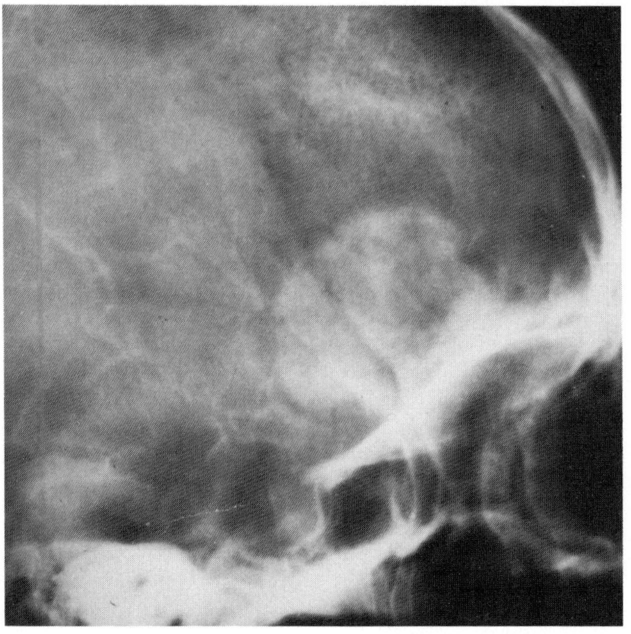

Fig. 62.40 Meningioma showing typical 'blush' or smear in venous phase. The tumour is growing from the floor of the anterior fossa.

Secondary deposits and even gliomas can on occasions show similar appearances, but there are suggestive angiographic and plain X-ray features to support the diagnosis in most cases of meningioma. The characteristic plain X-ray changes have been described in Chapter 59. The characteristic angiographic features are:

1. Evidence of a hypertrophied meningeal artery leading up to and supplying the tumour and filling in the early arterial phase.
2. Evidence of hypertrophied branches of the external carotid artery leading up to and supplying bone infiltrated by meningioma (Fig. 62.42A). Selective injection of the external carotid artery will often show the meningeal arteries and the pathological circulation in a meningioma better than selective internal carotid injection.
3. The site of the tumour, since meningiomas occur mainly in characteristic situations, e.g. the parasagittal region, the sphenoidal ridge, or the olfactory groove.
4. Invasion of arterial walls, usually evidenced by 'cuffing' or narrowing of a major artery.

One or other of these features may be present without the typical meningioma 'blush' or 'smear' and are in

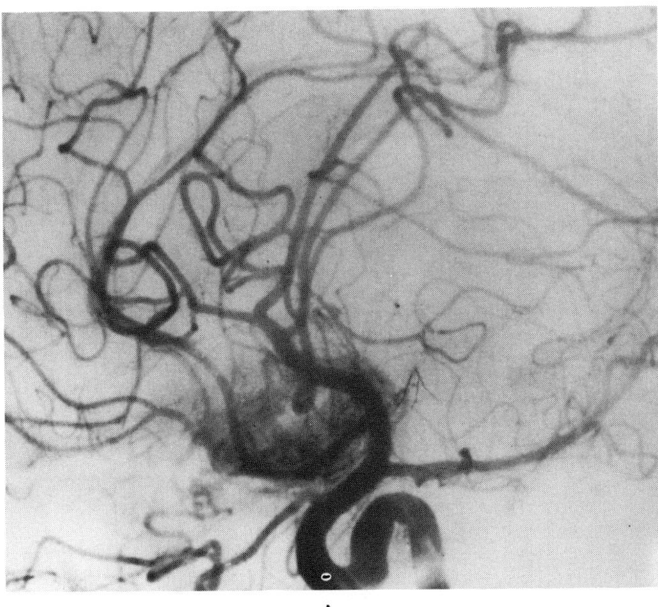

A

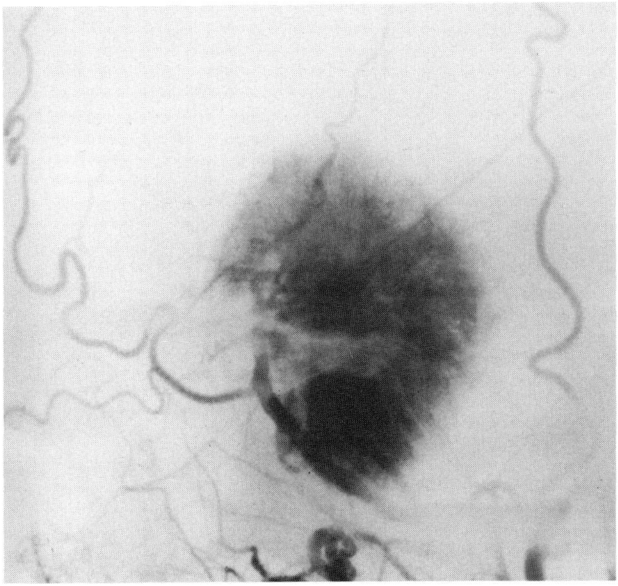

B

Fig. 62.41 (A) Selective internal carotid injection showing blood supply to sphenoidal ridge meningioma. (B) Selective external carotid injection showing larger supply from the external carotid and meningeal arteries. (Subtraction prints.)

themselves sufficiently good evidence for the diagnosis of meningioma to be suggested.

A small proportion of meningiomas will show no evidence of any of the angiographic features just described. In such cases there is no way of making a pathological diagnosis on the angiogram, although evidence of the tumour and its situation will still be demonstrated by the displacement of cerebral vessels.

As already noted, a parasagittal site should always raise the possibility of a meningioma. With parasagittal meningiomas it may be important to look for evidence of sinus involvement by the tumour. Meningiomas can invade the sagittal sinus and occlude it. A complete occlusion may be evident on a serial angiogram where the superficial cortical veins can be seen to drain not into the sagittal sinus but into a collateral circulation (Fig. 61.5). In doubtful cases or where the sinus is partially involved it may be necessary to perform a sagittal sinogram. As noted above, another angiographic feature seen with meningiomas and not with most other types of tumour is involve-

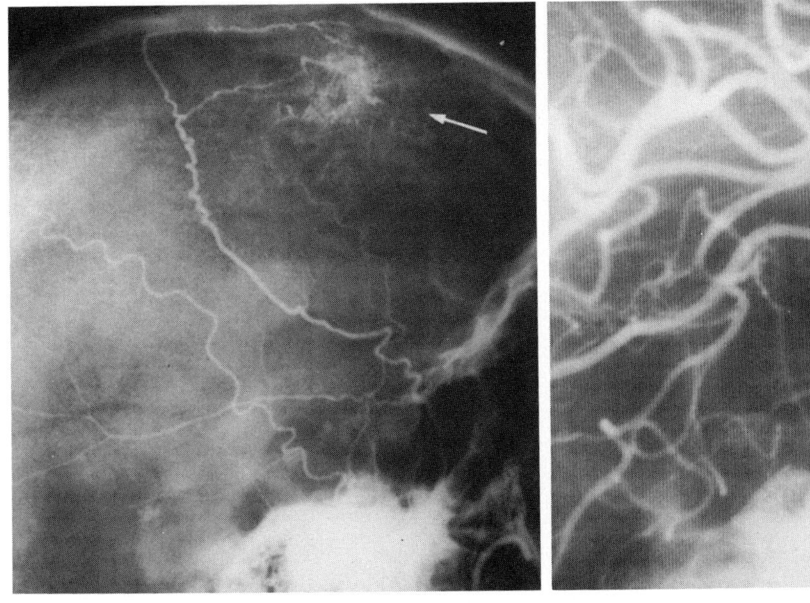

A

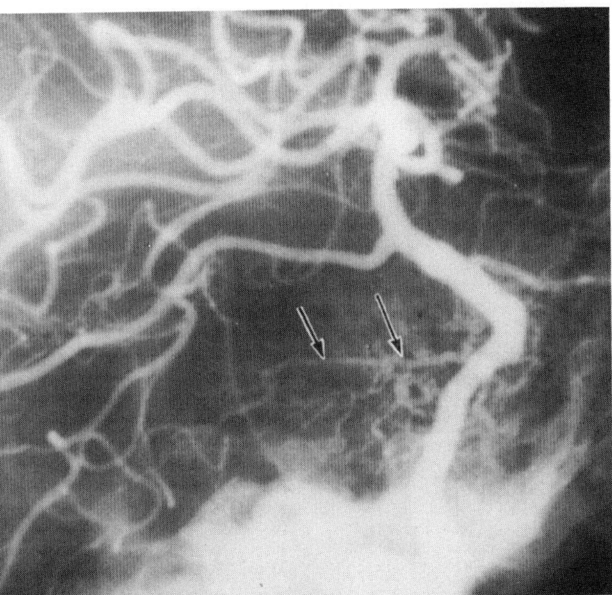

B

Fig. 62.42A Selective external carotid angiogram showing meningeal vessels supplying a meningioma (←). (B) Tentorial arteries supplying a basal meningioma (arrows).

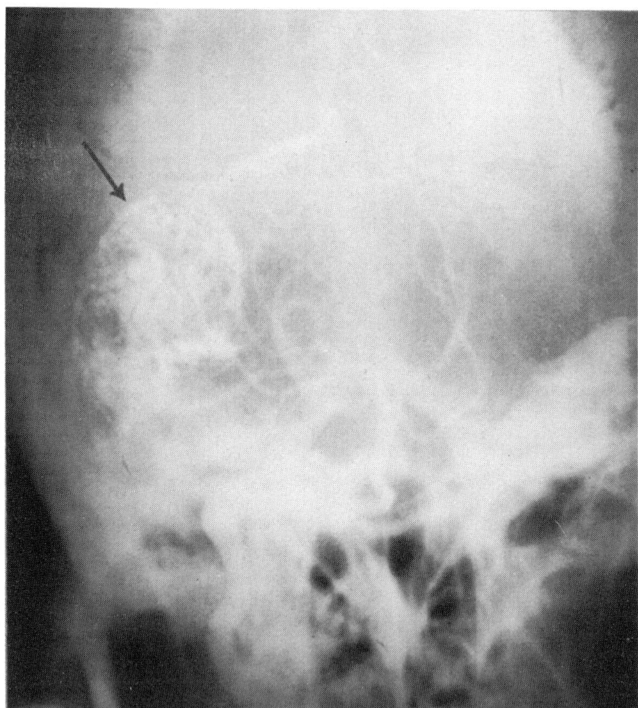

Fig. 62.43 Haemangioblastoma showing typical appearances (↘).

ment and invasion of arterial walls. This is most readily seen with sphenoidal ridge tumours involving the middle cerebral origin but has been identified in other situations.

Meningiomas in special sites. Intraventricular meningiomas are very rare but can occur within the lateral ventricle, usually on the left side and in the temporal horn. Presumably they are derived from cell rests during development of the brain. In these cases the tumour is supplied by the anterior choroidal artery and this vessel shows hypertrophy which can be recognized on the angiogram. Meningioma has also been described in the fourth ventricle, but this is extremely rare.

Meningiomas involving the tentorial hiatus and petrous apex may be supplied by hypertrophied small meningeal tentorial arteries arising directly from the internal carotid artery near its termination (Fig. 62.42B).

Hypertrophied anterior choroidal and tentorial arteries should always raise suspicion of meningioma but they are not diagnostic and can occur with other lesions such as glioma.

Haemangioblastoma. These tumours have always been associated in the literature with angioma of the retina (Lindau's disease). The association is in fact very rare whilst haemangioblastomas of the posterior fossa are relatively common. Of some 50 cases of haemangioblastoma reviewed by the author only three were associated with Lindau's disease. Whilst most examples of haemangioblastoma occur in the posterior fossa the tumour is also encountered in the spinal canal, and has even been recorded above the tentorium. The angiographic appearances are characteristic except in the predominantly cystic cases. The tumour is extremely vascular and when filled with contrast strongly resembles a

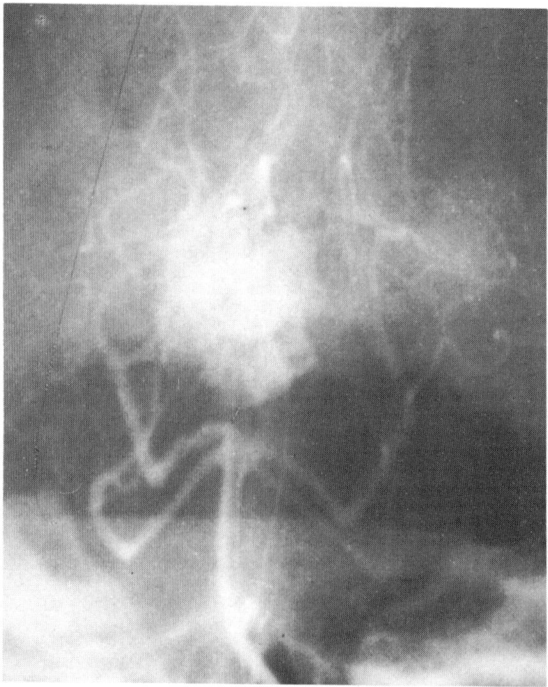

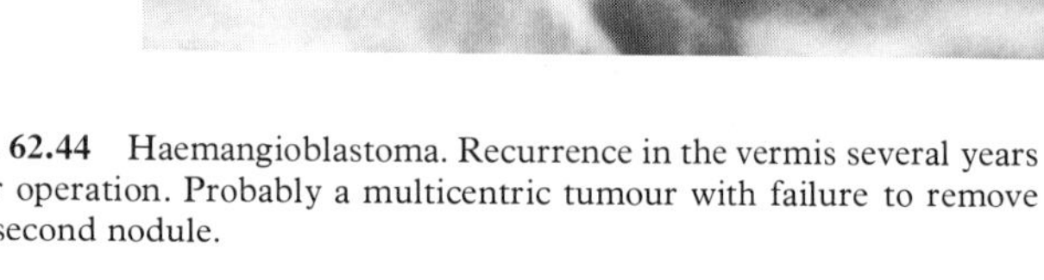

Fig. 62.44 Haemangioblastoma. Recurrence in the vermis several years after operation. Probably a multicentric tumour with failure to remove the second nodule.

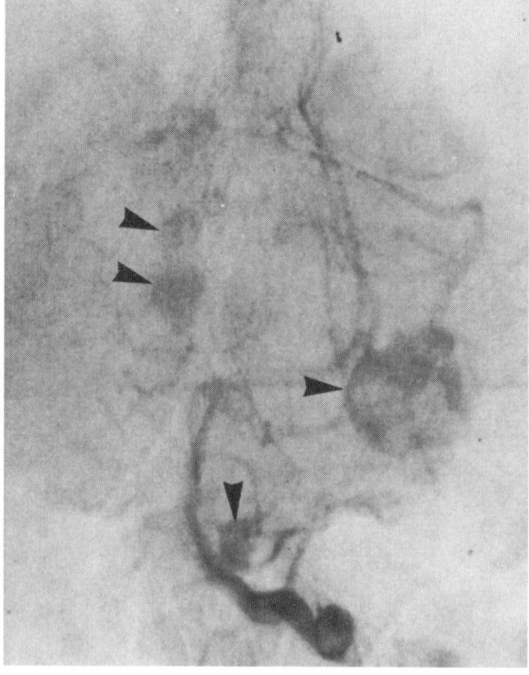

Fig. 62.45 Multiple haemangioblastoma nodules shown in the late arterial phase of an A.P. vertebral arteriogram. (Subtraction print.)

rounded angioma or occasionally an aneurysm (Figs 62.43 and 62.44). However, unlike the angioma there are no obvious large drainage veins. Smaller nodules appear as smears of contrast not unlike those seen in meningioma though appearing much earlier than the late capillary or venous phase (Fig. 62.45). The demonstration of a rounded and extremely vascular tumour in a cerebellar hemisphere or in the vermis should always suggest the diagnosis of haemangioblastoma.

Differential diagnosis is from an extremely vascular deposit. Cystic haemangioblastoma may show little evidence of vascularity but even in these cases there may be a vascular nodule in the wall of the cyst.

These tumours may be multicentric and it is vital to obtain first class subtraction prints of good quality vertebral angiograms if all the nodules are to be identified and removed (Fig. 62.45). We have encountered cases with as many as 11 separate nodules.

Acoustic neurinomas are usually non-vascular when small but a pathological circulation can frequently be demonstrated in large tumours (Figs 62.46 and 62.47). These tumours may also derive a blood supply from the external carotid artery which can be shown by selective external carotid angiography. In other cases a large acoustic tumour will show like any other angle tumour by displacement of the anterior inferior cerebellar artery and other vessels in the posterior fossa.

Choroid plexus papilloma and **ependymoma** are rare tumours which may occur in the fourth ventricle. **Meningioma** of the fourth ventricle is even rarer, but has been described. Angiography may demonstrate pathological vessels in these tumours, particularly if they have grown to a large size.

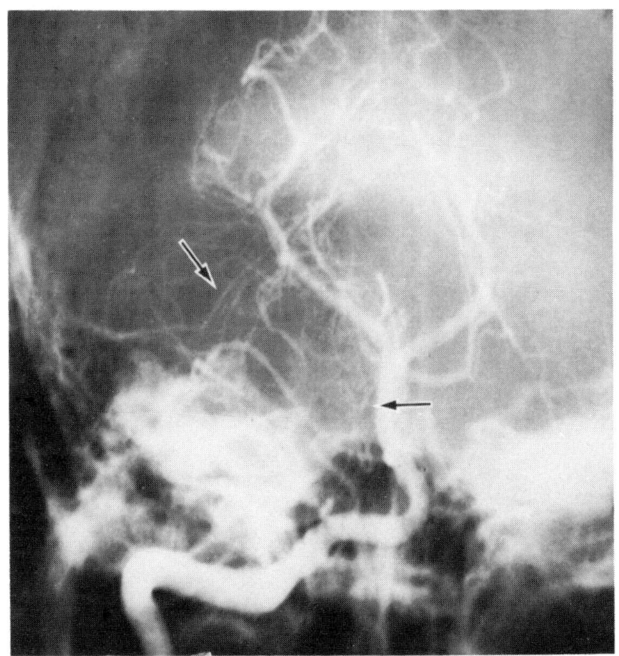

Fig. 62.46 Large acoustic neurinoma showing pathological circulation (arrows). Note the upward displacement of the anterior cerebellar artery, and also of the superior cerebellar and posterior cerebral origins.

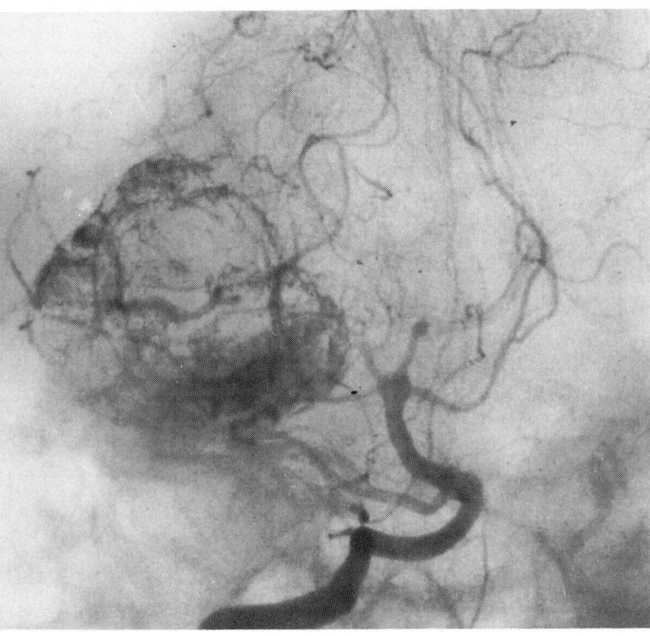

Fig. 62.47 Large vascular acoustic neurinoma showing pathological circulation. This was also supplied from the external carotid artery. (Subtraction print.)

Angiography with hyperventilation

This procedure has been used as a means of better demonstrating tumour circulation. It is well known that cerebral vessels are sensitive to carbon dioxide and oxygen concentrations in the blood. An increase of carbon dioxide tension will cause vasodilatation whilst the reverse effect is produced by an increase in oxygen tension.

If a patient is under a general anaesthetic the carbon dioxide content of the blood can be diminished and the oxygen content increased by hyperventilating the lungs. Normal cerebral arteries react in the way described, but pathological vessels such as those in a tumour circulation do not. Thus by performing an angiogram during hyperventilation it is claimed that the tumour circulation will stand out in a much more clear-cut manner owing to the relative shutdown of many normal small cerebral vessels. This procedure is possible only when the patient is under general anaesthetic, but it is useful in selected cases.

REFERENCES AND SUGGESTIONS FOR FURTHER READING

Alpers, B. J., Berry, R. G. & Paddison, R. M. (1959) Anatomical studies of the Circle of Willis in normal brain. *Arch. Neurol. Psychiat.*, **81**, 409–418.

Bull, J. (1969) Massive aneurysms at the base of the brain. *Brain*, **92**, 535–560.

DEBRUN, G., LEGRE, J., KASBARIAN, M. *et al.* (1979) Endovascular occlusion of vertebral fistulae by detachable balloons with conservation of the vertebral blood flow. *Radiology*, **130**, 141–147.

DI CHIRO, G. & WENER, L. (1973) Angiography of the spinal cord. *Journal of Neurosurgery*, **39**, 1–29.

DJINDJIAN, R. & MERLAND, J. J. (1978) *Superselective Angiography of the External Carotid Artery*. Berlin, New York: Springer Verlag.

EASTCOTT, H. H. G., PICKERING, G. W. & ROB, C. G. (1954) Reconstruction of internal carotid artery in a patient with intermittent attacks of hemiplegia. *Lancet*, **ii,** 994–995.

HASS, W. R., FIELDS, W. S., NORTH, R. R., KRICHEFF, I. I., CHASE, N. E. & BAUER, R. B. (1968) Joint study of extracranial arterial occlusions. *Journal of American Medical Association*, **203**, 961–968.

HOUSER, O. W., BAKER, H. L., RHOTON, A. L. & OKAZAKI, H. (1972) Intracranial dural A.V. malformations. *Radiology*, **105**, 55–64.

HUANG, Y. P. & WOLF, B. S. (1970) Differential diagnosis of 4th ventricle tumours from brain stem tumours in angiography. *Neuroradiology*, **1**, 4.

KRAYENBUHL, H. (1967) Cerebral venous and sinus thrombosis. *Clin. Neurosurg.*, **14**, 1–24.

KRAYENBUHL, H. A. & YASARGIL, M. G. (1968) *Cerebral Angiography*, 2nd edn. London: Butterworth.

LIE, T. A. (1968) *Congenital Anomalies of the Carotid Arteries*. Amsterdam: Excerpta Medica.

MONIZ, E. (1931) *L'angiographie Cerebrale*. Paris: Manson.

NEWTON, T. H. & POTTS, D. G. (eds) (1974) *Radiology of the Skull and Brain Vol. 2 Angiography*. St. Louis: Mosby.

PERRETT, G. & NISHIOKA, M. (1966a) Report on the co-operative study of intracranial aneurysms and subarachnoid haemorrhage. Section IV. Diagnostic value and complications of angiography. *Journal of Neurosurgery*, **25**, 98–114.

PERRETT, G. & NISHIOKA, M. (1966b) Report on the co-operative study of intracranial aneurysms and subarachnoid haemorrhage. Section VI. A.V. malformations. *Journal of Neurosurgery*, **25**, 467–490.

SCATLIFF, J. M., FOUSTINE, C. C. & RADCLIFFE, B. (1971) Vascular patterns in cerebral neoplasms and their differential diagnoses. *Roentgenology*, **6**, 59–69.

SUTTON, D. (1971) Skinner Lecture. The vertebro-basilar system and its vascular lesions. *Clinical Radiology*, **22**, 271–287.

SUTTON, D. & DAVIES, E. R. (1966) Arch aortography and cerebrovascular insufficiency. *Clinical Radiology*, **17**, 330–345.

TAVERAS, J. M. (1969) Multiple progressive intracranial arterial occlusions: a syndrome of children and young adults. *American Journal of Roentgenology*, **106**, 235–268.

TAVERAS, J. M. & WOOD, E. H. (1976) *Diagnostic Neuroradiology*, 2nd edn. Baltimore, Maryland: Williams & Wilkins.

PART 8

IMAGING

CHAPTER 63

COMPUTED TOMOGRAPHY—C.N.S. (1)

Historical

A new method of forming images from X-rays was developed and introduced into clinical use by the British physicist Godfrey Hounsfield in 1972, and is referred to as computed transmission tomography, computed tomography (CT), or computerized axial tomography (CAT). Many people regard this invention as the greatest step forward in radiology since the discovery of X-rays by Roentgen in 1895. It resulted in 1979 in the Nobel prize for Medicine being awarded jointly to Dr Hounsfield and Professor A. M. Cormack. Hounsfield's work was based on research into data retrieval and transformation. In the course of this work it became clear that there were many areas in which large amounts of information were theoretically available but where the technique of retrieval and presentation used were so inefficient that most of the available data were wasted. Hounsfield considered that this was particularly so in conventional X-ray examinations. A research programme was sponsored by the British Ministry of Health and by EMI Limited. The basic and revolutionary assumption was that measurements taken of X-rays transmitted through the body contained information on all the constituents of the body in the path of the beam. By using multidirectional scanning of the object multiple data were collected. Their interpretation required a mathematical solution using a computer to perform the calculations. This information could then be presented in a conventional raster form, and from these results a three dimensional picture could be produced. In practice the system developed was similar to the principle of tomography already widely used in radiology and in which pictures are presented as a series of 'slices'. After proving the principle Hounsfield spent several years developing the method clinically with Dr James Ambrose of the Atkinson Morley Hospital, London, using a prototype machine. The first report presented was at the British Institute of Radiology in April 1972 and news of the discovery spread rapidly. The first EMI production machines were installed in England and North America by 1973. So obvious and so vast was the potential of the method in cerebral work that by 1979 over 1000 of these expensive machines were in use, each costing about £250 000. Since 1973 North American, European, Israeli and Japanese commercial companies have produced alternative versions of the original CT scanner and a large competitive industry has developed. Whilst most of the early machines were dedicated head scanners, body scanners which are also capable of head scanning have now largely taken over and are established in clinical practice (see Ch. 65).

TECHNICAL ASPECTS

In computed tomography the X-ray output is collimated to a very narrow beam. After passing through the patient it is partially absorbed, and the remaining photons of the X-ray beam fall on radiation *detectors* instead of X-ray film. The detector response is directly related to the number of photons impinging on it and so to tissue density since a greater proportion of X-ray photons passing through dense tissues are absorbed than are absorbed by the less dense tissues. When they strike the detector the X-ray photons are converted to scintillations. These can be quantified and recorded digitally. The information is fed into a computer which produces different readings as the X-ray beam is traversed around the subject. Even in its original form this meant that the computer dealt with a vast number of digital readings. These can be presented as a numerical read out representing the absorption in each tiny segment of the section traversed. This information can also be presented in analogue form as a two dimensional display of the matrix on a screen where each numerical value is represented by a single picture element (pixel). The more modern machines have improved the resolution by diminishing the size of each pixel. The original EMI scanner worked with an 80×80 matrix. This was later upgraded to 160×160 matrix and the more modern machines can achieve 320×320 and even 520×520.

The first machines had only two detectors and used sharply collimated beams of X-rays. The more modern machines use a fan beam and multiple detectors. The original machines took 4½ minutes to perform a single tomographic slice. The present generation can obtain cuts in times varying from 1–20 seconds depending on the type of machine and programme used. These times will no doubt be reduced further in the future, and a prototype machine has now been designed capable of cardiac imaging in 1/60 second by using multiple X-ray tubes.

The early machines enclosed the patient's head in a water bag because of technical difficulties. These were rapidly overcome and all the present machines work with the patient's head or torso in air.

Further technical aspects are discussed in Chapter 65.

Data presentation

Most scanners now present the data obtained as an analogue display of each tissue slice on a cathode ray tube. Presentation is usually in the form of a Greyscale in which whiteness is proportional to the X-ray attenuation coefficient of tissue at each point of the scan. Thus radiopaque materials appear white and radiolucent tissue appears black. The range can be varied by changing the 'gate' or 'window' width (W) at will so that tissues within a *wide* range of densities or a *narrow* range can be evaluated. The central point or level (L) of the window can also be varied. In routine work the 'gate' width for brain work is 0–80 using the Hounsfield scale. Figure 63.1 shows the relative density on the Hounsfield scale of some normal body tissues. The Hounsfield scale is an arbitrary one with air at −1000 units and water at 0 units as fixed points. The numerical value assigned to the attenuation coefficient bears a linear relationship to the

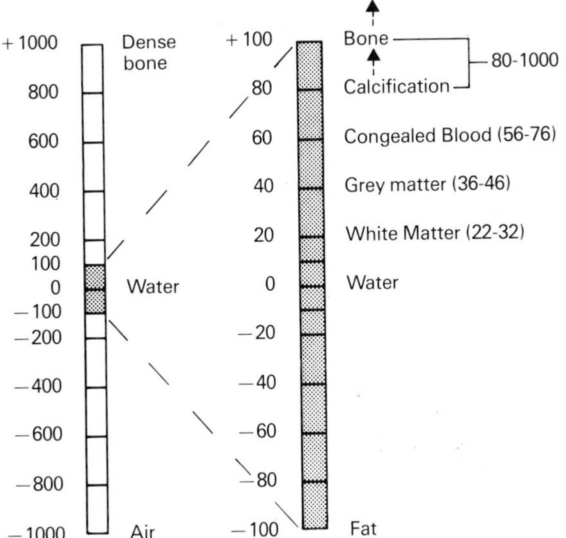

Fig. 63.1 Hounsfield's scale. The full scale on the left extends over 2,000 units. The expanded scale on the right extends over 200 units and includes all body tissues. Head scans are usually done routinely at a window level (L) of 34–40 and a window (W) covering 0–75.

electron density of the tissue concerned. It should be noted that 2 Hounsfield units are equal to 1 unit of the original EMI scale. Figures 63.17 and 63.34 show the effect of varying the window width on displays of individual scans.

In addition to the analogue display the machines as noted above also produce a digital print out. This is valuable in assessing certain cases and for research, but in routine practice is now little used, since modern display consoles have versatile facilities for obtaining such information directly.

Scan artefacts. With such a complicated apparatus using X-rays, sophisticated photon recording systems and computer programming, there are clearly many possible sources of error which can produce artefacts and erroneous results. The type of artefact seen on the final analogue picture can be classified into four types:

1. Noise
2. Motion artefacts
3. Artefacts due to high differential absorption in adjacent tissues
4. Technical errors and computer artefacts.

1. *Noise.* This can be defined as the degree of random statistical variation in the restructured X-ray picture and is equal to grain in a film. Noise is related to the contrast resolution of the scanner and is a very important measure of performance since the naturally occurring contrast between normal and pathological tissues is quite low. Noise depends on each of the following:

1. kV before and after patient filtration
2. Pixel width
3. Slice thickness
4. Subject size
5. Patient dosage
6. Detector efficiency.

Noise figures given without the conditions of measurements are of course worthless.

Patient exposure. It is clear from the above that contrast resolution (noise) is related to the number of photons detected at each measurement and therefore to radiation dose. Correct figures for this should be available for examination since some systems can deliver exposures in excess of 30 rad in a single CT study.

2. *Motion artefacts.* Movement of the patient's head results in some points appearing in different positions during the scanning cycle which will give false results. These are usually represented on the final picture as *linear artefacts* or streaking in rotate translate scanners. Since the head can rotate in any direction a variety of streak artefacts can be reproduced inside or outside the skull vault. Figure 63.2 shows an example of streak artefacts. Motion artefacts are of course less of a problem as scanning time has been progressively reduced.

With the rotate only type machines *ring artefacts* may be seen (Fig. 63.3).

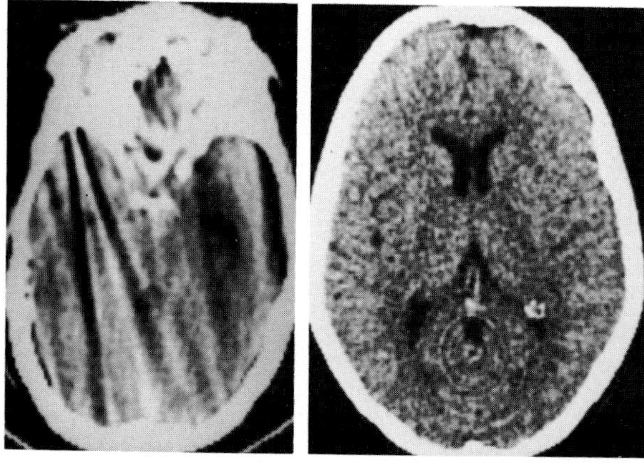

Fig. 63.2 *Fig. 63.3*

Fig. 63.2 Movement artefacts. Streaks due to movement with a rotate-translate scanner.

Fig. 63.3 Circular artefacts in the posterior fossa with a rotate only scanner.

3. *Differential absorption artefacts.* Where two tissues of greatly differing absorption are adjacent, e.g. bone and air, the computer tends to overshoot or overload producing linear artefacts again or streaking. Thus the very dense petrous bones sometimes combined with air in the ears can cause transpontine streaks obscuring the CP angle (Fig. 63.4). Surgical artefacts like clips, Holter valves, shunt reservoirs and metallic plates will also produce streaking, as will opaque contrast media such as Myodil. Reducing the scanning angle from 360° to 240° can help in decreasing this sort of artefact. Air in the ventricles will also produce streaking or overshoot at the air fluid level (Fig. 63.5). Computer overshoot may also produce a thin band of low density just internal to the skull, the so called 'false subarachnoid space'.

Partial volume phenomenon. Brain scan sections were usually performed at 13 mm width as standard. The newer machines have facilities for narrower sections, e.g. 10, 8 or 5 mm. These are particularly useful for improving resolution in difficult areas like the orbit. If a lesion such as a haematoma occupies only part of the thickness of the section then the view obtained will be an average for the whole of the 13 mm width. This phenomenon will affect the accuracy of the final image when dealing with small lesions or structures. Thus with tiny ventricles which are only partially included in the scan there will be a factitious reduction in size and extremely small ventricles may not be visualized. This so called 'partial volume effect' will be less with narrower sections, but must be borne in mind in interpreting standard sections which include tissues of widely differing density, e.g. bone and brain in the region of the petrous bones and skull base. Thus scans in the parasagittal region or through the petrous bones in the base of the skull will include the dense bone in part of the marginal sections and lead to false readings from this partial volume effect.

A single *surgical clip* does not normally present a major problem but multiple clips can interfere with the scan particularly when grouped close together (Fig. 63.6A). These problems are less marked with the newer, smaller matrices than with the older 80–80 and 160–160 matrices.

Air in the ventricles with the patient's brow up will produce a linear dense or white shadow at the air fluid level and a similar band of high reading about the margin of each frontal horn containing the gas (Fig. 63.5). Movement of the head during the scan where gas is present in the ventricles will produce alternating white and black zones around the ventricle which may degrade the areas below diagnostic levels.

Myodil in the ventricles does not normally create scan

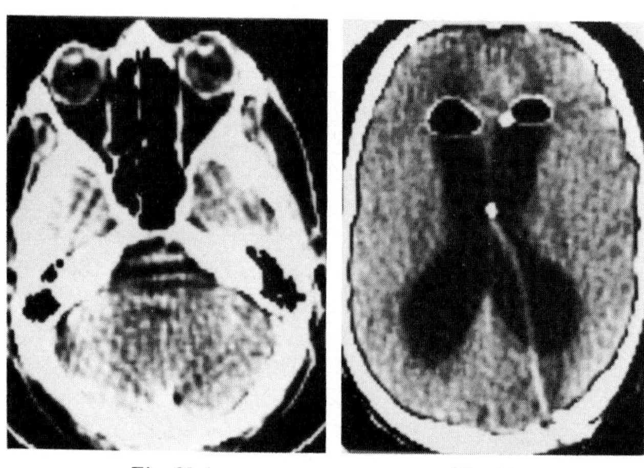

Fig. 63.4 *Fig. 63.5*

Fig. 63.4 Band artefact across brain stem.

Fig. 63.5 Air in ventricles producing overshoot and linear band at air fluid and air brain interfaces.

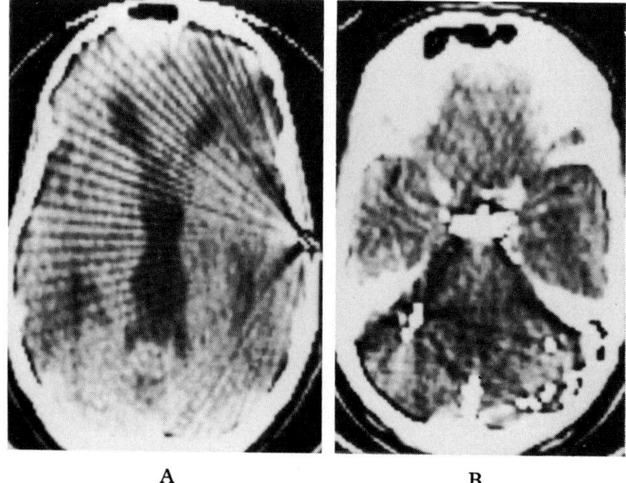

A B

Fig. 63.6A Linear streak artefacts from surgical clips (L34 W75). B Myodil in posterior fossa (L34 W100).

problems unless present in large amounts, but can be troublesome in the basal cisterns (Fig. 63.6B).

4. *Technical errors.* A high signal to noise ratio is necessary to a high quality scan. Image noise is defined as the degree of random statistical variation in the reconstructed X-ray picture. To overcome system noise increased photon flux is necessary. This of course results in increased dose and a compromise must be made in choosing the appropriate signal to noise ratio in order to achieve maximum resolution with minimum patient exposure since noise degrades the X-ray image. As the signal to noise ratio diminishes a mottled, compromised image results. This may also occur with improper tube detector elements or with faults in the tube, detectors or computers. Other technical errors such as changing the crystal photon multiplier technique during the scanning cycle can also produce linear artefacts. Further technical sources of error include incorrect use of window level and window width and faulty patient positioning.

Position of patient's head

Most brain scans are performed with the plane of section of the slices at 10° to 25° Reid's base line since this position was generally more comfortable for the patient with the original scanners and also gives better coverage of the posterior fossa (Fig. 63.7). Figures 63.8A to 63.8F illustrate the appearances of scans obtained in this way.

It is important to realize that the angle of section profoundly affects the apparent localization of a lesion or anatomical structure. Thus a lesion which appears anterior in the higher cuts may be in the parietal and not the frontal lobe. This is because the frontal lobe may be almost excluded from the highest sections, though it is well shown on the lower sections. Conversely the occipital lobes appear large and prominent in the higher sections but small in the lower section. The central fissure separating the frontal and parietal lobes becomes progressively more anterior on the higher sections. However, it is difficult to identify specific fissures and lobe margins on the CT scan.

Modern machines usually contain facilities for obtaining *coronal* and *sagittal* sections by computer reconstruction of the axial slices (Fig. 63.33). Alternatively direct coronal or oblique sagittal slices can be obtained with modern tilting gantries and slew tables.

Enhancement

Soon after the introduction of brain scanning Ambrose *et al.* (1973) showed that pathological lesions in the brain frequently accepted intravenous iodinated contrast media such as those used in pyelography in a manner different from normal brain.

Thus lesions not obvious on the simple scan could be revealed and many others enhanced by the contrast medium. The technique of contrast enhancement scanning has now become routine and has further extended the value of CT scanning.

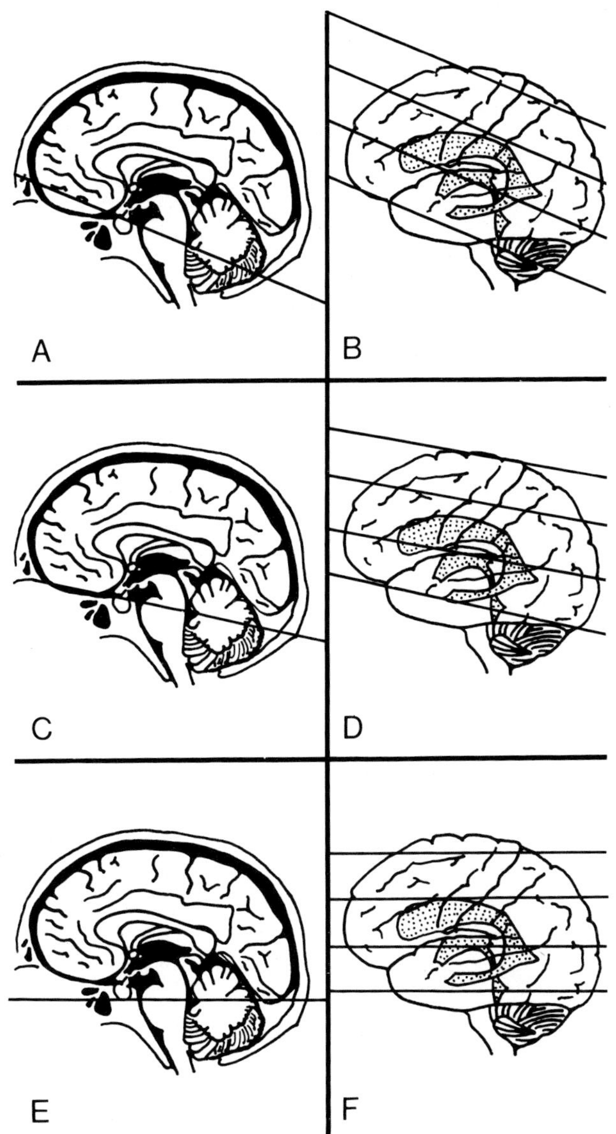

Fig. 63.7 The effect of angulation on scan sections. Planes of section superimposed on the midline and lateral views of the brain. A and B 257 to Reid's base line. C and D 10° to RBL. E and F parallel to RBL.

Different workers have varied the amount of contrast medium used. A dose equivalent to 60–80 ml of Conray or other contrast medium for an average adult given as a bolus is one that is widely accepted. It is usual to inspect the non-enhanced scan first and, if necessary, to proceed to injection of contrast followed immediately by the enhanced scan. It is not necessary to use enhancement in every case. Where the simple scan is normal and the clinical indications are vague it has been shown that the post-enhancement scan is most unlikely to add further information (Barrington and Lewtas, 1977).

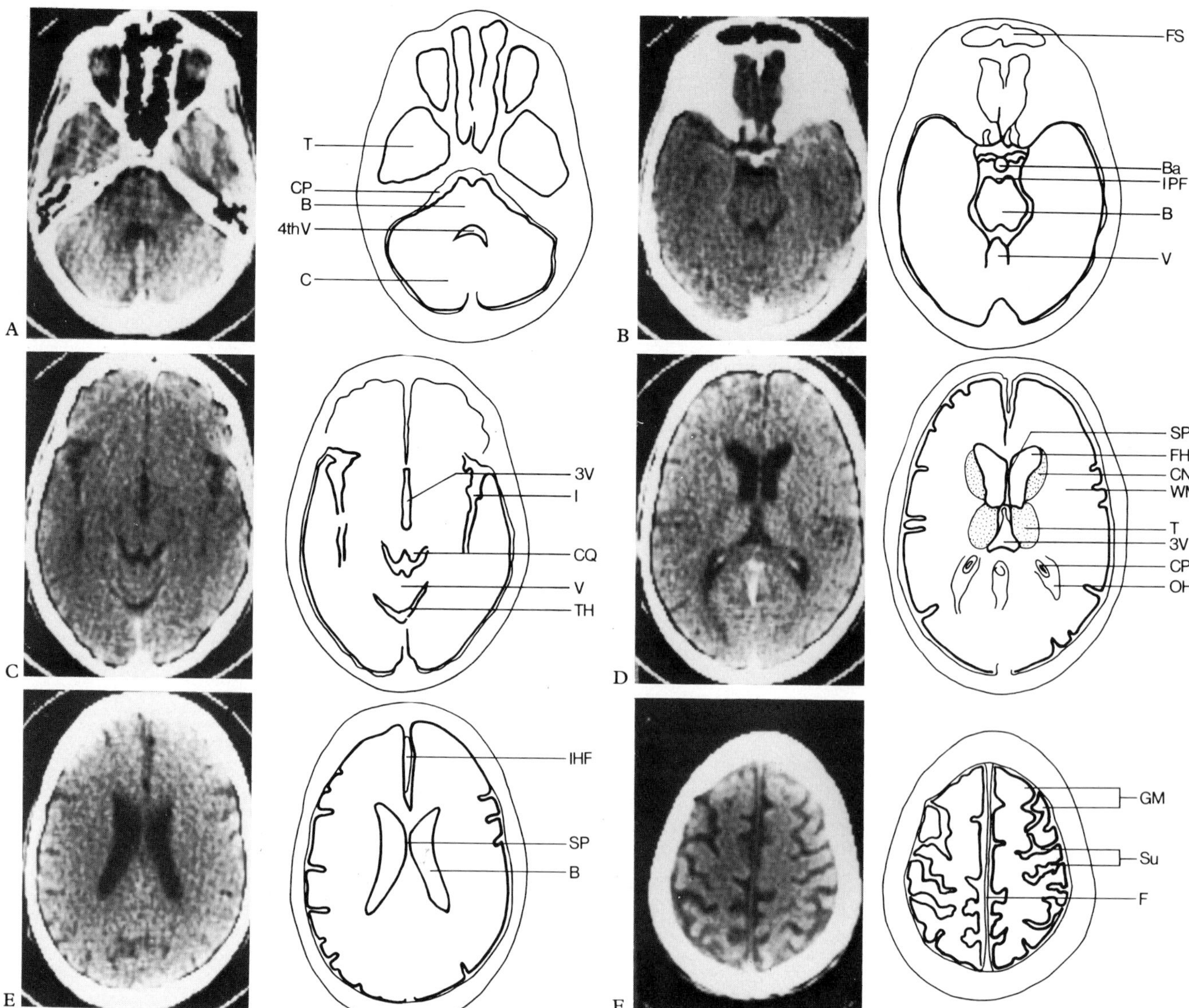

Fig. 63.8 Enhanced scan series in a patient with atrophy, to demonstrate normal anatomy (L34 W75). (A) T = temporal lobe. CP = cerebellopontine angle. B = brainstem. 4thV = 4th ventricle. C = cerebellum. (B) FS = Frontal sinus. Ba = basilar artery. IPF = interpeduncular fossa. V = vermis. (C) 3V = 3rd ventricle. CQ = corpora quadrigemina. TH = tentorial hiatus. (D) FH = frontal horn. SP = septum pellucidum. CN = caudate nucleus. T = thalamus. CP = choroid plexus. OH = occipital horn. WM = white matter. (E) IHF = interhemispheric fissure. B = body of lateral ventricle. (F) GM = grey matter. Su = sulci. F = falx.

Cisternography, Ventriculography and Myelography

The introduction of a safer water-soluble myelography agent in Amipaque (Metrizamide) led to the suggestion that this might be used for cisternography in CT scanning, and also for CT myelography. Following the introduction of Amipaque (3–5 g) by lumbar puncture, the medium is allowed to reach the head, either by diffusion or by deliberately tilting the patient under screen control until some enters the posterior fossa. The medium is well shown by CT scanning and the basal cisterns and sulci are well outlined (Fig. 63.9). Small tumours in the CP angle have been outlined by this technique when they were not obvious on the simple scan or obscured by artefact due to the dense petrous bones.

Normally some contrast will enter and outline the basal cisterns and fourth ventricle within 3 hours, but little or none enters the third and lateral ventricles and at 12 hours most of the contrast is over the cortex. In *communicating hydrocephalus*, however, the contrast will enter and linger in the lateral ventricles for 24 hours and longer, which correlates well with the findings at isotope cisternography. This enables the method to be used as a test for communicating hydrocephalus, parti-

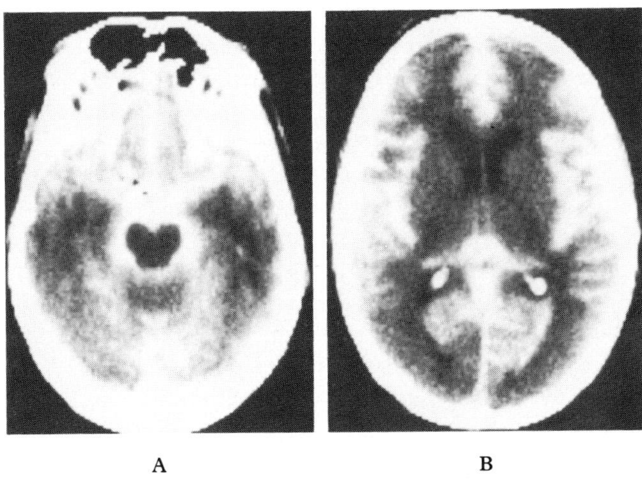

A B

Fig. 63.9 Amipaque cisternography.

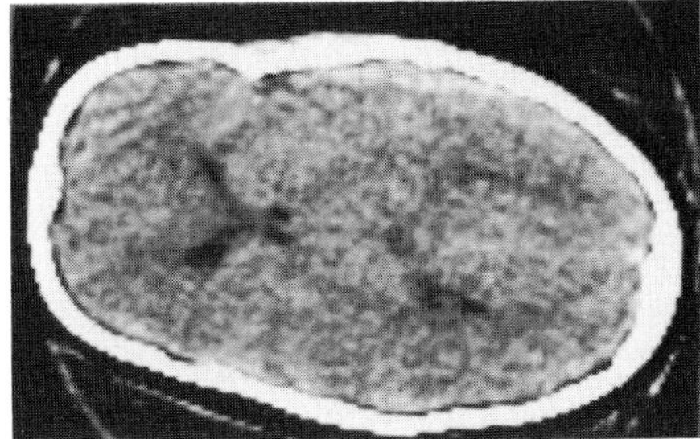

Fig. 63.10 Macrocephaly. The child's head was only fitted into the gantry in lateral position (L36 W80).

cularly for suspected *low pressure hydrocephalus*, which it is important to differentiate from atrophy as a cause of dementia.

The spinal cord is difficult to demonstrate routinely by CT because of the dense bone surrounding the spinal canal. However, with improvement of apparatus and software, routine visualization of the cord is theoretically possible. Hydromyelia and lipomas of the cord have been demonstrated as have some neurofibromas and meningiomas. After injection of the water soluble medium Metrizamide the cord can be routinely shown at all levels by CT.

CONGENITAL LESIONS

These may be divided into the following groups:

1. Lesions producing enlargement of the head
2. Other craniocerebral malformations
3. Phakomatoses
4. Miscellaneous.

LESIONS PRODUCING ENLARGEMENT OF THE HEAD

The cranium may enlarge because of enlargement of the brain, the cerebral ventricles, or the extracerebral spaces.

Enlargement of the brain (macrocephaly). This may occur in association with abnormal attenuation values in the cerebral substance, e.g. leukodystrophies or storage diseases. On the other hand no such alteration of attenuation values may be seen, in which case CT has the merit of excluding a treatable cause such as hydrocephalus, and a diagnosis of congenital idiopathic macrocephaly is made (Fig. 63.10).

Hydrocephalus may be communicating or non-communicating; this distinction depends on the normal direct continuity of the cerebral ventricles with each other and with the subarachnoid space. Although such a distinction cannot always be made at CT, the level of obstruction can be inferred from the extent of ventricular dilatation.

In childhood the large majority of cases are *obstructive*, due to aqueduct stenosis, the Dandy–Walker syndrome or arachnoid cysts. Up to one-third of cases may be of the *communicating* type; in such children the hydrocephalus is often secondary to subarachnoid haemorrhage or meningitis.

Hydrocephalus in *spinal dysraphism* is often associated with a Chiari type 2 malformation (caudal displacement of the pons, medulla, and part of the fourth ventricle). The hydrocephalus is generally not, however, the result of impaction of the hind brain in the foramen magnum, but of associated aqueduct stenosis; occasionally there is communicating hydrocephalus with occlusion of the ambient cistern.

Aqueduct stenosis is usually idiopathic; there is stenosis or occlusion of the aqueduct of Sylvius. It is therefore apparent at CT scanning that the hydrocephalus involves the third and lateral ventricles only (Fig. 63.11). The former is often markedly dilated; its suprapineal recess may be very enlarged, appearing as a

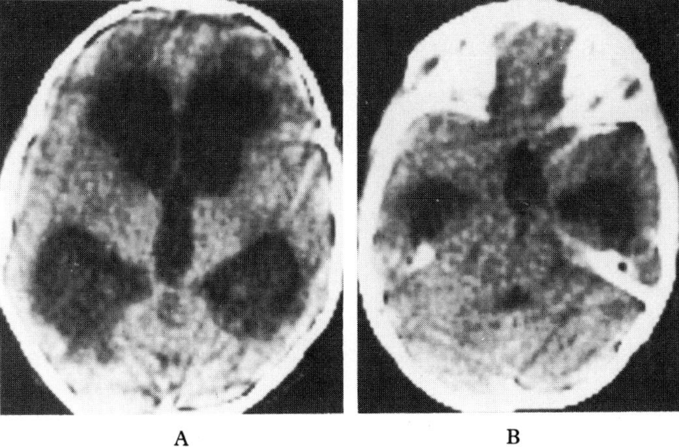

A B

Fig. 63.11 Acqueduct stenosis. Dilated lateral and third ventricles but small 4th ventricle.

rounded posterosuperior extension of cerebrospinal fluid attenuation, which is difficult, or even impossible, to distinguish from an arachnoid cyst. Anteriorly, the third ventricle can be seen extending down to or even into the sella turcica. The fourth ventricle is midline in position, but is low; this latter feature may be difficult to appreciate. It is essential in cases of suspected aqueduct stenosis to make certain that there is no other lesion, such as a midbrain or posterior fossa tumour. The skull vault is usually large and thin. Aqueduct stenosis usually presents in childhood, but may be seen for the first time in adult life. Some neurosurgeons will require ventriculography to confirm the diagnosis before treatment by ventricular shunting.

The Dandy-Walker syndrome has various forms, ranging from extensive malformation of the cerebellum to minor changes in the vermis (Fig. 63.12). It is considerably less common than aqueduct stenosis. Hydrocephalus occurs as a result of more or less complete membranous obstruction to the foramina of Magendie and Luschka, which causes a cystic dilatation of the fourth ventricle. The condition, which may be associated with other congenital anomalies such as meningocoele or defects in the corpus callosum, usually presents in early life, although occasional cases are seen in older children or young adults.

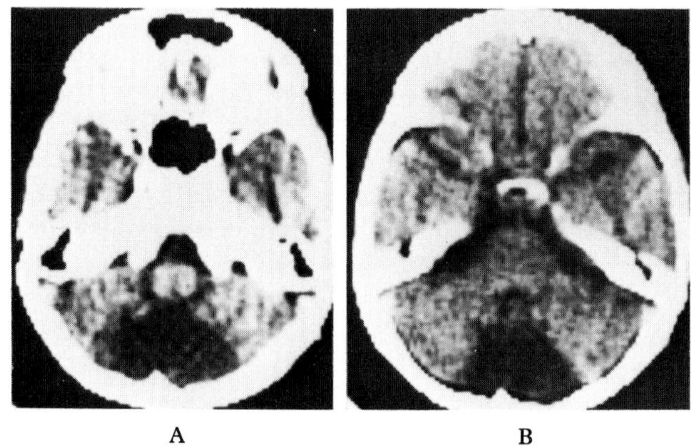

Fig. 63.12 Dandy-Walker syndrome.

CT features are those of a dysplastic cerebellum, often consisting of vestigial hemispheres only, surrounded by a very large cerebrospinal fluid space, limited superolaterally on either side by a straight line representing the tentorium. There is often enlargement of the posterior fossa, evidenced by bulging of the occipital bone, and the cystic infratentorial space separates the occipital lobes and may extend up almost to the lateral ventricles. Dilatation of the lateral and third ventricles is less marked, but the head is enlarged. The dysplastic cerebellum is the key feature in differential diagnosis from an arachnoid cyst or even a cystic tumour.

Arachnoid cysts. Although such cysts may occur anywhere, the classical locations are the suprasellar region, around the posterior end of the third ventricle, and in the middle and posterior cranial fossae. They appear at CT as collections, usually rounded or multilocular, of cerebrospinal fluid density, which may cause hydrocephalus. In each of the classic sites diagnostic confusion may arise:

1. Suprasellar cysts (Fig. 63.13) may be mistaken for dilated anterior third ventricles. The size and rounded configuration of the cyst suggest the correct diagnosis.
2. Posterior third ventricle cysts may mimic a dilated suprapineal recess, since the membrane between them and the ventricle may be extremely thin.
3. A cyst in the temporal fossa (Fig. 63.13C) may be confused with a tumour, e.g. an epidermoid, a chronic subdural haematoma or localized hydrocephalus of the temporal horn. Pneumoencephalography may be required to establish the correct diagnosis.

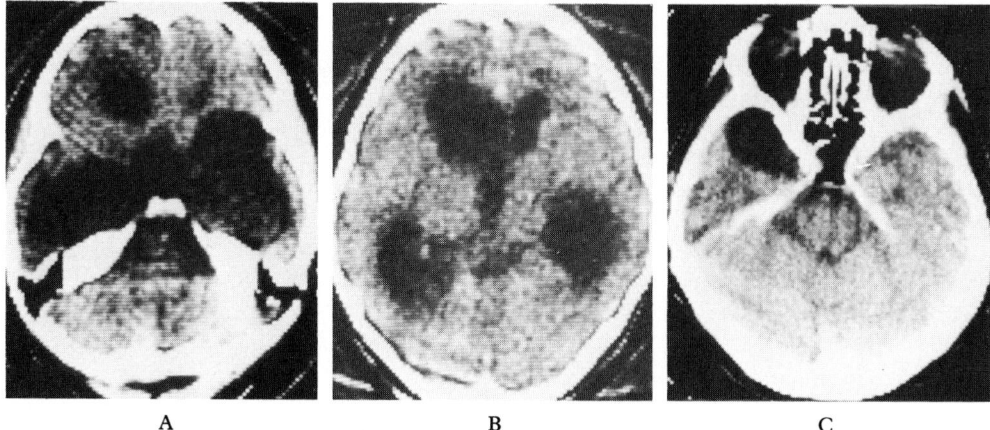

Fig. 63.13 Arachnoid cysts. A and B—Case 1: suprasellar midline arachnoid cyst shown in A with narrow 3rd ventricle displaced up in B and dilated lateral ventricles and temporal horns. C—Case 2: left anterior temporal arachnoid cyst (L36 W80).

Metrizamide CT cisternography may show delayed entry of the contrast medium into the cyst; this is strongly suggestive of the diagnosis.

In most cases of hydrocephalus which are not due to tumours, ventricular shunting is the definitive treatment. However, identification of an arachnoid cyst may enable more specific treatment.

Large *bilateral or unilateral extracerebral collections* may present with enlargement of the head. CT diagnosis depends on recognition of the normal cerebral structures compressed by large low attenuation areas subjacent to the cranial vault, which do not have the form of expanded cerebral ventricles. Distinction from gross hydrocephalus or a cerebral malformation may be vital for adequate treatment.

OTHER CRANIOCEREBRAL MALFORMATIONS

These include defects in cerebral development; encephalocoeles and meningeoceles; hamartomas.

Defects of cerebral development are extremely varied, but fortunately most of the types are rare. *Dysgenesis of the commisural plate* results in *malformation of the corpus callosum*, ranging from *complete agenesis* to minor anomalies. The characteristic abnormality at CT is separation of the medial borders of the lateral ventricles, between which the third ventricle may be seen extending upwards. Involvement of the posterior portion is commonly more severe than that of the anterior portion, and in partial dysgenesis, the anterior horns of the lateral ventricles may be normal. The occipital horns are frequently enlarged, possibly as a result of associated white matter hypoplasia. There may also be cystic dilatation of the suprapineal recess of the third ventricle. A *lipoma* may be present, seen at CT as a round or lobulated zone of density considerably less than that of the adjacent cerebrospinal fluid, with spots or streaks of marginal calcification anterolaterally; such a lipoma may be the only obvious manifestation of this malformation. *Lipoma of the corpus callosum* can often be diagnosed from the plain radiographic appearances (see Ch. 58).

Holoprosencephaly is a rare, more severe malformation, which involves both the brain and the facial structures, the cerebral manifestations. The cerebral ventricles are represented by a single cavity, often expanded posteriorly as a thin-walled sac. The falx cerebri is absent.

Hydranencephaly is the most severe form of cerebral dysplasia. The falx is present and the posterior fossa structures and basal ganglia usually appear relatively normal, but the upper part of the cerebrum is replaced by cerebrospinal fluid (Fig. 63.14). It may be impossible at CT to differentiate this condition from extreme hydrocephalus or massive bilateral extracerebral fluid collections.

Septo-optic dysplasia (de Morsier's disease) consists of

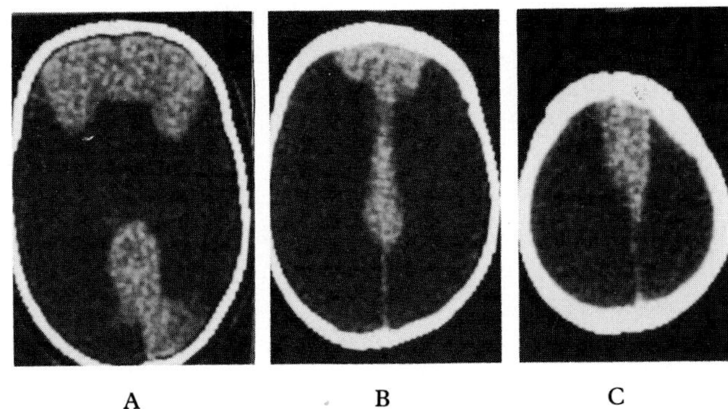

Fig. 63.14 Hydrancephaly (L36 W80).

defective development of the anterior optic pathways, with consequent hypoplasia of the optic nerves and chiasm and absence of the septum pellucidum. CT demonstration of optic nerve hypoplasia may be difficult, as the morphological changes may be minor. Absence of the septum pellucidum (which may also occur as an isolated defect) can be recognized however, since it is associated with absence of the normal invagination of the ventricular wall anteromedially.

The *Arnold Chiari malformation* has been discussed above.

Encephalocoeles and meningocoeles are usually evident clinically, but basal lesions, e.g. ethmoidal encephalocoeles, may only be identified radiologically. The contribution of CT is to show basal bone defects, to indicate the nature of the herniated structures and their relationship to adjacent portions of the brain and to demonstrate the commonly associated abnormalities such as hydrocephalus. Fronto-ethmoidal lesions may cause hypertelorism; coronal CT sections are frequently required to assess the relationships of the basal structures in this condition, especially when surgical correction is considered.

Hamartomas are congenital tumours, and include *dermoids*, *epidermoids* and *nasal gliomas* in addition to non-specific lesions. They may have intra- and extracranial components, and affect the cranium, usually with expansion of the diploic spaces. The fat-containing dermoids and epidermoids are characterized by low-attenuation values at CT, but these may not be lower than those of cerebrospinal fluid. Calcification is not uncommon in congenital tumours. The suprasellar region is one of the commonest sites for non-specific hamartomas. Lesions in this region are associated with precocious puberty, but vision is usually unimpaired. Since the attenuation values of these tumours are similar to those of brain both before and after intravenous contrast medium, they may be overlooked unless special attention is paid to this region; absence of the normal interpeduncular fossa and chiasmatic cistern may be the crucial observation.

PHAKOMATOSES

Included under this heading are the *neuroectodermal dysplasias*. There are numerous subdivisions and rare variations, but those of major radiological interest are *neurofibromatosis*, *tuberous sclerosis*, the *Sturge-Weber syndrome* and *Von Hippel-Lindau disease*. These hereditory conditions are characterized by the association of skin lesions with malformations and tumours which may involve any organ, but show a predilection for the nervous system. Tumour formation is not, however, a feature of the Sturge-Weber syndrome.

Neurofibromatosis (multiple neurofibromatosis; Von Recklinghausen's disease) is divided into *peripheral* and *central* types, of which the latter is of more neuroradiological interest. There are two main types of abnormality which may be demonstrated at CT—*developmental anomalies* and *tumour formation*.

Of the *developmental anomalies* of the skull and its contents, by far the commonest is dysplasia of the sphenoid bone (Fig. 63.15). The greater wing is often

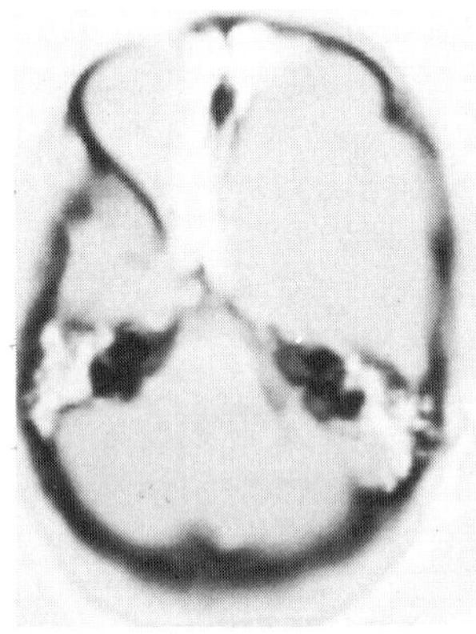

Fig. 63.15 Neurofibromatosis showing absence of sphenoid wing on the right. Reversal negative at wider window for bone detail (L10 W100).

completely absent, while both the lesser wing and the basisphenoid are commonly affected. CT shows a bony defect of variable size, sometimes involving only the region adjacent to the optic canal, more often an absence of the entire posterolateral wall of the orbit. The middle cranial fossa is expanded and the adjacent temporal lobe may herniate into the orbit, displacing the optic nerve and causing proptosis. The optic canal may also be large. It should be understood that both these anomalies are usually independent of any tumour formation. Asymmetry of the orbits, which may be abnormally large or small, is not uncommon; the ocular globe of the affected side is often expanded (buphthalmos), with loss of the normal regular shape.

The entire cranium may show hemihypertrophy or atrophy.

Approximately one-tenth of patients with neurofibromatosis are mentally retarded, and CT sometimes gives evidence of generalized or focal atrophy. Less commonly, heterotopic grey matter, cerebral hemihypertrophy or other malformations may be present.

Intracranial or intraorbital *tumours* are present in up to half of patients with the central form of this disease. The commonest is the optic nerve glioma, manifest at CT as fusiform but often rather bulbous widening and increased attenuation of the intraorbital portion of the nerve, with homogenous enhancement after intravenous contrast medium. Such a tumour may extend backwards to the optic chiasm, or may arise there. Further spread around the midbrain in the optic tracts has been observed. Intracranial extension, manifest as expansion of the chiasm, which comes to fill the interpeduncular fossa, is a grave prognostic sign, and should be carefully sought for when the patient is first seen and at subsequent examinations.

Optic nerve sheath meningiomas are rare tumours, but show an increased incidence in neurofibromatosis. They generally appear at CT as increased attenuation rather than expansion of the optic nerve, sometimes with calcification and with marked enhancement after intravenous contrast medium. As with optic nerve gliomas, intracranial tumour, expansion of the optic canal on the affected side and possible involvement of the opposite optic nerve should always be sought for.

Neuromas show a greatly increased incidence in neurofibromatosis, especially acoustic neuromas, whose characteristic appearances are described below.

The demonstration of bilateral acoustic neuromas is virtually pathognomomic of the systemic disease. Other cranial nerves may also be affected. In the plexiform neuroma of the fifth cranial nerve, all the soft tissues in the distribution of one or more divisions appear thickened; similar hypertrophy of the skin and subcutaneous tissues may, however, occur as an isolated phenomenon. Cutaneous and subcutaneous neuromas may be seen incidentally when CT examination is carried out for other reasons.

Cerebral and *intracranial meningeal tumours* also occur more commonly in neurofibromatosis, but their appearances are not specific for that disease.

Heavy calcification of one or more *choroid plexuses* is a rare but classical feature of the condition; it is said to indicate benign tumefaction.

Normal calcification in the pineal and choroid plexuses is regularly identified at CT scanning. Calcification in the *basal ganglia* is also readily identified (Fig. 63.16) whether idiopathic or secondary.

Tuberous sclerosis (epiloia; adenoma sebaceum; Bourneville's disease) is a complex syndrome with dominant inheritance characterized by the formation of multiple congenital tumour-like lesions in the skin, brain

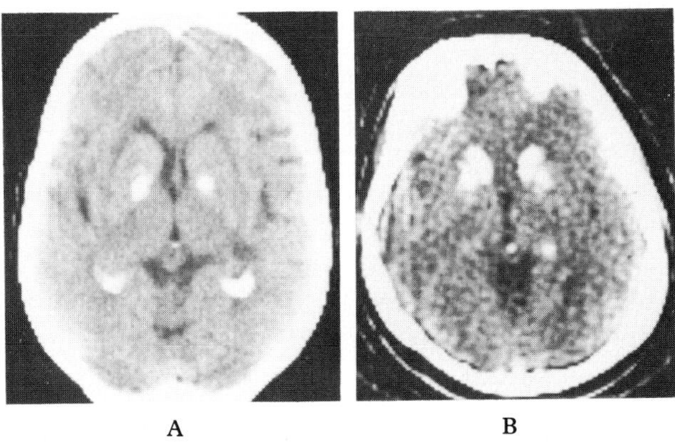

Fig. 63.16 Idiopathic calcification of the basal ganglia—two separate cases (L36 W80).

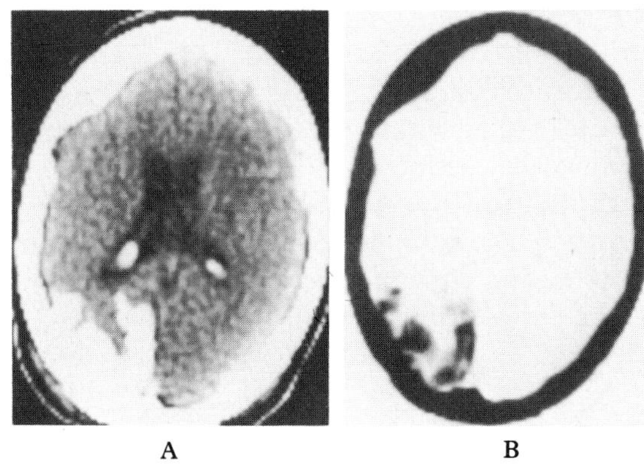

Fig. 63.17 A—Sturge-Weber syndrome. Occipital cortical calcification (L40 W75). B—Characteristic nature shown better at wide window (L200 W400).

and viscera (particularly the kidneys and lungs). Patients present with epilepsy, mental defect, or rarely with symptoms of raised intracranial pressure. In children with epilepsy the diagnosis is usually supected because of the cutaneous stigmata, but these may not be apparent in the early years of life. The role of CT scanning is to confirm the diagnosis, which is of importance as regards genetic counselling. The characteristic finding is of multiple, small, calcified foci in relation to the walls of the lateral ventricles. Occasionally, the nodules are only slightly denser than normal brain but become more apparent with intravenous contrast medium. Small areas of cortical dysplasia and more or less widespread cerebral atrophy may also be present. Plain radiography can be used to detect the calcified lesions, but only about half of those shown by CT are visible on the skull films; this is particularly true in the first few years of life.

About 15 per cent of patients with tuberous sclerosis subsequently develop intracranial tumours, often during adolescence. These are generally glial tumours; although normally of very low grade malignancy, they are occasionally glioblastomas. A characteristic feature is that they tend to develop in the region of the foramen of Monro; at CT they appear as rounded masses of slightly increased attenuation, often with adjacent flecks of calcification, causing obstructive hydrocephalus. Intravenous contrast medium causes little or no change, as is usually the case with low grade malignancy tumours. The combination of such a tumour and paraventricular calcification is virtually pathognomonic.

The **Sturge-Weber syndrome** consists of the combination of a cutaneous naevus, of 'port-wine stain' type, usually following the distribution of one or more divisions of the trigeminal nerve, a meningeal angiomatosis and calcification of the underlying cerebrum. Patients present with the cutaneous lesion, epilepsy and neurological deficits corresponding to the cerebral lesion. CT demonstrates calcification and atrophy of the affected portion of the cerebrum, often more extensive than suggested by plain skull films. The serpiginous nature of the calcification familiar from plain radiographs may be apparent only when the scans are viewed with a wide window width (Fig. 63.17). Enhancement of the affected portion of the brain may occur with intravenous contrast medium, but this is difficult to assess in the presence of heavy calcification. The skin lesion and the intracranial anomalies are usually on the same side, but one of the contributions of CT in this condition is the occasional demonstration of bilateral cerebral changes; this may be of importance if hemispherectomy is being considered because of intractable epilepsy.

Tumour formation is not a feature of this condition.

MISCELLANEOUS CONGENITAL CONDITIONS

Disease affecting the cranial bones include *craniosynostosis*, *fibrous dysplasia*, *achondroplasia* and certain *tumours*. There are, of course, numerous other rare conditions producing changes detectable by CT, but the demonstration of these changes is of little practical importance.

In *craniosynostosis* fusion of the sutures, with thickening of the vault both adjacent to the sutures and more widely can be shown by CT. Hydrocephalus may be present.

Fibrous dysplasia is manifest as simple thickening of the cranial vault and particularly the bones of the base and facial skeleton. In severe cases, the whole cranium is abnormally thick, with a bony texture which may vary from strikingly homogeneous to very irregular. Cysts may be present and when the rare complication of malignant transformation supervenes, irregular erosion may be apparent.

In *achondroplasia*, the craniofacial disproportion, due to the small skull base, is obvious. The commonest significant CT finding is associated communicating hydrocephalus.

Some developmental tumours, e.g. *epidermoids* may arise within the diploic space. They are seen at CT as low attenuation intraosseous expanding lesions, which may extend wither within the cranium or external to it. Intravenous contrast medium is usually without effect.

Metabolic and dystrophic diseases affecting the cerebrum include the storage diseases—*lipoidoses* and *gangliosidoses* and conditions with defective development of myelin, the *leukodystrophies*. The common finding at CT is abnormally low attenuation of the cerebral white matter. This may be generalized (e.g. in Tay-Sachs disease or spongiform degeneration), predominantly frontal (e.g. Alexander's disease) or occipital (adreno-leukodystrophy or Schilder's disease). Macrocephaly—enlargement of the brain and skull—may also be present (Alexander's disease, spongiform degeneration, Tay-Sach's disease), or there may be associated hydrocephalus (Hurler's disease, Hunter's disease). In adrenoleuko-dystrophy, the abnormal areas may show marginal enhancement with intravenous contrast medium.

Although characteristic, the white matter low attenuation is not specific and may be seen in other inherited disorders, e.g. *ocular myopathy*, or in acquired diseases such as *postinfective leukoencephalopathy*.

Porencephaly is generally the result of some pre- or perinatal vascular compromise, the end result of which is seen at CT as a rounded area of low attenuation, often apparently in contact or in continuity with a lateral ventricle, and sometimes with mass effect; the overlying portion of the skull vault may even be expanded. There are frequently associated atrophic changes, corroborative evidence of damage to the affected hemisphere.

Almost any form of *intracranial tumour*, particularly gliomas, cerebellar neoplasms and craniopharyngiomas, may be present at birth. Their CT features are those of acquired tumours, and are therefore described below under tumours.

INTRACRANIAL TUMOURS

Tumours within the skull may be either *intracerebral* or *extracerebral*—this distinction is extremely important with respect to treatment and prognosis. It cannot always be made with certainty on the basis of CT evidence alone, but in a large percentage of cases the scan, together with other invasive investigations as indicated in the individual case, can give vital pre-operative information. Classification and incidence of intracranial tumours is discussed in Chapter 56.

SUPRATENTORIAL TUMOURS

Intracerebral tumours encountered in the supratentorial compartment include:

Primary tumours
- glioma—astrocytoma
  - spongioblastoma
  - oligodendroglioma
  - microglioma
- ependymoma
- pineal tumours
- dermoid and epidermoid (these are more commonly extra-cerebral)
- intraventricular tumours—colloid cyst
  - papilloma of the choroid plexus
  - meningioma
- haemangioblastoma

Secondary tumours
- metastasis
- lymphoma

Gliomas. Tumours of the *glioma* series together with metastatic lesions are by far the commonest. The former are graded I–IV depending on the proportions of mitotic figures they show. Grades I and II are sometimes (incorrectly) called 'benign', while grades III and IV are termed 'glioblastomas'. As with cerebral angiography, the changes at CT reflect in a general fashion the degree of malignancy of the tumour (Figs. 63.18 to 63.23).

The commonest patterns are:

1. An ill-defined area of variably reduced attenuation lying anywhere within a cerebral hemisphere, compressing the ventricular system and displacing the midline structures. Large lesions often produce contralateral hydrocephalus. The low attenuation is often largely or exclusively confined to the cerebral white matter.

2. A similar area, but with patchily increased and decreased attenuation.

3. A well-defined, often rather rounded area of low attenuation, with nodules of less diminished attenuation within it. This pattern frequently represents a cystic tumour.

4. A more or less completely calcified lesion of any form, often irregular. Such a pattern is commoner with the less malignant tumours, and with oligodendrogliomas.

It may be difficult or impossible to differentiate the tumour itself from surrounding oedema, which is usually present. For this reason, intravenous contrast medium injection is indicated in all cases of suspected glioma. It is essential that postinjection scans should encompass the entire region which appears abnormal on the un-enhanced scans, since otherwise the presence of a relatively small tumour nodule in an extensive area of oedema may be overlooked.

Most gliomas will show some uptake of the contrast medium, often patchy or circumferential; this is related to breakdown of the blood-brain barrier rather than to tumour vascularity. More than 95 per cent of glioblastomas enhance with contrast medium, usually in a

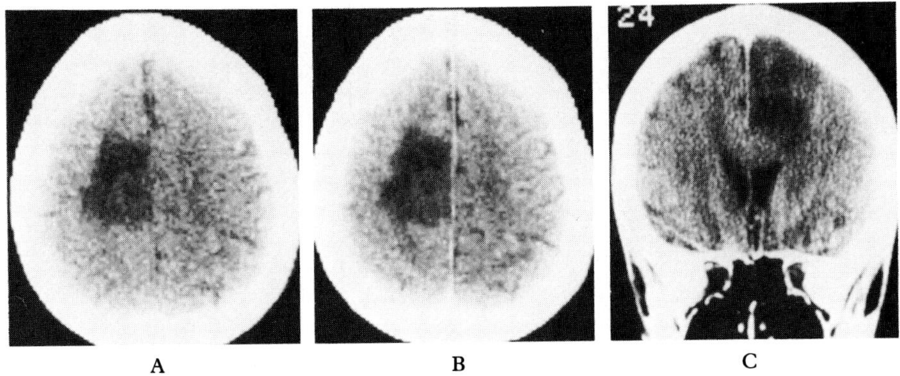

Fig. 63.18 Low grade glioma. A—Low attenuation left parasagittal area with no mass effect in axial cut. B—No enhancement after contrast. C—Coronal section shows slight mass effect depressing roof of L. lateral ventricle (L46 W80).

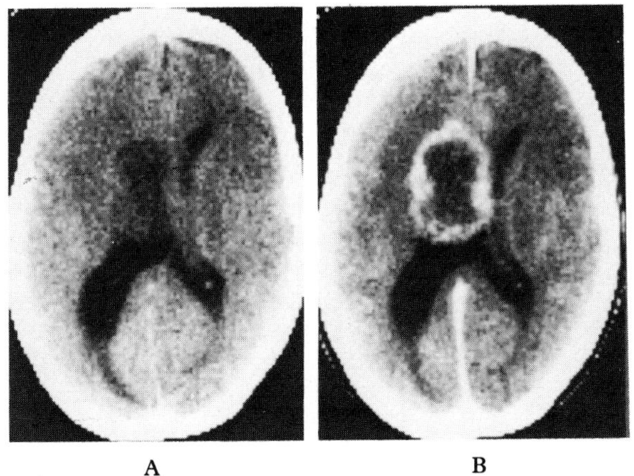

Fig. 63.19 Cystic glioma: A—before enhancement; B—postenhancement (L36 W80).

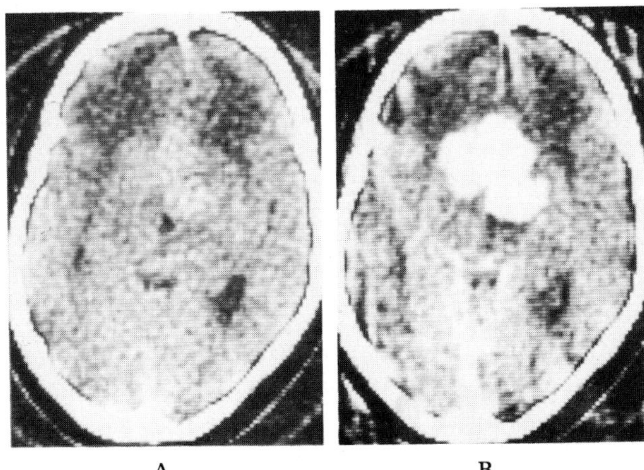

Fig. 63.20 Glioma involving the corpus callosum. High attenuation lesion enhancing strongly with contrast. Oedema of frontal lobes (L30 W80).

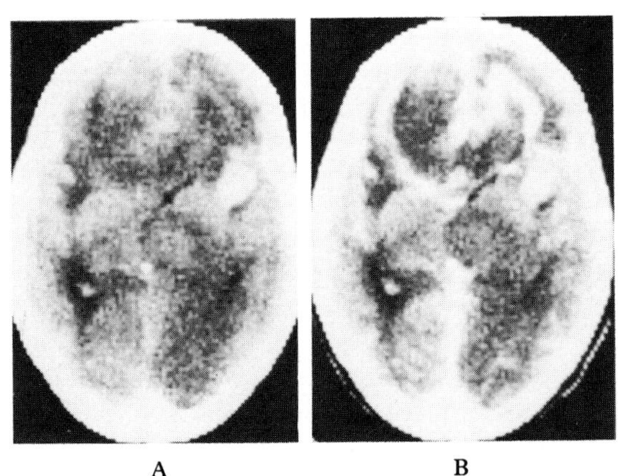

Fig. 63.21 Butterfly glioma involving corpus callosum and frontal lobes. Mixed attenuation lesion with serpiginous enhancement (L36 W80).

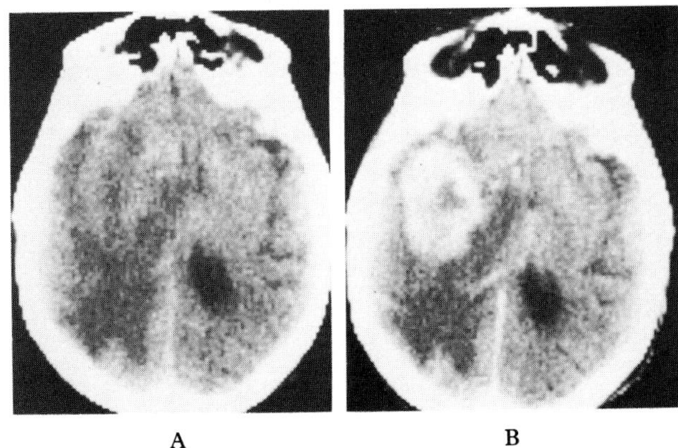

Fig. 63.22 Malignant glioma: A—mixed attenuation lesion with much oedema; B—marked enhancement after contrast (L30 W100).

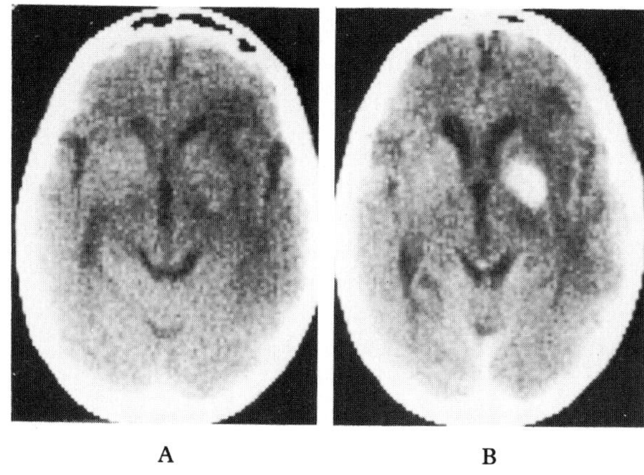

A B

Fig. 63.23 Microglioma: A—before; B—after contrast. Isodense tumour with some surrounding oedema but little mass effect. Strong enhancement after contrast (L38 W100).

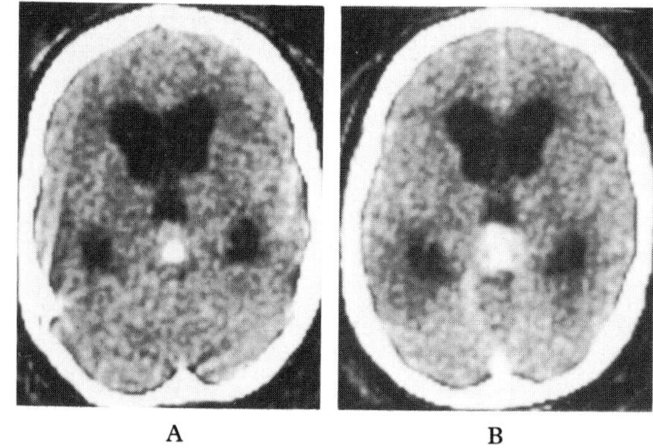

A B

Fig. 63.24 Pineal tumour: A—isodense mass with calcification indenting back of 3rd ventricle; B—enhancement after contrast (L36 W80).

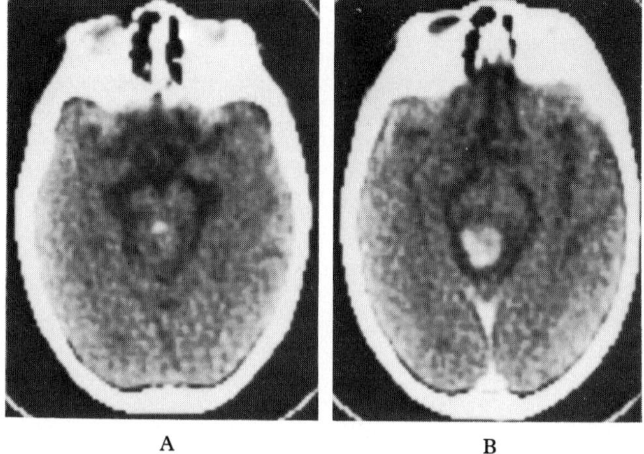

A B

Fig. 63.25A—Pineal tumour. Isodense mass with calcification projecting down onto brainstem. B—Enhancement with contrast (L34 W75).

strikingly irregular manner. Enhancement is least common and least marked in grade I astrocytomas (Fig. 63.18).

Completely normal scans, even without the use of contrast medium, are extremely rare in proven cases of glioma. This is in contrast to cerebral angiography and radioisotope scanning, both of which are not uncommonly negative or equivocal in the presence of extensive, low-grade, infiltrating tumours.

Interpretation of follow up CT examinations after surgery and radiotherapy of gliomas is complicated by the occurrence of radiation necrosis. This can give rise to masses of mixed attenuation, which may show marked contrast enhancement. Diagnosis of tumour recurrence must therefore be made with some caution in such cases.

The major difference between the CT appearances of *oligodendrogiomas* and those described above is the much greater incidence of calcification (more than 50 per cent), a fact which is related to their more indolent nature. In the low-grade tumours, calcification and some mass effect may be the only abnormalities at CT, since these lesions are not usually surrounded by extensive cerebral oedema and often show little or no enhancement.

Microgliomas are related to lymphomas and show an increased incidence in patients with deficient or suppressed immunity, such as those with renal transplants. They characteristically arise in the basal ganglia, but are commonly multifocal and appear at CT in one of two ways: as low-attenuation infiltrating lesions, showing little or no change after intravenous contrast medium, or as well-defined, rounded, high-attenuation nodules, showing marked enhancement. In the latter case, they may be difficult to distinguish from metastases or even granulomas (Fig. 63.23).

Pineal region tumours (often grouped together as 'pinealomas') may be of various histological types, e.g. germinoma, pinealocytoma and glioma, with corresponding variations in invasiveness, prognosis and CT appearances. Correlations between the histological and radiological features are rendered difficult by the fact that many of these lesions are treated by ventricular shunting and external radiotherapy, without biopsy. The commonest CT picture is of a rounded mass lesion of the same attenuation as the surrounding brain (or slightly higher), enclosing or adjacent to the calcified pineal gland (Figs. 63.24 and 63.25). The tumour bulges forwards into the dilated third ventricle, indenting its posterior end, and backwards into the quadrigeminal cistern, which is obliterated. There is often marked enhancement with intravenous contrast medium. Pineal tumours may also be of low or high attenuation; at operation some are found to be cystic, but the attenuation values may not indicate this fact. Surrounding oedema is characteristically absent.

Extension through the ventricular system, particularly into the suprasellar region, is an uncommon but characteristic feature of these tumours; they may present as suprasellar masses.

Dermoid and epidermoid tumours are, as noted above, more commonly extracerebral. Their characteristic features are therefore described below.

Colloid cyst of the third ventricle (paraphyseal cyst) occurs in one classical site: the posterior margin of the foramen of Monro. It therefore tends to cause obstructive hydrocephalus at an early stage and most patients present with symptoms of raised intracranial pressure when the tumour is relatively small. The CT appearances of this tumour are also characteristic: it is seen as a rounded area of raised attenuation, but without calcification, at the base of the septum pellucidum, without surrounding oedema, and unchanged after intravenous contrast medium (Fig. 63.26). This picture is so suggestive that most of these tumours are operated upon without further radiological investigation. Occasionally the cysts are isodense but the diagnosis should still be suggested.

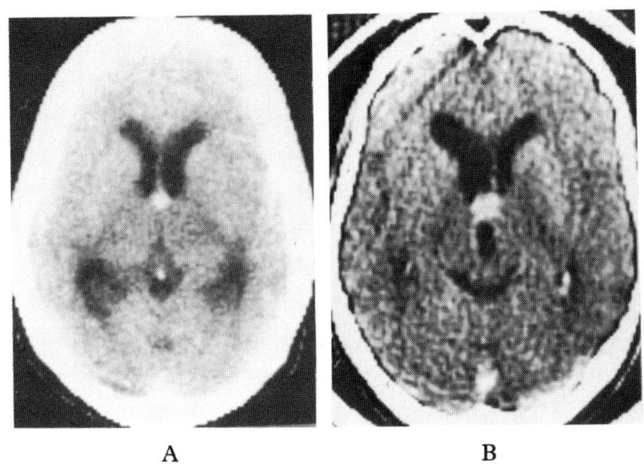

Fig. 63.26 Colloid cysts. Two separate cases. A—Case 1 unenhanced (L36 W80). B—Case 2 enhanced (L34 W75).

Papilloma of the choroid plexus usually arises in relation to the trigone or temporal horn of the lateral ventricle; the fourth ventricle is less commonly affected. It appears at CT as a rounded, well-defined mass of increased attenuation, occasionally calcified, which shows marked enhancement with intravenous contrast medium. Hydrocephalus is often present, and is commonly of marked degree; the temporal or occipital horns on the affected side may be loculated.

Intraventricular meningioma has appearances very similar to those of choroid plexus papilloma; the presence of oedema in the adjacent brain is more in favour of meningioma.

Ependymomas arise from the ependyma lining the ventricles and, depending on their maximum extension, may come to resemble either cerebral gliomas or intraventricular meningioma, but they are usually less regular in form and contrast enhancement than the latter.

Supratentorial haemangioblastomas are very rare, usually being seen in association with cerebellar lesions in von Hippel-Lindau disease. The characteristic appearances are described below.

Metastases. The site and form of metastases are highly variable (Figs. 63.27 to 63.30). They may be of reduced or increased attenuation, and the large majority show obvious enhancement with intravenous contrast medium. In general, there is no clear correlation

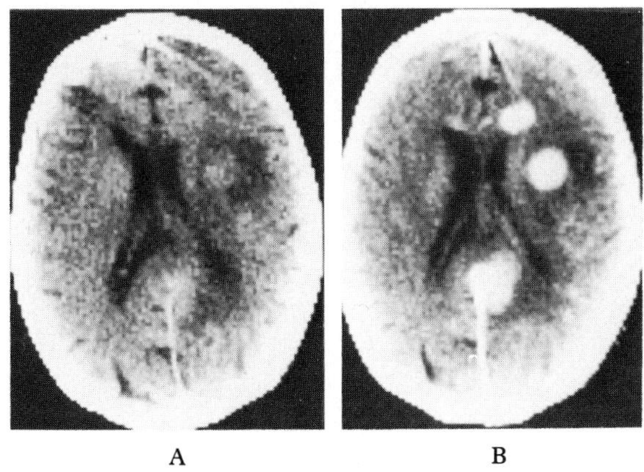

Fig. 63.27 Metastases. Three separate lesions, all isodense and enhancing strongly with contrast. Oedema around the larger secondaries (L40 W60).

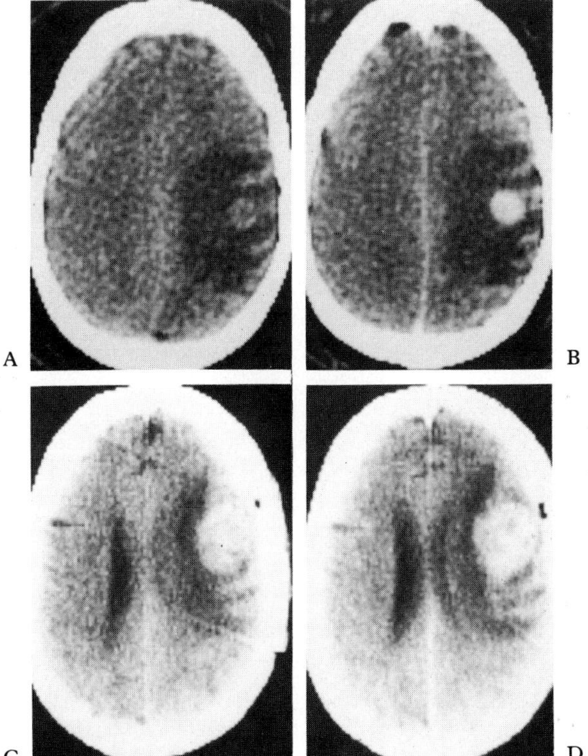

Fig. 63.28 A and B—Metastasis. Small isodense enhancing tumour with marked oedema (L36 W80). C and D—Secondary melanoma. Large high density tumour with some enhancement and much oedema (L36 W80).

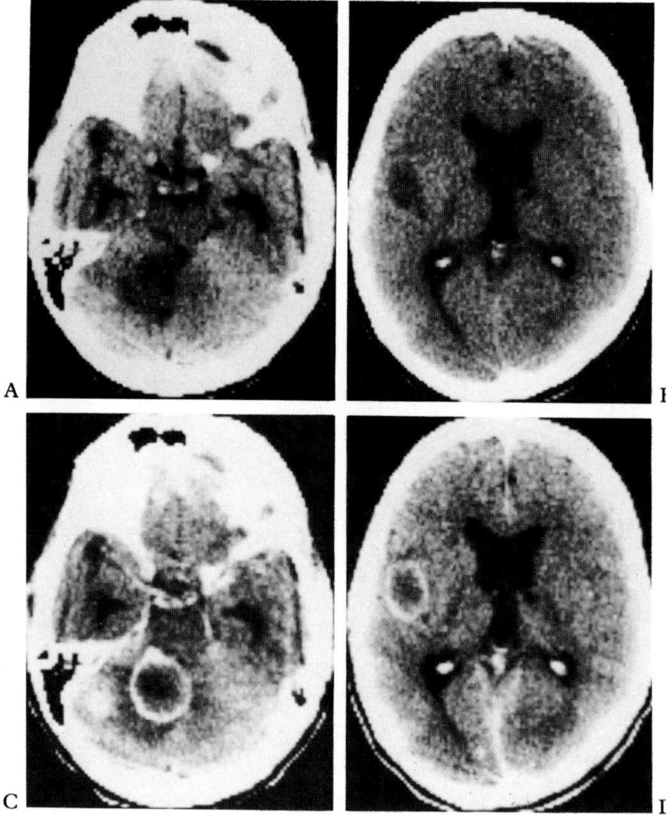

Fig. 63.29 A and B—Metastases. Two low density lesions, one in L. cerebellum and one in L. temporal lobe. C and D—After contrast there is ring enhancement of both tumours (L40 W80).

between CT appearances and histology. Haemorrhagic metastases are characteristic of malignant melanoma, while calcified lesions, although very rare, suggest primary colonic or osseous tumours. Associated cerebral oedema is often extensive and the association of a small, markedly enhancing tumour, even if solitary, with widespread oedema is strongly suggestive of a secondary deposit. The diagnosis is facilitated by the appropriate preceding history or by the demonstration of multiple lesions. Differential diagnosis includes primary malignant tumours and granulomas.

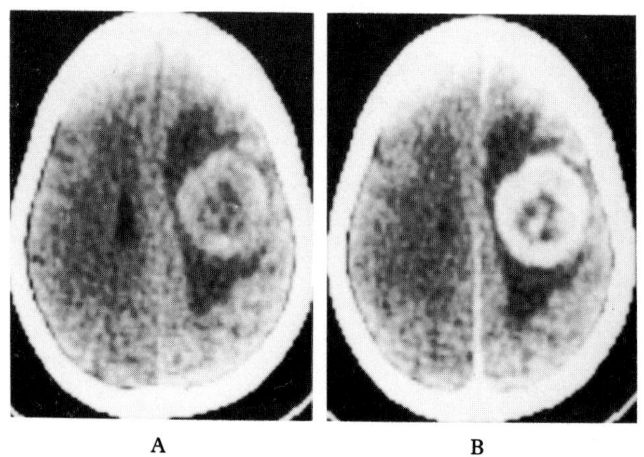

Fig. 63.30 Lymphoma. Mixed density lesion with marked enhancement (L34 W75).

EXTRACEREBRAL TUMOURS

Extracerebral supratentorial tumours include *meningioma*, *dermoid*, *epidermoid*, *pituitary adenoma* and *craniopharyngioma*. *Trigeminal neuromas* and *chordomas* may extend upwards from the posterior fossa, while *tumours involving the skull vault* occasionally expand inwards, affecting the brain. The latter phenomenon is seen with *osteochondroma* of the frontal sinus and with *ossifying fibroma* of the ethmoid or sphenoid sinuses. *Sarcoma* of the skull vault (most commonly seen in association with Paget's disease) can also extend intracranially, as can *myeloma*, in the form of a solitary plasmacytoma. *Extradural deposits* of carcinoma or reticulosis are rarely encountered, as is direct spread of primary or metastatic tumours of the skull base.

Certain benign lesions enter into the differential diagnosis of extracerebral tumours, e.g. *subdural haematoma*, *arachnoid cyst* and *giant aneurysm*. These are discussed below.

Meningiomas (Figs. 63.31 to 63.35) tend to arise in characteristic sites and this fact, coupled with their typical CT appearances, facilitates correct diagnosis. Many of the tumours arise in the parasagittal region, or

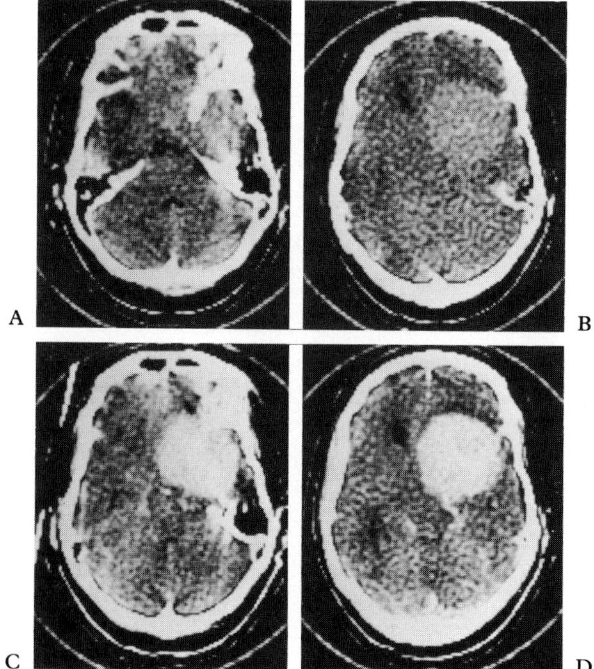

Fig. 63.31 A and B—Meningioma of sphenoidal ridge. Spherical high density lesion (L36 W75). C and D—Show marked enhancement. No significant oedema.

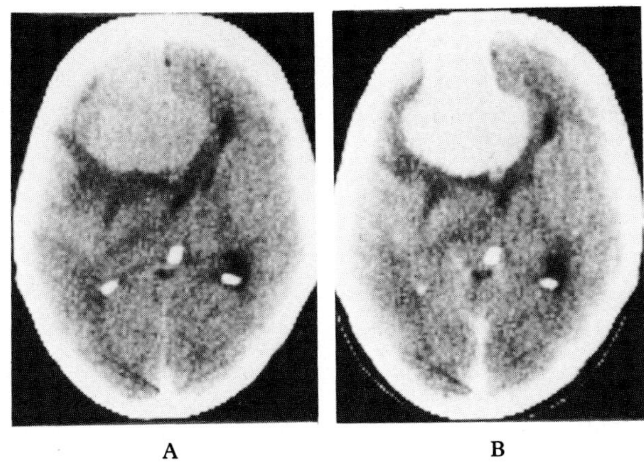

Fig. 63.32 A—Frontal meningioma. High density tumour with some surrounding oedema. B—Marked enhancement after contrast (L44 W80).

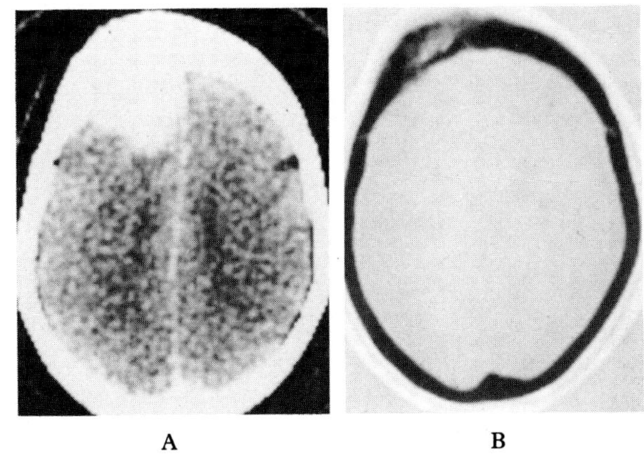

Fig. 63.34 A—Frontal meningioma with bone involvement. Enhanced view at (L36 W75). B—Reversal print at wide window to show the bone involvement (L80 W400).

over the cerebral convexities. The sphenoid ridge and the tuberculum sellae and cribiform plate area are also common sites. Less frequently, meningiomas arise from the cavernous sinus region or from the tentorium; in the latter case they may extend into both the supra- and infratentorial compartments. Meningiomas confined to the infratentorial region are discussed below.

Even before intravenous contrast medium, the CT scan shows very characteristic features in many cases of meningioma. The tumour usually appears as a well-defined rounded mass of increased attenuation, with H values 40–75. Calcification is present in about one-fifth of cases, with attenuation coefficients up to 300. Enhancement with intravenous contrast medium is well marked and clearly outlines the tumour. Cystic meningiomas do exist, but they are rare. The degree of surrounding oedema is very variable; although it is more commonly minimal or absent, up to 20 per cent of meningiomas will show moderate or very extensive oedema. Contralateral extension is an important complication of parasagittal tumours, and should be carefully sought for on the CT scan. Multiple tumours are seen in about 5 per cent of cases. Less typical are the lesions

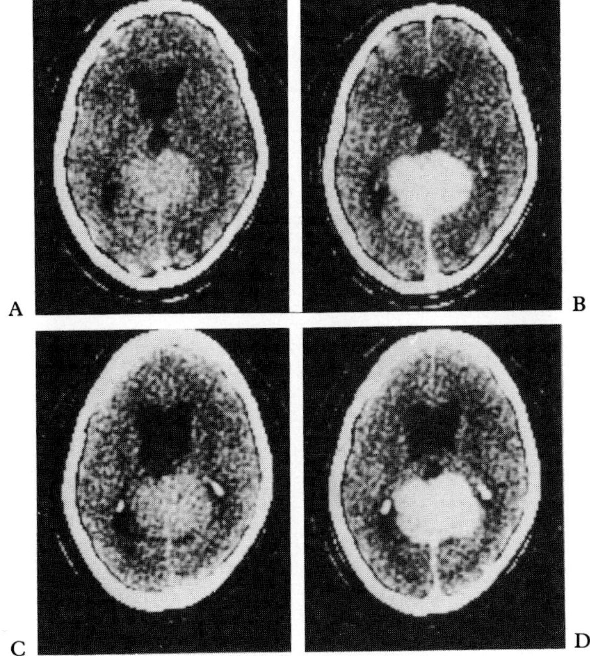

Fig. 63.35 Meningioma at the tentorial apex: A and B—before; C and D—after contrast (L36 W75).

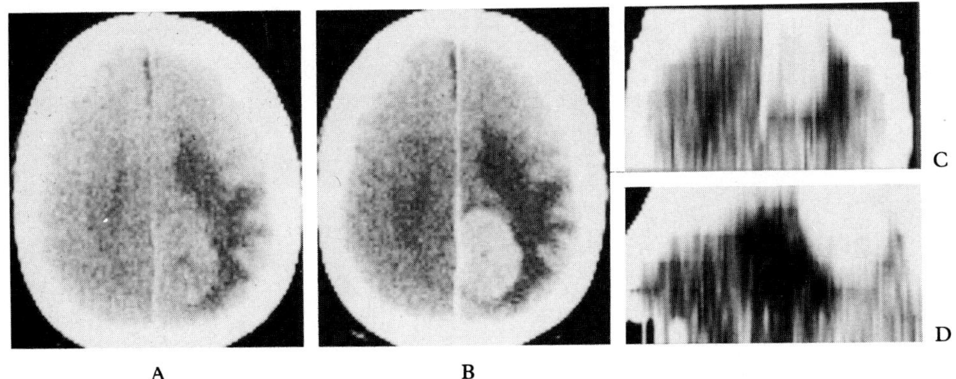

Fig. 63.33 A—Parasagittal meningioma. Tumour of slightly increased density with surrounding oedema. B—Marked enhancement (L36 W80). C—Coronal reconstruction. D—Sagittal reconstruction (L20 W40).

around the cavernous sinus, which tend to be of a more infiltrating, '*en plaque*' variety. At a stage when neurological abnormalities are prominent, tumours in this site may be difficult to distinguish from the normal slightly increased attenuation and contrast enhancement of the cavernous sinus. Some sphenoid ridge meningiomas may be totally of the *en plaque* variety, and manifest at CT only by thickening and increased density of the sphenoid bone on one side. Osseous changes should be sought (by viewing the CT picture with a wide window) in any case of suspected meningioma, as their presence further supports the diagnosis.

The differential diagnosis includes metastasis, glioma, pituitary adenoma and, very important in the case of basal lesions, giant aneurysm.

Epidermoid tumours are usually of low attenuation, often less than c.s.f., and fail to enhance with contrast medium (Fig. 63.36).

Pituitary adenomas. Clinically, pituitary adenomas may be divided into two major groups: (1) endocrinologically active tumours, which often cause only minor expansion of the pituitary and the sella turcica, and (2) inactive tumours, usually of chromophobe type, which present as mass lesions with visual problems. Characteristically a bitemporal hemianopia due to chiasmal compression is found and, less commonly, disturbances of eye movement. Paradoxically, eosinophil tumours producing acromegaly, not infrequently present in the second fashion.

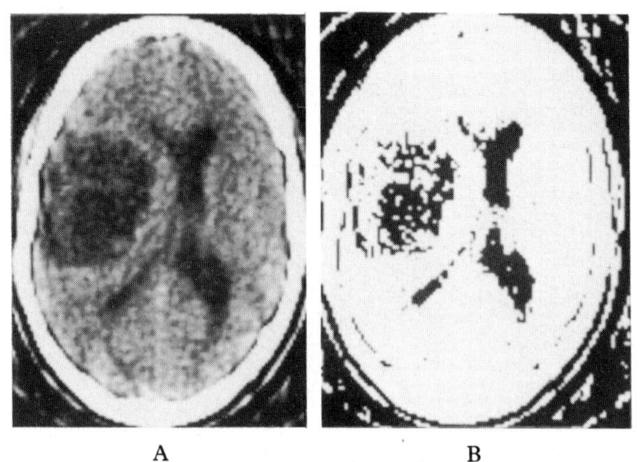

Fig. 63.36 A—Epidermoid (pearly tumour) in the left temporal region (L36 W80). B—Same case at L8 W1.

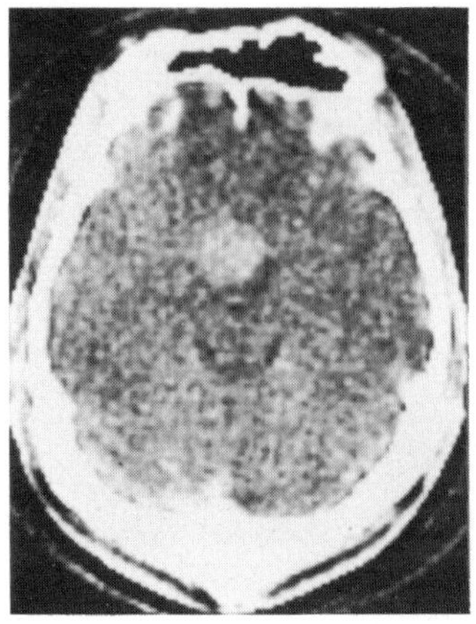

Fig. 63.37 Pituitary tumour; acromegaly with enhancing suprasellar mass (L36 W80). Note thick skull vault and large frontal sinuses.

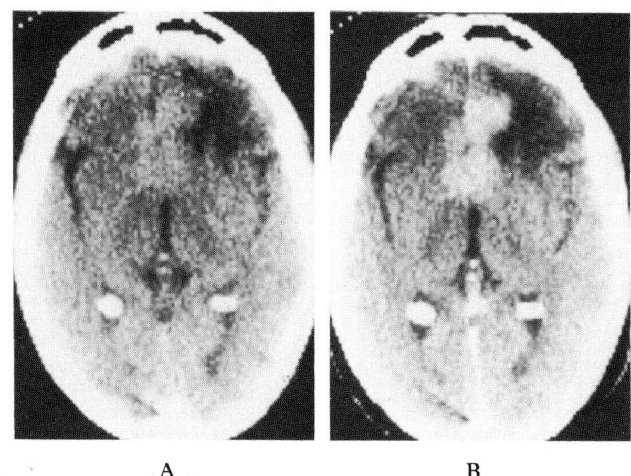

Fig. 63.38 Pituitary tumour with subfrontal extension on the right. The tumour enhances and there is peritumoral oedema (L36 W80).

CT has little part to play in the diagnosis of the first group of tumours, which is clinical and endocrinological, except to exclude any major intracranial extension.

Diagnosis of a large pituitary adenoma is frequently based on clinical data and the demonstration of a ballooned sella turcica by plain radiography. The role of CT is to confirm the diagnosis and to show the extent of the lesion. Enlargement of the sella turcica is usually obvious. A suprasellar extension can be demonstrated in the large majority of patients with visual deterioration (Figs. 63.37 and 63.38). Small tumours may merely efface the normal chiasmatic cistern and/or interpeduncular fossa; large chromophobe lesions may extend downwards into the basisphenoid, forwards towards the orbit, posterolaterally into the middle cranial fossae, and upwards to obliterate the third ventricle. Hydrocephalus is, however, uncommon. The tumours are generally more or less symmetrical. Multiple sections viewed at different window levels, possibly supplemented by coronal and/or sagittal sections or reconstructions, may be required to assess the full extent of a large tumour.

Suprasellar extension also occurs with eosinophil, and very rarely with basophil tumours. It is also seen occasionally with a prolactinoma. The CT features are indistinguishable from those of chromophobe adenomas.

Adenomas are usually rounded masses slightly denser than the surrounding brain, and showing obvious enhancement, generally rather homogeneous, with contrast medium. Low attenuation and apparently

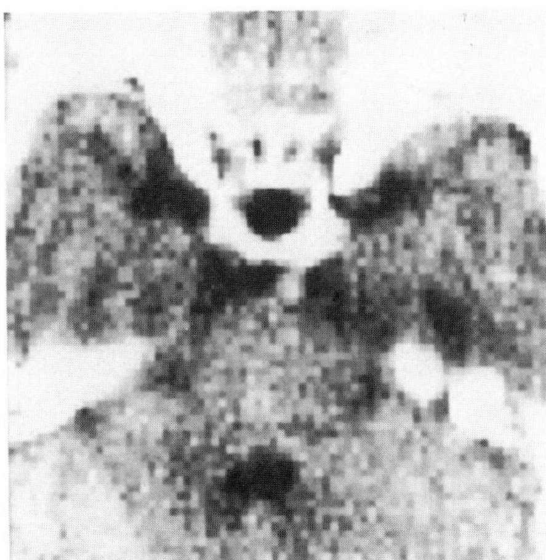

Fig. 63.39 Empty sella (L42 W80).

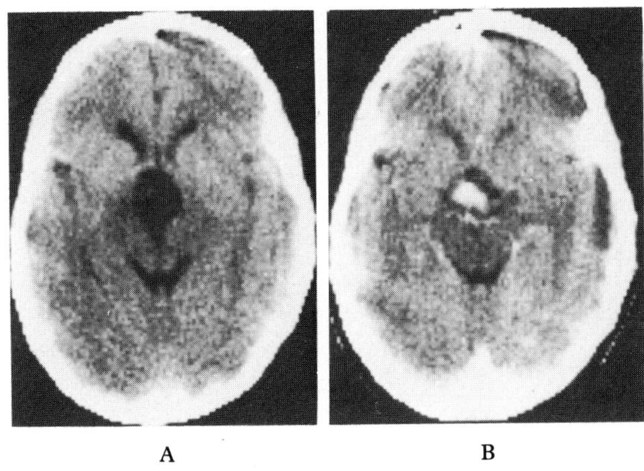

A B

Fig. 63.41 Craniopharyngioma. Cystic tumour with solid enhancing component (L34 W60).

cystic lesions are encountered, but calcification is distinctly rare.

Major considerations in differential diagnosis are suprasellar meningioma and aneurysm, but other lesions lying above the sella, e.g. craniopharyngioma, can simulate pituitary tumours. The combination of CT and plain film findings gives a high degree of diagnostic accuracy.

The *'empty sella' syndrome* may also occasionally simulate a pituitary adenoma, particularly as regards the plain film findings; some cases may arise as the result of involution of an adenoma. CT can suggest the diagnosis, by showing the sellar contents to be of cerebrospinal fluid attenuation (Fig. 63.39). However, caution should be exercised in suggesting this diagnosis by CT since averaging may occur from a large sphenoidal air sinus surrounding the sella, or from adjacent thick bony walls.

Craniopharyngioma (suprasellar cyst). Many of these tumours, which are probably developmental in origin, present in childhood. When this is the case, they are often manifest on plain skull films as suprasellar calcification. CT demonstrates a rounded, midline suprasellar mass, classically of low attenuation centrally, with a capsule, often calcified. The latter may enhance after intravenous contrast medium, but this is not universal.

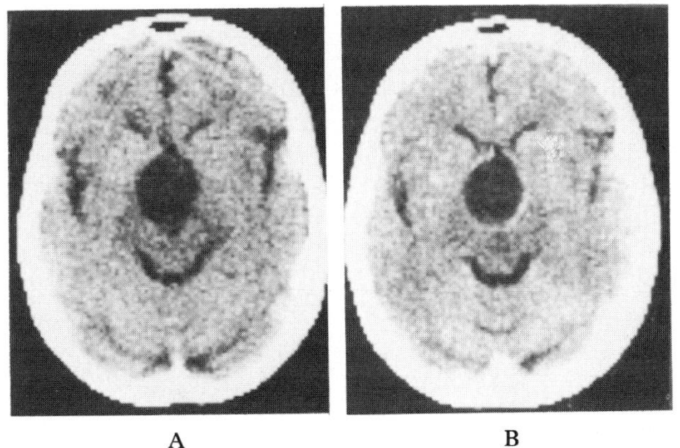

A B

Fig. 63.40 Craniopharyngioma. Cystic suprasellar mass with enhancing rim (L34 W60).

Although these appearances are very typical, a broad spectrum of combinations of attenuation characteristics may be seen (Figs. 63.40 and 63.41). Calcification is less common in adults.

Hydrocephalus is a not uncommon complication, usually due to obstruction at the foramen of Monro. A number of patients present with symptoms of raised intracranial pressure; a careful inspection of the suprasellar region should therefore be made in cases of unexplained hydrocephalus.

INFRATENTORIAL TUMOURS

Intracerebral tumours

These may be divided into *brain stem* and *cerebellar* tumours. This distinction can frequently be made at CT by noting the position of the fourth ventricle: brain stem tumours arise anterior to the ventricle and displace it posteriorly, while cerebellar tumours displace it forwards. Tumours alongside the fourth ventricle lie in the region of the cerebellar peduncles, but often prove to be extra-axial, lying in the cerebellopontine angle. Effacement of the ventricle occurs most commonly with cerebellar or fourth ventricular tumours.

Brain stem. The only common brain stem tumour is the *glioma*, which occurs mainly in children. This tumour may be difficult to identify until it is large; the cardinal signs at CT are alteration (especially reduction) of the attenuation characteristics of the medulla or pons, and expansion. The latter is manifest by posterior displacement and flattening of the fourth ventricle (Fig. 63.42) and obliteration of the cisterns around the brain stem. Hydrocephalus is uncommon. In general,

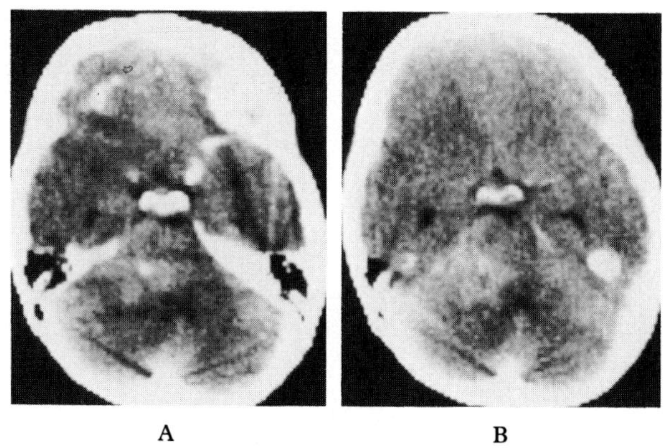

A B

Fig. 63.42 Brainstem glioma. Mixed attenuation lesion mainly on left displacing 4th ventricle backwards (L42 W80).

little change is seen with intravenous contrast medium, but irregular enhancement may occur.

Cerebellum and fourth ventricle. Tumours in these structures include:

primary: cerebellar astrocytoma
medulloblastoma
ependymoma
haemangioblastoma
dermoid
choroid plexus papilloma
colloid cyst
meningioma
secondary: metastases

Cerebellar astrocytomas are commonest in young males, as indeed are medulloblastomas and ependymomas. They are often of relatively low malignancy with a good prognosis if treated in childhood and represent the commonest type of primary intracranial tumour encountered in the posterior fossa. The large majority of these lesions are seen at CT as areas of low, or mixed high and low, attenuation, sometimes well defined, indicating cyst formation (Fig. 63.43) lying in one or other cerebellar hemispheres and often extending towards the cerebellar peduncles. Midline lesions, lying in the cerebellar vermis are not, however, uncommon. About two-thirds of these tumours show obvious enhancement after intravenous contrast medium, which may be homogenous, patchy or circumferential. Hydrocephalus is common and is often more marked with vermian lesions.

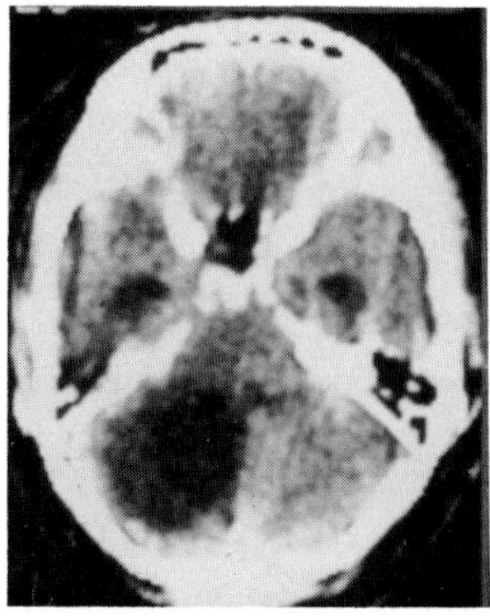

Fig. 63.43 Cystic glioma in left cerebellar hemisphere. Haemangioblastoma can present an identical appearance (L36 W80).

Medulloblastoma occurs particularly in young boys, arising in the region of the medullary velum, on the front of the vermis. They are usually therefore midline in position, often obliterating the fourth ventricle (Fig. 63.44). The large majority are rounded or lobulated lesions, denser than the surrounding brain, and showing generalized homogeneous or patchy enhancement. Hydrocephalus is common.

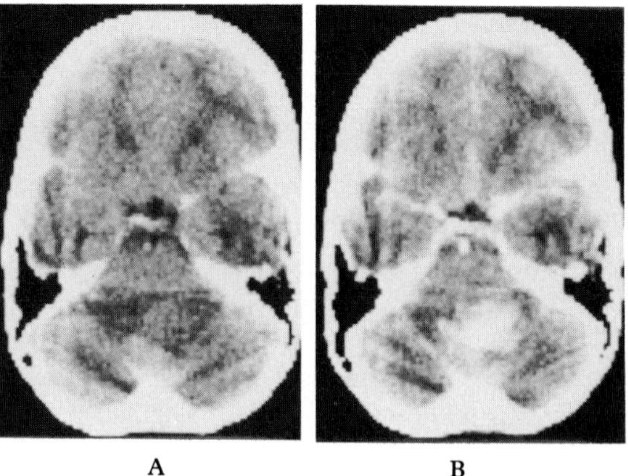

A B

Fig. 63.44 Medulloblastoma: A—isodense lesion obliterating 4th ventricle; B—strong enhancement after contrast (L36 W60).

Medulloblastomas are particularly likely to metastasise, via the cerebrospinal fluid. CT examination both at the time of initial diagnosis and at follow-up, should therefore include the entire cerebrum. Marked enhancement of the basal cisterns in known cases of medulloblastoma can represent extensive tumour seeding.

Ependymoma is a relatively uncommon tumour arising within the fourth ventricle, which is therefore usually obliterated, although an inferiorly placed tumour may cause dilatation of the upper part of the ventricle; this is a possible source of misdiagnosis as, for example, communicating hydrocephalus. The tumour resembles a medulloblastoma being of increased attenuation and showing homogeneous or patchy enhancement with intravenous contrast medium. Calcification is more suggestive of ependymoma. Hydrocephalus is commonly marked.

Haemangioblastomas may be either solitary, or multiple. Less commonly they occur as part of the von Hippel-Lindau syndrome, a phakomatosis characterized

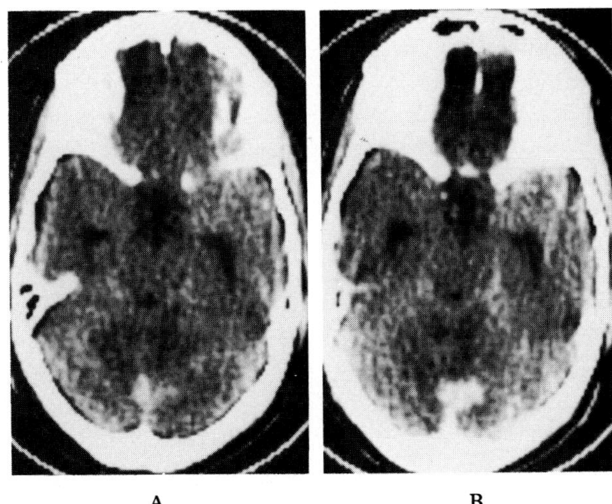

A B

Fig. 63.45 Haemangioblastoma. A—Low density area in vermis. Fourth ventricle displaced forwards. B—Enhancing nodule high in vermis beneath straight sinus (L34 W75).

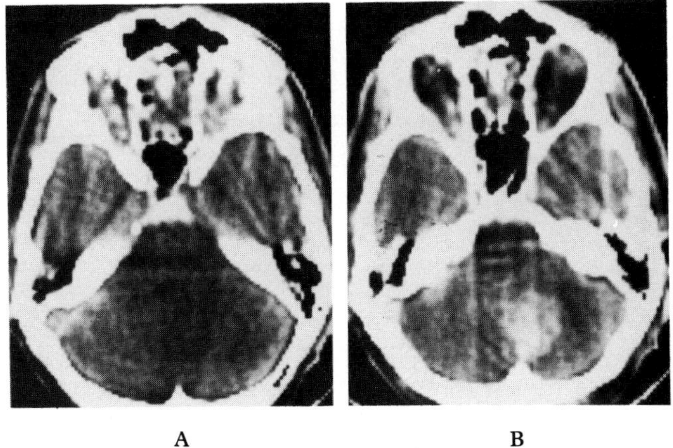

A B

Fig. 63.46 Haemangioblastoma. A—Low density area in vermis and right cerebellum. B—Large enhancing nodule.

by lesions in the eye, brain and spinal cord. Intracranial tumours are most common in the cerebellar hemispheres (Figs. 63.45 and 63.46), Before intravenous contrast medium, the haemangioblastoma appears at CT as a rounded area of reduced attenuation representing a cyst or local oedema. The enhancement pattern is typically that of a nodule but unless the nodule is actually in the section it may be missed. Small vascular tumours visible at angiography may not be shown by CT, but the cystic component is best shown by the latter. A solitary haemangioblastoma may be difficult to distinguish from a cerebellar astrocytoma or an infarct. There is frequently moderate or marked hydrocephalus.

Dermoid tumours of the cerebellum have the characteristic appearances described elsewhere. A specific though rare complication of dermoids in this region is infection via a cutaneous sinus; the lesion may then be indistinguishable from a cerebellar abscess.

Choroid plexus papilloma and *intraventricular meningioma* of the fourth ventricle are very rare; the existence of *colloid cysts* in this site is debated. The CT characteristics of these tumours are described above.

Metastases (Fig. 63.47) form the commonest type of cerebellar tumour seen in adults. They may be small at a time when clinical symptoms are marked, whereas cerebral metastases are often large. In such cases, surrounding oedema may be more marked than the tumour mass. The large majority lie in the cerebrellar hemispheres. They may be of decreased, mixed or increased attenuation, but virtually all show homogeneous, or less commonly patchy or ring enhancement. The appearances are non-specific and the differential diagnosis is based on the age of the patient, a history of prior neoplasia or the presence of multiple lesions. Hydrocephalus is commonly mild.

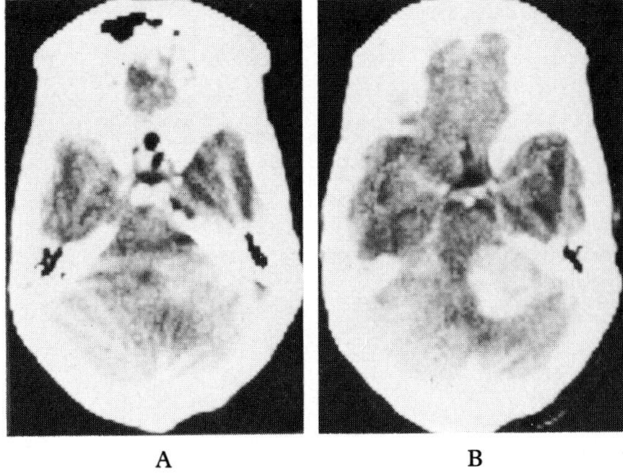

A B

Fig. 63.47 Secondary deposit. High density enhancing lesion in right cerebellum (L40 W80).

Extracerebral tumours

These include acoustic neuroma, meningioma, epidermoid chordoma, other cranial nerve neuromas (e.g. trigeminal and glossopharyngeal), glomus jugulare tumours and non-neoplastic masses such as basilar aneurysm.

Acoustic neuroma is a benign tumour. It is the commonest extracerebral tumour in the posterior fossa, and by far the commonest in the cerebellopontine angle, arising from the eighth cranial nerve. Its incidence is increased in neurofibromatosis, and the occurrence of bilateral tumours is virtually diagnostic of that disease. It may arise entirely within the internal auditory meatus, or extend into the posterior cranial fossa. Patients may present with hearing disturbances at a stage when the tumour is below 1 cm in diameter; demonstration of

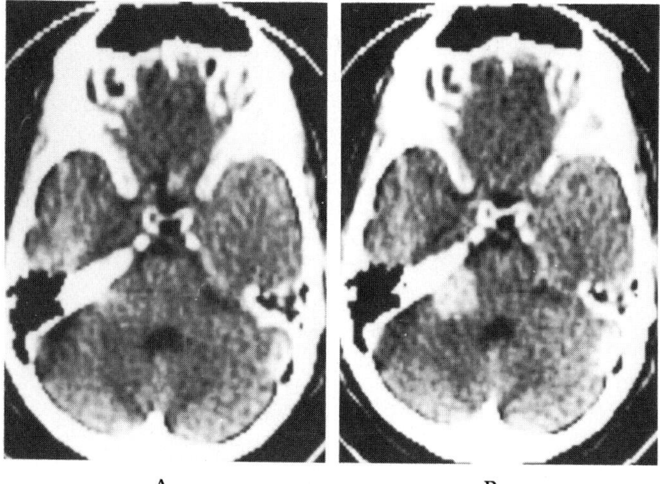

Fig. 63.48 Small acoustic tumour. Isodense lesion in left CP angle enhancing strongly after contrast (L34 W75).

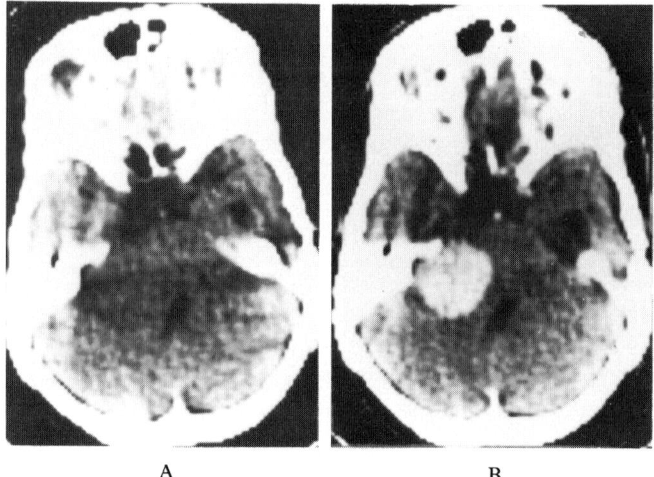

Fig. 63.49 A—Larger acoustic tumour. Low density mass in left CP angle. Note enlarged IAM. B—Strong enhancement after contrast (L36 W80).

such lesions by CT is unreliable, but diagnostic accuracy can be increased by scanning after intrathecal injection of Metrizamide (CT cisternography).

The neuromas are often poorly defined at CT (Figs. 63.48 and 63.49) being isodense with the adjacent brain, or with surrounding oedema. A small proportion (about 5 per cent) are denser than brain. Calcification is rare. The principal abnormality on the CT scan is often displacement or distortion of the fourth ventricle and this sign should be carefully sought in patients suspected of harbouring a neuroma. Intravenous contrast medium produces marked, homogeneous enhancement of a rounded mass in the anterolateral part of the posterior fossa, flattened laterally against the petrous bone, in the large majority of cases. The CT scan may also show widening of the internal auditory meatus on the affected side. A small proportion of these tumours are cystic. Large lesions may produce hydrocephalus, particularly in the elderly.

Meningiomas in the posterior fossa occur in the cerebellopontine angle (where clinically they may mimic acoustic neuromas) over the cerebellar convexity, particularly at its lateral angle, or growing from the undersurface of the tentorium. At CT, they are usually well-defined, rounded tumours of greater than brain attenuation and may be extremely dense if calcified. There is often peritumoral oedema. These tumours characteristically show marked homogenous enhancement with contrast medium (Fig. 63.50). Such lesions in the cerebellopontine angle may be distinguished from neuromas by their high precontrast attenuation; by calcification, if present; by a greater degree of enhancement after contrast medium; and by the fact that they are not centred on the internal auditory meatus. However, none of these differential features is invariable. A lesion over the cerebellar convexity, may be difficult to distinguish from an intracerebellar metastasis.

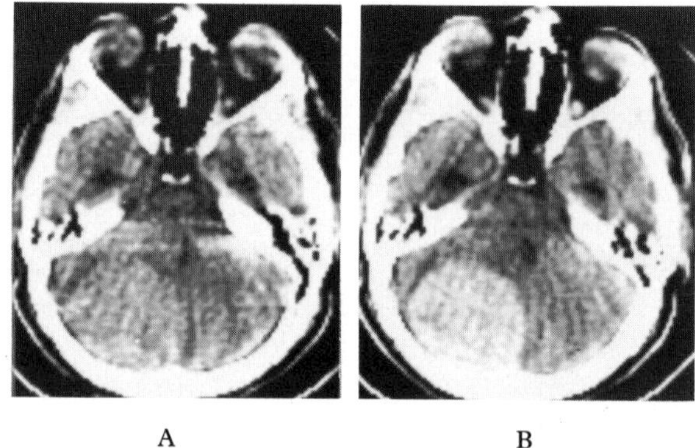

Fig. 63.50 Posterior fossa meningioma. High density mass with marked enhancement after contrast and arising over left cerebellar convexity.

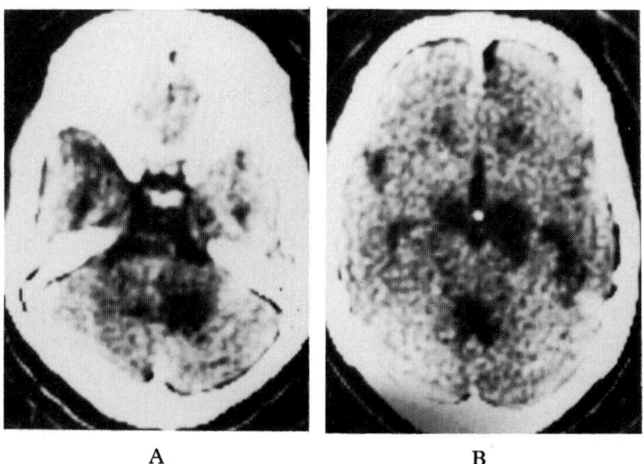

Fig. 63.51 Epidermoid in CP angle. Low density mass in left CP angle and extending into middle fossa (L36 W80).

Epidermoid tumours also characteristically occur in the cerebellopontine angle. They are typically of low attenuation, sometimes showing attenuation values less than those of cerebrospinal fluid and extend from the cerebellopontine angle cistern into the tentorial hiatus, in an irregular fashion (Fig. 63.51). However, some tumours are rounded, and apparently encapsulated. The capsule occasionally shows calcification. Contrast enhancement is usually absent or minimal.

Chordomas occur at either end of the spine, and these at the upper end extend into the posterior cranial fossa (Figs. 63.52 and 63.53). They are seen at CT as masses, often rather poorly defined, anterior to the brain stem, and characteristically showing calcification. However, many cases do not show calcification. Contrast enhancement is also variable, and may be marked or absent. Bone destruction in the region of the clivus may be apparent. An important differential diagnostic consideration is basilar artery ectasia.

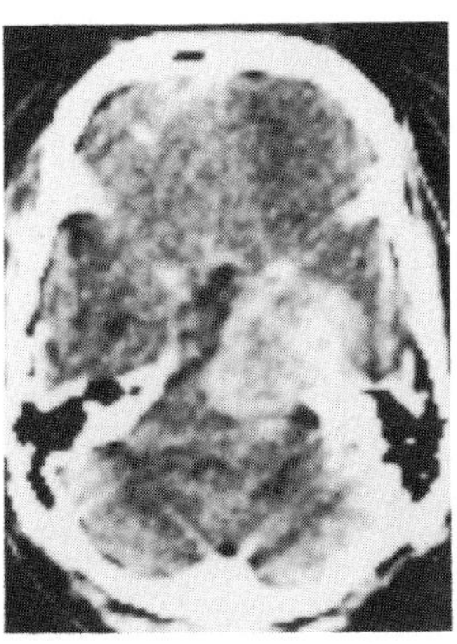

Fig. 63.54 Fifth nerve tumour with marked enhancement after contrast. The tumour at the petrous apex extends into both the middle and posterior fossae (L36 W80).

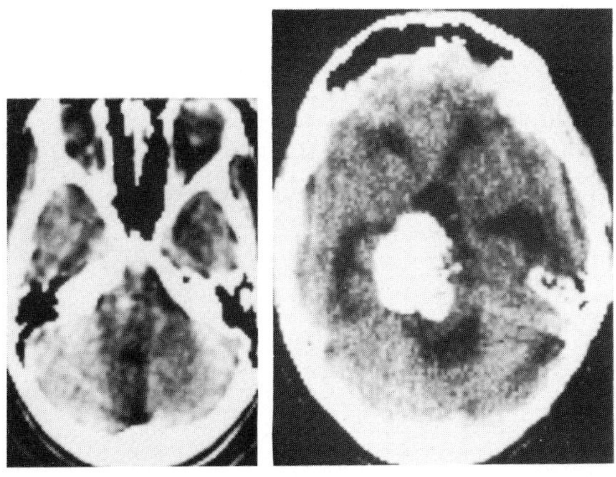

Fig. 63.52 *Fig. 63.53*

Fig. 63.52 Chordoma. Calcification anterior to the brainstem which is displaced backwards.

Fig. 63.53 Chordoma. Heavily calcified post operative recurrence extending up through tentorial hiatus (L44 W60).

Neuromas of the trigeminal or glossopharygeal nerves are very much less common than acoustic neuromas. Their CT appearances are similar, but it may be evident that they arise at a different level. Trigeminal neuromas, for example, may extend into the middle cranial fossa, and resemble a meningioma (Fig. 63. 52).

Glomus jugulare tumours are manifest at CT in two ways: basal bone destruction, centred on the jugular foramen, and rounded soft tissue masses which may extend intracranially from the base, or downwards into the upper part of the neck. The degree of contrast enhancement is frequently less than might be anticipated from the hypervascularity of these lesions.

REFERENCES AND SUGGESTIONS FOR FURTHER READING

See end of next chapter.

CHAPTER 64

COMPUTED TOMOGRAPHY—C.N.S. (2)

VASCULAR LESIONS

INTRACEREBRAL HAEMATOMA

Intracerebral haematomas may arise from so-called 'spontaneous' haemorrhage or be secondary to vascular lesions such as *angiomas* or *aneurysms*. Very rarely haemorrhage may be seen with *tumours* (1–2 per cent), and malignant melanoma deposits are particularly liable to haemorrhage. Occasionally also intracerebral haemorrhage is seen with *anticoagulants*, or with *blood dyscrasias*, though subdural haematomas are more common than intracerebral haemorrhage in the latter. Head *trauma* may also produce both subdural and intracerebral haemorrhage, most commonly in the temporo-parietal regions. These are discussed in detail below. Spontaneous haematomas are commonest in hypertensive, elderly patients and are probably due to rupture of a small atheromatous vessel. Because of the clear distinction between the high attenuation of extravasated blood and that of the surrounding brain, CT scanning is by far the most accurate radiological method of demonstrating these lesions. About one-third of intracerebral haemorrhages are *hypertensive* in origin. Of these some 60 per cent occur in the basal ganglia or centro-Sylvian areas; the remaining 40 per cent involve the pons (20 per cent), cerebellum (10 per cent) and less commonly, temporal, frontal, parietal or occipital lobes (Figs. 64.1–64.3). On CT the haemorrhage shows as an area of increased attenuation ranging from 50–100 Hounsfield units and is surrounded by a thin low attenuation ring which probably results from clot retraction. Haemorrhage can rupture into the subarachnoid space or ventricles (Figs. 64.4 and 64.5). In subarachnoid extension the normal low attenuation c.s.f. appears isodense with brain or has areas of increased attenuation. The mass effect depends on the size of the bleed. Tentorial herniation should be assessed by the degree of compromise of the quadrigeminal cisterns.

The ability to detect freshly clotted blood within the brain parenchyma and subarachnoid spaces is one of the most important diagnostic advances resulting from CT scanning. Congealed blood appears as an area of high attenuation as noted above. The absorption values increase with progressing haemoconcentration. A clot which is 48 hours old may develop slightly higher values than were present initially because of fluid loss from the clot.

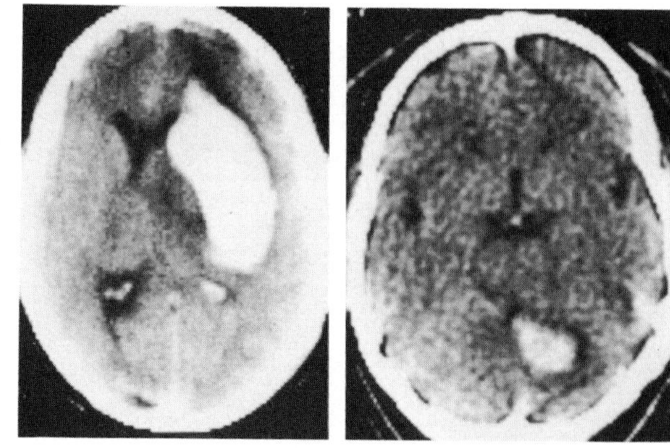

Fig. 64.1 *Fig. 64.2*

Fig. 64.1 Intracerebral haematoma. Massive right capsular haemorrhage (L36 W80).

Fig. 64.2 Right cerebellar haematoma (L36 W80).

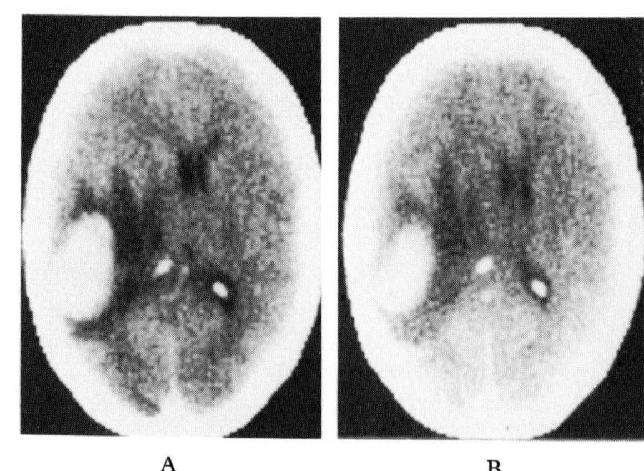

A B

Fig. 64.3 A—Left parietal haematoma with some surrounding oedema (L36 W80). B—Seven days later the haematoma appears smaller as the periphery becomes isodense (L36 W80).

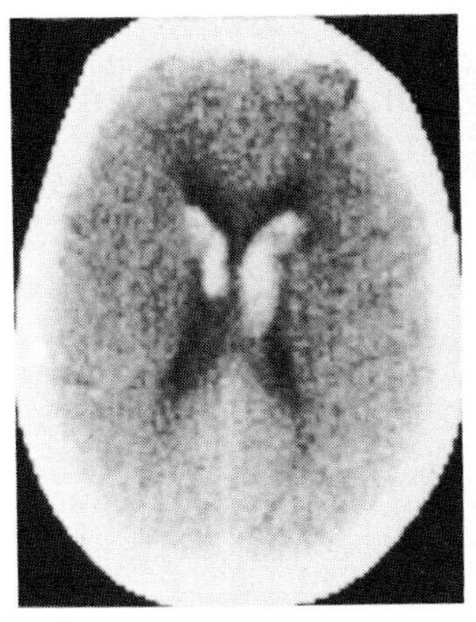

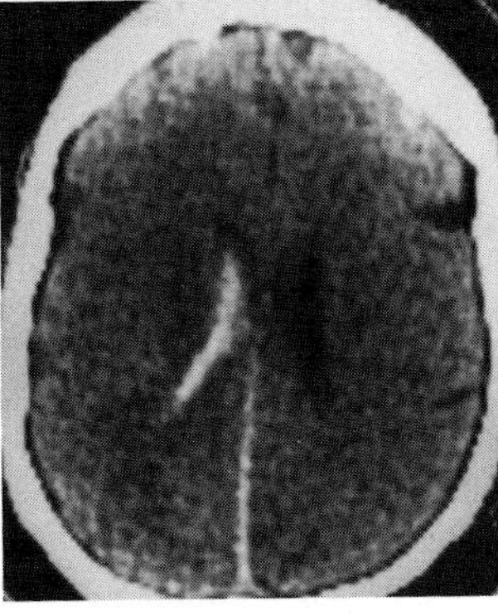

Fig. 64.4 *Fig. 64.5*

Fig. 64.4 Intraventricular haemorrhage (L36 W80).

Fig. 64.5 Intraventricular haemorrhage in L. lateral ventricle (L34 W75).

These high attenuation values were originally thought to be due to the presence of high atomic number (Z) elements within whole blood, i.e. calcium and iron. However, *in vitro* experiments have shown that their concentration is too low to make a significant contribution to the high values seen in clot. It is in fact the tightly packed haemoglobin molecules which are responsible for the high attenuation values. A blood specimen with 15 gm per cent haemoglobin has a Hounsfield number of approximately 50 units i.e. only slightly greater than grey matter. The 50 mg of iron present only contribute 7 per cent of the total value. A contracted clot, however, has a haemoglobin value of 30 gms per cent with an absorption value of approximately 80. The iron percentage here contributes about 4 units and the tightly packed haemoglobin molecules the rest of the increase. The base line for plasma is 24 units and each gram per cent of haemoglobin adds 2 units.

The high attenuation of intracerebral haematomas is seen directly from the time of haemorrhage. It slowly decreases over the subsequent weeks, until eventually a low-density cystic area remains. In the acute phase a spontaneous haematoma is surrounded by a thin line of lowered density and is usually solitary; it has less mass effect than a tumour of comparable size, but some lesions are surrounded by extensive oedema. It has already been noted that the majority of spontaneous hypertensive haemorrhages occur in the classical basal ganglia situation; since secondary haematomas may also occur in that position, the site of the lesion is unfortunately not a good clue to its aetiology.

Resolution of the haematoma takes place from the periphery (Fig. 64.3). Resolution of a clot at CT does not necessarily mean that the haematoma is absorbed but merely that it has become isodense with surrounding brain. Sometimes a ring of connective tissue forms around the site of a haemorrhage and then enhances following contrast. This ring surrounding a low attenuation area can be confused with abscess or tumour andcan only be differentiated by the history.

SUBARACHNOID HAEMORRHAGE

Subarachnoid haemorrhage from any cause (see Ch. 62) may be associated with a number of abnormalities in the CT scan. These include:

1. Intracerebral/intraventricular blood
2. Subarachnoid blood
3. Infarction/ischaemia
4. Hydrocephalus
5. Demonstration of the causative lesion (aneurysm, angioma or tumour)

1. The characteristics of intracerebral haematomas have been described above. The main indication that a haematoma may have arisen from a ruptured aneurysm is its basal situation near the circle of Willis. One-third of intracranial bleeds are secondary to ruptured aneurysms and a high proportion of ruptured aneurysms (30–60 per cent in different series) bleed into adjacent brain. CT is therefore helpful in identifying the site of the bleed if there is associated intracerebral clot. Haematoma in the septum pellucidum or corpus callosum can be taken as an indication of an anterior cerebral artery aneurysm bleed (Fig. 64.7B). A middle cerebral artery aneurysm can be recognized by fresh clot in the Sylvian cistern (Fig. 64.7B). Haematoma in the region of the external capsule may be hypertensive or may be from an internal carotid or middle cerebral artery aneurysm. Thus CT can be helpful in selecting the first vessel to be examined by angiography. If two or more aneurysms are shown the presence of intracerebral clot or of a low density area representing ischaemia secondary to spasm may identify the aneurysm which has bled. Occasionally the CT scan may be positive though the aneurysm is not shown by angiography. Conversely, if the CT study is negative soon after a presumed haemorrhage, the likelihood of showing a vascular lesion by angiography is reduced.

The presence of blood in both the cisterns and ventricles has a grave prognosis and is associated with a very high mortality. Blood in the cisterns only is associated with a serious though lesser mortality.

2. Extravasated blood may be identified anywhere in the subarachnoid space from its high attenuation. It is usually confined to the basal cisterns (Fig. 64.6). If the subarachnoid blood is localized, e.g. in the insula, this can be very helpful in identifying which of multiple aneurysms is responsible for the haemorrhage. Such extravasated blood can be demonstrated in about 90 per cent of cases during the first week after the haemorrhage, but during the second week this proportion falls to less than 40 per cent.

3. Low density areas representing infarcted or

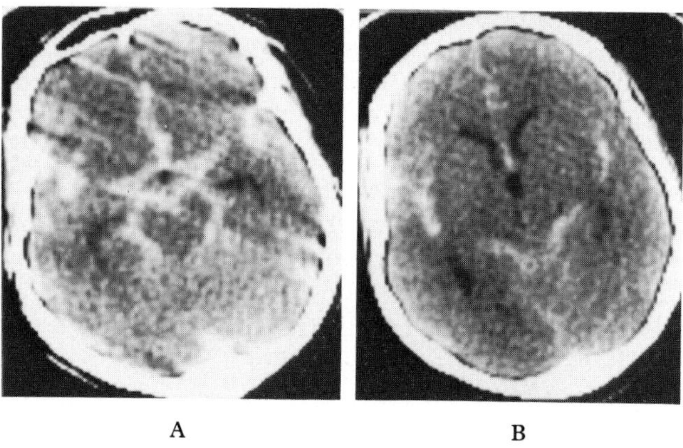

A B

Fig. 64.6 Subarachnoid haemorrhage. Congealed blood in the basal cisterns, insulae, and interhemispheric cleft (L34 W75).

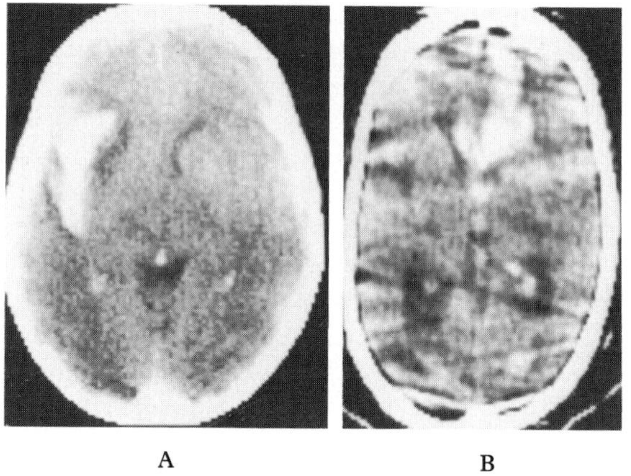

A B

Fig. 64.7 A—Subarachnoid haemorrhage. Clot in the left insula indicating a left middle cerebral aneurysm bleed. B—Subarachnoid haemorrhage. Clot in septum pellucidum and right medial frontal region indicating rupture of an anterior communicating aneurysm. There is also intraventricular clot. The lesions are recognizable despite movement artefact in a restless patient (L34 W75).

ischaemic brain are infrequently shown. It is thought that they are related to the arterial spasm which often accompanies subarachnoid haemorrhage.

4. Dilated ventricles are shown in 50 per cent of patients screened within 48 hours of a subarachnoid haemorrhage, since communicating hydrocephalus may develop quite rapidly, presumably due to blood and clot obstructing the c.s.f. flow. Posthaemorrhagic hydrocephalus also occurs in up to 20 per cent of cases; the initial examination is then of use as a baseline.

5. If the haemorrhage arises from an aneurysm, it is distinctly uncommon for the aneurysm to be visible, even after intravenous contrast medium. Angiomas, however, are shown before injection in more than 50 per cent of cases, and after contrast medium in more than 90 per cent. In the rare cases in which subarachnoid haemorrhage is a manifestation of a tumour, the main findings are those of the tumour itself, with an associated haematoma.

Aneurysms

The vast majority of cerebral aneurysms present clinically as subarachnoid haemorrhage. A smaller proportion present with oculomotor palsies or, if large and in an appropriate area, as suspected cerebral tumours. Thus a large basilar aneurysm can give rise to a brainstem syndrome and a large anterior communicating aneurysm can arouse suspicion of a suprasellar tumour.

The investigation of subarachnoid haemorrhage is discussed in Chapter 62 and CT scanning is the most important primary investigation in this condition. However, if surgery is to be undertaken angiography will also be required. The CT scan, by demonstrating the site of the bleed, can sometimes be followed by simple unilateral carotid angiography and obviate the necessity for four-vessel angiography in a seriously ill patient.

In patients with an oculomotor palsy the aneurysm, if large enough, will be demonstrated as a high density parasellar lesion on the simple scan, and this may enhance strongly and be clearly related to the circle of Willis on the postenhancement scan. Large aneurysms, i.e. those more than 1 cm in diameter, show up quite well at CT scanning as high-density rounded lesions at the base of the brain (Figs. 64.8 to 64.11). These enhance strongly after contrast injections. Since large aneurysms frequently contain thrombus, the enhancement usually involves only part of the lesion; paradoxically, a lesion showing marked enhancement in only one portion is more likely to be an aneurysm. Occasionally they show characteristic marginal calcification (Fig. 64.9). In an appropriate situation there may be a difficult differential diagnosis to be made, e.g. a large suprasellar aneurysm (Fig. 64.8) may simulate a suprasellar meningioma, craniopharyngioma or a pituitary tumour, and a large basilar aneurysm can simulate a clivus meningioma (Fig. 64.10). Basilar aneurysms can be

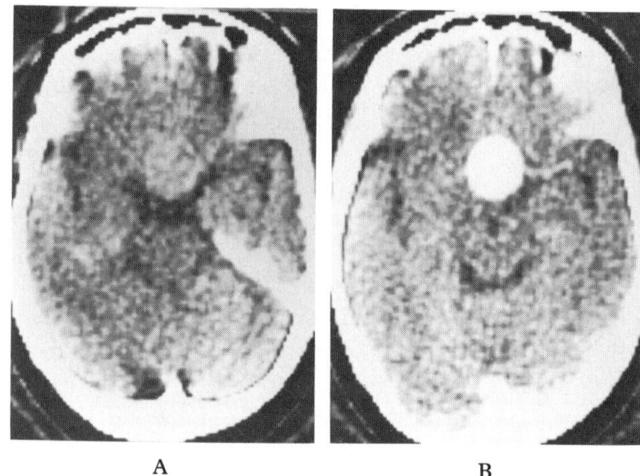

A B

Fig. 64.8 A—High density rounded mass in suprasellar region. B—The mass enhances strongly with contrast. Large aneurysm confirmed at angiography (L36 W80).

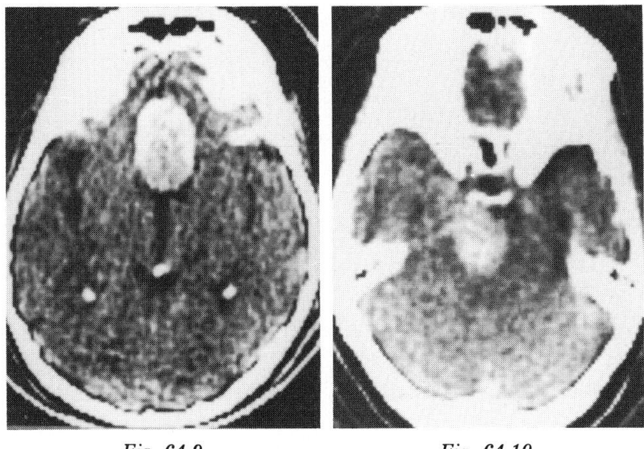

Fig. 64.9 *Fig. 64.10*

Fig. 64.9 High density suprasellar mass with marginal calcification. Large calcified anterior communicating aneurysm (L34 W75).

Fig. 64.10 High density rounded mass behind sella and extending into brain stem. Basilar aneurysm confirmed at angiography (L36 W80).

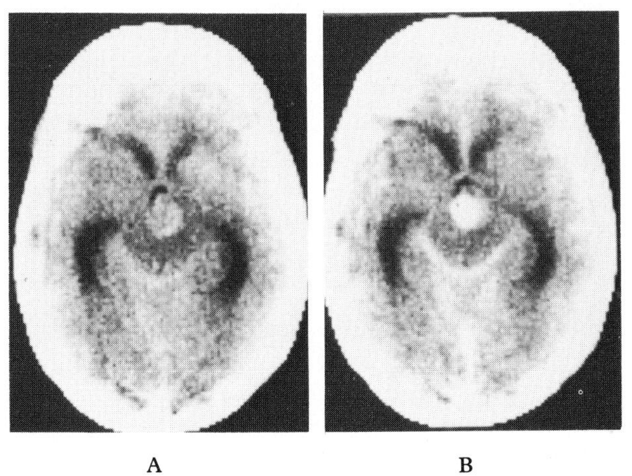

A B

Fig. 64.11 A—High density rounded mass projecting into third ventricle. B—The rounded mass enhances strongly with contrast. Basilar aneurysm projecting up into third ventricle confirmed at vertebral angiography.

fusiform or serpentine, and they sometimes show peripheral increased density representing calcification or mural thrombosis.

Angiomas

Angiomas or arteriovenous malformations involving the brain parenchyma or its overlying meninges may be well demonstrated by CT. A distinction must be made between those presenting with subarachnoid haemorrhage and those presenting with other symptoms. Patients with subarachnoid haemorrhage will usually show an intracerebral haematoma recognizable by its characteristic density and blood may also be shown in the basal cisterns, ventricles or sulci, as with a ruptured aneurysm. Direct evidence of the angioma may be seen near the site of the haemorrhage and will consist of features similar to those seen in patients without subarachnoid haemorrhage. This latter group of patients will show no obvious lesion in 10–20 per cent of cases. This happens where the lesion is relatively small and superficial. However, with the larger lesions the simple scan may show characteristic appearances. The most typical of these are serpiginous high density shadows suggesting thrombosed enlarged vessels or hypertrophied veins. Calcification may also be shown in a few cases which may be characteristically ring like or curvilinear and serpiginous. The exact appearance of the vessels in a large angioma will vary depending on the angle relative to the tomographic cuts. Usually tubular or vermiform shadows may be recognized when cut longitudinally and rounded or ovoid shadows when transected. The multiple vessels in a large lesion may give rise to a mottled appearance (Figs. 64.12 and 64.13).

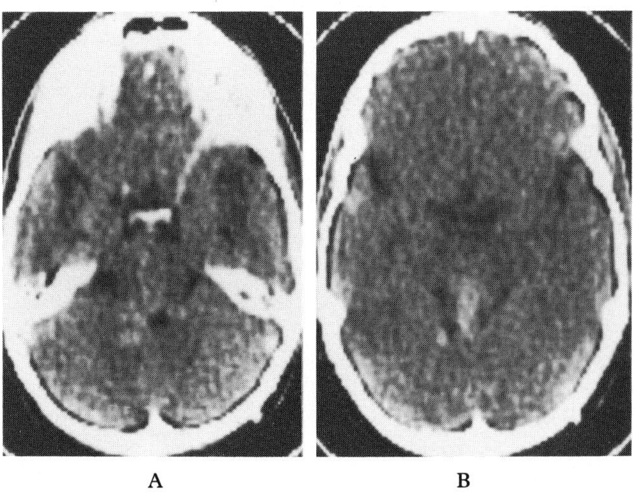

A B

Fig. 64.12 Irregular high density shadows in brain stem region. Brainstem angioma (L34 W75).

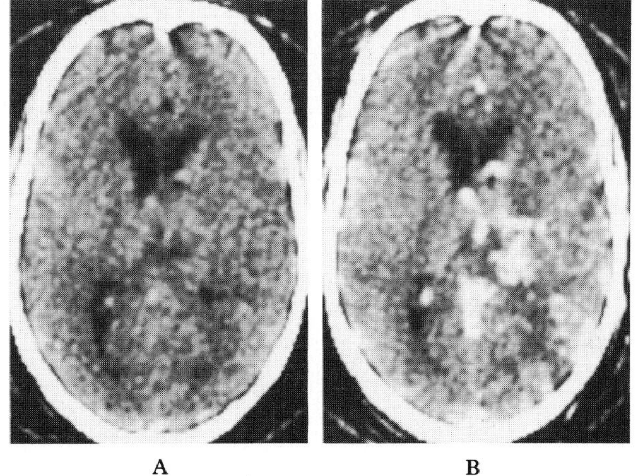

A B

Fig. 64.13 A—Irregular mixed density lesion in right medial parietal region with defects in right lateral ventricle. B—Multiple sinuous high density lesions seen after enhancement. Angiography confirmed giant angioma (L36 W90).

There may be low-density areas adjacent to or around the malformation, and adjacent areas of infarction may occur.

After the injection of contrast medium the appearances become more characteristic and the tortuous vascular shadows may be easily recognized (Fig. 64.12B). The large lesions may penetrate deeply into the brain in a wedge-shaped manner, though the majority will be superficial. Most angiomas produce little mass effect unless there has also been a large haemorrhage. Nevertheless, it is possible to mistake the appearances for gliomas or infarcts and the differential diagnosis should be borne in mind when the appearances are not characteristic.

Although the diagnosis of angioma may be certain on a CT scan, most of these cases will usually require angiography before surgery in order to define the exact anatomy of the feeding vessels and drainage veins.

Purely dural lesions are difficult to detect because of their proximity to the bony vault. A clotted angioma appears at CT as an area of high density often with adjacent area of low density and these may enhance with contrast to a varying degree giving rise to an erroneous diagnosis of tumour.

The rare cavernous intracerebral angioma, like a thrombosed angioma, may show clearly at CT but be invisible at angiography.

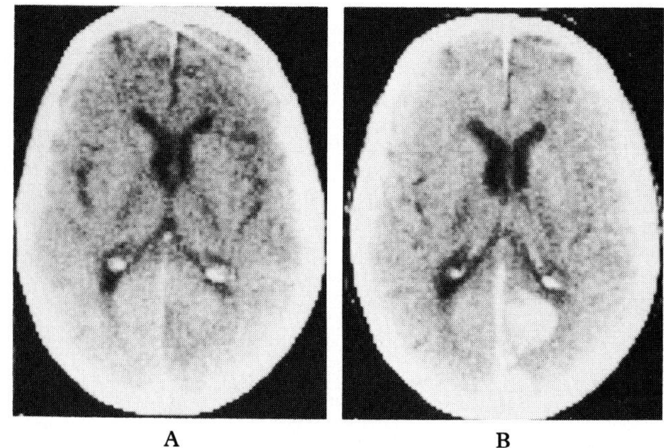

Fig. 64.14 Acute infarct. A—Doubtful low density lesion in right occipital region. No mass effect. B—Strong enhancement with contrast (L36 W80).

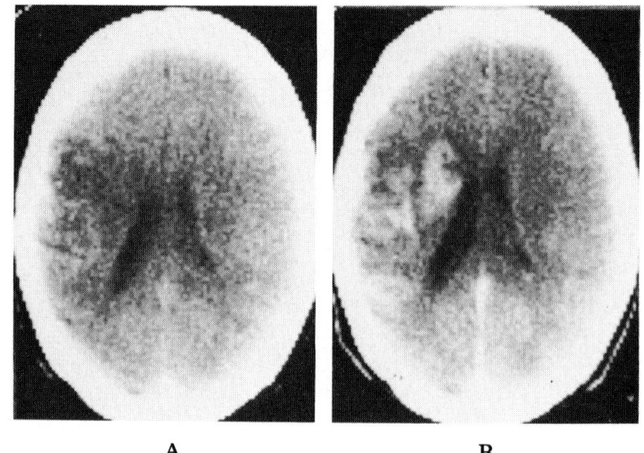

Fig. 64.15 Middle cerebral infarct. A—Mixed low density and isodense lesion in left parietal region. No mass effect. B—Patchy enhancement after contrast (L36 W80).

INFARCTS

Ischaemic infarction is due to interruption of the blood supply to a portion of the brain. It may be thrombotic or embolic, but the distinction cannot be made by CT scanning. The cardinal sign of infarction is an area of decreased attenuation within the cerebral substance. Typical locations are within the known territory of a major vessel (e.g. the middle or posterior cerebral arteries), or in the region of the basal ganglia and internal capsule. Infarcts are often triangular in shape, involving both the white and superficial grey matter, whereas oedema (around a tumour, for example) usually affects mainly the white matter. This area of diminished density may be seen as early as 6 hours after the onset of symptoms, but in many cases is not clearly visible during the first 24 hours. At first the margins of the infarcted area are poorly defined, although a few infarcts are clearly marginated from the outset. The density of the lesion becomes progressively lower over the succeeding weeks, until it approaches that of cerebrospinal fluid (Figs. 64.17 to 64.20). In the early stages there is often some swelling of the affected part of the brain but a major mass effect is rare and eventually there is loss of volume, with enlargement of the adjacent cerebrospinal fluid spaces in most cases. Complete healing is very rare.

Enhancement of an infarct may be seen after a few hours from the onset of symptoms, but is often not seen until some days have passed. Such enhancement may be around the lesion, suggesting hypervascularity of the adjacent brain, or within it, indicating a breakdown of the blood-brain barrier (Figs. 64.14 and 64.15). There is no clear relationship between the type of enhancement and the prognosis. It has been suggested that infarcts which flood with contrast medium will go on to marked necrosis. Since it is possible that the contrast medium may have a deleterious effect, administration in cases of obvious infarcts may in fact be contraindicated. Occasionally, in the acute stage, enhancement may be the only definite indication of ischaemia, the infarct itself being isodense with the surrounding brain (Fig. 64.14). Acute infarction is one of the very few situations in which contrast injection may show previously undetected lesions. The majority of infarcts will show enhancement at some stage during the first two weeks though some do not (Fig. 64.16A). The proportion showing enhancement is related to the dose of contrast medium, being low with

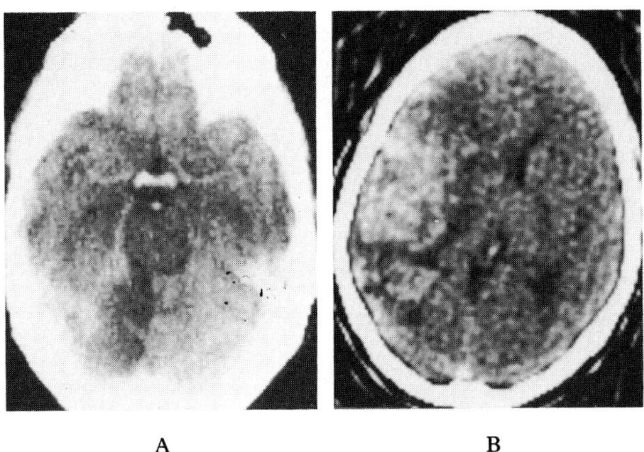

Fig. 64.16 A—Acute left cerebellar infarct. Low density area with no enhancement after contrast. B—Haemorrhagic infarct. Mixed high and low density lesion in left middle cerebral area. Slight mass effect. No contrast given (L36 W80).

a small bolus (50 ml) but high with the large dose technique (300 ml by drip infusion). After six weeks, however, persisting enhancement should suggest an alternative diagnosis.

A type of infarct whose appearances differ markedly from those described above is the uncommon haemorrhagic infarct. This is commoner with a major embolus. There is patchy increased density throughout the affected region, often with some mass effect (Fig. 64.16B). The ability to differentiate this type of infarct is important in its contraindication to the use of anticoagulant drugs. The CT appearances resemble those of a haemorrhage or haemorhagic contusion rather than a simple infarct.

Venous thrombosis, either spontaneous, or more commonly in association with an inflammatory process, may lead to infarction. In severe cases the white matter is predominantly affected, and the changes are often bilateral, showing as areas of diminished density. The affected central hemispheres are frequently swollen, and in severe cases may show marked contrast enhancement.

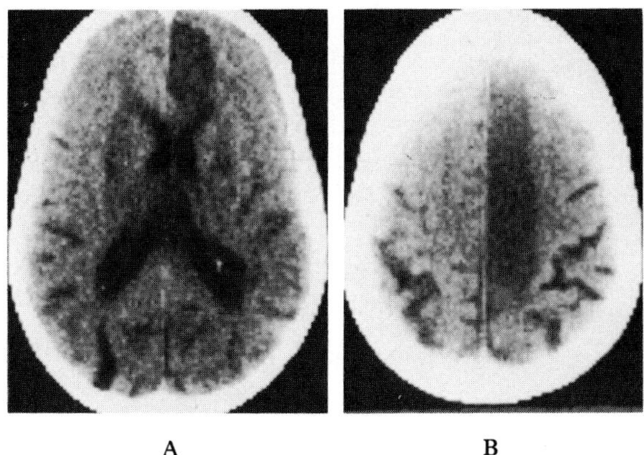

Fig. 64.18 Established right anterior cerebral infarct: low density area confined closely to right anterior cerebral territory (L36 W80).

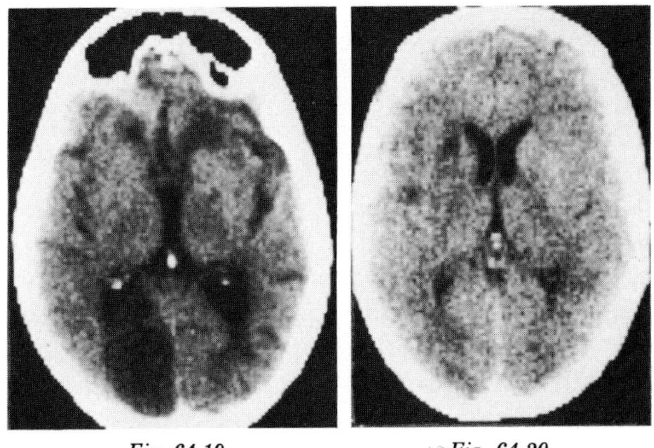

Fig. 64.19 Mature left occipital infarct (L40 W80).

Fig. 64.20 Small lacunar infarcts in left capsular region (L36 W60).

Angiography remains the only certain antemortem means of establishing the diagnosis.

Transient ischaemic attacks (TIAs) are generally regarded as due to small emboli arising from atheromatous plaques, which are most commonly situated at

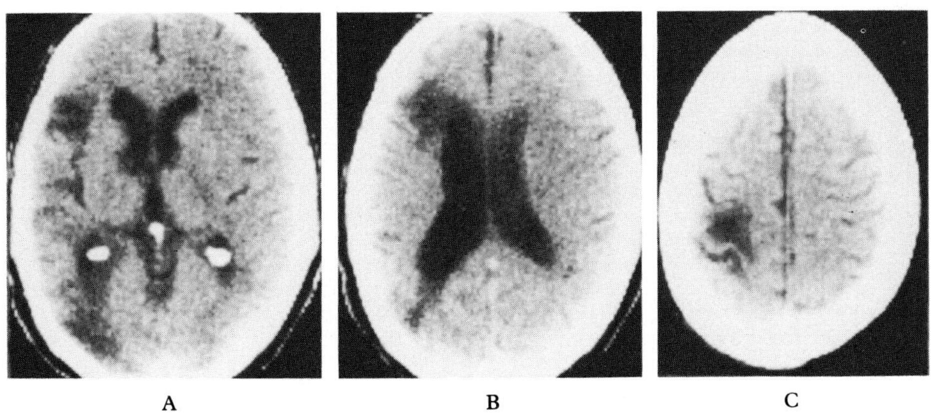

Fig. 64.17 'Watershed' infarcts at boundaries of the L. middle cerebral territory anteriorly and posteriorly (L36 W80).

the origin of the internal carotid artery. The causative lesions are usually well shown by angiography (see Ch. 62) and are amenable to surgical treatment. It is characteristic that the symptoms are transient until a major thrombosis supervenes and CT studies during the prodromal and TIA phase have proved negative. It appears that the cerebral lesion, though producing transient clinical symptoms, is insufficient in degree to produce detectable CT changes.

TRAUMA

Cranial trauma is a major problem in accident and emergency departments and in one series provided 10 per cent of the patients seen. It is also responsible for 150,000 hospital admissions per year in the UK.

It is not necessary for every patient who suffers a head injury, even with subsequent loss of consciousness, to undergo a CT scan. In the acute phase, the indications are similar to those formerly applied to cerebral angiography, i.e. deterioration of the patient's conscious level, with or without focal signs, for which no cause is otherwise apparent. Although CT scanning is quicker and carries a lower risk to the patient than cerebral angiography, local availability of the apparatus places a limitation on its use. When it is available, however, it should be regarded as the definitive, and frequently the only radiological investigation, other than plain skull radiographs. Hence sedation and/or general anaesthesia should be employed without hesitation when indicated, since the recently traumatized patient may be very restless.

Lesions encountered in the acute stages

Intracranial haematomas. These may be extradural, subdural or intracerebral. Subarachnoid or intraventricular haemorrhage may also occur.

Extradural haematomas are seen as biconvex high-density areas immediately subjacent to the vault (Fig. 64.21). They are most frequent in the frontoparietal regions, but may occur in the posterior fossa, when they are particularly likely to be missed if the CT scan is of poor quality. Occasionally less dense areas appear within them, perhaps due to unclotted blood, and if they should recur after surgery the classic shape may be lost. The lateral ventricles are characteristically displaced to the contralateral side, and there is usually some swelling of the affected cerebral hemisphere, although obvious oedema may not be apparent.

The appearances of **subdural haematomas** vary considerably, depending on their age, but also on other factors as yet unknown. The acute subdural haematoma, i.e. within 48 hours of the injury, can sometimes closely resemble the acute extradural lesion, but is more frequently concavoconvex, spreading over the surface of the cerebral hemisphere (Fig. 64.22). In the acute stage, the haematoma is usually of high density, often situated in the frontoparietal regions or middle cranial fossa, and associated with ipsilateral brain swelling. Subdural collections are generally of higher attenuation than brain for about two weeks, and after three to four weeks are of lower attenuation, eventually approaching that of c.s.f. (Fig. 64.25). However, between two to four weeks after injury, they pass through a stage when they are isodense with the underlying brain. Isodense haematomas (Fig. 64.23) present major problems in diagnosis, since the lesion is not directly visible, and it may be necessary to rely on indirect signs. These include ventricular or pineal displacement, and absence of visible sulci on the affected side; the former sign will, however, be absent in the not uncommon case of bilateral lesions. Squeezing together of the frontal horns, to give a 'rabbit's ears'

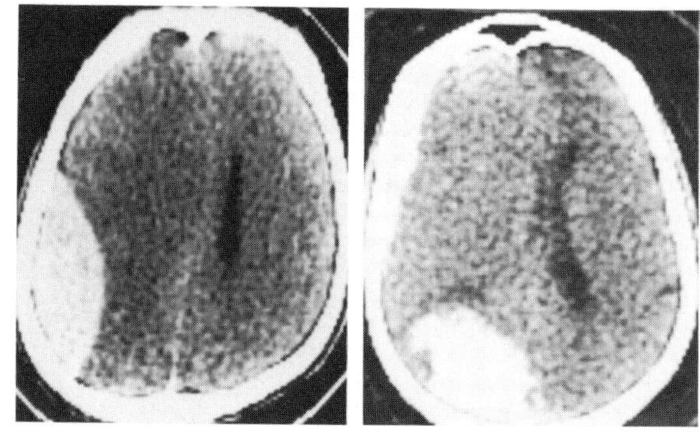

Fig. 64.21 *Fig. 64.22*

Fig. 64.21 Acute extradural haematoma. High density biconvex mass in left occipitoparietal region with mass effect following trauma (L34 W75).

Fig. 64.22 Acute subdural haematoma. High density peripheral lesion in left frontoparietal area. There is also a left occipital intracerebral haematoma. Both lesions followed rupture of a dural AV malformation (L36 W75).

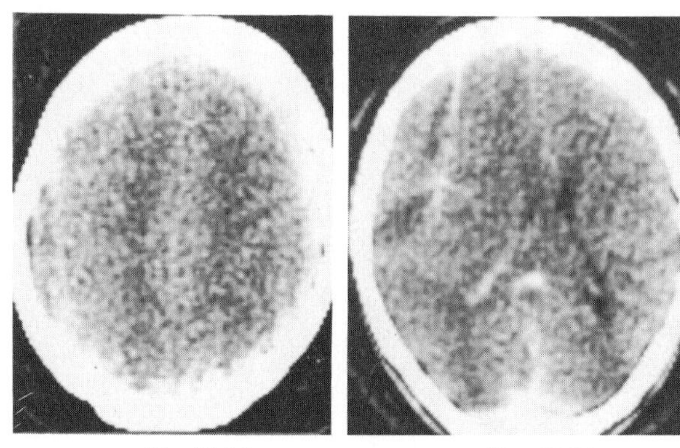

Fig. 64.23 *Fig. 64.24*

Fig. 64.23 Isodense subdural in subacute stage (L36 W75).

Fig. 64.24 Subacute subdural in left frontoparietal region. The lesion is largely isodense, but is better shown after contrast by enhancement of the capsule. Some mass effect (L36 W75).

appearance and effacement of the basal cisterns may suggest the diagnosis when bilateral isodense lesions are present. Intravenous iodinated contrast medium may help by causing enhancement of the capsule of such haematomas (Fig. 64.24) but this is not invariable. Recent studies with extra high-dose contrast injections have suggested that isodense subdurals can be identified by this technique since the surface of the brain is usually clearly identifiable. It has also been suggested that xenon enhancement can help in this problem. However, this is an expensive technique requiring general anaesthesia. Subdural haematomas of mixed density, probably indicating fresh bleeding into a chronic lesion, may be seen. With the patient in the supine position, the denser blood tends to sink to the posterior, dependent portion of the lesion, giving rise to a fluid level.

Very long-standing chronic subdural haematomas are invariably of low attenuation (Figs. 64.25 to 64.28). They may be associated with atrophy of the underlying brain and occasionally with expansion and thinning of the skull vault. They should not be confused with cases of post-traumatic hemiatrophy, in which the affected hemicranium is the smaller.

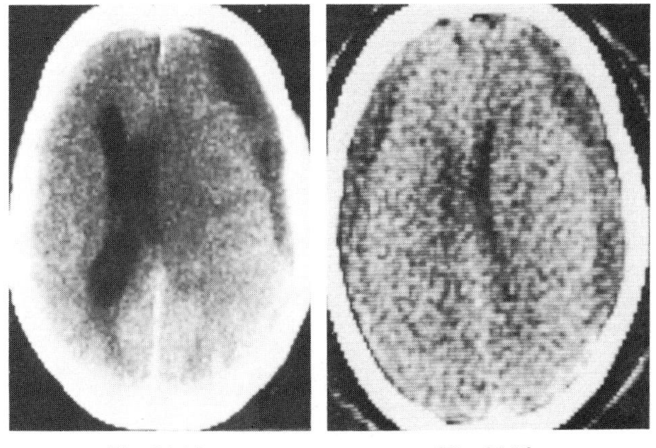

Fig. 64.25 *Fig. 64.26*

Fig. 64.25 Subdural haematoma three weeks after onset. The clot is largely absorbed and the subdural fluid is now of low density (L40 W80).

Fig. 64.26 Bilateral chronic subdural haematoma, larger on the right.

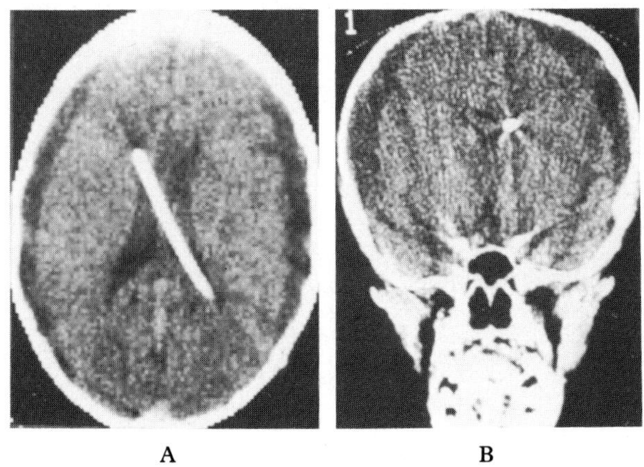

A B

Fig. 64.27 A—Bilateral subdural as a complication of shunt operation (L36 W80). B—Coronal view of same case (L28 W100).

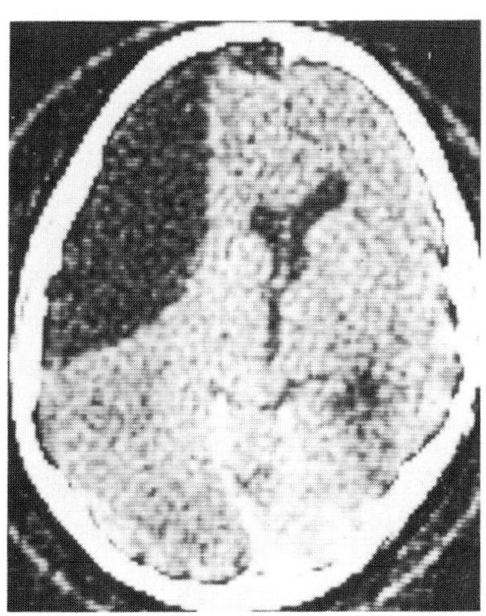

Fig. 64.28 Large chronic subdural haematoma with mass effect.

CT scanning is invaluable in the management and follow-up of both extra- and subdural haematomas, since it permits the detection of residual or recurrent lesions, of undiagnosed contralateral haematomas, or the presence of infection. The latter may be suggested by loculation of air within the haematoma cavity, by increase in density of the fluid contents, and by marked enhancement of the capsule.

Calcification of the capsule may occur in chronic lesions, with or without complications such as infection.

Traumatic **intracerebral haematomas** may be impossible to distinguish from spontaneous intracerebral haemorrhage, and in this context even the history may be unhelpful. The frontal and temporal lobes are classical sites, which are less commonly affected by spontaneous episodes. Both types are of high density, but traumatic bleeding is more frequently multifocal and in cases with a poor prognosis may be seen to involve the brain stem. It is also more commonly associated with low-density areas and brain swelling, even in the acute stages. The blood may extend to the ventricles or the subarachnoid space. Purely intraventricular haemorrhage is uncommon as a result of trauma. Subarachnoid haemorrhage is, however, relatively frequent, although often overlooked. It is commonly manifest as a line of high attenuation alongside the falx, especially posteriorly.

Retrobulbar or subperiosteal orbital haematomas are readily diagnosed in the context of head trauma as high density lesions within the orbits or applied to the bone. Without a history of head injury, the differential diagnosis is that of a retrobulbar mass.

It is also possible to demonstrate soft-tissue extracranial haemorrhage in the acute stage.

Cerebral contusion and oedema. Two types of cerebral contusion may be detected by CT scanning—haemorrhagic and non-haemorrhagic. The latter may be impossible to distinguish from focal cerebral oedema due to other causes.

Haemorrhagic contusion (Figs. 64.29 and 64.30) is commonly seen in the frontal and temporal lobes, although any part of the cerebrum, cerebellum or brain stem may be affected. It appears as a mass lesion of mixed high and low density not dissimilar from multifocal traumatic haemorrhage, but generally more diffuse; the area of swelling may be very extensive. The haemorrhagic areas may not be evident in the very acute stage, occurring only 24 hours or more later.

Non-haemorrhagic contusion (Fig. 64.31) cannot reliably be distinguished from cerebral oedema, but tends to be more focal and space occupying. Considerable enhancement may be seen with intravenous contrast medium; this does not occur with oedema.

Oedema may be focal or, more frequently, generalized, when it may be difficult to recognize, since the diminution in absorption coefficients may only be slight and ventricular compression difficult to assess. Since there is no well-defined lower limit of ventricular size, generalized brain swelling can often be identified in retrospect, when the ventricles have re-expanded to their normal size.

A normal scan in the acute and subacute phases does not necessarily entail a good prognosis; no abnormality may be apparent in cases with severe primary brain damage and 'axonal shearing', in whom the prognosis is very poor.

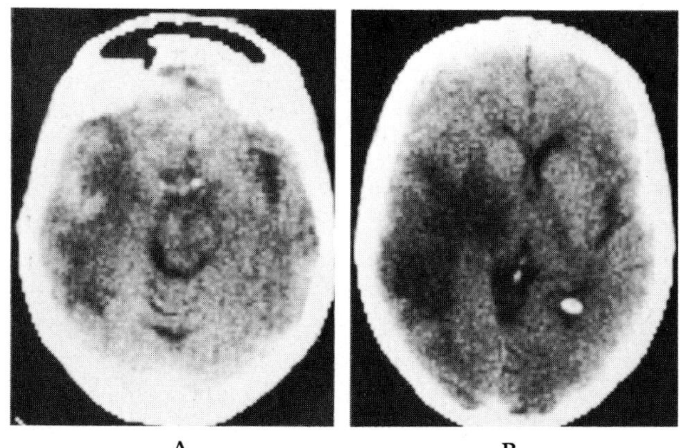

A B

Fig. 64.31 Cerebral trauma. Contusions in left temporal lobe (L36 W80).

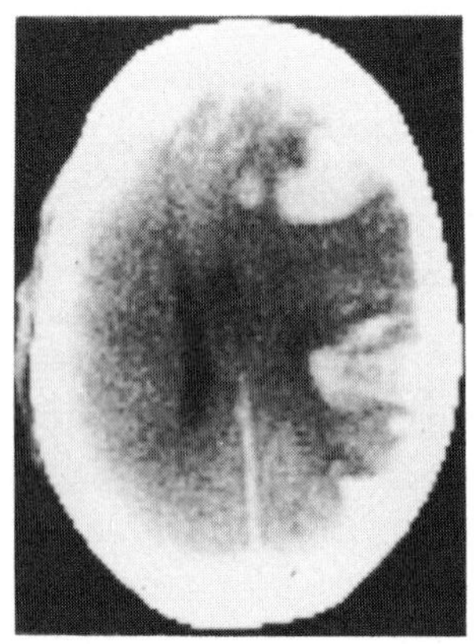

Fig. 64.29 Cerebral trauma. Contusions with multifocal haemorrhage (L44 W60).

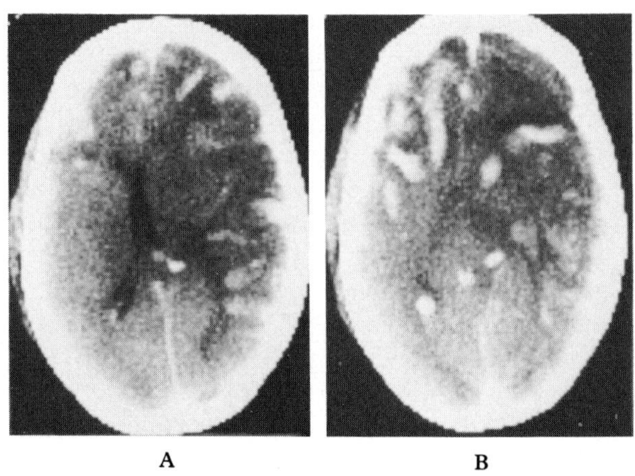

A B

Fig. 64.30 Cerebral trauma. Multifocal haemorrhagic contusions in both hemispheres (L40 W60).

Skull fractures

Fractures are, in most instances, best diagnosed by a combination of clinical features and plain radiography. However, basal fractures, which are often difficult to

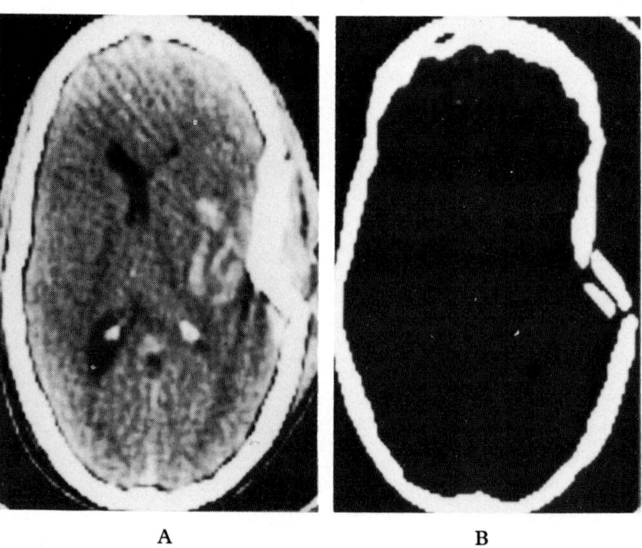

A B

Fig. 64.32 A—Depressed fracture right temporal region with underlying haemorrhagic contusions (L34 W75). B—Same case at higher level (L) to show bone detail (L128 W75).

demonstrate or to assess fully by these means may be shown very clearly by CT scanning.

Depressed fractures may be clearly demonstrated and their relationship to the underlying brain better shown than by plain X-ray films (Fig. 64.32). However, the chief value of the CT scan is in the assessment of underlying brain damage and haematoma formation.

Foreign bodies

Intracranial foreign bodies may be accurately localized by CT scanning. The value of the technique is in the demonstration of the position of the foreign body relative to and its effects on the intracranial structures features which cannot be seen on plain radiographs. Good demonstration of the relationships of metallic objects may however, be prevented by the resulting artefacts.

POST-TRAUMATIC SEQUELAE

These may include:

1. Cerebral infarction
2. Cerebral atrophy
3. Hydrocephalus
4. Complications (e.g. intracranial abscess).

1. **Cerebral infarction.** Vascular occlusion or spasm caused by trauma to the head or neck may cause cerebral infarction, the appearances of which are indistinguishable from those of cerebral infarction arising from thromboembolic lesions. Infarction can on rare occasions follow some weeks or months after trauma to the great vessels of the neck.

2. **Post-traumatic atrophy.** This can be focal or generalized. It may clearly reflect cerebral infarction, affecting a known vascular territory, or affect one cerebral hemisphere. If the latter occurs in infancy or childhood or from perinatal trauma the whole hemicranium may be underdeveloped. The appearances are those of cerebral atrophy. There is enlargement of the fissures and sulci and ventricular dilatation. Porencephalic cyst cavities may be present, whose communication with the ventricular system may or may not be obvious (Fig. 64.39).

3. **Hydrocephalus.** Ventricular enlargement commonly occurs in the subacute phase after head trauma. It may then resolve or become progressive and symptomatic. In the early stages, development of hydrocephalus may be difficult to distinguish from resolution of generalized cerebral swelling. Enlargement of the temporal horns strongly suggests the former, but further follow-up is indicated. For a general consideration of atrophy, hydrocephalus and their distinction, see below.

CT scanning is an excellent technique for non-traumatic monitoring of ventricular size.

INFECTIONS

Intracranial infections may be divided into abscesses, encephalitides and meningitides. The value of CT scanning is variable according to the type of lesion.

Abscesses may be pyogenic, tuberculous or fungal. *Pyogenic abscesses* are the most frequently encountered in clinical practice. They are often secondary to cardiac or aural disease, and may occur following chest infections or operations. They may occur anywhere in the brain or subdural space; the frontal and temporal lobes are commonly affected, the latter particularly when ear infection is present. Bilateral frontal abscesses clearly implicate the frontal sinuses as a source of infection. The CT may provide more direct evidence, by showing opaque sinuses or air cells, or bone defects. The CT scan will show an area of low density in the large majority of cases, and injection of intravenous contrast medium will demonstrate the abscess capsule as a thin-walled regular ring of enhancement (Fig. 64.33). Occasionally it may be

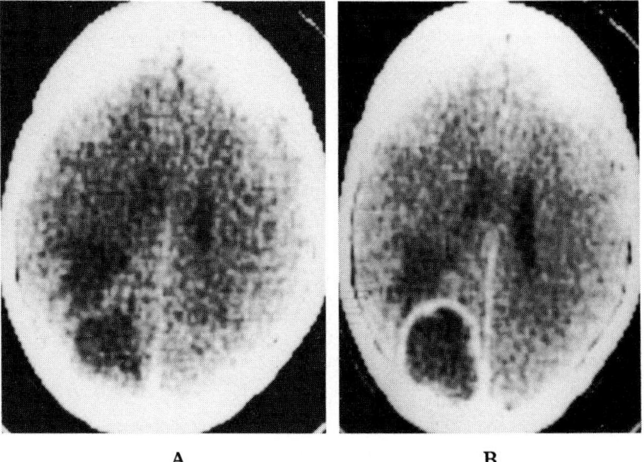

Fig. 64.33 Cerebral abscess. A—Low density lesions in left occipital region with some mass effect. B—After contrast there is a thin ring of enhancement round the abscess with oedema anteriorly (L34 W75).

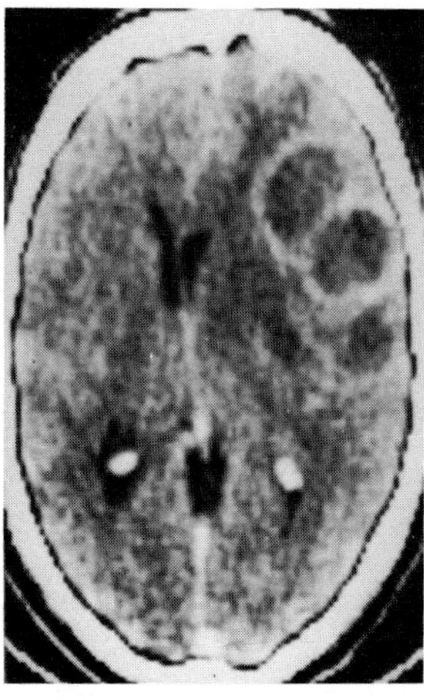

Fig. 64.34 Multiple abscesses in right frontoparietal area showing capsular enhancement after contrast (L34 W75).

clear that the lesion is multilocular (Fig. 64.34). The capsule may sometimes be seen as a ring of less reduced density before enhancement, but this is not a general feature of abscesses. Gas may be present adjacent to or within an abscess; it usually indicates that the cavity has been tapped, but in rare cases is present preoperatively, when it may indicate either infection with gas forming organisms or a fistulous connection with the exterior. There is usually some mass effect, but this may not be marked in relation to the extent of the oedema. Extension of the inflammatory process to the ventricular system is a bad prognostic sign. After successful tapping of the abscess, enhancement of the capsule is no longer seen. Subdural abscesses or empyemas are seen as areas of variable attenuation (usually reduced) adjacent to the skull vault, whose margins, and occasionally contents enhance markedly. Small lesions may be largely obscured by the overlying bone. When subdural empyemas are adjacent to the tentorium, coronal sections may be indicated to show whether the lesion is supra- or infratentorial.

Tuberculomata (Figs. 64.35 and 64.36) are commonly multiple and frequently follow a known episode of tuberculous meningitis. Once again, the lesions are usually of reduced density, but they may be isodense with brain and invisible before contrast, or very occasionally calcified. Enhancement occurs after intravenous contrast medium. Frequently there is a dense ring shadow which can simulate gliomas or pyogenic abscesses but this is not always seen. The appearance is characteristic of tuberculoma if there is central enhancement (target sign). Mass effect is not striking.

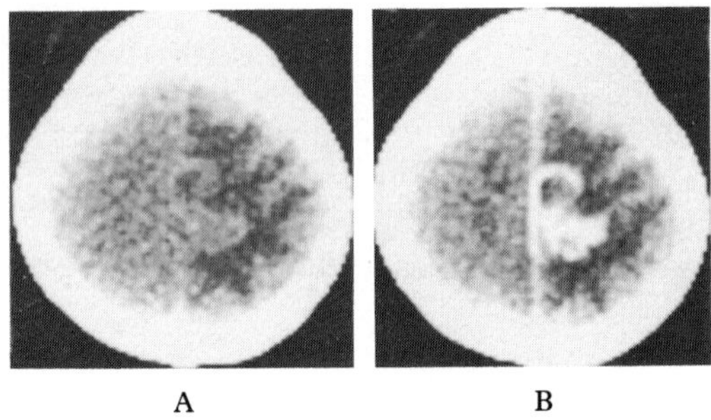

Fig. 64.35 Tuberculoma. A—Isodense lesion with surrounding oedema. B—Mixed enhancement after contrast (L36 W80).

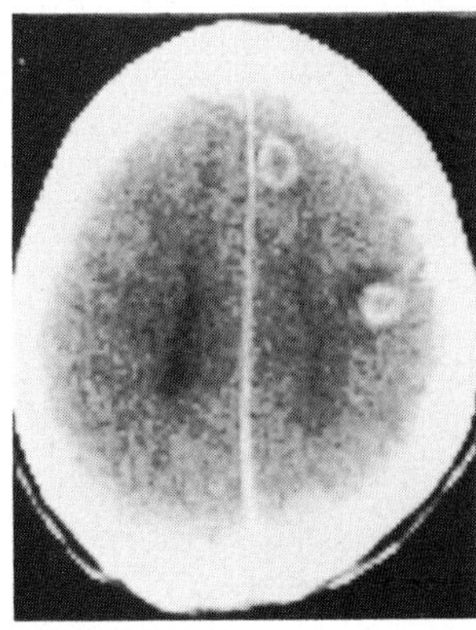

Fig. 64.36 Tuberculomata. Two small lesions with thick ring enhancement (L40 W80).

Fungal abscesses, caused by such organisms as Nocardia or Aspergillus, occur almost exclusively in patients receiving immunosuppressive drugs or steroids and they may be multiple. The CT appearances are similar to those of pyogenic abscesses, except that enhancement is more commonly homogeneous. The history is vital in suggesting the diagnosis and differentiating from tumour.

Hydatid cysts, although not strictly abscesses, may be considered here. They present as rounded homogenous low-density lesions without significant enhancement.

Encephalitis. Most types of encephalitis are associated with little or no change in CT appearances, although more or less extensive areas showing a slight reduction in density may be seen; their presence may only be appreciated by follow-up studies. *Herpes Simplex encephalitis* produces more definite reductions in density, affecting particularly the temporal lobes, and with some mass effect. Scattered lesions are typical and the lesions usually show no enhancement after contrast. Haemorrhage is occasionally seen. The changes are often bilateral though they may appear predominantly unilateral in the acute phase. This has resulted in misdiagnosis as tumours. Extensive necrosis of the involved portions of the cerebrum is a common late sequel. The same may occur with *Toxoplasma encephalitis*, in which condition there is usually associated calcification and often microcephaly. Gross cases in which the infection has been acquired in utero show marked cerebral atrophy with ventricles enormously dilated.

Progressive multifocal leukoencephalopathy is a viral infection, usually seen in patients with diminished resistance to infection. More or less widespread involvement of the white matter, with low attenuation and irregular enhancement, is seen. Focal lesions may simulate glioma. *Subacute sclerosing panencephalitis* is a sequel to measles infection; it also causes white matter low attenuation.

Pyogenic meningitis does not produce changes in the CT appearances, but *chronic granulomatous basal meningitis*, e.g. tuberculous or cryptococcal, may be associated with thickening of the basal meninges, which obliterate the basal cisterns and show marked enhancement with intravenous contrast medium injection. Similar changes may be observed in *sarcoidosis*. Such basal meningitides not uncommonly result in hydrocephalus; CT is invaluable for the detection of this complication. Cortical venous thrombosis also complicates meningitis; its appearances are described above.

Similar appearances to those seen in infective encephalitis may be observed in patients with clinical evidence of cerebral irritation in association with systemic infective illnesses or following vaccination; the latter are thought to have an allergic basis. Scattered or generalized areas of low density are seen to affect predominantly the periventricular white matter.

ATROPHIC AND DEGENERATIVE DISORDERS

Cerebral atrophy

Cerebral atrophy may be secondary to vascular disease, trauma, toxins and infection, but is generally idiopathic. The pathological features are those of a loss of substance which may affect the cerebrum (Fig. 64.37), cerebellum (Fig. 64.38) and brain stem. The CT appearances thus include:

1. Ventricular enlargement and 'rounding' of the ventricular angles
2. Increased prominence of the cerebral or cerebellar sulci
3. Increased size of the Sylvian and hemispheric fissures
4. Abnormally large basal cisterns
5. Reduction in size of the midbrain and pons.

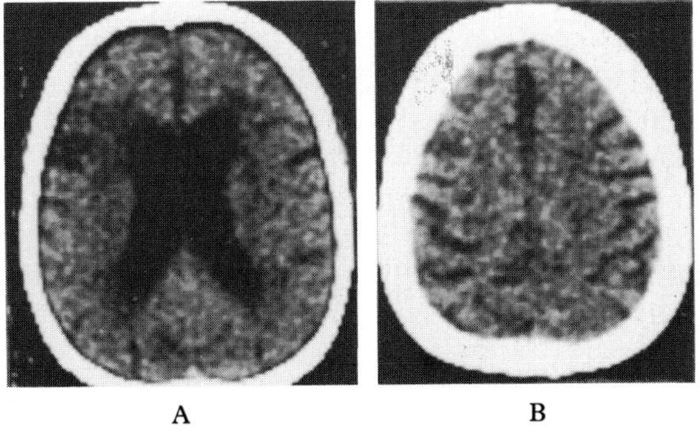

A B

Fig. 64.37 Generalized atrophy. A—Dilated lateral ventricle. B—Enlarged sulci and interhemisphere fissure (L36 W80).

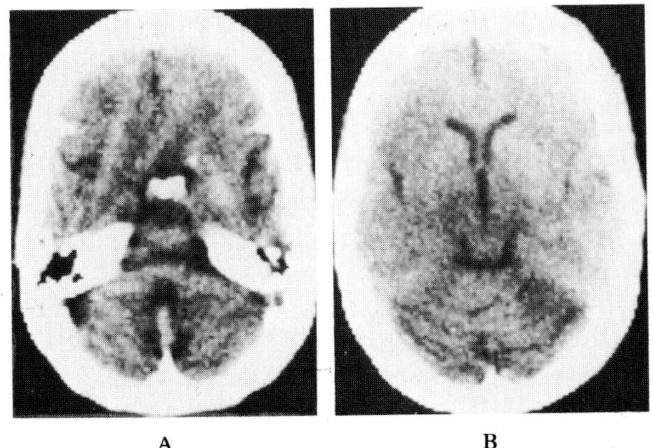

A B

Fig. 64.38 Cerebellar atrophy. A and B—widening of cerebellar sulci (L40 W80).

It is uncommon for an individual case to show all these features. Frequently the changes are focal rather than generalized. This is normally the case when atrophy follows a vascular or traumatic incident.

Ventricular enlargement. This affects particularly the frontal horns of the lateral ventricles (which lose their normal slit-like configuration), the bodies of the lateral ventricles, and the third ventricle. Enlargement of the temporal horns is uncommon and they are frequently not visible. Even with cerebellar atrophy, the fourth ventricle may not be obviously enlarged.

Sulci. Widening of the cerebral or cerebellar sulci is the hallmark of atrophy. It may be focal or generalized; focal changes suggest previous vascular or traumatic episodes (Fig. 64.39). Commonly, the wide sulci are

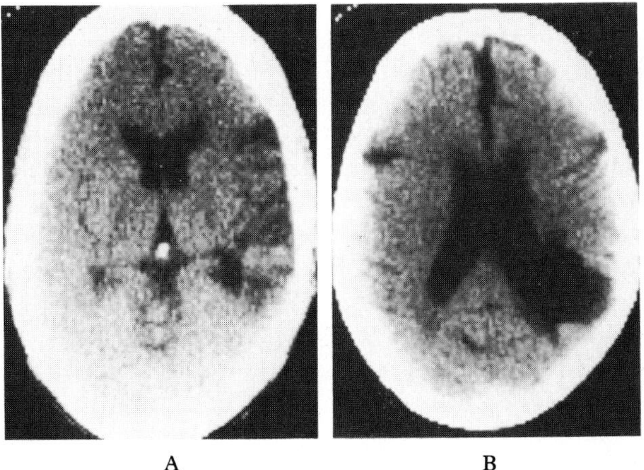

A B

Fig. 64.39 Post-traumatic atrophy. A—Focal atrophy in right parietal region. B—Focal atrophy with porencephalic cyst in right parietal region. Also some generalized atrophy (L36 W80).

limited to the frontal and/or parietal regions. Similar involutional changes are seen in normal elderly subjects. The borderline between normal and abnormal at any age is difficult to establish, and since different CT scanners show the sulci with variable clarity, a familiarity with the normal range of appearances of a given machine is essential. It should also be understood that there is only a loose correlation between 'atrophic' manifestations at CT and clinical signs, e.g. dementia.

Fissures. Widening of the fissures is also typical of atrophy, but may occur in hydrocephalus. It is commonly asymmetrical. When the interhemispheric fissure is widened, the changes are generally most marked anteriorly. In advanced cases, the falx may be seen clearly as a thin dense line in the cerebrospinal fluid between the hemispheres.

Basal cisterns. These may also be enlarged, especially when the brain stem is atrophic (see below).

Midbrain and pons. These structures are not infrequently smaller than normal in generalized atrophy and may be strikingly involved in such conditions as the Steele-Richardson syndrome.

Degenerative cerebral disorders

Certain specific diseases show cerebral atrophy on CT scanning. These include:

Parkinsonism. Cerebral atrophy is the most common CT finding. A small number of cases of post-encephalitic or idiopathic type will show infarcts or calcification in the basal ganglia. In the Shy-Drager subtype, where there is clinical involvement of the brain stem, this is also seen to be atrophic.

Striatonigral atrophy. Cavitation or lacunar infarction of the basal ganglia regions is also characteristic of this condition; atrophic changes may also be present.

Motor neurone disease. Some cases of this condition have also been described as showing typical atrophic changes.

Leukoencephalopathies. In this group may be included such rare entities of spongiform degeneration, Alexander's disease, metachromatic leukodystrophy, Krabbe's disease and sudanophilic leukodystrophy. The CT appearances reflect the pathological findings, which are of demyelination and gliosis affecting predominantly the white matter (Fig. 64.40). There is a reduction in density of the deep white matter. This may be focal, as in Schilder's disease (where the occipital region is affected) or, more commonly, generalized. The internal capsule, however, is often spared.

These appearances are characteristic, but non-specific, since similar changes may be seen in *encephalitis*, in association with *muscular dystrophy*, or in *hypertensive* and *nephrotic encephalopathy*. There is also a suggestion that white matter low attenuation may be seen more commonly in the elderly when the blood pressure is only mildly raised.

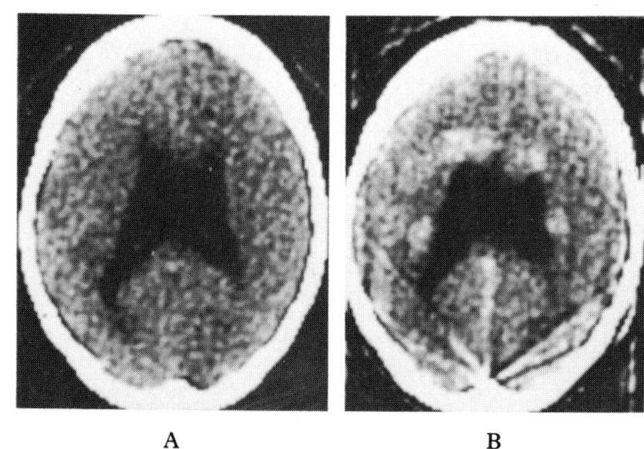

Fig. 64.41 Multiple sclerosis. A—Paraventricular low density areas. B—Enhancement after contrast (L40 W80).

Multiple sclerosis. Many patients with multiple sclerosis will show no abnormality on CT scanning, even in the acute stage. Paraventricular low-density areas have been described, however, and these may show marked enhancement (Fig. 64.41). About one-third of chronically-affected patients show these paraventricular low-density areas, and another third show atrophic changes.

Idiopathic epilepsy. Focal or generalized atrophic changes appear to be more common in patients with epilepsy than in the general population, particularly in the older age group. The relationship between focal changes and focal seizures or e.e.g. abnormalities is not close and the significance of these observations is not clear.

Migraine. Patients with a history of severe migraine also show an increased incidence of both focal and generalized atrophy. Again the significance of this finding is not clear.

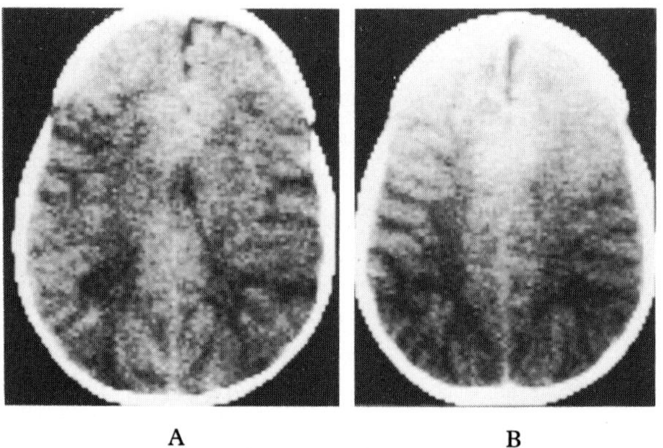

Fig. 64.40 Leukoencephalopathy. A and B—Reduced density of white matter (L34 W60).

COMMUNICATING HYDROCEPHALUS

It is important that cerebral atrophy should not be confused with communicating hydrocephalus. The former condition is usually not amenable to treatment, but surgery may produce striking improvement in patients with the latter. The CT features of this condition are:

1. Enlargement of the ventricles
2. Enlargement of the basal cisterns
3. Enlargement of the fissures
4. Periventricular low-density areas
5. Absence of enlarged sulci.

Enlargement of the ventricles. This is commonly more marked than in cerebral atrophy. The bodies and frontal horns are large and rounded, and the temporal horns are often clearly visible. The third ventricle is usually wide, but the fourth ventricle may not be definitely abnormal.

The basal cisterns. These may be prominent, but this is not a constant feature.

The fissures. The Sylvian fissures are often enlarged; the interhemispheric fissure is less commonly affected.

Periventricular low density areas. These may be observed in either obstructive or communicating hydrocephalus and are thought to indicate abnormal passage of cerebrospinal fluid through the ependyma into the white matter. They are usually most obvious around the frontal horns, where they may blur the ventricular outline.

Sulci. Widened sulci are only occasionally seen in this condition, except in association with enlargement of the Sylvian fissure.

It is clear from the foregoing that many of the CT features of cerebral atrophy are similar to those of hydrocephalus, and a difficult problem arises when even the clinical features do not enable them to be distinguished. The distinction is of importance because of the possibility of effective treatment of communicating hydrocephalus by ventricular shunting procedures. Pneumoencephalography and intrathecal isotope cisternography have been widely used for the differential diagnosis of these conditions. More recently Metrizamide (Amipaque) cisternography combined with CT has also been used (see Ch. 63, p. 1234).

THE SPINE

The value of CT examination of the spine is limited by several factors: the contrast and spatial resolution within the spinal canal; the length of the spine, which is much greater than that of the head, and difficulties of localizing the level to be scanned. However, with the 'scanogram' facilities on the most modern machines the latter problem has been largely resolved as has that of adjusting the alignment of the X-ray beam to the normal course of the vertebral column. For these reasons, spinal CT is used as an adjunct to myelography, rather than as a primary investigation.

Contrast resolution within the spinal canal is such that in most cases the spinal cord is only identifiable in the cervical region (where the subarachnoid space is largest) and little or no resolution of its internal structure is possible. Dilute Metrizamide is often injected before spinal CT, in order to increase the contrast discrimination between the cord and the c.s.f. This, of course, robs CT of its essentially innocuous character.

The indications for CT of the spine may be summarized as follows:

1. Investigation of vertebral column pathology. Here, the high contrast resolution of CT as compared with conventional radiographs makes it ideal for the demonstration of such lesions as osteolytic metastases. Moreover, any associated extraspinal soft tissue mass is also clearly shown; occasionally, intraspinal extension may also be visible.

2. Investigation of the nature of intramedullary space-occupying lesions. It may be possible to identify the contents of a spinal cord mass as fatty (thereby establishing the diagnosis of lipoma), solid (indicating a tumour, almost certainly of the glioma series) or fluid. In the latter case, the diagnosis rests between a cystic tumour or a hydromyelia.

In angiomas of the cord, scans after intravenous contrast medium may show an enhancing vascular lesion.

3. The value of scanning without intrathecal contrast medium in intradural-extramedullary or extradural lesions is currently a matter of debate and depends largely on the quality of the apparatus.

REFERENCES AND SUGGESTIONS FOR FURTHER READING

Ambrose, J. (1973) Computerised transverse axial scanning (tomography). Part 2—Clinical applications. *British Journal of Radiology*, **46**, 1023–1047.

Barrington, N. A. & Lewtas, N. A. (1977) Indications for contrast medium enhancement in computed tomography of the brain. *Clinical Radiology*, **28**, 535–537.

Bories, J. (ed.) (1978) *The Diagnostic Limitations of Computerised Axial Tomography*. Springer: Berlin.

Du Boulay, G. H. & Moseley, I. F. (eds) (1977) *Computerised Axial Tomography in Clinical Practice*. (1st European Seminar). Springer-Verlag: Berlin.

Gado, M. H., Phelps, M. E. & Coleman, R. E. (1975) An extravascular component of contrast enhancement in cranial computed tomography. *Radiology*, **117**, 589–597.

Gambarelli, J., Guerinel, G., Chevrot, L. & Mattei, M. (1977) *Computerised Axial Tomography*. Springer: Berlin.

Gonzalez, C. F., Grossman, C. B. & Palacios, E (1976) *Computed Brain and Orbital Tomography*. John Wiley and Sons: New York.

Greitz, T. & Hindmarsh, T. (1974) Computer assisted tomography of intracranial CSF circulation using a water soluble contrast medium. *Acta radiologica*, **15**, 497–509.

Gyldensted, C. (1976) Computed tomography of the cerebrum in multiple sclerosis. *Neuroradiology*, **12**, 33–42.

Hayward, R. D. *et al.* (1976) Intracerebral haemorrhage. *Lancet*, **i**, 1–4.

Hounsfield, G. N. (1973) Computerised transverse axial scanning (tomography). Part 1—Description of system. *British Journal of Radiology*, **46**, 1016–1022.

Huckman, M. S. *et al.* (1975) The validity of criteria for the evaluation of cerebral atrophy by computed tomography. *Radiology*, **116**, 85–92.

Lanksch, W. & Kazner, E. (eds) (1976) *Cranial Computerized Tomography*. Springer: Berlin.

Merino-de Villasante, J. & Taveras, J. (1976) Computerized tomography in acute head trauma. *American Journal of Roentgenology*, **126**, 765–778.

Naidich, T. P. *et al.* (1976) Evaluation of paediatric hydrocephalus by computed tomography. *Radiology*, **119**, 337–345.

New, P. F. & Scott, W. R. (1975) *Computed Tomography of the Brain and Orbit*, 2nd edn. Williams and Wilkins: Baltimore.

Sutton, D. & Claveria, L. E. (1977) Meningiomas diagnosed by scanning. A review of 100 intracranial cases. Springer-Verlag: Berlin. Du-Boulay, G. H. & Moseley, I. F. (eds) *Computerised Axial Tomography in Clinical Practice*, pp. 102–110.

Welchman, J. M. (1979) Computerised tomography of intracranial tuberculomata. *Clinical Radiology*, **30**, 567–573.

Yock, D. H., Marshall, W. (1975) Recent ischaemic brain infarcts at computed tomography. Appearances pre- and postcontrast infusion. *Radiology*, **117**, 599–608.

CHAPTER 65

COMPUTED TOMOGRAPHY—THE BODY

TECHNICAL ASPECTS

Technical aspects have already been discussed in the introductory part of Chapter 63 and the discussion is here extended.

DATA ACQUISITION

CT employs collimated X-rays directed only at the layer under investigation and radiographic film is replaced by either scintillation or ionization detectors. If a sufficient number of 'projections' or 'views' are obtained across the plane of interest then an image may be derived from the measurements of transmitted radiation. The original scanner made use of a simple collimated X-ray source and scintillation detector scanning together in a linear manner across the patient. During each linear scan some 250 observations were made of transmitted photons by the detector. The gantry supporting the X-ray tube and detectors then rotated or indexed at 1° intervals over 180° and the 'projections' repeated. This method requiring more than four minutes of scan time formed the basis for the 'rotate and translate' machine. Modifications to the method incorporating detector arrays and modified fans of collimated X-ray beams now permit much faster and more comprehensive data

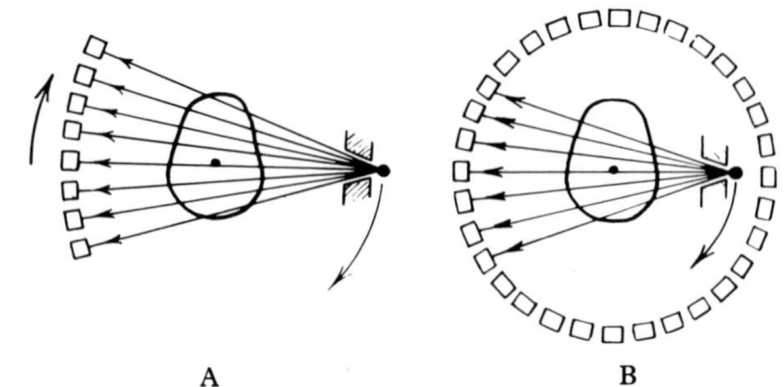

Fig. 65.2 Rotate only systems. (A) Fan beam and array of detectors. (B) Fixed ring of detectors. X-ray source within the ring.

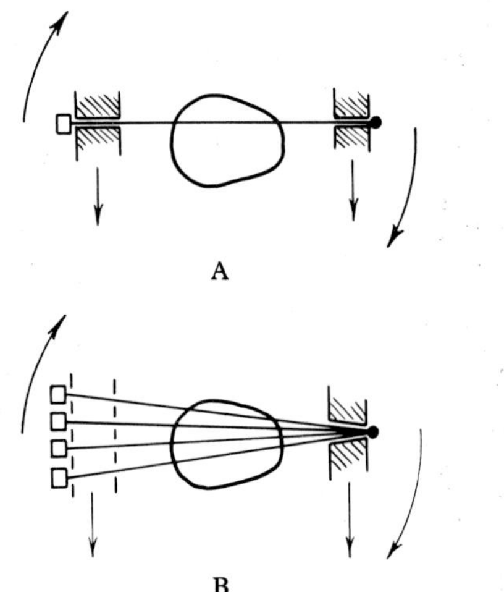

Fig. 65.1 Rotate and translate systems. (A) Single beam, single collimator. (B) Modified fan beam and an array of detectors.

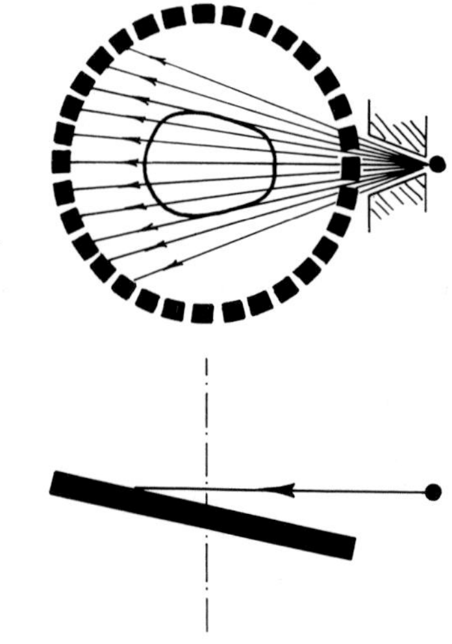

Fig. 65.3 Nutating geometry. Fixed ring of detectors. X-ray source outside the ring.

acquisition. Scan times for 'rotate and translate' units are now 5–20 seconds (Fig. 65.1). Various additional types of scanning motion have been employed incorporating true fan beams, fixed detector arrays and a variety of detector systems (Fig. 65.2). In those units employing a fixed ring of detectors the X-ray tube may be located either inside or outside the detector ring. In the latter it becomes necessary to oscillate the detector ring, a system referred to as 'nutating geometry' (Fig. 65.3). Scan times can now be reduced to 1–2 seconds. Efforts to overcome cardiac and vascular motion are currently under investigation in a number of centres and can involve costly and complex engineering. Slow scan times may still be desirable where an increased photon flux is required. Each design has advantages and disadvantages but all represent methods of collecting sets of transmission measurements across a body section of finite thickness.

The recorded transmission data, however it is acquired, must be processed by a suitable computer algorithm* in order to produce a precise mathematical reconstruction of the cross section. The basic principle of CT and the main methods of computing tomographic cross sections from transmission measurements have been comprehensively reviewed in the literature.

RESOLUTION

Each picture element (pixel) in the reconstruction has a cross sectional area which, depending on the particular machine characteristics and the area under investigation, may be 1·5 × 1·5 mm, 0·75 × 0·75 mm or even smaller. The size of the picture element is a measure of the spatial resolution. The depth or thickness of any section is determined by the collimation. It is usually 10–13 mm but may be reduced to as little as 2 mm. Volumes of tissue (voxels) so defined have computed numerical values dependent on their ability to attenuate X-rays. These numbers, which are very precisely related to the differences between the linear attenuation coefficients of the material scanned and water, are usually termed Hounsfield numbers (H) (see Ch. 63, Fig. 63.1).

DATA STORAGE AND INTERROGATION

The distribution of attenuation coefficients expressed as Hounsfield numbers may be stored on magnetic tape or 'floppy discs' (flexible, vinyl discs about 20 cm in diameter) and by digital to analog conversion be displayed as a grey level picture on a television monitor. High numbers, e.g. bone, are presented as white and low numbers, e.g. air, represented as black. The picture so produced has the unique property that it may be interrogated by the observer. Both the level on the Hounsfield scale (L) and the window width (W), may be varied and the whole dynamic range of body tissue thus explored. Hard copy or film obtained from the television display and selected by the observer represents only a fraction of the information contained within the numerically derived image.

**Algorithm:* A procedure for computation. From al-Khwarismi, a ninth century mathematician in the court of al-Mamun, son of Harun al-Rashid—the Arabian Nights' caliph of Baghdad.

MULTIPLANAR RECONSTRUCTION

The digital data derived from sequential transaxial sections can be used to provide reconstructions in planes other than the transaxial. Such alternative, computer-generated images obtained from the original block of digital information have, in the normal course of events, a lower resolution than the original transaxial sections. Considerable overlap of the transaxial sections is required to enable comparable resolution to be achieved in the reconstructed image. Such overlap inevitably incurs a radiation dose penalty. Nevertheless, multiplanar, rotating and 'walk through' displays are all possible by appropriate computed software programming. The objective value of such new conceptual information is still to be explored.

DENSITY DISCRIMINATION

Computerized tomography thus provides information about tissue density differences in a uniformly thin slice of tissue. Density discrimination of 1 part in 1000 may be achieved. The ability to discriminate tissue and the sensitivity to changes accompanying disease are functions of the signal to noise ratio. Noise is a measure of the fluctuation or uncertainty in transmission measurements due to the measuring system and also to the tissue under investigation. Total noise is not completely random and has a structure which can be defined mathematically and perhaps used as a means of characterizing tissue.

LIMITATIONS

Tissue composition

The linear attenuation coefficient of biological material contained in a voxel depends in a predictable and reproducible way upon the effective number of atoms (N), the effective atomic number (Z) of the material contained within the voxel together with the effective energy (E) of the main X-ray beam employed. The term 'effective' relates to the fact that no matter how small the computed volume of tissue it is unlikely to contain entirely homogeneous material. High and low density substances may contribute disproportionately to the derived Hounsfield number. This 'partial volume' effect becomes especially important when anatomical or disease process interfaces present within a section. Structural margins may be difficult to identify with precision and the accuracy of linear measurements is reduced. Interrogation of data with demonstration of different density ranges on hard copy may, under these circumstances, give rise to apparent changes in structural contour. It is important therefore in a sequential examination only to compare hard copy obtained at identical window widths and window levels.

Tissue characterization

A unique advantage of CT is its ability in some circumstances to distinguish heterogeneity of composition and pathological processes. This is particularly so in those lesions containing high (calcium) or low (fat) density material. Despite the ability to discriminate certain density differences, however, simple analysis of attenuation values does not yet permit precise histological characterization.

Attenuation values measured by CT are distributed in both magnitude and space. Distribution in magnitude can be described by the mean, standard deviation and skewness of the histograms of attenuation values. Other parameters, including analysis of gradients and autocorrelation functions, are required to describe spatial distribution. Current research is directed towards the special problems of tissue characterization.

Radiation dose

As a result of beam collimation and appropriate detector systems, CT has a high data retrieval per unit of radiation dose. An immutable relationship, however, exists between resolution or picture sharpness, density discrimination and radiation dose, enabling only compromise trade-offs to be made between these factors.

A 20-second scan on an EMI CT5005 using a 13 in (320 mm) reconstruction area results in a maximum skin entry dose to one section of 1·5 rad. Since radiation to one section results in scatter to adjacent tissue, examination of 8–10 adjacent 13 mm sections may increase the maximum entry dose at the centre section.

At a fixed dose as resolution improves the signal to noise ratio reduces and so the ability to see large low contrast objects deteriorates. Optimal conditions obviously depend on the size and contrast of the structure under investigation. Most structures within the abdominal cavity have very similar X-ray attenuation properties and are therefore dependent on surrounding low density fat for their contour delineation.

Any consideration of radiation dose must relate to information gained but measurement of dose under similar conditions of resolution, noise, slice thickness, scan field and scan diameter does permit some comparison of dose efficiency to be made.

Movement

Any movement, including breathing and other physiological movements during data acquisition will give rise to artefacts in the form of radiating streaks in the reconstruction. Such artefacts are particularly obtrusive when extremes of attenuation value such as air or metal are concerned. Even fast scanning times (1–2 seconds) cannot entirely counteract peristalsis or movement due to cardiac and vascular pulsation.

Reproducibility

Precise positioning and accurate reproducibility of a thin body section in all spatial co-ordinates presents significant problems. Careful external marking together with scanning radiographs enables reproducibility adequate for practical clinical purposes to be achieved. A precise numbering code which relates to bony anatomical levels is helpful with comparative studies.

CLINICAL ASPECTS—GENERAL

Computerized tomography is an imaging procedure where detailed information is obtained from thin transverse sections. Attention to patient preparation together with patient management during the CT examination is as important, if not more so, than with any other radiological procedure.

It is essential that the nature of the clinical problem is fully understood before the examination begins and that the circumstances of the investigation are as near ideal as possible. The role of the radiologist, whilst requiring technical skill, is directly concerned with clinical management. Dialogue with the referring clinician and a planned procedure are essential.

Patient preparation. Detailed preparation may vary according to the clinical situation but certain basic rules are important.

1. The nature and duration of the procedure should be explained to the patient.
2. Suspended respiration is important for body cavity examinations. Even for 10–20 second scans reassurance and adequate oxygenation can be helpful.
3. Sedation and analgesia are valuable in achieving stability of posture in children and difficult patients.

Abdominal preparation

1. A bulk-former administered for 24 hours prior to examination is essential to reduce intestinal gas.
2. Anticholinergic drugs are administered to reduce peristalsis, e.g. 30 mg propantheline i.m. 15 minutes beforehand or 0·1–0·25 mg glucagon i.v.

CONTRAST ENHANCEMENT

Oral

Opacification of the gastro-intestinal tract is frequently necessary to distinguish loops of bowel from pathological tissue or to identify the duodenal loop and the pancreatic head (Fig. 65.4). Gastrografin 5 per cent v/v 250 ml (20 mg iodine/ml) is then employed either some

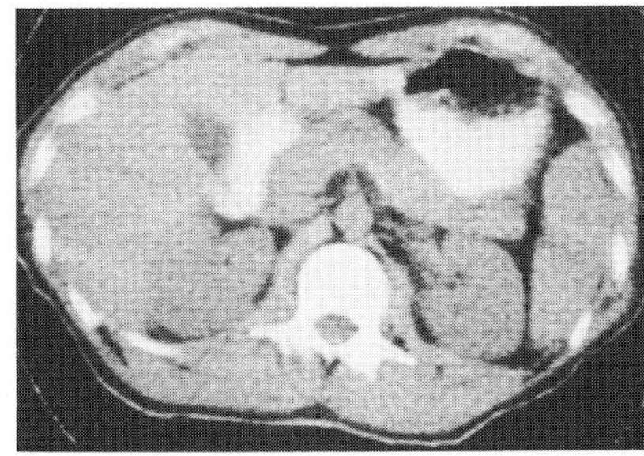

Fig. 65.4 Normal pancreas. Stomach and duodenum outlined by intra-oral contrast medium (Gastrografin). L+11. W200.

hours prior to or at the time of examination. The colon may also be demonstrated with Gastrografin but calcium phosphate administered orally for 2–3 days beforehand has also been employed.

Solu-Biloptin (2 g) can be added to the Gastrografin in order to demonstrate the gall bladder and in some cases the bile ducts.

Intravenous

Administration of iodine into the vascular system will raise the attenuation value of the blood by 10–15 EMI units (20–30 H) per mg/ml increase in iodine concentration at 120 kV_p. The linear relationship between Hounsfield units and iodine content of contrast solution has been demonstrated *in vitro*.

Current ionic intravenous contrast media are all very similar in their physical properties and, on an equiosmolar basis, their toxicity. For routine practical enhancement the particular nature of the contrast medium is unlikely to be of significance. Knowledge of the iodine content in mg/ml, and the total iodine administered, is of practical importance in order that optimal and reproducible studies may be devised.

Contrast enhancement of both normal and abnormal structures is influenced by the pattern of distribution of contrast medium in the intra- and extravascular spaces. This in turn depends on (*a*) vascularity of tissue under investigation; (*b*) dose of administered contrast; (*c*) renal excretion; (*d*) timing of scan; and in the special circumstances of the brain, (*e*) the blood/brain barrier. Iodine contrast material enters the extravascular spaces in most body organs with the exception of the normal brain and spinal cord. The extravascular distribution is a major component of the distribution volume. CT measures total iodine concentration in tissue and the resulting change of attenuation values depends on both intravascular and extravascular distribution. Contrast enhancement in the body makes use of the differing extravascular uptake of contrast as a means of tissue differentiation. The relationship between the blood pool, the extravascular space and renal excretion is a dynamic process.

Angio CT. Large blood vessels, both normal and abnormal, are demonstrated immediately following large doses of intravenous contrast. CT scans during the first circulation following rapid high-dose intravenous injection of contrast medium may be used to demonstrate not only the renal parenchyma but also the vascular bed of body organs (Fig. 65.5). Sequential studies of contrast movement may then be explored in selected sections.

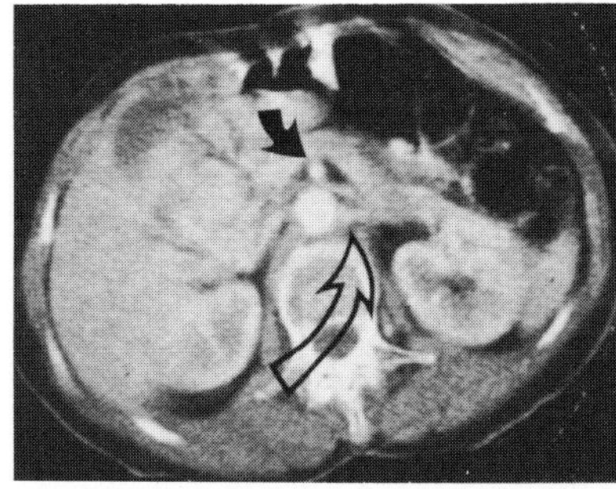

Fig. 65.5 Angio CT. Rapid high-dose intravenous injection of contrast medium demonstrating the aorta, superior mesenteric artery (↓), left renal artery (↑) and early filling of the renal cortex. L0 W200.

Water soluble iodine derivatives of organic compounds employed as contrast agents have acknowledged and well-recognized side effects ranging from minor reactions requiring no treatment, to death. Careful selection of patients is therefore required before contrast enhancement studies are undertaken and appropriate resuscitation facilities must be available during the examination.

Administration of intravenous contrast media. Three methods are available: (*a*) bolus; (*b*) drip infusion; (*c*) biphasic injection, i.e. half bolus, half infusion.

Elimination of contrast is much the same following all forms of injection from 30 minutes onwards. Many centres now employ bolus technique for routine conventional enhancement employing 21–42 g iodine. However up to 84 g have been used. There is no doubt that contrast studies are time-consuming and incur a penalty in both financial and radiation dose terms. A compromise between optimum enhancement, toxicity and economy is important.

If large volumes of contrast are to be used, the agent should be stored in a warm atmosphere to avoid cooling the patient and thereby risking motion artefacts.

Timing of the scan. Optimum timing of the CT scan depends upon the volume of intravenous contrast employed and the time taken to obtain the scan.

Fast scan times require a precise scheduling to ensure not only uniformity between patients but uniformity from one examination to another in the same patient.

Intrathecal

Myodil (pantopaque) though widely used for myelography is of little value in computed tomography because of its high density and its oily, non-miscible character.

Water-soluble contrast agents, in particular the non-ionic compound Metrizamide, have the distinct advantage of achieving a uniform concentration in cerebrospinal fluid and then diffusing throughout the subarachnoid space. The increased sensitivity of CT to tissue differences can then be used to demonstrate the much lower concentration of diluted contrast medium which may be detectable for up to 48–72 hours (Fig. 65.6). Such contrast may be employed to delineate not only morphological variations and the presence of pathological processes in the cerebrospinal fluid spaces of the spine and skull, but also used to explore the dynamics of the c.s.f. circulation.

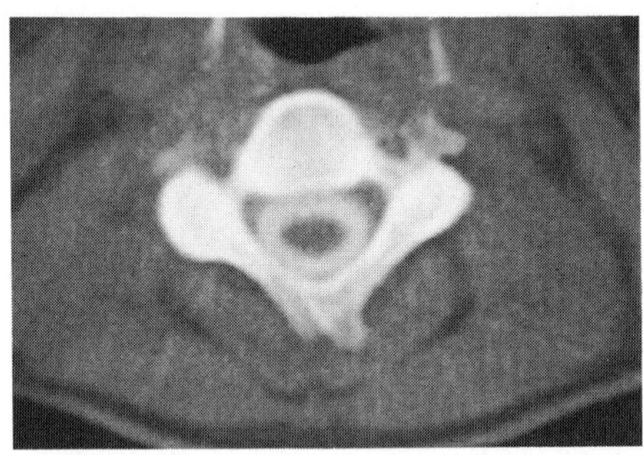

Fig. 65.6 CT myelogram. Water-soluble contrast medium is present in the subarachnoid space. Increased sensitivity of CT permits the demonstration of low concentrations of contrast medium. L+85 W400.

Inhalation

The potential value of xenon, atomic number 54, and krypton, atomic number 36, as inhalation contrast media has been explored. Krypton is less radio-opaque than xenon but less soluble in tissue and does not produce anaesthetic effects. The gases may prove of value both in lung and brain vasculature demonstration.

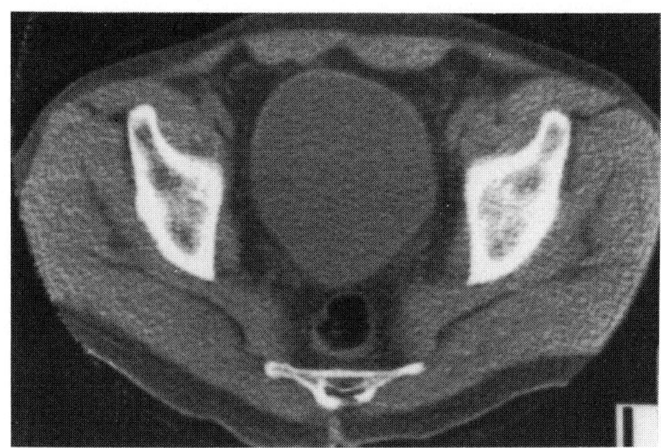

Fig. 65.7 CT pelvis. Normal urine (approximately 10 H) filling the bladder together with extravesical fat permit identification of the bladder wall. L+8 W200.

Per urethra

Both positive and negative contrast (carbon dioxide) may be employed per urethra in the bladder though urine itself in most circumstances is an effective contrast medium (Fig. 65.7).

Per vagina

Tampons are valuable vaginal markers and of value in identifying the uterine cervix (Fig. 65.8).

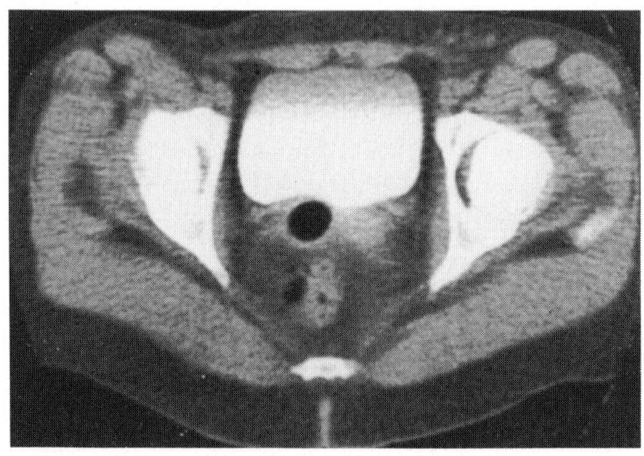

Fig. 65.8 CT pelvis. Negative contrast tampon in vagina permits localization of cervix. L+20 W200.

CLINICAL APPLICATIONS—REGIONAL

A. ABDOMEN

I. RETROPERITONEUM

1. Fascial planes

Normal appearances. Visualization of normal retroperitoneal structures depends very largely on the presence of fat planes creating sufficient contrast. In most patients the fascial planes which subdivide the retroperitoneal space are readily distinguished by CT. The most important planes are demonstrated by the anterior and posterior layers of Gerota's renal fascia and the lateroconal fascia (Fig. 65.9). The retroperitoneal space is thus subdivided into:

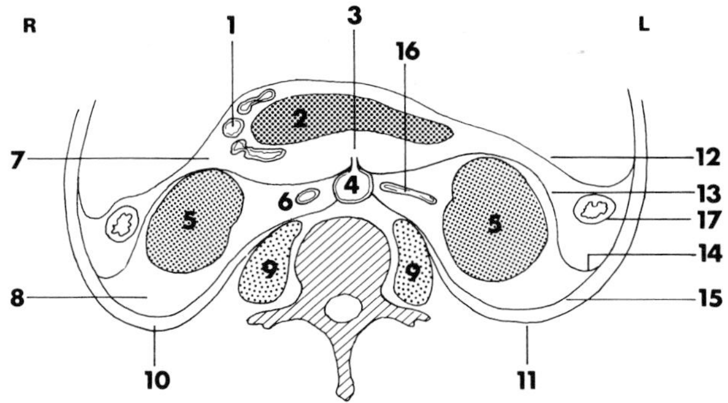

Fig. 65.9 Retroperitoneal structures. (1) duodenum; (2) pancreas; (3) superior mesenteric artery; (4) aorta; (5) kidney; (6) inferior vena cava; (7) anterior pararenal space; (8) perirenal space; (9) psoas muscle; (10) posterior pararenal space; (11) transversalis fascia; (12) peritoneum; (13) anterior pararenal fascia (Gerota's fascia); (14) lateroconal fascia; (15) posterior pararenal fascia; (16) left renal vein; (17) colon.

1. *Anterior pararenal space* limited anteriorly by the posterior parietal peritoneum, posteriorly by the anterior renal fascia and laterally by the lateroconal fascia. It contains the extraperitoneal gastrointestinal structures, i.e. the ascending and descending colon, the duodenum and the pancreas. It is potentially continuous across the midline.

2. *Perirenal space* which is cone-shaped vertically, encompasses the kidney and its investing fat and is limited by the anterior and posterior renal fascia. The perirenal spaces have no communication and their fat content is most abundant posterolateral to the lower pole of the kidneys.

3. *Posterior pararenal space* limited anteriorly by the posterior renal fascia and posteriorly by the transversalis fascia. This space which contains a thin layer of fat is open laterally and inferiorly and recognized on a conventional abdominal radiograph as the 'flank shadow'. There is a potential communication between the two posterior pararenal spaces via the anterior abdominal wall.

The retroperitoneal space is generally C-shaped with its convexity projecting anteriorly in the mid-line. This shape is a function of both the particular relationship of the abdominal walls one to another and their accommodation to the lordotic curvature of the lumbar spine. As a result, some retroperitoneal structures, e.g. body of pancreas and duodenal loop, lie significantly more anterior than some intraperitoneal viscera, e.g. spleen.

Role of CT in location of disease. The ability of CT to identify the compartments formed by the fascial planes assumes considerable importance in the accurate localization of retroperitoneal fluid collections and the understanding of spread of both infection and new growth.

Perirenal infection and fluid collections are usually detectable as areas of similar or lower attenuation than surrounding tissue in the posterolateral aspect of the perirenal space to which most are confined (Fig. 65.10). The anterior pararenal space is the commonest site of retroperitoneal infection. An abscess related to the pancreatic head tends to collect inferiorly and to the right but may remain confined to the anterior pararenal space displacing the kidney posteriorly. Large pancreatic abscess collections reach the flank by extending below the level of the vertically cone-shaped perirenal space thus gaining access to the posterior pararenal space without contamination of the intervening perirenal compartment (Fig. 65.11). Such collections in the posterior pararenal space are clearly delineated lateral to the psoas muscle displacing the kidney anteriorly and laterally.

Abnormalities of the psoas muscle either intrinsic or extrinsic due to spread of adjacent bone disease are well displayed. A psoas abscess enlarges the muscle outline and encloses an area of reduced or heterogeneous density. A hyperaemic abscess margin may enhance following CT angiography but the necrotic centre remains unchanged (Fig. 65.12).

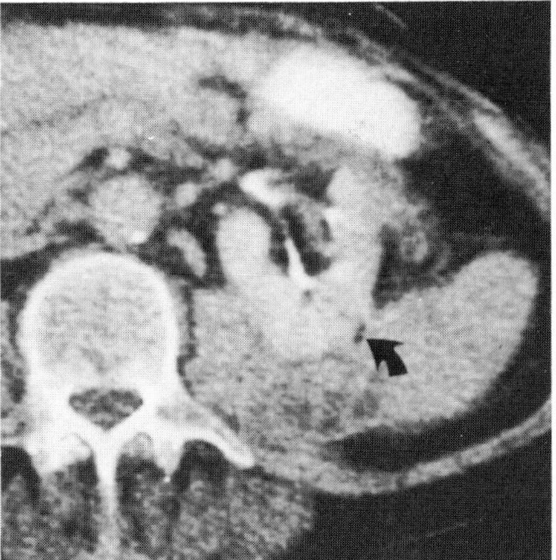

Fig. 65.10 Perirenal space abscess. Inflammatory tissue is detectable as multiloculated heterogeneous densities in the posterior aspect of the left perirenal space. Note gas loculus (↖) Kidney displaced anteriorly and rotated. L+15 W200.

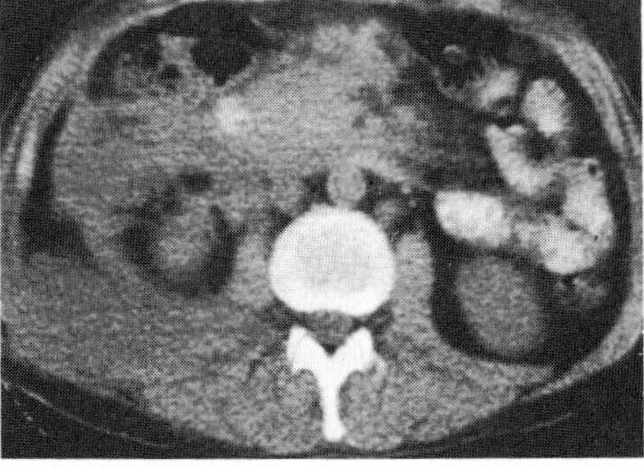

Fig. 65.11 Pancreatic abscess. Fluid is present in the right posterior pararenal space obliterating the outlines of the psoas and quadratus lumborum muscles. The intervening perirenal compartment is intact. L+5 W200.

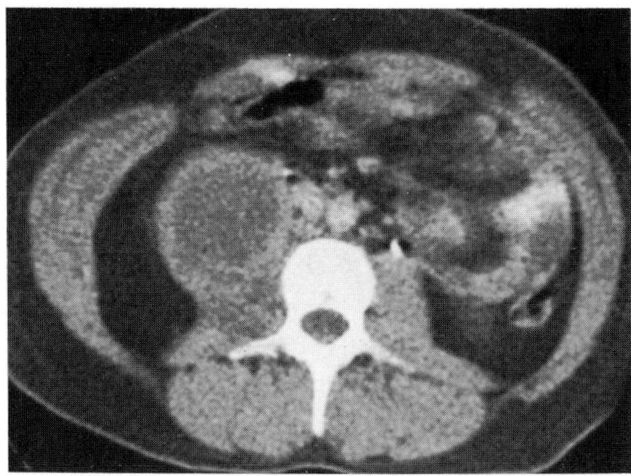

Fig. 65.12 Psoas abscess. Muscle outline is enlarged. The hyperaemic abscess margin is enhanced following CT angiography. The necrotic cavity remains unchanged. L+10 W200.

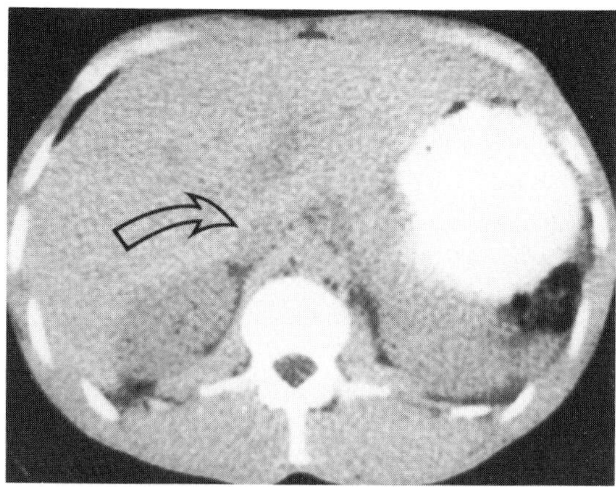

Fig. 65.14 Normal inferior vena cava (→). The intrahepatic portion of the IVC is detectable by its lower density compared to surrounding liver parenchyma. L+20 W200.

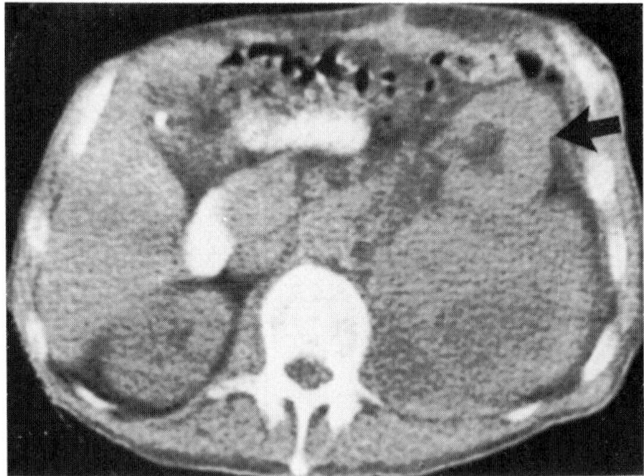

Fig. 65.13 Retroperitoneal sarcoma. Irregular mass of soft tissue density obliterating fascial planes. Note displacement of left kidney (←). L+20 W200.

Tumours of the retroperitoneal space are recognized by their mass effect and on occasion by secondary ureteral obstruction or displacement. The more malignant variety obliterate fascial planes (Fig. 65.13). Associated bone destruction is detectable at an early stage. Primary tumours together with metastatic and lymph node disease of the retroperitoneal space have no distinguishing infrastructure. They are usually differentiated by their anatomical location.

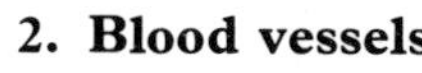

2. Blood vessels

Normal appearances. The abdominal aorta is invariably visualized as a homogeneous round structure just to the left of the midline. At the bifurcation it changes in shape and becomes flattened. The inferior vena cava to the right of the aorta is variable in shape depending upon the intrathoracic pressure and phase of respiration but frequently appears flattened or elliptical. Whilst the inferior vena cava is similar in density to the

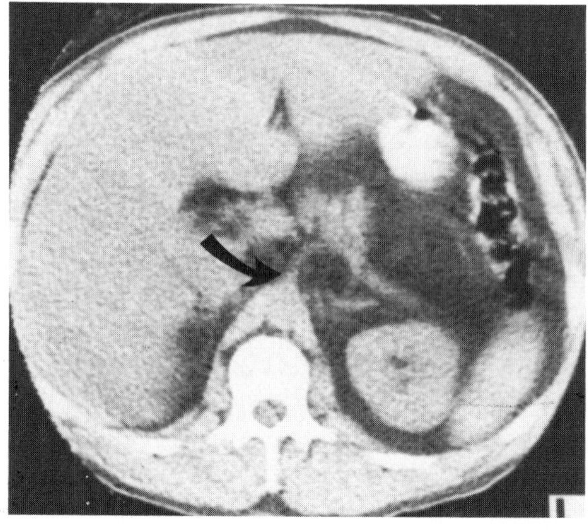

A

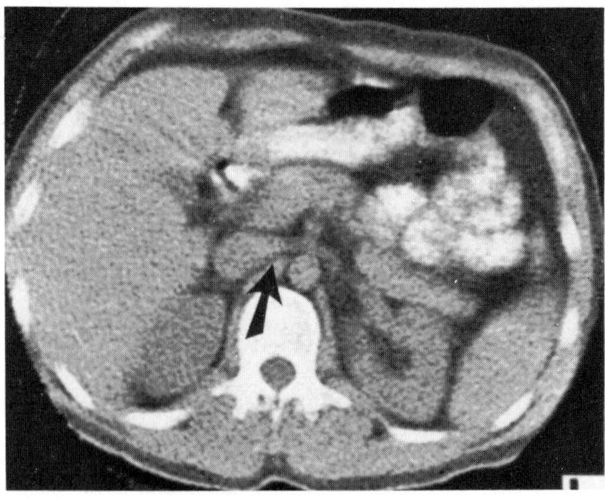

B

Fig. 65.15 Normal abdominal blood vessels. (A) Coeliac axis level (→). L+20 W200. (B) Superior mesenteric artery level. Note left renal vein entering inferior vena cava (↑). L+16 W200.

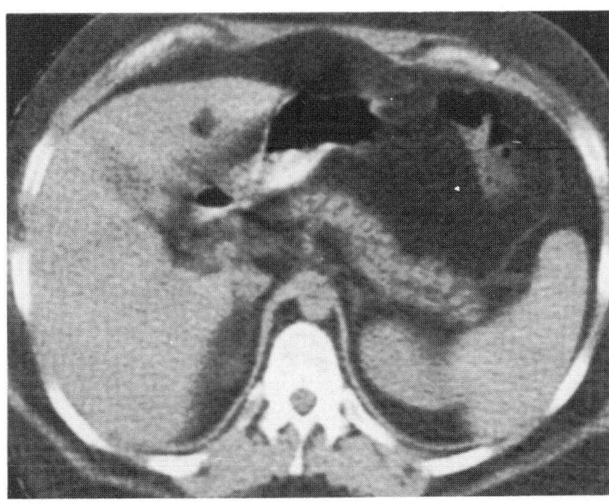

Fig. 65.16 Normal splenic vein. The vein is parallel to the posterior surface of the pancreas and separated from it by a fat plane. L+10 W200.

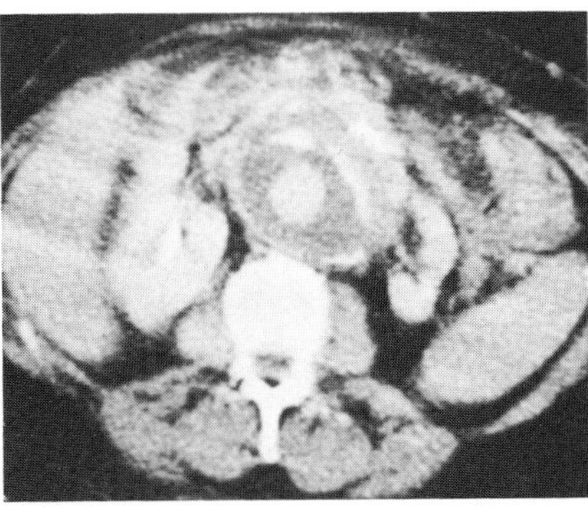

Fig. 65.17 Abdominal aortic aneurysm. CT angiography has demonstrated the true lumen surrounded by clot. Calcification is present in the aneurysmal wall. Note contracted left kidney. L+11 W200.

aorta its intrahepatic portion is often recognizable as an area of lower density compared to surrounding liver parenchyma (Fig. 65.14).

The major branches arising from the aorta together with various tributaries to the inferior vena cava are all identifiable in upper abdominal sections (Fig. 65.15) particularly where there is plentiful fat in the obese patient.

Normal vascular structures are valuable markers for intra-abdominal organs. The horizontal portion of the superior mesenteric artery is an important and reliable landmark for the posterior surface of the body of the pancreas. The superior mesenteric vein to the right of the corresponding artery passes between the uncinate process and the neck of the pancreas to join the splenic vein and form the portal vein. The splenic vein is closely applied to the posterior surface of the tail and body of the pancreas. It is important that the fat plane separating it from the pancreas should not be mistaken for the pancreatic duct (Fig. 65.16). The left renal vein crosses beneath the superior mesenteric artery anterior to the aorta and is more frequently identified than the shorter right renal vein (Fig. 65.15).

Role of CT in abdominal vascular disease. Calcification in the atheromatous aorta is frequent. Dilatation of the abdominal aorta due to aneurysm formation is easily detected and involvement of visceral branches identified. The true wall of an aneurysmal aorta unless calcified may, however, be indistinguishable from intraluminal blood. CT angiography is then necessary to display the true lumen. This is especially so in dissecting aneurysm and in the presence of intraluminal thrombi (Fig. 65.17).

A recently ruptured abdominal aneurysm is recognizable by the characteristic increased attenuation of fresh clotted blood, the distribution of which is limited by the fascial planes. Loss of the periaortic fat plane is an important sign of disease except in the very thin patient but is quite non-specific. Chronic leakage may appear as an inhomogeneous mass indistinguishable from a retroperitoneal tumour. The complementary roles of computed tomography and ultrasound considerably diminish the need for invasive arteriography and the non-traumatic demonstration of a normal aorta in a patient suspected of aneurysm formation is of considerable clinical value. Changes in renal morphology secondary to renal vascular involvement are readily detected.

3. Pancreas

Normal appearances. The facility to demonstrate the size, shape and position of the normal pancreas in the transaxial plane has revealed the very wide variation in pancreatic anatomy which exists and the unsuspected

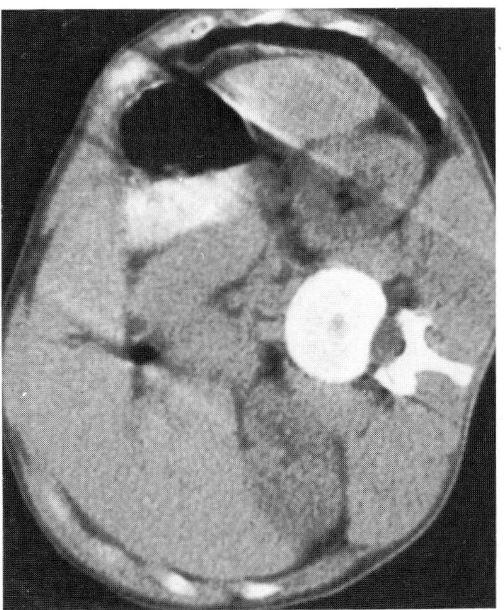

Fig. 65.18 Normal pancreas. Patient in lateral decubitus position. Note mobility and altered shape compared with pancreas in the supine position (Fig. 65.4). L+15 W200.

mobility of the organ in some patients. A comparison of the supine and decubitus positions during CT is of value in assessing individual mobility and flexibility (Fig. 65.18). Comparative studies of the fixed, cadaveric pancreas are of limited value.

The margins of the pancreas are readily identified except in the absence of normal fat planes. The margins are usually regular but lobulation is described in 20 per cent of normal patients and is related to obesity (Fig. 65.19).

The pancreas, which normally has a uniform and homogeneous density similar to liver and spleen at CT, usually lies in the upper retroperitoneal space with varying obliquity in relation to the long axis of the trunk. The number of 13 mm sections required to examine the entire pancreas may vary from 1 to 8. In thin patients, because of the shape of the retroperitoneal space discussed earlier, the pancreas may occupy an unexpectedly anterior situation.

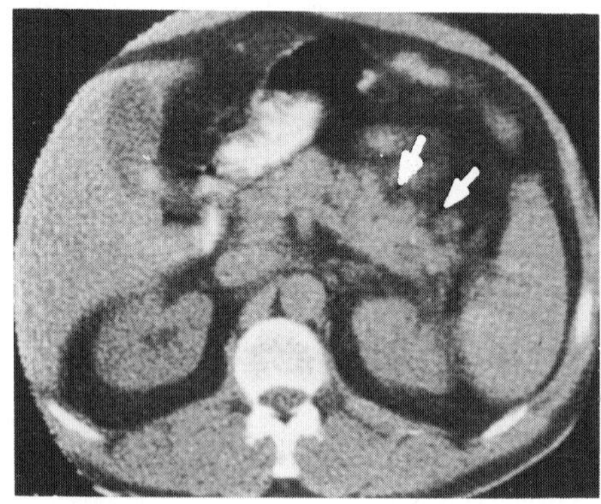

Fig. 65.19 Normal pancreas. Note lobulation of outline in obese patient. L+10 W200.

The pancreatic body is situated anterior to the superior mesenteric artery which is consistently visualized as a mid-line structure. It should be noted, however, that the craniocaudal level of the pancreatic body in the living may vary from L1 to L5. The body extends to the left with the left kidney and suprarenal gland as posteriorly related structures. The pancreatic tail is related to the splenic hilum.

The head of the pancreas anterior to the inferior vena cava lies medial to the second part of the duodenum and the uncinate process is often visualized posterior to the superior mesenteric vein. The junction of the left renal vein with the inferior vena cava, a venous complex visualized in 85 per cent of patients, can be a useful landmark for localizing the pancreatic head. The common bile duct lies to the right of this junction and the pancreatic duct anteriorly (Fig. 65.20).

Variations in the size of the pancreas are well recognized, particularly volume changes associated with senile atrophy. Apparent variations in size may result from

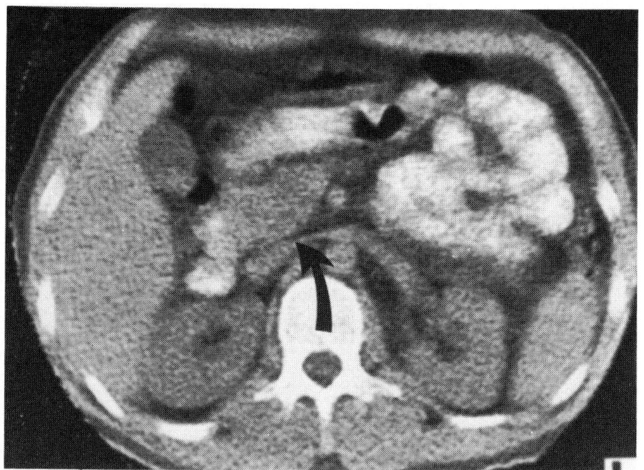

Fig. 65.20 Normal pancreas. The left renal vein/inferior vena cava complex (↑) localizes the pancreatic head. L+16 W200.

obliquity of section due to the 2:1 ratio of craniocaudal and anteroposterior diameters of the varying segments of the pancreas. Ratio measurements for evaluating the size of the pancreas have been suggested which relate the AP diameter of the pancreatic body to the transverse diameter of the vertebral body L2 and also to the AP diameter of the adjacent vertebral body. Both methods suggest that the AP diameter of the pancreatic body should be between one-third and two-thirds of the bony diameter. The ratio of normal AP diameters in the latter series was $0{\cdot}5 \pm 0{\cdot}11$ (mean SD ± 2 SD).

Role of CT in pancreatic disease. Increase in size, irregularity of outline, heterogeneity of density and loss of mobility all imply disease but none are specific to any particular disease entity. Some features such as calcification, intra- and extrapancreatic cysts and duct dilatation, are readily detectable and of value in the differentiation of diseased from normal pancreas. They may also contribute to the establishment of a definitive diagnosis.

Chronic pancreatitis. Chronic pancreatitis is a disease which progresses inexorably with loss of pancreatic tissue and eventual destruction. Nevertheless, 40 per cent of patients exhibit swelling of pancreatic tissue with accompanying calcification and 10 per cent may exhibit normal appearances. The principal diagnostic features of chronic pancreatitis encountered during CT are duct calculi, dilatation of the main pancreatic duct identified as an irregular line of decreased attenuation ('chain of lakes') and paraductal cysts which deform the surrounding parenchyma (Fig. 65.21). Obliteration of fascial planes, contour irregularity, changes in density and loss of mobility may also be encountered. These features, together with the presence of duct dilatation, make differentiation from carcinoma of the pancreas virtually impossible.

The demonstration of local cystic enlargement with associated calcification, particularly in patients with

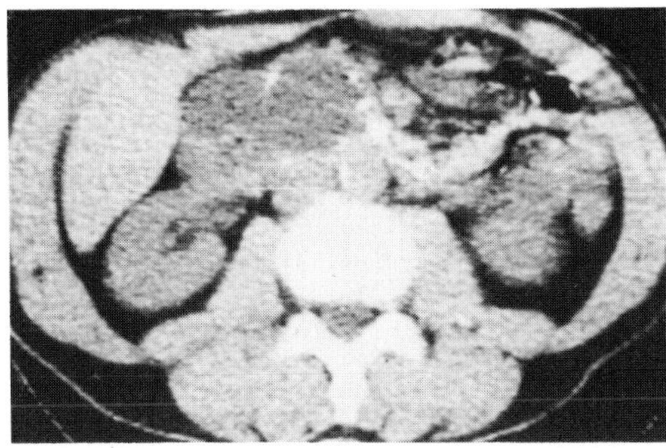

Fig. 65.21 Chronic pancreatitis. Paraductal cysts deform the pancreatic head. Note calcification. L0 W200.

relentless abdominal pain, or during clinical remission, can provide a valuable contribution to clinical management especially in preoperative assessment.

Acute pancreatitis. The appearances encountered at CT in this potentially recurrent disease vary with the extent of clinical recovery. In the acute phase the gland, due to oedema, may be diffusely swollen, irregular in outline and of heterogeneous density (Fig. 65.22). Following complete recovery the appearances may return to normal. The identification of characteristic pseudocysts with well-defined margins and low-density contents is important evidence in favour of the inflammatory nature of the disease. Demonstration of the extent and location of pseudocysts in relation to adjacent viscera is valuable preoperative information (Fig. 65.23).

Complications of acute pancreatitis are usually secondary to necrosis or haemorrhage but bleeding, rupture or infection may all affect a pseudocyst. Bleeding results in an increase of attenuation value (Fig. 65.24). Ascites due to rupture of a pseudocyst, lymphatic blockage or associated liver disease, is readily recognized by the presence of low-density fluid in the peritoneal spaces (Fig. 65.25).

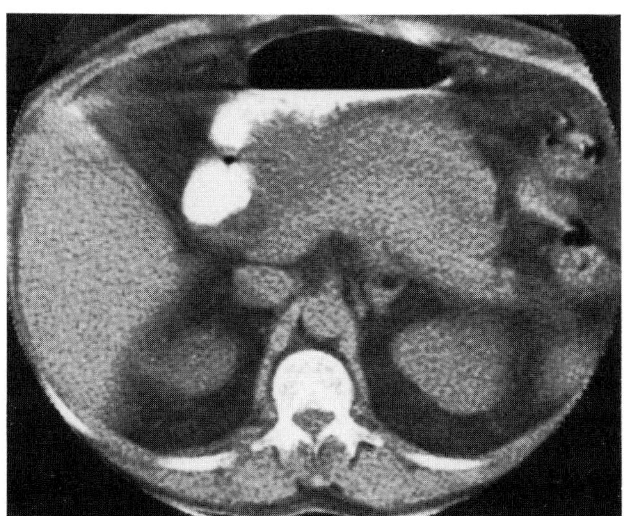

Fig. 65.22 Acute pancreatitis. Diffusely swollen gland irregular in outline and of heterogeneous density. Note displaced Gastrografin-filled stomach. L+25 W200

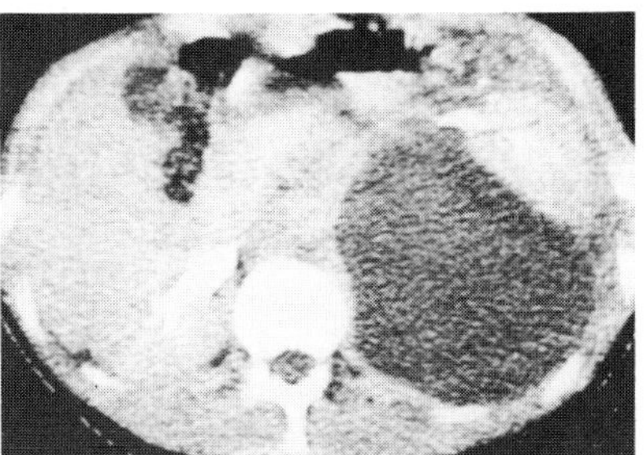

Fig. 65.23 Acute pancreatitis. Large pseudocyst with low attenuation contents displacing adjacent kidney. L+11 W100.

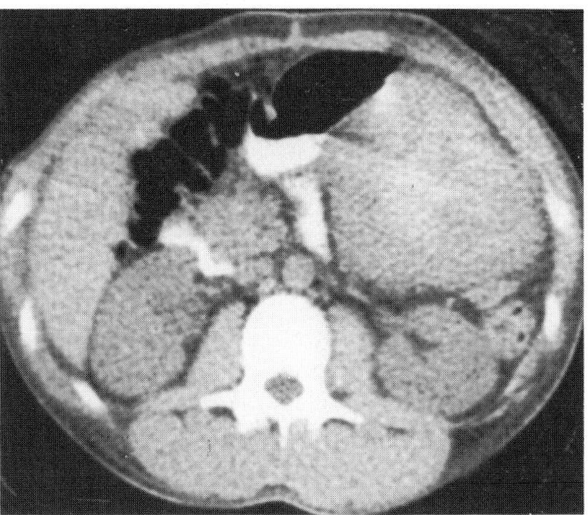

Fig. 65.24 Haemorrhagic pancreatitis. Bleeding has resulted in an increase of attenuation value in the pseudocyst. L+20 W200.

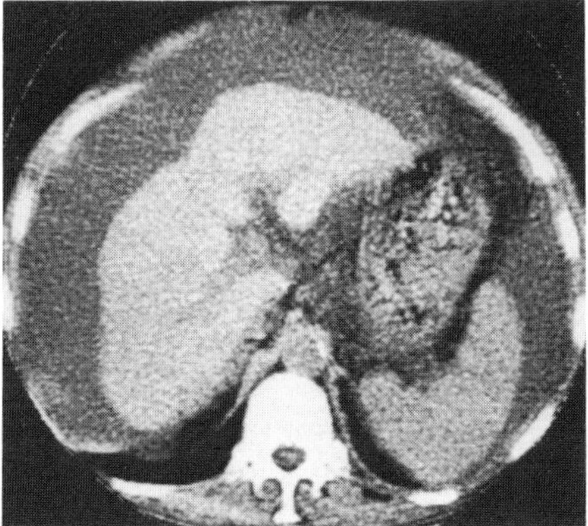

Fig. 65.25 Ascites. Low-density fluid is present in the peritoneal space displacing liver and spleen medially away from the costal margin. L −5 W200.

The location and contour of pancreatic abscesses may be recorded whilst the retroperitoneal extension of an inflammatory process can be logically defined and monitored by a study of the fascial planes (Fig. 65.11).

Neoplasms. Unfortunately patients rarely present with small pancreatic cancers. Symptomatology usually implies expansion of the gland and extension into peripancreatic tissue. Cancer of the pancreas is commonly identified at CT therefore as a solid, localized mass of varying density with distortion of local anatomy (Fig. 65.26). Local infiltration into the retropancreatic space may result in loss of the fat planes between the pancreas, superior mesenteric artery and surrounding viscera (Fig. 65.27).

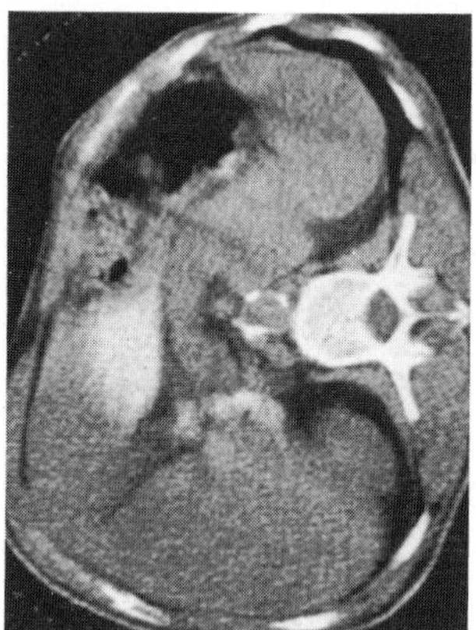

Fig. 65.26 Pancreatic carcinoma. Localized mass in the tail of the pancreas displacing adjacent viscera. Note calcified aorta. L+10 W200.

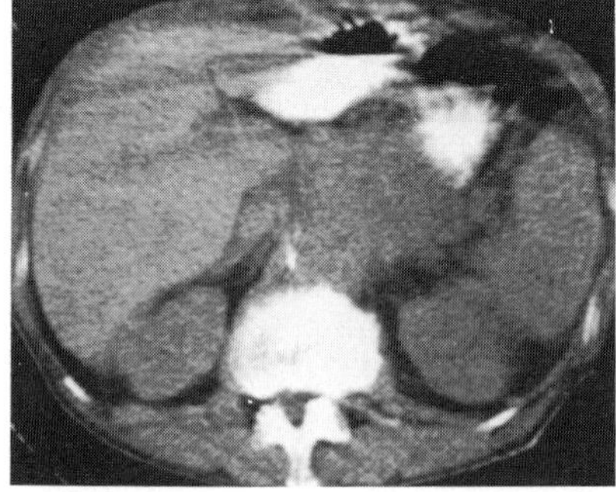

Fig. 65.27 Pancreatic carcinoma. Irregular mass involving the body of the pancreas and infiltrating the retropancreatic space obliterating fascial planes. L+5 W200.

Whilst the identification of pancreatic neoplasms in most published series has a high level of accuracy, usually more than 80 per cent, all authors agree that the majority of tumours so demonstrated are unresectable. Early cancers usually escape detection at conventional CT until the morphological changes are well-established or secondary events occur. CT angiography may have a contribution to make towards the early detection of vascular pancreatic tumours.

CT is not organ specific and therefore associated secondary changes may be detected in other organ systems, notably the liver and spine. Identification of hepatic metastases is improved by employing intravenous contrast to increase the attenuation of surrounding liver. Dilatation of the common bile duct and intrahepatic biliary tree may also be contributory evidence towards the establishment of malignancy (Fig. 65.28).

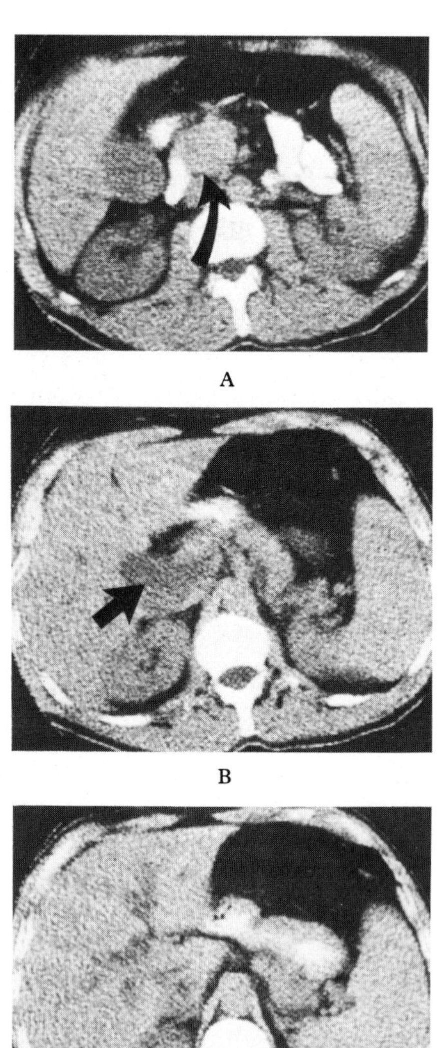

Fig. 65.28 Carcinoma pancreas with biliary duct obstruction (L+5 W200). (A) Well-defined tumour in the pancreatic head (↑). (B) Dilated common hepatic duct at the porta hepatis (↗). (C) Dilated intrahepatic bile ducts.

4. Kidneys

Normal appearances. The kidneys are well demarcated by CT as a result of the surrounding perirenal and renal sinus fat. Normal unenhanced renal parenchyma is slightly less dense (30–50 H units) than adjacent soft tissue structures (50–80 H liver and pancreas). Peripelvic fat is differentiated from a non contrast-filled renal pelvis by its characteristically negative attenuation value. The anterior, superior and posterior aspects of the renal outline and the margins of the parenchyma adjacent to the renal sinus are demonstrated significantly more clearly by CT than conventional radiology.

In most patients the renal vascular pedicle can be seen with the renal veins situated anterior to the renal arteries.

The left renal vein posterior to the superior mesenteric artery is notably longer than the right (Fig. 65.15).

The appearance of the nephrogram after intravenous contrast injection depends on the amount of iodine injected and the timing of the scan. During the late vascular/early nephrographic phase the enhanced cortex can be differentiated from the medulla (Fig. 65.5). Subsequent scans at one minute intervals demonstrate the nephrogram to increase in intensity for 4–5 minutes until the attenuation of renal parenchyma reaches 100–120 H. The collecting system is clearly seen as a result of the considerably enhanced attenuation values following contrast injection but detail is less precise than on conventional urography.

Role of CT in renal disease

Extrarenal abnormalities. The kidneys are easily displaced by enlargement of adjacent organs or by the presence of tumours, inflammatory masses or fluid collections (Fig. 65.29). Definition of the extent of disease by CT can be very accurate.

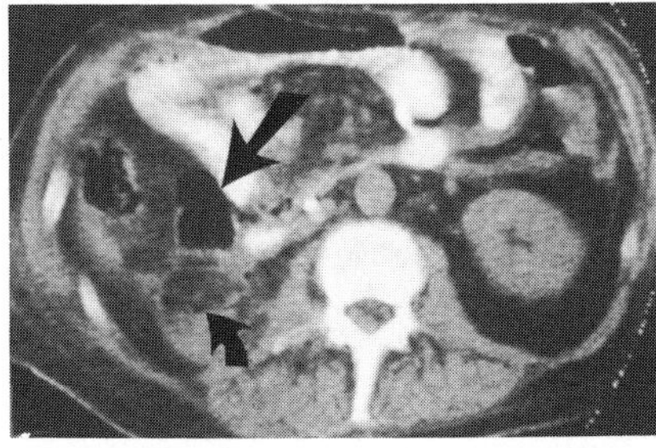

Fig. 65.29 Perirenal abscess. The multiloculated abscess on the right side contains gas of low attenuation (↙). L+35 W200.

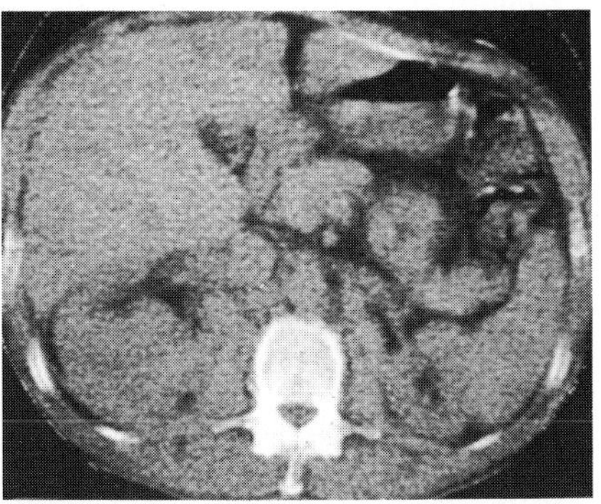

A

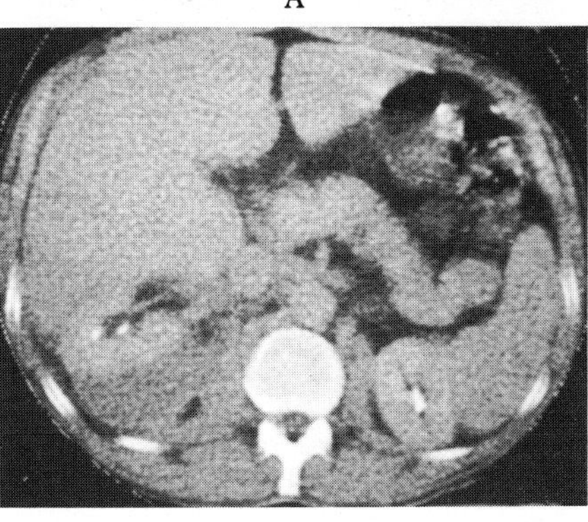

B

Fig. 65.30 Renal intracapsular haematoma (L+12 W200). (A) Pre-contrast enhancement. Haematoma, kidney and liver are all similar in density. (B) Post-enhancement. Displaced kidney has density increased. Haematoma now more clearly visualized on posterior aspect of right kidney.

The anterior pararenal compartment is the commonest site of extraperitoneal infection which arises mainly from primary lesions of the alimentary tract. Extraperitoneal perforations of the colon and duodenum together with haemorrhage or spread of pancreatic infection may all result in anterior pararenal masses with posterior displacement of the kidney.

Perirenal infections, haemorrhage or urinary extravasation obliterate the normal low attenuation of perirenal fat (Fig. 65.29). In the event of infection being due to a gas-producing organism then the extremely low attenuation of the gas is readily distinguished (Fig. 65.29) Perirenal abscess is most commonly found dorsolateral to the lower pole of the kidney where, as previously noted, fat is most abundant. The lower pole of the kidney in the early stages is then displaced anteromedially and rotated about its vertical axis. Subsequent compression of the renal pelvis may give rise to obstructive neprophathy and the infection may extend into other fascial planes. Intracapsular haematoma, even when isodense with adjacent renal substance, may be distinguished by enhancement of the renal parenchyma (Fig. 65.30).

Posterior pararenal collections of fluid, either inflammatory or haemorrhagic, displace the kidney anteriorly (Fig. 65.11). Rectosigmoid perforations enter this plane preferentially.

Renal mass lesions. CT has the ability not only to detect mass lesions but also to differentiate between cystic and solid processes. It may also delineate the extent of tumour spread to adjacent structures.

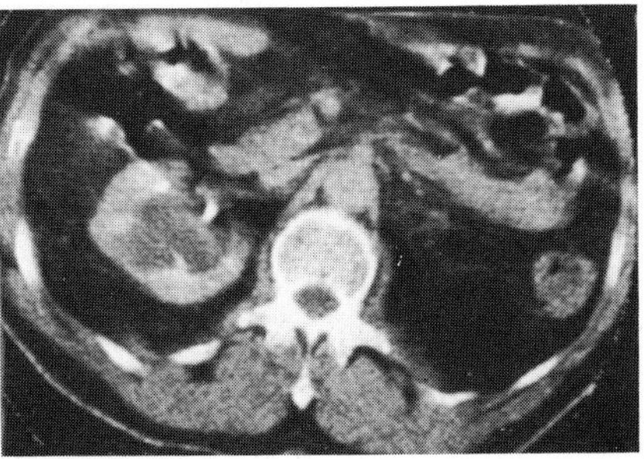

Fig. 65.31 Benign renal cyst. Well-defined, low density, intrarenal cyst on the right side following contrast enhancement. Note left nephrectomy. L+5 W200.

Renal masses are detectable in three ways: a change in normal renal contour, distortion of the collecting system or a difference in density from normal renal parenchyma.

Benign *renal cysts* are round or oval with well-defined margins and have a uniform attenuation near to that of water (O H) unless contaminated with blood, pus or contrast medium. The uncomplicated renal cyst does not enhance following intravenous contrast injection but becomes more clearly defined against the background of enhanced renal parenchyma (Fig. 65.31). The thin wall of the benign cyst is frequently discernible. A significant incidence of unsuspected solitary or multiple benign cysts has been detected in patients undergoing CT examinations for other reasons. Small intrarenal cysts in familial polycystic disease are detectable at a stage before renal enlargement or calyceal deformities are apparent by conventional techniques. Characteristic appearances can be seen even in the presence of grossly impaired renal function. Associated hepatic, splenic and pancreatic cysts may also be found (Fig. 65.32).

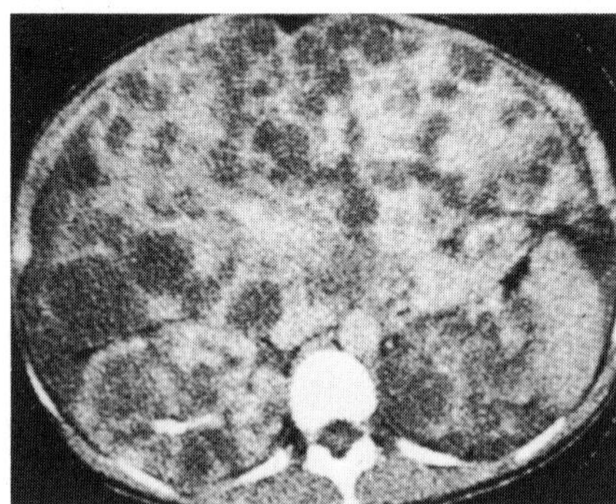

Fig. 65.32 Polycystic disease. Multiple cysts in kidneys and liver. L+10 W100.

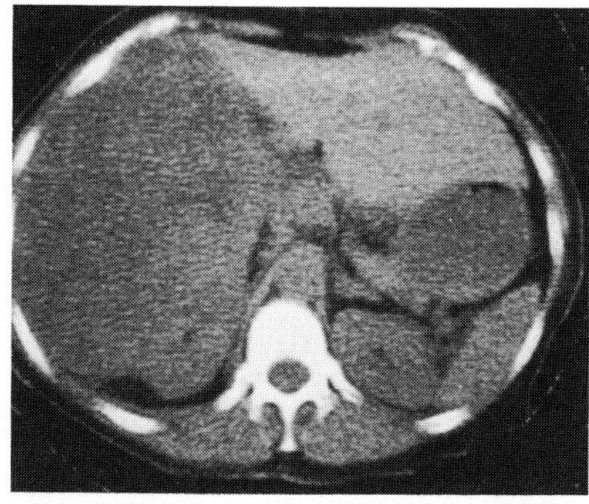

A

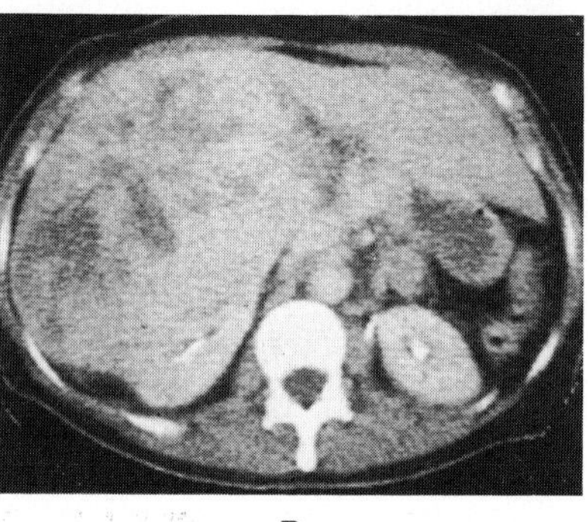

B

Fig. 65.33 Hypernephroma (L0 W200). (A) Precontrast enhancement. (B) Postcontrast enhancement. Apart from areas of necrosis within the tumour the general attenuation of the mass has increased to the same level as adjacent renal tissue.

Solid *renal tumours* have attenuation values which approximate to the value of normal renal parenchyma (30–50 H) though large neoplasms may be heterogeneous with areas of lower density (0–20 H) as a result of necrotic or cystic change within the tumour (Fig. 65.33). Enhancement of renal tumours following intravenous contrast injection reflects the distribution of contrast in the blood pool and the extracellular spaces and is usually less than that of normal functioning renal tissue. Renal neoplasms are often poorly delineated from normal parenchyma. The thick, irregular wall of a cystic neoplasm can usually be differentiated and confirmed by intravenous contrast and the increased sensitivity of CT enables calcification not otherwise visible to be detected In addition to invasion of surrounding fascial planes, metastatic disease in retroperitoneal lymph nodes, liver, axial skeleton and opposite kidney may all be detected.

Histological differentiation of renal tumours by CT is not possible though very low attenuation values (−40 to −180 H) within a renal mass might suggest an angiomyolipoma (Fig. 65.34). Attenuation values slightly greater than normal renal parenchyma can be produced by blood within a cystic or necrotic tumour. CT may provide a definitive diagnosis in lesions which show a mixed echo pattern on ultrasonography but are hypovascular at conventional nephrotomography.

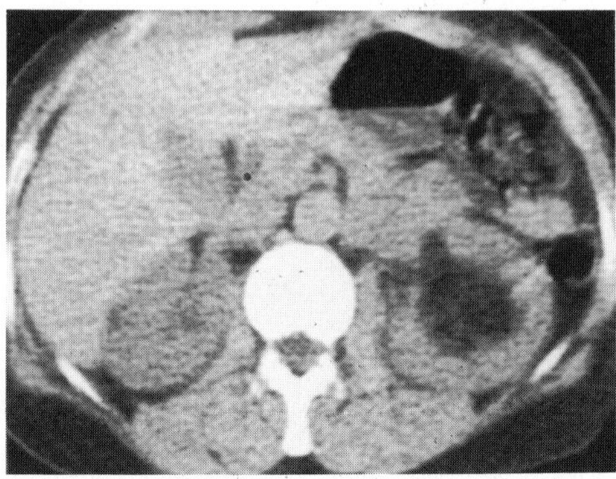

Fig. 65.34 Angiomyolipoma. Mass in the left renal hilum has an attenuation value of −40 indicating a high fat content. (L+20 W200.)

It is clear that CT cannot replace conventional excretion urography nor ultrasonography in the demonstration of renal tumours but is complementary to these imaging methods.

Impaired renal function. The conditions responsible for non-visualization of renal parenchyma often require invasive and potentially hazardous investigations for further evaluation. The ability of CT to interrogate soft tissue densities together with its increased sensitivity in the detection of low iodine concentrations permits additional information to be gained in a non-invasive manner.

Differentiation between agenesis and a small non-functioning contracted kidney is important. CT enables the renal vascular pedicle and any residual renal tissue to be identified. In renal hypoplasia minimal degrees of function not detected on either excretion urography or dynamic isotope studies may be identified (Fig. 65.35).

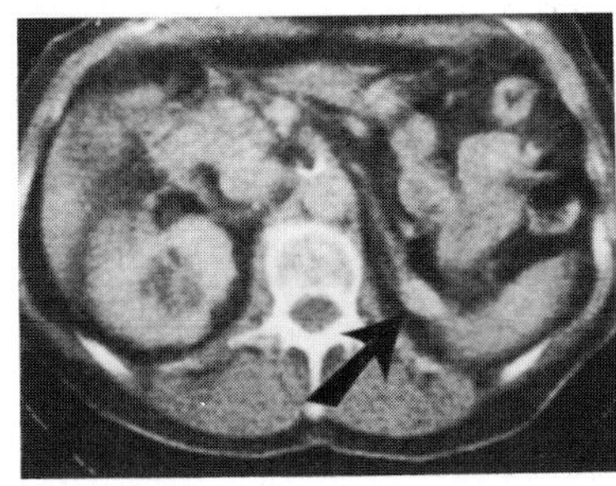

Fig. 65.35 Small contracted kidney on the left side increased in density after contrast enhancement (↗). Left renal vein well visualized. Note irregular medial margin of pyelonephritic kidney on right side. L0 W200.

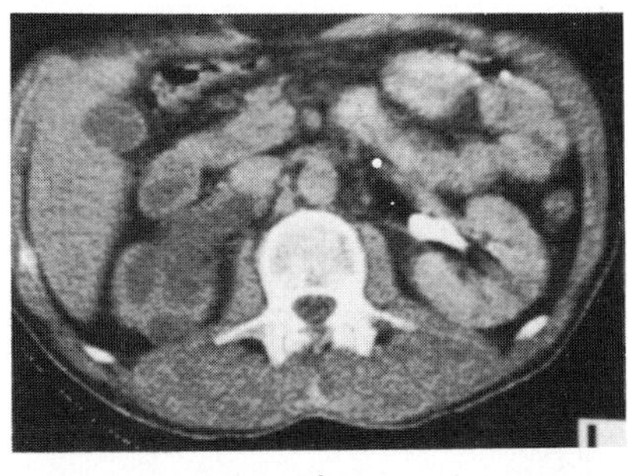

A

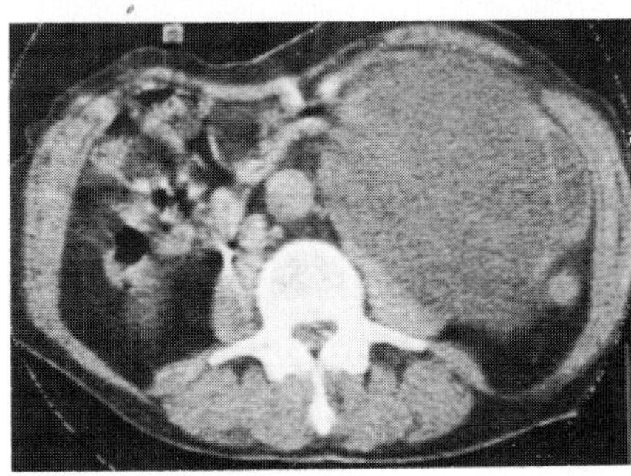

B

Fig. 65.36 Hydronephrosis (L +5 W200). (A) Dilated pelvis and calyces within a small, non-functioning kidney on the right side due to distal obstruction by retroperitoneal tumour. (B) Massive dilatation of the renal pelvis with minimal residual renal function on the left side secondary to pelviureteric junction obstruction.

The hydronephrotic kidney has a characteristic appearance irrespective of its size. It is recognized as a well defined, sometimes lobulated structure of urine density (0–15 H) unless contaminated. A peripheral enhancing rim of tissue may be seen even in the absence of detectable renal excretion by conventional urography. In addition to the presence of hydronephrosis the mechanism of the obstructing agent, e.g. retroperitoneal fibrosis, enlarged peritoneal nodes or primary tumour, can be demonstrated (Fig. 65.36).

In acute renal failure resulting from parenchymal disease, CT is of value in excluding remediable obstruction of the lower urinary tract and the quantifiable nature of the image permits its use in the evaluation of renal failure.

Solitary kidneys. The absence of renal tissue and the renal vascular pedicle provides definitive evidence in suspected congenital absence of the kidney (Fig. 65.35).

Monitoring of the nephrectomy patient is ideally carried out by CT. It is a safe, non-invasive method for assessing the postoperative complications of renal bed infection, monitoring tumour recurrence and evaluating the contralateral kidney.

In the evaluation of morphology and function following renal transplantation a gradual decrease in the volume of the transplanted kidney indicates chronic rejection while an abrupt increase in volume may herald acute rejection. Severe oedema in a rejected kidney may result in a much reduced density on the CT examination. The formation of a lymphocyst following

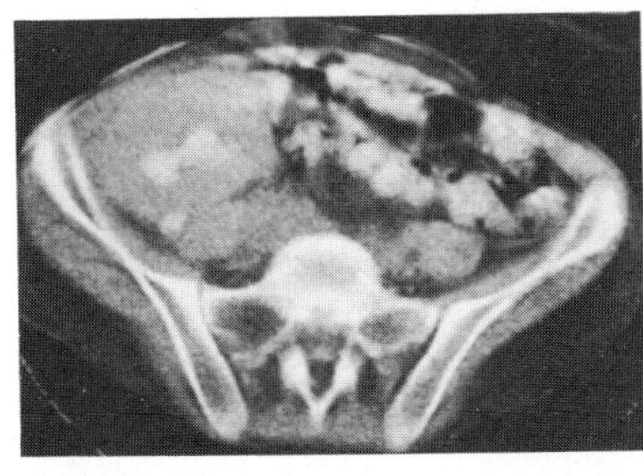

A

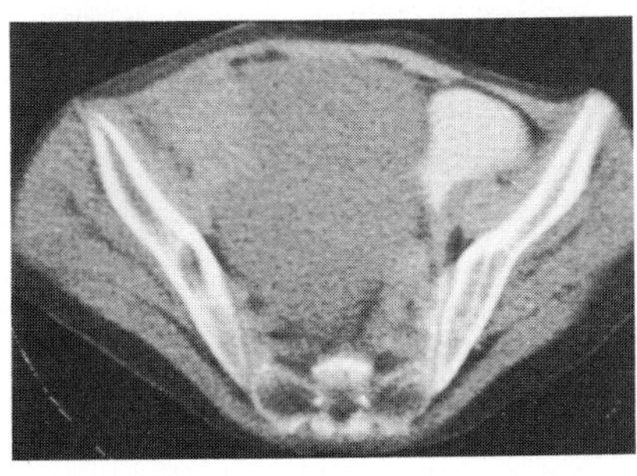

B

Fig. 65.37 Lymphocele following renal transplant. (A) Dilated pelvicalyceal structure of transplanted kidney in the right iliac fossa (L0 W200). (B) Large lymphocele of low attenuation arising in the pelvis and displacing contrast-filled bladder to the left. L+8 W200.

renal transplantation is readily detected by the characteristic appearance of a well-defined juxta renal mass of water density (Fig. 65.37).

5. Adrenal glands

Normal appearances. The normal adrenal glands are detectable in 85 per cent of normal CT examinations. Both glands are triradiate in shape with a body lying anteriorly and the medial and lateral limbs posteriorly. The right adrenal gland is anterior and superior to the right kidney and immediately posterior to the inferior vena cava and right lobe of the liver. The proximity of the right adrenal gland to the junction of the intra- and extrahepatic portions of the inferior vena cava together with its similarity in density can make identification difficult in some patients (Fig. 65.38). The lateral posterior limb of the right gland is shorter and at a more caudal level than the medial limb.

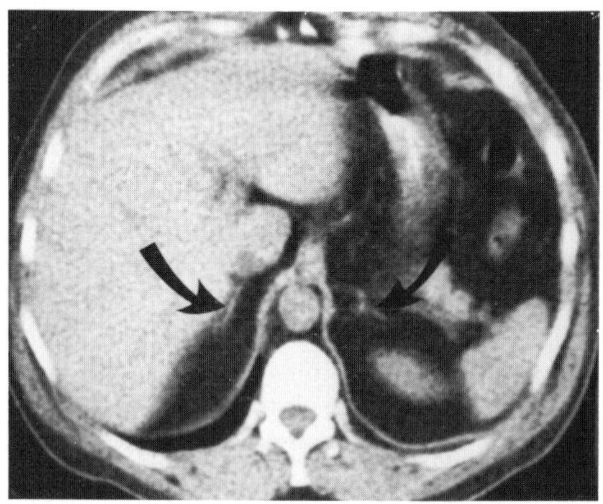

Fig. 65.38 Normal adrenal glands. The right gland is immediately posterior to the inferior vena cava and right lobe of the liver (→). The left gland is superior and anterior to the upper pole of the left kidney (←) L+20 W200.

The left adrenal gland is superior and anterior to the left kidney. It has a larger body than the right and is usually 1 to 1·5 cm in length. The posteriorly situated medial and lateral limbs are 0·5 to 1 cm long with the lateral limb often slightly longer. The left gland is more variable in position than the right. Its ventral surface is in contact with the tail of the pancreas and the splenic vein.

The density of the adrenal glands is similar to that of adjacent abdominal organs. Inadequate visualization is usually due to reduction in retroperitoneal fat, failure to suspend respiration completely and artefacts due to local bowel gas motion. The gland is best seen where retroperitoneal fat is abundant.

Role of CT in adrenal disease. CT is of value not only in detecting the presence of adrenal masses and differentiating between solid and cystic lesions but also in evaluating adrenal hyperplasia (Fig. 65.39).

Adrenal mass lesions are recognized by enlargement and distortion of the margins of the gland (Fig. 65.51B). The relationship of the splenic vascular pedicle on the left side is important and enables masses arising from the adrenal gland to be differentiated from those arising from the pancreas. Masses located posterior to the splenic vascular pedicle arise from the adrenal gland whereas pancreatic masses are located anteriorly (Fig. 65.26).

Mass lesions 1 cm in size are detectable but whilst cysts and fat may be readily differentiated and calcification is usually well delineated, most tumours do not give rise to any characteristic changes in attenuation. Extension of adrenal tumour into the hepatic retroperitoneal space, however, together with metastatic disease in the axial skeleton or liver may be detected (Fig. 65.54).

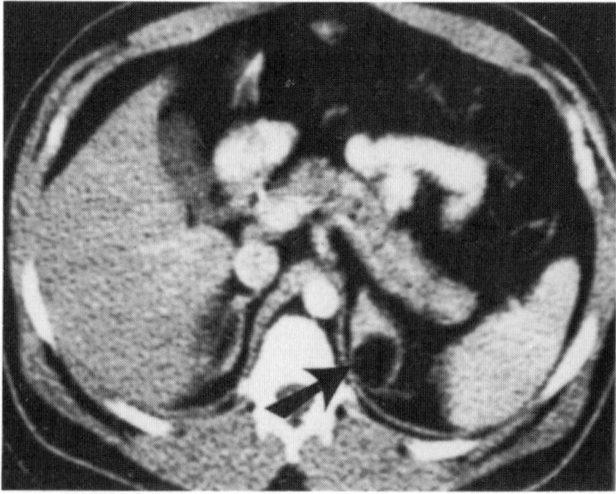

Fig. 65.39 Hyperplasia of adrenal glands in Cushing's syndrome with cystic enlargement on the left side (↗). L+15 W200.

An important contribution to clinical management is the lateralization of adrenal enlargement. CT alone will not permit histological differentiation but the findings combined with the results of clinical and biochemical investigations reduces considerably the need to employ invasive investigative methods.

6. Lymph nodes

Normal appearances. Infrastructure of lymph nodes cannot be distinguished by CT. A definition of abnormality must therefore be made on increased size and altered shape. The degree of confidence with which enlarged nodes are distinguished varies from site to site. Normal sized nodes in the lymphographic area are reliably identified only when outlined with lymphographic contrast medium (Fig. 65.40). It is generally accepted that nodes above 1·5 cm in diameter are abnormal but in the retrocrural region very small differences in size can be detected. In this space normal

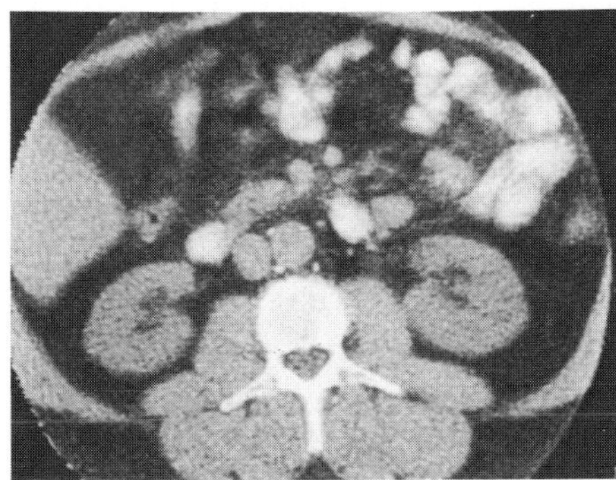

Fig. 65.40 Normal para-aortic lymph nodes outlined with lymphographic contrast medium. L+10 W200.

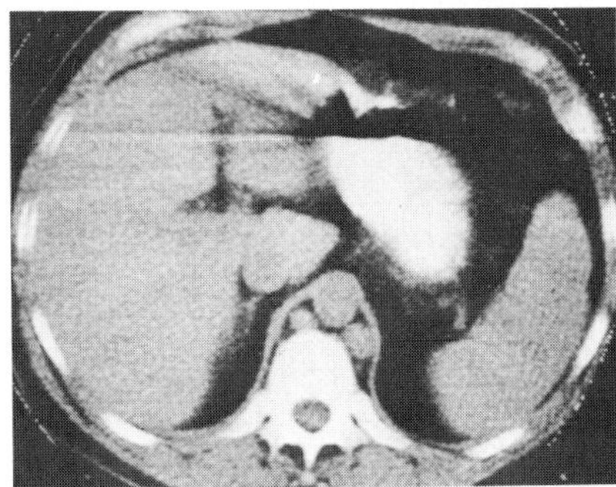

Fig. 65.41 Retrocrural lymph node enlargement. Discrete bilateral nodes in non-Hodgkin's disease. L+11 W200.

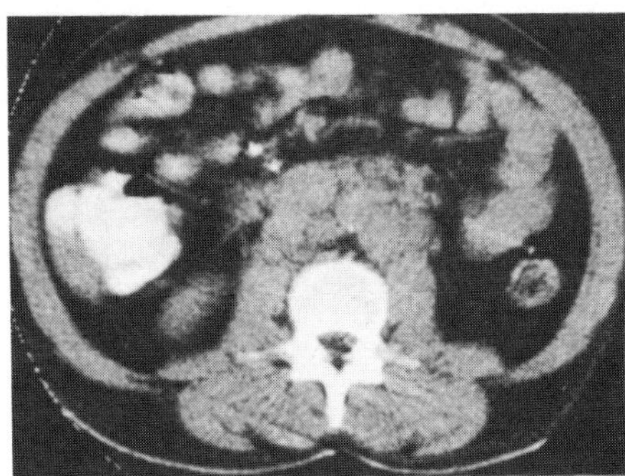

Fig. 65.42 Para-aortic lymph node enlargement obscuring the contour of aorta and inferior vena cava. L+15 W200.

structures, e.g. azygos and hemiazygos veins, cannot be differentiated from normal lymph nodes but discrete densities above 6 mm in diameter in patients with lymph node disease can be shown to represent abnormal lymph nodes (Fig. 65.41). In other areas where anatomy is more variable, e.g. mesenteric and coeliac regions, the degree of confidence in deciding whether nodes are enlarged is much less. As nodes enlarge in the para-aortic distribution the contour of the aorta and inferior vena cava may become obscured and even obliterated (Fig. 65.42).

Role of CT in lymph node disease. The factors which affect treatment and prognosis in lymph node disease are anatomical distribution and cell type. Current radio- and chemotherapeutic regimes used for example in the treatment of patients with lymphoma and testicular tumours, rely on accurate evaluation of the anatomical regions involved by disease. Clinical examination and lymphography are often unreliable for this purpose and many centres undertake staging laparotomy for apparently localized disease.

Lymphoma. The lymphomas are classified into two groups, Hodgkin's disease and non-Hodgkin's disease. In non-Hodgkin's disease the histopathology is broadly subdivided into favourable (nodular) and unfavourable (diffuse) groups. The anatomical distribution of lymphoma is outlined in Table 65.1.

Table 65.1 Anatomical distribution of lymphoma (%)

	HD	Non-HD
Spleen	37	41
Liver	8	14
Marrow	3	15
Para-aortic nodes	25	49
Mesenteric nodes	4	51

In Hodgkin's disease, where staging is usually made by the Ann Arbor classification (Table 65.2), a staging laparotomy and splenectomy may be necessary to determine whether the spleen is involved. In many centres patients between 15 and 65 years and below stage IIIa are subjected to laparotomy. Surgery is less frequently carried out in the evaluation of non-Hodgkin's disease because of the associated hypogammaglobulinaemia.

Table 65.2 Ann Arbor clinical staging classification of HD

Stage	
I	Involvement of single lymph node region or extralymphatic site
II	Involvement of two or more lymph node regions or extralymphatic sites on same side of diaphragm
III	Involvement of lymph node regions or extralymphatic sites on both sides of diaphragm which may be accompanied by splenic involvement
IV	Diffuse or disseminated involvement with or without lymph node involvement
	A without and B with general symptoms

From Kadin, M. E. *et al.*, 1971. *Cancer*, **27**, 1277–1294.

If the aim of initial investigation is to assess the extent of abdominal disease, CT provides a non-invasive means of visualizing all the abdominal lymph node areas. When CT is compared with lymphography the former has definite advantages. The technique demonstrates not only the distribution of disease shown by lymphography but also permits detection of additional enlarged lymph nodes within the lymphographic field (Fig. 65.43) together with further enlarged nodes in areas not covered by the examination (Fig. 65.44). An increase of 24 per cent in detectable disease by CT over lymphography has been demonstrated in patients with lymphoma. Mesenteric lymph nodes are involved in more than one-half of patients presenting with non-Hodgkin's lymphoma (Table 65.1). Such involvement is detectable by CT when clinical examination and other tests are normal. Enlarged mesenteric nodes are distinguished from loops of bowel by the use of oral contrast medium (Fig. 65.44). Extranodal disease in bone and soft tissue is readily identified but detection of splenic involvement is unfortunately unreliable.

When radiological investigation is directed towards the pathological diagnosis, then lymphography with its better spatial resolution will of course permit a contributory evaluation to be made of the lymph node infrastructure.

Repeat CT examinations can be performed easily, enabling the response of the disease to treatment as indicated by reduction in bulk to be monitored satisfactorily (Fig. 65.45). Residual disease after initial treatment or the full extent of relapsed disease can then be accurately assessed.

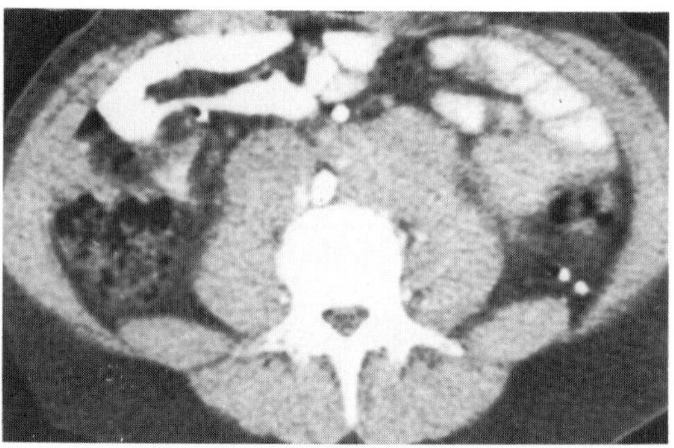

Fig. 65.43 Para-aortic lymph node enlargement. Note mass of nodes not opacified by lymphangiographic contrast medium. L+20 W200.

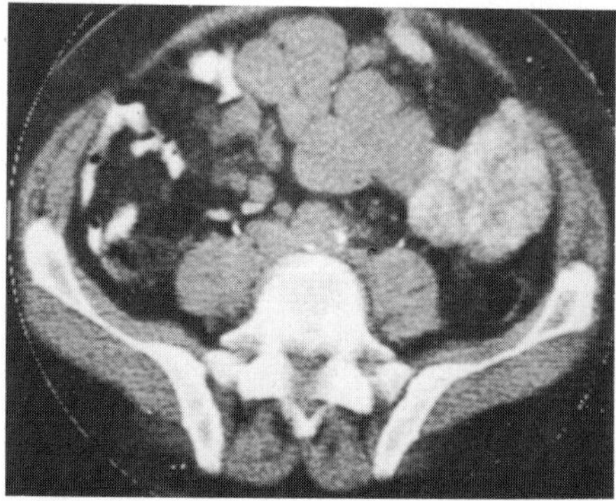

Fig. 65.44 Mesenteric lymph node enlargement. Discrete node enlargement distinguished from bowel loops by orally administered contrast medium. L+3 W200.

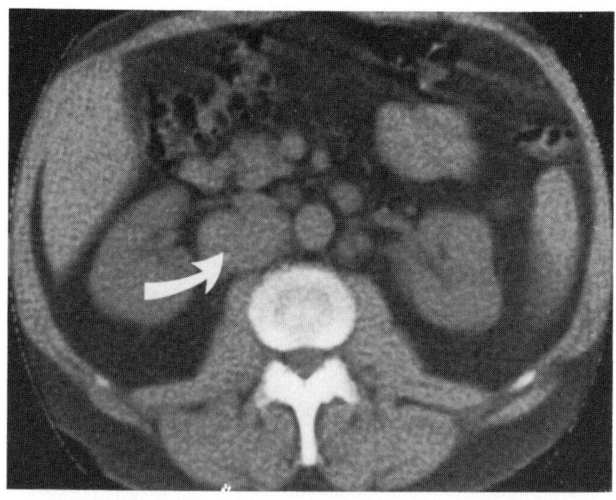

A

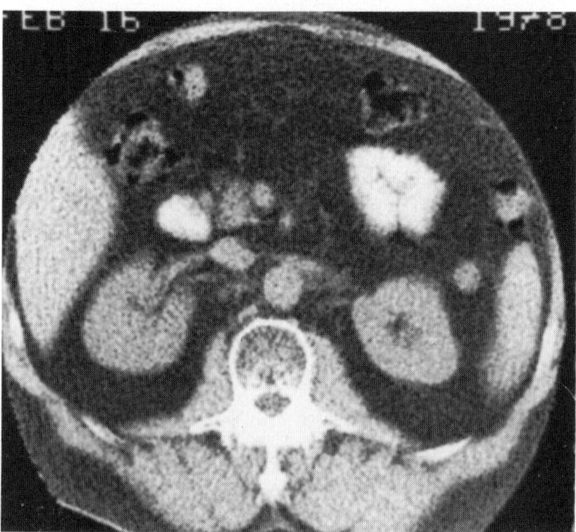

B

Fig. 65.45 Right para-aortic lymph node mass (→) in diffuse histocytic lymphoma (L+20 W200). (A) Pretreatment. (B) Post-treatment.

The unique ability to detect occult abdominal disease in patients in complete remission is of considerable value in predicting the course of the disease and indicating when and where further treatment is necessary. An estimate of the size of involved nodes and of bulk disease allows better delineation of radiotherapy fields.

The ability of CT to aid in staging lymphoma according to the Ann Arbor classification (Table 65.2) is unfortunately limited because of its inability to detect splenic disease reliably. CT does not at present therefore eliminate the need for laparotomy in the staging of Hodgkin's disease but its superiority over lymphography and its ability to detect otherwise unsuspected disease in patients in relapse or remission make it the primary non-invasive investigation of abdominal disease in patients with lymphoma.

Testicular tumours. Testicular tumours metastasize initially to the para-aortic region and lymph node enlargement is not infrequently bilateral. Associ-

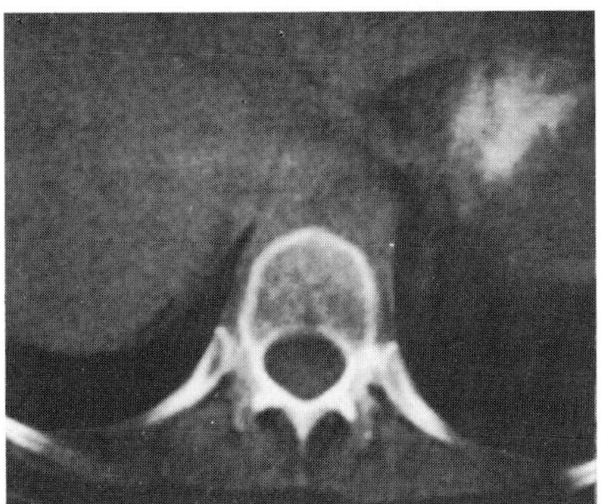

Fig. 65.67 Normal thoracic spine. L+80 W400.

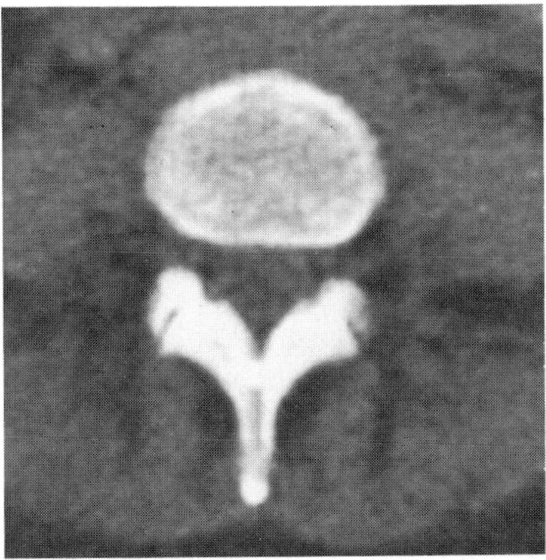

Fig. 65.69 Normal lumbar spine intervertebral disc level. Note indistinct corticomedullary boundary zone and intervertebral foramina. L+80 W400.

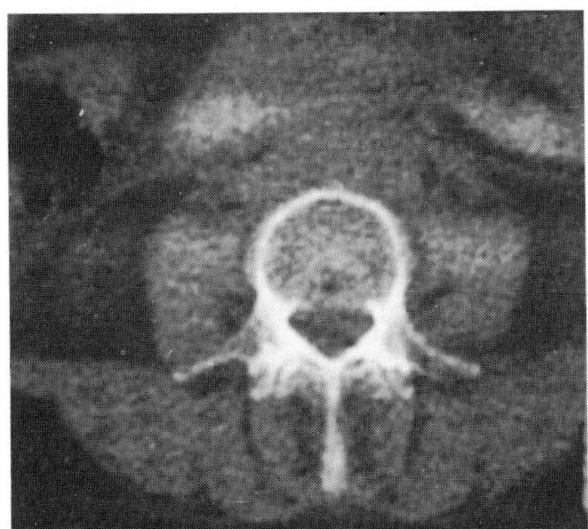

Fig. 65.68 Normal lumbar spine mid-vertebral body. Note clearly defined corticomedullary junction. L+60 W400.

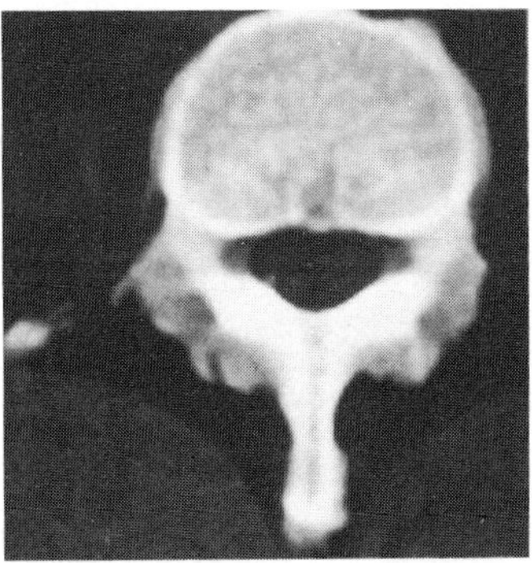

Fig. 69.70 Anatomical specimen lumbar spine. Note effect of tilt with apparent loss of left transverse process. L+55 W400.

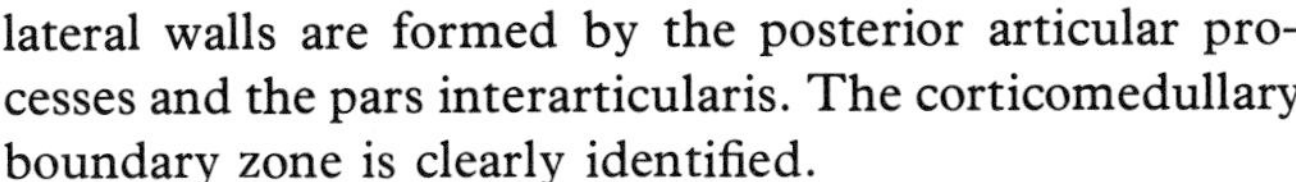

lateral walls are formed by the posterior articular processes and the pars interarticularis. The corticomedullary boundary zone is clearly identified.

Lower segment of vertebral body. The bony ring of the spinal canal is discontinuous due to the intervertebral foramina. The superior articular facets of the adjacent caudal segment form the dorsal margins of the intervertebral foramina and are therefore ventrally situated at the apophyseal joints. The inferior articular facets and laminae form the dorsal margin of the spinal canal which at this level is at its most capacious.

Intervertebral disc level. The corticomedullary boundary zone is not identifiable and the bony margin is indistinct, particularly anteriorly. The lateral walls of the spinal canal are discontinuous due to the intervertebral foraminae (Fig. 65.69).

Despite the obvious advantages afforded by CT there are significant constraints limiting its full exploitation.

(i) Anatomical

Spinal curvature due to scoliosis, kyphosis or lordosis results in significant variation of the anatomical features displayed in one section of finite thickness. Caution must therefore be exercised in the interpretation of apparent bony abnormality displayed in single sections (Fig. 65.70).

(ii) Radiological

The accurate positioning, registration and reproducibility of thin sections in all spatial co-ordinates in different patients or the same patient on different occasions can present problems. A number of techniques to improve anatomical registration are currently available. These consist of remote radiographic control, opaque markers and exploitation of the CT X-ray source in conjunction with a moving table top and patient (Scannergram). Careful use of these techniques will enable reproducibility adequate for practical clinical purposes though further study is required to enable detailed comparison of attenuation values.

The 'partial volume' effect can in addition make the precise identification of boundaries or edges difficult. Higher resolution or reduced section thickness can contribute towards their more accurate definitions.

The role of CT in diseases of the bony spine

(i) Bone disease

In those circumstances where the diagnosis is available from plain films, CT offers both an additional dimension and an analysis of adjacent soft tissue structures. In the early stages of bone destruction by either primary or secondary disease conventional radiology may reveal only minimal trabecular disturbance. CT is then capable of delineating clearly the area of bony abnormality (Fig. 65.71A). Restricted sectional thickness precludes its use however as a screening technique.

In the evaluation of mestastatic disease, skeletal isotope scanning followed by conventional radiology of abnormal areas so demonstrated is a realistic and economic approach. False-positive isotope scans of the spine may occur due to degenerative joint disease of intervertebral or costovertebral origin. Plain radiographs may be unhelpful; CT at the appropriate level is then of practical value in differentiating between metastatic and degenerative joint disease even when the two are coincident (Fig. 65.71B).

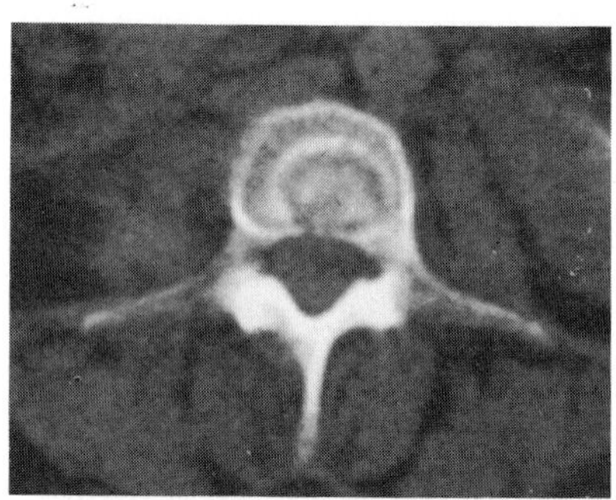

A

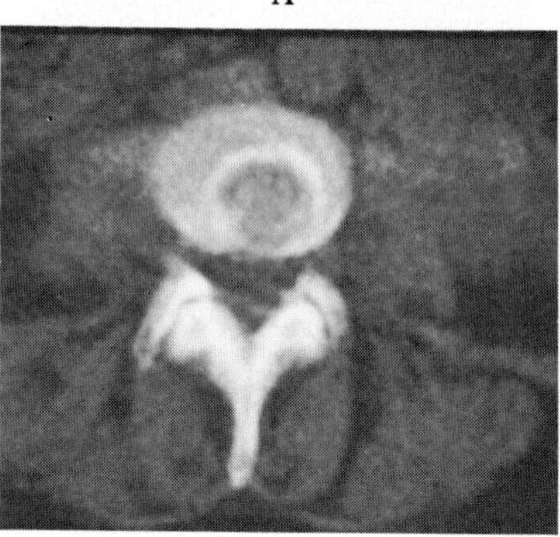

B

Fig. 65.71 (A) Vertebral body metastasis of mixed lytic and sclerotic type. Minimal trabecular disturbance on plain radiograph. L+88 W400. (B) The same patient. Note associated apophyseal joint disease. L+88 W400.

(ii) Joint disease

The role of apophyseal joint disease in the pathogenesis of back pain is speculative but there is little doubt that osteoarthrosic outgrowths from the apophyseal joints not only inhibit movement but frequently project into the intervertebral foraminae and compress their contents. Such outgrowths may also project into the spinal canal and give rise to spinal stenosis. The value of CT lies in its unique ability to display the angulation and articular surfaces of the apophyseal joints and the extent of new bone growth (Fig. 65.74).

(iii) Intervertebral disc disease

Prolapsed intervertebral disc material unless calcified does not have sufficient density discrimination to be visualized in the spinal canal with conventional CT. Schmorl's nodes or herniations of disc material through defective end-plate cartilage are however detectable and readily distinguished from intrinsic intravertebral bone defects (Fig. 65.73). Sagittal reconstruction of digital data with overlapping sections may provide further information but attention must be directed towards the inevitable increase in radiation dose.

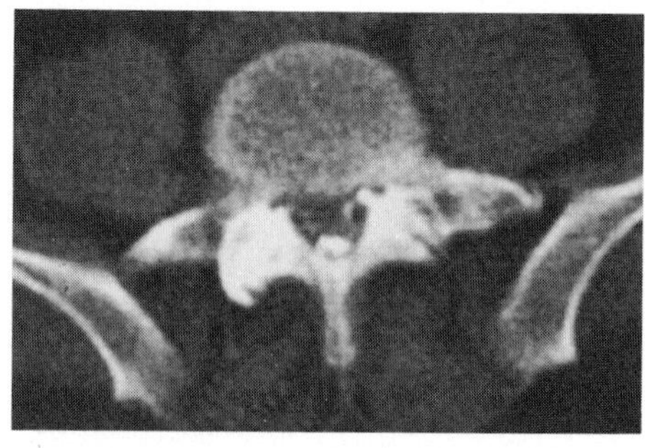

Fig. 65.72 Apophyseal joint disease. Note new bone growth and residual myodil in the spinal canal. L+8 W400.

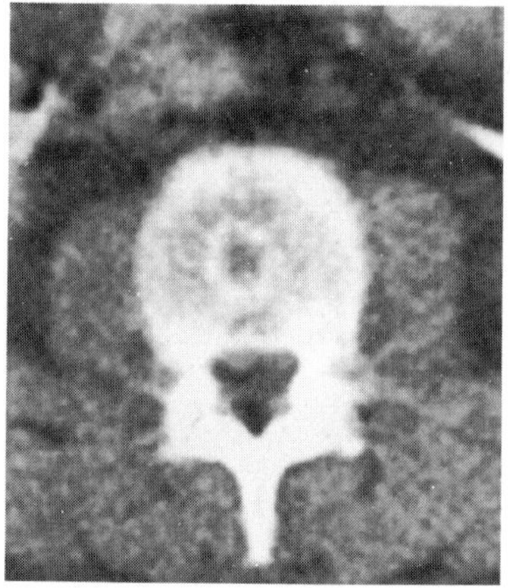

Fig. 65.73 Schmorl's node. L+80 W400.

(iv) Trauma

The role of CT in the assessment of spinal injury is concerned specially with the demonstration of fractures

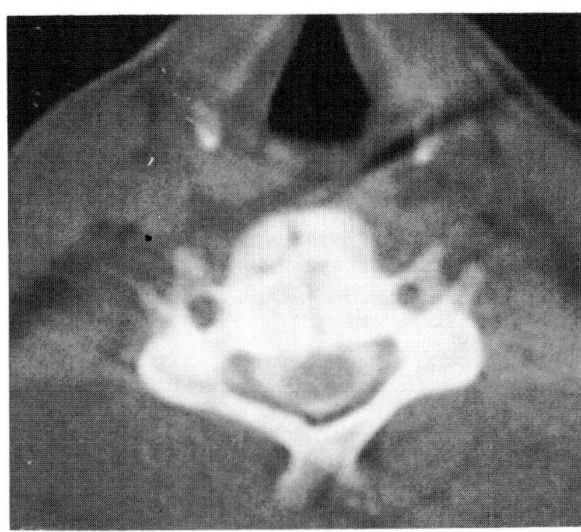

Fig. 65.74 Fracture cervical spine. Note sagittal plane of fracture with encroachment of bone on spinal cord. Metrizamide is present in the subarachnoid space. L+70 W400.

in the transaxial plane and their effect on neural tissue in the spinal canal (Fig. 65.74). Valuable information can be gained about the extent of fracture and associated joint stability.

(v) Diseases affecting the spinal canal

Alterations in cross-sectional area of the spinal canal are sometimes detectable from careful inspection and linear measurement of plain radiographs obtained under controlled conditions but no conventional radiograph can demonstrate the true shape of the spinal canal. CT enables the total cross sectional area including shape to be explored and also permits accurate evaluation of those factors contributing to both primary and secondary canal narrowing.

Spinal stenosis secondary to degenerative disease in the lumbar spine is either localized or segmental. The canal can assume a trifoliate shape as a result of bone change adjacent to the apophyseal joints (Fig. 65.75).

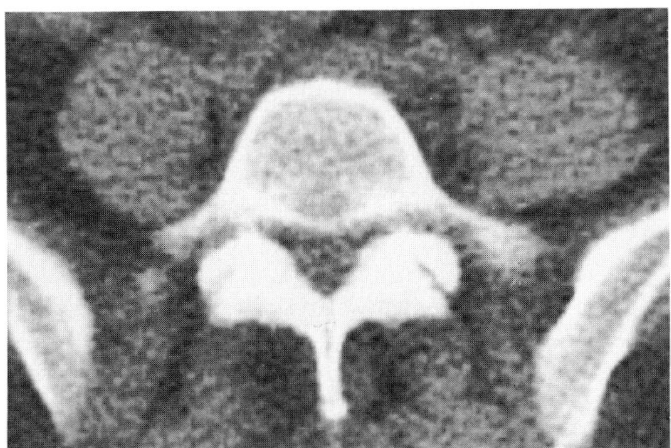

Fig. 65.75 Spinal canal stenosis secondary to degenerative disease. Note trifoliate canal. L+80 W400.

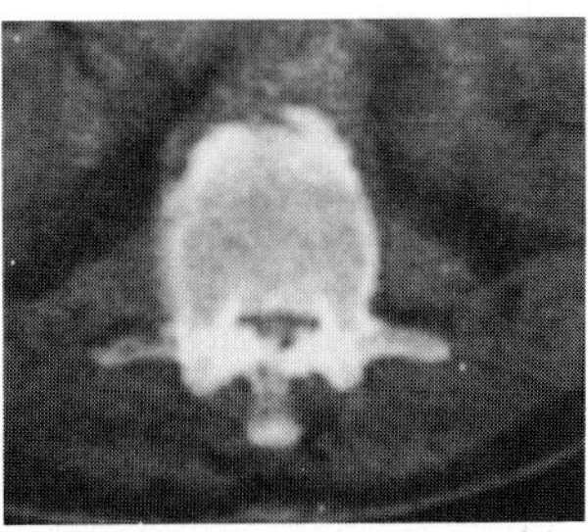

Fig. 65.76 Achondroplasia with extreme spinal canal stenosis and pedicular shortening. L+40 W400.

Achondroplasia presents an extreme example of developmental spinal canal stenosis with premature fusion of the neural epiphyseal plates resulting in pedicular shortening and narrowing of the entire canal (Fig. 65.76).

SPINAL CORD AND NEURAL TISSUE

Normal appearances. Significant statistical fluctuations occur in the quantitative data relating to the near isodense spinal canal contents. Spatial resolution and density discrimination with existing radiation dose levels are such that identification of neural tissue without contrast material in the spinal canal is unreliable. Higher resolution using limited areas of reconstruction together with addition of numerical data may enable the spinal cord to be recognized in the cervical region where the subarachnoid space is at its widest. Identification of the cord in the thoracic canal, however, can only be made with certainty by employing contrast medium in the subarachnoid space. Experimental studies suggest that inhalation of high atomic number xenon can by virtue of its lipid solubility enhance normal neural tissue and render it detectable.

CT myelography

Computer assisted myelography refers to the study of water soluble contrast medium in the spinal subarachnoid space by CT. Metrizamide (Amipaque) a non-ionic glucose amide with molecular weight 789·1, is a very suitable water-soluble contrast agent containing three iodine atoms. It has low osmolality and in a concentration of 170 mg iodine per ml it is isotonic with c.s.f. It has been extensively used as a conventional myelographic agent and as a means of studying c.s.f. flow and the intracerebral absorption pathways (see Ch. 59 and Ch. 63).

Metrizamide is detectable in the spine by CT in much lower concentration than would be possible by conventional radiology because of the greatly increased sensitivity of CT. When introduced by the lumbar route, metrizamide appears in the thoracic spine in one hour and in the cervical and cerebral subarachnoid spaces in one to two hours. The pattern of movement and diffusion of water-soluble contrast medium depends on a variety of factors including c.s.f. circulation, body cavity pressures and diffusion into neural tissue. Evidence suggests that metrizamide enters the neural tissue of the spinal cord transiently during the first hour after subarachnoid injection.

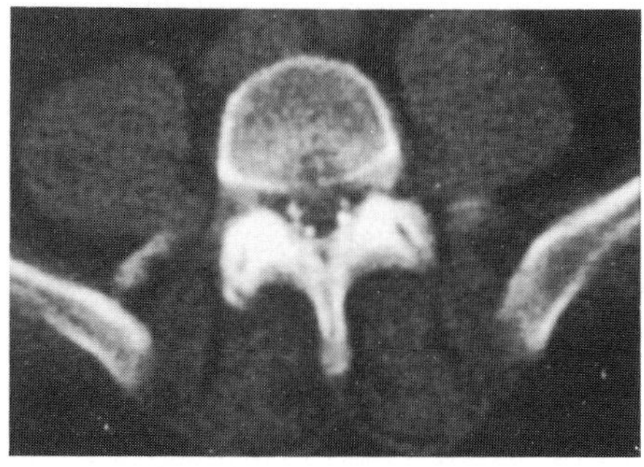

Fig. 65.77 Contrast-filled root pockets in the lumbar spine. Note apophyseal joint disease. L+110 W400.

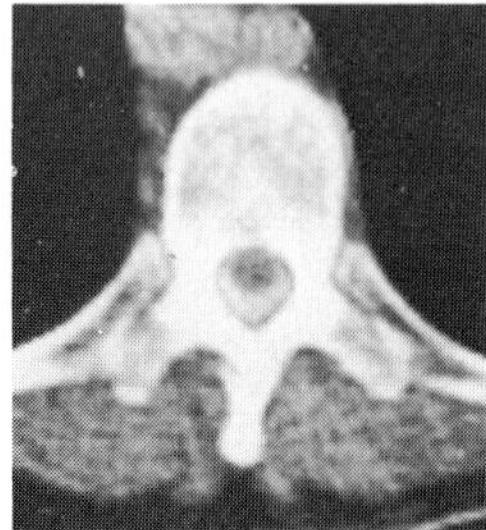

Fig. 65.78 Normal thoracic spinal cord anteriorly located during computed myelography. L+41 W200.

The normal c.s.f. space is demonstrated by CT as a continuous ring of increased attenuation surrounding the spinal cord or nerve roots (Fig. 65.6). The contrast-filled root pockets are identifiable in the lumbar spine (Fig. 65.77). The dorsal spinal cord is anteriorly located during computed myelography (Fig. 65.78) supporting the belief that this is the situation under physiological conditions.

Role of CT in diseases affecting spinal neural tissue

(i) Extramedullary. The aim of both conventional myelography and computer assisted myelography is the demonstration of the site and extent of lesions within the spinal canal and of their relationship to neural tissue, the meninges and the spinal canal itself. Herniated discs can displace dura, subarachnoid space and root pockets (Fig. 65.79).

In the evaluation of trauma, spinal cord deformity and distal atrophy are important not only as parameters of clinical management but also as prognostic indicators (Fig. 65.74). Acute haemorrhage is reliably detected as a high attenuation abnormality due to accumulation of haemoglobin.

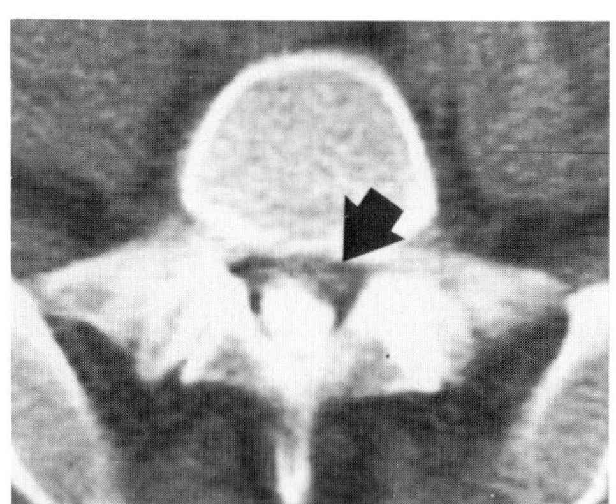

Fig. 65.79 Herniated intervertebral disc (↓) displacing contrast-filled subarachnoid space and root pockets. L+100 W400.

The configuration of the spinal canal is well displayed by conventional CT but computer assisted myelography is clearly necessary to evaluate the effects of spinal stenosis on neural tissue.

(ii) Intramedullary. Since cord contour is clearly delineated during computed myelography, expansion of cord is detectable (Fig. 65.80). In syringomyelia associated tonsillar herniation is also identifiable although its precise extent may be difficult to evaluate (Fig. 65.81).

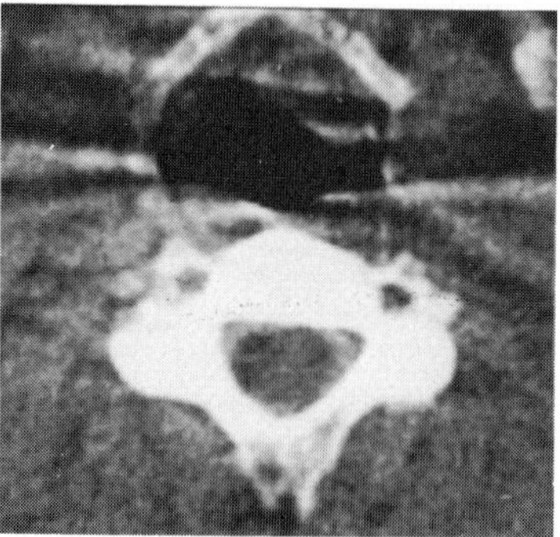

Fig. 65.80 Syringomyelia. Both spinal cord and bony canal are expanded. L+35 W200.

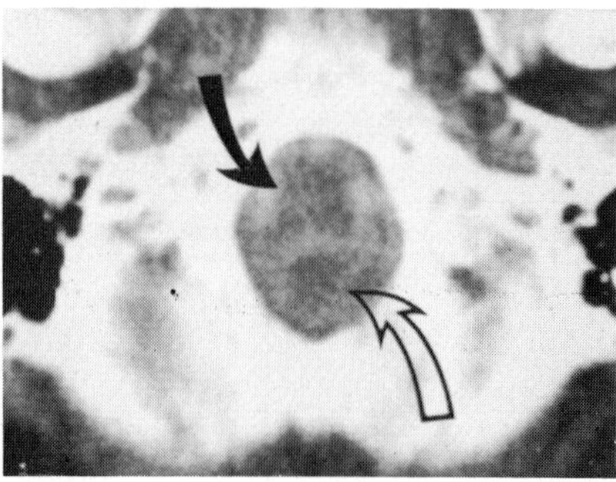

Fig. 65.81 Chiari type I malformation. Note expanded cord (↘) and cerebellar tonsillar herniation (↖) at the foramen magnum. L+35 W200.

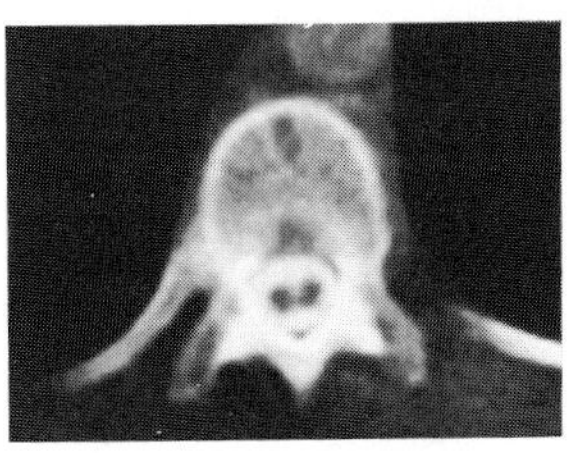

Fig. 65.82

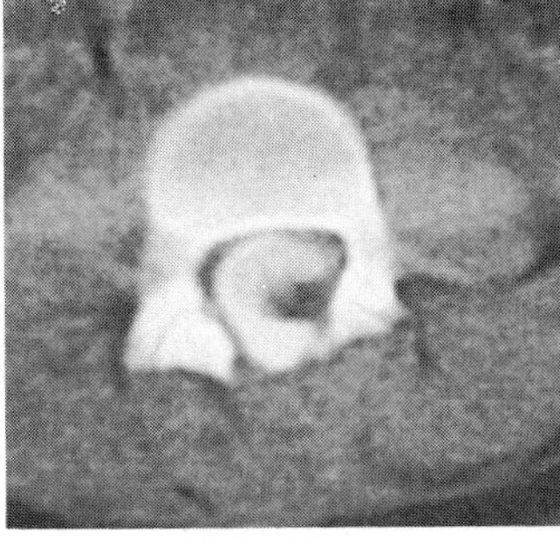

Fig. 65.83

Fig. 65.82 Diastematomyelia. Note divided cord demonstrated by CT myelography. L+100 W400.

Fig. 65.83 Spinal dysraphism with tethered cord, occult meningocele and intramedullary lipoma. L+86 W400.

Cord cavitation and variation in cord calibre have also been demonstrated.

In the presence of spinal dysraphism, CT is of particular value in the demonstration of a diastematomyelic septum (Fig. 65.82) and of the tethered cord with any associated embryonic tumour (Fig. 65.83).

A unique advantage of computed myelography is its ability to determine the heterogeneity of composition of pathological processes, a quality exploited successfully in the brain. This is of particular importance in the tumours containing high (e.g. calcium) or low (e.g. fat) density material (Fig. 65.83). Intravenous contrast enhancement has been employed to demonstrate vascular abnormalities within the spinal canal. The limited sectional thickness afforded by CT limits its role as a screening procedure but does permit segmental exploration in depth.

Fatty embryonic tumours can extend from an intramedullary location to within the pelvic cavity (Fig. 65.84).

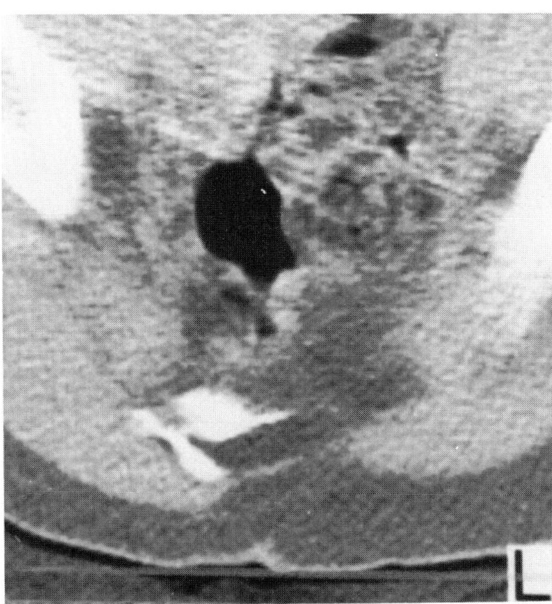

Fig. 65.84 Intramedullary lipoma extending from the lumbar spinal canal into the pelvic cavity on the left side. L+40 W400.

C. FACIAL STRUCTURES AND PARANASAL SINUSES

Normal appearances. The structures of the face, paranasal sinuses, skull base and postnasal space are all clearly visualized in the transaxial section (Fig. 65.85). Most general purpose CT scanning units also permit the presentation of data in the coronal section either by patient positioning in the scanner aperture or by reconstruction of digital data acquired from contiguous

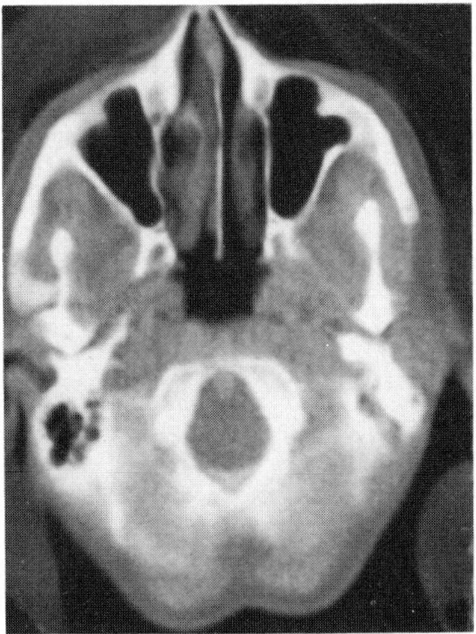

Fig. 65.85 Normal maxillary antra. Note infratemporal and pterygoid fossae. L+10 W400.

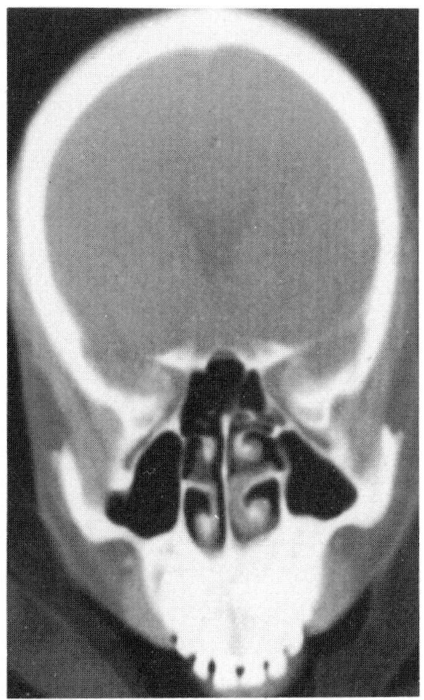

Fig. 65.86 Normal coronal section of maxillary antra. L+10 W400.

transaxial sections. If the head can be sufficiently extended with the patient either supine or prone, coronal sections may be achieved with optimal resolution (Fig. 65.86). Reconstruction of digital data requires a significant overlap of sections to achieve similar resolution.

Coronal sections are particularly valuable in the assessment of palatal, orbital and intracranial extension of paranasal sinus disease. In the transaxial section display of the posterolateral walls of the maxillary antra together with the soft tissue structures of the infra-temporal and pterygopalatine fossae, anatomical regions difficult to identify by conventional radiology, is particularly important (Fig. 65.85).

The normal nasopharynx is quadrilateral in shape and the Eustachian tubes are identified as air-filled linear structures directed obliquely and posteriorly from the fossae of Rosenmuller (Fig. 65.87).

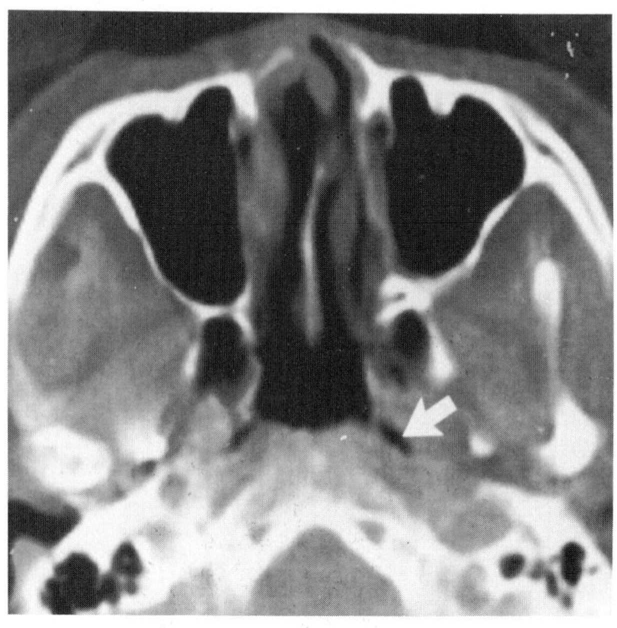

Fig. 65.87 Normal nasopharynx. Note air-filled Eustachian tube (↙). L+30 W400.

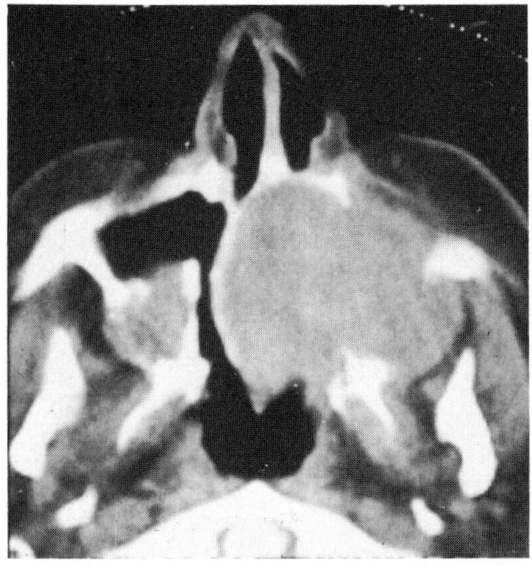

A

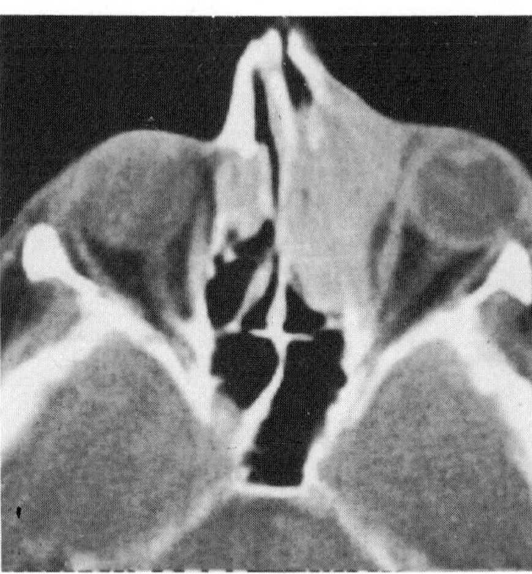

B

Fig. 65.88 (A) Bilateral carcinomata maxillary antra. Extension into infratemporal fossae on both sides. L+15 W200. (B) Ethmoidal carcinoma with extension into the orbit as an extraconal mass. Note displacement of medial rectus muscle and globe of the eye. L+1 W200.

Role of CT in paranasal sinus disease

Malignant disease. Conventional radiology, including complex movement tomography, will often reveal bony destruction and accompanying soft tissue mass lesions. Soft tissue involvement, however, can be extensive before bone destruction is identified. CT can detect soft tissue components of invasive tumours not only by revealing their expanding contour but also by providing evidence of fascial plane obliteration. Early and accurate assessment of tumour extension may therefore be made (Fig. 65.88). In particular, extension of tumours into the infratemporal fossa may only be revealed clinically by the onset of trismus by which stage tumour involvement is often extensive and treatment possibilities restricted. The facility to identify the full extent of disease, to plan treatment and to monitor the response to treatment, are major assets of CT.

Necrosis and abscess formation in tumours are identified as areas of low attenuation within the soft tissue mass (Fig. 65.89). The mean attenuation values, however, of malignant lesions fall within the normal soft tissue range represented by local muscle and tissue characterization is therefore not possible. Contrast enhancement is of little value since most tumours in the

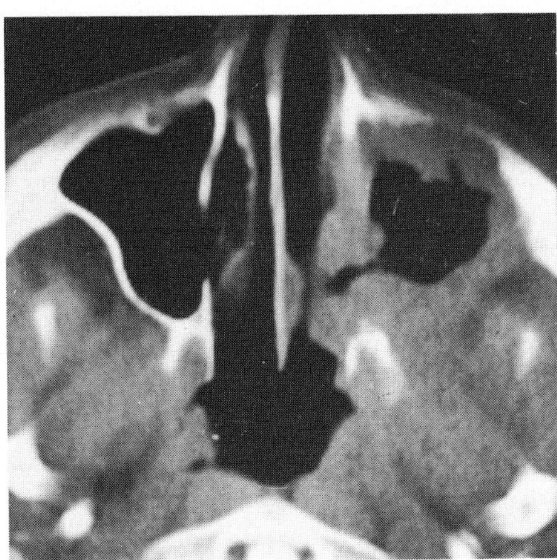

Fig. 65.89 Carcinoma antrum with central necrosis. Note posterolateral bone destruction and extension of tumour into infratemporal fossa. L+40 W400.

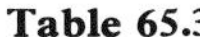

Table 65.3

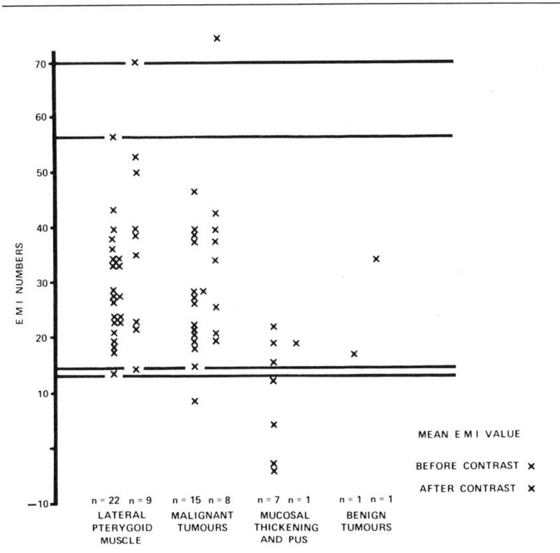

paranasal region are relatively avascular and, as discussed earlier, the blood/brain barrier plays no part. Perivascular tumours may show some evidence of enhancement (Table 65.3).

The CT assessment of minor degrees of bone erosion in the paranasal sinuses can be impaired by the partial volume effect. In these circumstances, conventional tomography is an essential, complementary examination.

Inflammatory disease. The mean attenuation values of paranasal sinuses containing pus or retained secretions range from below the lower level for normal soft tissue to the upper limit (Table 65.3). Inflammatory disease cannot therefore be separated easily from neoplasia when there is no evidence of soft tissue extension beyond the sinus cavity (Fig. 65.90). The presence of low attenuation values in some inflammatory situations due to increased water content in retained secretions may be a helpful sign of differentiation.

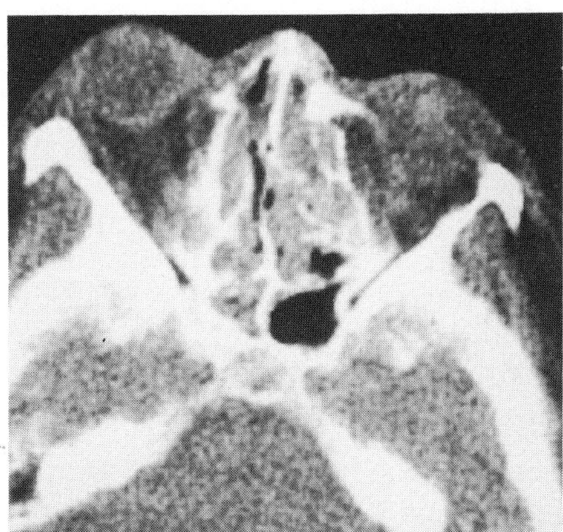

Fig. 65.90 Pansinusitis. No evidence of bone destruction. L+1 W200.

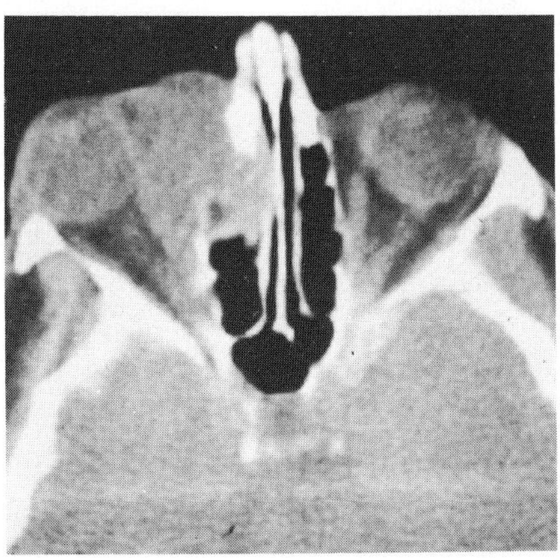

A

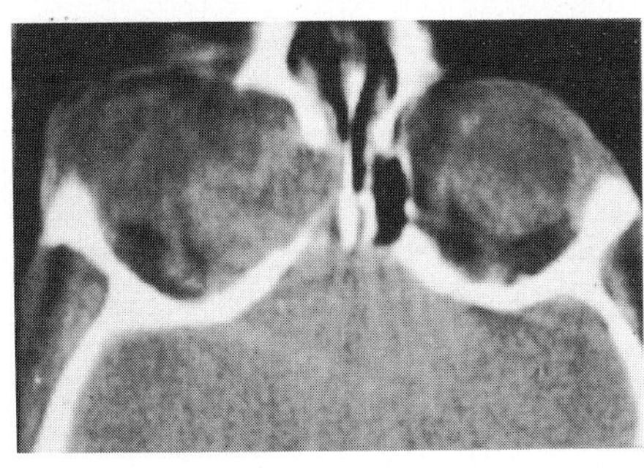

B

Fig. 65.91 Ethmoidal mucocele (L+6 W200). (A) Transaxial section. (B) Coronal section.

CT sections in transaxial and coronal planes demonstrate clearly the size and extent of associated mucoceles (Fig. 65.91). In the case of the ethmoidal mucocele, its relationship to orbital contents and the extent of any associated proptosis can be assessed. The technique is clearly important in the evaluation of unilateral proptosis.

D. THORAX

LUNG

Normal appearances. *Anatomical considerations.* The whole dynamic scale of tissue densities is present in each CT section of the thorax. Interrogation of the grey-scale image at a variety of window levels and window widths is therefore necessary to witness the full range of anatomical structures (Fig. 65.92).

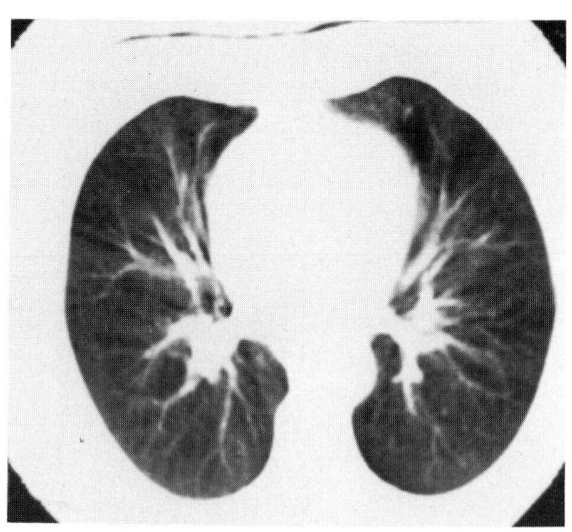

A

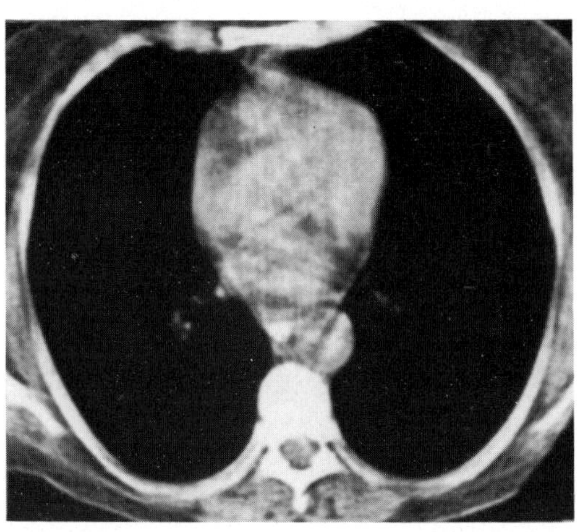

B

Fig. 65.92 Normal thorax. (A) Low window level demonstrating lung fields. L−320 W400. (B) High window level demonstrating mediastinal structures. L+20 W200.

The pulmonary vessels are clearly visible against aerated lung and can be traced to the periphery of the lung field. Secondary and frequently tertiary order bronchi can also be identified. The radial distribution of pulmonary arteries from the hila results in the differential 'sampling' of the vessels in transaxial sections. At the lung apices and bases, vessels pass obliquely through the thin sections whereas at central level a greater degree of arborization is encountered (Fig. 65.93). Apparent discontinuities in arborizing structures should not be interpreted as evidence of occlusive disease. Reference must always be made to sequential sections.

The dome of the diaphragm obtrudes into the basal sections to a varying degree and may, as a result of the partial volume effect, give rise to apparent increase in density at the centre of the lung field (Fig. 65.94).

Physiological considerations: Respiratory phase. The density of lung in a CT section is strongly dependent upon the respiratory phase. In expiration there is a striking increase in density particularly in the dependent part of the lung. Whilst the change is likely to be the result of inadequate alveolar inflation, the effect of any related variations in perfusion might also be considered (Fig. 65.94).

Suspended respiration is necessary to obtain optimal scanning conditions. Most patients can hold their breath for 20 seconds or more during full inspiration, which also provides optimal conditions for reproducibility regardless of posture. Occasionally preliminary hyperventilation or even oxygenation may be helpful to patients with respiratory difficulties. Neutral or expiratory phases of respiration are not easily reproducible

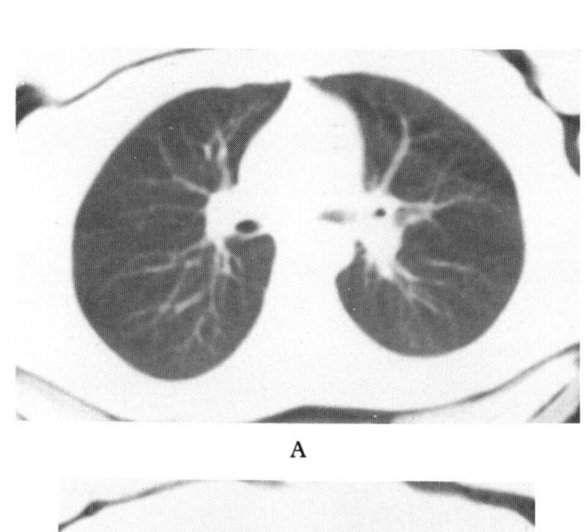

A

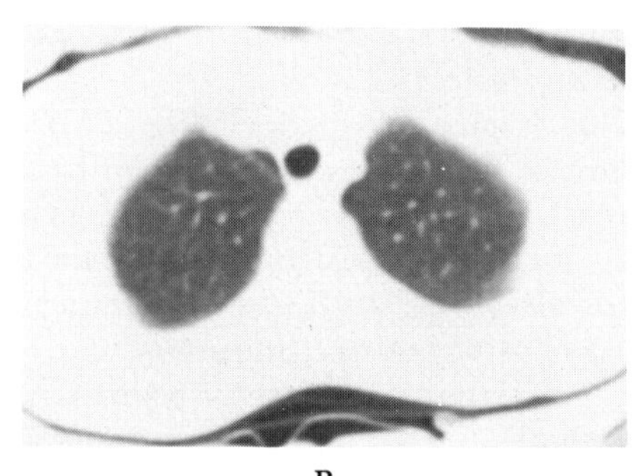

B

Fig. 65.93 Normal pulmonary vascularity. (A) Hilar level. L−320 W400. (B) Apical level. L−320 W400.

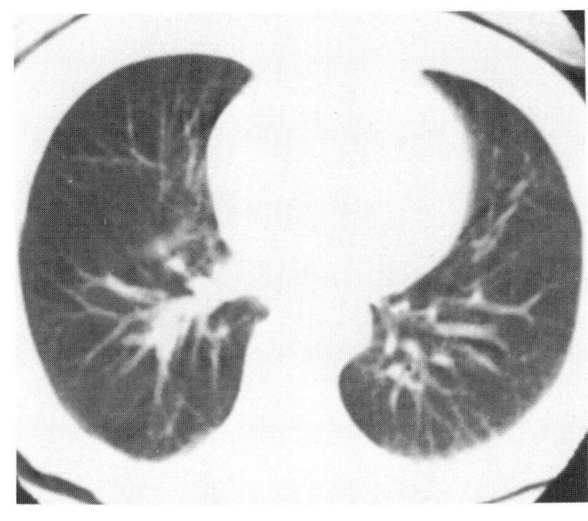

A

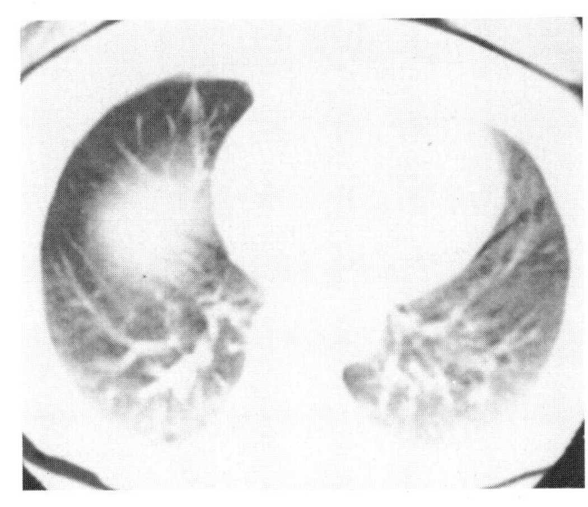

B

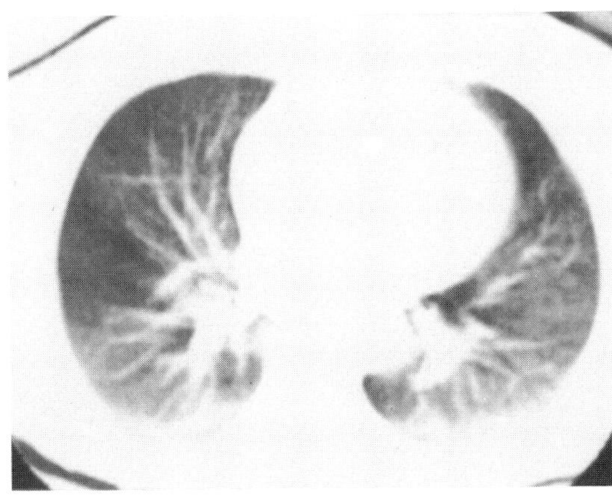

C

Fig. 65.94 Normal lungs. L −320 W400. (A) Inspiration. (B) Expiration. Note intrusion of diaphragm dome into right lung base section. (C) Expiration at higher level demonstrating increase in density in the dependant lung.

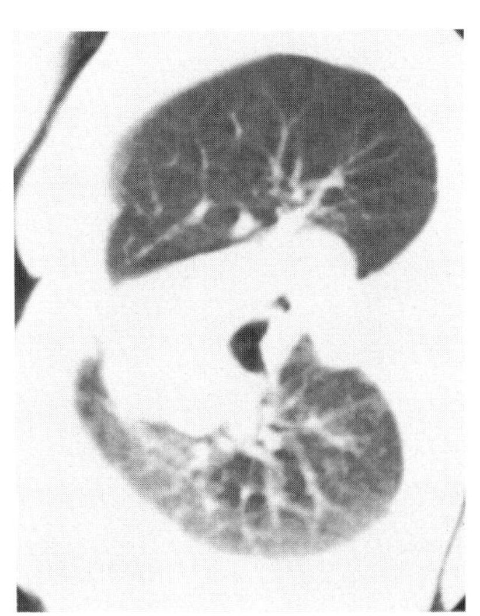

Fig. 65.95 Normal lung fields. Patient in right lateral decubitus position. Note change in pulmonary vessels in dependent lung together with 'splinting' of upper lung in expiration. L −320 W400.

and do not provide the best circumstances for breath holding.

Posture. The influence of gravity on pulmonary vessel calibre is well demonstrated by CT. Dependent vessels are notably larger whatever the position of the patient (Fig. 65.95). In the supine position the gravity gradient is from apex to base.

Posture also results in compression of the dependent lung, most noticeable during expiration (Fig. 65.95). In the lateral decubitus position the uppermost lung is in a state of relative inspiratory apnoea with diminution in the vascular component. This upper lung 'splinting' may be used to advantage in patients whose breath holding capacity is limited.

Role of CT in diseases affecting the lungs and pleura

Patterns of disease. Conventional radiological investigations usually reveal the anatomical distribution of lobar or sublobar disease. CT is of value in confirming such disease and has a particular role in the identification of segmental atelectasis (Fig. 65.96). The cross-sectional nature of the image makes it possible, for example, to identify alveolar disease as predominantly in the outer third of the lung fields (Fig. 65.97).

Identification of occult disease

Nodular

Computerized axial tomography is a very sensitive technique for the identification of single, unsuspected nodules over 3 mm in diameter but is relatively insensitive to the presence of nodules less than 3 mm. It is of

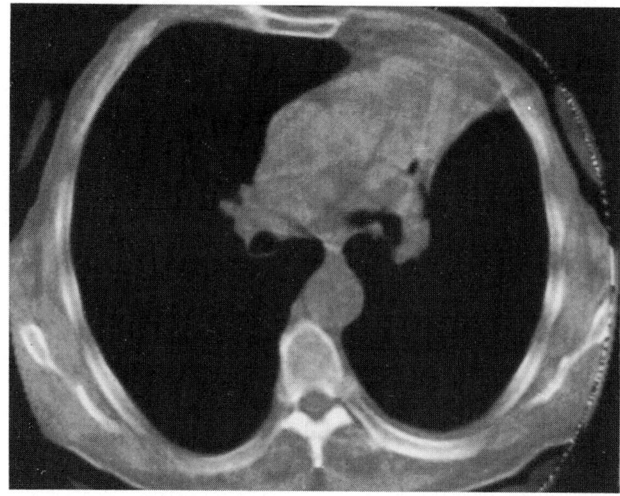

Fig. 65.96 Left upper lobe collapse. Note asymmetry of thoracic cavities. L + 20 W400.

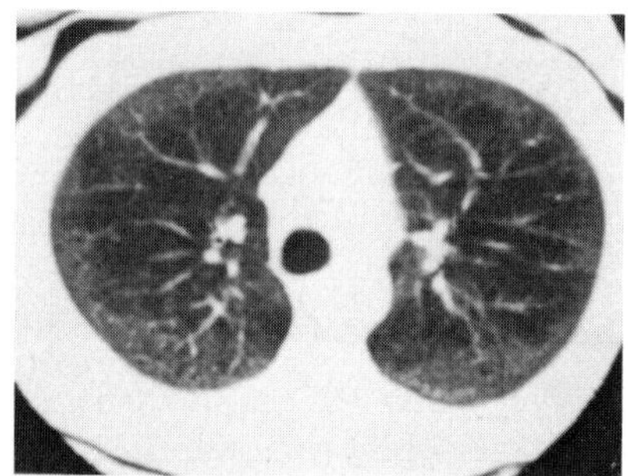

Fig. 65.97 Fibrosing alveolitis. Note increased alveolar density in outer third of the lung fields. L − 325 W400.

particular value in the detection of nodules in the costophrenic, retrocardiac and retrosternal regions in addition to the periphery of the lung fields where conventional radiographs and lung tomography are relatively insensitive (Fig. 65.98).

More nodules are detected by CT than by conventional chest radiology or even whole lung tomography. Most metastatic disease of the lungs affects the outer third of the lung fields and the majority of metastases are subpleural. Despite the improved sensitivity of CT a proportion of nodules may still go undetected. In addition there is a lack of specificity, particularly in those lesions less than 3 mm with a result that many small nodules (up to 60 per cent) are later found to be unrelated granulomata indistinguishable by CT from malignant metastatic disease. The potential incidence of false positive and false negative results does not at present enable CT to replace conventional tomography but only to complement it.

Interstitial parenchymal disease

Most parenchymal disease is best evaluated by conventional radiology. Interstitial fibrosis may, by con-

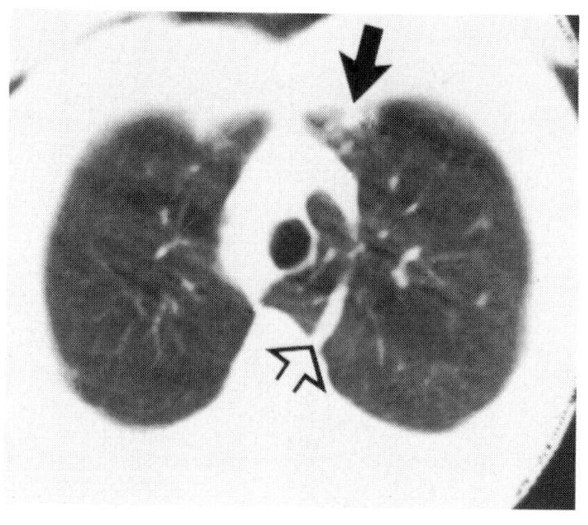

A

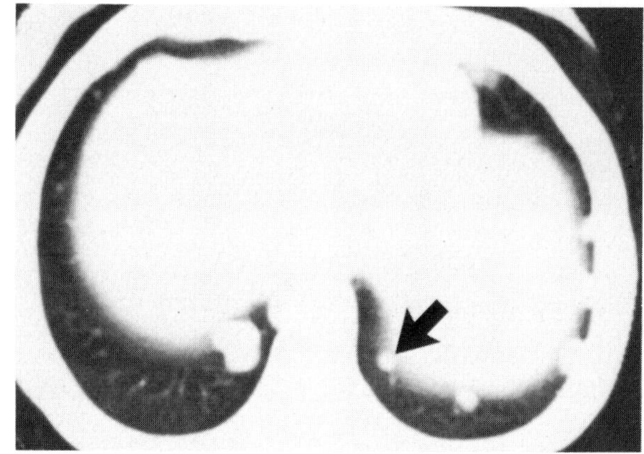

B

Fig. 65.98 Occult nodular metastases. (A) Periphery anterior segment right upper lobe (↓). (Note azygos lobe (↑). L −320 W400. (B) Posterior costophrenic sulci. (↙) L − 250 W400.

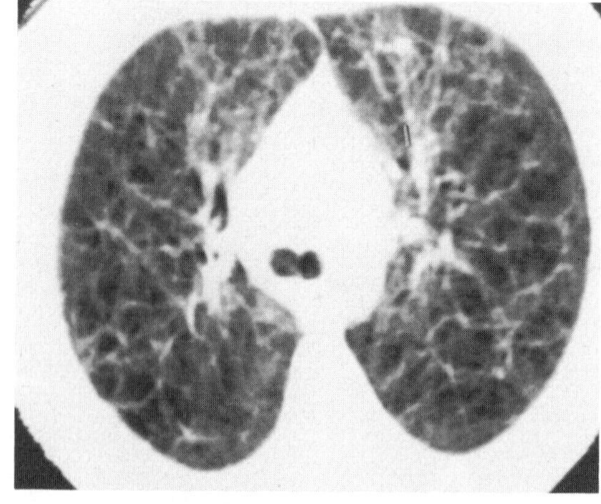

Fig. 65.99 Congenital emphysema with multiple bullae. L − 350 W400.

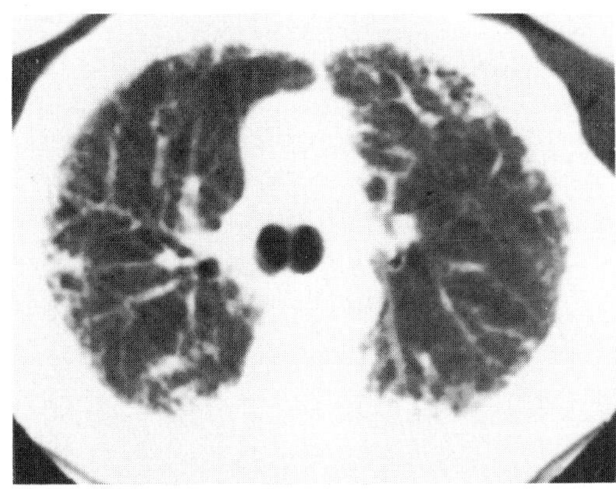

Fig. 65.100 Interstitial fibrosis with compensatory emphysema. Note loss of normal physiological response due to lack of lung compliance. L−320 W400.

ventional chest radiography, appear to affect the whole lung field, but by CT is observed to be predominantly in the outer third (Fig. 65.97). Bullae are clearly demonstrated with increased sensitivity to local areas of emphysema before the formation of bullae (Fig. 65.99). Such areas remain unaltered with changes in posture. Lack of compliance in the lung results in a loss of the normal physiological responses previously described (Fig. 65.100).

Pleural disease

Differentiation between pulmonary and pleural disease may influence clinical management significantly, particularly in the identification of loculated pleural collections (Fig. 65.101). Early identification of pleural and chest wall involvement in parenchymal disease is possible. Pleural plaques which may contain calcium and are often associated with asbestosis are visualized tangentially and can be seen to extend circumferentially (Fig. 65.102).

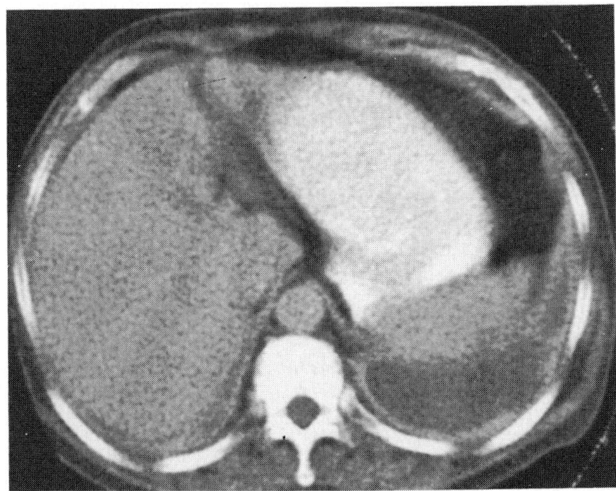

Fig. 65.101 Loculated left pleural effusion. L+30 W200.

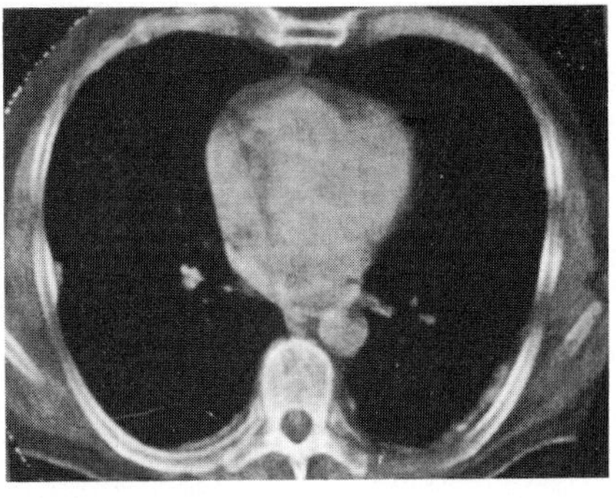

A

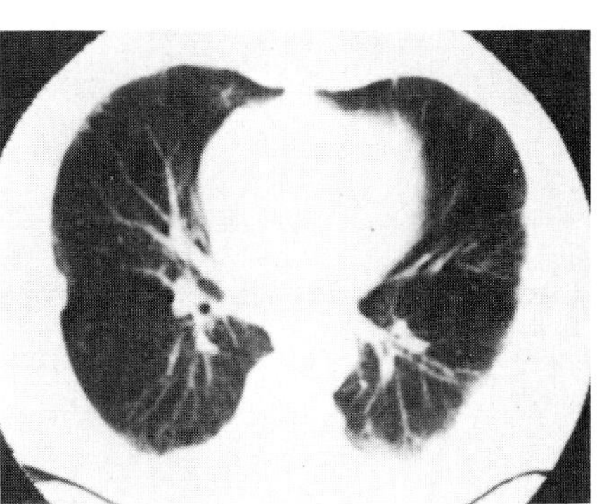

B

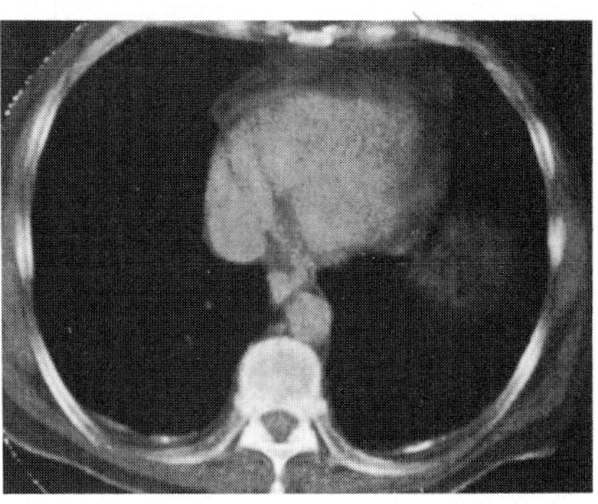

C

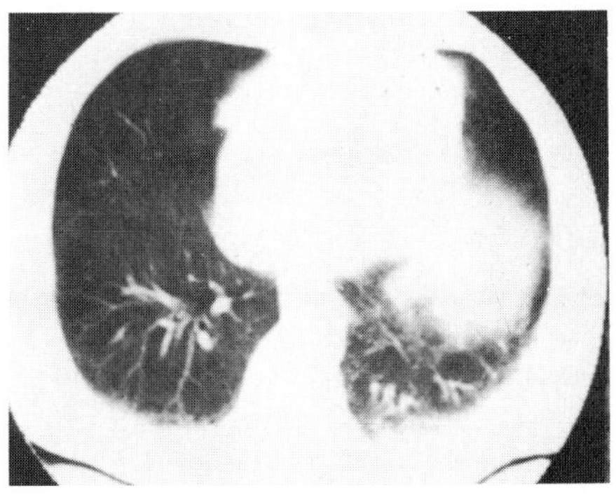

D

Fig. 65.102 Asbestosis (A–D). Demonstrating interstitial fibrosis and pleural plaques with calcification at different window levels. L+14 W400 (A and C). L−330 W400 (B and D).

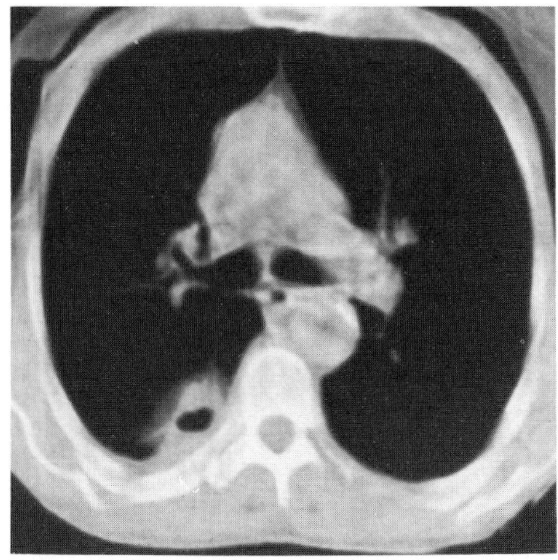

A

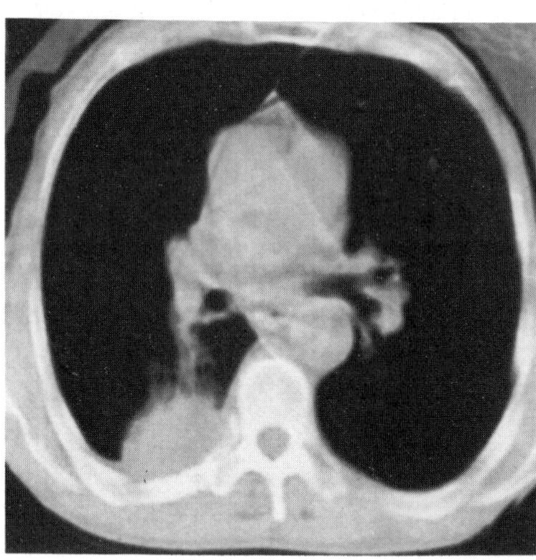

B

Fig. 65.103 (A and B) Bronchial carcinoma in right paravertebral gutter demonstrating cavitation and spread to hilum and chest wall. L −55 W400.

Evaluation of the pulmonary nodule

The principal role of CT in the evaluation of the pulmonary nodule is in excluding multiplicity within the constraints of detectability, in determining the degree of malignancy and in contributing to staging procedures before treatment is instituted.

The benign pathological character of a pulmonary nodule can be inferred primarily by the detection of calcium and the lack of growth over a two-year period. Other signs relating to marginal character and density are unreliable. Cavitation is detectable at an early stage but may not necessarily indicate malignancy. Spread to hilum, pleura or chest wall together with involvement of lymph nodes is important pretreatment staging information (Fig. 65.103).

Treatment planning together with monitoring of both single and multiple nodules after treatment are most readily undertaken by CT.

MEDIASTINUM

Normal appearances. An understanding of the normal vascular structures of the mediastinum in cross-section is essential to permit a logical analysis of abnormal mediastinal masses. The unique ability of CT to identify small density differences in the cross-section allows the

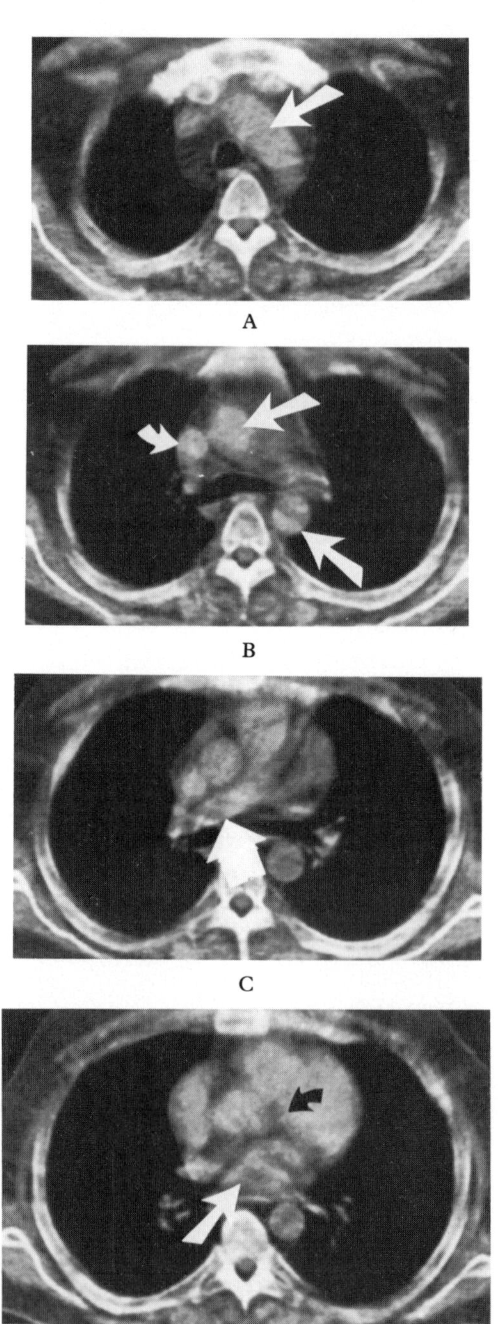

A

B

C

D

Fig. 65.104 Mediastinal anatomy demonstrated in patient with Cushing's syndrome. Note increased fat content giving rise to apparent mediastinal widening on plain radiograph (L+20 W200). (A) Aortic arch (↙). (B) Ascending (↙) and descending (↖) limbs of aortic arch and superior vena cava (↘). (C) Intrapericardial right pulmonary artery (↖). (D) Left atrium (↗) superior pulmonary veins, and interventricular septum (↙).

demonstration of some structures not previously detectable by conventional techniques. Cardiac and vascular pulsation can result in overlying artefacts and loss of marginal definition.

CT angiography, i.e. high dose intravenous contrast with first circulation studies, is of considerable value in the better definition of major vessels. An excess of fat in the mediastinum, e.g. in Cushing's syndrome, may allow identification of vascular structures without contrast enhancement (Fig. 65.104).

The following normal features of the mediastinum are of particular importance:

Aortic arch (Fig. 65.104A and B)
The ascending limb of the aortic arch lies anterior to the trachea and anterolateral to the superior vena cava. The descending limb is closely related to the oesophagus which may also contain air.

Right paratracheal stripe
The interface between the right upper lobe and the right lateral wall of the trachea is represented by the 'right paratracheal stripe' on a conventional chest radiograph.

Pulmonary arteries (Fig. 65.104C)
The main pulmonary artery lies to the left of the ascending limb of the thoracic aorta. The intrapericardial portion of the right pulmonary artery passes posterolaterally between the superior vena cava and the intermediate bronchus. CT offers a unique opportunity to make direct measurement of the diameter of the vessel. The left pulmonary artery has a short intrapericardial course and passes posterolaterally anterior to the left main bronchus which may be displaced by it.

Pulmonary veins (Fig. 65.104D)
The superior and inferior pulmonary veins draining into the left atrium on the posterior aspect of the heart lie caudal to the pulmonary arteries and anterior to the oesophagus.

Cardiac chambers (Fig. 65.104D)
The approach to cardiac scanning is dealt with separately but even a conventional CT scan of 2–18 seconds may permit some cardiac chambers to be identified, particularly the left atrium posteriorly and the ventricles at the diaphragmatic surface. The interventricular septum is recognizable as a linear structure of fat density passing obliquely from the left anteriorly towards the inferior vena cava posteriorly on the right side.

Diaphragmatic crura (Fig. 65.41)
The diaphragmatic crura are clearly identified by CT as curvilinear structures of varying thickness demarcating the aortic hiatus. The right crus is longer and frequently thicker, particularly in males, than the left. The retrocrural space contains, in addition to the aorta, lymph nodes and the azygos vein. Localized thickening of the right crus should not be mistaken for lymph node enlargement.

Azygo-oesophageal recess (Figs. 65.93A and 65.109).
The right lower lobe lies in intimate relationship with the posterior wall of the right main bronchus and the oesophagus and azygos vein medially. The azygo-oesophageal recess created in the mediastinum by the right lower lobe is known as the space of Holzknecht. Enlargement of carinal nodes may be identified at an early stage by their intrusion into this easily recognized space.

Aortopulmonary window (Figs. 65.93A and 65.109)
The aortopulmonary window between the descending aorta and the left pulmonary artery is recognized on CT by the protrusion of a portion of the left lower lobe into its posterior aspect. Hilar node enlargement or changes in pulmonary artery calibre can obliterate this recess at an early stage in their development.

Role of CT in mediastinal disease

Evaluation of mediastinal mass
The location, size, contour and extent of mediastinal masses whether tumourous or vascular are usually well demonstrated. CT in the transverse plane frequently permits a clearer identification of abnormalities otherwise partially obscured in conventional radiographs, e.g. retrosternal (Fig. 65.98A) or retrocrural (Fig. 65.41) areas. Whilst histological characterization is not possible, some information about the consistency of a mass can often be determined by variations in its attenuation

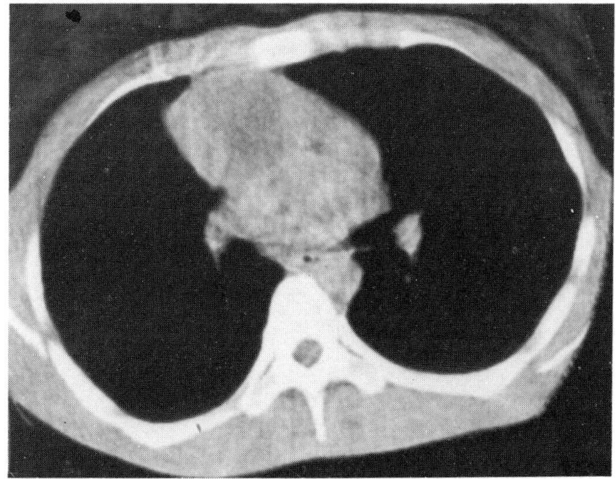

Fig. 65.105 Necrotic lymph node mass in anterior mediastinum. Hodgkin's disease of mixed cellularity type. L0 W200.

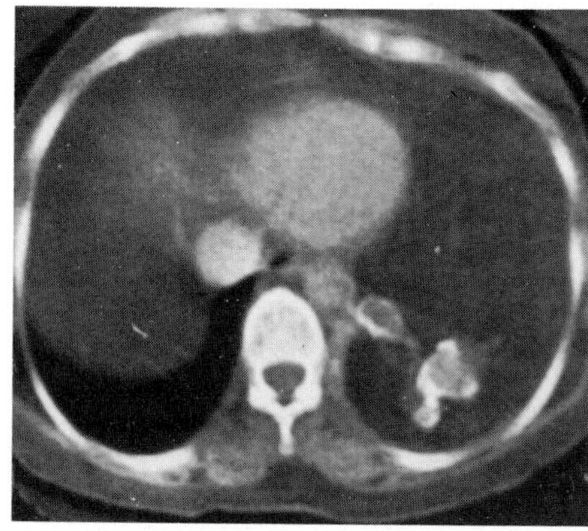

Fig. 65.106 Lipodermoid. Anterior mediastinal mass of fat density containing calcific deposits posteriorly. L0 W200.

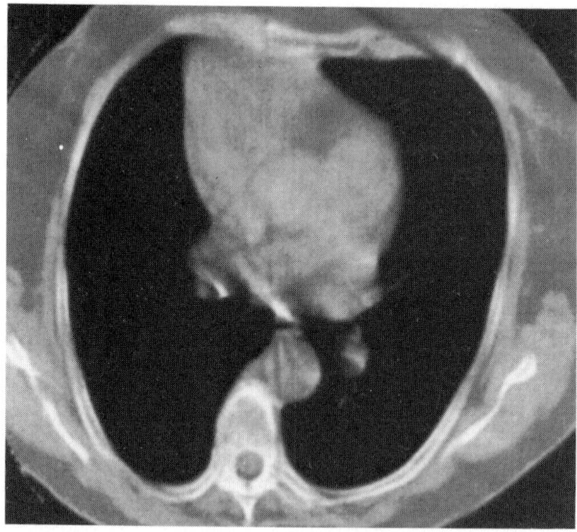

A

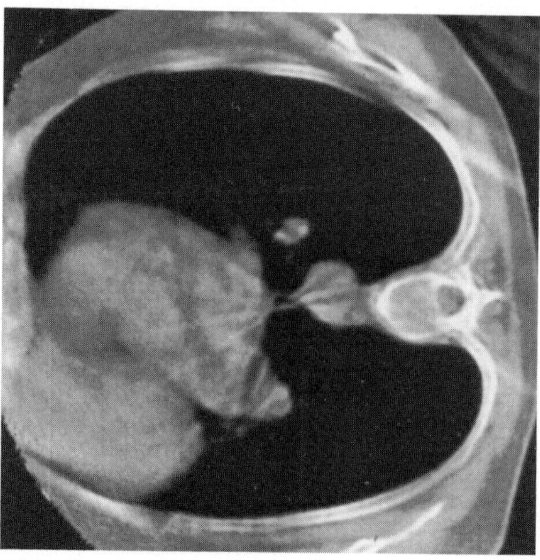

B

Fig. 65.107 (A and B) Pericardial cyst. Note displacement in lateral decubitus position. L −10 W400.

characteristics, i.e. density (Fig. 65.105). Fat and calcification are easily detected and may permit a positive diagnosis of lipoma or dermoid (Fig. 65.106) to be established in situations where only a soft tissue mass is visible by conventional techniques. Alteration in shape of a mass by change in posture suggests fluid content and may also reveal a consistent relationship of the mass with an anatomical structure, e.g. pericardial cyst (Fig. 65.107).

CT angiography enables normal and ectatic vessels to be identified and the lumen of an aortic aneurysm to be differentiated from perivascular thrombus and the false lumen of a dissection (Fig. 65.108).

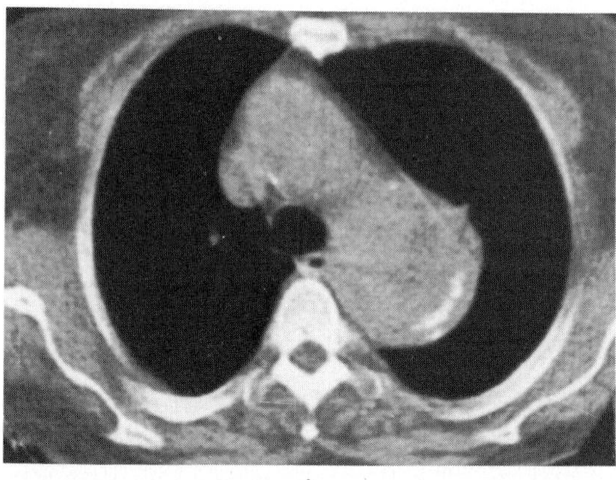

A

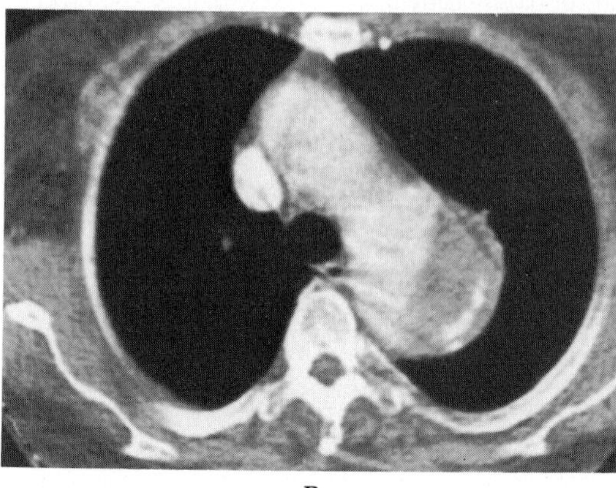

B

Fig. 65.108 Dissecting aortic aneurysm (L+10 W200). (A) Precontrast enhancement. (B) Postcontrast enhancement. Note double lumen.

Evaluation of hilar mass

The hilum is frequently involved in mediastinal disease and the usual problem on a conventional radiograph is the distinction of a true hilar mass from an enlarged vessel. CT demonstrates normal pulmonary vessels well (see above) and reveals in transverse section enlarged mediastinal lymph nodes at an early stage, particularly those presenting in the azygo-oesophageal recess and the aortopulmonary window (Fig. 65.109).

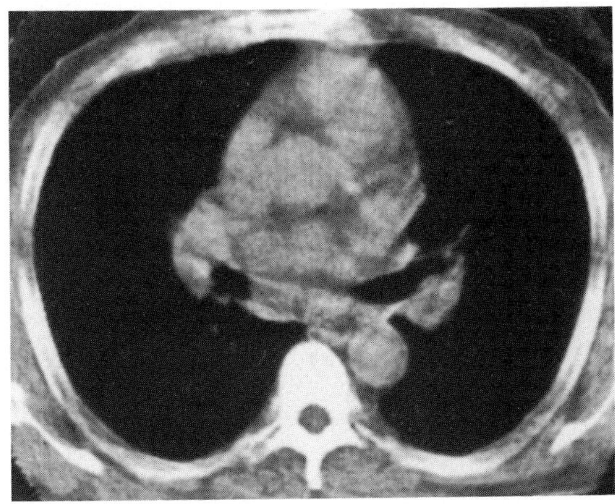

A

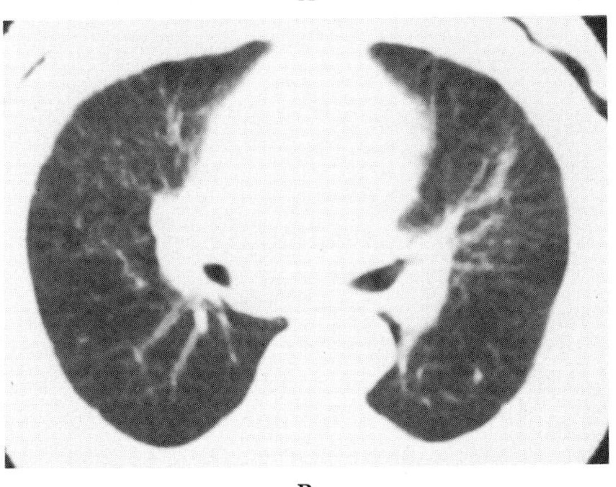

B

Fig. 65.109 (A and B) Sarcoidosis. Lymph node enlargement affecting both hila and encroaching on the azygo-oesophageal recess and aorto-pulmonary window. L+10 W200 (A). L −320 W400 (B).

Evaluation of paraspinal mass

It has been noted previously that an advantage of CT is its ability to demonstrate the whole range of biological tissue densities. In the study of paraspinal disease therefore both soft tissue and bone can be studied together (Fig. 65.103).

HEART

CT imaging of the heart is presently available only in specialized research centres. The constraints which govern the availability of cardiac imaging by CT are related to the provision of a resolution sufficient to visualize coronary arteries, a density discrimination sufficient to visualize myocardial infarcts and a scan time sufficiently short to avoid cardiac movements.

The provision of all the ideal requirements simultaneously is at present impractical. Tube technology and radiation dose set the limits. As a compromise, improved density discrimination can be gained at the expense of resolution and scan time or alternatively density discrimination can be sacrificed to gain resolution and a better scan time.

In general, cardiac images obtained from present scanners (Fig. 65.110) can be improved significantly by minimizing heart motion and by the use of intravenous contrast media. The latter can be used to visualize both cardiac chambers and myocardial infarcts. Several technological approaches are currently under review.

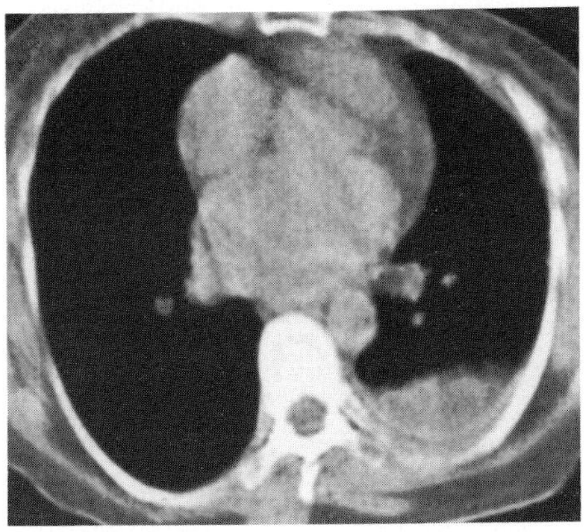

Fig. 65.110 Mitral valve disease demonstrating enlarged left atrium and posterior pleural effusion. L0 W200.

1. Gating and the gathering of data over several cardiac cycles.
2. Very long scan times relying on the image in diastole being nearly stationary and the image in the remainder of the cardiac cycle blurred.
3. Very fast scan times with multiple X-ray tubes and image intensifying chains to obtain multiple, simultaneous cardiac sections, i.e. a real time mode. This technique is referred to as Dynamic Spatial Reconstruction (DSR).

CHEST WALL

In each cross-sectional image only part of each rib is seen obliquely depending on its angulation. It is often impossible to be certain precisely which rib or ribs are being displayed. The advantage of CT lies in its ability to detect any associated soft tissue mass related to rib or arising independently in the thoracic wall (Fig. 65.111).

BREAST

Two main types of breast are likely to be recognized by CT:

1. Normal postmenopausal involuting breast in which periductal fibrous stroma is defined clearly against a background of fat density.
2. Mammary dysplasia in which fibrous stroma is replaced by lobulated areas of increased density.

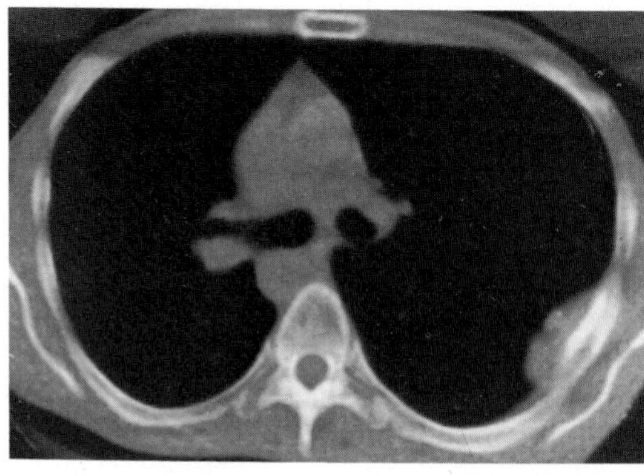

A

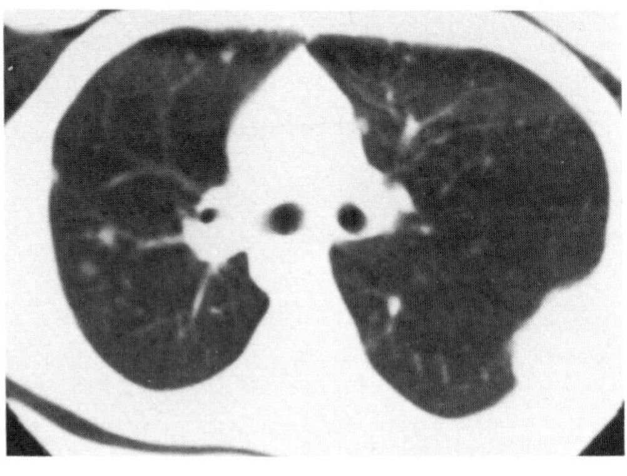

B

Fig. 65. 111 (A and B) Hodgkin's disease of rib. Note pleural involvement and hilar node enlargement. L +20 W400 (A). L −320 W400 (B).

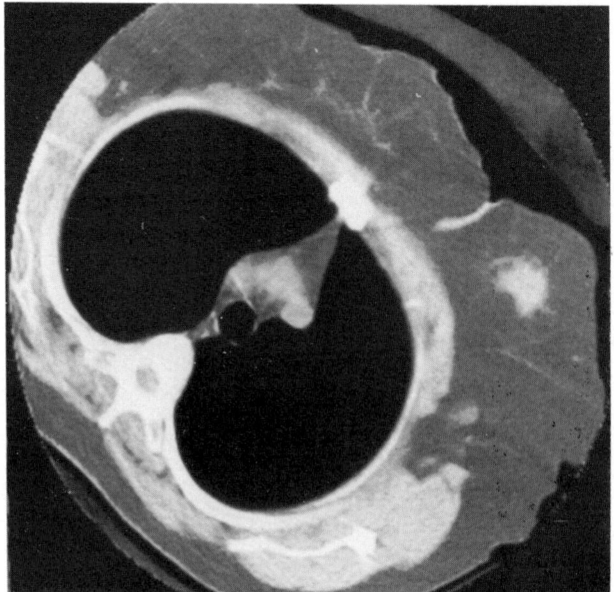

Fig. 65.112 Carcinoma breast and axillary lymph nodes. L −20 W200.

Cysts can be recognized as rounded, well-defined zones of lower density and solid masses are detectable as areas of relatively homogeneous increased density. Microcalcification may be typically 300 μm in diameter. Such a small quantity of calcium is insufficient to influence the attenuation value of a voxel and is therefore less well detected than by mammography.

The use of intravenous contrast enhancement may influence the detection rate of breast malignancy but at the present with conventional scanners CT is less successful than mammography in detecting carcinoma.

Only those axillary and internal mammary lymph nodes which are palpable are detectable by CT. It is impossible to distinguish malignant deposition from reactive hyperplasia (Fig. 65.112).

E. MUSCULO-SKELETAL SYSTEM

Normal appearances

Bone. The cross-sectional image provided by CT of both tubular bone and the axial skeleton permits direct visualization of the trabecular space. The quantitative nature of the image then provides a basis for measurements of bone mineral. Such measurements are independent of subcutaneous fat and unrelated to bone contour. Attenuation values alone can be used as a measure of mineral content but the presence of fat within the medullary cavity may, as a result of the partial volume effect, introduce errors. Dual energy scanning, by separating high and low atomic number elements, viz. calcium and fat, can overcome some of these errors. CT therefore provides a very precise means of making measurements of both bone mass and bone mineral in trabecular and cortical bone.

Muscle

CT has enhanced significantly the ability of the radiologist to visualize and study the morphology of normal musculature. Most muscle groups related to the appendicular and axial skeleton are identifiable in the cross-sectional image. The number of individual muscles clearly detectable by CT increases with age and with obesity as a result of increased deposition of fat in interstitial tissue.

Whilst variations in muscle bulk might be anticipated as a result of differences in age and sex, changes in muscle density are observed less frequently and related usually to ageing. No significant differences in density are detectable between the sexes or between the two sides of the body.

CT is not organ-specific and therefore each body section displays the appropriate muscle groups which provide valuable markers of anatomical level.

ROLE OF CT IN MUSCULO-SKELETAL DISEASE

Bone

The clarification of equivocal changes observed in conventional bone radiographs (Fig. 65.63) together with the precise delineation of associated soft tissue masses are the most important factors in the clinical management of potential bone malignancy (Fig. 65.113). Benign soft tissue tumours are usually homogeneous, well-defined and result in displacement of local fat planes. Malignant masses are evidenced by irregular invasive margins and obliteration of local fat planes (Fig. 65.114). Heterogeneity of composition can be helpful in the characterization of tissue, particularly where fat or calcium are present, but in histological terms, tissue specificity by CT is low. CT angiography can be contributory in demonstrating hypervascular regions (Fig. 65.12).

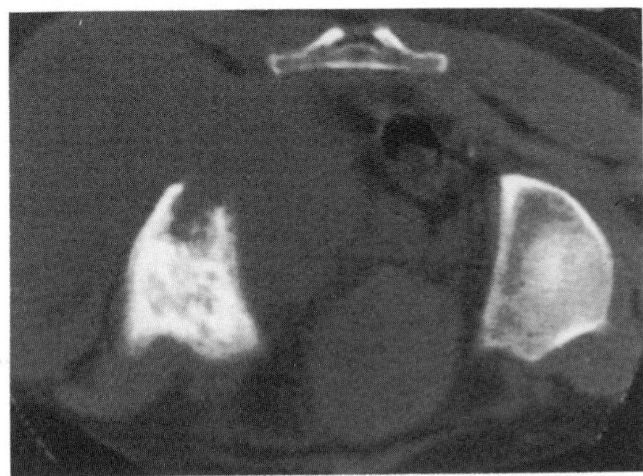

Fig. 65.113 Paget's sarcoma arising from the right ischial spine. Soft tissue mass extends from the buttock into the pelvic cavity. L+115 W400.

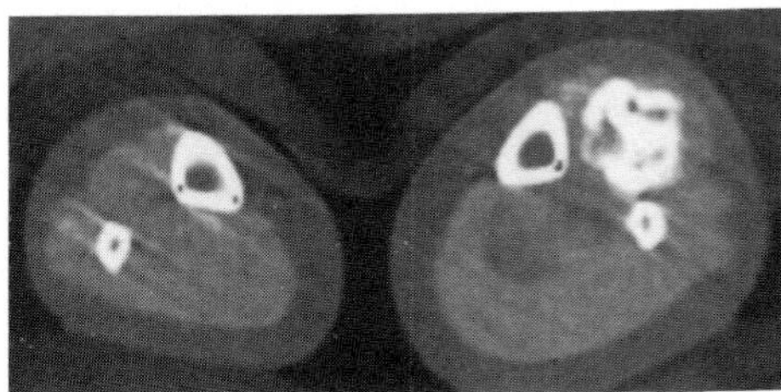

Fig. 65.114 Soft tissue sarcoma lower leg. Calcification is present within the mass. No bone involvement. L+25 W400.

The ability to visualize the medullary cavity of bone enables some observations to be made concerning intramedullary spread of bone tumour. The differentiation of tumour spread from inflammatory change is, however, difficult to achieve and changes in intramedullary density should be interpreted with caution when histological evidence is lacking.

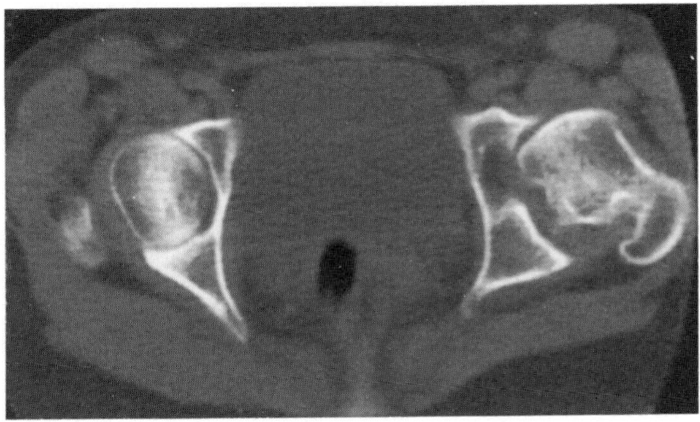

Fig. 65.115 Congenital dislocation of the hip in an adult. Note shallow acetabulum. L+80 W400.

The role of CT in treatment planning and monitoring has been emphasized in other situations but is a particularly important consideration in bone and soft tissue tumour management.

CT of joint disease is of most value in those situations where the partial volume effect is least obtrusive. In the knee and smaller joints, very thin sections (2 mm) are necessary to reduce the partial volume effect but reduction of section thickness results in increased noise and difficulties of reproducibility.

In the pelvis, the hip and sacro-iliac joints are readily accessible to conventional CT and the transverse section is particularly applicable to these sites. At the hip joint the femoral head, acetabulum and long axis of the femoral neck are demonstrable (Fig. 65.115). Alterations in femoral neck disposition, including anteversion, are readily detected. Position, shape and size of the acetabulum are well displayed in cross section, indicating a role for CT in the evaluation of congenital dislocation and hip joint trauma.

Muscle

Neither intrinsic muscle disease nor neuromuscular disease gives rise to specific CT appearances. Loss of bulk or deprivation of fat are features observed in those conditions leading to muscle atrophy (Fig. 65.116).

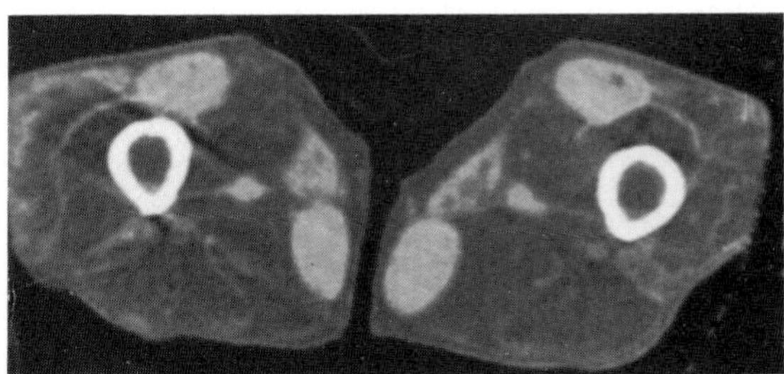

Fig. 65.116 Muscular dystrophy. Note fat replacement of normal muscle tissue in all muscle groups. L0 W200.

F. INTERVENTIONAL CT

CT can be used to guide biopsy procedures and certain therapeutic techniques, e.g. drainage of abscesses and percutaneous nephrostomies, in a similar manner to the use of ultrasound.

The advantages of CT relate to the anatomical detail provided in the cross sectional image and the facility with which the needle or cannula can be identified and localized on the section. The disadvantages concern the availability of equipment and the use of ionising radiation.

REFERENCES AND SUGGESTIONS FOR FURTHER READING

General

ABRAMS, H. L. & MCNEIL, B. J. (1978) Medical implications of computed tomography ('CAT scanning'). *New England Journal of Medicine*, **298,** 255–261, 310–318.

BROOKS, R. A. & DI CHIRO, G. (1976) Principles of computer assisted tomography (CAT) in radiographic and radio-isotope imaging. *Physics in Medicine and Biology*, **21,** 689–732.

GERHARDT, D. & VAN KAICK, G. (eds) (1979) *Total Body Computerised Tomography*. Thieme: Stuttgart.

HOUNSFIELD, G. N. (1973) Computerised transverse axial scanning (tomography)—Part I: Description of system. *British Journal of Radiology*, **46,** 1016–1022.

ISHERWOOD, I. (1979) Contrast enhancement in brain and body. In *Medical Imaging* (ed. L. Kreel). H.M. & M. Publishers: Aylesbury.

KREEL, L. (ed.) (1979) *Medical Imaging*. H. M. & M. Publishers: Aylesbury.

New indications for computed body tomography—Society for Computed Body Tomography (1979) *American Journal of Radiology*, **133,** 115–119.

PULLAN, B. R., RUTHERFORD, R. A. & ISHERWOOD, I. (1976) Computerised transaxial tomography. In *Medical Images: Formation, Perception and Measurement*. pp. 20–38. John Wiley: New York.

PULLAN, B. R., RITCHINGS, R. T. & ISHERWOOD, I. (1980) Quantitative aspects of computed tomography. In *Radiology of the Skull & Brain, Vol. VI* (ed. T. H. Newton & D. G. Potts). C. V. Mosby Co.: St. Louis.

Whole Body Computed Tomography (1977) *Radiologic Clinics of North America*, **15.**

WITTENBERG, J., FINEBERG, H. V., BLACK, E. B., KIRKPATRICK, R. H., SCHAFFER, D. L., IKEDA, M. K. & FERRUCCI, J. T. (1978) Clinical efficiency of computed body tomography. *American Journal of Radiology*, **131,** 5.

Atlases

An Atlas of Axial Transverse Tomography and its Clinical Applications. TAKAHASHI, S. (1969) Springer-Verlag: Berlin.

A Cross Sectional Anatomy. EYCLESHYMER, A. C. & SCHOEMAKER, D. M. (1970) Appleton-Century-Crofts: New York.

Cross Sectional Anatomy—Computed Tomography and Ultrasound Correlation. CARTER, B. L., MOREHEAD, J., WOLPERT, S. M., HAMMERSCHLAG, S. B., GRIFFITHS, H. J. & KAHN, P. C. (1977) Appleton-Century-Crofts: New York.

An Atlas of Cross Sectional Anatomy—Computed Tomography, Ultrasound, Radiography, Gross Anatomy. Ed. KIEFFER, S. A. & HEITZMAN E. R. (1979) Harper & Row: Hagerstown.

Abdomen

Abdominal Imaging (1979) *Radiologic Clinics of North America*, **17(1).**

HAAGA, J. & REID, N. E. (1978) *Computed Tomography of Abdominal Abnormalities*. C. V. Mosby Co.: St. Louis.

MEYERS, A. M. (1976) *Dynamic Radiology of the Abdomen—normal and pathological anatomy*. Springer-Verlag: New York.

Blood Vessels

MONCADA, R., REYNES, C., CHURCHILL, R. & LOVE, L. (1979) Normal vascular anatomy of the abdomen on computed tomography. *Radiologic Clinics of North America*, **17,** 25–37.

Pancreas

FAWCITT, R. A., FORBES, W. St. C., ISHERWOOD, I., BRAGANZA, J. & HOWAT, H. T. (1978) Computed tomography in pancreatic disease. *British Journal of Radiology*, **51,** 1–4.

HAAGA, J. R. & ALFIDI, R. J. (1977) Computed tomography of the pancreas. *Radiologic Clinics of North America*, **15,** 367–376.

ISHERWOOD, I. & FAWCITT, R. A. (1979) Computed tomography of the pancreas. In *The Exocrine Pancreas*, ed. H. T. Howat & H. Sarles. W. B. Saunders: London.

SHEEDY, P. F., STEPHENS, D. H., HATTERY, R. R., MACCARTY, R. L. & WILLIAMSON, B. (1977) Computed tomography of the pancreas. *Radiologic Clinics of North America*, **15,** 349–366.

Kidneys

FORBES, W. St. C., ISHERWOOD, I. & FAWCITT, R. A. (1978) Computed tomography in the evaluation of the solitary or unilateral nonfunctioning kidney. *Journal of Computer Assisted Tomography*, **2,** 389–394.

HATTERY, R. R., WILLIAMSON, J. B., STEPHENS, D. H., SHEEDY, P. F. & HARTMAN, G. W. (1977) Computed tomography of renal abnormalities. *Radiologic Clinics of North America*, **15,** 401.

SAGEL, S. S., STANLEY, R. J., LEVITT, R. G. & GEISTE, G. (1977) Computed tomography of the kidneys. *Radiology*, **124,** 359–370.

Suprarenals

BROWNLEE, K. & KREEL, L. (1978) Computerised axial tomography of normal suprarenal glands. *Journal of Computer Assisted Tomography*, **2,** 1–10.

KOROBKIN, M., WHITE, E. A., KRESSEL, N. Y., MOSS, A. A. & MONTAGUE, J. P. (1979) Computed tomography in the diagnosis of adrenal disease. *American Journal of Radiology*, **132,** 231.

Lymph Nodes

BEST, J. J. K., BLACKLEDGE, G., FORBES, W. St. C., TODD, I. D. H., EDDLESTON, B. CROWTHER, D. & ISHERWOOD, I. (1978) Computed tomography of abdomen—staging and clinical management of lymphoma. *British Medical Journal*, **2,** 1675–1677.

HUSBAND, J. E., PECKHAM, M. J., MACDONALD, J. J. & HENDRY, W. F. (1979) The role of computed tomography in the management of testicular teratoma. *Clinical Radiology*, **30,** 243–252.

KREEL, L. (1976) The EMI whole body scanner in the demonstration of lymph node enlargement. *Clinical Radiology*, **27,** 421–429.

Liver and Biliary System

FAWCITT, R. A., FORBES, W. St. C., ISHERWOOD, I., MORRIS, A. I., MARSH, M. N. & TURNBERG, L. (1978) Computed tomography in liver disease. *Clinical Radiology*, **29,** 251–254.

MORRIS, A. I., FAWCITT, R. A., WOOD, R., FORBES, W. St. C., ISHERWOOD, I. & MARSH, M. N. (1978) Computed tomography, ultrasound and cholestatic jaundice. *Gut*, **19,** 685–688.

RITCHINGS, R. T., PULLAN, B. R., LUCAS, P. B., FAWCITT, R. A., BEST, J. J. K., ISHERWOOD, I. & MORRIS, A. I. (1979) An analysis of the spatial distribution of attenuation values in computed tomographic scans of liver and spleen. *Journal of Computer Assisted Tomography*, **3,** 36–39.

STANLEY, R. J., SAGEL, S. S. & LEVITT, R. G. (1977) Computed tomography of the liver. *Radiologic Clinics of North America*, **15,** 331–348.

Pelvis

HODSON, N. J., HUSBAND, J. E. & MACDONALD, J. S. (1979) The role of computed tomography in the staging of bladder cancer. *Clinical Radiology*, **30,** 389–395.

SEIDELMANN, F. E., REICH, N. E., COHEN, W. N., HAAGA, J. R., BRYAN, P. J. & HAVRILLA, T. R. (1977) Computed tomography of the seminal vesicles and the seminal vesicle angle. *Journal of Computer Assisted Tomography*, **1,** 281–285.

Spine

FORBES, W. St. C. & ISHERWOOD, I. (1978) Computed tomography in syringomyelia and the associated Arnold Chiari Type I malformation. *Neuroradiology*, **15,** 73–78.

ISHERWOOD, I. & ANTOUN, N. M. (1980) CT scanning in the assessment of lumbar spine problems. In *The Lumbar Spine and Back Pain*, ed. M. Jayson. Pitman Medical, pp. 247–264.

ISHERWOOD, I., FAWCITT, R. A., FORBES, W. St. C., NETTLE, J. R. L. & PULLAN, B. R. (1977) Computed tomography of the spinal canal using metrizamide. *Acta Radiologica Diagnosis*, Supp, 355, 299–305.

ISHERWOOD, I., FAWCITT, R. A., NETTLE, J. R. L., SPENCER, J. W., & PULLAN, B. R. (1977) Computed tomography of the spine. In *Computerised Axial Tomography in Clinical Practice*, ed. G. du Boulay & Moseley. Springer Verlag: Berlin, pp. 322–335.

RESJO, I. M., HARWOOD-NASH, D. C., FITZ, C. R. & CHUANG, S. (1978) Computed tomographic metrizamide myelography in spinal dysraphism in infants and children. *Journal of Computer Assisted Tomography*, **2,** 549–558.

RESJO, I. M., HARWOOD-NASH, D. C., FITZ, C. R. & CHUANG S. (1979) CT metrizamide myelography for intraspinal and paraspinal neoplasms in infants and children. *American Journal of Radiology*, **132,** 367.

Cranio-Facial Structures

FORBES, W. St. C., FAWCITT, R. A., ISHERWOOD, I., WEBB, R. & FARRINGTON, T. (1978) Computed tomography in the diagnosis of diseases of the paranasal sinuses. *Clinical Radiology*, **29,** 501–511.

HESSELINK, J. R., NEW, P. F. J., DAVIS, K. R., WEBER, A. L. & ROBERSON, G. H. & TAVERAS, J. M. (1978) Computed tomography of the paranasal sinuses and face—Parts I & II. *Journal of Computer Assisted Tomography*, **2,** 559–576.

Thorax

HEITZMAN, E. R., GOLDWIN, R. L. & PROTO, A. V. (1977) Radiologic analysis of the mediastinum utilising computed tomography. *Radiologic Clinics of North America*, **15,** 309–329.

ISHERWOOD, I. & BEST, J. J. K. (1980) The use of computed tomography in lung disease. In *Recent Advances in Respiratory Medicine*, ed. D. Flenley. Churchill Livingstone: Edinburgh.

KATZ, D. & KREEL, L. (1979) Computed tomography in asbestosis. *Clinical Radiology*, **30,** 207–213.

MCLOUD, T. C., WITTENBERG, J. & FERRUCCI, J. T. (1979) Computed tomography of the thorax and standard radiographic evaluation of the chest—a comparative study. *Journal of Computer Assisted Tomography*, **3,** 170–180.

PULLAN, B. R. & BEST, J. J. K. (1980) Computed tomographic scanning of the heart. In *Recent Advances in Cardiology, Vol.* 8. Ed. Hamer & Rowlands. Churchill Livingstone: Edinburgh.

ROBB, R. A. & RITMAN, E. L. (1979) High speed synchronous volume computed tomography of the heart. *Radiology*, **133,** 655–662.

SCHANER, E. G., CHANG, A. E., DOPPMAN, J. L., CONKLE, D. M., FLYE, M. W. & ROSENBERG, S. A. (1978) Comparison of computed and conventional whole lung tomography in detecting pulmonary nodules: a prospective radiologic-pathologic study. *American Journal of Radiology*, **131,** 51–54.

Breast

BEST, J. J. K., ISHERWOOD, I., ASBURY, D. L., HARTLEY, G., GEORGE, W. D. & SELLWOOD, R. A. (1978) Computed tomography of the breast. *Clinical Oncology*, **4,** 173–178.

CHANG, C. H. J., SIBALA, J. L., FRITZ, S. L., DWYER, S. J. & TEMPLETON, A. W. (1979) Specific value of computed tomographic breast scanner (CT/M) in diagnosis of breast diseases. *Radiology*, **132,** 647–652.

Musculo-Skeletal System

BALCKE, J. A., TERMOTE, J. L., PALMERS, Y. & CROLK, D. (1979) Computed tomography of the human skeletal system. *Neuroradiology*, **17,** 127–136.

BERGER, P. E. & KUHN, J. P. (1978) Computed tomography of tumours of the musculo-skeletal system in children. *Radiology*, **127,** 171–175.

ISHERWOOD, I., RUTHERFORD, R. A., PULLAN, B. R. & ADAMS, P. H. (1976) Bone mineral estimation by computer assisted transverse axial tomography. *Lancet*, **2,** 712–715.

LEVINE, E., LEE, K. R., NEFF, J. R., MAKLAD, N. F., ROBINSON, R. G. & PRESTON, D. F. (1979) Comparison of computed tomography and other imaging modalities in the evaluation of musculo-skeletal tumours. *Radiology*, **131,** 431–437.

Proceedings: International Workshop on Bone and Soft Tissue Densitometry using Computed Tomography (1979) San Francisco, California. *Journal of Computer Assisted Tomography*, **3,** 847–862.

Interventionalist CT

HAAGA, J. R., REICH, N. E., HAVRILLA, T. R. & ALFIDI, R. J. (1977) Interventional CT scanning. *Radiologic Clinics of North America*, **15,** 449–456.

CHAPTER 66

RADIOISOTOPE IMAGING

Radioisotope imaging has now become an essential radiological technique. The obvious physical similarities of dealing with ionizing radiation, and interpreting two dimensional images of the body are important, but familiarity with the anatomy of the organs being studied is more important; and radiologists' familiarity with physiological studies, e.g. in the cardiovascular system, the intestinal tract and the urinary tract, is frequently underestimated and undervalued. But the most important reason for embracing radioisotope imaging into radiology is the radiologist's unique ability to advise his colleagues on the appropriate investigations of the clinical problem. Few isotopic investigations can be interpreted without a first-hand study of the relevant radiographs.

The rapid advances that continue to be made in developing radiopharmaceuticals and recording techniques make it impossible to give a comprehensive account of all the possibilities that exist. The aim of this chapter is to outline the principles involved and provide an introduction to the applications that are of general radiological interest.

ISOTOPES AND RADIOACTIVITY

An elementary knowledge of the following terms in general use is necessary in order to understand the techniques.

A nuclide is a species of atom with characteristic properties that are determined by:

1. Atomic number, which is the number of nuclear protons.

2. Atomic mass, numerically equal to the sum of nuclear protons and neutrons.

3. Energy state.

In the notation used to identify a nuclide fully, the atomic mass is written as a superscript of the atomic symbol, and the atomic number as a subscript on the same side, e.g. ${}^{2}_{1}H$ for hydrogen and ${}^{131}_{53}I$ for iodine.

Isotopes of an element are nuclides with the same atomic number, and therefore the same chemical and biological behaviour, but different mass number and often different energy state, e.g. ${}^{197}Hg$ and ${}^{203}Hg$ are isotopes of mercury and ${}^{123}I$, ${}^{125}I$ and ${}^{131}I$ are isotopes of iodine.

Radionuclides and radioisotopes are radioactive varieties, but the terms are often interchanged with nuclides and isotopes in practice. Most radionuclides are made artificially and all disintegrate spontaneously, emitting one or more of the following radiations:

1. Alpha particle, consisting of two protons and two neutrons. It has high energy and poor penetration, causes intense local biological damage, and has no medical uses.

2. Beta particle, which is a negatively charged electron. It has high velocity and high energy, and is absorbed easily, giving a high radiation dose to adjacent cells.

3. Positron, which is the same as a beta particle except that it carries a positive charge. Its range is only 1 mm or so, and as it comes to rest it combines with an electron. Both are annihilated and a pair of gamma photons is emitted in exactly opposite directions.

4. Gamma photon, which is electromagnetic wave radiation of high penetrating power.

Gamma emission is often accompanied by obligatory beta emission. Some nuclides emit a gamma photon a variable interval after beta emission by the parent nuclide. During this interval they are said to be *metastable* and this is indicated by writing 'm' after the atomic symbol, as in ${}^{99}Tc^{m}$ and ${}^{113}In^{m}$. Thus ${}^{99}Mo$ decays by beta emission to ${}^{99}Tc^{m}$ which in turn decays by gamma emission to ${}^{99}Tc$ with a half-life of six hours. ${}^{99}Tc^{m}$ and ${}^{99}Tc$ are *isomers* of each other.

The energy is measured in electron volts (eV) and the spectrum of energies is constant for each isotope. The important peaks in the spectrum can be identified by their energies, e.g. 140 keV for ${}^{94}Tc^{m}$, 160 keV for ${}^{123}I$, 93, 185, 300 and 394 keV for ${}^{67}Ga$.

The radioisotopes that are used most commonly in diagnostic work are gamma emitters. In some circumstances positron emitters can be used, e.g. ${}^{64}Cu$, ${}^{11}C$ and ${}^{15}O$. Each positron is short lived, and combines with a free electron and is annihilated, producing two gamma photons, each of 0·511 MeV at 180° to each other.

Coincidence counters are used to detect these photons giving depth independent collimation.

High energy beta emitters such as ^{32}P have been used to localize superficial tumours, e.g. in the eye and skin, but they are not used in scanning deep structures because the beta particles are absorbed too readily. Alpha particles are emitted only by naturally occurring isotopes such as ^{226}Ra, which have no place in diagnostic studies.

Radioisotopes that are used in scintigraphy always form part of a chemical compound that is tolerated by the patient, and either is pharmacologically inert, or is given in too small a quantity to have any effect, e.g. ^{131}I-labelled albumen, ^{75}Se-methionine, $^{99}Tc^{m}$ diethylene triamine penta-acetate (DTPA).

Radioactive disintegration

A single radioactive atom may disintegrate at any time and whether it does so at any particular time is a matter of chance. However, if the total number of unstable atoms is large, the fraction of the total number that is disintegrating at any given instant can be estimated and is known as the decay constant. The half-life of a nuclide is the time taken for its activity to fall by one half, e.g. 120 days for ^{75}Se, and 6 hours for $^{99}Tc^{m}$. The decay constant is related to the half-life expression.

$$\text{Decay constant } (\lambda) = \frac{0{\cdot}693}{\text{half-life } (T_{\frac{1}{2}})}$$

The activity given to the patient is measured in millicures or microcuries. By definition, a curie is the activity of 1 g of ^{226}Ra or $3{\cdot}7 \times 10^{10}$ disintegrations per sec.

The absorbed *dose* of radiation is measured in rads (1 rad = 100 ergs per g of tissue). Some of the important factors in considering radiation dose are:

1. The unit of measurement, the rad, does not take into account the total mass of absorbing tissue.
2. Some tissues absorb radiation more readily than others, e.g. at a photon energy of 70 keV bone absorbs about four times as much radiation as soft tissues.
3. The sensitivity of different tissues to radiation is variable, e.g. rapidly dividing cells such as those in the bone marrow are much more sensitive to a given dosage than less rapidly dividing cells, such as those of liver or muscle.
4. The location of the radioisotope is crucial. Iodine-labelled albumen microspheres trapped by the pulmonary capillaries gives a much higher dose to the adjacent pulmonary capillaries than the same isotope absorbed by thyroid colloid gives to thyroid cells.
5. Excretion of the radiochemical causes a biological decay as well as a physical decay. This is not always a simple matter, e.g. ^{197}Hg is excreted by the kidney in two stages, one taking a few hours, the other much longer. The effective half-life is linked to the physical half-life and biological half-life by the expression:

$$\frac{1}{T_{eff}} = \frac{1}{T_{biol}} + \frac{1}{T_{phys}}$$

The International Commission on Radiation Units and Measurements have recommended the adoption of an International System of consistent units for use in all branches of science (S.I. Units). The S.I. unit of activity is the becquerel (Bq) equal to one nuclear transformation per second ($3{\cdot}7 \times 10^{10}$ Bq = 1 CI). The S.I. unit of absorbed dose is the grey (Gy) equal to one Joule per kilogram (1 Gy = 100 rads).

METHODS OF RECORDING RADIOACTIVITY

SCANNING

The conventional **linear scanner** consists of:

1. Detector and collimator

The detector is a crystal of sodium iodide containing thallium iodide as an activator. Gamma photons striking the detector are converted indirectly into light quanta, which are led off into a photomultiplier. Here a corresponding small-voltage pulse is produced and the number of pulses is proportional to the original activity. The whole is surrounded by a thick lead collimator, which has a number of hexagonal holes between the crystal and the source. These holes are directed on a small area, so that only desired radiation from the source is recorded, the remainder being absorbed by the lead walls of the collimator. When high-energy gamma photons are being recorded, e.g. ^{198}Au at 410 keV, the lead walls of the collimator must be correspondingly thicker to absorb all the unwanted gamma photons because their penetrating power is greater. This increases the mechanical problems of designing the instrument.

The detector is moved to and fro mechanically across the field being scanned. The size of the field and the rate of scanning can be varied to suit the conditions of the examination. Most commercial scanners have two linked detectors so that anterior and posterior views, or both lateral views, can be taken at the same time.

2. The display

The voltage pulses from the photomultiplier are recorded permanently in one or more of these ways.

(a) A dot diagram, in which the density of dots per unit area is proportional to the number of pulses coming from the photomultiplier. The range of dot densities may be represented in colour.

(b) A similar diagram made by a light spot on an unexposed X-ray film. A reduction of 5 : 1 image size is a convenient way of recording a whole skeletal scan on conventional sized X-ray film.

(c) In colour on a television monitor.

(d) Facilities may be available for electronic subtraction so that two radionuclides can be used and the contribution of either subtracted from the combined image. Thus, the image of the pancreas (selenomethionine) can be shown to good advantage by subtracting the image of the liver (colloid) from that of liver plus pancreas (selenomethionine).

Areas of significant activity are located anatomically by recording convenient surface markings on the scan.

Gamma camera

The gamma camera has a stationary detector which records activity over the whole of its field simultaneously.

Scintillations are recorded on an oscilloscope and photographed directly by a polaroid camera or on X-ray film. A predetermined number of scintillations is recorded, e.g. 500 000 for brain, or all scintillations in a given time are recorded, e.g. 10 minutes for pancreas scintiphoto. It is convenient to record rapid sequences with a camera that changes its frames automatically, and videotape recording offers the additional facility of replaying to extract maximal information. The gamma camera can be used for all applications of a linear scanner in addition to the possibilities opened up by the above features.

Its most useful practical applications are that the images are produced rapidly so that additional views can be done more readily; more patients can be examined; and serial changes in total organ activity (dynamic studies) such as the heart, kidney, pancreas, can be recorded. The initial disadvantage of having a small image is overcome with familiarity.

Large field of view cameras use 37 photomultiplier tubes to view a useful field of 39 cm and are invaluable for lung scanning and abdominal scanning. Also they are useful in skeletal scanning particularly with tracking devices that enable the final skeletal image to be unified.

Rapid sequence (dynamic) studies: use of computers

In its simplest form a rapid series of images can be obtained by pulling films from the polaroid pack of the gamma camera as quickly as possible. Alternatively the oscilloscope images can be photographed with a 35 mm camera using a predetermined time lapse of a few seconds between each frame. Both these methods may give useful results, but suffer from the relative disadvantage that the optimum timing of the sequences often become clear after the series has been completed.

This difficulty is overcome by recording the information using a dedicated computer. Variable time intervals are predetermined for succeeding frames which can be re-played in cine mode. Also frames can be summated over any selected time interval, e.g. in cardiac and renal studies. Regions of interest can be selected and time-activity curves generated, e.g. for renography. Similarly in cardiac images, curves can be generated over the ventricles and used to estimate the interventricular transit time.

Computers are used for smoothing curves and images, background subtraction, and quantitating functional parameters of individual organs such as the kidneys.

Tomography

The aim of isotope tomography is similar to that of radiographic tomography, and a focusing collimator is used so that activity in a selected plane is in focus while activity in other planes is smeared into background. Usually there is an upper and a lower probe producing six separate images in each passage. The greatest use of the technique is in brain scanning.

Positron camera (positron emission tomography)

Two opposing crystals are used to detect the annihilation photons, which are used to define the line of the original interaction. The image is reconstructed in a number of planes so the distribution of radionuclide is plotted accurately. This type of system requires virtually no collimation, is not depth dependent and is inherently tomographic. Its full utilization awaits the greater availability of positron emitting isotopes.

AVAILABLE ISOTOPES

Nearly every organ in the body can be investigated by means of radionuclide scanning. The most important considerations in choosing an isotope apart from its efficiency in detecting abnormalities, are the radiation dose to the patient and the possible need to repeat the examination.

A suitable isotope has the following properties:

1. *Relatively short half-life.* The activity is then greater for a given radiation dose, improving the sensitivity without increasing radiation hazard.

2. *Absence of beta emission.* Beta rays are absorbed readily, and increase the radiation dose without being available for scanning.

3. *Absence of positron emission.* Except when a positron camera is being used positrons increase the radiation without being available to the conventional gamma scanner.

4. *Suitable gamma energy.* Below 100 keV there is too much tissue absorption and scatter. High-energy gamma photons, e.g. ^{198}Au at 410 keV, are able to penetrate the septa of the collimator, thereby interfering with the record. Most of the isotopes used for scanning have gamma emission below 300 keV. Suitable collimators must always be used.

5. *Suitable pharmaceutical.* The isotope must be incorporated into a pharmaceutical compound that is not toxic, and either: (a) is inert, e.g. ^{99}Tc^{m} albumen or ^{113}In^{m} chloride; or (b) has no measurable pharmacological effect in the dose given, e.g. ^{99}Tc^{m} diethylene triamine penta-acetate, a chelating agent.

The biological fate of the pharmaceutical is important also. Whenever possible it is better to avoid compounds that are accumulated in organs not under investigation. ^{99}Tc^{m} pertechnatate is widely used for brain scanning, but it is accumulated by the thyroid and excreted into the gut by the salivary glands and the gastric mucosa. Thus it is impossible to avoid incidental accumulation outside the organ of interest in all instances. It should be kept to a minimum by proper choice of compound and by blocking vicarious uptake when possible, e.g. by giving potassium iodide before giving labelled iodide for lung scanning, etc. ^{99}Tc^{m}-DTPA is an alternative choice for brain scanning, with the advantage of no thyroid uptake and the disadvantage of renal excretion, leading to urinary tract radiation.

6. *High specific activity*. The activity required should be contained in as little as possible of the pharmaceutical for the reasons given already.

7. *Purity*. The pharmaceutical must be chemically pure and the radioisotope should be as free as possible of contamination by other isotopes or radionuclides.

ADVERSE REACTIONS

Fortunately, adverse reactions to radiopharmaceuticals are uncommon and have been estimated at about one in 10 000 investigations. These include some that may be due to the patient's anxiety rather than to the agents used. Reactions due to the agents may take the form of *fever* and *rigor*, e.g. following one of the colloid preparations containing gelatin; *urticaria, bronchospasm* or even *cardiovascular collapse* due to a true idiosyncrasy to any compound; *aseptic meningitis* following intrathecal ^{131}I-labelled albumen. *Death* has been recorded after ^{131}I-labelled macroalbumen injection and, although it is excessively rare, it seems that severe pulmonary arterial hypertension may predispose to it. Clinical evidence of this condition must therefore be regarded as a contraindication to lung scanning. Adverse reactions are much less common than they are after the use of radiographic contrast agents, but this should not be allowed to induce complacency. A room in which scanning is being carried out should have the same facilities for treating reactions as one in which contrast agents are being used.

Activity in human milk

After use of ^{131}I radioactive tracers, there is a hazard due to the accumulation of free iodide in the thyroid of the breast-fed infant. It persists for at least one week after a lung scan and for at least two days after a renogram. The hazard following placental localization immediately before delivery depends on the dosage used and may be so small that no restrictions are needed.

Gallium-67 also is secreted to a significant degree by the lactating breast and is a hazard to the infant.

CENTRAL NERVOUS SYSTEM

The advent of transmission computed tomography (CT) has had a profound effect on the use of isotope brain scanning. Where CT is available it has become the investigation of choice for the great majority of intracranial problems, and its uses are discussed in detail in Chapters 63 and 64. In these circumstances isotope scanning has a subsidiary role. Elsewhere, if CT is not available, isotope scanning has a more important primary role and the main aspects of its application will be discussed.

Scanning is a reliable way of showing the site and size of many intracranial lesions. Sometimes the pathology of the lesion can be predicted from its topography, but this is unusual.

The isotopes in general use are:

1. ^{99}*Tc*^{m} *as sodium pertechnetate*, which is eluted from a ^{99}Mo generator and is ideal because of its short half life (6 hr), and low single energy gamma emmission (140 keV). The scan is done one hour after intravenous injections of 5 to 10 mCi. Two hundred milligrams of potassium perchlorate is given by mouth to diminish choroid plexus activity.

2. ^{113}*In*^{m} which is eluted from a ^{113}Sn generator and also has a short half-life (1·7 hr) and mono-energetic gamma emmission (393 keV). Its main advantage over ^{99}Tc^{m} is the relatively long half-life of the generator, which only needs to be placed ever four to six months rather than every week. Also there is less interference from vascular activity in the soft tissues, particularly over the posterior fossa. For brain scanning it is made up as the *diethylene triamine penta-acetate (DTPA)* and many find the preparation needed a marked disadvantage. Its high gamma energy is more suited to a linear scanner than a gamma camera.

3. ^{99}*Tc*^{m} *DTPA*. This compound is less taxing to prepare than ^{113}I^{m} DTPA and has the advantages of both technetium and DTPA. Its use is becoming more widespread.

Anterior, posterior and both lateral scans are done and may be supplemented with oblique and superior projections. In the normal scan there is a high activity over the base of the skull and the neck muscles because of their vascularity. A less marked activity is seen over the vault which is most obvious posteriorly. Small lesions near these areas are easily obscured and can be difficult to detect. This is especially true of lesions in the posterior fossa and it may be helpful to scan these in the plane of the reversed Townes' view. High vascularity of the torcula is a useful landmark in this projection. Intracranial lesions are likely to be shown if they are vascular and/or destroy 'the blood-tissue barrier' so that the radionuclide carrier diffuses into the lesion.

TUMOUR

Parasellar and *posterior fossa* lesions are often obscured by normal uptake and tumours in these sites can usually be shown more accurately by other methods unless they are large, e.g. craniopharyngioma. On the other hand superficial hemisphere tumours such as frontal, parasagittal and occipital tumours are readily detected. The size of all tumours is crucial and tumours less than 1·5 cm in diameter cannot be detected reliably.

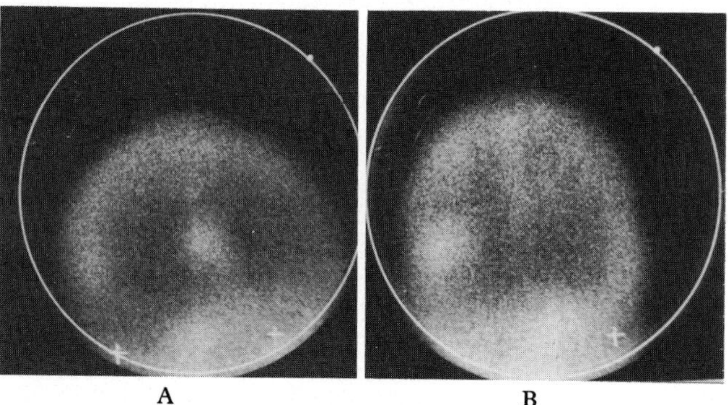

Fig. 66.1 Cerebral glioma. Pertechnetate scan: (A) R. lateral. (B) Anterior projection, showing a spherical peripheral lesion.

The more vascular tumours, e.g. *meningiomas* and most *gliomas* (Fig. 66.1), have a greater activity than avascular tumours, e.g. *acoustic neuroma*, *optic nerve glioma*, *pituitary tumours*, and *oligodendrogliomas*. *Gliomas* cannot be separated into their histological types from the scan appearances. The majority of *acoustic neuromas* can be detected despite their relative avascularity.

Some tumours, even large ones, are difficult to detect because they fail to concentrate the isotope selectively, or they do so at an unusual rate. If a negative scan is associated with a high suspicion of tumour it is an advantage to do a further scan at four to six hours. The nature of some lesions can be determined by studying their relationship to anatomical landmarks. Lesions that straddle the falx or tentorium are likely to be *meningiomas*. Tumours of the corpus callosum have a central high activity in all projections and are nearly always *gliomas*.

Multiple lesions are more commonly due to *metastases* (Fig. 66.2) than to any other cause such as multiple infarcts, but many metastases are of course single at the time of investigation. Scanning is not an entirely satisfactory screening method in suspected cerebral tumour because tumours that are small, avascular, or inaccessible will not be shown by conventional techniques. However positron emission tomography (*vide supra*) shows considerable promise in this field.

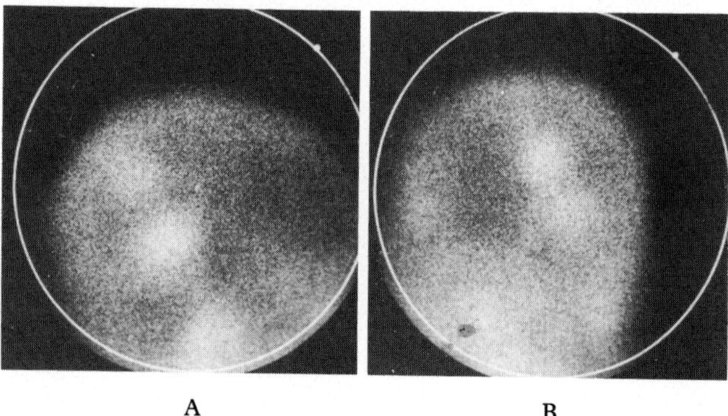

Fig. 66.2 Cerebral metastases. Pertechnetate scan: (A) R. lateral. (B) Posterior projections, showing multiple lesions.

The investigation of *late onset epilepsy* is often an important clinical problem because of the possibility of underlying tumour, yet full neuroradiological investigation is rigorous and often unrewarding. Although there are reservations about the value of scanning as a screening test to exclude a lesion, it is often held in this particular instance that a normal scan, supported by a normal electroencephalogram may justify deferring exhaustive radiological tests and awaiting clinical developments.

Rapid sequence studies of intracranial masses may help to indicate the nature of the lesion. *Arteriovenous malformation* characteristically produces high activity in the early arterial phase. Meningiomas tend to show up earlier than other tumours.

Finally it should be noted that *cerebral abscesses* can be shown and their progress under treatment followed by scans.

VASCULAR LESIONS

Cerebral infarcts become positive during the first week but the greatest incidence of positive scans is during the third week after a full stroke. The abnormality corresponds to the region supplied by the involved artery (Fig. 66.3), and a large abnormality corresponds to an extensive neurological deficit. Transient ischaemia and partial strokes are much less likely to be positive. This is in marked contrast to a stroke due to haemorrhage into a tumour which will be positive from onset. In stroke a positive scan carries a poorer prognosis for recovery, but an improvement in serial scans is a good prognostic sign. Rapid sequence studies will show unilateral low activity followed by increased activity in a healing infarct. Asymmetrical activity may be also shown in severe carotid artery stenosis, but there will be no positive infarct.

There is high uptake in *cerebral haemorrhage* and in the surrounding oedema, and in *arteriovenous malformation*, but *aneurysms* are not shown unless they are relatively large or have bled into surrounding tissues. Arteriovenous malformations that are large or near the surface usually give rise to an area of high activity, but if they are small or deep they are less easy to detect. Sequential studies highlight the lesion by showing high activity in the very early images, followed by a decline of activity and a reappearance with subsequent cardiac cycles.

HEAD INJURIES

All *external head injuries* are liable to have increased radioactivity. Craniotomies and fractures are liable to be positive for weeks or months. The importance of confirming suspected *extradural or subdural haemorrhage* needs no emphasis. Radiopharmaceuticals diffuse into

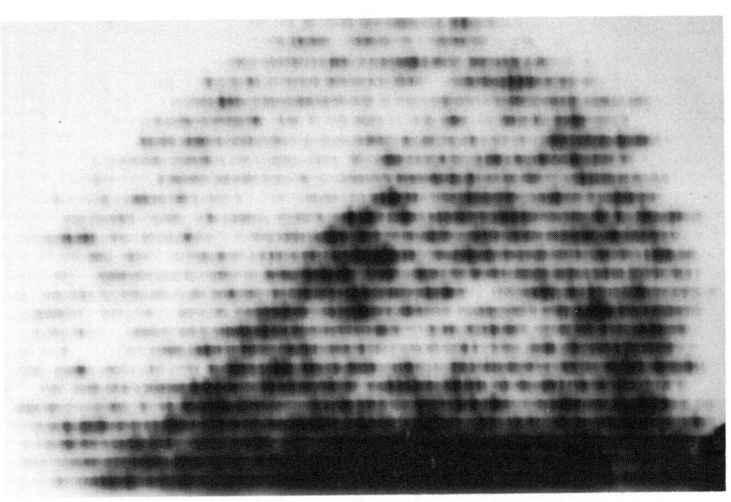

A

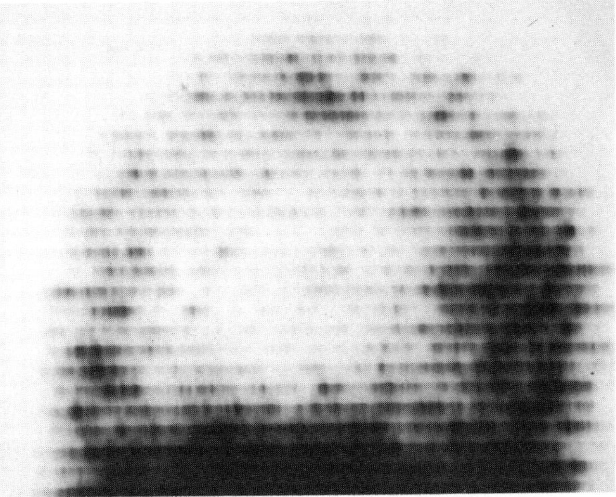

B

Fig. 66.3 Cerebral infarct. Pertechnetate scan: (A) l. lateral. (B) Anterior projections. The abnormal activity occupies the territory of the left middle cerebral artery.

these lesions according to physical laws and are removed slowly. Typically in *chronic haematoma* there is a crescentic uptake at the periphery of the cranium when viewed tangentially, as in an anterior or posterior scan. The uptake is more diffuse in the lateral projection and the abnormality may be overlooked. The appearances are similar in *extracranial haematoma* or laceration except that the activity lies outside the line of the vault as judged from the normal side. Similar appearances in *Paget's disease* and *hyperostosis* can be differentiated from the radiographs. Scanning is less reliable in detecting acute subdural haematoma, especially if it is bilateral. Rapid sequence studies typically show a non-crescentic peripheral defect.

In *intracranial contusion* the abnormal uptake is more central than in subdural haematoma, and a scan is a useful means of differentiation. In cases of intracerebral haematoma, a variable amount of the uptake is in surrounding oedema. The resolution of deep lesions can be followed by serial scanning.

CEREBROSPINAL FLUID

The dynamics of the cerebrospinal fluid can be studied after injection of a suitable radioactive substance by lumbar puncture or by cisternal puncture. Several compounds have been proposed since the original studies with ^{131}I-labelled albumen, but the most satisfactory of these is ^{111}In-diethylene-triamine-penta-acetic acid (DTPA). Anterior and lateral images of the cranium are obtained at 2 hours and at suitable intervals during the next 48 hours. In the normal the early scans show high uptake over the basal cisterns and the Sylvian fissures, and the later scans show gradual transport of activity over the vertex, as well as a progressive fall in basal activity as the labelled compound is absorbed by the Pacchionian corpuscles of the superior sagittal sinus. There is no recognizable ventricular activity. The absence of intracranial activity raises the possibility of either a spinal canal obstruction or an incorrect injection, either subdural or epidural. The scan of the spine may show a characteristic accumulation of activity adjacent to the level of the puncture, and in the case of extradural injection there will be confirmatory early excretion of DTPA in the urine.

The commonest application of cisternography is in the detection of suspected *communicating hydrocephalus*, e.g. following meningitis or subarachnoid haemorrhage. The resorption of c.s.f. is impaired and the ventricles become dilated. The cisternogram shows high intraventricular activity, with little or no activity over the vault. The abnormality may be unilateral or asymmetrical, and becomes more severe with time. The importance of recognizing the condition is that substantial clinical improvement may follow a bypass shunt operation. Isotope cisternography is well tolerated by these patients and it does not give rise to the clinical deterioration that may follow air encephalography.

Localized *cerebral atrophy* may give rise to focal accmulation of radioactivity over the cortex of the brain.

Porencephalic cysts are recognized as out pouchings from the ventricular system.

In the case of *non-communicating hydrocephalus* the movement pattern is either normal or shows obstruction in the region of the basal cisterns. In these cases also c.s.f. shunt operation may re-establish normal flow. Another cause of obstruction at the level of the basal cisterns is the *Dandy Walker malformation* in which the fourth ventricle is enlarged and obstructed because of atresia of its foramina. In this condition, the fourth ventricle can be shown isotopically only by direct injection into a lateral ventricle.

Other important applications of isotope cisternography are

1. Investigation of the patency of c.s.f. shunts.

2. Detection of c.s.f. fistula, usually into the nasal cavity following trauma. Multiple pledglets of cotton wool may be placed at predetermined points in each nasal cavity and their radioactivity counted after a suitable interval in order to determine the most likely site of the fistula.

Cisternography is discussed in further detail in Chapter 57.

THE LIVER

COLLOID SCINTIGRAPHY

Colloid particles labelled with $^{99}Tc^{m}$ are taken up by the cells of the reticulo-endothelial system after intravenous injection. In an adult, between 80 and 90 per cent of administered activity is accumulated in the liver. Most of the remainder is accumulated in the spleen, and a small amount accumulated in the lymphatic system and in the red marrow.

Alternatively, millimicrospheres of albumen (less than 10 μ) can be labelled with $^{99}Tc^{m}$ and are distributed similarly. In children a greater proportion is accumulated in the red marrow. Scanning begins within a few minutes of injecting 2 to 3 mCi of $^{99}Tc^{m}$ colloid. Anterior, lateral or oblique, and posterior views should be done in order to show as much of the liver as possible, and it is convenient to do a left lateral or posterior view of the spleen at the same time. The normal liver is roughly triangular, with curved margins following the contours of the diaphragm and the rib cage. The lower edge is oblique, and often has a gallbladder impression in its lateral third. Also there is a cleft between the right and left lobe, and this accentuated in the lateral supine projection. The highest activity is over the right lobe and falls gradually towards the margin. There are many variations of shape, the most common being a Reidl's lobe; variations in position due to alteration of the level of the right dome of the diaphragm are common also. Respiratory movement causes some irregularity of the margins particularly in linear scans.

A *large* liver may be found in malignant disease, early cirrhosis, sarcoidosis, amyloid disease, haemochromatosis, etc. A *small* liver is most commonly due to cirrhosis but sometimes it is a normal variant and of course can be due to hypoplasia or partial hepatectomy.

The commonest abnormality is diminished activity and this may be localized or diffuse. A *localized defect* is created by any lesion that does not contain reticulo-endothelial cells, provided it is large enough to come within the resolution of the camera or scanner. Generally lesions near the surface are easier to detect than deeper lesions and the best resolution that can be obtained is usually about 2 cm (Fig. 66.4).

Metastasis is one of the commoner causes of a defect

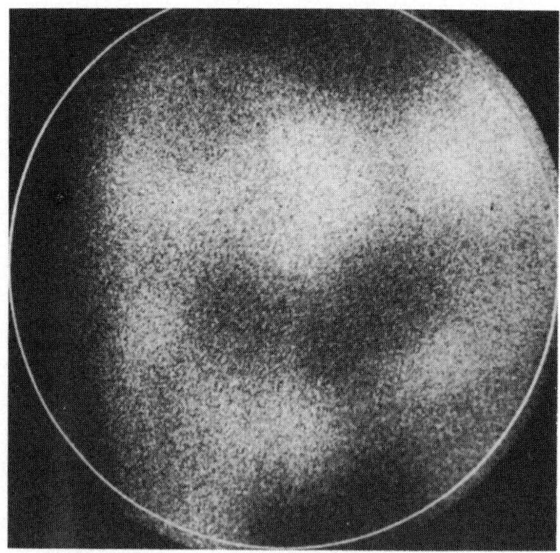

Fig. 66.4 Liver metastases. $^{99}Tc^{m}$-S colloid scan. Anterior projection. The liver is large and contains many defects caused by the metastases.

and the accuracy of detection can be as high as 90 per cent of patients. Unsuspected metastases can be detected more reliably by scanning than by biochemical tests or inspection at laparotomy. *Primary neoplasms* of the liver (Fig. 66.5), *lymphoma*, and *angioma* can create similar defects.

Among the non-neoplastic causes of defects, *abscess* and *cyst* are encountered more often than *haematoma*, *arterio-venous malformation* and localized *ischaemia*. *Hydatid cysts* are detected twice as commonly as from radiographic calcification (Fig. 66.6). If the liver has been included in a radiotherapy treatment field, e.g. to the left kidney, a characteristically angular defect is found, corresponding to the treatment field (Fig. 66.7).

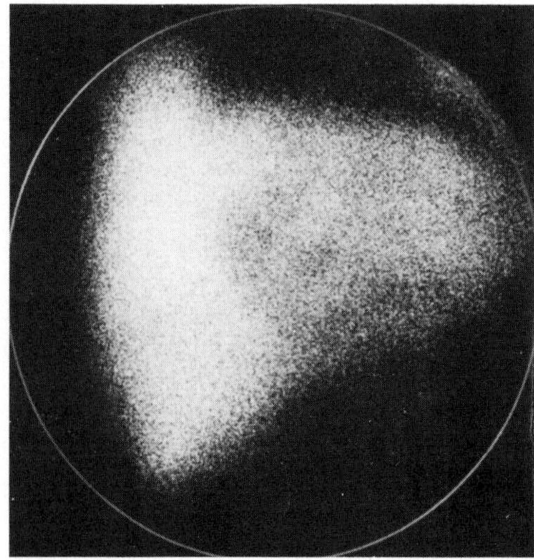

Fig. 66.5 Bile duct carcinoma. $^{99}Tc^{m}$-S colloid scan. Anterior projection. There is a diffuse defect in the L. lobe, which was found to contain a bile duct carcinoma. Part of the defect is caused by dilated obstructed bile ducts.

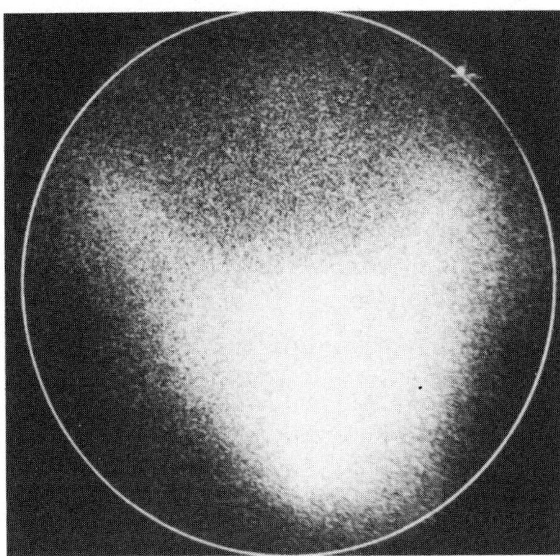

Fig. 66.6 Hepatic hydatid cyst. $^{99}Tc^{m}$-S colloid scan. R. lateral projection. There is a large crescentic defect in the upper third of the liver.

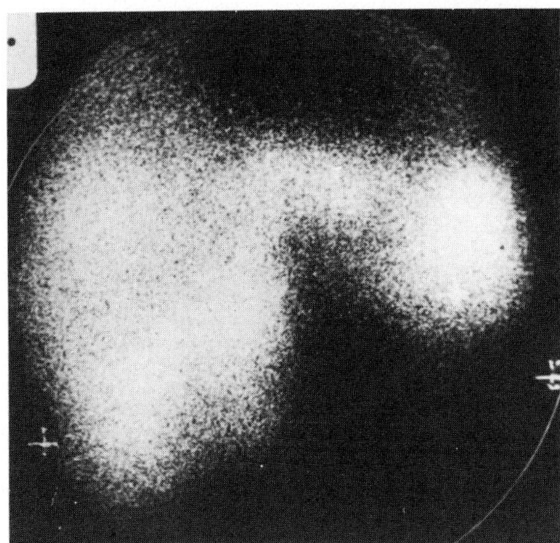

Fig. 66.7 Radiation defect. $^{99}Tc^{m}$-S colloid scan. Anterior projection. There is an angular defect in the L. lobe of the liver corresponding to the field of treatment of a Wilms' tumour of the L. kidney. Note that splenic activity is not impaired.

Multiple lesions are usually due to metastases, though hepatoma is sometimes multifocal and abscesses and cysts may be multicentric also.

Diffusely low activity is recognized by random variations in activity due to low accumulation and by comparison with other structures. Thus recognized accumulation over the vertebral bodies is an indication of poor hepatic accumulation. Usually this is due to *diffuse hepatocellular failure* but occasionally it is found in *extensive metastasis*. The poor accumulation of activity is due to reduced availability of nuclide or decreased capacity of liver to extract it. Thus it may occur:

1. If too little is given.
2. In diffuse hepatic disorder, e.g. cirrhosis, reticulosis.
3. In diminished hepatic perfusion, e.g. cirrhosis, portal vein thrombosis.
4. If there is increased competition from an enlarged spleen, e.g. myelosclerosis, portal vein occlusion, or the skeleton (Fig. 66.8).

In occlusion of the hepatic veins (*Budd-Chiari syndrome*) (Fig. 66.9) there is a marked fall in hepatic activity except for a localized island of relatively high activity in the caudate lobe. The caudate lobe has an independent venous drainage into the vena cava which preserves its function and accounts for the characteristic appearance.

Defects in the margin of the liver may be made by adjacent lesions, e.g. carcinoma of the right kidney, tumour of the right adrenal, cyst of the lesser sac, carcinoma of the stomach, hydronephrosis and subphrenic abscess. The correct diagnosis in these cases can only be made with the aid of the clinical features and conventional radiography.

Combined techniques may be helpful:

1. Lung and liver scanning is useful in localizing right subphrenic abscess.
2. The relative affinity of primary liver cell carcinoma for ^{75}Se-methionine can be used to distinguish defects from liver cell carcinoma from those due to metastases, and from the unexplained non-neoplastic defects sometimes found in cirrhosis.
3. A combination of ultrasonic and isotopic scanning

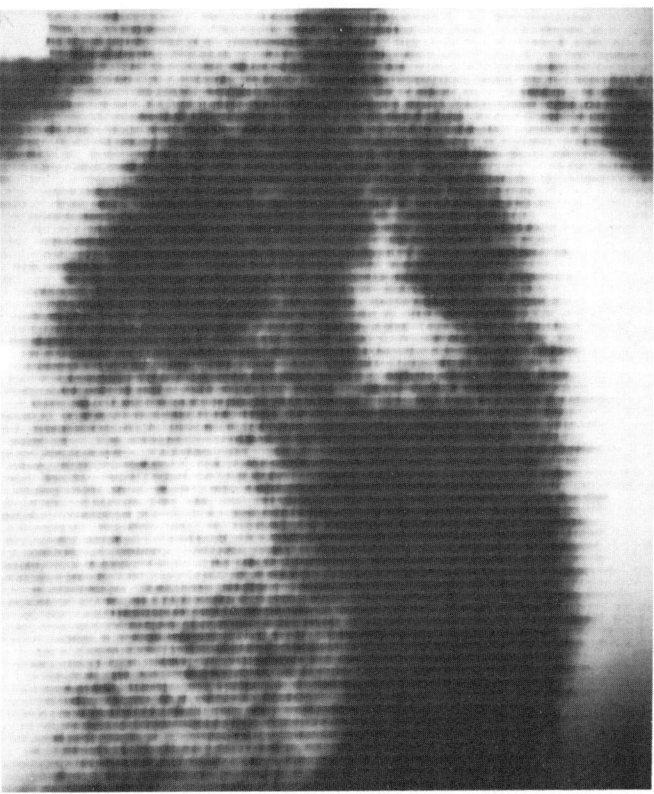

Fig. 66.8 Diffuse hepatic abnormality in a child. $^{99}Tc^{m}$-S colloid scan. Anterior projection of trunk. There is virtually no activity in the liver; but there is high activity in the skeleton and in the grossly enlarged spleen.

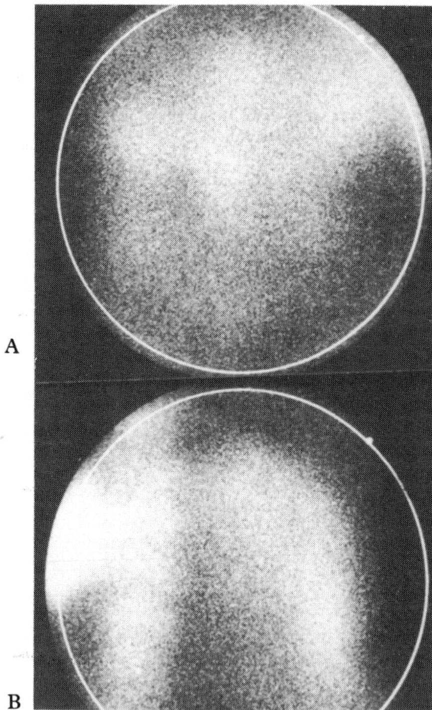

Fig. 66.9 Budd-Chiari syndrome. ^{99}Tc-S colloid scan. Above, anterior; below, posterior projections. There is impaired hepatic activity except in the caudate lobe. Note the increased vertebral activity—an indication of poor hepatic uptake.

has a greater diagnostic accuracy than either test alone and is particularly useful in distinguishing transonic cysts and abscesses from solid tumours.

4. CT of the liver has the great advantage of obligatory demonstration of adjacent structures and lesions, and is a useful adjunct to isotope scanning in evaluating conflicting information and in diagnosing parahepatic masses.

The main applications of colloid scanning are:

1. The investigation of hepatomegaly or upper abdominal mass.
2. The pre-operative assessment of carcinoma, especially in the gut.
3. The follow up of known liver tumours after operation or chemotherapy.
4. The investigation of clinically suspected lesions, e.g. hydatid cyst, amebic abscess where combined scanning is an essential preliminary to aspiration; hepatoma, complicating cirrhosis.
5. The investigation of suspected subphrenic abscess.

BILIARY TREE SCANNING

Rose Bengal is a dye excreted by the biliary system; and by ^{131}I labelling, it was developed as an agent for determining biliary patency, particularly in the investigation of suspected biliary atresia in the new born. ^{131}I has the dual disadvantage of a photon energy that is too high for efficient gamma camera imaging, and the constraint of low administered activity because of its radiation body burden. Other radiopharmaceuticals have been developed to overcome these disadvantages, and the most promising of them is a ^{99}Tc^{m} labelled imino-diacetic acid derivative (^{99}Tc^{m}-HIDA), that is concentrated by the hepatocytes. After food restriction for two hours, 2–4 mCi are injected intravenously and visualized by serial gamma camera images of the upper abdomen at 15 min intervals (Fig. 66.10).

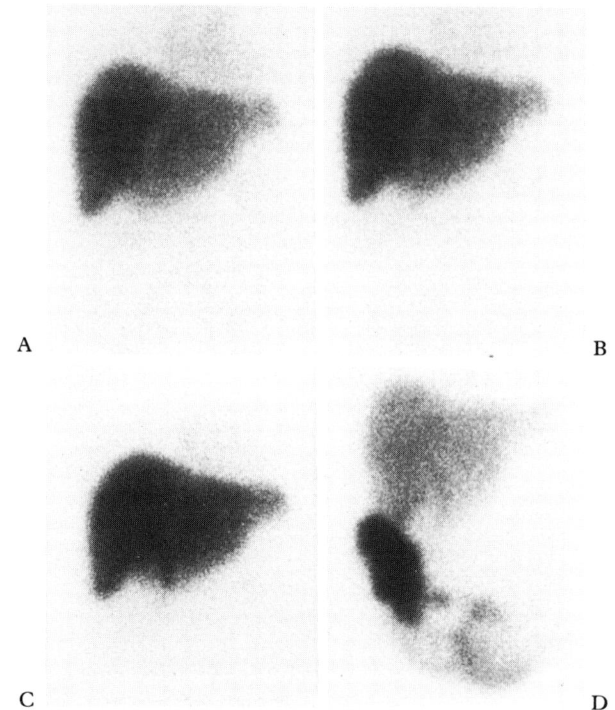

Fig. 66.10 ^{99}Tc^{m} dimerthy IDA. Serial images at 7 min, 15 min, 80 min and 270 min, showing transit of radioactivity through the liver into the small gut and ascending colon. The gallbladder is not shown, indicating there is cystic duct obstruction.

In the *normal* the biliary tree and gall bladder are visualized at 30 min and the gut at 60 min. If there is no gut activity at 60 min, further images are taken up to 5 hours, followed by a final image at 24 hours. In *hepatocellular* disease or *cholestasis* without obstruction there is a delay in transit, but gut activity is always present even when the biliary tree is not shown well. In *biliary obstruction* there is no gut activity even at 24 hours. Distended ducts are identifiable in congenital intrahepatic dilatation (Caroli's disease) as well as in choledocal cyst and sometimes in biliary obstruction.

The most important application of this test is in the evaluation of jaundice. In the majority of instances clinical and biochemical evaluation enables medical causes to be distinguished from 'surgical' causes of jaundice. The

HIDA test is indicated in the remainder. One disadvantage is that it is less reliable when the serum bilirubin is greater than 5 mg per cent. However, substitution compounds have been developed and the most useful of these is iso-butyl IDA which is reliable even with high bilirubin levels, probably because of its low renal excretion at these levels.

A number of alternative compounds that can be labelled with $^{99}Tc^{m}$ have been proposed for biliary scanning. None of them is used as widely as the derivatives of iminodiacetic acid, which they resemble physiologically, and the best known is *pyridoxylideneglutamate*. Up to 5 mCi is injected intravenously and within 15 min the gall bladder is demonstrated and within 30 min there is activity in the gut. Varying degrees of delay are experienced in hepatic disorders and the most reliable indicator of biliary obstruction is total absence of gut activity up to 24 hours. This compound, like IDA compounds, is most useful when the serum bilirubin is greater than 3·0 mg per cent and intravenous cholangiography is unreliable.

Partial obstruction of the extrahepatic biliary tree may mimic congenital dilatation or may cause delayed appearance of gut activity with absent gall bladder activity. The place of HIDA scanning along with ultrasound of the bile duct and CT of the liver and pancreas is becoming well established early in the diagnostic strategy of problem jaundice.

The detection of *biliary atresia* is obviously important in infancy and the IDA compounds have the same advantages as in adults over ^{131}I Rose Bengal.

Finally, in *acute cholecystitis* failure to show the gall bladder is a useful discriminating feature from other conditions, e.g. acute pancreatitis. Further, the gall bladder may fail to fill in some cases of *chronic cholecystitis* even when common bile duct is not obstructed.

KIDNEYS

RENOGRAPHY

Traditionally ^{131}I-*o*-hippurate is used for renography. Its high extraction ratio (90 per cent) by the tubule cells, and virtually nonexistent glomerular excretion make it very suitable. The constraints imposed by the physical properties of ^{131}I have been mentioned already and are overcome to a large extent by the use of cyclotron produced ^{123}I where this is available.

In probe renography, a collimated scintillation counter is centred over each kidney, either by using a small preliminary injection of labelled hippurate to locate the kidneys, or by using the anatomical landmarks. The upper pole of each kidney lies deep to the twelfth rib, the left being 1 cm or so higher than the right. Each probe touches the skin and is centred 5 cm from the midline. Other probes can be placed over the heart and the bladder if required. The record begins immediately after an intravenous injection of Hippurate. ^{131}I-*o*-hippurate is removed almost entirely in one passage through the kidney, by the tubule cells, and is not re-absorbed. It is convenient to consider the events in each nephron separately. The quantity of Hippuran in its lumen depends on the concentration in the blood, the blood flow to the nephron, and the ability of the nephron to extract it. Hippuran accumulates in the lumen of the nephron and then in the renal pelvis until the head of the radionuclide column reaches the pelvi-ureteric junction. Then it drains along the ureter, and the quantity in the nephron falls. At the same time smaller quantities are being extracted from the circulation until there is none left. At any one time, the activity in the nephron represents the balance between these events, and the activity in the whole kidney is the sum of the activity in all the nephrons. These events are represented by the standard renogram which has the following features (Fig. 66.11).

1. *The first phase*, a sharp rise (AB) within 30 s of injection. This represents vascular radioactivity within the vessels of the kidney and adjacent structures. The latter can be shown even after nephrectomy.

2. *The second phase*, a slower rise (BC) in the next 3 to 5

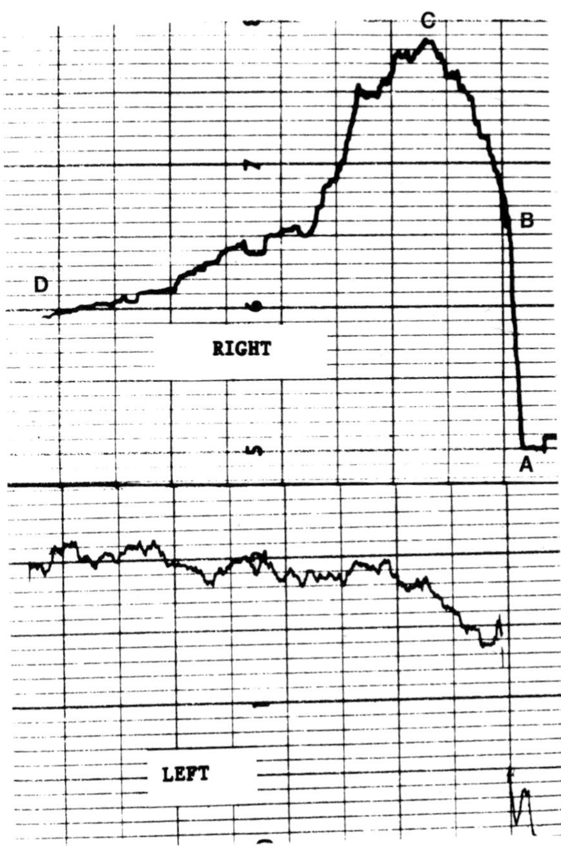

Fig. 66.11 ^{131}I-*o*-hippurate renogram. Above, normal R trace. For explanation, see text. Below, impaired drainage L. kidney. The peak cannot be identified and the third phase continues to rise slowly.

min. It represents the dominance of nephron accumulation, and the slope of the curve is related to the rate of accumulation. Thus the slope is steep during a diuresis, but is decreased in renal tubular failure, impaired renal perfusion from renal artery stenosis (Fig. 66.12), shock, and dehydration.

3. *The peak* (C), which is normally sharp, because the rate of transit through all the nephrons is roughly the same. The peak is rounded where transit is unequal, e.g. in diffuse vascular or parenchymal disease. The peak is sharper in diuresis than in dehydration.

4. *The transit time* (AC), is usually 3 to 5 min. It is relatively longer when the urine flow rate falls, e.g. in dehydration, shock, ischaemia (Fig. 66.12), and renal failure; and it is relatively shorter in a diuresis.

5. *The third phase* (CD), is a roughly exponential fall over the next 20 min or so. It represents the dominance of ureteric drainage over the relatively small accumulation that takes place at this stage. The fall is abnormally slow whenever drainage from the pelvis is impaired (Figs. 66.11 and 66.13), whether from ureteric obstruction, hydronephrosis, or severely reduced urine flow rate. As the degree of impaired drainage increases so the curve becomes flatter, until in the more severe cases, e.g. calculus obstruction, it does not fall at all but continues to rise.

Diethylene-triamine-penta-acetate (DTPA) is excreted entirely by glomeruli and is the compound of choice for measuring glomerular filtration rate. When labelled with $^{99}Tc^{m}$ ($^{99}Tc^{m}$-DTPA) it is particularly suitable for studying renal function and excretory pathways by means of the gamma camera.

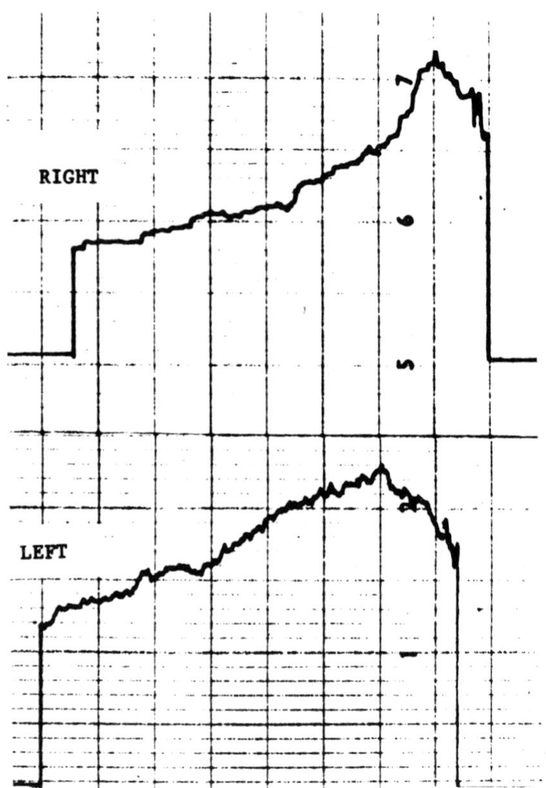

Fig. 66.12 L. renal artery stenosis. ^{131}I-Hippuran renogram. The R trace is normal. The L trace is rounded, its transit time increased and the slope of its third phase decreased.

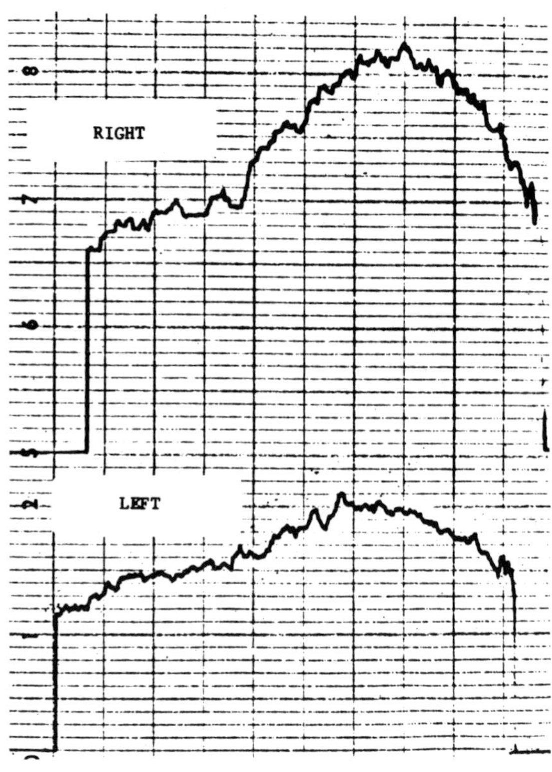

Fig. 66.13 Obstructive uropathy with bilateral hydronephrosis or hydro-ureter. ^{131}I-Hippuran renogram. Both R and L traces are similar, with rounded, delayed peaks and decreased slope in the third phase. Note the similarity between these traces and that of the L. kidney in Figure 66.12.

Gamma camera renography

The patient sits with his back to the camera so that the kidneys are at the centre of the field and the heart at its upper end. After intravenous injection data are recorded for 30 min by a small computer. Collection periods can be of equal length (20 sec each) or shorter during the early phase, e.g. (1 sec each) and longer during the third phase (30 sec each). A summed image of the whole study is produced and regions of interest are described over each kidney as well as over the heart or liver, a background area and the bladder. Time activity curves are for qualitative assessment, but some form of background subtraction is necessary for quantitative assessment.

Whichever region is chosen to represent non-urinary-tract background the inherent errors in the technique amount to about 10 per cent.

Deconvolution

The renogram traces the change in renal activity with time and depends on the rate of input and rate of drainage, both of which are changing continuously. These factors make quantitative comparison of renograms inaccurate and *deconvolution* is a mathematical technique used to overcome the difficulties. Briefly the data collected from the renogram are manipulated to create a theoretical curve that would be produced if the radioactive input to the kidney were in the form of a single impulse. The need for ^{131}I-HSA is dispensed with. The ratio of the initial heights of the curves from each kidney is a useful comparison of renal functions, and the time taken for the activity to fall to half its maximum value is a useful basis for quantitative comparisons.

Diuresis renography

The evaluation of a dilated urinary tract or enlarged renal pelvis can be difficult and renography under deliberate diuresis has been found valuable. Essentially, impaired drainage that disappears during diuresis is regarded as less significant than persistently impaired drainage. Diuresis can be produced by ensuring a high fluid intake before the renogram, by giving a diuretic to a well hydrated patient 5 min before the hippuran, or by giving a diuretic during the third phase of the renogram.

Clinical value

From the above it is obvious that an accurate pathological diagnosis is unlikely from a consideration of the renogram alone. But if the altered physiology that the renogram represents is interpreted in conjunction with clinical, biochemical and urographic findings, it can be used to investigate many problems in children and adults.

1. *Obstructive uropathy and nephropathy.* Excretion urography is the primary technique for diagnosing the cause of urinary tract obstruction, and renography enables the functional effect of the obstruction on the renal parenchyma, as well as the degree of obstruction, to be measured. This can help to judge the optimum time for surgery, and to monitor post surgical recovery. Also the diuretic techniques (*vide supra*) are useful in assessing suspected obstruction at the pelvi-ureteric junction.

2. *Reflux uropathy.* In children renographic abnormality is a useful discriminator between those who are likely to need surgical treatment, and those who are not.

3. *Acute renal failure.* The aim is to distinguish obstructive uropathy from parenchymal failure. In the former the traces are asymmetrical with greater evidence of impaired drainage on the obstructed side. In the latter traces are symmetrical and rise slowly. Usually CABBS technique is needed for best results in renal failure, but even then there is enough overlap to require considerable caution in interpreting results.

4. *Hypertension.* In unilateral renal ischaemia the trace on the side of the lesion is lower and flatter and the peak is later and less sharp. Differences of less than 20 per cent are not significant. Renography and urography together can be used to select the patients for renal arteriography, which remains the only way of showing the arterial anatomy. However, the whole strategy of investigating hypertension is influenced by the likelihood that surgery will only be needed in a very small proportion of cases.

5. *Pregnancy.* It is normal to find rounding of the peak and impaired drainage as early as the first trinester, and the changes are more marked on the right. They begin to return to normal immediately after delivery, some change persists into the puerperium.

Relatively mild urinary tract symptoms are not uncommon in pregnancy. Sometimes potentially serious urinary tract disease such as hydronephrosis or calculus may present in, or be exacerbated by pregnancy. It is desirable on the one hand not to postpone necessary investigations of these conditions, and on the other not to expose the foetus to unnecessary radiation hazards. Some have found the renogram a useful adjunct to clinical judgement and favour postponing urography if the renogram is within normal limits.

6. *Anuria following transplantation.* There are many causes of anuria or oliguria after transplantation, and the renogram is abnormal in most. In the normal course of events it is low rounded and flat. In renal artery occlusion, only a background trace is obtained; with ureteric occlusion or leakage the delay in drainage is greater than normal; with rejection there is progressive deterioration of function.

RENAL SCANNING

Renal scans define the size and position of the kidneys and locate parenchymal defects. Scanning gives some information about overall function and is particularly useful in the presence of renal failure or hypersensitivity to contrast agents. Most of the renal blood perfuses the cortex, where the scanning agents in common use are extracted by the renal tubule cells or by the glomeruli. These compounds are:

1. *Chlormerodrin*, a diuretic labelled with ^{197}Hg. A posterior image was taken two hours after intravenous injection. The activity administered was limited by the radiation dose and this diminished the quality of the image.

2. *Technetium compounds.* These can be given in greater activity, thereby improving the quality of the image, and have superseded chlormerodrin. The pertechnetate ion passes through the kidney without being trapped or excreted and can be used to determine vascularity of the

kidney by taking rapid sequence images after injection. $^{99}Tc^{m}$ DTPA can be given in larger activities than for renography, and used to study the vascularity and morphology of the kidney. $^{99}Tc^{m}$-labelled dimethyl-tetraethylene-penta-acetate (DTPA) is extracted by the glomeruli and can be used to estimate the glomerular filtration rate. However sufficient is retained within the cortex, particularly from the compounds commercially available, to produce satisfactory images. More recently $^{99}Tc^{m}$ dimercaptosuccinic acid (DMSA) has been developed because it has the advantage of being stable, easily prepared and giving a good image of renal parenchyma (Fig. 66.14). It differs from DTPA in that it is not excreted well enough to be used for visualizing the collecting system. The relative activities of the kidneys reflect their relative functions accurately.

3. ^{131}I-*o*-hippurate. Hippuran is extracted by the renal tubules and its use in renography has been described already. After intravenous injection of 200 μCi, serial images are taken every 5 minutes for 20 minutes or so. Valuable information can still be obtained when renal function is considerably impaired, and delayed studies up to 24 hours are then useful.

The normal image is formed by the functioning cortical tissue, and corresponds well with the radiographic renal outlines. This correlation is important in studying congenital abnormalities. Thus in horse-shoe kidney the scan shows whether the isthmus contains functioning renal tissue; and in lobulate kidneys or fused kidneys, the demonstration of functioning renal tissue is important in making the distinction from a renal mass.

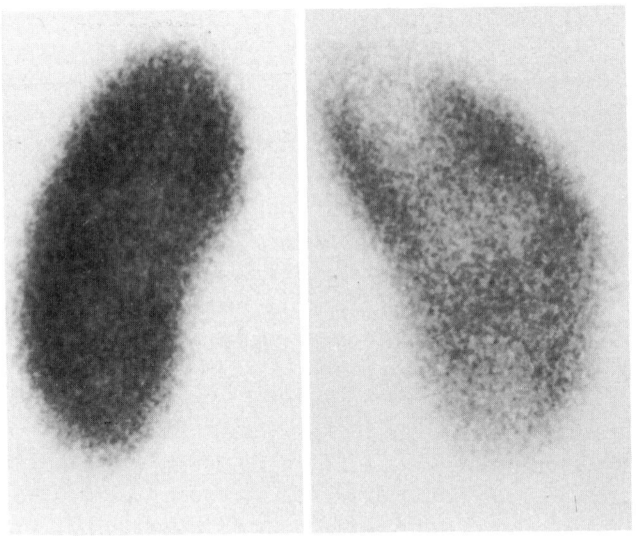

Fig. 66.14 R. hydrocalycosis. $^{99}Tc^{m}$-DMSA scan. Posterior projection. The L image is a normal cortical image. On the R there are defects that correspond to dilated calyces.

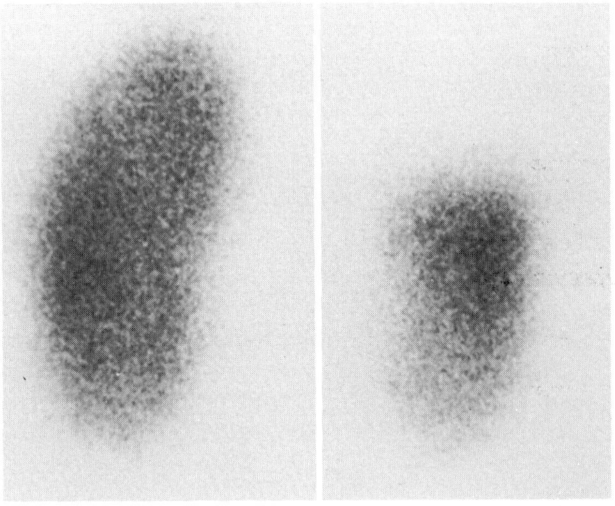

Fig. 66.15 R. renal cyst. $^{99}Tc^{m}$-DMSA scan. Posterior projection. Normal L image. There is a non-specific deficit in the upper half of the right kidney due to a cyst.

The commonest *abnormality* in a renal scan is a defect, and this may be caused by any lesion that destroys or displaces the renal cortex. It is exceptional to find increased activity, which has been recorded only in functioning renal tubule cell adenoma, or in localized compensating hypertrophy.

Tumours

In a static image there are no features to distinguish *carcinoma*, *cyst* (Fig. 66.15), *haematoma*, *arteriovenous fistula*, etc. Rapid sequence studies show the relatively increased vascularity of carcinomas and fistulae, compared with cysts and haematomas. However, some carcinomas are relatively avascular. In general, scanning can be used to confirm a suspected mass or to assess a dubiously abnormal urogram. If the lesion can be shown to be transonic as well as avascular it is logical to proceed to cyst puncture. Thus the combination of isotopic and ultrasonic scanning can be used to determine the choice of confirmatory investigation. It should be borne in mind that small defects in the centre of the kidney are likely to be obscured by surrounding tissue, and even at the margin of the kidney the limit of resolution is 1 cm.

Infection

In *chronic pyelonephritis* the activity is irregular and diminished (Fig. 66.16) particularly where the urogram shows evidence of cortical scarring. In other chronic infections such as *tuberculosis* the size of the defect

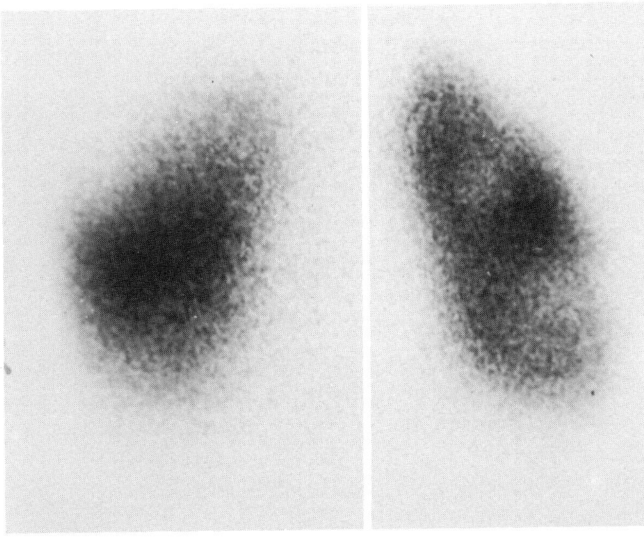

Fig. 66.16 Chronic pyelonephritis. $^{99}Tc^m$-DMSA scan. Posterior projection. There is diffusely low activity over the l. upper pole; and there are focal deficits extending to the renal margin in the right upper and lower poles. The abnormalities in Figures 66.14–16 are non-specific and these images are concerned with the distribution of remaining renal function rather than the nature of the lesion.

depends on the extent of the disease. Often it is greater than would be suspected from the urogram, which is useful information in planning conservative surgery. In *acute pyelonephritis* localized defects can be shown in a substantial number of patients even when the urogram is normal. Usually these defects resolve but may persist if the infection is severe.

Vascular lesions

A *renal artery occlusion* from any cause leads to an absent image. In unilateral *renal artery stenosis* the ischaemic kidney is small with impaired activity. In the presence of severe arterial disease in the contralateral kidney, its pattern of uptake also will be abnormal. Segmental arterial occlusion will cause a segmental defect. Static imaging gives less information about vascular lesions than renography.

Trauma

A *renal contusion* causes generalized depressed function or localized filling defects, and can be shown when the only urographic evidence of injury is delayed excretion. Usually urography is the keystone for the management of renal injuries, and scanning, ultrasound and arteriography are rarely required supplements. Scanning is a useful test for monitoring recovery from the injury.

Obstructive uropathy

In *primary pelvic hydronephrosis* the quality of the image with DMSA reflects the degree of impaired function, but a normal image does not indicate that renal function will remain good. In acute and chronic obstructive uropathy, DMSA scanning is only an adjunct to conventional urography and renography.

Renal transplantation

The commonest problem is to determine whether anuria or oliguria is due to *rejection*, *acute tubular necrosis*, *renal artery occlusion*, *ureteric leak* or *obstruction*, etc. No single test is adequate to make this distinction in every case, but isotopic studies have the advantage that they are simple to perform, can be repeated frequently and in the majority of cases make the diagnosis without recourse to serial urography, arteriography or ureteric catheterization.

The most widely used technique is to follow the passage of $^{99}Tc^m$ DTPA through the transplanted kidney in anterior view. Data are recorded at 1 to 5 sec intervals and can be analysed to show whether there is arterial obstruction, ureteric obstruction, or leakage etc. In tubular necrosis the accumulation will be poor and there

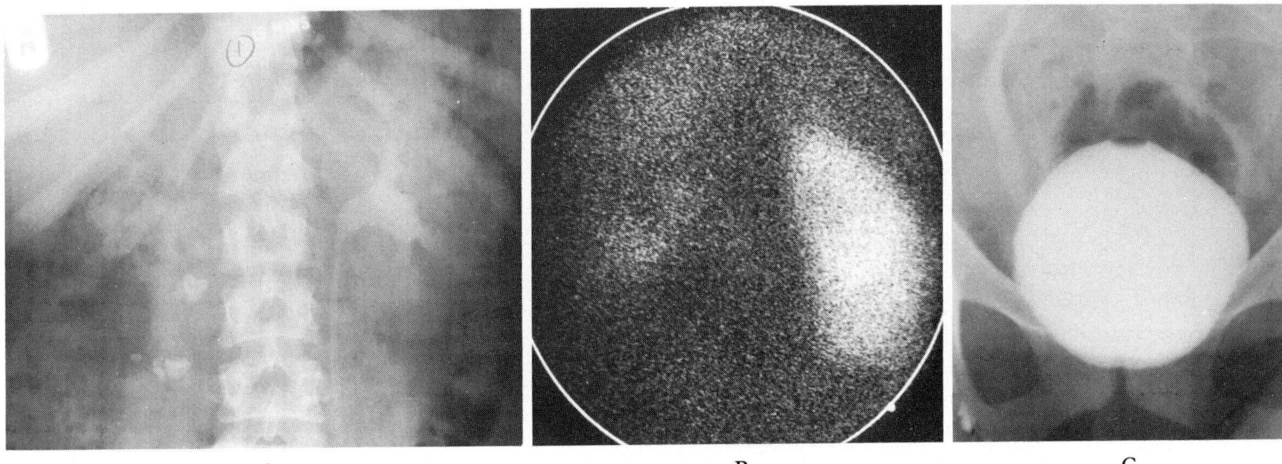

A B C

Fig. 66.17 (A) Excretion urography. There is no apparent function in the R. kidney. (B) $^{99}Tc^m$-DTPA scan. The image is reversed to correspond with the urogram. There is minimal R. renal function. (C) Micturating cystourethrogram. There is R. vesico-ureteric reflux.

are theoretical advantages in using ^{131}I-hippuran which is excreted by glomerular filtration. However the greater administered activity of ^{99}Tc^{m} DTPA usually overcomes this difficulty. Serial studies are useful in distinguishing the sudden deterioration of acute tubular necrosis, from the progressive deterioration of rejection, with its poorer prognosis. Renal uptake of ^{99}Tc^{m} colloid or ^{67}Ga is an indication of rejection.

Finally it is important to bear in mind that serial investigations may be used to gain maximum information in any one case (Fig. 66.17).

Radionuclide cystography

The traditional way of detecting ureteric reflux is by contrast fluorography, with its attendant disadvantages of urethral catheterization and prolonged fluorography. The latter can be overcome by instilling 1 mCi of ^{99}Tc^{m} pertechnetate or sulphur colloid in saline into the bladder, and viewing the abdomen with serial gamma camera images. In some instances this technique is more sensitive than contrast cystography in detecting ureteric reflux but does not avoid the need for catheterization. An alternative but less sensitive test is to view the abdomen at the end of a standard renogram when radio activity has cleared the kidneys; and await spontaneous micturition. This test has the major advantage of being well tolerated in addition to not requiring catheterization.

PANCREAS

Methionine, labelled with ^{75}Se in place of a sulphur atom is the only radionuclide widely available for scanning the pancreas. After intravenous injection, ^{75}Selenomethionine is accumulated in sites where there is a high turnover of amino acids, and this may be due to enzyme synthesis (pancreas), protein synthesis (liver), or hormone synthesis (thyroid, parathyroid). The highest concentration of activity occurs in the pancreas and the pancreatic juice shows maximum activity one to four hours after injection. However, because of its greater bulk the liver accumulates three times as much radioactivity as the pancreas. The physical half-life of ^{75}Selenomethionine is 120 days but because of the complicated metabolic fate of injected selenomethionine several fractions can be identified each with a different biological half-life. Thus 42 per cent of the injected activity has a biologica half-life of 220 days. The greatest organ dose is to the liver.

Many special techniques have been devised for enhancing the activity within the pancreas but the most satisfactory preparation is to give the patient a meal before he comes to the department and to give a protein supplement (Complan) at the time of the injection. It is helpful to begin by doing a standard colloid liver scan. Three to four microcuries of selenomethionine per kg body weight are then injected intravenously. Four or more sequential camera images are then done within the next hour because the pancreas background ratio is greatest at about 30 min. It is a help to separate the pancreas from the liver by raising the patient's left side 10 degrees and tilting the scanning head 15 degrees cephalad. Alternatively two linear scans can be done of the upper abdomen, one in the antero-posterior projection and another in the tilted projection. The colloid liver image can be subtracted electronically from the combined liver and pancreas image to give an uncomplicated view of the pancreas.

Digital subtraction is more reliable than analogue subtraction but both are imperfect because:

1. The hepatic distribution of colloid and methionine are different

2. ^{99}Tc^{m} activity in the skeleton and stomach causes artefacts

3. One of the photopeaks of ^{75}Se coincides with that of ^{99}Tc^{m}.

In most cases an experienced observer can dispense with subtraction images.

The normal pancreatic image lies slightly obliquely across the midline and below the liver which partly overlaps it. Pancreatic excretion is not uniform and it is important to obtain sequential images wherever possible in order to clarify the distribution of activity throughout the whole gland (Fig. 66.18). Some activity occurs in the duodenal loop and in the duodenojejunal flexure, especially after 1 hour from the biliary excretion, pancreatic secretion and cellular accumulation. These foci of activity modify the shape of the pancreatic image and may contribute to so called horse-shoe and sigmoid shapes that are described.

The sensitivity of a normal image is said to be as high

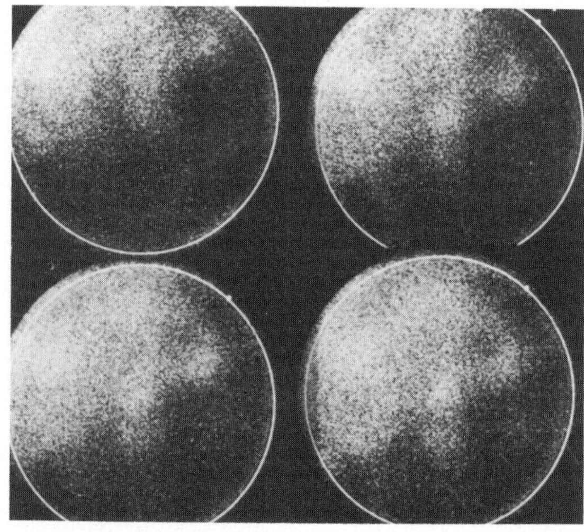

Fig. 66.18 Normal pancreas. ^{75}Se-methionine scans. Four sequential anterior images during the first hour after injection. Note (a) pancreatic activity is uneven, (b) the distribution of pancreatic activity changes slightly, (c) there is considerable activity in the liver.

segment where the clinically significant thrombi are likely to be.

c. fibrinogen uptake in arthritic knees may complicate the interpretation.

Alternatively the radiopharmaceutical being given for a lung scan can be divided into two equal amounts that are injected synchronously into a dorsal pedal vein in each foot, with compression of superficial veins at the ankle. Rapid sequence images of the limbs and abdomen can be taken to show the whole venous drainage including the inferior vena cava. Delayed transit, filling defects and asymmetric pattern are indications of abnormality and the technique has many obvious advantages. The lung scan is then done in the usual way.

SKELETAL SCANNING

It is the mineral component of bone that is important in scanning. The chief mineral is a complex crystal of hydroxy apatite containing calcium, phosphate and hydroxyl ions. The crystals are formed from solution and when they are newly formed they dissolve and re-crystallize spontaneously and rapidly. At this stage ions in surrounding solution exchange with ions on the surface of the crystal and there is some exchange with the deeper layers of the crystal. As the bone becomes mature, e.g. compact bone, there is much less exchange with surrounding solution. Radionuclides that exchange in this way are used in skeletal scanning, and the uptake of radionuclide is affected by the blood supply and mineral turnover of the bone. As these are closely inter-related it is not always possible to determine the dominant influence on radionuclide uptake.

The following radiopharmaceuticals are available for skeletal scanning:

1. *Technetium-labelled phosphate complexes*

Pertechnetate that has been reduced to technetium ion by the stannous ion can be used to label phosphate complexes that are then taken up in the skeleton. Several compounds have been developed, among them pyrophosphate, polyphosphate, ethylenehydroxy diphosphonate (EHDP) and methylene diphosphonate (MDP). The main advantages shared by all these compounds are the low radiation dose to the patient, the relatively low cost, and the greater detection efficiency because of the appropriate gamma energy. The blood clearance of all these compounds is more rapid than that of other compounds during the first hour or so after injection but the rate of clearance then falls and there is still a considerable blood background even at six hours. This is a relative disadvantage compared with compounds like strontium and there is the further disadvantage that there is often some uptake in extraskeletal tissues such as liver and muscle. The major excretion of these compounds is by the renal

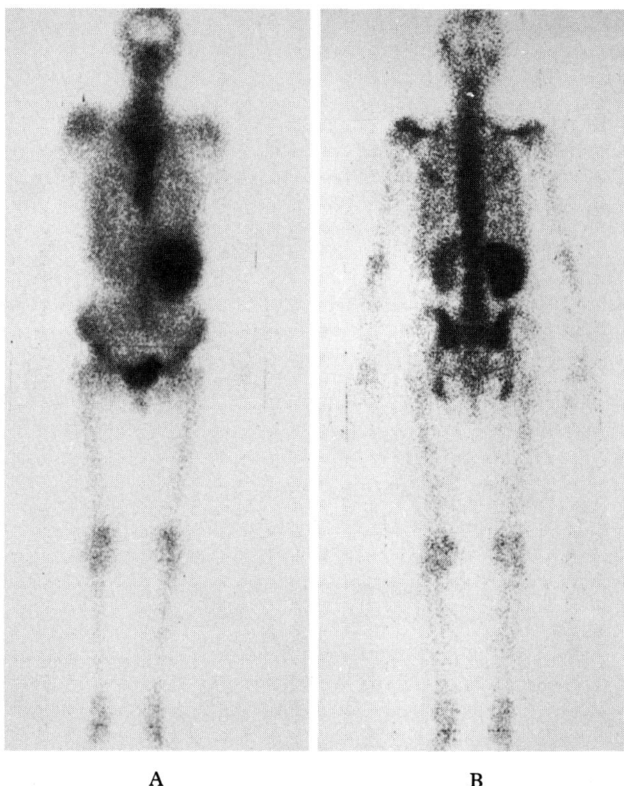

Fig. 66.26 Normal skeletal scan. Incidental hydronephrosis $^{99}Tc^{m}$-DMP scan. (A) Anterior and (B) posterior projections show symmetrical skeletal activity. Note excreted activity in the urinary tract, especially over L. kidney. Excretion urography showed L. hydronephrosis.

tract and both a nephrogram and pyelogram can be shown (Fig. 66.26).

The usual administered activity is 10mCi and it is advisable to wait at least three hours before scanning. The minute quantity of tin administered is well within the margins of safety.

Technetium-labelled fluorophosphate has also been developed but is probably less useful than the other phosphate compounds.

2. *Fluorine*

Fluorine-18 is usually given intravenously and is cleared more rapidly than other compounds. Also there is a higher ratio between skeletal activity and tissue activity as well as between abnormal bone activity and normal bone activity. Bone has a very high affinity for fluorine probably because hydroxy apatite is converted to fluorapatite. The main disadvantage of fluorine is that its short half-life (two hours) make it unsuitable for widespread use, and its relatively high gamma energy is not ideal for imaging. It is excreted by the kidney. The optimum time for scanning is about two hours after intravenous injection.

3. *Strontium*

$^{87}Sr^{m}$ and ^{85}Sr are calcium analogues that are taken up rapidly by the skeleton. Their physical characteristics are less satisfactory than those of the $^{99}Tc^{m}$ compounds which have superceded them.

4. *Other agents*

Gallium, indium and rare earth elements are among those that have been proposed for skeletal scanning but their applications have not been developed sufficiently to replace the $^{99}Tc^{m}$ compounds.

Both linear scanners and gamma cameras can be used for skeletal scanning. The better resolution of gamma cameras is superior for detecting lesions in ribs and other bones near the surface but the linear scanner is more efficient at detecting deeper lesions such as those in the pelvis. Whichever instrument is used it is important to give adequate radioactivity in order to achieve better sensitivity.

In a normal $^{99}Tc^{m}$ skeletal scan (Fig. 66.26) there is symmetry about the midline and a smooth graduation of activity along the spine. The lower lumbar vertebrae are shown better in anterior projections whereas the upper dorsal vertebrae are shown better in posterior projection. There is greater activity over growing epiphyses than elsewhere. Symmetrical activity is noted in both sacro-iliac joints. Detail is seen better in younger patients but it can be influenced by the size of the patients, the compound used and the interval after injection. The renal tract and bladder are identified easily. Occasionally abnormalities in the renal tracts can be predicted from the scan but it is an unreliable way of assessing the renal tract. Assymetry may be produced over the shoulder of the dominant side by scoliosis or a joint undergoing weight-bearing stress. There is often increased activity over both shoulder joints in older patients. Activity may be seen in vascular calcification, normal and abnormal breast tissue, operation scars, the liver (with polyphosphate), and occasionally over a mastectomy because of reduced absorption of gamma rays by the soft tissues.

Abnormally high activity is a non-specific feature influenced by:

a. Blood supply. Vascular lesions have high activity, especially in the phase immediately after injection.

b. Bone mineral activity. The greatest activity is in freshly mineralized osteoid and high activity will occur therefore in response to a variety of neoplastic and other stimuli.

c. Cellular content. Fibrocytes and histiocytes have an avidity for MDP and *fibrous dysplasia* and *histiocytosis* have positive scans (Fig. 66.27).

Abnormally low activity is rare but can occur in acute *bone infarction*, to be followed by high activity during healing; or in total bone destruction from any cause.

These processes can be detected earlier by scanning than by conventional radiography. Even so, longstanding sclerotic lesions that are metabolically inactive will have a normal scan. There is an overall false negative rate of 5–10 per cent.

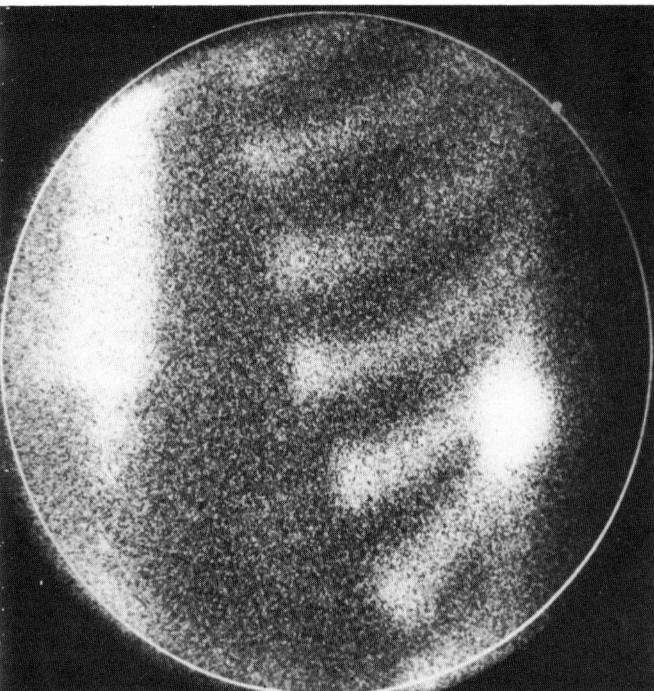

Fig. 66.27 Histiocytosis of L. 7th rib. $^{99}Tc^{m}$ MDP scan showing intense activity over the lesion.

Many benign lesions accrue radioactivity. In *Paget's disease* (Fig. 66.28) there is good correlation between scan and radiograph except when the lesion is too small to be detected by the scan. Occasionally in a patient known to have Paget's disease elsewhere, a negative radiograph is accompanied by a positive scan. In florid Paget's disease some fall of activity can be detected under the influence of calcitonin. There is a diffusely high uptake at *fracture sites* especially where callus is prominent, and in osteoporosis (Fig. 66.29). Other non-neoplastic lesions over which high uptake has been observed are *osteomyelitis*, *rheumatoid arthritis*, *osteoarthrosis*, *fibrous dysplasia* and *hyperostosis frontalis interna*. The variety of these lesions emphasizes the need for radiographic and clinical correlation in interpreting a lesion accurately.

Malignant tumours both osteolytic and osteoblastic, *primary* (Fig. 66.30) and *secondary* (Fig. 66.31) also produce high activity. Metastases from primary bone tumours also may accumulate high activity (Fig. 66.32).

Detection of metastases is the widest application for skeletal scanning. Occult metastases occurs in up to 30 per cent of patients with carcinoma of the breast and the likelihood of metastasis is greater when the tumour is large. The significance of such metastases is that the prognosis is as poor as it is with clinically apparent metastasis. Similarly, in carcinoma of the prostate the scan may be abnormal before the radiograph. Where clinical symptoms are accompanied by normal or dubiously abnormal radiographs the scan is a reliable way of detecting

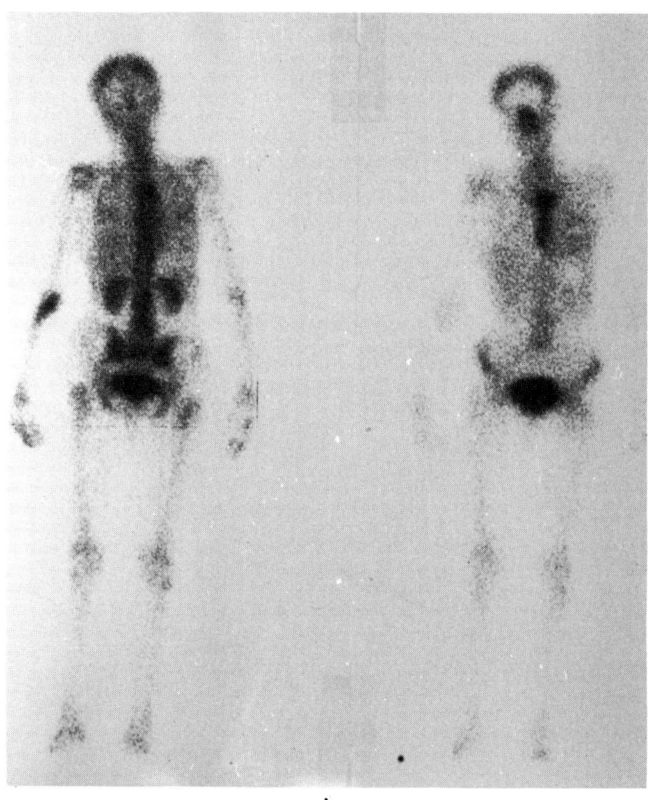

A

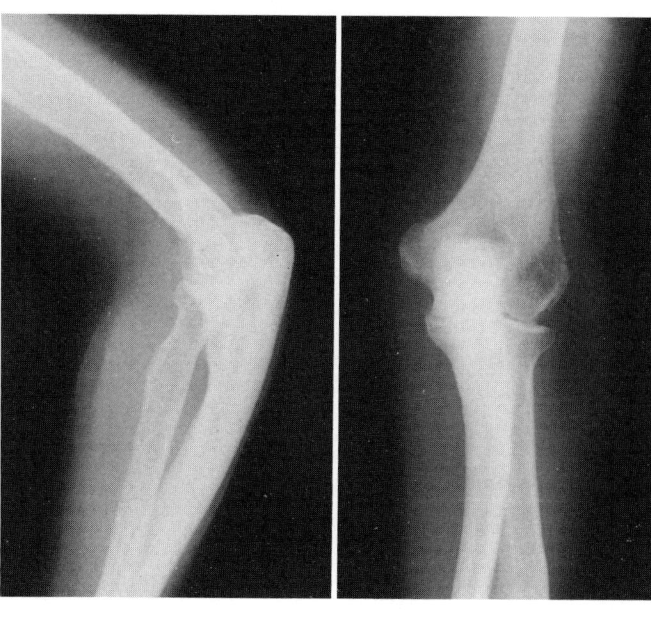

B

Fig. 66.28 Paget's disease. $^{99}Tc^{m}$-DMP scan. (A) Anterior and posterior projections show symmetrical activity apart from high activity below Rt. elbow. (B) Radiographs show Paget's disease of Rt. ulna.

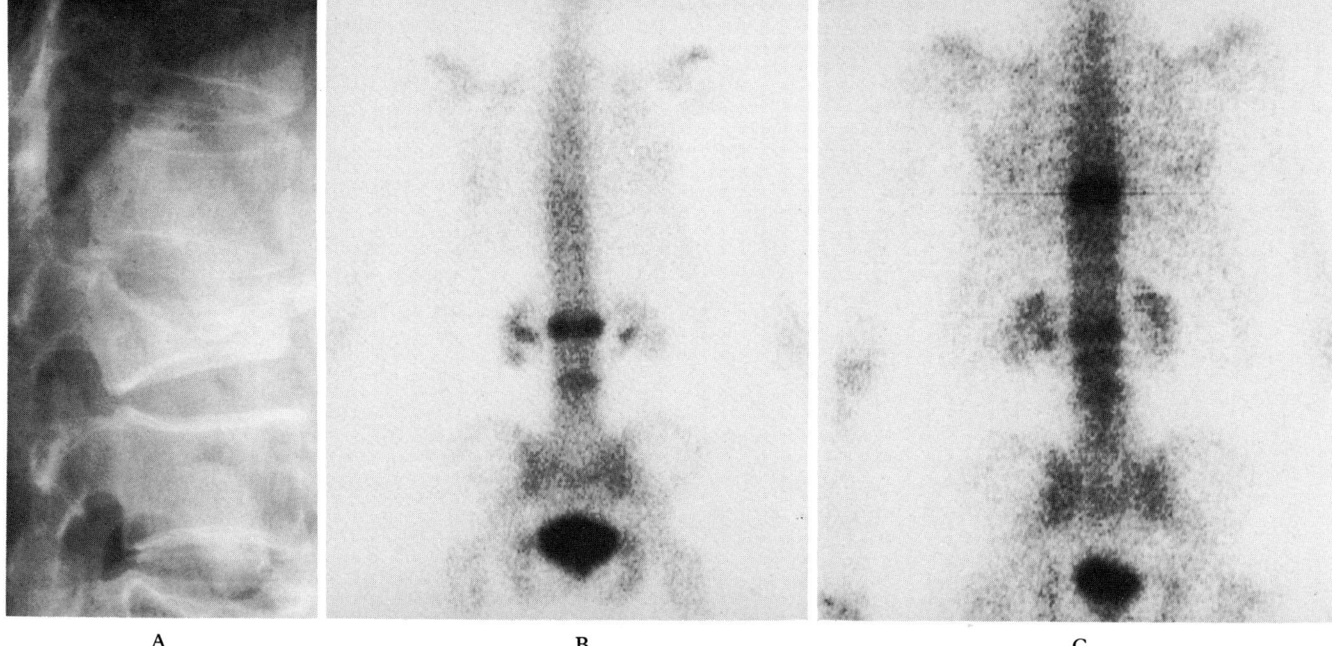

A B C

Fig. 66.29 Osteoporosis. (A) Lateral radiograph showing wedging of L.V.1. (B) $^{99}Tc^{m}$ MDP scan showing increased activity over L.V.1 and over L.V.3. (C) Six months later; the activity over L.V.1 and L.V.3 is less and there is increased activity over a recently collapsed mid-dorsal vertebra.

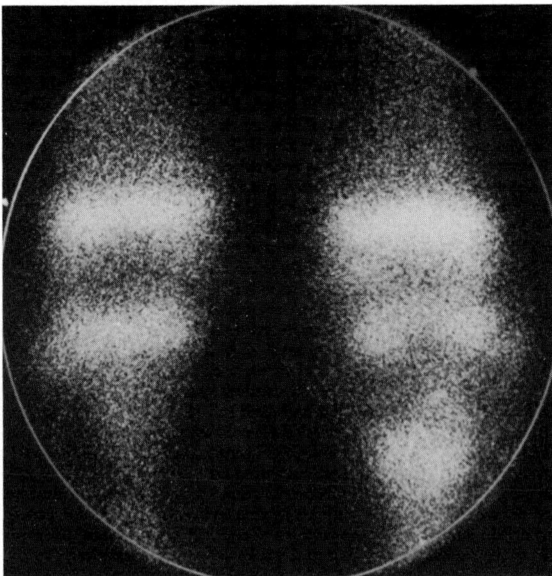

Fig. 66.30 Osteosarcoma of tibia in a child. $^{99}Tc^{m}$-DMP scan of knees. Note the normal high activity over the epiphyses and the abnormal high activity over the Lt. upper tibia.

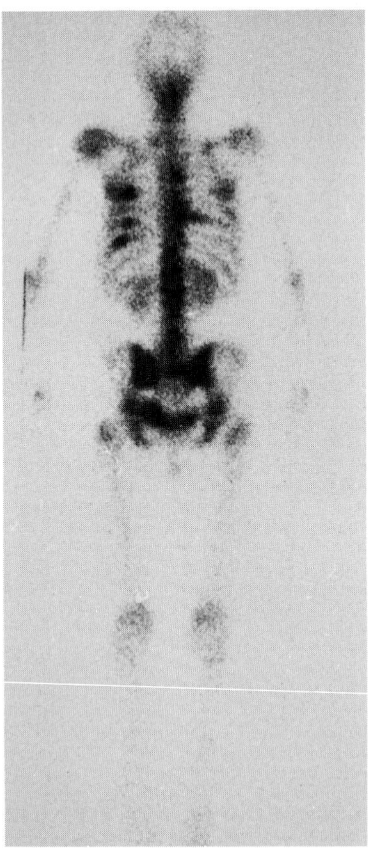

Fig. 66.31 Metastatic carcinoma. $^{99}Tc^{m}$-DMP scan. Posterior view. There is increased activity over many ribs at the sites of metastases. Note the normal high activity over the shoulders, especially the right.

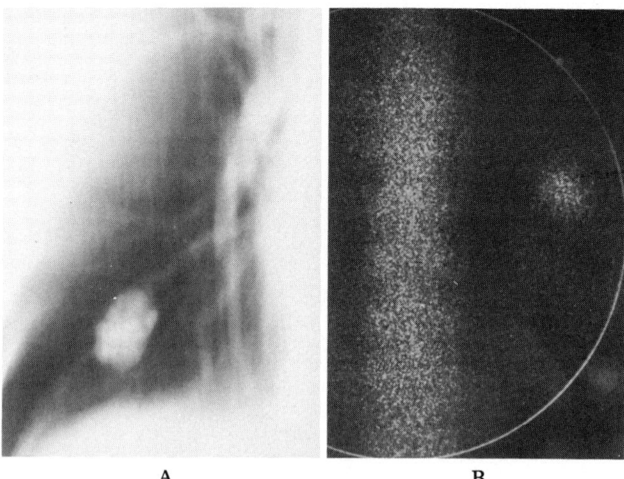

Fig. 66.32 Pulmonary metastasis from osteosarcoma. (A) Tomogram; Rt. lower lobe showing ossification in a metastasis. (B) $^{99}Tc^{m}$-DMP scan, posterior view of Rt. lung showing increased activity in the lesion.

metastasis. Positive scans may be due to benign lesions in patients known to have primary carcinomas and it is important to radiograph all abnormal areas in order to confirm that there is no benign abnormality such as osteo-arthrosis or osteophytosis. Occasionally unsuspected lymphoma may be detected in the skeleton. In *acute osteomyelitis* the scan becomes positive much earlier than the radiographs and is an invaluable initial investigation. The skeletal distribution of the activity helps to distinguish osteomyelitis from cellulitis which has a more diffuse distribution. Exceptionally, fulminating osteomyelitis is associated with raised intraosseous pressure and impaired perfusion leading to a falsely negative scan. Occult distant foci and recurrence of activity in *chronic osteomyelitis* are well detected by scanning. In primary bone tumours the role of scintigraphy is well defined. Certainly the abnormalities are often larger than other investigations would suggest but the significance of this is uncertain. When lesions are treated by radiotherapy a fall in activity occurs and this may persist for a considerable time.

Total body scanning is an efficient way of displaying the extent of polyarthrosis and may be used to monitor the progress of the disease though clearly local radiographs will be necessary to assess the nature of any changes.

GALLIUM AND INDIUM

Gallium-67 scanning

Gallium-67 citrate is a widely used tumour-seeking agent. ^{67}Ga is produced by cyclotron and decays by electron capture with a physical half-life of 78 hours. It emits gamma photons at four discrete energies, 93 keV (45 per cent), 184 keV (24 per cent), 296 kev (22 per cent) and 388 keV (7 per cent). The first three of these are suitable for imaging with either a rectilinear scanner or a gamma camera. After intravenous injection ^{67}Ga citrate binds with the serum protein, with a half-life in the blood of 12 hours. During the first 24 hours about 10 per cent of the activity is excreted by the kidneys and during the next five days about 25 per cent is excreted via the bile into the gut. Some is accumulated in the liver, spleen, bone marrow skeleton and normal breast tissue, and its biologic half-life is two to three weeks. The usual activity is 1–3 mCi. A suitable aperient is given to clear the colon on the following day and scans are done at 24, 48, 72 hours. The total body radiation dose is 0·2 to 0·3 rad/mCi.

In a normal scan there is some uptake in nasopharynx, the axial skeleton (including the sternum) the shoulder joints, the liver and spleen, as well as in the gut. Serial scans identify the changing pattern of the latter. In the female, activity in the breasts is not uncommon and is particularly likely during lactation, and prolactinaemia due to pregnancy, pituitary adenoma, some bronchial carcinomas, renal failure and many drugs.

Gallium is bound within the cells to lysozomes probably by displacing calcium and magnesium. Gallium scans are positive in a large variety of neoplasms and in many inflammatory lesions.

Current treatment of the *lymphomas* is intense and the initial assessment of the extent of the disease and continuing assessment during its treatment are a vital part of management. The most important role of ^{67}Ga scanning is in this assessment. Its greatest accuracy is in the mediastinum (Fig. 66.33), where the extent of known disease can be determined accurately and the presence of occult lesions can be detected. In the abdomen its overall accuracy is less but can still produce useful evidence of

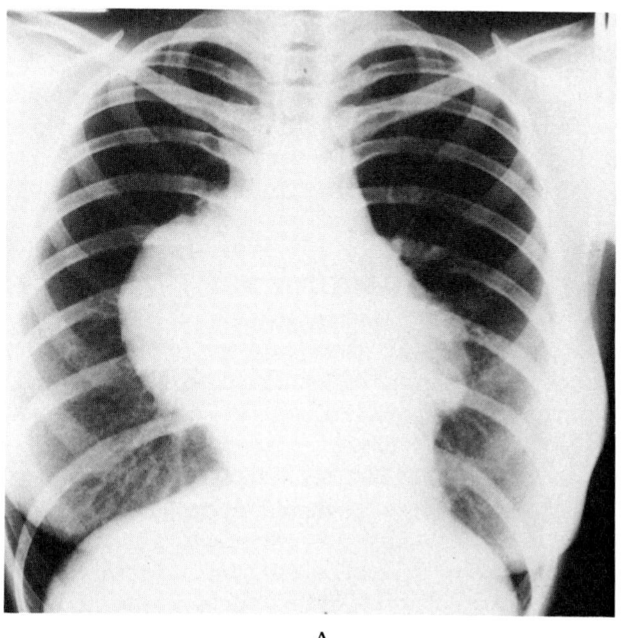

A

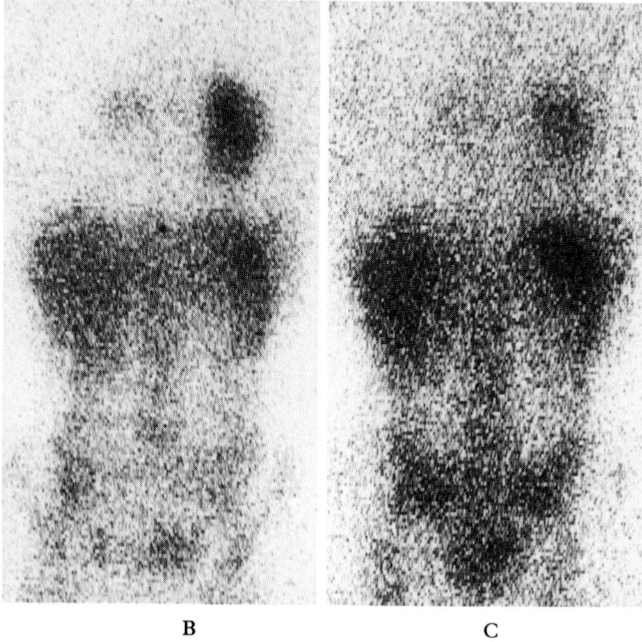

B C

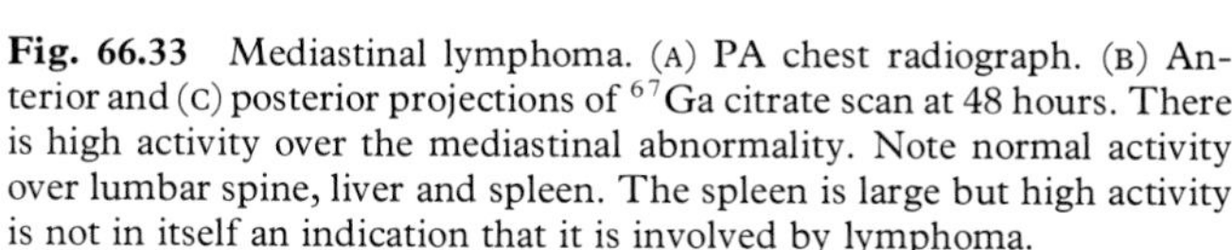

Fig. 66.33 Mediastinal lymphoma. (A) PA chest radiograph. (B) Anterior and (C) posterior projections of ^{67}Ga citrate scan at 48 hours. There is high activity over the mediastinal abnormality. Note normal activity over lumbar spine, liver and spleen. The spleen is large but high activity is not in itself an indication that it is involved by lymphoma.

involved nodes when considered alongside lymphography. Gallium scanning is more accurate in lymphocyte predominant Hodgkin's disease than in the other lymphomas but in all it is a very reliable method of following the results of treatment and detecting recurrent disease. The incidence of false positives is so low that increased activity in an irradiated region is very significant and the gallium scan may indeed be the only non-invasive index of recurrence.

Increased uptake of ^{67}Ga has been described in many other tumours, e.g. *carcinoma of the bronchus, oesophagus, colon, breast, thyroid, malignant melanoma, cerebral metastases,* etc. However, the reliability is not high enough for any useful clinical application and is further diminished by the fact that certain non-malignant lesions notably *sarcoidosis* and *cerebral infarcts* are well-known to accumulate ^{67}Ga. It may be rather more helpful in detecting *liver cell carcinoma* in some instances. When there is a defect in a liver colloid scan demonstrable increased activity with ^{67}Ga is a strong pointer towards liver cell carcinoma. Confusion is most likely to arise from *liver abscess* or metastasis from *melanoma* but the clinical circumstances will usually be distinctive.

The affinity of certain inflammatory and infective

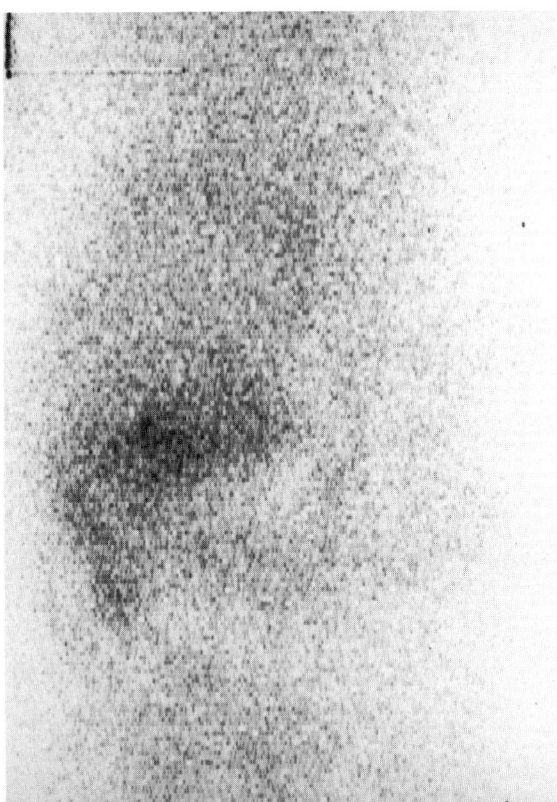

Fig. 66.34 Post-operative sub-hepatic abscess. ^{67}Gallium citrate at 24 hrs. There is some colonic activity and a focus of increased activity over the abscess.

lesions for ^{67}Ga citrate has already been mentioned as a disadvantage. This can be turned to advantage, however, when there is a high clinical suspicion of infection, e.g. pyrexia of unknown origin or suspected *subphrenic abscess* (Fig. 66.34). The technique is highly reliable and it is usually possible to distinguish liver and spleen activity from the activity in the abscess. It is more reliable than the standard radiological techniques and is probably more reliable than ultrasonic scanning in the left subphrenic area. It is an advantage to use both techniques in doubtful instances.

Indium

1. ^{113}Indium^{m} is produced from a ^{113}Sn generator which has a half-life of 115 days. ^{113}In has a half-life of 1·7 hours and its main emission peak is 393 keV, making it more suitable for a linear scanner than a gamma camera. Ionic ^{113}I^{m} is bound to transferrin, with a half-life of 8–10 hours after which it becomes localized in bone marrow. There is no significant excretion by the kidneys or the gut. If the plasma transferrin is saturated with iron indium is unable to bind to it and is excreted by the kidneys.

Colloid preparations of ^{113}In^{m} are used to scan the liver and particle preparations to scan the lungs.

2. ^{111}In is cyclotron produced, has a half-life of 2·8 days and emits gamma photons at 173 and 247 keV. Indium DTPA chelate is now the compound of choice for encephalography and cisternography, because the relatively long half-life enables satisfactory images to be produced at 48 and 72 hours. The counting statistics are much better than with ^{131}I-labelled albumen and are comparable with those of ^{99}Tc^{m}-labelled albumen. The risk of asceptic meningitis is much less than with other compounds.

Indium-111 is also used for isotope lymphography.

3. Indium-111 has been used to detect tumours, both in the ionic form and attached to bleomycin. The tumour specificity of the latter is in doubt, as there is evidence to suggest that the indium becomes attached *in vivo* to transferrin in the same way that ionic indium is attached.

CARDIOLOGY

Developments in the management of coronary artery disease have brought to the fore the need for objective methods of measuring regional myocardial perfusion and of detecting myocardial ischaemia.

Acute myocardial infarct scintigraphy

The ideal compounds are those that are taken up by myocardial infarcts giving a positive image. The most useful complex is ^{99}Tc^{m} pyrophosphate, a bone-scanning agent which monitors the transfer of calcium into the infarct. The optimum time for scanning is 90 minutes after intravenous injection of 10 mCi of ^{99}Tc^{m} pyrophosphate. Anterior views of the precordium are essential and may be supplemented by left anterior oblique and lateral views. In the normal there is symmetrical activity about the midline over the sternum and ribs. The activity is increased over an infarct (Fig. 66.35) and the size of the abnormal area is related to that of the infarct. Abnormal activity can be detected within 12 hours of infarction and is maximal during the next 7 days. Then it returns slowly to normal. Persistent or increased activity suggests an extension of the infarct.

False negative results are uncommon unless the infarct is on the diaphragmatic surface of the heart and usually occur if the scan has been done too soon after infarction or too late after infarction. Some infarcts are too small to be detected, but others are so large that there is insufficient collateral circulation round their margins to deliver radionuclide. Unexpected positive scans may be obtained from *sternal* and *rib fractures* due to external cardiac massage, *multiple skeletal metastasis*, *carcinoma of the breast*, etc. These should be eliminated by careful radiographic and clinical assessment.

The main applications of this form of scanning are:

1. In the assessment of obscure chest pain
2. Suspected myocardial infarction where the e.c.g. is

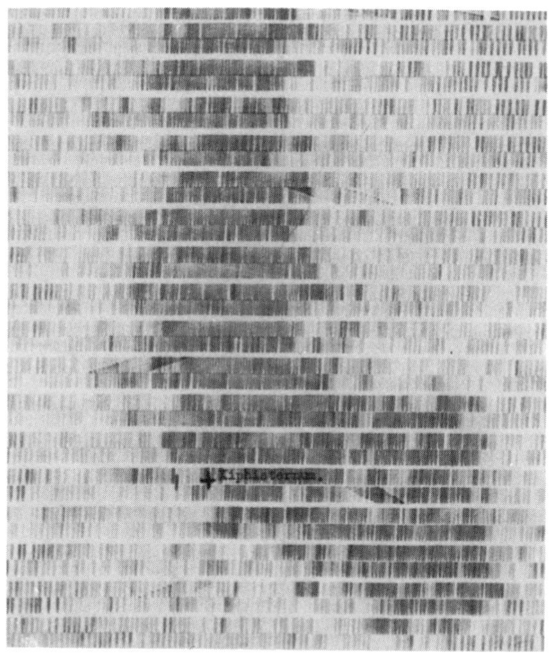

Fig. 66.35 Myocardial infarction. $^{99}Tc^{m}$-pyrophosphate scan of praecordium. There is normal sternal activity, and abnormal high activity to the left of the lower sternum, in a large myocardial infarct.

already known to be abnormal, or where serum enzymes are elevated for other causes

3. In the assessment of unstable angina.

The latter application is an important development as a positive scan may be encountered in severe angina before there is evidence of overt infarction. Patients especially at risk can be selected for energetic treatment.

Myocardial perfusion scanning

The compounds used are analogues of potassium, the most promising being thallium-201. Its main radioactive disintegration are from characteristic X-rays at 69 to 83 keV and it is concentrated in normal myocardium rather better than potassium. Myocardial activity is flow dependent and a normal pattern is a uniform horse-shoe or doughnut shape with a central zone of diminished activity representing the left ventricular cavity. Usually the wall of the right ventricle cannot be identified. A myocardial infarction creates a corresponding defect. In the normal myocardial blood flow increases uniformly during exercise, but in coronary artery insufficiency the increase in blood flow is much less especially when the lumen of the arteries is reduced to 50 per cent. If the scan is repeated after exercise on a treadmill myocardial ischaemia is shown by deficient zones which were not present on the rest scan (Fig. 66.36). Deficient zones present at rest and after exercise indicate infarction. These tests help to distinguish myocardial pain due to infarction from that due to ischaemia, and from chest pain that is not myocardial in origin.

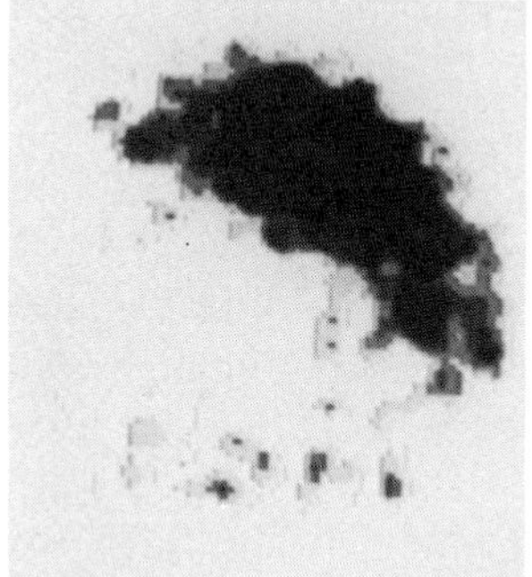

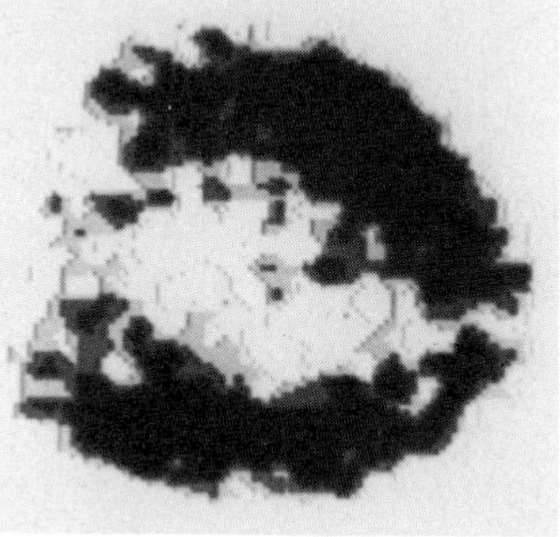

Fig. 66.36 Myocardial ischaemia. ^{201}Thallium citrate. Left. Anterior image after exercise showing a large inferior defect. Right. 3 hours later, at equilibrium. Normal image. Thus there is exercise induced transient myocardial ischaemia.

Coronary artery perfusion scanning

The use of this technique is severely limited by the fact that the radioactive tracer is injected directly into the coronary circulation at the time of angiography. One to two millicuries of $^{99}Tc^{m}$ microspheres (10 to 40 μ) are injected into the left coronary artery and a similar activity of $^{113}In^{m}$ microspheres or ^{131}I microspheres are injected into the right coronary artery. The scan is done immediately. Defects are caused by myocardial scarring or infarction, but severe stenosis can cause streaming and gives rise to irregular activity. There is good correlation between these defects and areas of abnormal ventricular contraction demonstrated by contrast ventriculography.

Flow studies

Xenon-133 dissolved in saline is injected into the coronary artery after coronary angiography. Xenon diffuses rapidly into the parenchyma of the heart, and its washout rate is directly proportional to the myocardial blood flow. If this washout is measured by rapid sequence images using a gamma camera crystal on which regions of interest can subsequently be selected, it is possible to generate curves from which the myocardial blood flow can be calculated in ml per min per 100 g.

$^{81}Kr^{m}$ has been developed in the research field for studying myocardial perfusion. Unfortunately it is delivered to the coronary sinuses via a catheter which limits its application to patients already being catheterized, but its brief half life permits moment-to-moment perfusion changes to be perceived, and it has promising applications in the assessment of coronary artery lesions and the follow up of by-pass grafting.

Multiple gated images

Data acquired and analysed by computer can be reconstituted to form cine film of a cardiac cycle. The method of choice is to label red cells *in vivo* by giving stannous monofluorophosphate intravenously followed in 30 min

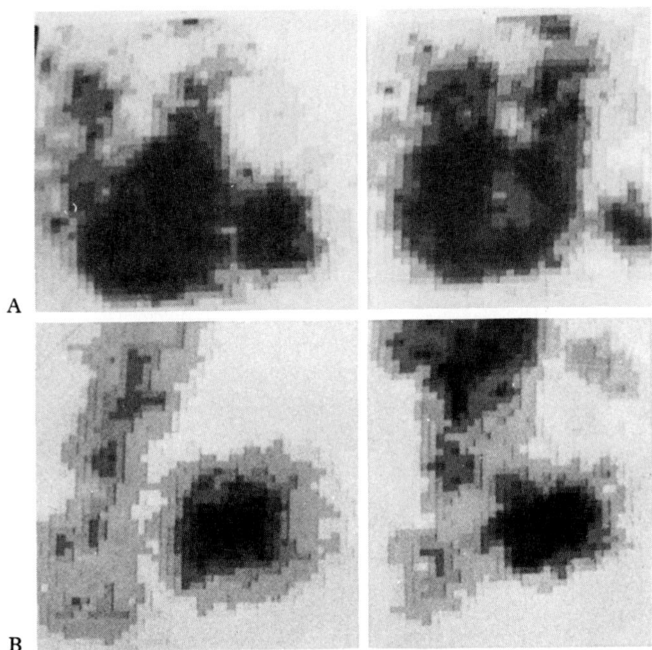

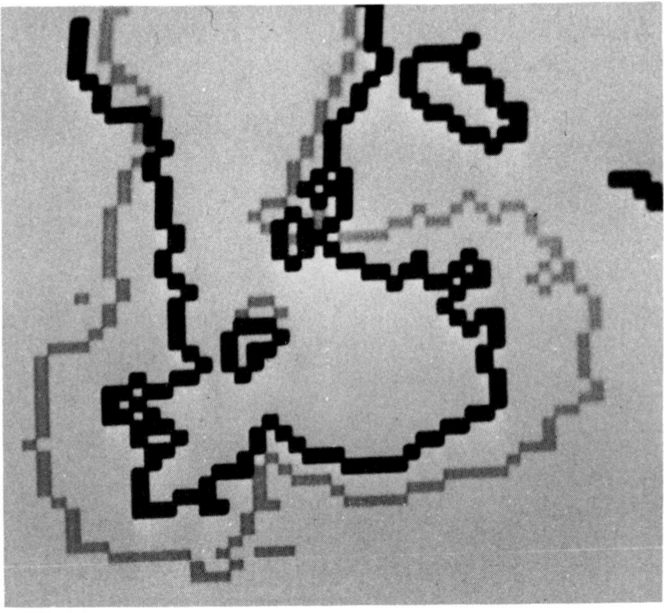

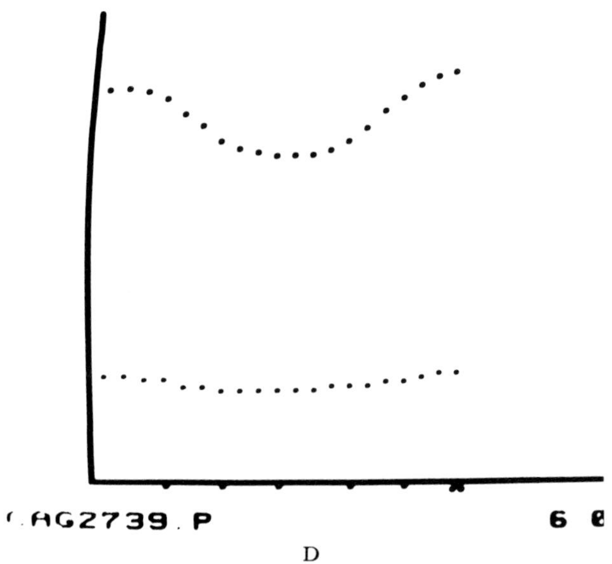

Fig. 66.37 (A) Isotope cardiogram: left, end diastolic frame; right, end systolic frame. There is good contraction of the left ventricle. (B) Isotope cardiogram in L anterior oblique projection showing poor contraction of a dilated L ventricle. (C) End systolic (dark) and end diastolic (light) edges have been drawn by the computer. (D) L ventricular activity curve generated by completing a region of interest in B. The ejection fraction was 30 per cent.

by 10–15 mCi $^{99}Tc^{m}$ as sodium pertechnetate. In the L anterior oblique projection, with an E.C.G. linked to the computer data are stored over some 500 cardiac cycles. The R–R interval is divided into a series of 60 msec intervals and the data from corresponding intervals in successive cycles are summed to form a single image sequence. This sequence is displayed in cine mode, so that the ventricular contraction pattern can be analysed in detail (Fig. 66.37). Regions of *ventricular dyskinesia* and *aneurysm* can be detected safely and accurately. Ventricular volume is proportional to ventricular count rate and volume changes can be demonstrated by drawing a region of interest round the ventricle and generating a curve showing change of volume. End systolic (ES) and end diastolic (ED) count rates are read from the curve and if the background activity (B) is estimated during systole in the extra-ventricular area of the region of interest, the *ejection fraction* is given by the formula:

$$\frac{ED - ES}{ED - B}$$

Electrocardiogram-linked myocardial function studies

At equilibrium, the count rate over any given region is proportional to the volume containing the tracer. If a blood pool tracer such as $^{99}Tc^{m}$ albumen is used, that volume is the volume of circulating blood in the region of interest. Following the injection of this tracer into the circulation rapid sequence images over the heart may be gathered at intervals as short as 50 milliseconds. By linking the record to a synchronous e.c.g. record it is possible to build up images of the cardiac outline during systole and diastole so that end diastolic volumes and stroke volumes can be calculated. Movement of the myocardial wall can be charted by computer, which indicates those areas in which the count rate does not differ significantly between systole and diastole. Good correlation has been claimed between this method and contrast ventriculography and if these findings are substantiated the technique, although expensive, will be a very important hazard free advance in the assessment of patients with myocardial disease.

Rapid sequence isotope cardiography

The quality of the images obtained by the above technique is good enough to identify individual heart chambers and valuable information can be obtained about the flow of blood within the heart. In congenital heart disease the sequence of filling may indicate atrial septal defect, or Fallot's tetralogy, or transposition of the great vessels, etc. Time intensity curves over individual chambers and over the lung fields can be used to detect intracardiac shunts and in the best hands shunts as small as 1:2 pulmonary:systemic ratio have been detected. In acquired heart disease the signs of obstruction and incompetence at the usual valve sites can be shown and filling defects due to intracardiac myxoma have been identified.

These cardiological techniques have not yet stood the test of time in the way that contrast techniques have, but apart from intracoronary injection, they are essentially non-invasive and can be repeated without hazard even in seriously ill patients. They are useful in the following circumstances:

1. *In myocardial disease.* True myocardial disease can be distinguished from other diseases with similar symptoms and infarction or threatened infarction can be distinguished from ischaemia. This is particularly important when the e.c.g. is already abnormal because of an earlier infarction. In known myocardial disease the regional function of the myocardium can be measured and this is often a vital step in the management especially when surgery is being contemplated. The results of surgery and medical treatment can be monitored without hazard.

2. *To monitor the progress of disease* both before and after surgery. Frequent contrast studies are not practicable whereas repeated non-invasive tests are free from physical hazard. The radiation hazard, though small will have to be considered when serial studies are being done, especially in congenital heart disease.

3. *As a screening test.* In the newborn it is important and sometimes difficult to distinguish suspected congenital heart disease from respiratory disorders and it would be of considerable benefit if a simple test enabled the more hazardous tests to be avoided in seriously ill infants. In adults rapid sequence isotope angiography has been used as an early line of investigation of mediastinal enlargement, in order to distinguish aneurysm from solid tumours.

THYROID

The thyroid gland arises from the thyroglossal duct which extends caudally from the pharynx to the neck. The adult gland lies in front of the thyroid cartilage, but may lie anywhere from the base of the tongue along the line of the thyroglossal duct. A normal gland consists of two lobes joined by a central isthmus from which a small pyramidal lobe occasionally arises, usually on the left.

The ability of the thyroid gland to trap iodine or iodine analogues such as $^{99}Tc^{m}$-pertechnatate form the basis of a large number of thyroid function tests, as well as of thyroid scanning. The details of thyroid function tests are beyond the scope of this chapter which will be confined to the uses of thyroid imaging.

The isotopes in common use for thyroid scanning are:

1. ^{131}I. This was the first compound to be used and is still very popular. Its main disadvantage is the relatively high radiation dose which makes it unacceptable for paediatric use. The usual activity in an adult is 50 μCi.

2. ^{125}I. Its main disadvantage is the lower energy of its emission. This is not usually a problem in thyroid scanning except when the thyroid is retrosternal.

3. ^{123}I. This is the most suitable radionuclide physically. It has a relatively short half-life and a low radiation dose. Unfortunately it is produced by cyclotron, has a half-life of 13 hours and tends to be contaminated by other iodine isotopes.

4. $^{99}Tc^{m}$. The pertechnatate ion is trapped by the thyroid in a similar way to iodine, because they are analogues, but the pertechnatate ion does not take part in any further synthesis and this is a relative disadvantage. The usual activity given to an adult is 2·5 mCi. Technetium differs from iodine in that the stomach is the critical organ for absorbed dose. Scanning begins 20 minutes after intravenous injection.

Whichever isotope is used, careful clinical assessment is important preliminary to all thyroid scanning. This includes palpation of the neck to ensure that all palpable masses are included in the area of the scan. Because the thyroid is such a small organ good resolution is vital, and in order to achieve a satisfactory resolution below 1 cm it is usually necessary to use a 3-in crystal with a high resolution collimator. Alternatively a gamma camera using a pinhole collimator or converging collimator should be used.

The normal thyroid image shows two lateral lobes linked by a narrow isthmus. Occasionally the isthmus may not be visible, or it may constitute the bulk of the gland. A pyramidal lobe arising from the isthmus is sometimes found.

Ectopic gland

Thyroid tissue may occur anywhere along the line of the thyroglossal duct and usually there is then no functioning thyroid tissue in the normal site. The absence of normally sited thyroid and the presence of abnormally sited thyroid can be shown convincingly by scanning. It is equally important to show normal thyroid uptake in the thyroglossal fistula. A lateral scan may be the best way of showing the upper part of the neck and the region of the foramen caecum.

Retrosternal thyroid

Sometimes the thyroid is situated in the superior anterior mediastinum and may appear as a retrosternal mass on a chest radiograph. Usually it is attached to cervical thyroid tissue but may be the only functioning thyroid tissue present. It is less active than normal thyroid and ^{131}I is the preferred scanning agent. A retrosternal thyroid that becomes cystic does not always take up ^{131}I. The nature of a retrosternal mass sometimes remains uncertain despite exhaustive radiological investigation, and a positive scan is an important and simple discriminatory test.

Thyroid nodules

In a *hot nodule* the activity is greater than that of the surrounding thyroid tissue. Usually this is due to *autonomous thyroid tissue* and there may be clinical signs of thyrotoxicosis. Less commonly it may be due to *hyperfunction of normal thyroid* tissue in a gland that has been damaged by surgery or radiation etc. Rarely it is due to *anatomic variant*. Alternatively the activity over a nodule may be equal to that in the remainder of the gland and these nodules are rarely significant clinically. It is very rare for *carcinoma* to accumulate as much activity as surrounding tissue but authentic cases have been reported. A *cold nodule* is one in which there is a defect of activity corresponding to the palpable nodule. The more important possibilities are *adenoma*, which may be cystic or solid, and *carcinoma*. About 35 per cent prove to be adenomas and the scan itself is not a satisfactory discriminatory test. Further studies using selenium uptake and gallium uptake have not proved satisfactory, and alternative methods have included ultrasound technique and cyst puncture. Other causes of cold nodules include focal *thyroiditis*, *abscess*, *reticulosis*, *parathyroid adenoma*.

Carcinoma of the thyroid

Carcinoma of the thyroid may be:

1. Well-differentiated papillary, follicular or mixed. This is the commonest type. In the majority of patients, metastases take up ^{131}I provided normal thyroid tissue is ablated.
2. Poorly differentiated. These are commoner in older people and have a poor prognosis. Metastases rarely take up ^{131}I.
3. Medullary carcinoma. About 5 per cent of thyroid carcinomas are medullary and may be hormonally active. They tend to be familial and to be associated with other endocrine tumours. Metastases do not take up ^{131}I.

Over half of all carcinomas of the thyroid produce a cold nodule on a scan, and carcinoma is the commonest cause of such a nodule. Occasionally the thyroid scan is normal in carcinoma of the thyroid. Thus the scan is not an absolute discriminator of carcinoma of the thyroid but helps to determine the probability especially if the nodule is cold. Further attempts to confirm the diagnosis have been made using ^{75}Se-methionine which is disappointing, and ultrasonic scanning to detect cysts, which is more promising.

^{131}I scanning is very helpful in detecting metastases from known thyroid cancer. About three quarters of well differentiated metastases will show some uptake of radioiodine following total ablation of normal thyroid tissue by surgery and/or a large dose of ^{131}I. Serial body scans are used to locate metastases, determine the activity required to treat them and follow their response to treatment.

Thyroiditis

1. Chronic thyroiditis (Hashimoto's thyroiditis) is relatively common and causes an enlarged hard gland in patients who are asymptomatic or mildly hypothyroid or hyperthyroid. The scan appearances may vary from absent uptake to diffusely increased uptake.
2. Reidl's thyroiditis is rare and mimics carcinoma so that the diagnosis is usually made after operation.
3. Acute and subacute thyroiditis are usually diagnosed clinically and the scan appearances are not important.

ADRENAL GLANDS

The clinical syndromes associated with tumours of the adrenal glands are usually distinctive and in most cases radiological investigations are directed to locating the tumour, and its metastases if it is malignant. Among the problems that occur are the location of aldosterone secreting *adenomas* (*Conn's tumours*) because these are usually very small, and the distinction between adrenal cortical adenoma and hyperplasia. The development of scanning techniques to apply to these problems is based on the uptake of cholesterol by the adrenal cortex, so that labelled cholesterol is used to detect physiological changes in the glands. At first ^{131}I was used as the labelling agent, but most recently ^{79}Se-cholesterol is used with the advantage of lower radiation hazard. 1 mCi or so is administered intravenously and images are taken daily for 5 days. Initially there is hepatic and biliary as well as adrenal activity, but the latter gradually becomes dominant, the R adrenal activity being slightly higher than the L. The demonstration can be improved by computer enhancement and by doing a renal scan to aid localization.

Increased cortical function gives rise to increased activity and in *Cushing's syndrome* the asymmetry of adenoma is distinct from the bilateral abnormality of *hyperplasia*. In Conn's tumour there is intense localizing activity on the side of the lesion, but probably beyond the confines of the tumour itself. Activity is diminished on the side of any tumour that does not metabolize cholesterol, e.g. carcinoma. Also it is diminished in the presence of a *medullary tumour*, when the clinical syndrome will usually have led to venography or arteriography.

INTESTINAL TRACT

1. Salivary glands

Pertechnetate is secreted by the salivary glands and suitable images can be obtained with a gamma camera during an hour or so after intravenous injection. Suitable time intervals are 2, 4, 8, 12, 20, 30 and 60 minutes. The activity is symmetrical over the glands but often higher over the submandibular gland. Activity usually reaches a peak in the glands between 10 and 20 minutes and in the buccal cavity between 20 and 40 minutes. Decreased activity is found in all neoplasms, except Warthin's tumours in which the activity is increased and in areas of focal destruction of acinar tissue. Scanning is a useful supplement to sialography in the investigation of suspected neoplasm, and in the assessment of sialectasis, xerostomia and Sjogren's syndrome.

2. Stomach

The stomach is the target organ following the administration of pertechnatate because of secretion by the chief cells of the gastric mucosa. Gastric activity due to free pertechnatate can be a pitfall for the unwary in any technique using a $^{99}Tc^{m}$ compound. Following partial gastrectomy, residual gastric mucosa can be detected by scanning.

3. Ectopic gastric mucosa

Meckel's diverticulum is notoriously difficult to detect but if it contains gastric mucosa, abdominal scanning at intervals from 30 minutes to 2 hours after injection of sodium pertechnetate is a very reliable method of detection. It is more reliable and has less radiation hazard than barium studies.

The oesophagus sometimes contains ectopic gastric mucosa that gives rise to peptic ulceration. This also can be shown by $^{99}Tc^{m}Ox$ scanning.

THE SPLEEN

$^{99}Tc^{m}$-S colloid is the agent of choice for spleen scintigraphy, because of the ease of preparation and the speed of examination. The high activity in the adjacent liver is not usually a disadvantage, except when it is important to detect ectopic or accessory splenic tissue, in recurrence of hypersplenism after splenectomy. The agent of choice is then ^{51}Cr-labelled heat-damaged erythrocytes, which are sequestered in the spleen. This agent can be used also for physiologic studies of the splenic function.

The size of the spleen is best determined from the lateral view, and is normally less than 100 cm^2. Splenic enlargement can be shown on occasion before it is detectable clinically.

Cysts, tumours, abscesses of the spleen create cold areas but these causes cannot be differentiated from each other. Defects may be caused by deposits of reticulosis, but unfortunately relatively large lesions may be overlooked, and the value of spleen scanning in these conditions is less than was at one time thought. Metastasis to the spleen is not common but may occur in advanced disease. Scanning helps to distinguish liver from spleen as a cause of a left upper quadrant mass.

Splenic injury will cause defects in the image due to haematoma or separation of the splenic moieties in more severe injury. When the clinical indications do not call for immediate splenectomy the conservative management is considerably aided by serial scanning.

LYMPHATIC SYSTEM

Direct lymphography is an exacting technique which provides an unequalled demonstration of the distribution and pattern of the lymphatics and lymph nodes.

Subcutaneous injection of labelled colloid particles into the webs of the toes has been used to show pelvic and abdominal lymph nodes and into the rectus sheath to show the internal mammary nodes.

PARATHYROID GLANDS

Selenomethionine is taken up by the parathyroid and thyroid glands, as well as by the pancreas and liver. Relative parathyroid accumulation is improved if thyroid accumulation is suppressed by sodium iodide, or Lugol's iodine.

Parathyroid activity is at its highest 20 to 40 minutes after intravenous injection of 250 microcuries of ^{75}Se, and the scan should therefore be done during this time. Normal parathyroid activity is too similar to that of surrounding tissues for it to be detectable, but some adenomas and hyperplasias can be recognized.

The value of the present technique is severely limited by the number of false negatives and false positives that occur. Multiple sampling of the neck veins to estimate their content of parathyroid hormone, and inferior thyroid arteriography are more reliable.

THE TESTES

Usually the clinical differentiation between *orchitis* and *torsion* is clear cut but as the management is fundamentally different it is useful to have a reliable discriminatory test.

The patient is placed under a gamma camera with the scrotum resting on a supporting bandage. 5 mCi $^{99}Tc^{m}$ pertechnetate is injected intravenously and a perfusion study is done followed by a static image. Increased activity on the side of the lesion favours an inflammatory cause whereas decreased activity indicates torsion. The test can be used to follow the post-operative recovery of acute torsion.

REFERENCES AND SUGGESTIONS FOR FURTHER READING

AGNEW, J. E., MAZE, M. & MITCHELL, C. J. (1976) Review article. Pancreatic scanning. *British Journal of Radiology*, **49**, 979–995.

BEKERMAN, C., GENANT, H. K., HOFFER, P. P., KOZIN, F. & GINSBERG, M. (1976) Radionuclide imaging of the bones and joints of the hand. *Radiology*, **118**, 653–659.

BERQUIST, T. H., NOLAN, N. G., STEPHENS, D. H. & CARLSON, H. C. (1976) Specificity of ^{99m}Tc-pertecnetate in scintigraphic diagnosis of Meckel's diverticulum. *Journal of Nuclear Medicine*, **17**, 465–469.

BONTE, F. J., PARKEY, R. W. & GRAHAM, K. D. (1974) A new method for radionuclide imaging of myocardial infarcts. *Radiology*, **110**, 473–474.

DUNLOP, J. A., MCLANE, R. C. & ROPER, J. J. (1975) The retained gastric antrum. *Radiology*, **117**, 371–372.

DUSZYNSKI, D. O., KUHU, J. P., AFSHANI, E. & RIDDLESBERGER, M. M. (1975) Early radionuclide diagnosis of acute osteomyelitis. *Radiology*, **117**, 337–340.

EGE, G. N. (1976) Internal mammary lymphoscintigraphy. *Radiology*, **118**, 101–107.

FRANKEL, R. S., RICHMAN, S. D., LEVENSON, S. M. & JOHNSTON, G. S. (1975) Renal localization of gallium-67 citrate. *Radiology*, **114**, 393–397.

FRICK, M. P., LOKEN, M. K., GOLDBERG, M. E. & SIMMONS, R. L. (1976) Use of ^{99m}Tc sulphur colloid in evaluation of renal transplant complications. *Journal of Nuclear Medicine*, **16**, 181–183.

GEORGE, E. A., CODD, J. E., NEWTON, W. T., HAIBACH, H. & DONATI, R. M. (1976) Comparative evaluation of renal transplant rejection with radioiodinated fibrinogen, ^{99}Tc^{m} sulphur colloid and ^{67}Ga-citrate. *Journal of Nuclear Medicine*, **17**, 175–179.

GESLIEN, G. E., PINSKY, S. M., POTH, R. K. & JOHNSON, M. C. (1976) The sensitivity and specificity of ^{99}Tc^{m}-sulphur colloid liver imaging in diffuse hepatocellular disease. *Radiology*, **118**, 115–119.

GORIS, M. L., DASPIT, S. G., WALTER, J. P., MCRAE, J. & LAMB, J. (1977) Applications of ventilation lung imaging with ^{81m}krypton. *Radiology*, **122**, 399–403.

HANELIN, L. G., USZLER, J. M. & SOMMER, D. G. (1975) Liver scan 'Hot Spot' in hepatic veno occlusive disease. *Radiology*, **117**, 637–638.

JENNER, R. E., CLARKE, M. B. & HOWARD, E. R. (1976) Liver and gall-bladder imaging with ^{99}Tc^{m} DHTA and ^{99}Tc^{m} PG. *British Journal of Radiology*, **49**, 852–857.

KENNY, R. W., ACKERY, D. M., FLEMING, J. S., GODDARD, B. A. & GRANT, R. W. (1975) Deconvolution analysis of the scintillation camera renogram. *British Journal of Radiology*, **48**, 481–486.

KIRCHNER, P. T., JAMES, A. E., REBA, R. C. & WAGNER, H. N. (1975) Patterns of excretion of radioactive chelates in obstructive uropathy. *Radiology*, **114**, 655–661.

LAVENDER, J. P. (Ed.) (1978) Clinical and experimental applications of Krypton 81^{m}. *British Journal of Radiology*.

LAVENDER, J. P., EVANS, I. M. A., ARNOT, R., BOWRING, S., DOYLE, F. H., JOPLIN, G. F. & MACINTYRE, I. (1977) A comparison of radiograph and radioisotope scanning in the detection of Paget's disease and in the assessment of response to human calcitonin. *British Journal of Radiology*, **50**, 243–250.

LEVENSON, S. M., WARREN, R. D., RICHMAN, S. D., JOHNSTON, G. S. & CHABNER, B. A. (1976) Abnormal pulmonary gallium accumulation in *P. carinii* pneumonia. *Radiology*, **119**, 395–398.

LISBONA, R. & ROSENTHALL, L. (1977) Observations on the sequential use of ^{99}Tc^{m} phosphates complex and ^{57}Ga imaging in osteomyelitis, cellichitis, and septic arthritis. *Radiology*, **123**, 123–129.

MAILIN, T. R., MOORE, J. S. & SHAFER, R. B. (1976) Evaluation of the posterior flow study in brain scintigraphy. *Journal of Nuclear Medicine*, **17**, 13–16.

MCIVOR, J., ANDERSON, D. R., BRITT, R. P. & DOVEY, P. (1975) Comparison of ^{125}I-labelled fibrinogen uptake and venography in the detection of recent deep vein thrombosis in the legs. *British Journal of Radiology*, **48**, 1013–1018.

MERRICK, M. V. (1975) Review article—bone scanning. *British Journal of Radiology*, **48**, 327–351.

NISHIYAMA, H., SODD, V. J., ADOLPH, R. J., SAENGER, E. J., LEWIS, J. J. & GABEL, M. (1976) Intercomparison of myocardial imaging agents ^{201}TI, ^{129}Cr, ^{43}K, ^{81}Rb. *Journal of Nuclear Medicine*, **17**, 880–889.

O'REILLY, P. H., SHIELDS, R. A., TESTA, H. J. (1979) *Nuclear Medicine in Urology and Nephrology*. Butterworths, London.

PARKEY, R. W., BONTE, F. J., STOKELY, E. M., LEWIS, S. E., GRAHAM, K. D., BUJA, L. M. & WILLERSON, J. T. (1976) Acute myocardial infarction images with ^{99m}Tc-stannous pyrophosphates and ^{201}TI: a clinical evaluation. *Journal of Nuclear Medicine*, **17**, 771–779.

PATERSON, A. H. G. & MCCREADY, V. R. (1975) Review article—tumour imaging radiopharmaceuticals. *British Journal of Radiology*, **48**, 520–531.

PATERSON, A. H. G., TAYLOR, D. M. & MCCREADY, V. R. (1975) A clinical comparison of the tumour imaging radiopharmaceuticals ^{67}Gallium citrate and ^{111}Indium-labelled bleomycin. *British Journal of Radiology*, **48**, 832–842.

RIGO, P., STRAUSS, H. W. & PITT, B. (1975) The combined use of gated cardiac blood pool scanning and myocardial imaging with ^{43}K in the evaluation of patients with myocardial infarction. *Radiology*, **115**, 387–391.

ROSENTHALL, L., SHAFFER, E. A., LISBONA, R., PARE, R. (1978) Diagnosis of hepatobiliary disease by ^{99m}Tc-HIDA cholescintigraphy. *Radiology*, **126**, 467–474.

SCHEIBEL, R. L., MOORE, R., KORBULY, D., OVITT, T. W., PAYNE, J. T., TUNA, N. & AMPLATZ, K. (1975) Regional myocardial blood flow measurements in the evaluation of patients with coronary artery disease. *Radiology*, **115**, 379–386.

SECKER WALKER, R. H., RESNICK, L., KUNZ, H., PARKER, J. A., HILL, R. L., POTCHEN, E. J. (1973) Measurement of L ventricular ejection fraction. *Journal of Nuclear Medicine*, **14**, 798–802.

SILBERSTEIN, E. B. (1976) Causes of abnormalities reported in nuclear medicine testing. *Journal of Nuclear Medicine*, **17**, 229–232.

SNOW, J. H. (1979) Comparison of scintigraphy, sonography and computed tomography in the evaluation of hepatic neoplasm. *American Journal of Roentgenology*, **132**, 915–918.

SORENSON, S. G., HAMILTON, G. W., WILLIAMS, D. L., RITCHIE, J. L. (1979) R wave synchronised blood pool imaging. *Radiology*, **131**, 473–478.

SUBRAMANIAN, G., MCAFEE, J. G. & BELL, E. G. (1971) New ^{99}Tc^{m}-labelled radiopharmaceuticals for renal imaging. *Nuclear Medicine*, **12**, 399.

TER-POGOSSIAN, M. M., PHELPS, M. E., HOGGMAN, E. J. & MULLANI, N. A. (1975) A positron-emission transaxial tomograph for nuclear imaging (PETT). *Radiology*, **114**, 89–95.

TRONCONE, L., GALLI, G., SALVO, D., BARBARINO, A. & BONOMO, L. (1977) Radioisotopic study of the adrenal glands using ^{131}I-19-Iodocholesterol. *British Journal of Radiology*, **50**, 340–349.

WACKEN, F. J., SCHOOL, J. B., SOKOLE, E. B., SAMSON, G., NIFTRIK, G. J. C., LIE, K. L., DUIRER, D. & WELLENS, J. J. J. (1975) Non-invasive visualisation of acute myocardial infarction in man with thallium-201. *British Heart Journal*, **37**, 741–744.

WILLERSON, J. T., PARKEY, R. W. & BONTE, F. J. (1975) Acute sub-endocardial myocardial infarction in patients. Its detection by technetium ^{99}m stannous pyrophosphate myocardial scintigrams. *Circulation*, **51**, 436–441.

WILLIAMS, E. S. (1974) Adverse reactions to radiopharmaceuticals. *British Journal of Radiology*, **47**, 54–59.

WYBURN, J. R. (1974) Human breast milk excretion of radionuclides following administration of radiopharmaceuticals. *Journal of Nuclear Medicine*, **2**, 115–117.

CHAPTER 67

ULTRASOUND (1) PRINCIPLES: GENERAL: CARDIAC

Ultrasound is a form of energy which consists of mechanical vibrations occurring at a frequency too high to be detected by the human ear. Human beings can hear sound of frequencies up to 20,000 cycles per second (1,000 cycles per second = 1 kilohertz = 1 KHz); sound generated at frequencies above this level is therefore ultrasound. Frequencies of between 1 and 15 MHz (one megahertz = one million hertz = one MHz) are used in medicine. Ultrasound differs from X-radiation in that it does not produce ionization.

Generation of ultrasound. Ultrasound is produced and detected by transducers which are substances that have the property of being able to convert one form of energy into another (Fig. 67.1). Transducers are made of materials which are mechanically deformed when an electric voltage is applied to them. This is the direct piezo-electric (pressure-electric) effect. The degree of mechanical deformation is directly proportional, within the limits of the material, to the magnitude of the applied voltage. In addition, if a mechanical stress is applied to a piezo-electric material, a voltage will be generated across it in direct proportion to the applied stress. This is known as the converse piezo-electric effect (Fig. 67.1). Quartz is a naturally occurring crystal which is piezo-electric. A group of artificial materials, known as polarized polycrystalline ferroelectrics have strong piezo-electric properties, examples of which are lead or calcium barium titanate. The transducer substance most frequently used in medical ultrasonic apparatus is lead zirconate titanate, a polarized solid solution with very strong piezo-electric effects.

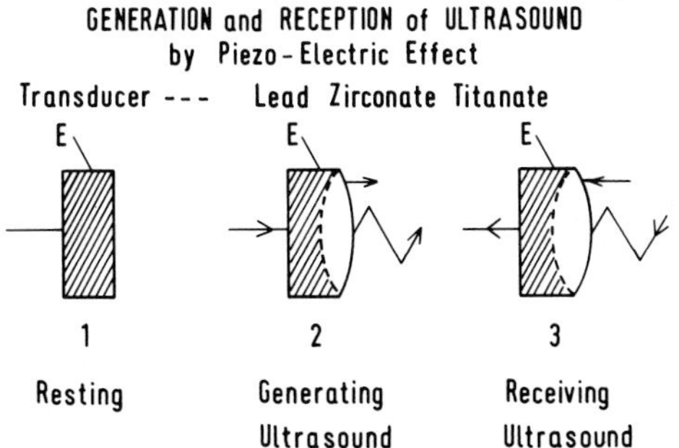

Fig. 67.1 Generation and reception of ultrasound.
1—The transducer (hatched) coated with conducting material is in a resting phase.
2—A voltage (→) is applied to the transducer surface. The transducer resonates in response and it produces ultrasound from its surface (⁄\/↗) (direct piezo-electric effect).
3—A pulse of ultrasound (⁄\/↙) strikes the surface of the transducer which resonates as a result. A voltage (←) is generated on the transducer surface (converse piezo-electric effect).

In medical diagnosis a narrow beam of ultrasound is used; it is generated by a disc of lead zirconate titanate excited by two electrodes, one on each parallel surface of the disc. The disc resonates at its fundamental frequency depending on its size and the properties of the piezo-electric material. The thinner the disc generally speaking, the higher the frequency of the generated ultrasound. Ultrasound waves are produced from both surfaces of the disc. In order to produce a directional beam the transducer disc is mounted at one end of a cylindrical tube into which are incorporated materials which damp down the ultrasonic waves arising from the back surface of the transducer. The tube, damping material and transducer with its electrical connections are known as the probe. The beam of ultrasound is focussed either by using a concave surfaced transducer disc or by placing the ultrasonic equivalent of an optical lens over the flat surface of the transducer. Weak focussing to about 10 centimetres is most frequently used in medicine. The probe functions also as a receiver of the returning ultrasound echoes. These set the transducer vibrating and the voltages generated on its surface are amplified and used to produce a signal on a cathode-ray oscilloscope. Transducer discs are between 1 and 2 centimetres in diameter and about 1 millimetre thick.

Ultrasound may be generated as a continuous beam; for this, two transducers mounted side by side are required, one to produce and the other to receive back the ultrasound (Fig. 67.2). This method is used to detect movement by the Doppler effect such as blood flowing in an artery or vein or the fetal heart. Ultrasound may

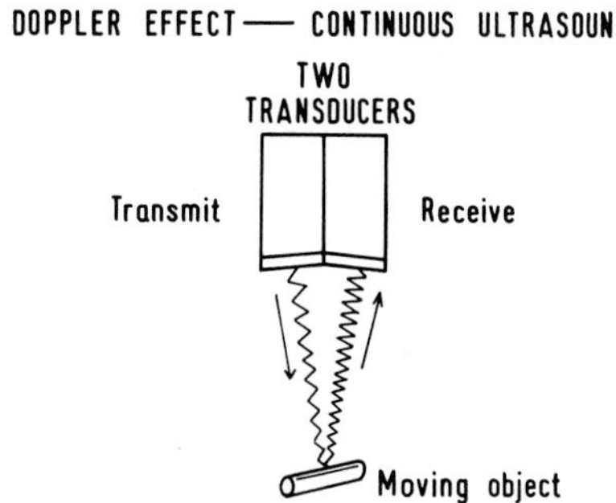

Fig. 67.2 Doppler effect. Two transducers are mounted side by side and inclined towards each other. One transmits and the other receives the continuous ultrasound beam reflected from a moving object. The reflected ultrasound is at a different frequency from that of the generated ultrasound.

also be generated in very short pulses repeated at a high rate. This technique is known as the pulse-echo method and it is used to produce static sectional images of internal structures or time-position tracings of the movement of certain internal structures such as the valves of the heart.

Frequency and wave length. The frequency at which ultrasound is generated is inversely proportional to the wave length of the beam. The frequency affects the passage of ultrasound through the soft tissues. The higher the frequency, the less will the beam penetrate into the body but the resulting image will be sharp in outline. The converse also applies; the longer the wavelength, the greater the penetration into the body but the sharpness of the image will be reduced. Thus a compromise has to be reached to ensure adequate penetration of the beam into the patient and at the same time produce optimal sharpness of the resultant image. In addition ultrasound can only differentiate between two interfaces close together if there is a distance of more than half the wavelength of the incident beam between them. It is important therefore to use wavelengths of 1·5 millimetres or less so that interfaces separated by 0·75 millimetres can be visualized. For abdominal work frequencies of around 2 megahertz (2 MHz) are suitable.

Attenuation of ultrasound. As the ultrasonic pulse passes through the soft tissues it loses intensity. This is due to spread of the energy over an area and absorption in soft tissues. Absorption of ultrasound in the soft tissues leads to the echoes from deeper structures being displayed at a less intensity than those arising from more superficial structures. To combat this, swept-gain (time-gain control) has been introduced. Swept-gain intensifies echoes from the deeper structures and when properly adjusted ensures that the echoes of equal amplitude from superficial and deep structures are all displayed at similar intensities.

ULTRASONIC TECHNIQUES AND DISPLAYS

The technique employed for diagnostic purposes and the several systems for the display of the returning echoes are described below.

PULSE ECHO TECHNIQUE

Ultrasound is generated in pulses of microsecond length at a repetition rate of 500 to 1000 pulses per second. Between each pulse the transducer is resting for sufficient length of time to ensure the returning echo can be detected before the next pulse is due to be generated.

DISPLAYS

1. A-Scan

In this type of display the echoes are recorded as vertical deflections of the spot on the cathode ray oscilloscope (Fig. 67.3A). These deflections may be upward or downward. The echoes arising from the contact of the transducer on the skin surface are displayed at the left end of the baseline of the cathode ray oscilloscope. The distance of the other signals along the baseline is proportional to the distance of the echoing surface from

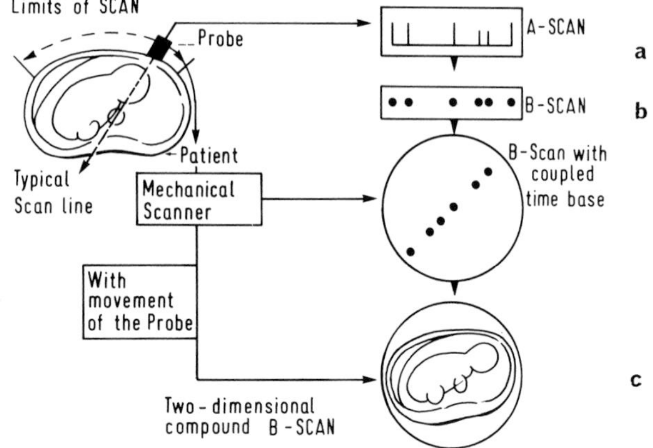

Fig. 67.3 Ultrasonic displays. The probe is applied to the surface of the pregnant abdomen (top left). The various displays on the cathode ray oscilloscope demonstrating the echoing surfaces are shown on the right side: **a**—A-scan (probe stationary); **b**—B-scan (probe stationary); **c**—compound B-scan. The probe has been moved across the skin surface (see text).

the skin. The apparatus can be accurately calibrated. Therefore the depth of the echoing surfaces can be measured from the skin and the distance between successive echoing surfaces will give the dimensions of internal structures. The height of the deflection produced by each echo is proportional to the intensity of the echo signal; the greater the height the stronger the echo and vice-versa.

2. B-Scan

This is also known as the brightness modulation display. In this the echoes are displayed as bright dots along the baseline of the cathode ray oscilloscope (Fig. 67.3B) instead of the vertical deflections used in the A-scan. In modern compound B mechanical scanning apparatus the time base or baseline on the cathode ray oscilloscope follows exactly the direction of the ultrasonic beam as it passes through the patient (coupled time base, Fig. 67.3C). As the probe is moved across the skin surface, the small dots on the cathode ray oscilloscope summate to build up a sectional picture of the interfaces over a width of about 1 centimetre in the line of movement of the probe (Fig. 67.3C). This image is recorded by photographing the cathode ray oscilloscope either by using a time exposure onto Polaroid film as the picture builds up or by observing or photographing the image on a long persistence tube (Wells, 1977; Barnett and Morley, 1974) or the monitor display when a scan converter is employed.

1. **Bistable display.** In many present day standard compound B-scan apparatuses, an echo will produce a dot on the cathode ray oscilloscope when its strength is strong enough but echoes of greater strength will not produce an increase in brightness of the dot. There is a threshold below which no signal will be demonstrated and above which all echo signals no matter their strength, will be demonstrated by equal brightness of the dot. This is known as the bistable display. Therefore information about the quality or strength of the echoes which is obvious on observing the different heights or amplitudes of the echo signals on the A-scan is being lost on the compound B-scan.

2. **Grey-scale display.** In more recent scanners, cathode ray oscilloscopes are being used in which the brightness of the dots is proportional to the strength of the returning echoes, i.e. the brighter the dot the stronger the echo. Pictures on Polaroid film or, better still, negative film will show differing brightness of the dots and therefore differing parts of the scan picture, according to the strength of the echoes, will range through shades of grey to white. This is the basis of the grey-scale recording and more information about the structures in the area of the examination is obtained by this method. Scan converters with television display have now been introduced which produce similar recordings more easily. A scan converter is a non-direct view storage tube raster scanned by an electron gun and viewed on a television monitor. Scan converters are now rapidly coming into use but they are expensive compared with the earlier bistable display system.

3. Time-position (M-mode) display

This display is used to record the movement of structures within the body particularly the heart. It is developed from the B-scan. As the line of moving bright dots deriving from the echoes arising from the various moving structures within the heart is swept across the face of the cathode-ray oscilloscope by a second slow speed time-base generator, a recording may be made of the trace of their movement by photographing it onto Polaroid film using a time exposure (Fig. 67.4). A longer and therefore a more certain recording onto lengths of ultraviolet sensitive or photographic paper may be made by using a strip chart recorder (Fiegenbaum, 1976).

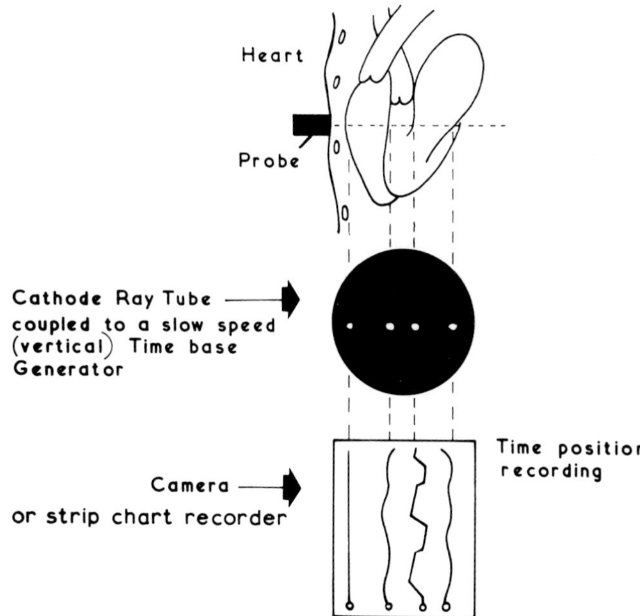

Fig. 67.4 Time-position (M-mode) display. The coupled slow speed time base generator is required when the tracing is to be recorded onto Polaroid film. It is not needed when the tracing is recorded by the use of a strip chart recorder which employs a fibre-optic system (see text).

4. Real-time display

All the techniques described above result in a static display. However, if sequential ultrasonic pictures are produced at a rate of about 40 frames a second on a non-storage display, an impression will be given to the observer's eye of an instantaneous and continuous grey-scale picture of a section of the patient in which anatomy and movement can be observed. These images are generated by the so-called real-time scanners. The pictures are not in fact real-time or instantaneous; they are delayed by a time interval which varies with the picture frame rate and the depth of the structures examined within the body. The delay is likely to be about 1/40th second. This degree of delay is so small that it is in effect equivalent to real-time and does not normally have any clinical significance. The technique is very useful to assist rapid searching of the area of interest such as the pancreas or uterus, and also for analysis of the anatomy and movements of the heart and other structures. This technique also enhances observation in certain

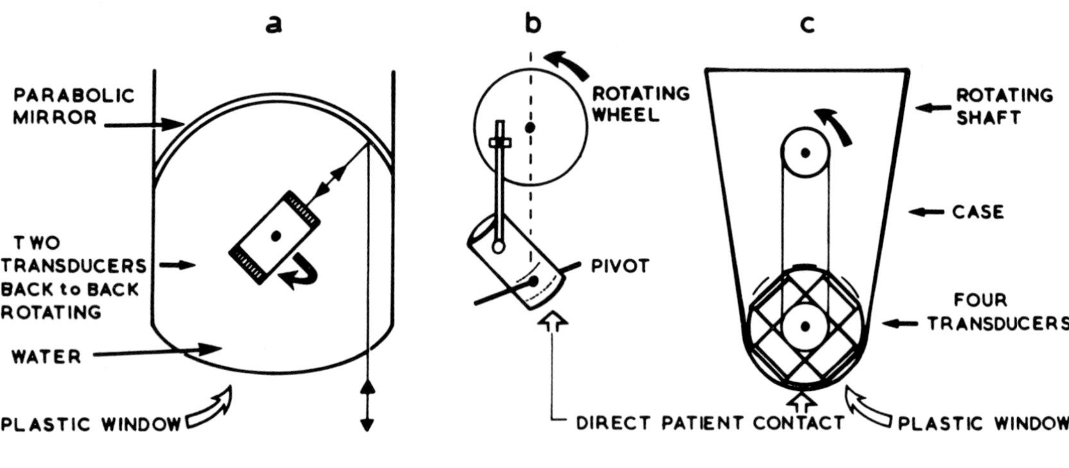

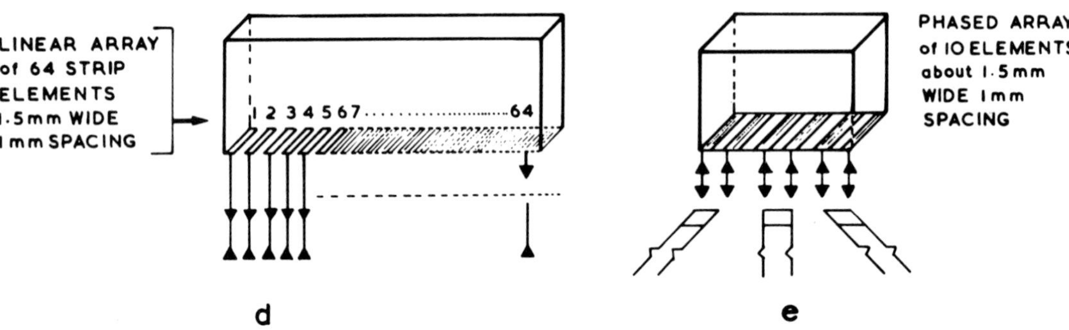

Fig. 67.5 Current types of real-time scanners.
a—Rotation of two transducers in a waterbath, the ultrasound being reflected off a parabolic mirror.
b—Single transducer mechanically rocked on its face.
c—Rotation of multiple transducers sequentially activated.
d—Linear array of transducers sequentially activated.
e—Phased array of transducers activated with serial delay (see text).

circumstances; every radiologist is aware of the fact that the eye is more attracted to an object that moves than one that is stationary. Real-time images are best recorded onto videotape but they may also be photographed from the monitor either directly or by a stop frame method to present a static picture. Several types of real-time scanner have been developed. They depend on either mechanical movement of one or more transducers or sequential electronic switching of multiple electrical transducers (Fig. 67.5).

1. **Mechanical real-time scanners** (a) Continuous sector scans are produced by a single transducer rotating in a waterbath and the ultrasonic beam is reflected off a mirror. The waterbath has a plastic face which is applied to the patient's oil-covered skin (Fig. 67.5A).

(b) A single transducer is rocked pivoting on its face through an angle of about 60° and it is activated at a rate of about 20 frames a second (Fig. 67.5B).

(c) Four transducers are mounted at the points of a cross. The cross is rotated behind a thin flexible plastic shield which is applied directly to the patient's oil-covered skin. As each transducer sequentially comes opposite to the skin surface it is activated producing sector scans at a rate of 15 frames a second. The scanning arc is about 90°. As each transducer leaves the area of the scan surface it is switched off (Fig. 67.5C).

2. **Electronic real-time scanners** (a) **Linear array.** A line of up to 64 small transducers is assembled along a length of about 10–15 centimetres (Fig. 67.5D). The transducers are sequentially activated starting at one end and sweeping the ultrasound beam from one end of the array to the other. This produces a tomogram the length of the array. By activating the transducers sequentially in blocks of four (i.e. transducers 1–4, followed by 2–5, then 3–6, etc.), at a rate of 30–80 frames a second, lateral resolution is increased though it remains poor.

(b) **Phased arrays.** An array of small transducers is assembled and they are activated in sequence with slightly differing delays so that the ultrasound beam emerges at an angle to the transducer face. The subsequent transmitted pulses are delayed less with the effect that the beam is nearer to being emitted perpendicular to the transducer face [Fig. 67.5E( )]. In a later pulse there is no delay and at this point in time the beam is perpendicular to the transducer face [Fig. 67.5E( )]. A further delay in the opposite direction is then introduced which ensures that the beam is swept in a direction opposite to its starting direction [Fig. 67.5E( )]. Thus by repetition of the pulses with varying sequential delays, arc or sector scans are electronically produced without the use of moving parts. 90° fields can be examined. These phased array real-time scanners are very expensive.

DOPPLER EFFECT TECHNIQUES

When an ultrasound beam echoes off a stationary surface the frequency of the reflected beam is the same as that of the generated beam. On the other hand, if the surface from which the ultrasound is being reflected is itself in motion, then the reflected ultrasound will be at a different frequency from that of the generated ultrasound. The latter is called the Doppler effect. The shift in frequency can be amplified and either impressed on a loudspeaker to produce an audible signal or recorded by a frequency spectrum analyser or rate meter (Wells, 1977). Continuous wave ultrasound is usually used in these circumstances. Two transducers are required (Fig. 67.2), the transmitting one being placed by the side of the receiving transducer and they are inclined towards each other so that the echoes are received from a relatively large specified depth range. Improvement in the precision of the depth information can be achieved by using pulsed Doppler systems, now being introduced.

PROBE MOVEMENTS IN B-SCANNING

Various types of probe movements are used to produce B-scan pictures (Fig. 67.6).

1. *Linear* (Fig. 67.6A). The probe is held vertically while it is moved in a straight line over the skin surface. This technique is useful for quick searching and it is also essential for demonstrating minute anatomy such as the branches of the upper lumbar aorta.

2. *Arc* (Fig. 67.6B) In an arc scan a similar movement of the probe is made but the probe is always kept at right angles to the skin surface.

3. *Sector* (Fig. 67.6C). To produce a sector scan the probe is rocked around its distal end which is held stationary on the skin surface. Thus a wedge of tissue is examined with its apex at the probe-skin surface contact point. This method has proved of great value in examining the liver and also in structures where the point of entry of the ultrasonic beam is restricted by adjacent gas containing organs such as the intestines.

4. *Compound* (Fig. 67.6D) Compound scanning is a complex combination of linear, arc, and sector scanning as the probe is slid over the skin surface. It presents the beam at right angles to the multitude of interfaces in the scan line as frequently as possible. It therefore tends to write in as much detail of the interfaces as possible but it may obscure minute anatomy, such as arteries or veins, which become overwritten by reverberant echoes.

In order to produce the best quality pictures it is often of value to use combinations of these scanning techniques, such as linear for one part of the scan and sector for another.

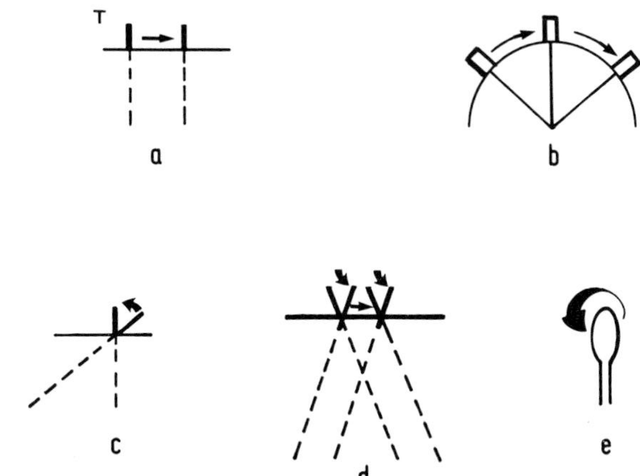

Fig. 67.6 B-scan probe movements. Probe (T) movements used to produce B-scan pictures.
a—linear; **b**—arc; **c**—sector; **d**—compound; **e**—radial (see text).

5. *Radial* (Fig. 67.6E). Another technique is the compound radial scan which is produced when a specially designed probe is rotated about a fixed point within or near the part to be examined. It is useful for the examination of the prostate or the uterine cervix (Barnett and Morley, 1974) but it is a technique which is not generally available.

ULTRASONIC POWER AND INTENSITY

The unit used to express ultrasonic power is the watt. A power of one watt is equivalent to a rate of flow of energy of one joule per second.

The intensity of the ultrasound is equal to the quantity of energy flowing through that area in unit time and it is expressed as watts per square centimetre. The absolute value of ultrasonic intensity is important when considering possible biological effects. More frequently it is advantageous to measure the ratio between two intensities particularly if the level of one intensity is used as a reference level for other intensities. This is the basis on which ultrasonic diagnostic apparatus is calibrated and the reference intensity level is either the maximum or minimum of the apparatus. As the electrical methods used in diagnostic ultrasound have evolved from those employed in radar and audible sound, the decibel notation is used to compare the output power levels. The decibel notation is best understood by considering an example. If the maximum output intensity level of an apparatus is P_1 and if the intensity of the output is reduced to a level P_2, a measure of this new intensity level relative to the maximum power level of the apparatus is the ratio P_2/P_1. This measure of P_2 is expressed in decibels by taking the logarithm and multiplying by 10 thus:

$$\text{Intensity } P_2 \text{ in decibels (relative to } P_1) = 10 \log_{10}\left(\frac{P_2}{P_1}\right)$$

The factor 10 is introduced here because it is convenient to work in tenths of a bel which is the unit used as a power ratio in audible sound. It is most important to realise that ultrasonic intensity calibrated in decibels is not an absolute measure but an expression of the intensity relative to an arbitrary reference level which will vary from apparatus to apparatus. The reference level can be maximum or minimum output. When it is maximum level, maximum power is 0 dB and a lesser power would be expressed as a negative value, say -20 dB. Similarly, if the reference level is the minimum, all other power levels would be greater and would be expressed as positive values, i.e. say $+20$ dB. It is meaningless to express an absolute value of any intensity level in decibels unless a reference level is quoted (Wells, 1977). As the reference level will vary, decibel levels on one machine cannot be expected to produce the same results on another machine, particularly one of different manufacture. Though it is not possible to equate the results for similar decibel settings on two different machines, similar changes in echo patterns should result from the same changes in decibel settings, e.g. filling in the speckled echo pattern of the placenta with an intensity increase of 10 dB (McDicken, 1976).

ULTRASOUND IN MEDICAL DIAGNOSIS

The value of ultrasound in medical diagnosis depends on the following properties:

1. It can be transmitted at a constant speed through the soft tissues of the body; the mean velocity in human soft tissues is 1,540 metres per second.

2. Soft tissue boundaries or interfaces within the body can be detected by ultrasound. When a pulse of ultrasound strikes a boundary between two structures of differing acoustical impedence (a product of the density of the tissue and the speed of ultrasound in it) part of the pulse will be reflected back from the boundary as an echo and part will pass on to reflect off a deeper boundary or to be absorbed. The ultrasound pulse striking an interface obeys the law of light in that the angle at which the reflected echo leaves the interface is dependent on the angle of incidence of the pulse to the interface. It is only when an echo reflects off the interface at or nearly at right angles will it be possible for the probe to detect it.

3. The echo returning from the interface can be detected, processed and displayed as a signal on the face of a cathode ray oscilloscope. These echo displays can be used to produce a pictorial image of the part or a tracing of the movement of structures within the beam.

4. With suitable calibration, ultrasound can be used to measure the depth from the skin surface and dimensions of anatomical structures or pathological masses within the body.

5. Ultrasound can differentiate between solid masses (tumours) and fluid-containing masses (cysts).

6. Ultrasound is non-invasive and does not usually cause patient discomfort.

7. Ultrasound is harmless to patients, fetus and staff at the intensities normally used for diagnostic purposes. Therefore examinations can be repeated with safety and the method can be used in pregnancy.

Limitations in use of diagnostic ultrasound

1. Ultrasound will not pass through gases at the frequencies used for diagnostic purposes. This is a severe limitation to its use in the thorax and abdomen.

2. Air has to be excluded between the transducer face and the skin. For this purpose oil is usually placed on the skin; either liquid paraffin, olive oil or commercial preparations may be used. There are occasions when a waterbath can best be employed as a couplant between transducer and patient.

3. Ultrasonic examinations can be time-consuming; this affects both radiologist and technician time.

4. Skill derived from training and practice is required to perform the examinations and to interpret the results.

5. The apparatus is not yet as reliable or stable in performance as radiological apparatus.

APPLICATIONS OF ULTRASONIC TECHNIQUES IN MEDICINE

General considerations. Diagnostic ultrasound is a non-invasive technique which gives information about soft tissues and this information may be unobtainable by other non-invasive methods, an example being the demonstration of fetal life in early pregnancy (Robinson, 1972). More often it adds information about a lesion that has already been detected by palpation or some other imaging technique such as radiology. An example of this is the ability of ultrasound to differentiate between those masses which are solid tumours and those which contain fluid such as cysts. Ultrasound is thus complementary to clinical examination, biochemistry, haematology, diagnostic radiology, isotope imaging techniques, and CT scanning.

Ultrasound will demonstrate the outline of various organs or pathological mass lesions. It may also give information about the composition of a structure by analysis of the echoes that arise from within it. If ultrasound is transmitted easily through a lesion and no echoes arise within it, it is said to be *transonic*. This occurs in a cyst.

On the other hand, if multiple echoes arise from within the lesion it is said to be *echogenic*. This is the case with tumours. Benign masses usually have well-defined margins whereas malignant lesions may have poorly defined margins.

Ultrasound may also be used to determine the depth of a lesion from the surface and the dimensions of space-occupying lesions because the apparatus can be calibrated accurately. This may be of considerable value for radiotherapy planning. By examining the patient serially it can be determined whether a lesion is increasing or decreasing in size with time.

Detection of fluid. Until the introduction of computerized tomography, ultrasound was the only non-invasive diagnostic method capable of differentiating between a deep mass which is composed of fluid such as a cyst or hydronephrosis, and one which is a solid tumour. Fluid is the ideal medium for transmitting ultrasound and no echoes arise from within a single cavity fluid-containing mass. There are, however, multiple interfaces within a tumour between the various histological parts of it and between tumour and blood vessels. An A-scan directed through a fluid-containing mass will show no echoes where it passes through the mass but if it is a solid tumour, multiple echoes will arise from within it (Fig. 67.7). A mass which is solid in some parts and cystic in others will show the characteristic echo patterns of a tumour in some places and a cyst in others. Both cysts and benign tumours will have sharp outlines but the posterior margin of a cyst will be a sharp high-intensity white line. If a mass contains fluid the ultrasound beam will not be attenuated as it passes through it. Therefore ultrasound penetrating to the tissue behind the cystic mass will be at high intensity and will produce high intensity echoes posterior to it (Fig. 67.11). If the mass is a solid tumour the ultrasound beam will be attenuated by passage through it and relatively few echoes will arise behind the mass (Fig. 67.13). Another helpful method of differentiation is to put the power intensity of the apparatus to a high setting. If the mass is fluid-containing it will stand out as a 'transonic' area against a white background which has filled in with echoes (Fig. 67.30). If the mass is a solid tumour on the other hand it will also fill in with echoes. It must be realised though that at high power intensity, echoes from soft tissues between the transducer and the mass will reverberate into the image of the mass. If the mass is small (1–2 cm in diameter) this will make differentiation as to whether it is cystic or solid impossible. If the mass is a larger fluid-containing structure, the reverberant echoes will show as a thick white line anteriorly, the margin of which parallels the surface of the body.

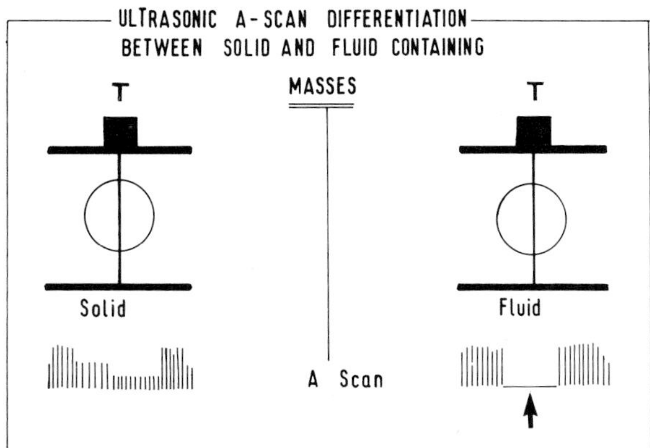

Fig. 67.7 Ultrasonic differentiation between solid and fluid containing masses. The two circles represent two masses within the body, one solid and one fluid containing. A beam of ultrasound is directed vertically through each mass from a transducer (T) above. The corresponding A-scan display is depicted below each mass. Multiple echoes arise within the solid mass whereas no echoes occur (arrow) as the beam passes through the fluid containing mass.

Soft tissue measurement. Calibration of ultrasonic apparatus allows direct measurement of soft tissues to be made by an A-scan technique or by measurement of the B-scan image photographed onto film. The depth of a lesion from the surface of the skin and the dimensions of a structure can be determined accurately. By serial examination it can be demonstrated whether a lesion is increasing in size or not. These features can be of considerable help in determining the management of patients or assisting in the performance of needle biopsy of a mass or aspiration of an abscess. They can also contribute to the planning of radiotherapy fields and the selection of the most suitable electron beam energy values for the treatment of breast carcinoma without damaging the underlying lung. The latter is determined on the measurement of the anterior chest wall thickness.

URINARY TRACT

Method of examination. It is important that intravenous urography films be available at an ultrasonic examination as this gives information about the position and obliquity of the kidneys as well as the size and position of renal masses. It is essential to ensure that any abnormality shown by ultrasound corresponds to that demonstrated on the intravenous urography films. The right kidney can be shown behind the liver with the patient in the supine position (Fig. 67.8). Routine examination of the kidneys is performed with the patient lying comfortably prone on a pillow. The level of the iliac crests is marked on the skin centrally as an anatomical reference point and oil applied to the skin. Longitudinal and transverse scans are made at 1 cm intervals. The first longitudinal scan should aim at showing the length of the kidney and is best performed at about 5–7 cm from the midline in an adult patient. The angle of scan relative

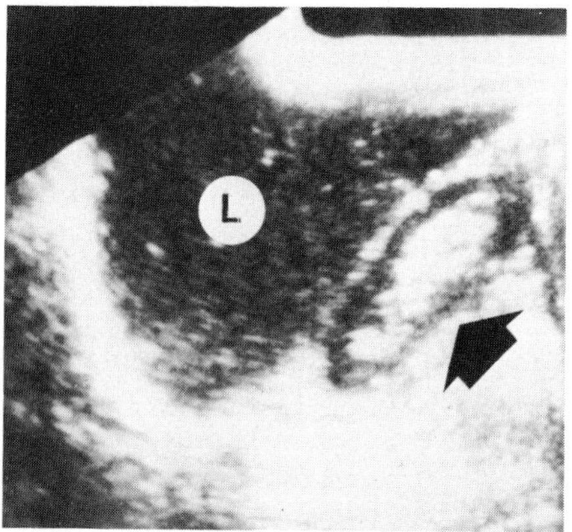

Fig. 67.8 Normal right kidney. Normal right kidney, scanned from in front, is well seen (arrow), its lower pole being inclined forwards. L = liver.

to the long axis of the spine may have to be adjusted to coincide with the obliquity of the kidney as shown on the intravenous urogram to ensure that the scan traverses the full length of the kidney. The whole of the kidney is examined by serial scans on each side of the first orientation scan. Serial transverse scans are then made from about 2 cm above the iliac crest until the kidneys have been fully outlined. Most examinations are best performed on suspended inspiration as this provides better accessibility to the upper pole. Occasionally the lower pole of the kidney or a renal mass is obscured in these circumstances by the iliac crest; examination in suspended expiration can then be helpful. Bladder examinations are performed with the patient supine and the bladder full of urine or saline. Longitudinal and transverse scans are performed and angulation of the probe into the pelvis is frequently necessary. The use of a waterbath may considerably assist examination of neonates and young children especially for the kidneys.

Normal appearances. On the longitudinal scan the renal outline is ovoid and sharply defined. Centrally placed within it is a dense thick linear echo pattern produced by the calices and renal pelvis (Fig. 67.9A). The renal parenchyma is generally free of echoes but on some newer machines a fine echo pattern may be seen especially if enhanced by computer processing. If the kidney is duplex or has a bifid pelvis the central echo line is divided into two, the upper part being less extensive than the lower. On transverse section the kidney outline is circular with a rounded collection of echoes within it produced by the calices. The latter is central at the poles but towards the medial side at the hilum (Fig. 67.9B). The average normal kidney is 11–12 cm long, 5–6 cm broad and 3–4 cm in antero-posterior diameter.

Renal masses. The most frequent use of ultrasound in renal disease is to determine whether a mass shown on intravenous urography is a cyst or a tumour. The ultrasonic characteristics of these lesions are the same as cysts or tumours elsewhere (see p. 1345). The renal outline is usually enlarged with a bulbous upper or lower pole. The central caliceal echoes are compressed or displaced and if the mass is a malignant neoplasm, they may be destroyed locally. A cyst will have a sharp outline; its margin is frequently a curved thin white line particularly on the side opposite to that on which the transducer is applied (Fig. 67.10). The echoes deep to a cyst are of high intensity (Fig. 67.11). On the other hand a malignant neoplasm is poorly defined on all surfaces and the echoes deep to it are of lower intensity than those adjacent to them (Figs 67.12 and 67.13). In elderly patients in whom it would be undesirable to carry out invasive radiological investigations and in whom the renal mass presents as an incidental finding, ultrasound diagnosis is sufficiently accurate to warrant avoiding renal arteriography or puncture. In younger patients, particularly those with symptoms re-

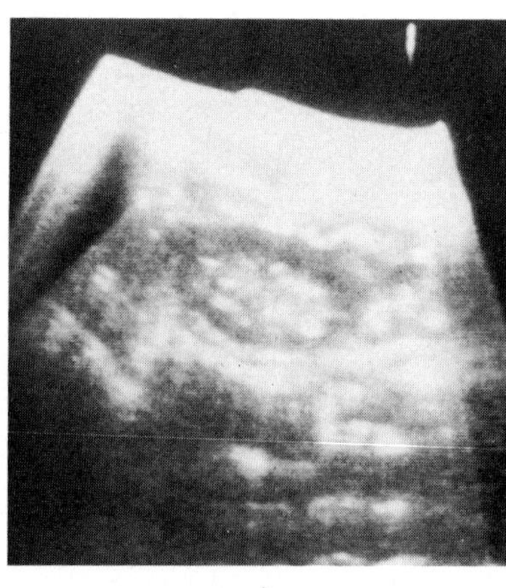

A

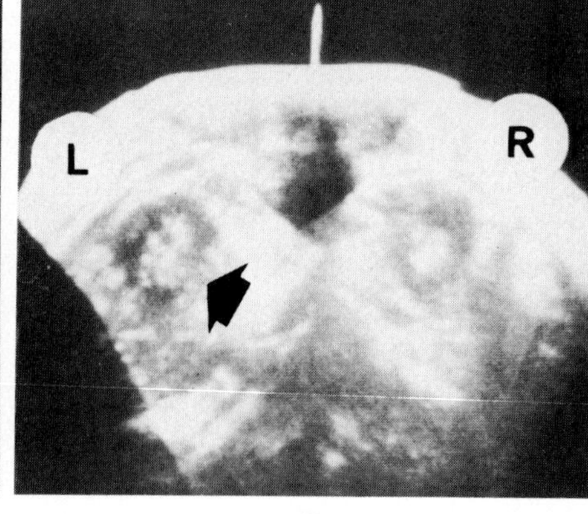

B

Fig. 67.9 Normal kidney. Patient prone.
(A) Longitudinal scan. The kidney is a well-defined oval organ with a central complex of echoes arising from the calices and renal pelvis.
(B) Transverse scan through the renal pelvis of the left kidney, the echo complex being eccentric towards the medial side (arrow). The scan of the right kidney is through the lower pole, the central echo complex being central in position (L = left, R = right).

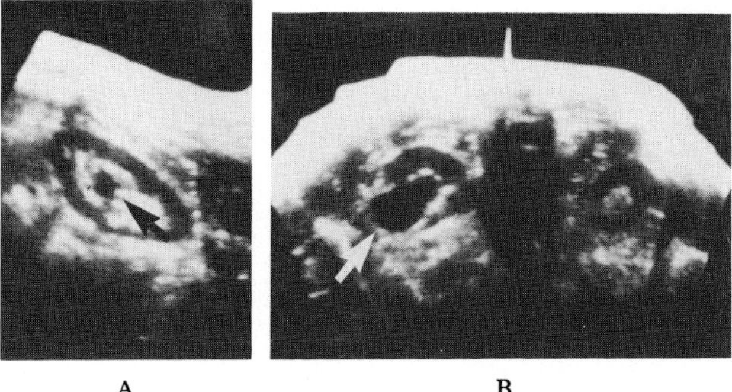

Fig. 67.10 Cyst of left kidney.
(A) Longitudinal scan. A small rounded transonic area in the central echo complex is produced by the medial part of the cyst (arrow).
(B) Transverse scan shows the cyst has a sharply defined white line around it and it bulges the outer surface of the kidney (arrow).

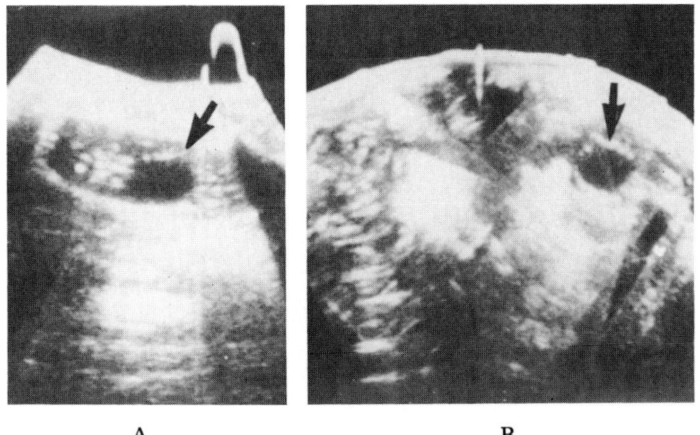

Fig. 67.11 Cyst lower pole of right kidney.
(A) Longitudinal scan. Transonic area in lower pole (arrow) with sharp posterior wall and lack of attenuation of ultrasound shown by high intensity echoes deep to the cyst. Calices displaced.
(B) Transverse scan. The cyst (arrow) has sharp anterior and posterior walls.

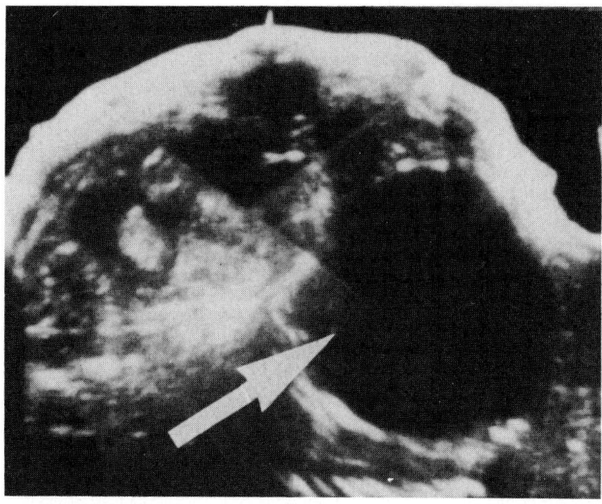

Fig. 67.13 Renal cell carcinoma of right kidney. Transverse scan. The huge tumour was necrotic (arrow) and appeared to be transonic but it attenuated the ultrasound. This indicated that the mass was in fact solid. Note low intensity echoes behind the mass.

lated to the renal lesion, ultrasound should be used as an indicator of the next desirable radiological investigation. If ultrasound demonstrates a cyst, the next radiological examination indicated is cyst puncture; if a tumour is shown by ultrasound, renal arteriography is indicated next. Using ultrasonic methods alone the accuracy of differentiating tumour from cyst ranges in reported series from 75 per cent to 96 per cent. When taken in conjunction with the other diagnostic techniques the accuracy for renal masses becomes nearly 100 per cent. Ultrasound is especially valuable in avascular tumours and when a non-functioning kidney has been shown by intravenous urography.

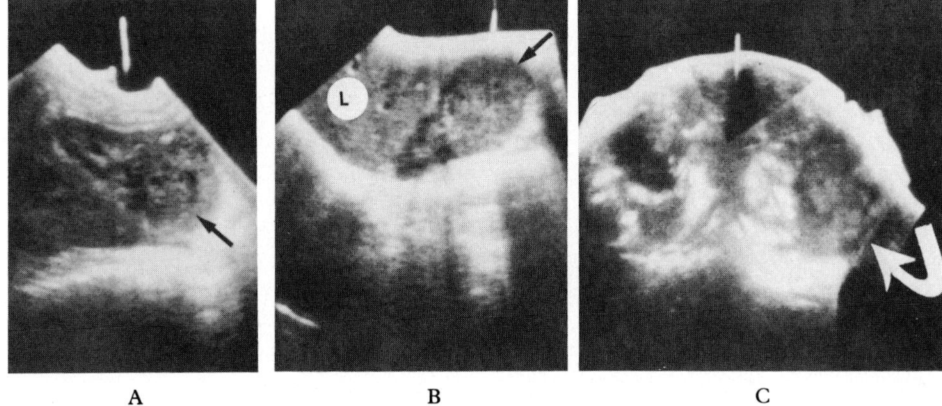

Fig. 67.12 Renal cell carcinoma of right kidney.
(A) Prone longitudinal scan. The lower pole of the kidney is bulbous. The central echo pattern is destroyed and the mass (arrow) contains multiple echoes arising from within the tumour. The outline of the mass is poorly defined.
(B) Supine longitudinal scan of same patient. The tumour was so large that it could be demonstrated easily on scanning from the front (arrow). L = liver.
(C) Transverse scan. The tumour mass (arrow) is large and has an ill-defined edge.

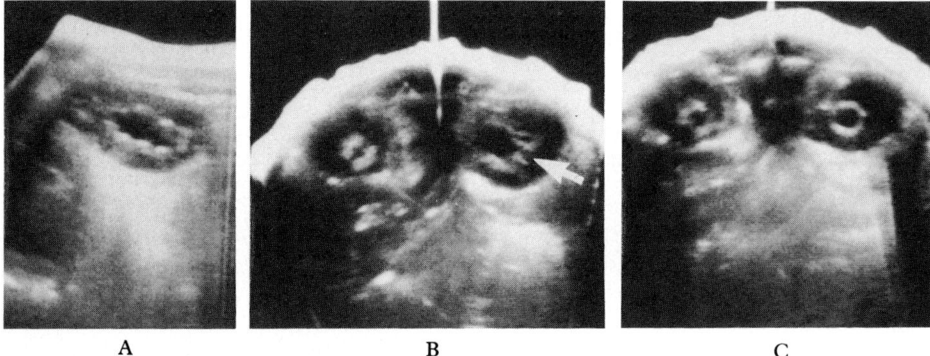

Fig. 67.14 Bilateral hydronephrosis. Patient 20 weeks pregnant.
(A) Longitudinal scan. Right kidney. Dilatation of the renal pelvis and calices produces a transonic area in the centre of the caliceal echoes.
(B) Transverse scan through right renal pelvis. The dilatation of the pelvis produces a crescentic disposition of the central echo complex (arrow).
(C) Transverse scan at a higher level than (B). The circular pattern of the central echo complex indicates dilatation of the upper pole calices.

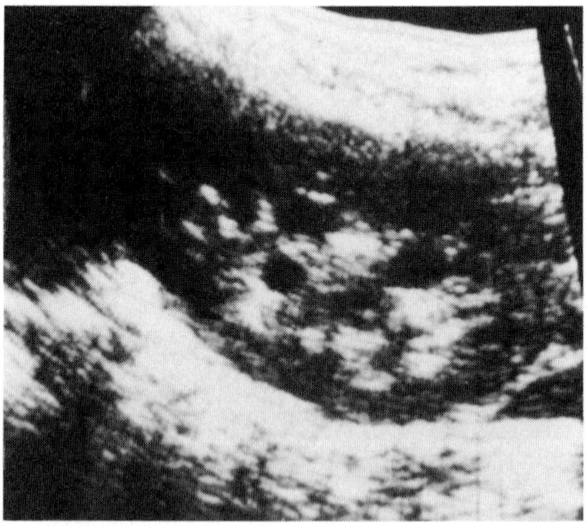

Fig. 67.15 Hydronephrosis. Multiple large transonic areas within the central echo complex of the kidney indicate dilatation of the calices peripherally and therefore an advanced hydronephrosis. (Courtesy of the Ultrasonic Unit, Western Infirmary, Glasgow.)

Hydronephrosis. The earliest sign of hydronephrosis is separation of the central kidney echoes by a transonic area produced by the distension of the renal pelvis and calices with urine. On longitudinal section this produces an oval ring; in the transverse section a circular ring or 'c' sign is apparent (Fig. 67.14), the latter occurring at pelvis level and the former at the renal poles. When the calices dilate further more peripheral large transonic areas (Fig. 67.15) are seen which may be separated by coarse septa and the kidney may be enlarged. As the renal pelvis dilates a round transonic area may be seen medially produced by the dilated pelvis. The dilated upper end of the ureter may be revealed if the obstruction is below the pelvi-ureteric junction.

Polycystic kidneys. The kidneys are enlarged, frequently with a lobulated outline. Multiple small and large transonic areas are seen within them distorting the

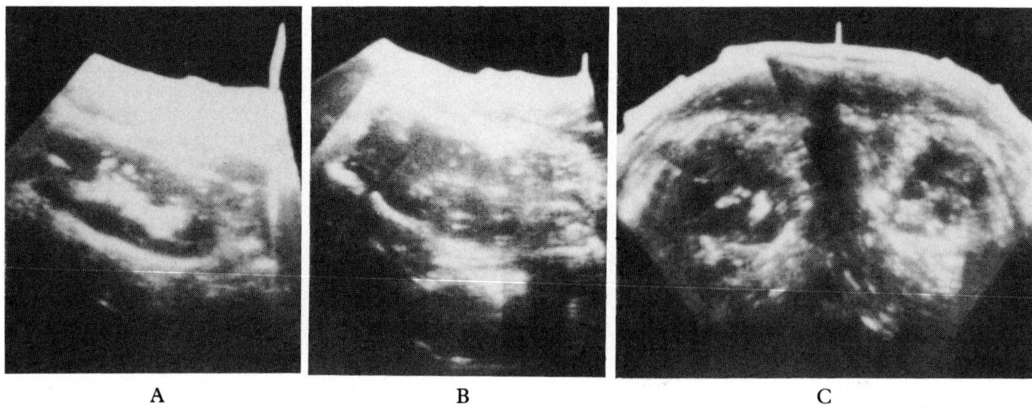

Fig. 67.16 Polycystic kidneys. Longitudinal scans.
(A) Right kidney. The cysts produce indentations on the central echo complex and transonic areas in the upper and lower poles.
(B) The left kidney is enlarged and lobulated in outline, multiple cysts being shown.
(C) Transverse scan. Both kidneys are enlarged and lobulated with multiple transonic areas distorting the central echo complex.

calyceal echo pattern. The lesion is bilateral (Fig. 67.16). The septa between the cysts in polycystic disease are usually fine. Ultrasound is very accurate in demonstrating polycystic disease, as it is also in showing multiple cysts in one kidney. The liver and pancreas should also be examined in order to detect cysts in these organs which may co-exist with polycystic disease of the kidneys.

Perinephric fluid. Collections of fluid (blood, pus, urine) around the kidney are shown as transonic areas against the normal renal outline and the latter is frequently displaced from its normal position (Fig. 67.17).

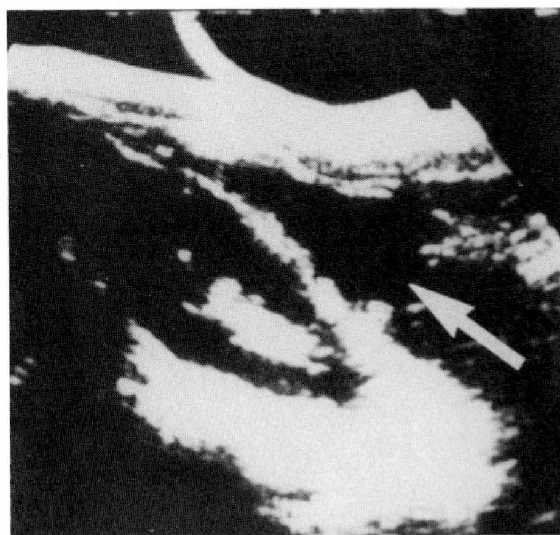

Fig. 67.17 Perinephric abscess. Prone longitudinal scan of right kidney. The kidney lower pole is displaced forwards by the transonic posterior perinephric abscess (arrow). (By courtesy of Dr Stanley Bennett, Truro.)

Renal calculus. If large enough, a renal calculus appears as a high echogenic area within a calix or renal pelvis. Particularly if linear scanning is used, an echo-free band may extend deep from the highly echogenic area produced by the stone indicating absorption of the ultrasonic beam by the dense stone. This ultrasonic 'shadowing' can be virtually the only sign of a stone if the stone itself is within an echogenic area. The principle is the same in the diagnosis of a gallstone (Fig. 67.39).

Renal transplants. In the specialized field of renal transplantation, ultrasound has a part to play particularly in the recognition of rejection and perirenal fluid collections.

Bladder

Radiological and cystoscopic methods of investigation allow for high accuracy in the diagnosis of lesions of the bladder, especially tumours. However ultrasonic examination can reveal infiltration of the bladder wall and surrounding pelvic cavity with neoplasm (Barnett and Morley, 1971). The mass of the tumour projecting into the fluid-filled bladder lumen is revealed fairly easily (Fig. 67.18). The width of the base of the tumour is shown and destruction or thickening of the adjacent bladder wall by tumour infiltration will be revealed. Displacement of the bladder by pressure from pelvic masses can be shown. The prostate size and volume can be calculated (Fig. 67.19).

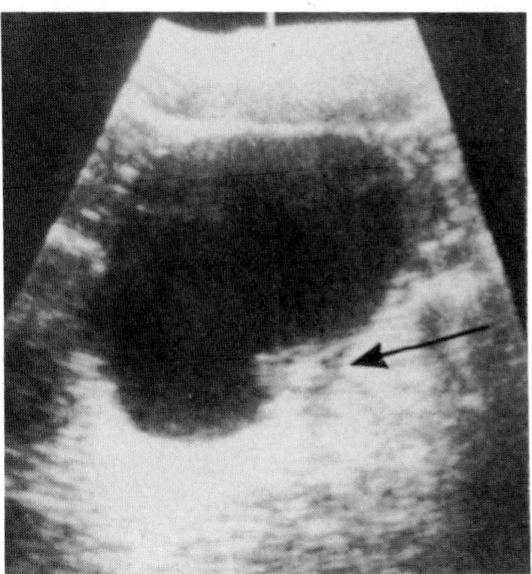

Fig. 67.18 Transitional cell carcinoma of left side of bladder. Transverse scan. The tumour (arrow) encroaches on the bladder lumen. It is wide-based and infiltrates the bladder wall and perivesical tissues.

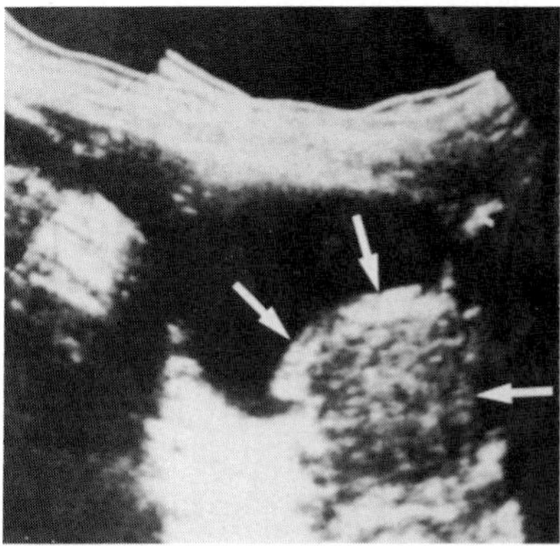

Fig. 67.19 Enlarged prostate. Longitudinal scan. The mass of the enlarged prostate (arrows) indents the bladder base. The prostatic area is filled with multiple echoes. (Courtesy of the Ultrasonic Unit, Western Infirmary, Glasgow.)

ULTRASONIC VASCULAR ANATOMY OF THE UPPER ABDOMEN

Hepatic veins. Usually the right, middle and left hepatic veins drain into the inferior vena cava just below the diaphragm but there is variation in their actual entry point into the inferior vena cava. They are demonstrated most readily on parasagittal scans of the liver. Tracing the veins to the inferior vena cava is time consuming and unnecessary when basic patterns and principles are recognised. Hepatic veins drain towards the inferior vena cava near the diaphragm and they will increase in size as they approach the diaphragm and the right atrial/inferior vena caval junction (Fig. 67.20). Portal veins become smaller as they pass peripherally within the liver. The same applies to bile ducts which become visible when they are

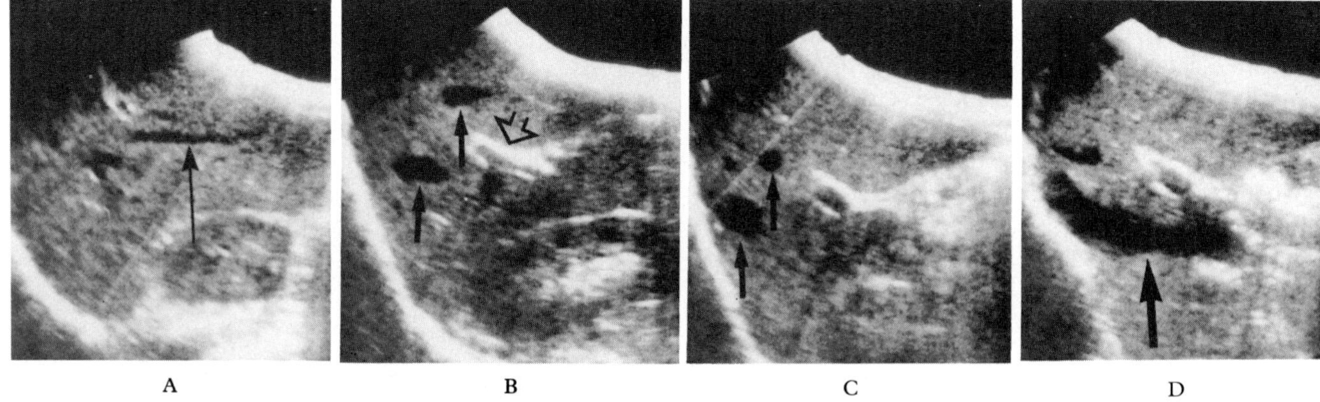

Fig. 67.20 Normal liver and hepatic veins. Longitudinal scans. (A) 8 centimetres; (B) 6 centimetres; (C) 5 centimetres; (D) 4 centimetres from the midline. The hepatic veins (small arrows) converge posteriorly on the inferior vena cava (large arrow in D). A portal vein branch is indicated by the open arrow in (B). The kidney is visible posteriorly in (A) and (B).

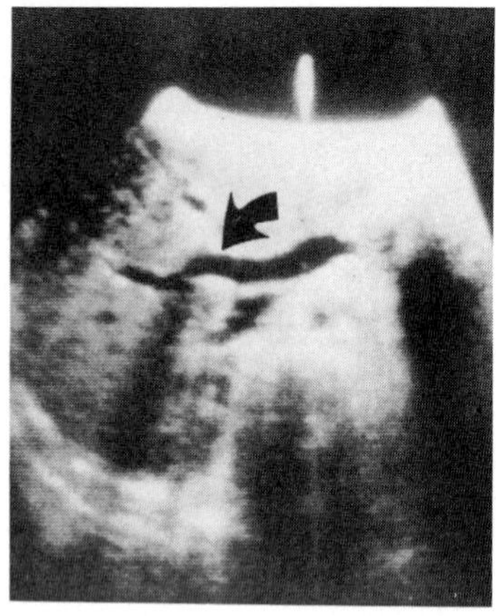

Fig. 67.21 Splenic and portal vein. Transverse scan. Case of hepatitis. The splenic vein courses across the upper abdomen and enters the portal vein (arrow). The right branch of the portal vein continues into the right lobe of the liver. The left branch of the portal vein is seen in the cross-section more anteriorly. The inferior vena cava is posterior to the portal vein.

dilated. Hepatic artery branches in the liver are not visualized. All large vascular channels near the diaphragm are considered to be hepatic veins. On transverse section the angle formed by hepatic vein branches above a plane through the porta hepatis points superiorly or supero-medially. Below this plane the angle formed by both portal and hepatic veins is similar.

Portal system of veins. The large portal vein branches traverse the liver transversely. They are therefore best demonstrated in transverse sections (Fig. 67.21) but they are also seen end-on in the parasagittal sections. The portal vein branches converge inferiorly on the porta hepatis and therefore the angle subtended by their branches points inferiorly or infero medially.

The portal vein is immediately anterior to the inferior vena cava (Fig. 67.22) and at this level the right branch extends from it horizontally into the liver. The caudate lobe of the liver may be interposed between the portal vein

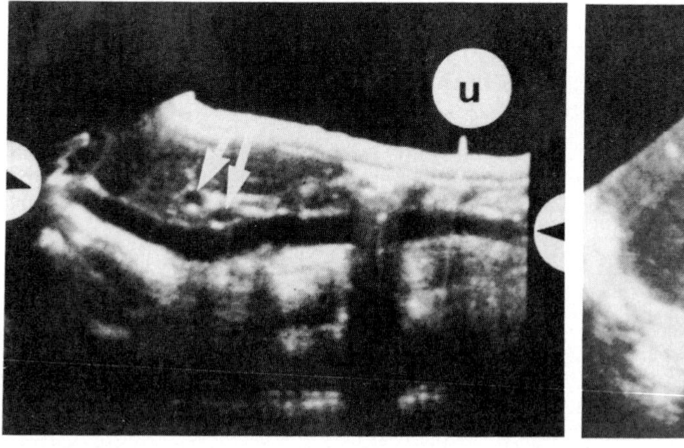

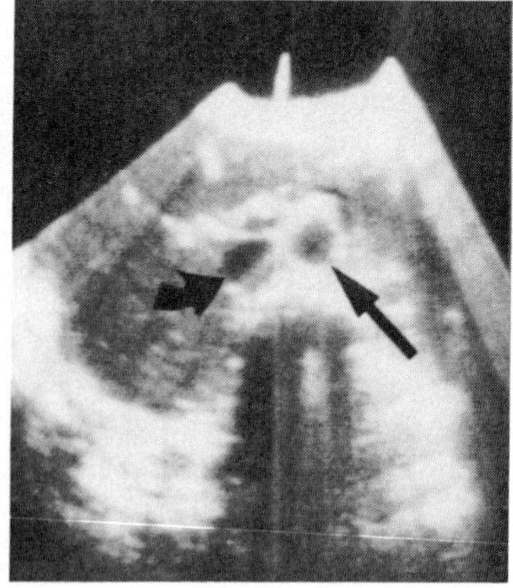

Fig. 67.22 Inferior vena cava and portal vein.

(A) Longitudinal scan. On this scan the inferior vena cava is unusually well demonstrated—it appears as a well-defined transonic line (black arrows) in front of the spine. Note that it inclines forwards at its upper end where it enters the right atrium. u = umbilicus. Portal vein and its left branch (white arrows).

(B) Transverse scan. The inferior vena cava (curved arrow) and aorta (straight arrow) are side by side in front of the spine. The portal vein is in front of the inferior vena cava.

and the inferior vena cava. The left portal vein branch is narrower than the right and it extends into the left lobe from the main portal vein. The extrahepatic part of the portal vein is shown on parasagittal and transverse sections. The splenic vein joins the portal vein from the left side and the superior mesenteric vein enters the portal vein inferiorly in front of the aorta. It is worth noting that venous channels change size between scans taken on expiration and inspiration. The large portal veins are surrounded by high intensity echoes and hepatic veins are not.

Renal veins. In transverse section the outline of the inferior vena cava is oval above the entrance of the renal veins. The right renal vein entry into the inferior vena cava is shown by a prolongation of the right posterolateral outline of the inferior vena cava. The left renal vein enters the left anteromedial aspect of the inferior vena cava and its outline is prolonged in this direction. The continuation of the left renal vein may be seen between the superior mesenteric artery and the aorta. Inferior to the entry of the renal veins the inferior vena cava decreases in size, a change best seen on the longitudinal scan.

Major arteries to the viscera. Renal, hepatic and splenic arteries can be seen in transverse sections; the inferior mesenteric artery has been shown on longitudinal

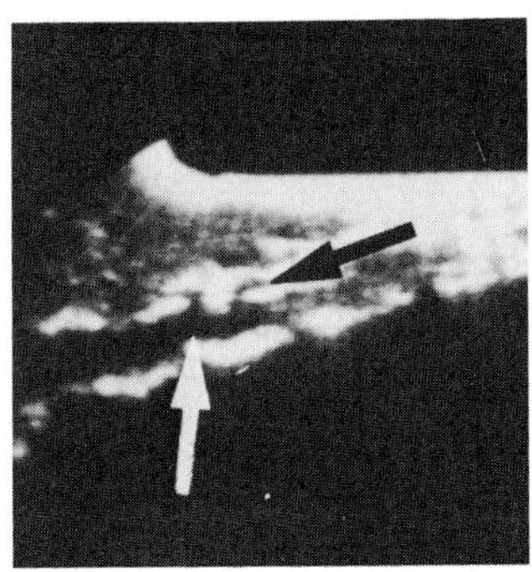
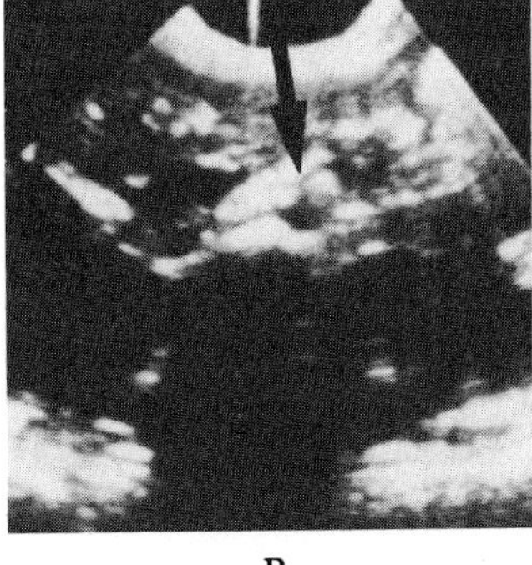

A B

Fig. 67.23 Coeliac axis and superior mesenteric artery.
(A) Longitudinal scan. The coeliac axis (white arrow) arises from the front of the aorta caudad to the superior mesenteric artery origin (black arrow).
(B) Transverse scan. The coeliac axis (arrow) is seen arising from the aorta and dividing into the hepatic and splenic arteries.

sections and the coeliac axis and superior mesenteric artery can be demonstrated on both transverse and longitudinal scans (Fig. 67.23A and B). The coeliac axis may be shown as a 'bubble-like' distortion or slit from the anterior surface of the aorta and on the transverse section it may be shown branching into hepatic and splenic arteries (Fig. 67.23B). This occurs at about the same level as or just above the junction of portal and splenic veins. The main hepatic artery is anterior to the portal vein and

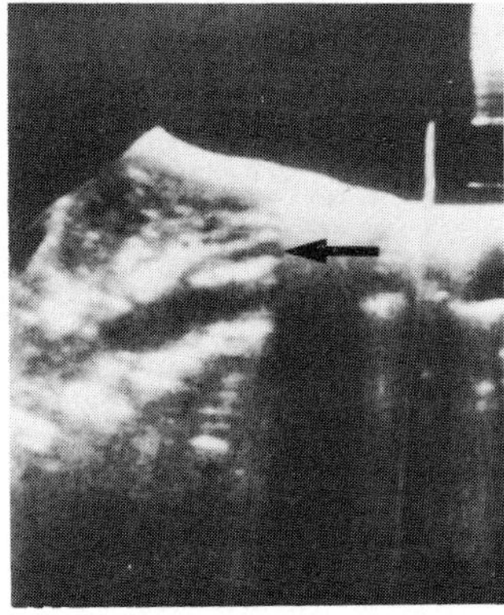
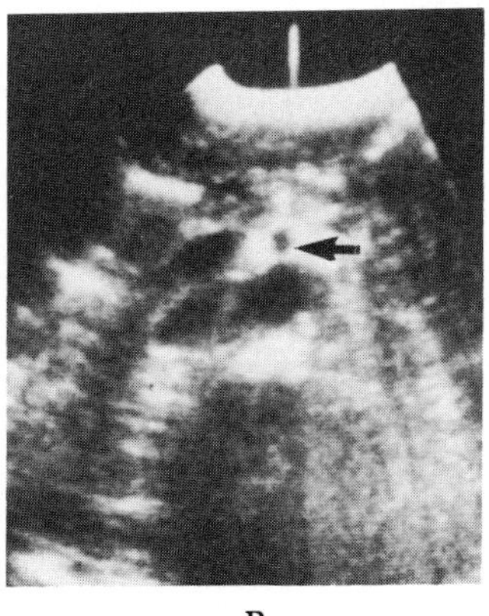

A B

Fig. 67.24 Superior mesenteric artery.
(A) Longitudinal scan. The artery (arrow) arises from the front of the aorta.
(B) Transverse scan. The artery (arrow) appears as a black dot in front of the aorta.

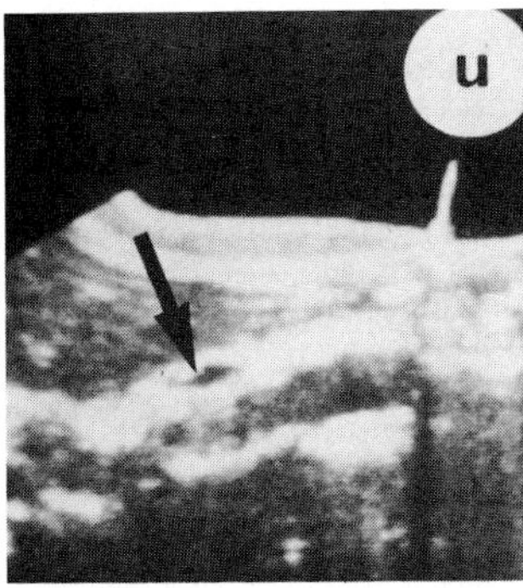

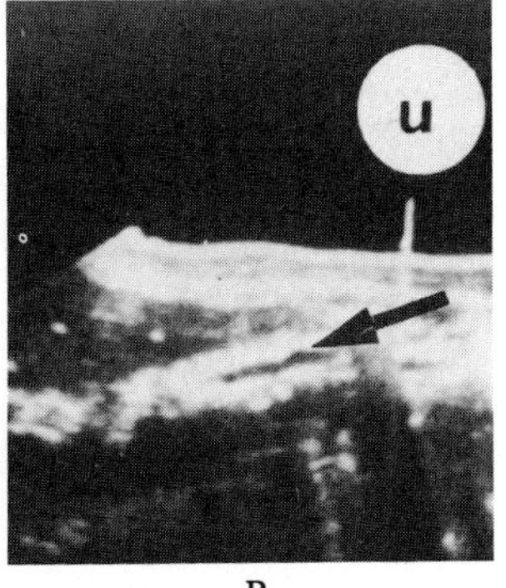

A B

Fig. 67.25 Inferior mesenteric vein. Longitudinal scans.
(A) 0·5 cm to left of midline the confluence of the splenic and portal veins is seen (arrow) in front of the aorta.
(B) 2 cm to left of midline. The inferior mesenteric vein (arrow) courses upwards to join the splenic vein. u = umbilicus.

it may appear as a small rounded area touching the portal vein.

The superior mesenteric artery arises from the aorta just distal to the coeliac axis. On transverse scans it may produce a 'bubble-like' distortion of the anterior aortic wall but the artery is most frequently seen as a rounded black dot anterior to the aorta (Fig. 67.24B). The renal arteries arise from the postero-lateral aspect of the aorta at about superior mesenteric artery level. The right renal artery passes between the vertebra and inferior vena cava. On the longitudinal scan, the coeliac axis and superior mesenteric arteries can be shown arising from the anterior surface of the aorta (Fig. 67.23A). The coeliac axis passes anteriorly and upwards whereas the superior mesenteric artery courses inferiorly. The superior and inferior mesenteric veins (Fig. 67.25) can be demonstrated entering the splenic vein.

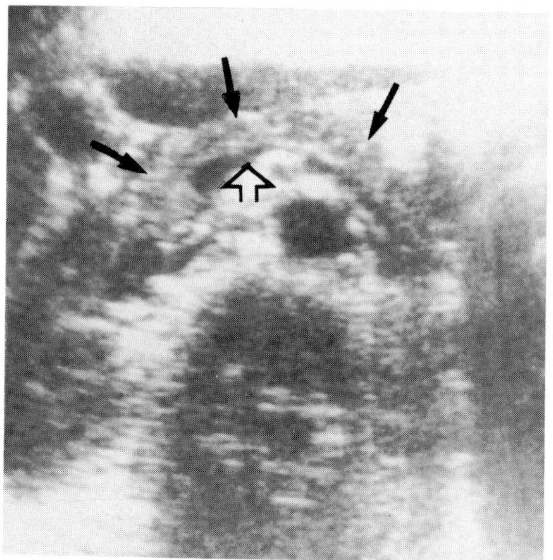

A

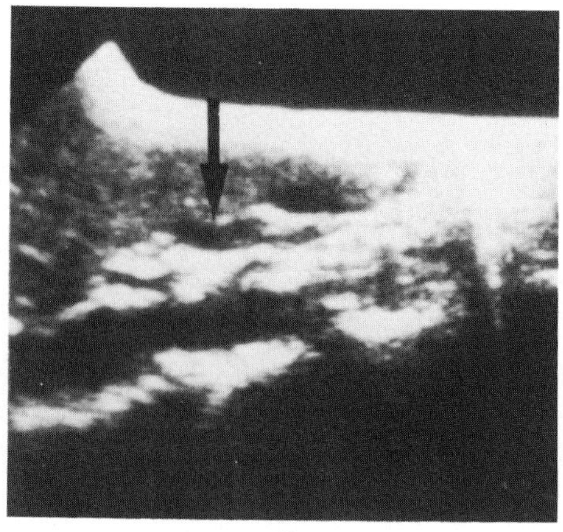

B

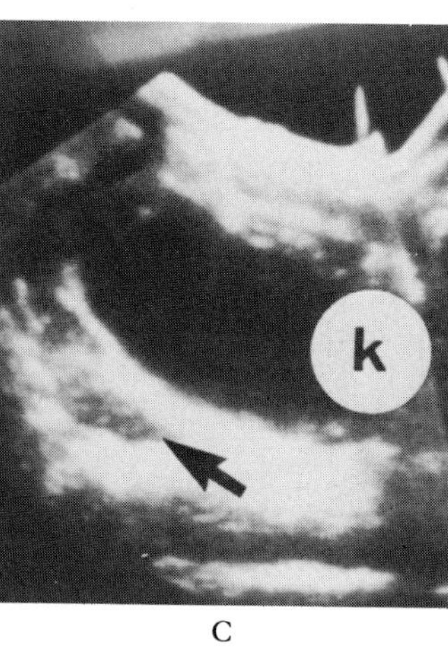

C

Fig. 67.26 Normal pancreas.
(A) Transverse scan. The pancreas is crescentic in shape (arrows) and is in front of the superior mesenteric artery and splenic vein (open arrow).
(B) Longitudinal scan. The pancreas (arrow) is situated in front of the coeliac axis and superior mesenteric artery.
(C) Longitudinal scan (prone). The tail of the pancreas (arrow) is situated in front of the kidney (k). (In this patient the kidney is hypertrophied.)

PANCREAS

Localization of the pancreas. The anatomical landmarks described above can give good localization to the expected site of the pancreas. However, it must be borne in mind that there is a variation both in its degree of obliquity and in its posterior relationships in different individuals. The body and tail are usually in front of and just below the splenic vein. The neck is in front of the confluence of splenic and portal veins and in front of and above the origin of the superior mesenteric artery (Fig. 67.24). The head is in front of the proximal part of the portal vein and lateral to the inferior vena cava.

Normal pancreas. Careful scanning will demonstrate the normal pancreas in a good proportion of cases. It is 1–3 cm in anteroposterior diameter and crescentic in shape when seen in transverse section. Multiple fine echoes arise from its substance. The head is in close relationship to the inferior vena cava and the body arches over the aorta at the level of the origin of the superior mesenteric artery (Fig. 67.26A). The tail extends to the upper part of the anterior aspect of the left kidney and is

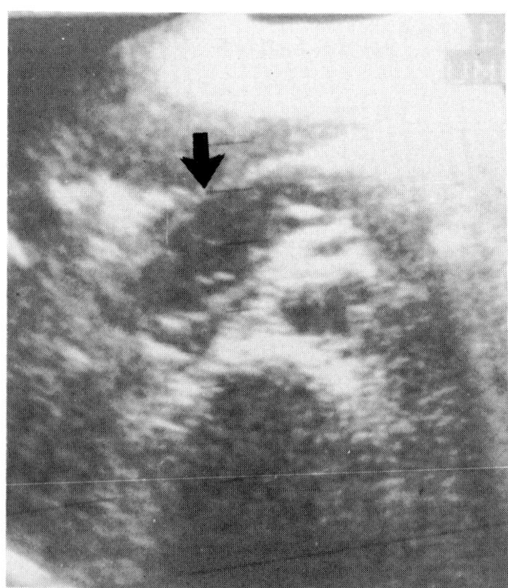

A

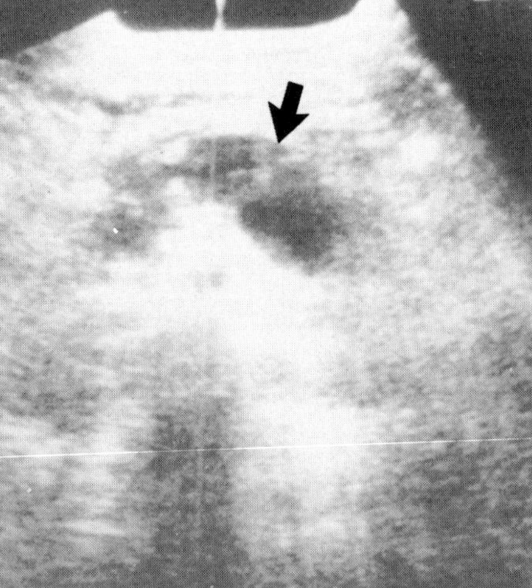

B

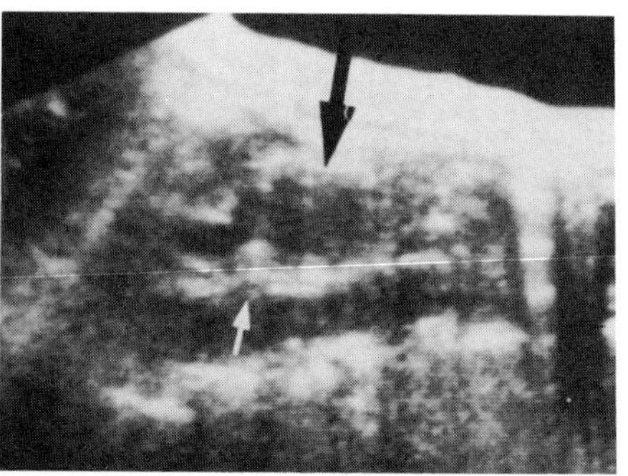

C

Fig. 67.27 Acute pancreatitis. Transverse scans. The pancreas is enlarged and transonic.
(A) The region of the head is especially affected (arrow).
(B) Another patient. The whole of the pancreas is grossly enlarged (arrow).
(C) Pancreatic carcinoma. Longitudinal scan. The enlargement of the pancreas produces a mass with echoes in it (black arrow) situated in front of the superior mesenteric artery origin from the aorta (white arrow).

best seen in prone scans of the kidney (Fig. 67.26C). On longitudinal scans, the body is shown in the angle between the left lobe of the liver and aorta and lies in front of the origin of the superior mesenteric artery (Fig. 67.26B). Its upper border is about level with the coeliac axis. The whole pancreas is seldom shown on one transverse section. With grey-scaling the pancreas contains multiple fine echoes. The pancreatic duct has been shown ultrasonically.

Pancreatitis. In acute pancreatitis the organ is enlarged and oedematous. Ultrasonically, it is shown best on transverse scans. The pancreatic outline is enlarged and relatively transonic compared with the surrounding soft tissues.

Solid pancreatic masses. Chronic pancreatitis and carcinoma produce solid masses and it is not possible to differentiate between them ultrasonically at the present time. These conditions are shown as enlargement of the organ (Fig. 67.27). Enlargement of the head is shown as a comma-shaped mass to the right of and in front of the inferior vena cava with the comma's tail level with the superior mesenteric artery in front of the aorta. Tumours of the body cause enlargement of the pancreas in front of the aorta and extending to the left side. Enlargement of the tail is frequently obscured by the gas in the stomach.

Abscesses and pseudocysts. Pancreatitis may result in abscess or psuedocyst formation. These are revealed ultrasonically as small or large, well-defined, rounded, transonic areas in the line of the pancreas and extending forwards from it. They frequently contain areas of high echogenicity due to debris within them (Fig. 67.28). It is not possible to differentiate between abscesses and cysts. In a series of 15 surgically proved pseudocysts, ultrasound correctly diagnosed 13 (Hancke, 1976).

Guidance for percutaneous needle biopsy. Once a pancreatic mass has been located by B-scanning, the optimum site, direction and depth for needle puncture for biopsy can be demonstrated. This is done by using a special transducer with a central hole in it for insertion of the needle along the ultrasound beam down to the mass. An A-scan display is employed for this part of the procedure and with this method carcinoma, if present, can be demonstrated without surgical exploration.

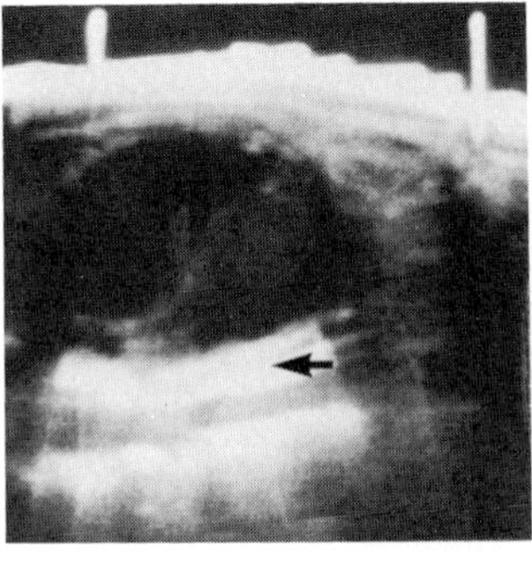

A

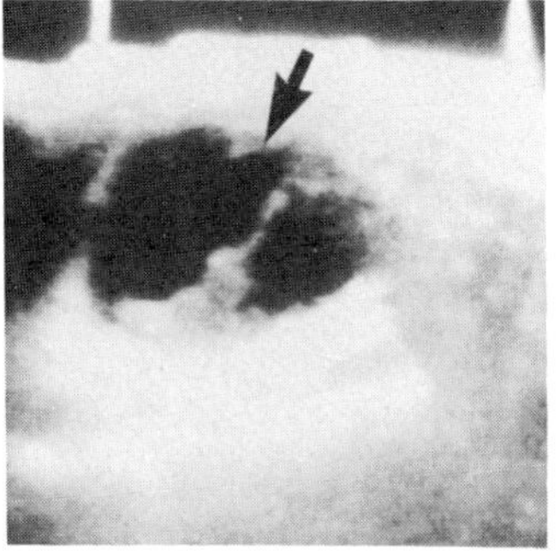

B

Fig. 67.28 Pancreatic pseudocyst. Longitudinal scans.
(A) Low power. The pseudocyst is shown as a large transonic mass in front of the aorta and superior mesenteric artery (arrow).
(B) High power. The outline of the cyst is better seen (arrow) and a septum and echoes are shown within it.

LIVER

Up to the time of the introduction of grey-scaling in about 1972, the technique of ultrasonic examination was aimed at demonstrating the outlines of anatomical structures and pathological states. To this end compounding of the transducer movement was employed in order to present the ultrasonic beam at right angles to as many interfaces as possible with the object of taking advantage of the specular reflection that occurred at the surfaces. This was a very successful method for showing the outline of the organs and pathological masses. Any information gained at the same time about the echo pattern arising from the internal structure of the organ was taken as a bonus. Grey-scaling introduces the ability to record the high and low amplitude echoes arising from the structure of an organ together with any pathological process in it, as well as delineating the outline. Echoes arising from the fine structure of tissues do not have a simple specular relationship to the tissue constituents but they occur in all directions. Compounding is therefore not required to display them. They are best shown by employing linear and sector scanning by which technique each element of tissue is interrogated only once. Thereby incidental movement of the tissues and inaccuracy of sound velocity lead to only slight distortion of the image without blurring of detail (Taylor and Hill, 1975). This applies particularly to the examination of the liver.

Method of examination. The close relationship of the costal margin to the gas-containing colon and stomach makes it difficult to examine the liver by ultrasound. The ultrasound beam has to enter the liver through the restricted space between these structures. Oil is applied to the skin of the upper abdomen. A longitudinal scan is made in the midline (sagittal) plane followed by serial scans parallel to it at 1 cm intervals until the whole of the liver area has been covered. Each scan is performed in deep inspiration. Sector and linear scanning are the transducer movements best suited for liver examination and compounding is kept to the minimum (Taylor and Hill, 1975). The probe is placed on the skin just below the costal margin and angled as acutely as possible towards the head. It is rotated at a constant rate through an arc pivotting on the transducer face until it is vertical and the scan is continued then down the abdomen as a simple linear scan. The latter part of the scan permits the aorta and inferior vena cava to be visualized (Fig. 67.20). Transverse scans can also be of value and they may be performed

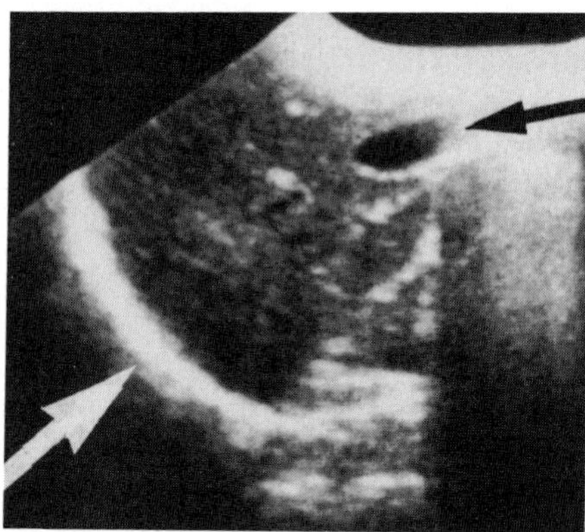

Fig. 67.29 Normal liver and gallbladder. Longitudinal scan. The gallbladder appears as a well-defined oval transonic organ (black arrow) anteriorly. The diaphragm produces the curved line (white arrow) posteriorly.

in several ways. Serial linear scans may be made across the upper abdomen between the costal margins terminating or starting with sector scanning into the liver at the right end of the scan. This is the best method, which gives the most information. Alternatively linear scans may be made as described with additional compounding across the rib cage. Linear scans made across the upper abdomen just below and parallel to the costal margin with the transducer angled upwards may also be of considerable value—these are known as subcostal scans. On occasions scanning through an intercostal space may also be of value.

The main causes of failure to obtain a satisfactory examination of the liver are obesity and gas in the colon. The ideal patient for liver examination has a concave upper abdomen on inspiration. In obese men particularly, the protuberant upper abdomen prevents adequate transducer skin contact. Gas in the colon and stomach will also stop the ultrasound beam entering the liver.

Normal appearances. The appearances vary with the plane of section. The liver parenchyma is shown as evenly distributed fine echoes. The diaphragm is revealed as a thin white curved line, convex superiorly and posteriorly limiting the liver outline (Figs 67.20 and 67.29). The inferior surface of the liver is inclined at varying angles downwards and it may be either concave or straight. The antero-inferior and left lateral liver edges have an acute angled outline. Normal intrahepatic bile ducts, either intra- or extrahepatic are not demonstrated but the gallbladder is usually seen anteriorly towards the right side (Fig. 67.29). The inferior vena cava is shown as a black strip posteriorly to the right of the midline continuous superiorly with the right atrium (Fig. 67.22). The aorta is seen to the left of the midline and the superior mesenteric artery and coeliac axis may be identified. The portal vein passes upwards in front of the inferior vena cava to enter the porta hepatis where it divides usually into right and left branches. These can be traced as they divide and become smaller as they pass peripherally. Hepatic veins enter the inferior vena cava superiorly. They are shown as linear transonic structures directed posteriorly and superiorly (Fig. 67.20). A *Riedl's lobe* can be identified when a column of liver tissue is shown to extend down from the inferior surface on the lateral side.

LOCALIZED ABNORMALITIES OF THE LIVER

Abscess. An abscess may be intrahepatic or subphrenic. It is shown as a rounded transonic area which may be surrounded by a rim of high intensity echoes or apparently

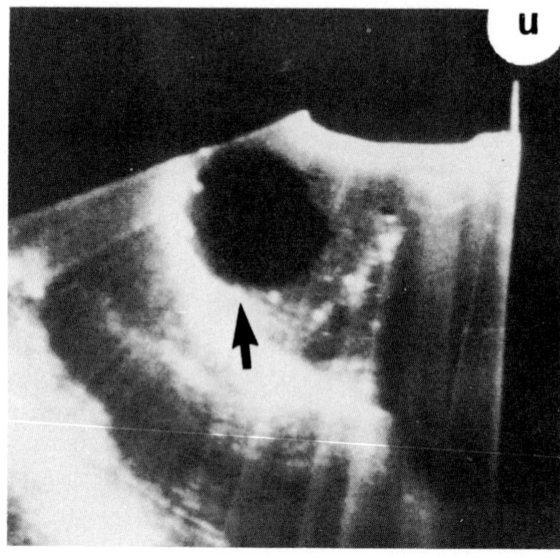

A

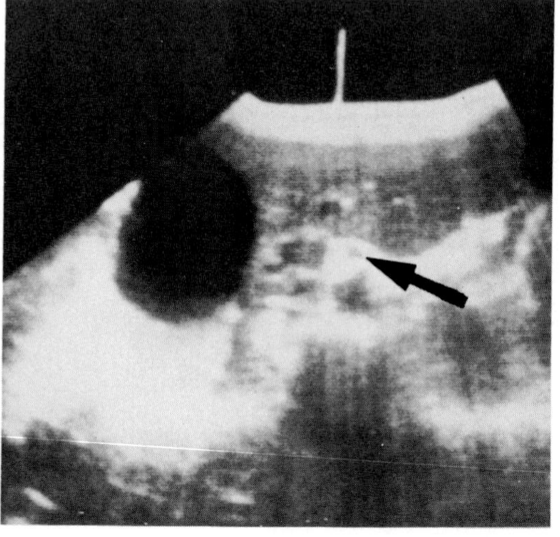

B

Fig. 67.30 Liver abscess.
(A) Longitudinal scan. The abscess is revealed as a large transonic mass, lobulated in outline (arrow) adjacent to the diaphragm. u= umbilicus.
(B) Transverse scan. The abscess is situated in the right lobe. It does not attenuate the ultrasound. Superior mesenteric artery (arrow) in front of aorta.

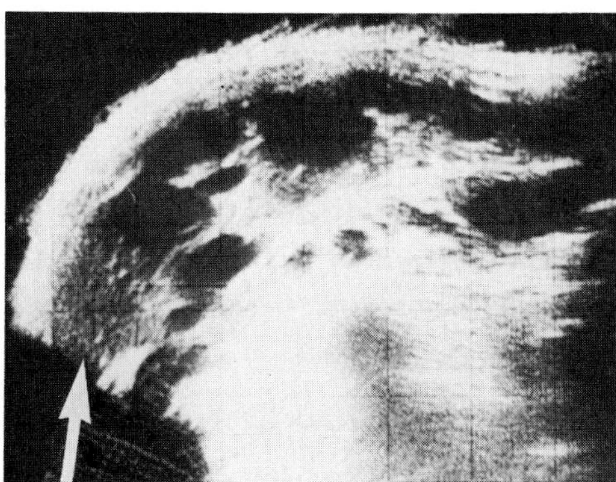

Fig. 67.31 Polycystic disease of the liver. Transverse scan. The liver is enlarged filling most of the upper abdomen. The only normal liver (arrow) is on the right side. The rest of the liver is filled with multiple transonic areas due to the cysts which do not attenuate the ultrasound.

normal liver substance (Fig. 67.30). The latter is the case particularly with amoebic abscesses. More than one abscess may be present.

Cyst. Hydatid cysts have a similar appearance to abscess cavities but they are not surrounded by a rim of high intensity echoes. A characteristic occasionally seen is the presence of a daughter cyst within the main cyst, i.e. a cyst within a cyst. Hydatid cysts may be single or multiple.

In polycystic disease the liver may be considerably enlarged. It will contain in places multiple rounded transonic areas with fine septa between them produced by compressed liver substance (Fig. 67.31). Occasionally polycystic disease of the kidneys will co-exist.

Haematoma. Subcapsular haematoma of the liver usually results from trauma. It is shown ultrasonically as a transonic area which is well defined and at the periphery of the liver (Fig. 67.32).

Malignant neoplasm. The malignant neoplasm may be primary or metastatic and if the latter, it may be solitary or multiple. The transonic appearances of primary or metastatic tumours are the same. The ultrasonic appearances vary widely, the commonest being a fairly well-defined area in which the echo amplitude is less than that of the surrounding liver parenchyma (Fig. 67.33). If the lesions are multiple, the liver will be enlarged and the acute angles of its edges become rounded. Some metastatic tumours, particularly from colonic primaries, produce higher intensity echoes (Fig. 67.34) than the surrounding liver and some will consist of areas of high echogenicity together with relatively transonic areas. In some conditions, such as Hodgkin's disease or metastases from bronchial carcinoma, the metastases are very transonic. McArdle (1976) found that the most common appearances of metastases were (1) echogenic nodules (2) a transonic area within an echogenic parenchyma.

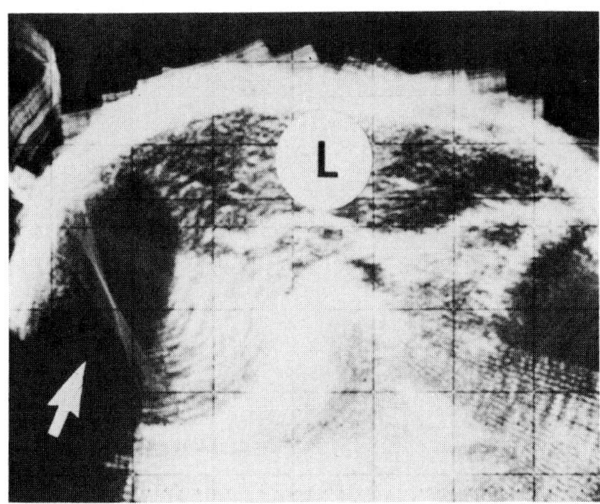

Fig. 67.32 Haematoma of liver. Transverse scan. The right-sided haematoma produces a well-defined transonic mass (arrow) in the right flank. L = liver.

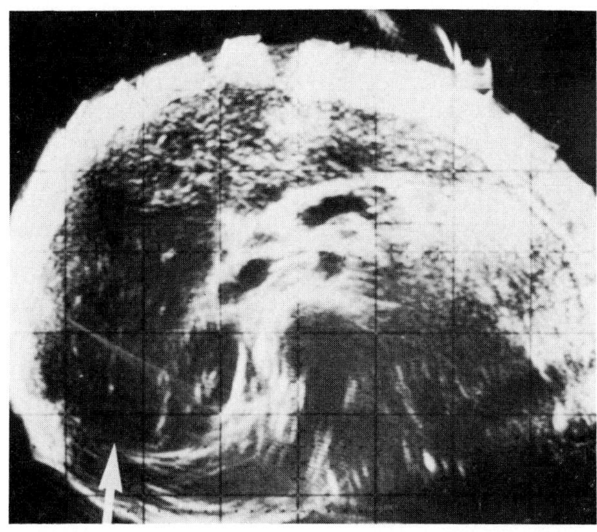

Fig. 67.33 Primary carcinoma of liver. Transverse scan. The carcinoma has produced a large poorly-defined transonic area (arrow) in the right lobe of the liver.

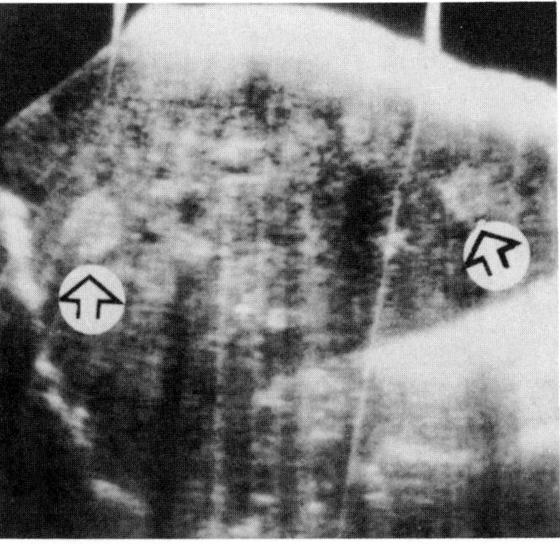

Fig. 67.34 Multiple liver metastases. Longitudinal scan. The liver is enlarged and there are multiple areas of high echogenicity (arrows), scattered through it indicating metastases. Primary tumour in large bowel.

DIFFUSE LIVER DISEASE

Cirrhosis. Mountford and Wells (1972) have shown that the echoes returning from cirrhotic livers are of higher amplitude than those from normal livers and that cirrhotic livers can be identified by an A-scan technique. Others have claimed that if the liver is severely affected by cirrhosis, multiple high level echoes will be unevenly scattered through the liver on B-scan examination. The ultrasound beam may be so attenuated that the deeper parts of the liver can only be examined if the frequency of the ultrasound beam is lowered. In these cases, the portal vein may be enlarged together with the spleen.

Fatty infiltration may produce high intensity echoes throughout the liver more uniform in distribution than with cirrhotic livers. If right heart failure is also present, the hepatic veins may be dilated.

Hepatitis. In viral hepatitis and drug-induced jaundice, the biliary tract will be normal in calibre but there may be increased periportal echoes.

Diagnostic accuracy of ultrasound in liver disease

The accuracy will vary very considerably with the experience of the operator and how advanced the pathology is. Ultrasound is superior to isotopes in demonstrating liver normality. It is slightly inferior to isotopes in detecting space-occupying lesions but once a lesion is detected it can determine whether it is a tumour or an abscess or cyst.

BILIARY TRACT

In jaundiced patients with a serum bilirubin exceeding 3 mg/dl (50 μmol/l), oral and intravenous cholangiography are not likely to be successful. In these patients ultrasound has a place in differentiating between intra- and extra-hepatic causes of jaundice. If the jaundice is due to intrahepatic causes the liver scan is likely to be normal and the biliary tract is unlikely to be dilated.

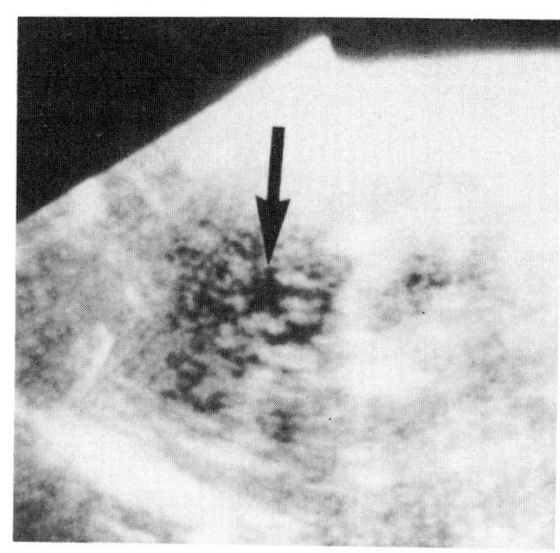

Fig. 67.36 Biliary obstruction. Multiple dilated ducts converging centrally (arrow) are characteristic of dilated bile ducts.

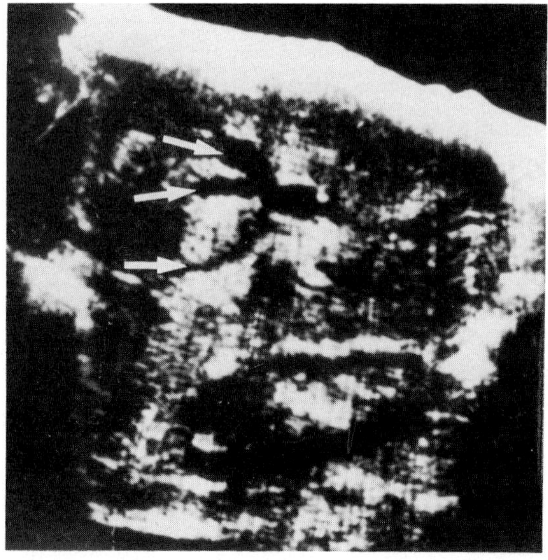

Fig. 67.35 Biliary obstruction. Dilated intrahepatic bile ducts arising from obstruction of common bile duct. Three ducts (arrows) converge on a central duct, an appearance characteristic of dilated bile ducts. (Courtesy of Dr D. Cosgrove, Royal Marsden Hospital, London.)

In patients with extrahepatic obstruction of the ducts the appearances will vary with the site and type of obstruction. In high obstruction of the common bile duct such as is produced by carcinoma of the common bile duct itself, dilatation of the intrahepatic bile ducts may be shown (Figs 67.35 and 67.36). If the obstruction is low in the common bile duct, dilatation of the gallbladder and common bile duct may be seen as well (Fig. 67.37).

Once the gallbladder has been outlined, its size may be determined. If it contains a stone a group of high intensity echoes may be shown within it with a line of ultrasonic shadowing behind it (Figs 67.38 and 67.39). The common bile duct is located to the right of the midline and when dilated it appears as a well-defined transonic

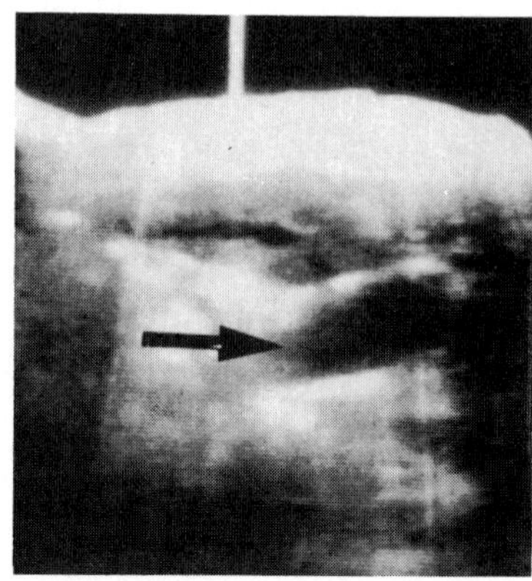

Fig. 67.37 Obstruction of lower end of common bile duct. The common bile duct is very dilated (arrow) and it runs transversely across the upper abdomen. A dilated intrahepatic duct is also shown. Cause of obstruction was a stone in the common bile duct.

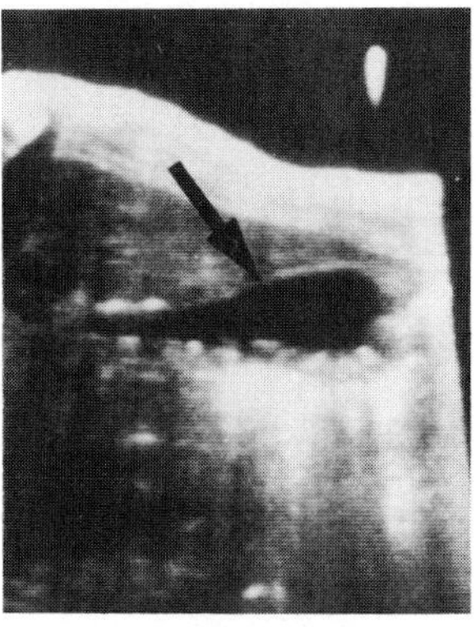

Fig. 37.38

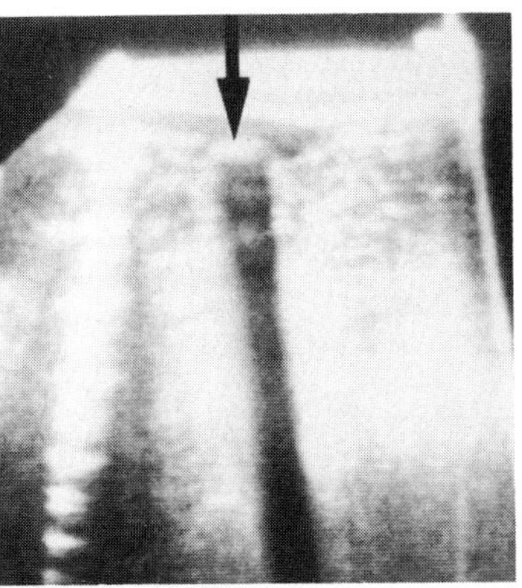

Fig. 67.39

Fig. 67.38 Dilated gallbladder containing gallstones. Longitudinal scan. The dilated gallbladder (arrow) contains multiple small gallstones which lie along its posterior wall, some of which produce ultrasonic shadowing.

Fig. 67.39 Gallstone. Longitudinal scan. The gallstone is revealed as a small area of high echogenicity anteriorly (arrow) and extending posteriorly from it is an 'ultrasonic shadow' (black line) produced by high attenuation of the ultrasound by the dense gallstone. The gallbladder is not dilated.

line extending downwards from the porta hepatis in front of the portal vein. Sometimes the dilated common bile duct may take a more horizontal course. The shadow of a stone may be shown within it or evidence of enlargement of the head of the pancreas indicating the possible cause of the obstruction. Dilated intrahepatic bile ducts are usually well shown as transonic tubular structures converging in a stellate pattern on the porta hepatis and decreasing in size towards the liver periphery (Figs 67.35 and 67.36).

In an analysis of 50 patients with proven dilated bile ducts, Laing *et al.* (1978) showed the following characteristic changes which allowed differentiation between portal veins and dilated bile ducts.

1. Alteration in the anatomic pattern adjacent to the main right portal vein segment and the main portal vein bifurcation.
2. Irregular walls of dilated bile ducts.
3. Stellate confluence of dilated bile ducts.
4. Acoustic enhancement of dilated bile ducts.
5. Peripheral bile duct dilatation.

Taylor (1977) claims a correct diagnosis by ultrasound in 64 of 66 patients with extrahepatic obstruction and that an intrahepatic cause of cholestatic jaundice was correctly predicted in a further eight patients.

SPLEEN

At the present time ultrasonic examination of the spleen has little to offer. The enlarged spleen can be recognised and it is noteworthy that few echoes arise from within it. It is therefore important to be aware of this fact when considering the differential diagnosis of transonic lesions in relation to the left kidney. Occasionally a cyst within the spleen may be encountered.

ADRENAL GLANDS

The normal adrenal gland is difficult to image ultrasonically and a special approach to it is necessary. Sample (1977) describes a technique which involves placing the patient in a lateral decubitus position. Oblique scans are made in the longitudinal axis of the kidney with the transducer angled to align the kidney and the aorta in the scanning plane. Using this approach Sample claimed to demonstrate the normal adrenal gland as a separate distinct structure in 85 per cent of attempts; the success rate was equal for right- and left-sided glands. Others have not approached this success rate but the method has proven to be of value (Sample, 1978) in demonstrating mass lesions which produce changes in outline of the gland ranging from a single convex margin to complete roundness. The lesions likely to be shown are carcinoma, adenoma, cyst, pheochromocytoma and hyperplasia but small intraglandular aldosterinomas are not likely to be visualized at the present time.

ASCITES

It is not possible to distinguish ultrasonically between ascitic fluid, blood or pus in the peritoneum. The fluid collects posteriorly in the paracolic gutters and can be identified either by the A-scan or compound B-scanning. As little as 500 ml can be detected. As further quantities of fluid collect it separates the intestines and passes between the liver and abdominal wall (Fig. 67.40). In non-malignant causes of ascites the intestines float forwards but if the cause is a malignant tumour the intestines may be bound to the posterior abdominal wall.

ABDOMINAL AORTA

A common clinical problem is whether a pulsatile abdominal mass is transmitting pulsations from a normal aorta behind it or whether an aortic aneurysm is present. Ultrasound will readily distinguish between the two. The maximum diameter of the normal lumbar aorta is 3·5 cm (Fig. 67.41). An aorta wider than this is aneurysmal (Fig. 67.42). Aneurysms can be shown with accuracy and their dimensions measured—serial measurements will reveal whether the aneurysm is increasing in size with time. The presence of thrombus on the aortic wall can be shown (Fig. 67.43) and also extension of the aneurysm down the iliac arteries.

PERIPHERAL ARTERIES

Most of the major arteries of the body can be visualized by arteriography. Arteriography however is invasive and is not free of hazard or discomfort to the patient. In recent years attention has been applied to methods for

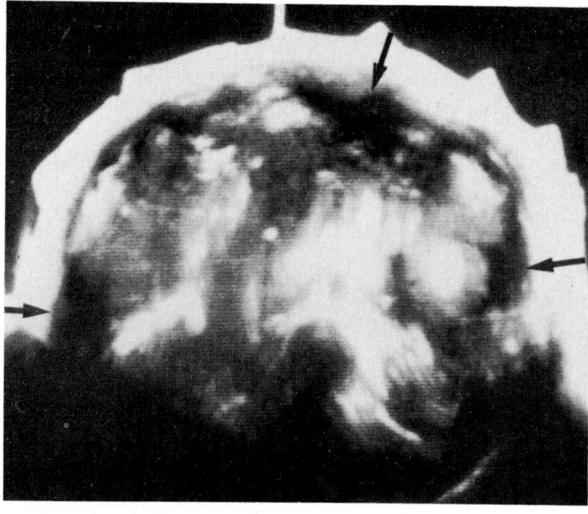

A

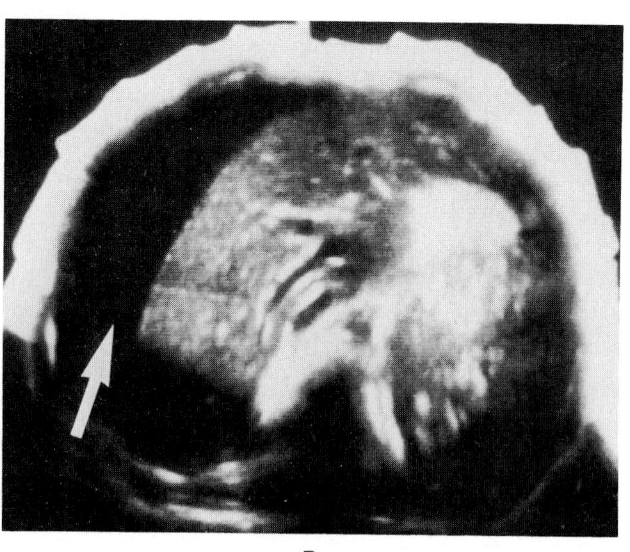

B

Fig. 67.40 Ascites. Transverse scans.
(A) At umbilical level. The transonic fluid (arrows) separates the intestines and higher in the abdomen (B) separates the liver and abdominal wall.

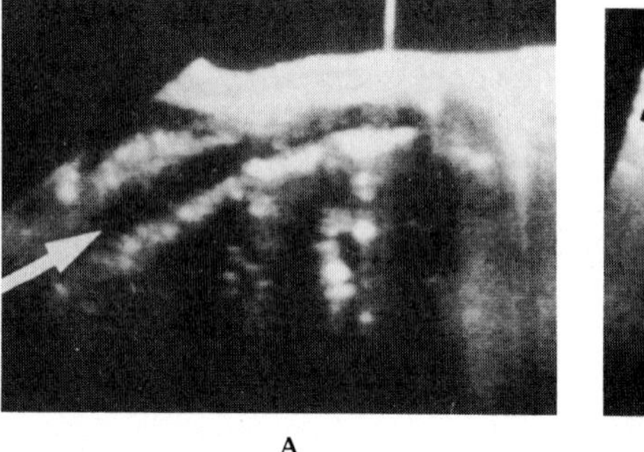

A B

Fig. 67.41 Normal aorta.
(A) Longitudinal scan. The aorta is seen as a thin transonic line (arrow) in front of the spine and tapering distally. (B) Transverse scan. The aorta is circular in outline (arrow).

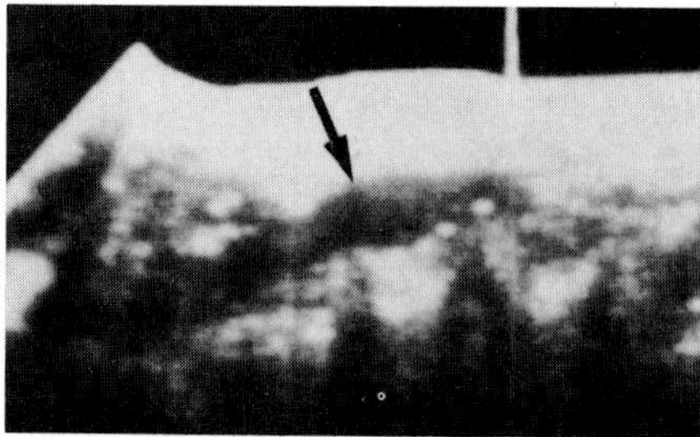

Fig. 67.42 Small fusiform aneurysm of abdominal aorta. There is a bulge of the aortic lumen producing lack of parallelism of the walls at the site of the small aneurysm (arrow).

the non-invasive investigation of disease of the peripheral arteries.

Ultrasonic methods have been in the forefront of these non-invasive procedures and they have had considerable success. They are:

1. use of a B-scanner
2. techniques using the Doppler Effect.

B-scanning. A high frequency transducer is needed of either 5 or 10 MHz (Gompels, 1979), the latter producing the higher definition of the arteries but its use is limited to the more superficial arteries. The arteries most frequently studied are the carotid, superficial femoral and popliteal arteries, to demonstrate stenoses due to atheroma and also aneurysms.

Doppler techniques. Two Doppler techniques are used: (1) continuous wave; (2) pulse echo systems.

(1) *Continuous wave Doppler techniques.* By this method blood flow either arterial or venous can be detected transcutaneously and recorded onto tape through a loudspeaker or as a waveform produced through a frequency analyser. Reduced or absent blood flow distal to an arterial stenosis or block, and abnormal blood flow produced by superficial malignant tumours can be demonstrated.

(2) *Pulse-echo Doppler imaging techniques.* This method is really a combination of the Doppler effect used to detect blood flow combined with the principle of the B-scanner employed to plot the source of the Doppler signals in space. The ultrasound is produced in rapidly repeated short pulses and the echoes recorded through a mobile artery and vein imaging system (MAVIS). Thus superficial arteries and veins are imaged and they are displayed as antero-posterior, lateral and cross-sectional images. High resolution real-time ultrasonic scanners are also available to demonstrate superficial arteries. Both these apparatuses can also record blood flow. Arterial

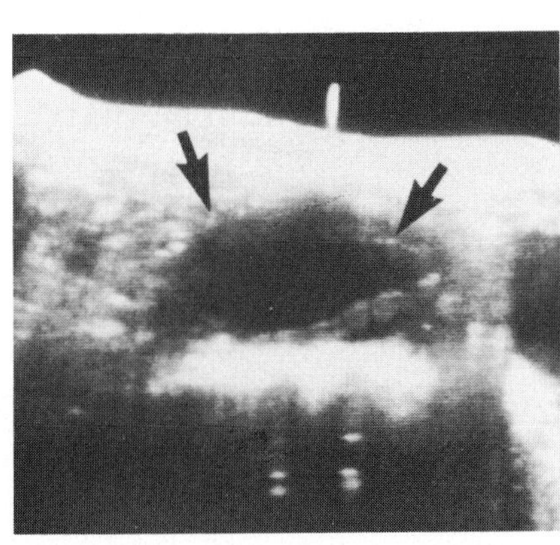

A

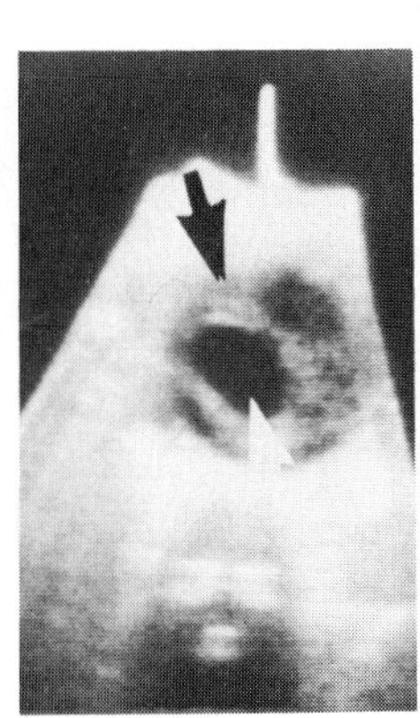

B

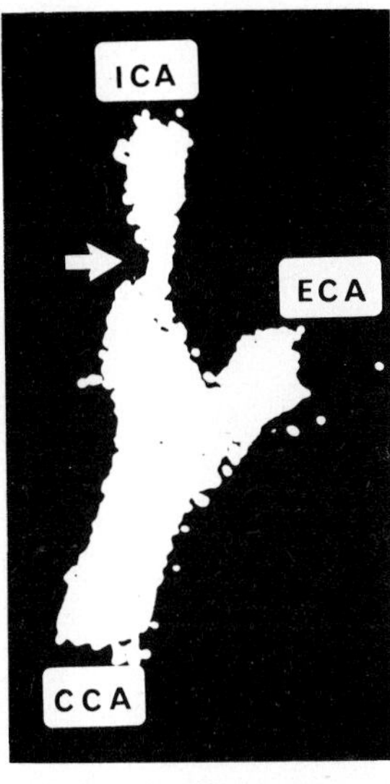

C

Fig. 67.43 Abdominal aortic aneurysm.

(A) Longitudinal scan. The aneurysm appears as an oval transonic mass (arrows) with echoes along its edges inferiorly (right arrow) produced by thrombus.

(B) Transverse section. The transonic lumen (white arrow) of the dilated aorta is eccentric and surrounded by thrombus (black arrow).

(C) Carotid artery. Antero posterior. Typical picture produced by the Mobile Artery and Vein Imaging System (MAVIS). Localized stenosis (arrow) of the internal carotid artery. The external carotid artery is not occluded; its distal portion merely passes out of the plane of examination. CCA—common carotid artery. ICA—internal carotid artery. ECA—external carotid artery.

stenoses, blocks and arteriosclerosis can thus be visualized transcutaneously (Fig. 67.43C) (Baird *et al.*, 1979).

All these methods are capable of further development and have considerable promise for the future.

THE RETROPERITONEUM

The presence of gas in the intestine tends to reduce the usefulness of ultrasound in imaging the para-aortic glands. However, if they are over 3·0 cm in diameter they may be visualized but this represents advanced adenopathy. The enlarged glands will be seen as small echo-containing well-defined masses adjacent to the aorta. Larger masses of glands will surround the aorta or even displace it forwards so that there is a space between it and the spine. One of the commonest causes of para-aortic lymphadenopathy is some form of lymphoma. When the adenopathy is recognized it is important to examine the liver, porta hepatis and spleen to image the extent of the disease. Pelvic adenopathy can also be visualized. One of the objects of visualizing the retroperitoneal adenopathy is to stage the lymphoma or testicular seminoma and another is to monitor the effects of radiotherapy.

THYROID GLAND

The thyroid gland may be scanned ultrasonically with the use of a B-scanner either:

1. By direct skin contact of the transducer.
2. Through a water bath.

It may also be imaged by real-time scanning.

Ultrasonic examination of the thyroid may:

1. Show the size and shape of the gland; this is important information for radiotherapy planning and for demonstrating the response of a lesion to radiotherapy.
2. Show the presence of and internal echo pattern of nodules. Though a positive differential diagnosis cannot yet be made, certain ultrasonic features may indicate the likelihood of a lesion being benign or malignant.
3. Show the presence of and nature of cysts (a clearly defined area with no echoes in it).
4. Aid the direction of biopsy needles.

Hales *et al.* (1978) state that while malignant thyroid disease is most frequently shown as a well-defined localized area with moderate to low level echoes in it, non-malignant cases show similar appearances and therefore a clear diagnosis of cancer cannot be made on the basis of echo patterns alone. On the other hand the accuracy of diagnosing cysts of the thyroid is near 100 per cent provided that care is taken to avoid overlooking low level echoes.

THE ORBIT AND EYE

Ultrasonic examination of the eyes has been practised for about 20 years. A-scan methods were used in the first place but latterly methods employing B-scanners have been developed. Purpose built specialized B-scan apparatus has been produced using either direct transducer contact with the eye or ultrasonic beam transmission into the eye through a waterbath. Standard B-scan apparatus can also be used (Sutherland and Forrester, 1974).

Technique. The patient is examined recumbent. A watertight open-ended plastic bag is suspended over and sealed around the orbit and the eye anaesthetized with local anaesthetic. The plastic bag is filled with an adequate amount of warm saline through which the eye is scanned. A 5–10 MHz transducer is necessary to produce the high definition required of the examination. The transducer is placed so that its face is about 5·0 cm from the cornea. Three to five parallel scans are made transversely separated by a distance of about 2 mm. Both eyes should be examined at the same time for comparison purposes.

Normal appearances. The outline of the globe is shown together with the surfaces of the cornea, the anterior chamber, the lens, the vitreous and the retina. The retro-orbital tissues including the fat, the optic nerve and the lateral rectus muscle can be identified (see Ch. 52, p. 996).

Clinical value. Ultrasonic examination of the eye is of most value when the interior cannot be evaluated by the use of conventional optical methods such as the ophthalmoscope because the anterior media are opaque or there is haemorrhage into the vitreous. It also has an important place in the investigation of the retro-orbital tissues (Sutherland and Forrester, 1974). It is particularly indicated (Coleman and Smith, 1978) in the assessment of retinal or choroidal detachments and trauma when the media are opaque, localization of foreign bodies and the diagnosis of retro-ocular tumours. It has also proved its value in the diagnosis of orbital lesions producing proptosis (Sutherland, 1978) and it will reveal tumours, inflammatory lesions, post-traumatic lesions and muscle swelling in dysthyroid ophthalmopathy.

CARDIOLOGY

Except for a small area to the left of the sternum, the lungs and pleura cover the anterior aspect of the heart. It is by passing the ultrasound beam through this bare area that the heart can be examined and echocardiography performed (Fig. 67.44).

Method. The patient lies supine on a couch and electrocardiography leads are attached. Oil or proprietary gel is applied to the skin and the probe placed over the third or fourth intercostal space in the parasternal region. The probe is rotated until the kicking movement of the echo from the anterior cusp of the mitral valve is obtained at a depth of about 6–8 cm from the anterior chest wall. Slight downward inclination of the probe from this position usually allows echoes from the posterior cusp to be obtained. If the examination is not successful with the patient lying flat, rotating him to the left will frequently produce a good examination. The mitral valve echo is used as a landmark and from it echoes from many other intracardiac structures can be obtained. By adjusting the beam direction upwards and to the right the echoes from the base of the aorta and aortic valve are obtained. By rotating the beam downwards and to the right from the mitral valve position, echoes from the tricuspid valve cusps may be detected, especially in a patient with a large right ventricle. Downward and outward inclination of the beam from the mitral valve position especially if the patient is rotated towards the left side will enable the interventricular septum to be displayed and also the posterior wall of the left ventricle. The latter is distinguished from the left atrial wall by the fact that the left ventricular posterior wall moves forwards in ventricular systole; the left atrial wall moves backwards in ventricular systole. A recently introduced technique is to sweep the ultrasound beam slowly downwards and to the left from the aortic valve, through the mitral valve position and on down the central line of the left ventricle to the apex, making a continuous slow speed recording on the strip chart recorder (Fig. 67.45). This method particularly helps determining the relationship of the aortic walls to the interventricular septum and anterior cusp of the mitral valve. It also demonstrates the contractility of the left ventricular walls and may identify areas of infarction. The pulmonary valve is the most difficult valve to examine. It may be demonstrated by rotating the probe upwards and to the left from the mitral valve position. If the pulmonary valve is not demonstrated in this probe position, then repeating the procedure with the probe placed one intercostal space higher may be more successful.

Occasionally an alternative approach to the heart through the upper abdomen or suprasternal notch can be useful if the conventional approach fails.

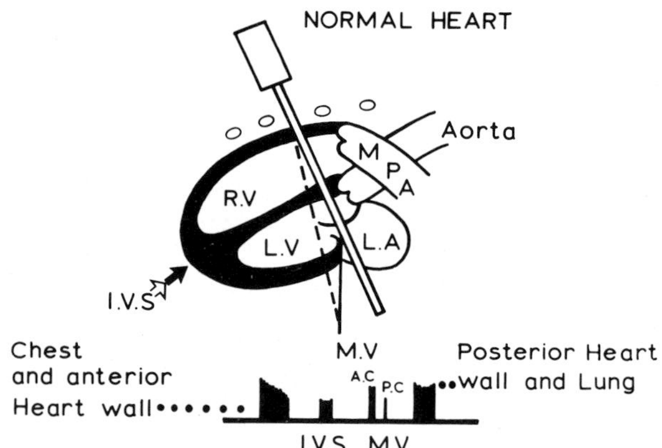

Fig. 67.44 Echocardiography. Diagram of longitudinal section of heart to show path of ultrasound beam (two parallel lines) through an appropriate intercostal space onto the anterior cusp of the mitral valve. The resultant echoes on the A-scan are displayed below. The dotted line indicates the deflection of the ultrasound beam often necessary to examine the posterior mitral valve cusp.

AC—anterior mitral valve cusp. IVS—interventricular septum. LA—left atrium. LV—left ventricle. MPA—main pulmonary artery. MV—mitral valve. PC—posterior mitral valve cusp. RV—right ventricle. T—transducer on anterior chest wall.

(Reproduced with permission from 'Recent Advances in Radiology and Medical Imaging—6'. Ed. Lodge and Steiner.)

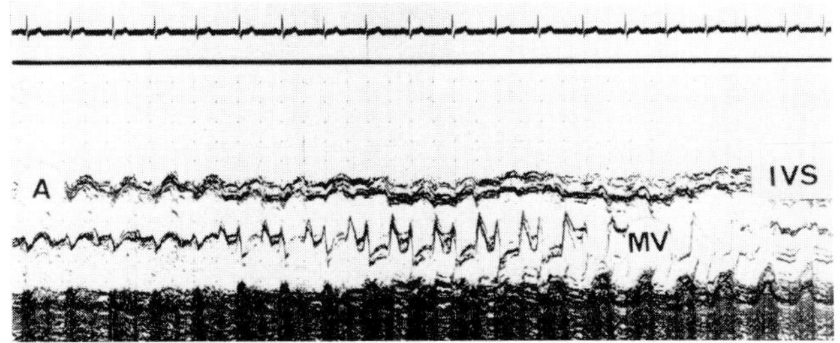

Fig. 67.45 Slow sweep echocardiogram. The transducer is slowly rotated downwards from the aorta (A), through the mitral valve (MV) to the left ventricle, thus displaying a longitudinal section of the left side of the heart. Note the continuity between the anterior wall of the aorta and the interventricular septum (IVS) and the posterior aortic wall and the anterior mitral valve cusp.

For adults it is best to use a transducer which is focussed to about 9 cm and has a frequency of about 2·25 MHz. Shorter focussed transducers may enhance the examination of the more superficial parts of the heart.

NORMAL APPEARANCES

Mitral valve. The normal mitral echocardiogram is shown in Figure 67.46. Upward deflection of the echocardiogram trace is produced by the movement of a structure towards the anterior chest wall and *vice-versa.* An electronic grid consisting of vertical lines of small dots is superimposed on the trace (Fig. 67.47). The vertical distance between each dot represents one centimeter in the patient and the horizontal spacing between each column of dots half a second in time. Using this grid the depth of a structure within the patient and its rate of movement can be measured (Fig. 67.47B). The 'A' peak (Fig. 67.46) is produced by left atrial contraction. This is followed by ventricular systole, the onset of which is shown by rapid descent of the trace of the movement of the anterior cusp through position B to position C, the position of maximal closure of the valve. As ventricular contraction continues, the trace rises slowly to position D, the C–D slope being produced by the forward movement of the whole valve ring during ventricular systole. As the ventricle dilates in early ventricular diastole the valve cusps open widely, position E being the position of maximal opening of the anterior cusp of the mitral valve. During early ventricular diastole and under the influence of various haemodynamic factors, the mitral valve partially closes and the trace from the anterior cusp descends to position F frequently in two stages. The initial slope will be fairly slow until position F_0 is reached, then it speeds up to position F. The slope

E
F_0
A A
AC B D F B
PC C C

A

A E
C D F

B

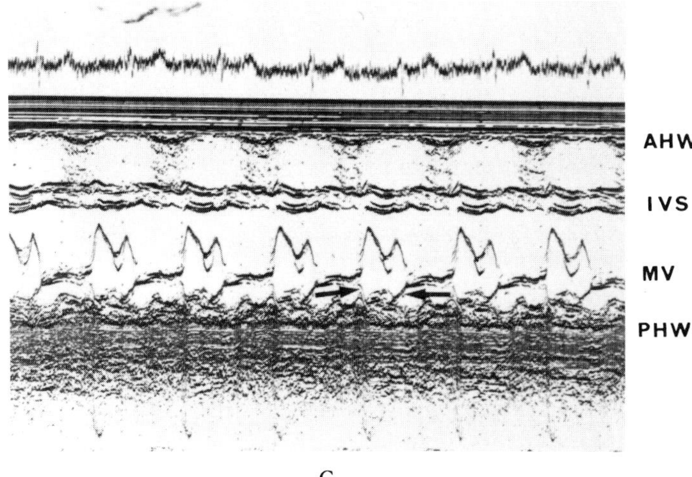

C

Fig. 67.46 Normal mitral valve echocardiogram.

(A) Diagram. A.C—anterior cusp. P.C—posterior cusp. Upward deflection of the trace is produced by a structure moving towards the anterior chest wall and downward deflection by a structure moving in the reverse direction. The peak A represents atrial systole. After this the trace descends through position B to position C at which point the valve is closed in early ventricular systole. The slope C–D is produced by the whole mitral valve structure moving forwards during ventricular systole and it includes the period of isovolumetric contraction. The peak E is produced by the valve opening fully in early ventricular diastole. The E–F_0–F slope, known as the 'diastolic slope' represents the partial closure of the valve during early ventricular diastole following which the valve cusps remain partially open until the next atrial contraction occurs. In ventricular diastole the posterior cusp movement is opposite to that of the anterior cusp but the posterior cusp movement is of less amplitude (see text).

(B) Anterior cusp movement displayed by strip chart recorder, the echocardiogram being annotated as in (A).

(C) Anterior and posterior cusp (arrows) movement in same patient as (B). A.H.W—anterior heart wall. I.V.S—interventricular septum. MV—mitral valve. PHW—posterior heart wall.

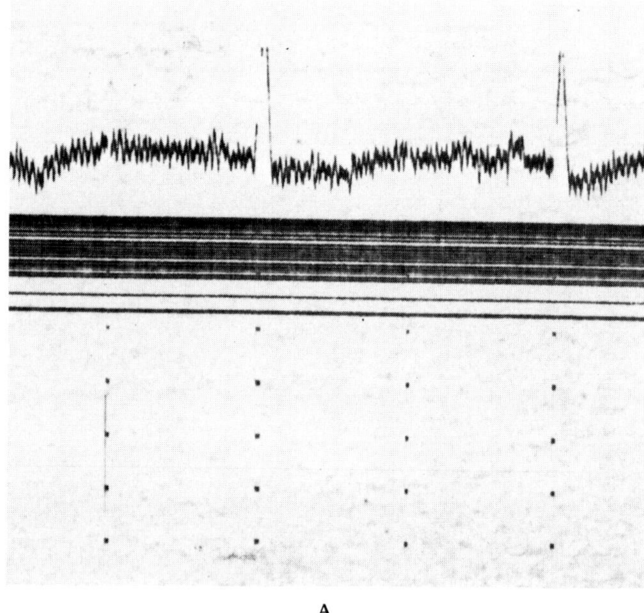

A

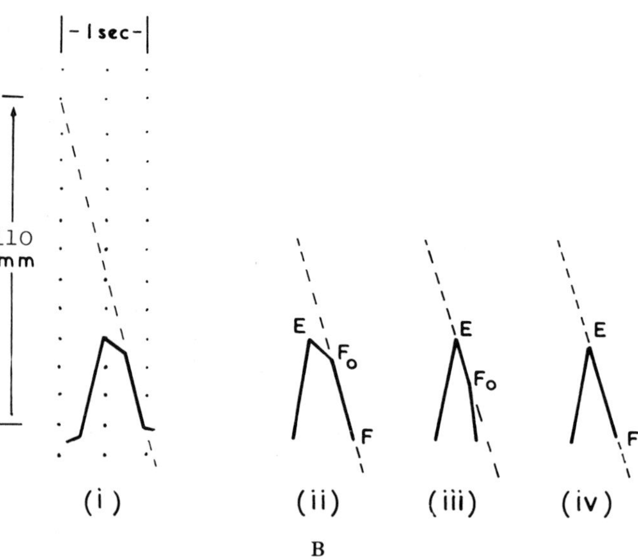

B

Fig. 67.47 Echocardiogram. Time/depth graticule and its use in measurement.

(A) Vertical lines of dots are sequentially impressed as a background onto the echocardiogram and are used for measurement purposes. The vertical distance between the dots represents 1 cm within the patient. The time between successive lines of dots is 0·5 second.

(B) Method of measuring the diastolic closure rate of the anterior cusp of the mitral valve. (i) The slope of the trace of diastolic closure is prolonged upwards until this line intersects one vertical line of dots and downwards until it intersects the second line of dots. The height of the first intersection point above the second one determines the speed of movement of the anterior cusp in 1 second; in this case 110 millimetres per second. The diastolic slope may be measured in three differing ways. (ii) E–F_o. (iii) F_o–F. (iv) E–F. Unfortunately there is no international agreement as to which should be utilized. The author prefers F_o–F. If this is not possible E–F is taken.

E–F is known as the 'diastolic slope'. The cusps then remain partially open for a variable time until the next atrial contraction occurs when the cycle starts again. The movement of the posterior cusp of the mitral valve is a mirror-image of the anterior cusp in ventricular diastole (Fig. 67.46C); the amplitude of movement of the posterior cusp is less than that of the anterior cusp. The two cusps are in apposition during ventricular systole.

Tricuspid valve. The normal tricuspid valve echocardiogram is similar to that of the mitral valve (Fig. 67.48).

Aorta and aortic valve. The aorta is shown as two parallel echo lines which move forwards in ventricular sytole and backwards in ventricular diastole (Fig. 67.49). Between them a midline echo arises from the closed aortic valve cusps in late ventricular systole and in ventricular diastole. During ventricular systole a rectangular box-like echo trace is produced by the forward movement of the echocardiographically anterior aortic cusp (right coronary cusp) and the backward movement of the echocardiographically posterior cusp (posterior non-coronary cusp). The left atrial cavity is shown behind the aorta.

Left ventricular cavity. The interventricular septum is revealed as a thick undulating column of echoes between the right and left ventricles (Fig. 67.50). The posterior left ventricular wall is seen as two parallel lines in front of the lung echo pattern and separated from each other by low amplitude echoes. The inner endocardium and outer epicardium account for the parallel lines. The left ventricular muscle thickens during ventricular systole.

Pulmonary valve. Only the movement of the posterior leaflet of the pulmonary valve can be recorded. It is a tracing difficult to obtain and its study does not often contribute much to the management of the patient.

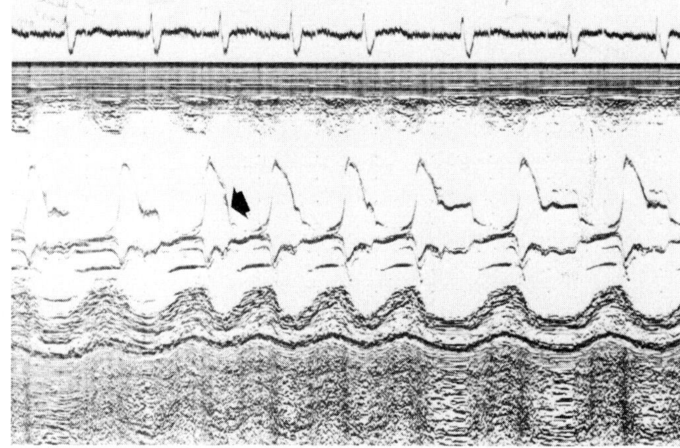

Fig. 67.48 Echocardiogram of normal tricuspid valve well seen in a patient with a dilated right ventricle. The tricuspid valve cusp movements are similar to those of the mitral valve and they produce a comparable echocardiogram trace (arrow) to that of the mitral valve.

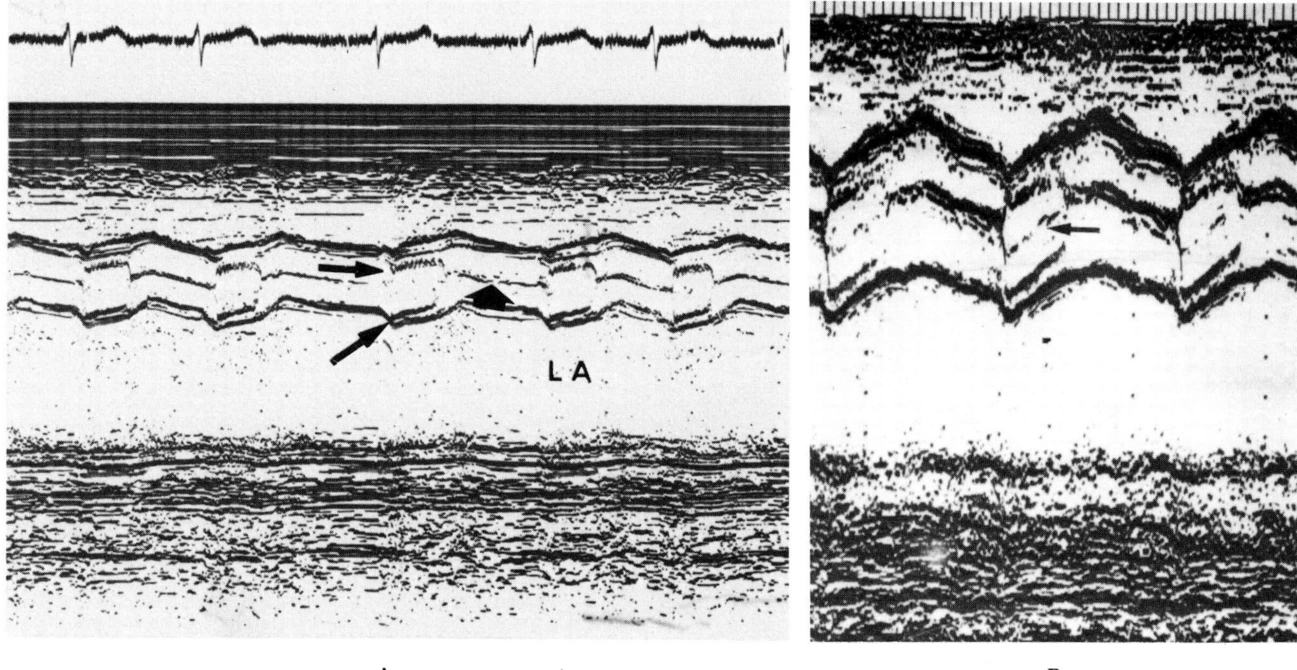

Fig. 67.49 Echocardiogram. Normal aorta and aortic valve.
(A) The aortic root moves forwards in ventricular systole and backwards in ventricular diastole. The aorta is shown as two parallel lines. The aortic valve cusps produce a box-like pattern in ventricular systole while the cusps are open (arrows). In late ventricular systole and in ventricular diastole the cusps close and they produce a single line echo central in the aorta (flat arrow) (see text). The left atrium (LA) is behind the aorta and the outflow tract of the right ventricle in front of the aorta. The fluttering of the anterior aortic cusp is a normal phenomenon.
(B) An echo (arrow) produced by the third (left coronary) aortic valve cusp may be demonstrated between the other two cusps.

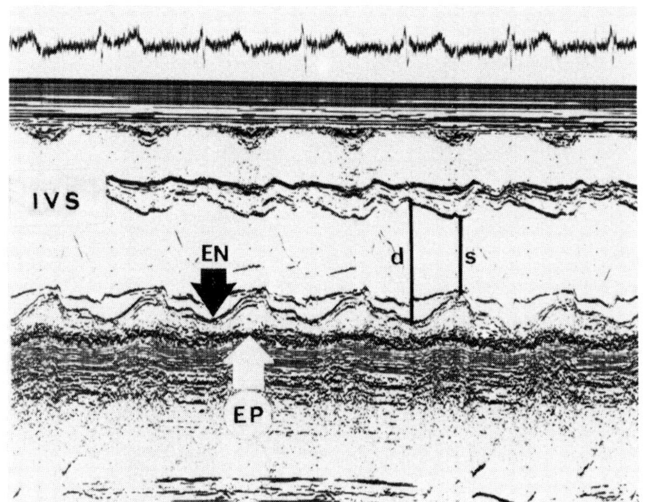

Fig. 67.50 Echocardiogram of normal left ventricle. The posterior left ventricular wall and interventricular septum (IVS) are clearly seen. They converge during ventricular systole and diverge during ventricular diastole. EN—endocardium. EP—epicardium. Systolic (s) and diastolic (d) internal diameters of left ventricle.

Causes of failure to obtain an echocardiogram

There are many causes of failure to obtain a satisfactory echocardiographic examination. The main ones are obesity, muscular anterior chest wall, emphysema, sternal depression, tachycardia, previous left-sided thoracotomy particularly after mitral valvotomy, and a mobile uncooperative child.

ABNORMALITIES DEMONSTRATED BY ECHOCARDIOGRAPHY

MITRAL VALVE

Mitral stenosis. In mitral stenosis the rigidity of the valve cusps, fusion of the commissures and the resultant narrowing of the valve orifice cause the two cusps to move in the same direction, the more mobile cusp being the anterior one. In early ventricular diastole both cusps move forward, the anterior cusp reaching maximum opening at point E. Throughout ventricular diastole the anterior cusp slowly moves backwards producing a slow diastolic slope which continues either till the next atrial contraction (Fig. 67.60B) or if no atrial contraction occurs, until the onset of ventricular systole when the valve closes (Fig. 67.51). During ventricular diastole the posterior cusp parallels or nearly parallels the movement of the anterior cusp. The movement of the anterior cusp is measured to assess the severity of the stenosis (i.e. the diastolic slope—the flatter the slope the more severe is the stenosis—Fig. 67.51) and also the mobility of the cusp (the height of point E above point C). A thick cusp echo will indicate fibrosis or calcification (Fig. 67.52).

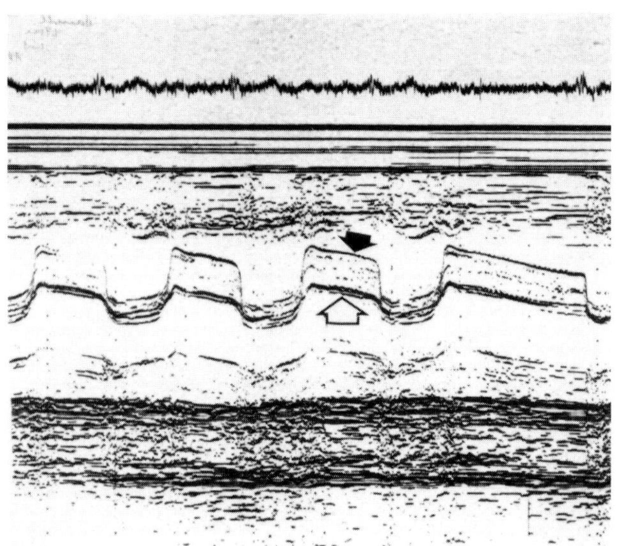

Fig. 67.51 Echocardiogram. Mitral valve—mitral stenosis. Patient in atrial fibrillation. The slow diastolic slope of the anterior cusp (black arrow) is well seen. The posterior cusp (open arrow) moves forwards and parallels the movement of the anterior cusp in ventricular diastole. The valve cusps are only slightly thickened.

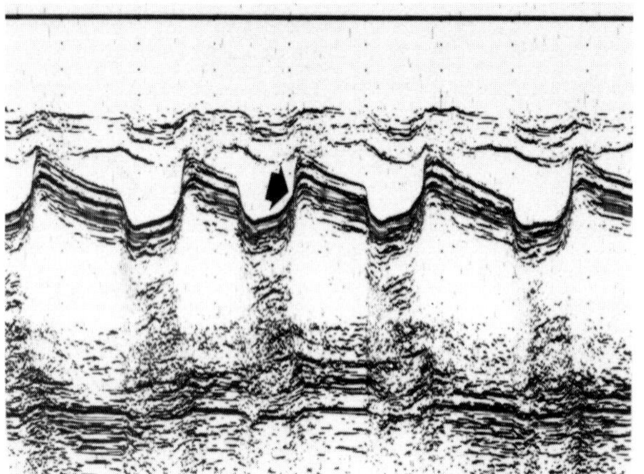

Fig. 67.52 Echocardiogram. Mitral valve—mitral stenosis. Patient in atrial fibrillation. The valve cusps (arrow) are thickened and calcified and produce high intensity echoes.

False mitral stenosis. The slow diastolic slope of mitral stenosis is not specific to the diagnosis of mitral stenosis. It will be present in any condition which leads to a slow filling rate of the left ventricle such as hypertrophic cardiomyopathy or aortic stenosis. The distinguishing feature is the movement of the posterior cusp in ventricular diastole; in organic mitral stenosis this is parallel to the movement of the anterior cusp whereas it is in the opposite direction in conditions producing a slow filling rate of the left ventricle. Unusual cases of organic mitral stenosis are being reported in whom the posterior mitral valve cusp moves backwards in ventricular diastole. These must be distinguished by identifying other signs of organic mitral stenosis such as thickening of the anterior cusp echo.

Mitral regurgitation. Most patients with mitral regurgitation echocardiographically have normal mitral cusp movement. Some will have a fast ventricular diastolic slope and high amplitude of anterior cusp movement; these features merely indicate a high blood flow through the valve and will also be seen in such conditions as ventricular septal defect and patent ductus arteriosus. However, some causes of mitral regurgitation can be demonstrated such as prolapse of the posterior cusp (Fig. 67.53), rupture of the chordae tendineae and vegetations resulting from subacute bacterial endocarditis (Ross, 1978).

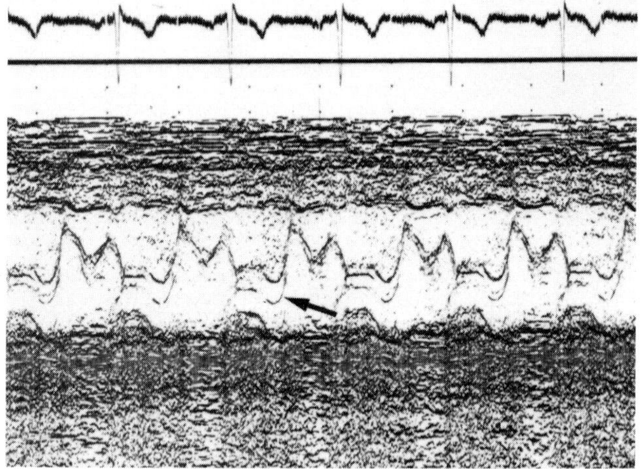

Fig. 67.53 Echocardiogram. Mitral valve—prolapse of the posterior mitral valve cusp. In late ventricular systole the posterior cusp moves backwards (arrow) to a greater extent than the anterior cusp. The echocardiogram otherwise is normal.

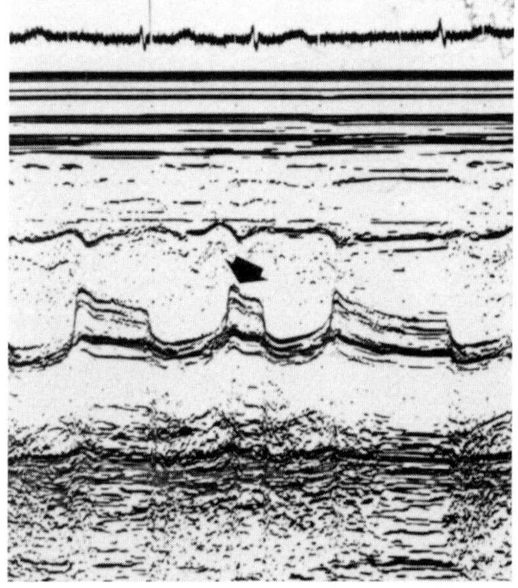

Fig. 67.54 Echocardiogram. Mitral valve—combined mitral stenosis and regurgitation with dominant regurgitation. The dominant regurgitation produces a short but rapid diastolic slope (arrow) at the commencement of ventricular diastole, otherwise the echocardiogram is the same as mitral stenosis. Atrial fibrillation.

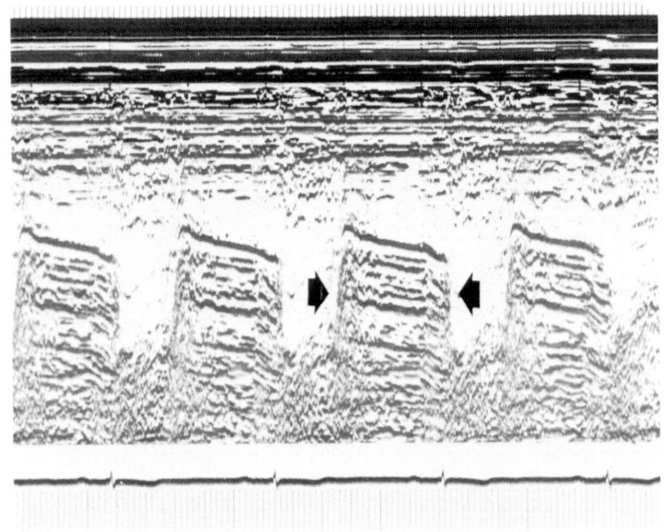

A

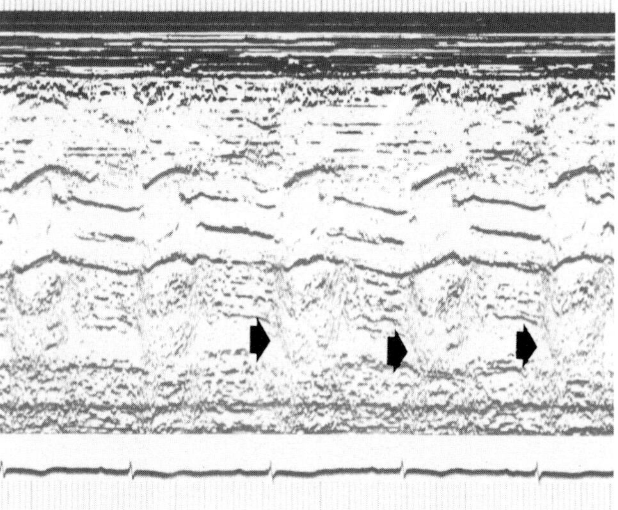

B

Fig. 67.55 Left atrial myxoma.

(A) Mitral valve echocardiogram. In ventricular diastole the tumour produces multiple echoes behind the anterior cusp of the mitral valve (arrows) and the diastolic slope is slow.

(B) Aortic valve echocardiogram. The tumour produces echoes within the left atrium: it is close to the aortic wall in ventricular diastole but in ventricular systole the tumour moves further back (arrows) into the left atrium.

Combined mitral stenosis and regurgitation. Frequently mitral stenosis and regurgitation co-exist. When stenosis is the dominant lesion the echocardiographic pattern is that of mitral stenosis. If the regurgitation is dominant, the diastolic slope immediately after the 'E' point is relatively rapid for a short-time interval after which the diastolic slope assumes the usual form of mitral stenosis (Fig. 67.54).

Left atrial myxoma. These patients present with signs of intermittent mitral valve obstruction or systemic embolism. The tumour, arising on a pedicle from the interatrial septum herniates into the mitral valve orifice in ventricular diastole. The presence of the tumour in this position reduces the diastolic slope of the anterior cusp and also produces multiple echoes deep to this cusp (Fig. 67.55). In ventricular systole the tumour returns to the left atrium where it can give rise to echoes behind the aorta. Echocardiography is a very sensitive method of detecting left atrial myxoma: the signs may however be confused with a left atrial thrombus or multiple echoes from a calcified mitral valve.

Mitral valve movement in aortic regurgitation. In patients with aortic regurgitation the anterior cusp of the mitral valve in ventricular diastole is suspended between two streams of blood, one from the mitral valve and the other regurgitating through the aortic valve. This streaming sets up a vibration or 'fluttering' movement of the anterior cusp and occasionally the posterior cusp as well (Fig. 67.56). Usually there is also a slow anterior cusp diastolic slope and there may be early closure of the mitral valve, the latter being due to regurgitant blood from the aorta prematurely raising the diastolic pressure in the left ventricle above that of the left atrium. The left ventricle will be dilated if significant regurgitation is present. Early diastolic fluttering of the left ventricular side of the interventricular septum may also be seen in aortic regurgitation (Fig. 67.57).

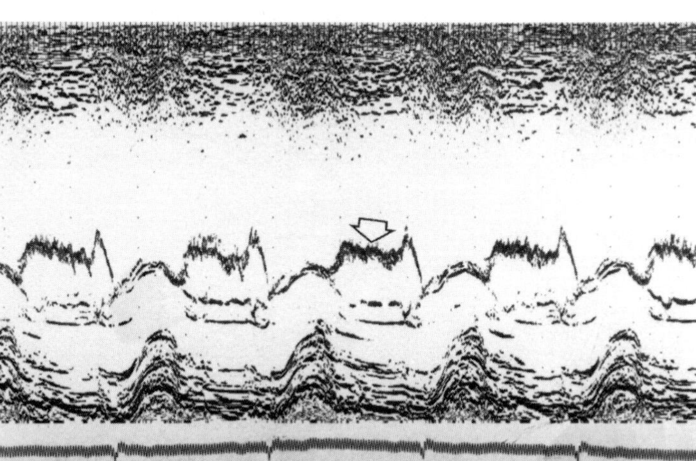

Fig. 67.56 Echocardiogram. Mitral valve—aortic regurgitation. The left ventricle is dilated. There is coarse fluttering of the anterior cusp (arrow) of the mitral valve in ventricular diastole and the diastolic slope is slow. The posterior cusp moves backwards during ventricular diastole.

Hypertrophic obstructive cardiomyopathy

In this condition there is asymmetrical hypertrophy of the walls of the left ventricle, the interventricular septum being thicker than the posterior wall. In the normal heart the ratio of the thickness of the septum to the posterior wall is about unity whereas in hypertrophic cardiomyopathy it will exceed 1·3. There is also a slow diastolic

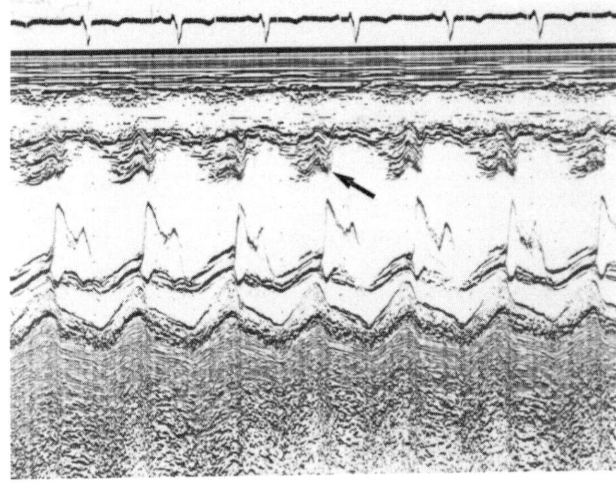

Fig. 67.57 Echocardiogram. Mitral valve—aortic regurgitation. The mitral valve cusp movement is normal except for minor fluttering of the anterior cusp in ventricular diastole. The left ventricular outflow tract is dilated. There is volume overload of the left ventricle shown by excessive movement of the left ventricular side of the interventricular septum. The aortic regurgitation also produces fluttering of the left ventricular side of the septum in early diastole (arrow).

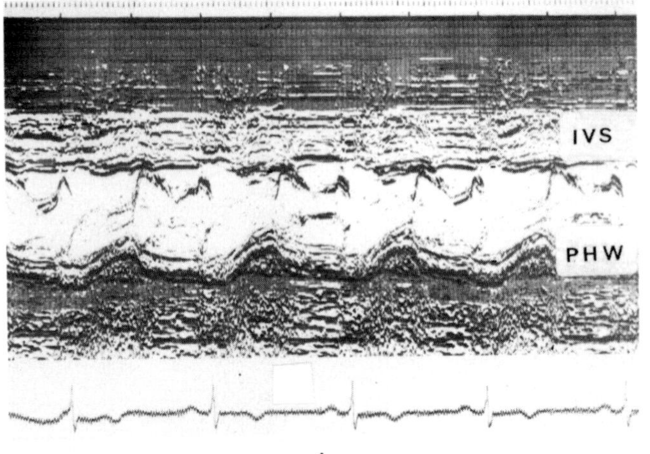

A

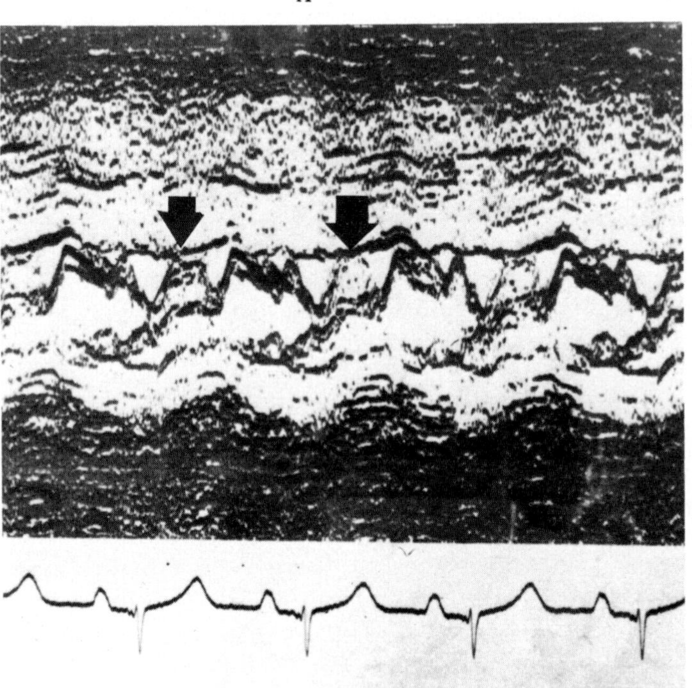

B

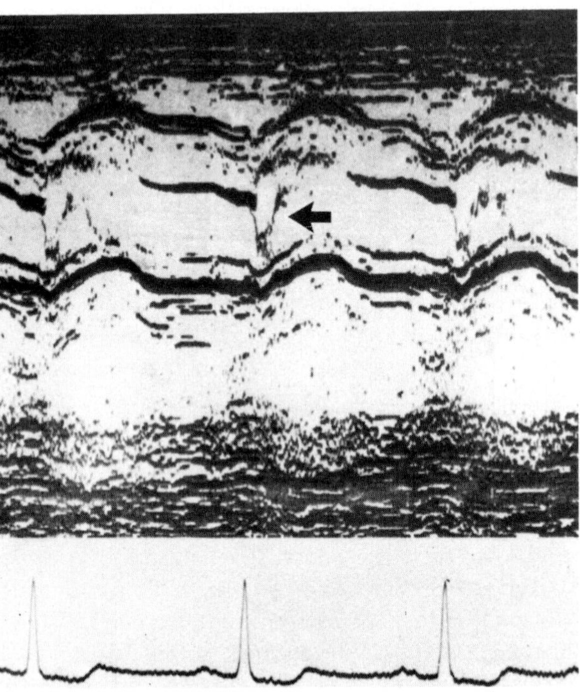

C

Fig. 67.58 Echocardiogram. Mitral valve. Two cases of hypertrophic cardiomyopathy.

(A) Hypertrophic cardiomyopathy (non-obstructive). The interventricular septum (IVS) is very thickened compared with the posterior wall of the left ventricle (PHW). The mitral valve anterior cusp contacts the septum in early ventricular diastole and the diastolic slope is slow.

(B) Hypertrophic obstructive cardiomyopathy. In this condition the findings are the same as in (A) but in addition there is anterior motion (arrow) of the anterior cusp of the mitral valve during ventricular systole.

(C) Same case as in (B). The obstruction produced by the anterior movement of the anterior mitral valve cusp against the interventricular septum leads to early partial closure of the aortic valve (arrow). (By courtesy of Dr David Shaw, Exeter.)

slope of the anterior cusp of the mitral valve due to reduced compliance of the ventricular wall leading to a slow ventricular filling rate. When outflow tract obstruction is present there will be forward movement of the anterior cusp against the interventricular septum in early or mid ventricular systole—so-called S.A.M. or systolic anterior motion (Fig. 67.58).

AORTIC VALVE AND AORTA

Aortic stenosis. Calcific aortic stenosis will be revealed by the presence of high intensity echoes arising from the aortic valve cusps within the lumen of the aorta. In addition, the cusps will move poorly or one may not move at all (Fig. 67.59).

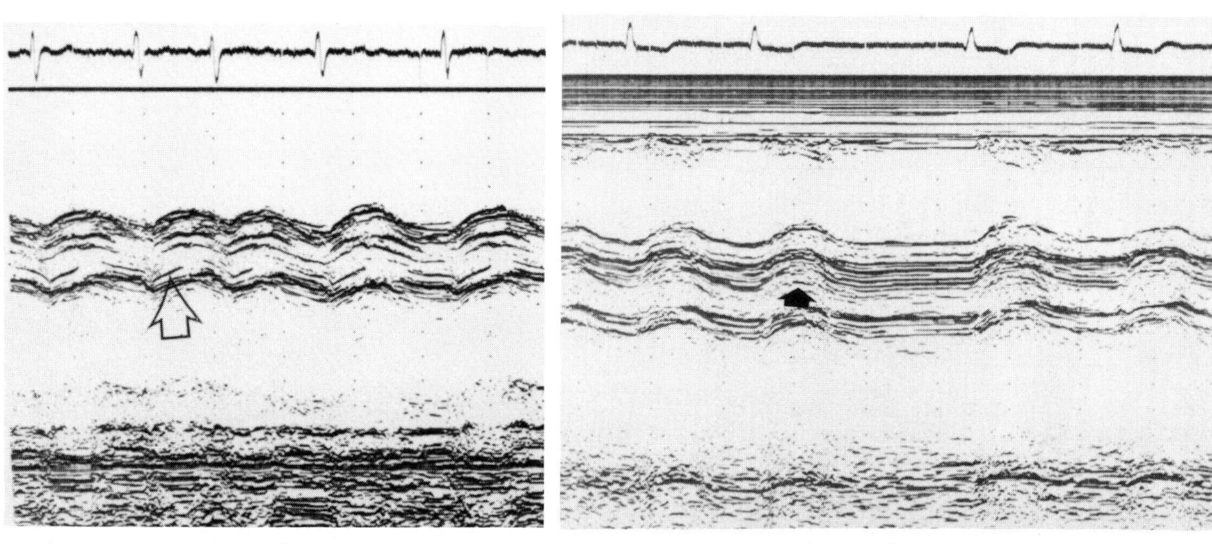

Fig. 67.59 Echocardiogram. Aortic stenosis.
(A) The anterior (right coronary) cusp is thickened; it hardly moves and it produces dense echoes. The posterior (left non-coronary) cusp (arrow) opens almost fully. The left atrium is large in this patient.
(B) In another patient the calcification in the aortic valve cusps produces high intensity echoes and there is minimal cusp movement (arrow). The left atrium is large.

Dissecting aneurysm of the aorta. If the dissection involves the ascending aorta just above the aortic valve, splitting of the normal single linear echoes from the anterior and posterior walls of the aorta into double lines may be demonstrated (Ross, 1978).

Pericardial effusion

When fluid collects in the pericardial sac, it will separate the parietal pericardium from the heart wall. No echoes will be seen where the fluid is present. Thus in pericardial effusion the echoes arising from the anterior chest wall and the anterior heart wall and also from the lung and the posterior heart wall will be separated by transonic areas due to the pericardial effusion. The heart wall will be seen as an undulating echo pattern separated by a clear transonic band from the chest wall and lung echoes (Fig. 67.60). A pericardial effusion will not be seen posterior to the left atrium because the pericardial space is obliterated by the insertion of the pulmonary veins (Fig. 67.60).

Left ventricular volume and function studies

The outline of the normal left ventricle is a prolate ellipse and therefore its volume can be calculated by cubing the shortest diameter. This diameter is obtained by measuring the distance between the posterior surface of the interventricular septum and the endocardial surface of its posterior wall at a point just distal to the mitral valve (Fig. 67.50). If this measurement is made in ventricular systole and in ventricular diastole the difference in the left ventricular volumes will represent the ventricular stroke volume and from this the ejection fraction and also the cardiac output can be calculated. These calculations are accurate to about 15 per cent only so long as the long diameter of the left ventricle is twice the short diameter. Once this relationship is altered such as occurs in left ventricular enlargement, these calculations become inaccurate.

Congenital heart disease

The value of echocardiography in the diagnosis of congenital heart disease has become more apparent in recent years. In the normal person there is continuity between the anterior wall of the aorta and the interventricular septum as well as the posterior aortic wall and the anterior cusp of the mitral valve.

If the aorta overrides the septum as in Fallot's tetralogy, the echoes for the aortic anterior wall will be in front of those from the septum. If the whole aorta is displaced forwards as in transposition of the great arteries and double outlet right ventricle the continuity between the

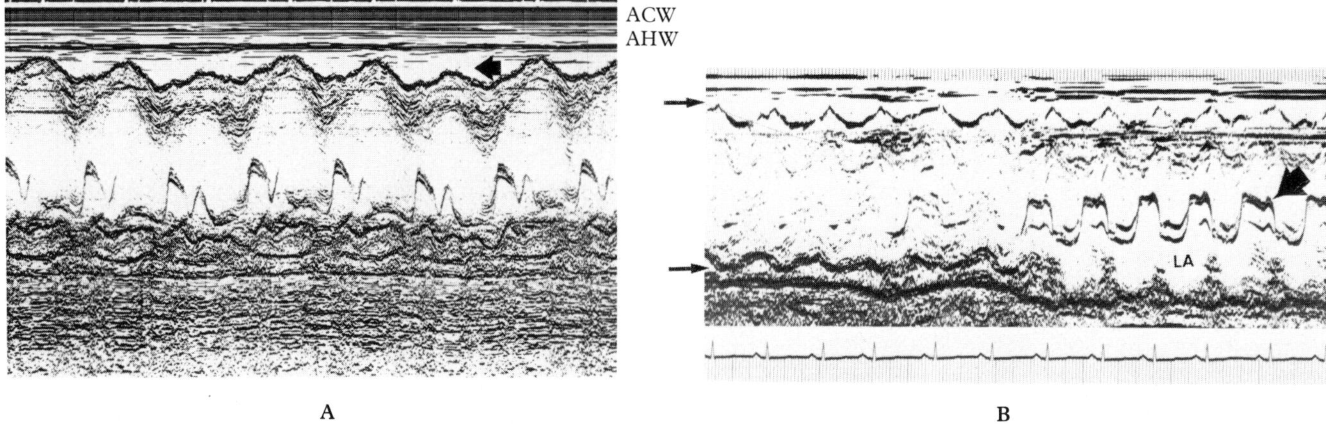

Fig. 67.60 Echocardiogram. Pericardial effusion.
(A) The pericardial effusion produces an echo-free area (arrow) between the anterior chest wall (ACW) and the anterior heart wall (AHW), the contraction of the latter being clearly demonstrated.
(B) Anterior and posterior pericardial effusion (small arrows). As the transducer is rotated from left ventricle up to left atrium (LA) it is demonstrated that there is no pericardial effusion posterior to the left atrium. The patient also suffers from mitral stenosis and is in sinus rhythm. The diastolic slope of the anterior cusp of the mitral valve is slow and there is an 'A' wave (large arrow). The posterior mitral valve cusp is also seen; it parallels precisely the movement of the anterior cusp.

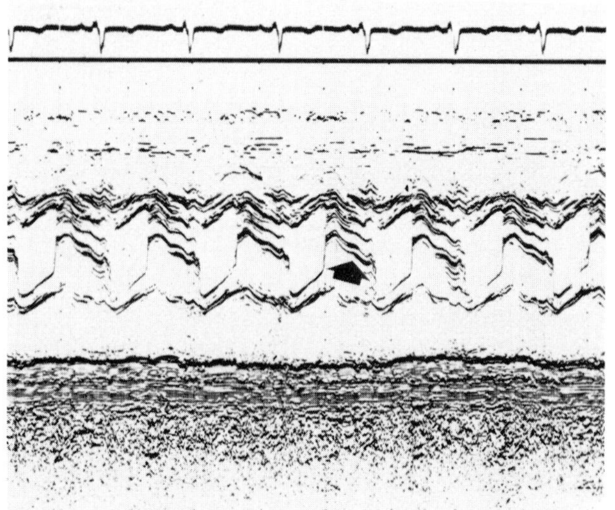

Fig. 67.61 Echocardiogram. Aortic valve—bicuspid aortic valve. The aortic cusps open normally. The anterior cusp is smaller than the posterior cusp and as a result the echo produced by the closed cusps in ventricular diastole is eccentric (arrow) to the aortic walls. The cusps in this case are also redundant as shown by the production of multiple echoes.

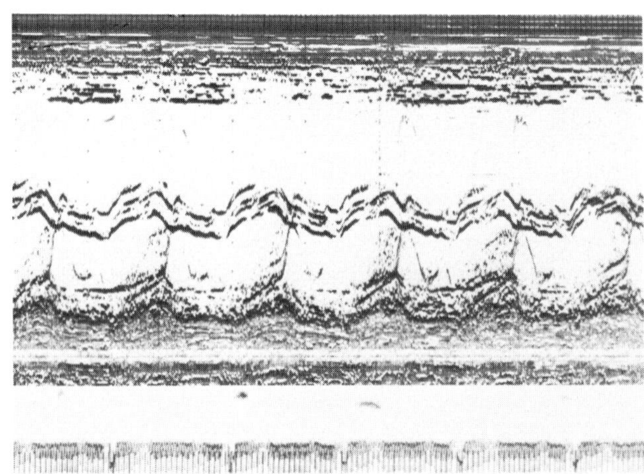

Fig. 67.62 Echocardiogram. Left ventricle—volume overload of right ventricle due to atrial septal defect. During ventricular systole and diastole the interventricular septum and posterior heart wall move forwards and backwards synchronously. The right ventricle is large and the left ventricle small.

posterior wall of the aorta and the anterior cusp of the mitral valve will be lost. If the aortic valve is bicuspid, the echoes from the cusps may be eccentric (Fig. 67.61). In patients with volume overload of the right ventricle such as occurs in atrial septal defect, total anomalous venous drainage and tricuspid regurgitation, the movement of the interventricular septum will become synchronous with that of the posterior heart wall (Fig. 67.62) instead of their movements being opposed to each other as in normal persons or patients with volume overload of the left ventricle (Fig. 67.56). Ultrasonic 'contrast medium' may be introduced into the blood passing through the heart and great vessels by injecting rapidly small quantities of 5 per cent dextrose or normal saline through a catheter introduced into the heart with its tip proximal to the area of interest. The rapid injection produces cavitation at the tip of the catheter and the microbubbles so produced give rise to multiple echoes within the blood stream on echocardiography. In this way echoes from anatomical structures can be confirmed and also transposition of the great arteries and intracardiac shunts, such as a ventricular septal defect, revealed in neonates. A suprasternal position of the transducer is best in neonates for this particular examination.

REAL-TIME EXAMINATION OF THE HEART

Real-time scanning has recently introduced a new dimension into cardiological assessment. Its ability to demonstrate cross-sections of the heart is unique to non-invasive techniques. By this method the normal anatomy can be shown in a different plane; chamber function can be studied and the relationship of the great vessels to each other and the ventricles demonstrated. The movement of the cusps of the various valves are revealed in remarkable detail, especially the mitral and aortic valves and disease of these valves demonstrated such as stenosis and calcification. The method is of considerable value in assessing ventricular wall movement, particularly of the left ventricle and identifying areas of dyskinesia arising from coronary artery disease. In congenital heart disease the method is very valuable in revealing the size and position of the ventricles and great arteries to show or exclude transposition of the great arteries. It will assist in the diagnosis of hypoplastic left ventricle in neonates and may save expensive angiocardiography examination. The interventricular septum is outlined with considerable accuracy by real-time scanning and therefore the method is of help in the diagnosis of single ventricle and the cardiomyopathies. Pericardial effusion is detected with accuracy. In addition real-time scanning may be used to assist in selecting the best position and direction of the transducer to obtain an optimum M-mode echocardiogram. Real-time scanning of the heart is a rapidly advancing field of investigation. As the quality of the apparatus and therefore the clarity of the picture advances, so the method will find wider application in the future.

REFERENCES AND SUGGESTIONS FOR FURTHER READING

BAIRD, R. N., LUSBY, R. J., BIRD, D. R., GIDDINGS, A. E. B., SKIDMORE, R., WOODCOCK, J. P., HORTON, R. E. & PEACOCK, J. H. (1979) Pulsed doppler angiography in lower limb arterial ischaemia. *Surgery*, **86**, 818–825.

BARNETT, E. & MORLEY, P. (1971) Ultrasound in the investigation of space-occupying lesions of the urinary tract. *British Journal of Radiology*, **44**, 733–742.

BARNETT, E. & MORLEY, P. (1974) *Abdominal Echography*. Ultrasound in the diagnosis of abdominal conditions, pp. 7–8. Butterworths, London.

COLEMAN, D. J. & SMITH, M. E. (1978) Retinal and orbital detachments. In de Vlieger, M., Holmes, J. H., Kazner, E., Kossoff, G., Kratochwil, A., Kraus, R., Poujol, J. & Strandness, D. E. (eds.) *Handbook of Clinical Ultrasound*, pp. 857–862. John Wiley & Sons, New York.

FIEGENBAUM, H. (1976) *Echocardiography*, 2nd ed. Lea & Febiger, Philadelphia.

GOLDBERG, B. B. (1977) *Abdominal Gray Scale Ultrasonography*. John Wiley & Sons, New York.

GOMPELS, B. M. (1979) High definition imaging of carotid arteries using a standard commercial ultrasound 'B' scanner—a preliminary report. *British Journal of Radiology*, **52**, 608–619.

HALES, I., JELLINS, J. & PUSSELL, S. (1978) The role of ultrasound in diagnosis of thyroid tumours. In Hill, C. R., McCready, V. R. & Cosgrove, D. O. (eds.) *Ultrasound in Tumour Diagnosis*, pp. 67–92. Pitman Medical, London.

HANCKE, S. (1976) Ultrasonic scanning of the pancreas. *Journal of Clinical Ultrasound*, **4**, 223–229.

LAING, F. C., LONGDEN, L. A. & FILLY, R. A. (1978) Ultrasonic identification of dilated intrahepatic bile ducts and their differentiation from portal venous structures. *Journal of Clinical Ultrasound*, **6**, 90–94.

MAKLAD, N. F. & WRIGHT, C. H. (1978) Grey scale ultrasonography in the diagnosis of ectopic pregnancy. *Radiology*, **126**, 221–225.

MCARDLE, C. R. (1976) Ultrasonic diagnosis of liver metastases. *Journal of Clinical Ultrasound*, **4**, 265–268.

MCDICKEN, W. N. (1976) *Diagnostic Ultrasonics: Principles and Use of Instruments*, p. 80. Crosby, Lockwood, Staples, London.

MOUNTFORD, R. A. & WELLS, P. N. T. (1972) Ultrasonic liver scanning: the A scan in the normal and in cirrhosis. *Physiology, Medicine and Biology*, **17**, 261–269.

ROSS, F. G. M. (1978) In *Recent Advances in Radiology—6* (in press). Churchill Livingstone, Edinburgh.

SAMPLE, W. F. (1977) A new technique for the evaluation of the adrenal gland with grey scale ultrasonography. *Radiology*, **124**, 463–469.

SAMPLE, W. F. (1978) Adrenal ultrasonography. *Radiology*, **127**, 461–466.

SUTHERLAND, G. R. (1978) The contribution of echography in the diagnosis of proptosis. *British Journal of Radiology*, **51**, 116–121.

SUTHERLAND, G. R. & FORRESTER, J. (1974) B-scan ultrasonography in ophthalmology. *British Journal of Radiology*, **47**, 383–386.

TAYLOR, K. J. W. (1977) Ultrasonic investigation of the hepatobiliary system and the spleen. In Wells, P. N. T. (ed.) *Ultrasonics in Clinical Diagnosis*, 2nd edn., pp. 97–113. Churchill Livingstone, Edinburgh.

TAYLOR, K. J. W. (1978) *Atlas of Gray Scale Ultrasonography*. Churchill Livingstone, Edinburgh.

TAYLOR, K. J. W. & HILL, C. R. (1975) Scanning techniques in gray scale ultrasonography. *British Journal of Radiology*, **48**, 918–920.

WELLS, P. N. T. (1977) *Ultrasonics in Clinical Diagnosis*, 2nd edn. Churchill Livingstone, Edinburgh.

CHAPTER 68

ULTRASOUND (2): OBSTETRICS AND GYNAECOLOGY

OBSTETRICS

Ultrasound has made its greatest contribution to medicine in the field of obstetrics. This is largely because the pregnant uterus is easily accessible to ultrasonic examination. Ultrasound may also be used in pregnancy to examine for suspected disease of other systems, such as the urinary tract or biliary tract, when the use of radiology is contraindicated because of the pregnancy.

EQUIPMENT AND TECHNIQUE

Equipment for obstetric work should be able to present A-scan and B-scan grey-scale display modes simultaneously and also have the facility to record in the Time Position (TP) mode. It should be possible to display the B-scan in different degrees of magnification. Delay and expansion features on the A-mode are desirable when seeking moving echoes such as those from the fetal heart. A measuring facility using caliper displays on the A- and B-scans combined with a digital read-out are essential. A real-time scanner is also required.

Most work can be done using a transducer of 2–2·5 MHz but for fine detail a transducer of higher frequency (e.g. 3·5 MHz) is useful. The selection of transducer is partly determined by the characteristics of the machine such as its output power and sensitivity and partly by the patient's size.

Permanent records can be made on Polaroid, 70 mm or X-ray film using appropriate adaptors or a multiformat camera back. Polaroid film is expensive but convenient when measurements have to be made directly from the picture, e.g. crown-rump and circumferential measurements.

The patient presents with a bladder well-filled with urine. This is important particularly when examining a case of early pregnancy as it is the only means of displacing the gas-containing bowel at this stage and thus allowing access of the ultrasound beam to the uterus behind the bladder. A partly filled bladder will suffice in the later stages of pregnancy as the uterus itself will have displaced the intestines, and even a partly filled bladder will give the ultrasound beam better access to the lower pole of the uterus and the region of the cervix.

The patient lies supine with a pillow behind her knees to increase her comfort. It is important to explain the procedure and its safety aspects to the patient to put her at ease. Oil is applied to the skin of the abdomen and the apparatus positioned. It is advantageous to conduct the examination as quickly as possible compatible with efficiency, especially in the later stages of pregnancy. Many of these patients are unable to lie on their backs for any length of time because of the development of hypotension with consequent feelings of dizziness or faintness. This is due to reduction of the venous return to the heart from compression of the inferior vena cava by the gravid uterus. When this happens the patient must be turned on to her side to relieve the pressure on the inferior vena cava. Recovery is usually rapid but the examination time is prolonged and the lie of the fetus usually altered. Unfortunately the symptoms often recur rapidly when the patient resumes the fully supine position and it may be difficult to complete the examination at the same session.

Serial longitudinal and transverse scans are made as a routine and the spacing will vary with the size of the uterus. In early pregnancy closely spaced scans possibly 0·5 to 1 cm apart are necessary particularly when searching for the heart beat. Late in pregnancy wider spacing 2 to 3 cm apart is appropriate. Judgement of optimal spacing comes with experience of ultrasound examination. Oblique and inclined scanning planes may be necessary. By raising the transducer off the skin surface, marker signals can be made on the scan. It is a practice of some workers to mark the sites of the symphysis pubis, umbilicus and xiphisternum on the longitudinal midline scan and the umbilical level on all other scans. These markers allow ready clinical correlation and easier comparison on serial scans.

ULTRASONIC APPEARANCES OF THE NORMAL UTERUS

The normal non-pregnant uterus is seen behind the full bladder as a smooth, pear-shaped, relatively transonic area on the longitudinal scan (Figs 68.1 and 68.2). Inferiorly the anterior and posterior surfaces of the cervix are parallel and there is usually a central white line representing the echoes from the cavity of the canal (see Figs 68.6 and 68.7). Above the canal the body widens up to the fundus which is convex in outline superiorly. The body is slightly tilted forwards on the cervical canal in the normal uterus. If this forward tilt is excessive the uterus is *anteverted* and if the body and canal are in line or if the body is tilted backwards the uterus is *retroverted* (Fig. 68.3). If the interface between the endometrium on the anterior and posterior walls is at right angles to the ultrasonic beam a line of echoes will be seen in the midline of the uterus (Figs 68.2 and 68.4). On transverse section the uterus is oval, rounded or diamond-shaped, wider in transverse diameter above than below. When the uterus is inclined forwards it may be necessary to tilt the transducer upwards in order to achieve a satisfactory scan. The size of uterus will vary from patient to patient and particularly between nulliparous and multiparous women, being larger in the latter. The uterus is about 8 cm long, 5 cm in width and 3 cm in depth. The normal ovaries can also be shown and are best displayed on the transverse scan (Fig. 68·5).

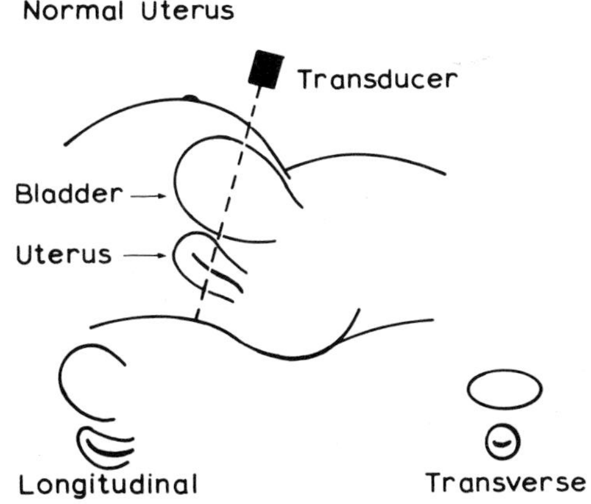

Fig. 68.1 Diagram indicating the position of the ultrasound transducer, the patient's abdominal wall, bladder and uterus.

ULTRASONIC APPEARANCES IN PREGNANCY

The shape of the pregnant uterus varies. Most commonly it is egg-shaped, being wider near the fundus than inferiorly (Fig. 68.6). In some patients it may be flat from before backwards (Fig. 68.7) and in that case it is usually wide from side to side. In others it may be very rounded with its widest diameter centrally (Fig. 68.8). The lower end is cone-shaped, usually concave on its antero-inferior wall where it is impressed by the full bladder (Fig. 68.8). The cervix is shown as three parallel lines behind the bladder, and their uterine end denotes the site of the internal os (Figs 68.6 and 68.7).

The fetus in early pregnancy. The uterus is shown to be enlarged and the decidua fills the uterine cavity with multiple fine echoes within which is the *gestation sac*. The gestation sac is seen as a well-defined rounded or oval transonic area within the decidua. It may be seen about 5 weeks after the first day of last menstrual period and should certainly be seen at 6 to 7 weeks (Fig. 68.9). Frequently a rim of high intensity echoes surrounds the gestation sac (Fig. 68.10). As pregnancy develops the gestation sac increases in size and by about 10 weeks it occupies most of the uterine cavity. At about 6 or 7 weeks a collection of echoes is seen within the gestation sac

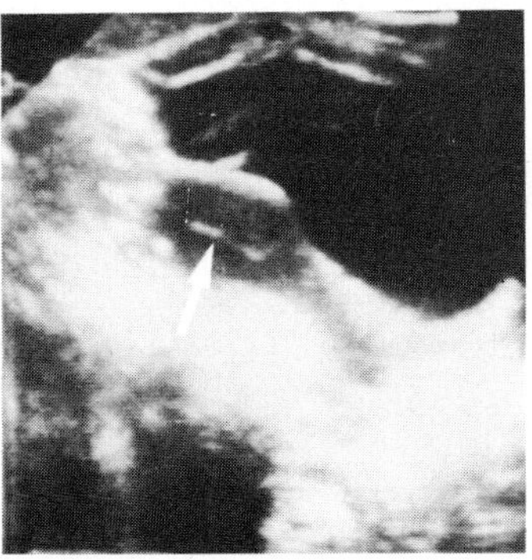

Fig. 68.2

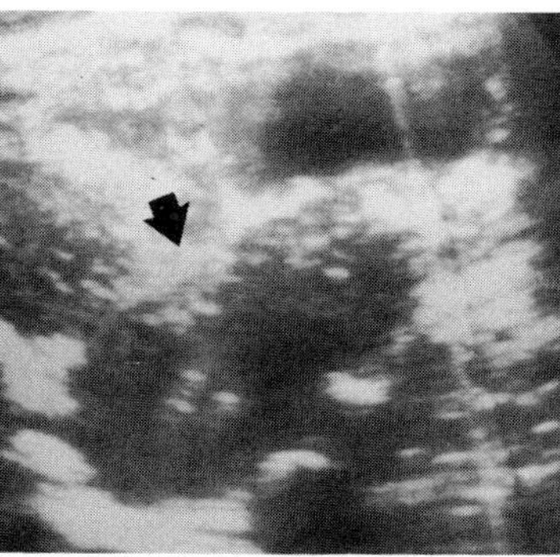

Fig. 68.3

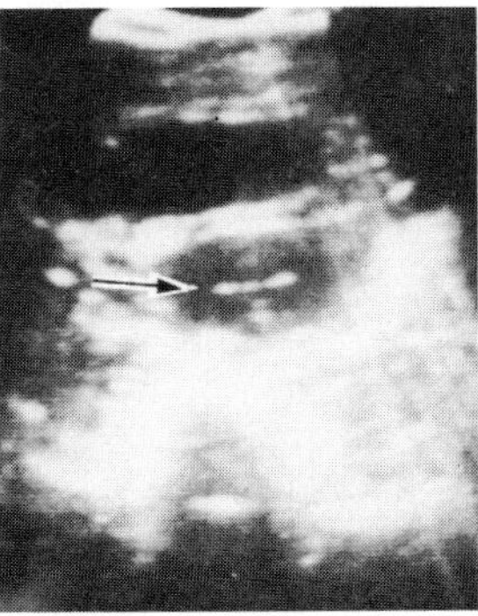

Fig. 68.4

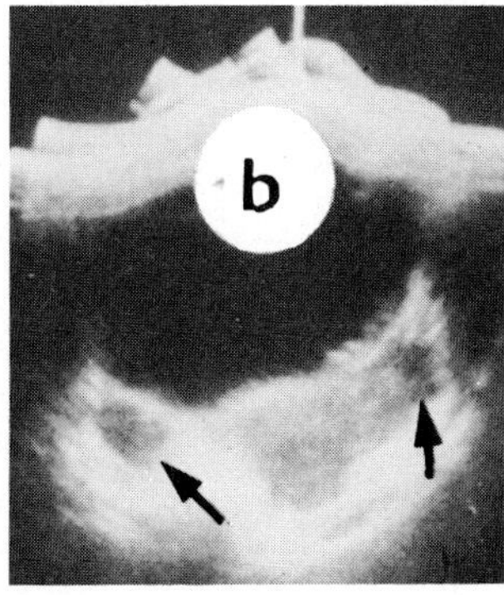

Fig. 68.5

Fig. 68.2 Longitudinal scan showing the structures indicated in Figure 68.1. The arrow indicates the uterine cavity.

Fig. 68.3 Retroverted uterus (arrow). Longitudinal scan.

Fig. 68.4 Uterine cavity (arrowed) shown on transverse scan.

Fig. 68.5 Transverse scan showing the ovaries (arrowed), on each side of the uterus, behind the filled bladder **(b)**.

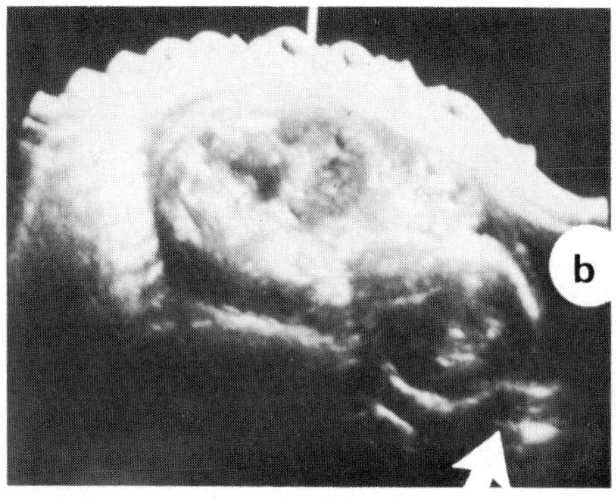

Fig. 68.6

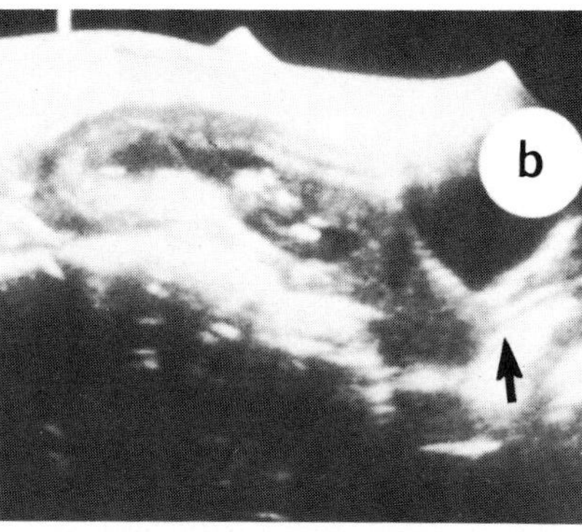

Fig. 68.7

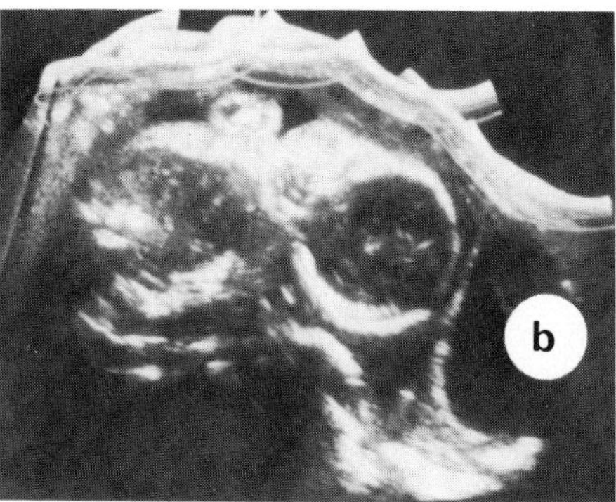

Fig. 68.8

Fig. 68.6 Pregnant uterus. Longitudinal section. The cervical canal is seen as three horizontal parallel echo lines (arrow) behind the bladder **(b)**.

Fig. 68.7 Flat uterus. Longitudinal scan. The antero-posterior diameter of the uterus is narrow. The lower end is indented anteriorly by the filled bladder **(b)**. Arrow points to cervix.

Fig. 68.8 Rounded uterus. Longitudinal scan. The anterio-posterior diameter of the uterus is wide. The lower end is indented anteriorly by the filled bladder **(b)**.

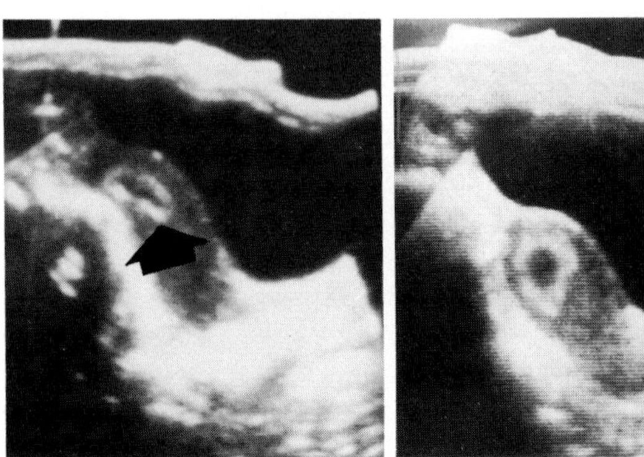

Fig. 68.9 *Fig. 68.10*

Fig. 68.9 Early pregnancy. Longitudinal scan. 6½ weeks menstrual age. The uterus is enlarged. It contains a small gestation sac shown as an eccentric black line surrounded by a thin zone of dense echoes (arrow).

Fig. 68.10 7-week pregnancy. Longitudinal scan. Enlarged uterus containing a well-formed gestation sac which has a highly echogenic rim. No fetal node visible on this scan.

produced by the developing embryo, an appearance referred to as the '*fetal node*' (Fig. 68.11). By about 8 weeks a localized area can be identified in which the echoes between the gestation sac rim and the uterine wall are wider than elsewhere and this represents the site of development of the placenta (Fig. 68.14). By about 14 weeks the fetal head can be identified and the midline structures of the brain demonstrated (Fig. 68.12). The fetal body at this stage is well-formed.

The *fetal heart beat* can be identified soon after the fetus is demonstrated within the gestational sac. It is demonstrated by careful scanning along the length of the fetus while watching the A-mode display for a definite to-and-fro sideways moving echo coming from heart structures as they move towards and away from the probe and pulsating at a rate faster than the maternal heart beat. Parallel scans moving the scanning frame a few millimetres at a time may be necessary to pick up the fetal heart beat. If the caliper dots are placed on the fetal node on the B-scan the corresponding echoes can be identified

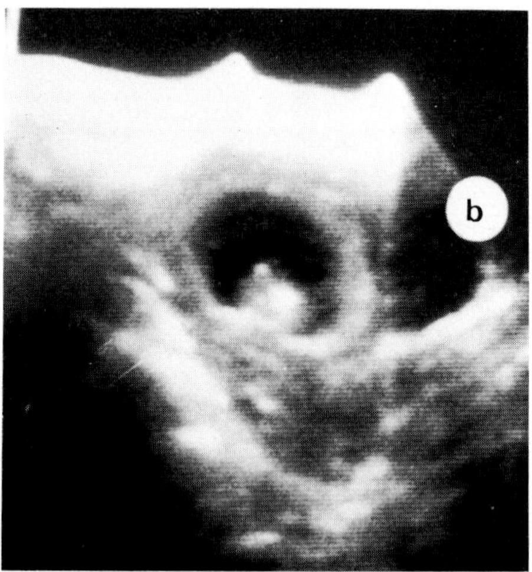

A

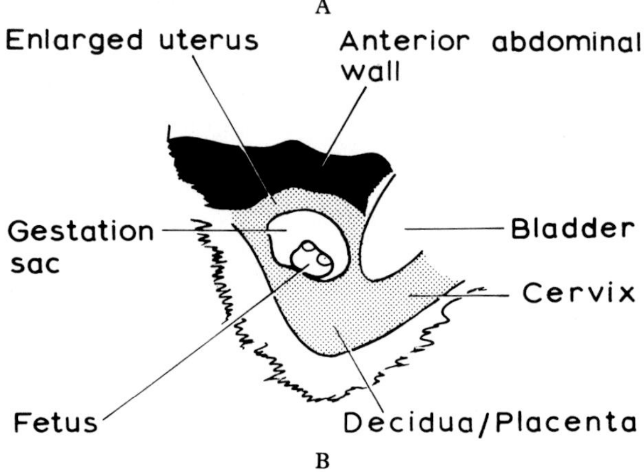

B

Fig. 68.11 Early pregnancy. (A) Longitudinal scan. 9 weeks menstrual age. The gestation sac is large at this stage and the fetus (fetal node) is shown as an oval collection of echoes within it. **b** = bladder. (B) Diagram of (A).

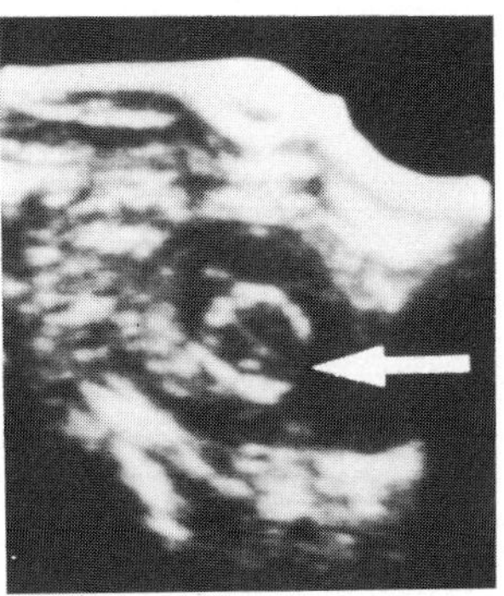

Fig. 68.12 Fifteen-week pregnancy. Longitudinal scan showing skull with midline echo (arrow).

echoes with a central line of echoes produced by the falx cerebri. This line may traverse the whole length of the skull or only part, according to the position of the skull and the relationship of the ultrasonic beam to the falx (Fig. 68.14). Sometimes the facial bones and orbits may be recognized (Fig. 68.15). The body is shown as an elongated well-defined structure in longitudinal section (Fig. 68.16) and rounded in transverse section (Fig. 68.25).

The spine is shown in longitudinal section as two parallel rows of echoes separated by a transonic line (Figs 68.17 and 68.18). In transverse section the transonic spinal canal is seen surrounded by an echogenic ring produced by the vertebral body and neural arch (Fig. 68.19). The rib cage is shown by a series of parallel echogenic lines (Fig. 68.20) when the ribs are imaged along their length; and as dark lines distal to them when either the technique of linear scanning is used or with linear array real time scanners (Fig. 68.21). In these circumstances the ribs themselves cast an acoustic shadow where the ultrasound beam is reflected from its first point of reflection from the ribs. The surface of the limb (Fig. 68.22) may be outlined and the central bones seen as a central echo within the limb outlined (Fig. 68.23). The major joints (knees and elbows), fingers and toes may also be seen.

Details of some intrafetal anatomical structures can be identified. The bladder is seen as a transonic club-shaped structure arising from the pelvis (Figs. 68.16 and 68.24).

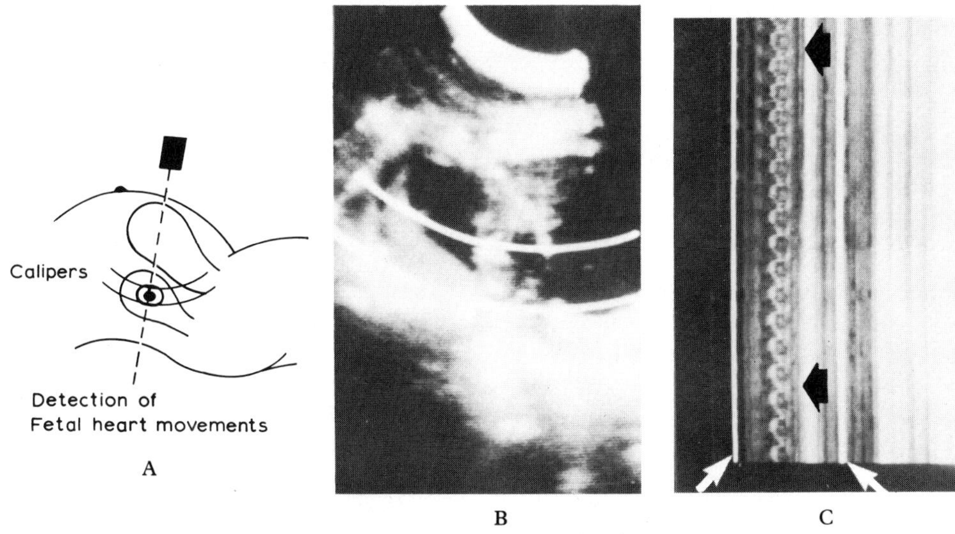

Fig. 68.13 Detection of fetal heart movements. (A) Diagram illustrating method. The fetal node within the gestation sac is identified in the routine manner. An A-scan is made through the fetus and the electronic calipers placed one anterior and one posterior to the fetus (Robinson, 1972). (B) Actual 'B'-scan with caliper lines written in. (C) The fetal heart movements are written out on the time-position mode. Caliper markings (white arrows). Fetal heart movements (black arrows).

on the A-scan. It then becomes easy to recognize the moving echoes from the heart (Fig. 68.13). The beating heart can also be seen directly on real time scanning from about 7 weeks onwards.

The fetus in late pregnancy. As the uterus enlarges and the fetus grows, more detail of the fetal anatomy can be outlined particularly if an adequate amount of amniotic fluid is present. The amniotic fluid is transonic and there is good contrast between it and the fetus to reveal detail of the latter. If the amniotic fluid is sparse, recognition of fetal anatomy is made more difficult. In the last weeks of pregnancy the amniotic fluid tends to be absorbed. The best fetal detail is seen between about the 26th and 36th weeks of pregnancy. The outline of the head is shown as a circle or oval of well-defined high intensity

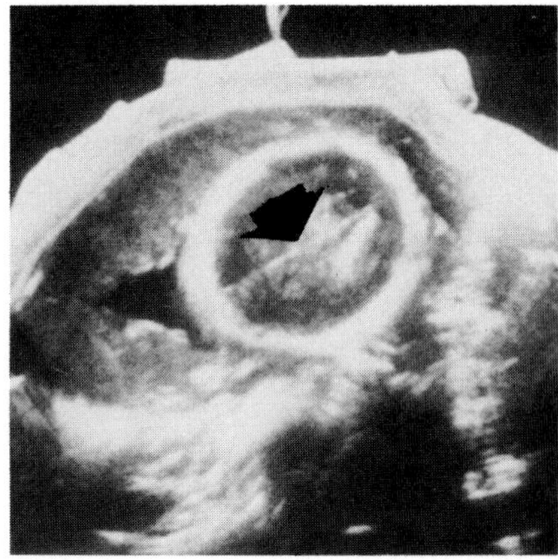

Fig. 68.14 Normal fetal skull. 34 weeks maturity. Transverse scan showing midline echo (arrows) across circle of skull outline.

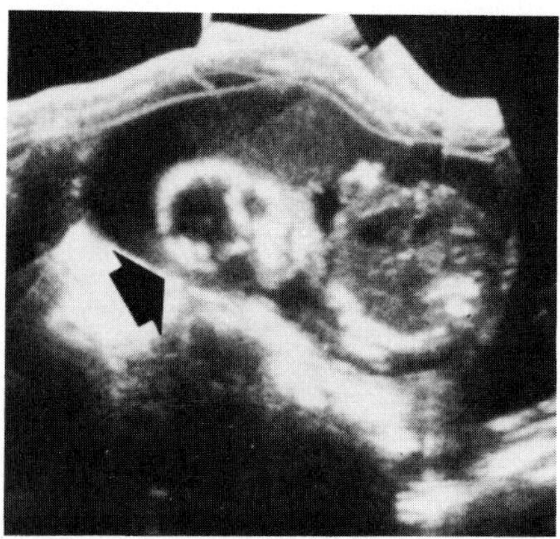

Fig. 68.15 Normal fetal skull, orbits and facial bones. 23 weeks maturity. Longitudinal scan. Breech presentation. The skull, orbits and facial bones can be clearly seen (arrow).

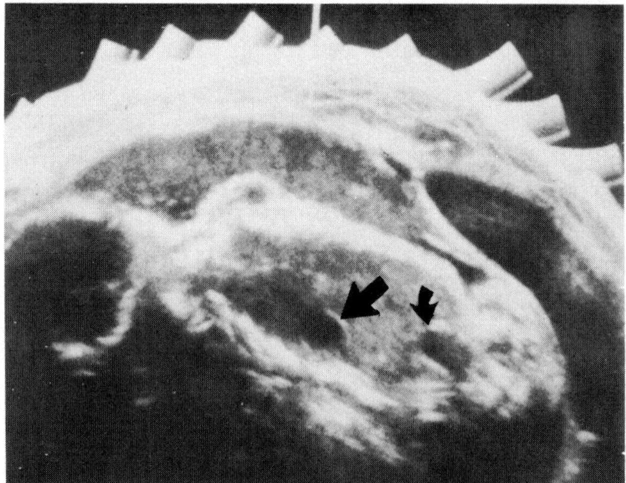

Fig. 68.16 Fetal body. Longitudinal scan. 32 weeks maturity. Breech presentation. The body is seen as an elongated structure. Fetal bladder (curved arrow) and fetal stomach (large arrow) demonstrated.

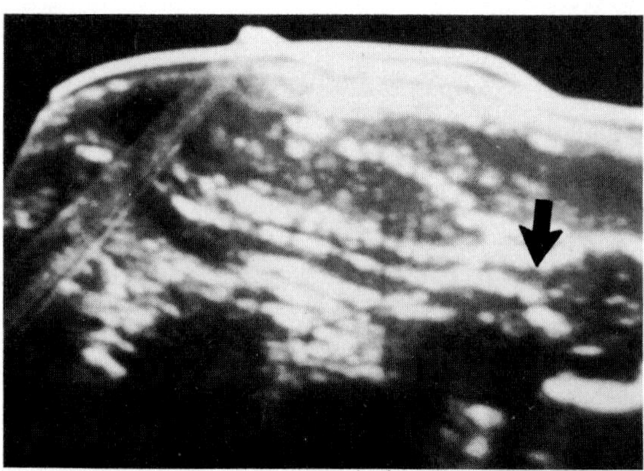

Fig. 68.17 Longitudinal scan of the fetal spine, almost in the coronal plane. The arrow indicates the site of the foramen magnum.

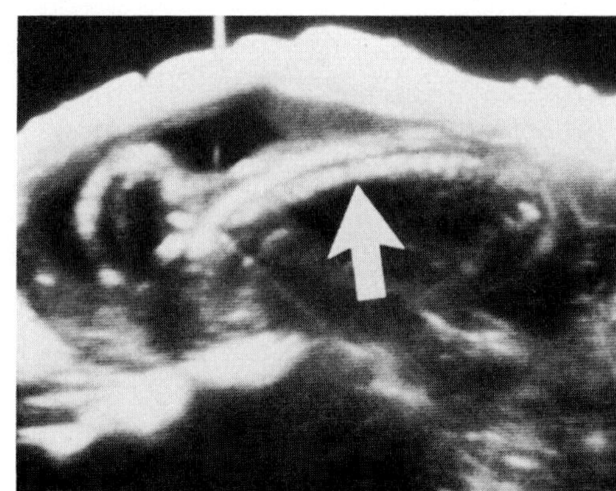

Fig. 68.18 Longitudinal scan of the fetal spine in the sagittal plane.

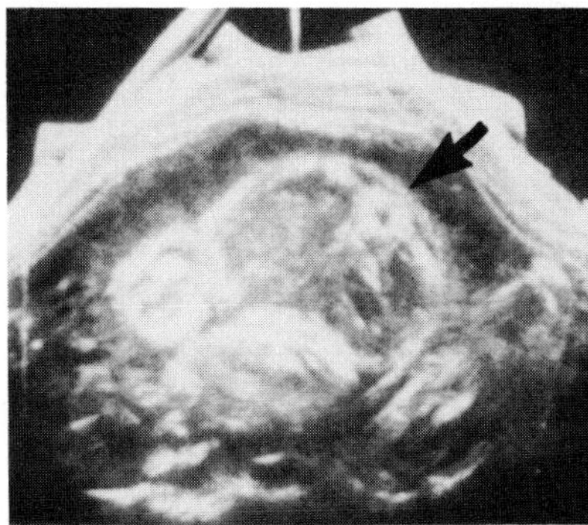

Fig. 68.19 Fetal spine. Transverse scan. The spinal canal is seen as a transonic dot (arrow) surrounded by the neural arch and vertebral body.

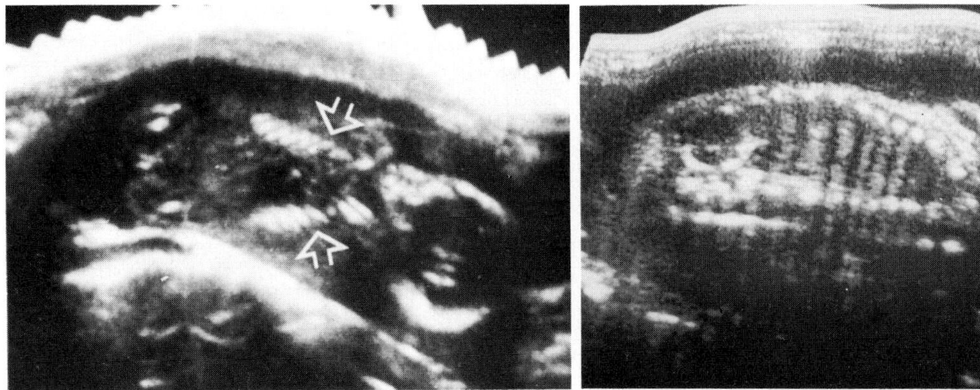

Fig. 68.20 Fetal ribs. Longitudinal scan at 30 weeks maturity. The rib echoes are seen on each side of the thorax.

Fig. 68.21 The 'bright-up' effect in the intercostal spaces is shown.

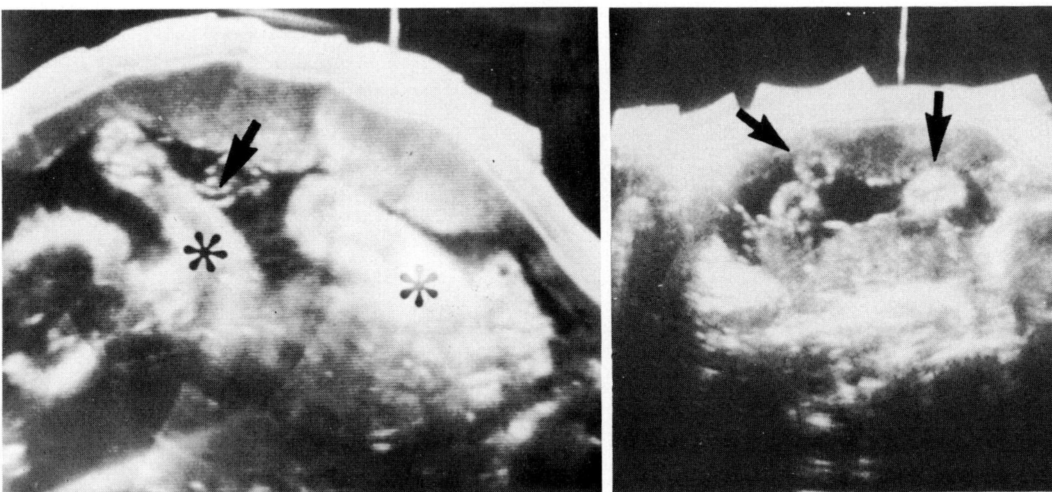

Fig. 68.22 Fetal limbs. Breech presentation. An arm and a leg are shown (stars). In addition the umbilical cord is seen (arrow).

Fig. 68.23 Fetal limbs seen in cross section. The bones can just be discerned as central echoes in the legs.

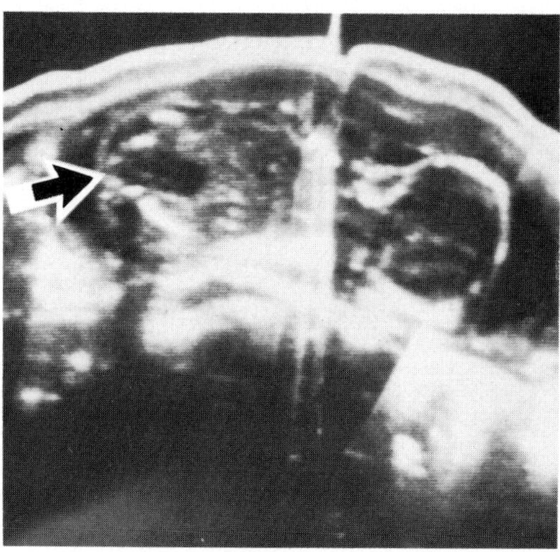

Fig. 68.24

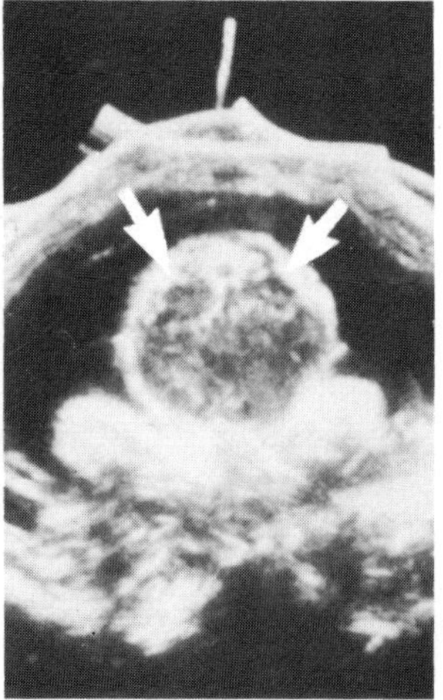

Fig. 68.25

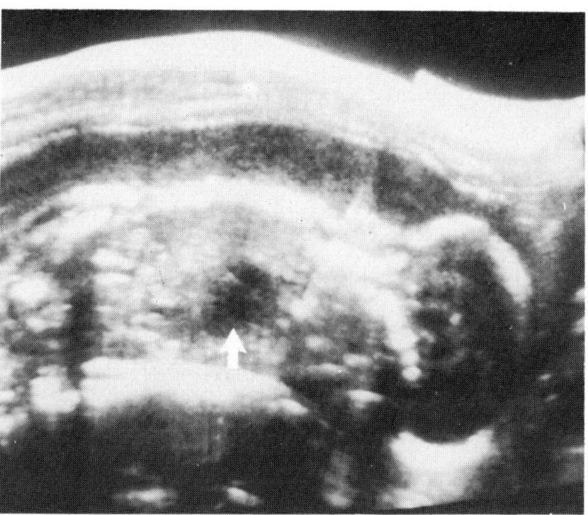

Fig. 68.26

Fig. 68.24 Fetal bladder. Longitudinal scan at 32 weeks maturity. Vertex presentation. The bladder appears as a transonic structure (arrow) arising from the pelvis.

Fig. 68.25 Fetal kidneys. Transverse scan. The kidneys (arrows) can be seen on each side of the spine.

Fig. 68.26 Fetal heart. Longitudinal scan of fetus. The transonic cardiac cavity set well down in the thorax is arrowed.

The kidneys can be identified on each side of the spine (Fig. 68.25). The heart is shown as an oval transonic area in the thorax (Fig. 68.26). It has a longitudinal central line of echoes in it representing the septum. Recognition of a cardiac cavity indicates the direction in which the ultrasound beam must be directed to detect the heart beat. From the heart a transonic line passing in front of the spine represents the aorta (Fig. 68.27). Many other intrafetal structures have been identified such as the liver, fluid-filled stomach (Fig. 68.16), intestines, the umbilical vein (Fig. 68.28), etc. Tortuous parallel echo lines in the amniotic fluid represent the umbilical cord (Fig. 68.29). All these fetal structures can also be observed on real-time scanning.

Fetal lie and presentation. The lie, presentation and position of the fetus can be difficult to determine clinically, especially in an obese or unco-operative patient. Scanning will demonstrate the relation of the fetal to maternal structures allowing an accurate assessment of lie, presentation and position in these cases. The definition of these parameters has been given before (Ch. 47) and examples are shown in Figure 68.30.

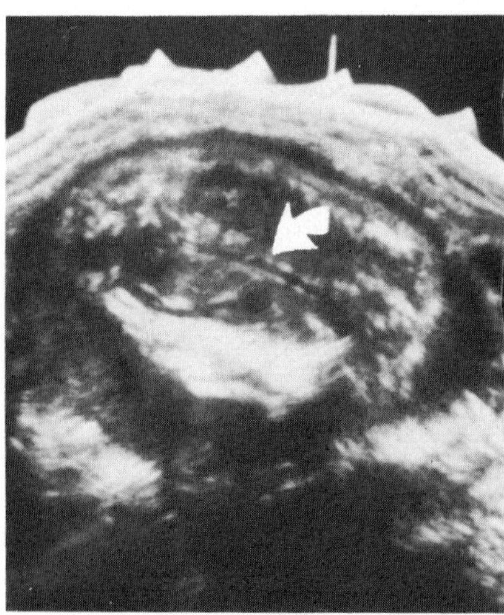

Fig. 68.27

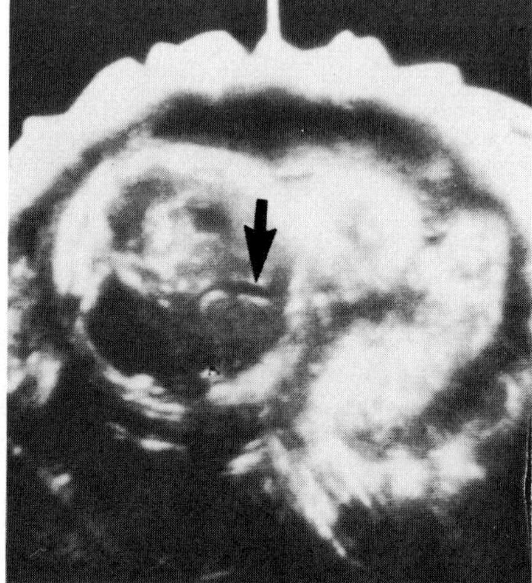

Fig. 68.28

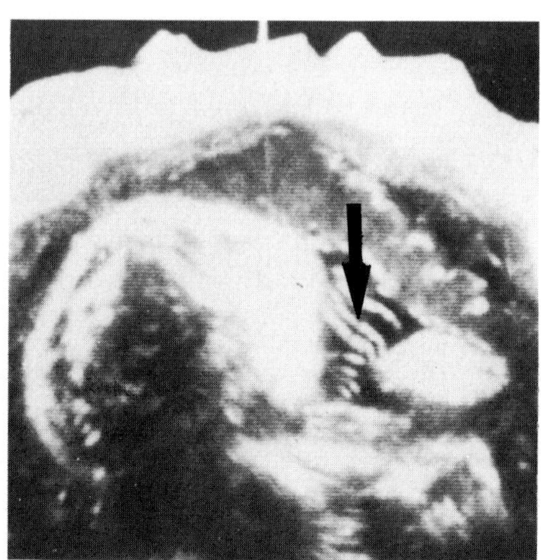

Fig. 68.29

Fig. 68.27 Fetal aorta. Longitudinal scan. The aorta is shown as a transonic line (curved arrow) directed lengthwise from thorax to abdomen. It can be seen to pulsate on real-time scanning.

Fig. 68.28 Fetal umbilical vein. Transverse scan. The umbilical vein (arrow) is identified as a transonic line extending anteriorly to the umbilicus.

Fig. 68.29 Umbilical cord. Tortuous parallel lines (arrows) arise from the umbilical cord. Transverse section.

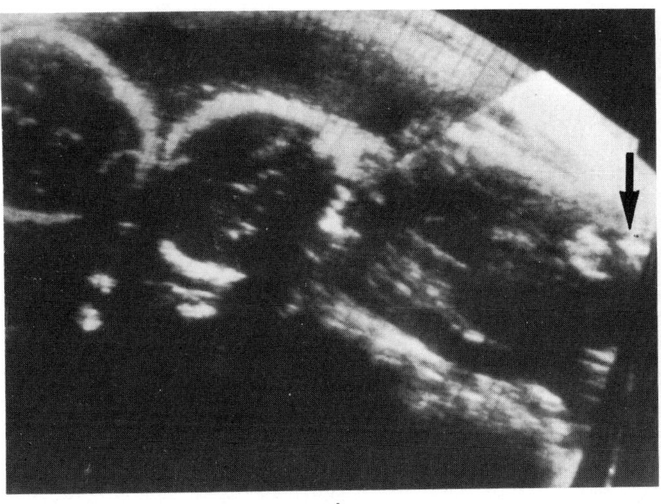

A

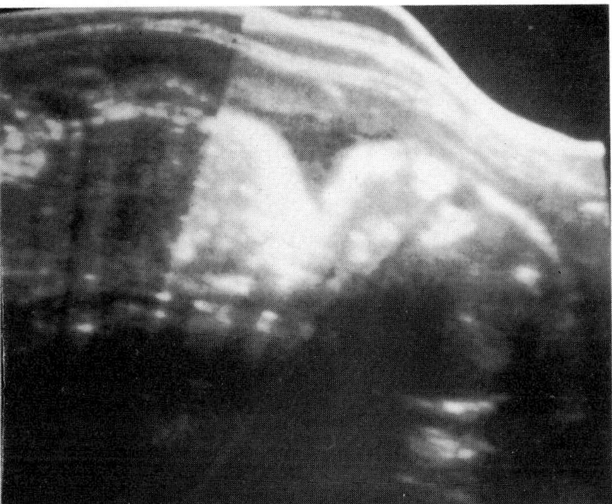

B

Fig. 68.30 (A) Twin pregnancy (note the two heads) with the lower twin presenting by the breech (arrow). Longitudinal scan. (B) Vertex presentation, head in the occipito-posterior position. Longitudinal scan. (C) Transverse lie. The fetus is lying across the uterus with the head to the right and the body to the left side. Transverse scan.

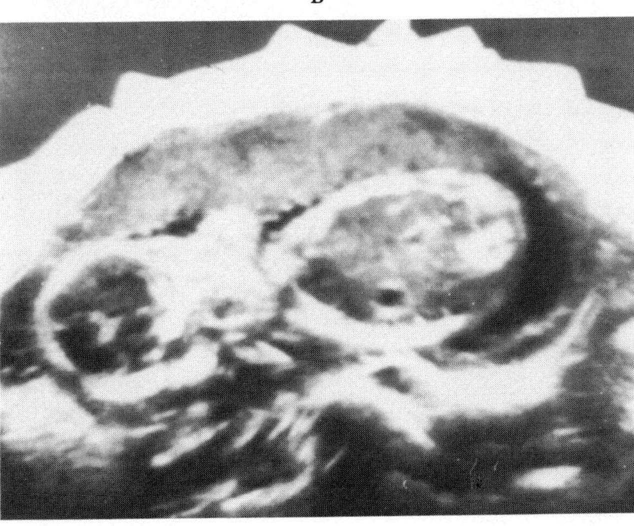

C

Fetal pulsations. By the use of the Doppler effect incorporated into small machines specially designed for use in obstetrics, pulsation from various vascular structures can be located because they produce characteristic sounds on the loudspeaker. Blood flow in the maternal femoral arteries should first be detected to ensure that the apparatus is working satisfactorily, and blood flow in the mother's aorta should be located to demonstrate that the ultrasound beam is penetrating to the back of the uterus. The probe should be held vertically and moved across the abdomen in closely placed parallel lines separated by the width of the transducer so that the whole of the uterus is searched. Fetal pulsations may be detected by this method at 10 weeks maturity but they should definitely be heard at 12 weeks. The 'galloping' sound of the fetal heart will be heard at 12 weeks and later, a swishing noise from blood flow in the umbilical artery will be heard. Fetal pulsations are at a higher rate than the maternal rate and may normally be between 120 and 160 beats per minute. The placenta may also be located by the Doppler method.

Fetal respiratory movements. Intrauterine fetal respiratory movements can be detected by the use of either of two blind ultrasonic methods which do not employ real-time scanning and also by real-time scanning. In each blind method the fetal heart pulsations are detected initially and this ensures that the ultrasonic beam is traversing the fetal chest wall. The ultrasound beam is then directed slightly away from the site at which the fetal heart sounds have been heard. In one method the fetal respiratory movements are recorded by means of a modified A-scan apparatus with a standard pen-recorder (Boddy and Robinson, 1971). This method has the disadvantage of not being generally available. The other method is to use one of the commonly available obstetrical Doppler apparatuses and listen to the characteristic sounds as amniotic fluid is drawn into and expelled from the fetal thorax. The sounds may be recorded onto tape or onto a frequency analyser. A low-pitched sound is heard at a frequency of between 30 and 70 a minute and is present between 55 and 90 per cent of the time. Fetal hiccuping may also be heard. The respiratory movements of the fetal thorax can also be observed on real-time scanning.

MULTIPLE PREGNANCY

At all stages of pregnancy, the possibility of multiple pregnancy must be borne in mind and carefully checked for at scanning. If care is not taken, it is quite possible to fail to demonstrate in the first trimester one or both of the fetal nodes in the presence of two gestation sacs. In the

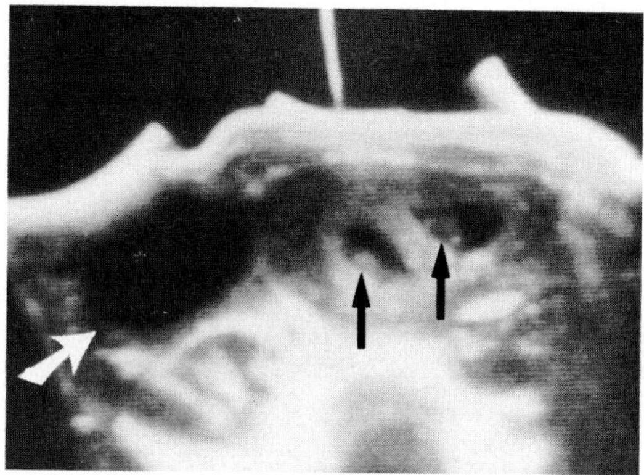

Fig. 68.31 Twin pregnancy. 10 weeks maturity. Transverse scan. The enlarged uterus is shown containing two gestation sacs each with a fetal node in it (black arrows). An ovarian cyst is also present on the right side (white arrow).

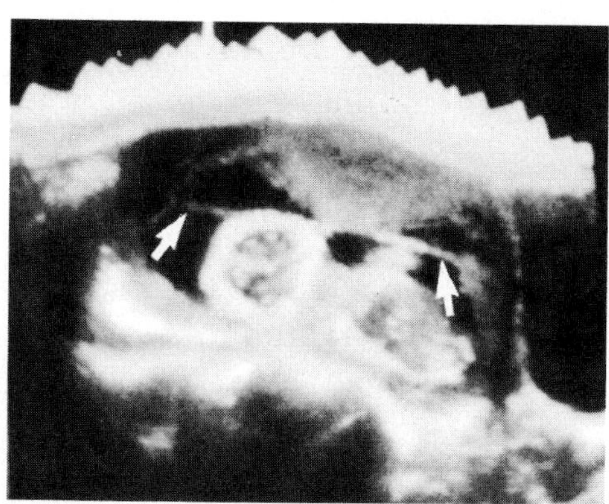

Fig. 68.32 Twin pregnancy. Two amniotic cavities. Longitudinal scan. 20 weeks maturity. On this scan the septum (arrows) dividing the amniotic cavities is clear, a fetus lies in the posterior sac and a placenta anteriorly.

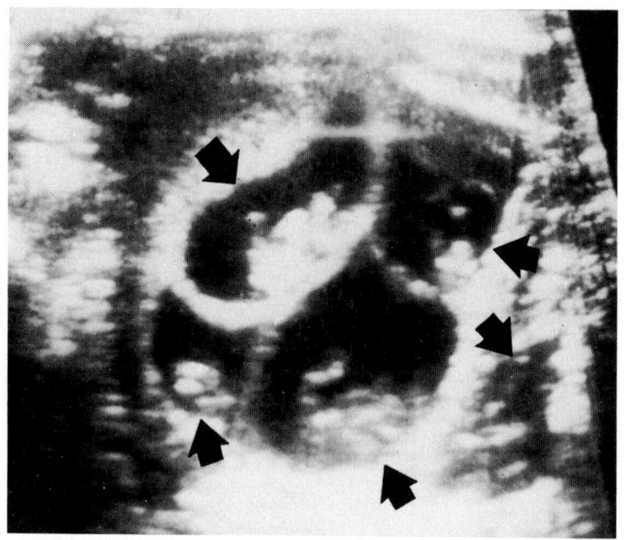

Fig. 68.33 Quintuplet pregnancy. Each arrow indicates a node-containing gestation sac.

second and third trimesters fetal movement can make the diagnosis difficult. This difficulty can be minimized by carrying out the examination expeditiously. Real-time scanning can assist in the diagnosis of multiple pregnancy. At all stages the uterus will be larger than would be expected for dates.

First trimester. Two or more gestation sacs will be shown with a fetal node in each (Fig. 68.31). Twin sacs have been detected as early as $5\frac{1}{2}$ weeks of amenorrhea and they may also be identified later in pregnancy (Fig. 68.32). Campbell and Dewhurst (1970) successfully diagnosed a quintuplet pregnancy at 9 weeks (Fig. 68.33 shows a similar case). Twin pregnancies diagnosed in the first 14 weeks of pregnancy are about twice as common as the expected incidence of 1 in 80 pregnancies. Approximately 30 per cent result in a singleton at a term while about 20 per cent miscarry entirely. Most of the failures are due to one or both gestation sacs representing an anembryonic pregnancy (Robinson and Caines, 1977).

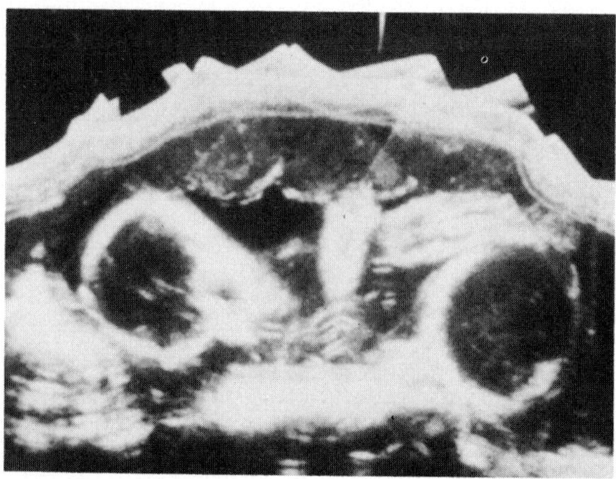

Fig. 68.34 Twin pregnancy, 30 week maturity. Two fetal heads are present, one in the fundus and one in the lower pole of the uterus.

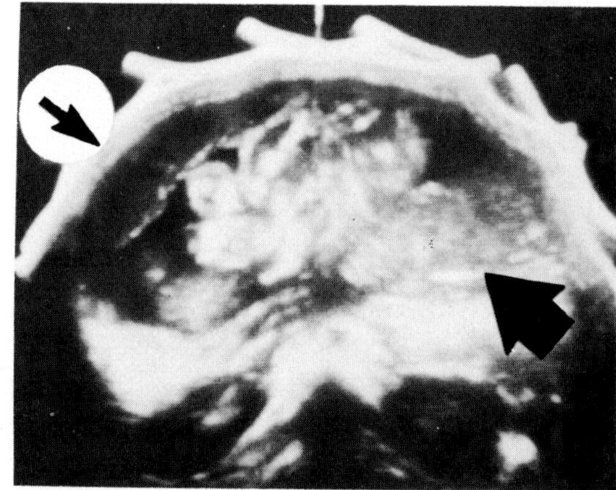

Fig. 68.35 Twin pregnancy. Two placentae. Transverse scan. One placenta is anterior on the right side (small arrow) and the other posterior on the left side (large arrow).

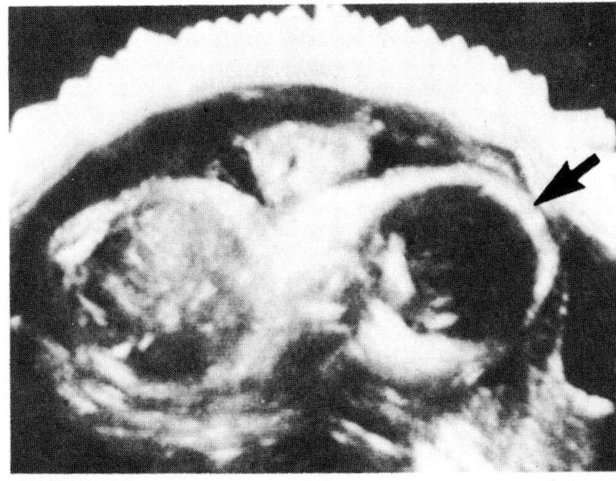

A

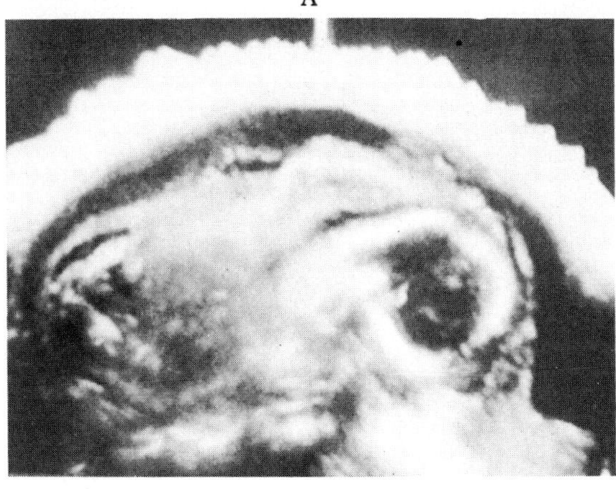

B

Fig. 68.36 Curled fetus. Longitudinal scans, 32 weeks maturity. Vertex presentation. (A) Two centimetres to right of midline. The head (arrow) and cross section of the body are close together and could be misinterpreted as representing two heads. (B) Adjacent midline scan demonstrates continuity between head and body proving that only one fetus is present.

Second and third trimesters. The diagnosis rests on detecting two or more fetal heads and bodies. The presentation of twin fetuses may be similar, i.e. both cephalic, breech or transverse, but they can also be opposite to each other. Once the diagnosis of twins is strongly suspected it is convenient to confirm it by so positioning the apparatus that both heads are shown on one scan (Fig. 68.34). When more than two fetuses are present it is often not possible to demonstrate all the heads on a single scan. Careful and methodical examination with a Doppler apparatus should reveal two fetal hearts beating at different rates. In twin pregnancies, two placentas are frequently present (Fig. 68.35). If a single fetus lies very curled up in the uterus a section scan may show the head and a cross-section of the body lying side by side, an appearance which can simulate a twin pregnancy (Fig. 68.36). Care must be taken to differentiate between the two by showing continuity in the case of the curled fetus between the head and body on an adjacent parallel scan.

MONITORING OF EARLY PREGNANCY AND DETECTION OF ITS COMPLICATIONS

Ultrasound is the only diagnostic technique which gives direct information on the well-being of the fetus in the first trimester and therefore it has an important role in the assessment of early pregnancy. This applies particularly to patients who have a history of threatened or recurrent abortion. Three techniques have recently been introduced to differentiate reliably between normal and abnormal early pregnancy. These are:

1. Fetal heart beat identification
2. Crown rump length measurement
3. Gestational sac volume.

Fetal heart movement (Robinson, 1972). The method for the identification of the fetal heart beat in early pregnancy has already been described. The earliest identification of the fetal heart movement has been given as 6 weeks and 2 days and Robinson (1973b) found no false results in 200 cases who had 7 weeks or more amenorrheoea. A positive finding of fetal cardiac pulsation allows conservative treatment of a threatened abortion. A negative result on the time-position study is an absolute indication that the fetus is dead. Difficulty with the examination may arise from fetal movement and therefore careful searching is important. Definite diagnosis of fetal death should only be made after meticulous and even repeated examination. Fetal heart movements can also be demonstrated at this stage of pregnancy by real-time scanning which has an additional advantage of showing fetal movements at the same time.

Measurement of crown-rump length (Robinson, 1973; Robinson and Fleming, 1975). It is possible to demonstrate the fetal echoes within the gestational sac on the B-scan display during the period from 6 to 12 weeks of gestation. By systematically scanning the uterus longitudinally and transversely, using multiple close parallel scans it is possible to demonstrate the cephalic and caudal ends of the fetus. Accuracy in this may be obtained if the two ends of the fetus as shown on the preliminary scans are marked on the mother's skin or located by real-time scanning (Fig. 68.37). The scanning plane should be

ULTRASONIC Crown-Rump Length measurement
BASIC STEPS

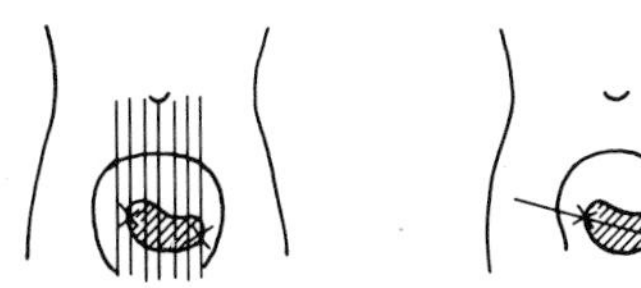

Serial longitutinal Section Scans

Transverse [Skewed] Scan along Fetal length

Fig. 68.37 Measurement of crown–rump length. Diagram illustrating method. Serial longitudinal scans locate each end of the fetus. A transverse (skewed) scan is then made along the length of the fetus (Robinson, 1973*a*; Robinson and Fleming, 1975).

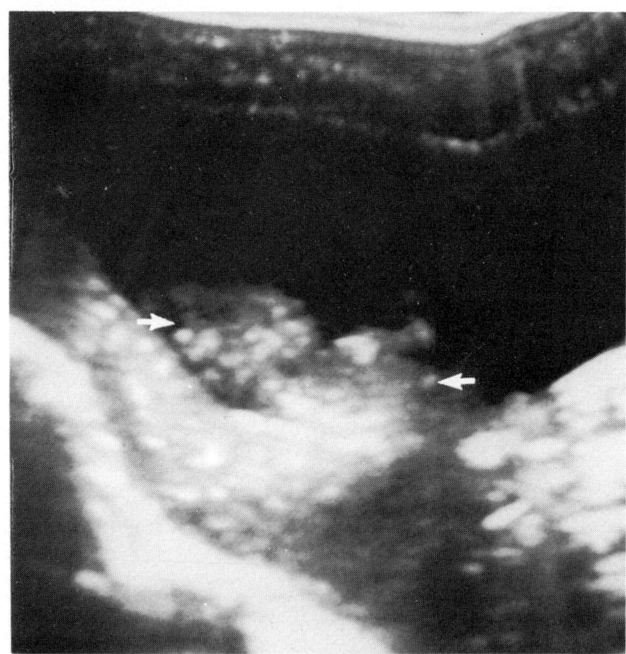

Fig. 68.38 11-week pregnancy. The length from the crown to the rump (arrows) is measured (Robinson, 1973*a*).

rotated in order to scan along the long axis of the fetus. When optimum definition in longitudinal section is obtained (Fig. 68.38) its length, excluding limbs may be measured directly from the monitor with the calipers

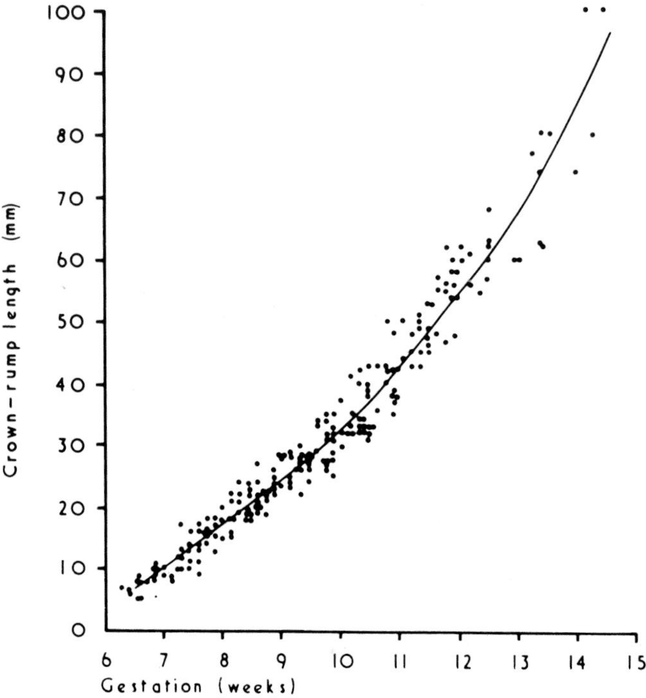

Fig. 68.39 Graph of crown–rump length plotted against fetal maturity. (Robinson, 1973*a*. Reproduced by permission of the author and the editor of *British Journal of Obstetrics and Gynaecology*.)

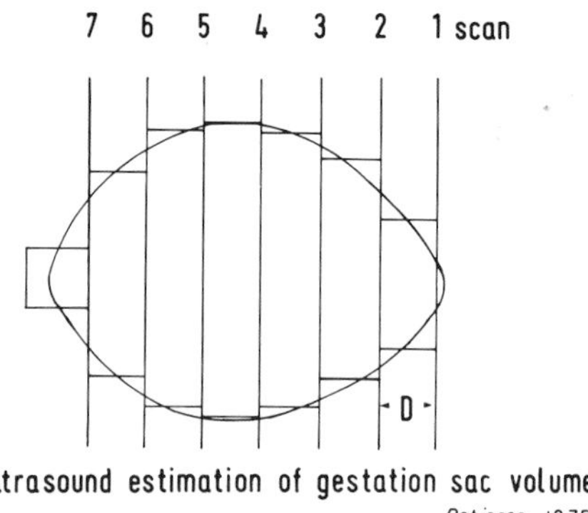

Fig. 68.40 Measurement of gestation sac volume. Diagram (Robinson, 1975). Parallel scans are made across the gestation sac at 1·0 or 0·5 cm intervals. The volume of these sections is summated to obtain the total volume of the gestation sac (see text).

(calibrated for an ultrasound speed of 1540 inches per second) provided the long axis of the fetus is not too far from the vertical. When it lies nearly horizontal the fetal image may be measured by calipers, or in some machines has to be photographed and measured directly. The photographed image measurement has to be corrected in order to allow for magnification within the imaging system. Tables indicating maturity have been published by Robinson (1973*a*) (Fig. 68.39). It is possible by this method to predict maturity in 95 per cent of cases to within 4 to 7 days with a single measurement and to within 2·7 days if three independent measurements are made. The method is applicable from the 7th to 14th week of pregnancy.

Estimation of gestation sac volume (Robinson, 1975a). This requires the use of a planimeter. Several parallel scans are made across the sac at measured intervals. The volume between each scan can be calculated using the planimeter to measure the area of the sac and then multiplying this by the space between the scans (Fig. 68.40). Summating the volumes between each section gives the total volume of the gestation sac within 10 per cent. The mean volume measures from 1 ml at 6 weeks to 100 ml at 13 weeks. The method is applicable from 5 to 14 weeks of pregnancy.

DIAGNOSIS OF ABNORMALITIES OF EARLY PREGNANCY

Most, but not all of the pregnancy failures considered in this section occur in the first trimester. Those in which the maternal cervix is still closed at the time of examination were classified by Robinson (1975*b*) into four groups:

1. Missed abortion
2. Anembryonic pregnancy (syn: blighted ovum)
3. Live abortion
4. Hydatidiform mole.

In addition the conditions of *complete* and *incomplete*

abortion and of *ectopic pregnancy* are considered in this section.

Missed abortion. These account for about 45 per cent of cases of early pregnancy failure. In some of these cases the fetus may be seen and the crown–rump length measured: in others the fetal echoes are formless (Fig. 68.41). Most important, however, is that in no case can the fetal heart beat be detected on T–P mode, nor any fetal movement be seen on real-time scanning. At delivery the fetus is frequently macerated accounting for the poor definition of the echo image. The trophoblast can continue to function after the fetus dies so that it is possible to have a positive pregnancy test in association with a dead fetus. Most fetuses appear to die at about eight weeks but the abortion can be delayed on an average by another four to five weeks during which time the gestation sac can continue to increase in size.

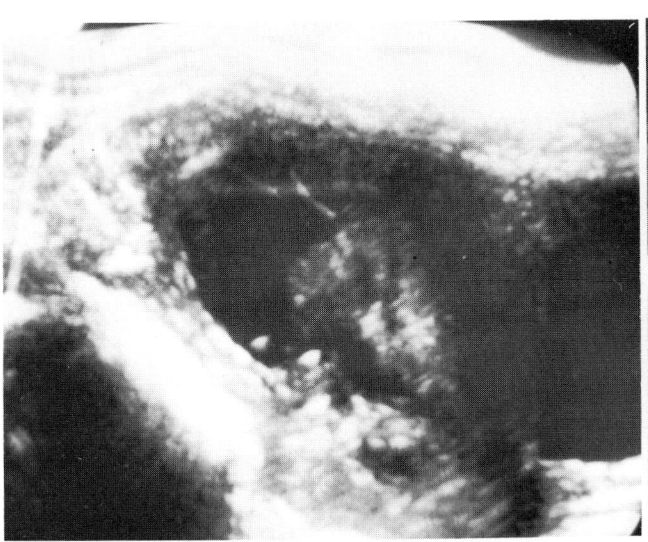

Fig. 68.41

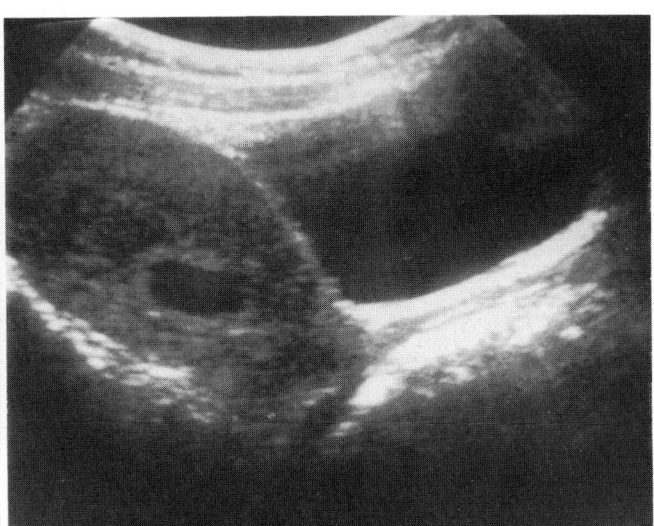

Fig. 68.42

Fig. 68.41 Missed abortion. The fetal echoes here are formless and no fetal heart beat could be found.

Fig. 68.42 Anembryonic pregnancy. There is a gestation sac, but no fetal node which should be present given the known duration of amenorrhoea (9 weeks).

Anembryonic pregnancy (blighted ovum). Anembryonic pregnancy is a situation which inevitably leads to abortion. The condition is as common as missed abortion. The diagnosis is restricted to those pregnancies in which a gestation sac can be outlined ultrasonically but which cannot be shown to contain a fetus either by ultrasonic examination (Fig. 68.42) or in the aborted products of gestation. The only measurement that is ultrasonically possible is gestation sac volume. If the sac is 'small for dates' and does not contain a fetus, a diagnosis of anembryonic pregnancy can be made with reasonable certainty. However, in some such patients the sac will be small because of mistaken dates and the pregnancy will not be far enough advanced to allow ultrasonic detection of the fetus. It has been shown that a fetal node can always be demonstrated ultrasonically if the gestation sac volume is 2 ml or more. If the gestation sac volume is 5 ml or less, it will increase in volume by more than 100 per cent in one week. Using ultrasonic criteria alone, the diagnosis of anembryonic pregnancy may be made when:

1. A gestation sac volume of 2·5 ml or over is shown on any single examination but in which no fetus can be demonstrated.
2. If the gestation sac is less than 2·5 ml in volume, and it fails to increase by at least 75 per cent in one week.

Live abortion. An abortion is considered to be live if:

1. Fetal heart movements are shown by ultrasound a few days prior to spontaneous abortion, or
2. The fetus, when aborted, is not macerated and has a crown–rump length compatible with the period of amenorrhoea.

Live abortions may be subgrouped into *early*, which occur before the 12th week and *late* if the abortion occurs at a later date. The incidence of live abortion is much less than missed abortion or anembryonic pregnancy, and represents about 11 per cent of the cases. In the early group the fetal heart movements and crown–rump lengths are normal, but gestation sac volume is on or below the second standard deviation of the mean for the period of amenorrhoea. These patients therefore have a low sac/fetus ratio and this low ratio is found in only 5 per cent of pregnancies which subsequently progress normally. In the late group (4 per cent of cases) no abnormal findings are detected ultrasonically, but these are associated with an incompetent cervix (i.e. the classical mid-trimester abortion).

Hydatidiform mole. This condition is uncommon in Europe but relatively frequent in the Far East. It occurs in 1 in 2,000 pregnancies in Europe. The uterus is usually large for dates and it contains no fetal parts on the B-scan and no fetal pulsations can be detected by the Doppler technique. The uterus is filled with multiple fine echoes of varying echogenicity which decrease in intensity or disappear as the ultrasonic power level is reduced. This characteristic was emphasized in the past when bistable displays were used but it is not of much importance in making the diagnosis if a scan converter grey-scale display is being employed (Fig. 68.43). Multiple small transonic areas may be seen scattered within the fine echoes in the uterus due to collections of blood or larger 'cystic' areas in the tumour (Fig. 68.44). These patients usually have high human chorionic gonadotrophin (HGG) levels in the urine. It is important to recognize that the echoes produced by the normal placenta are identical to those arising from hydatidiform mole and therefore extreme caution must be taken to exclude normal pregnancy. If a single transonic area is shown within the uterus, the suspicion of normal pregnancy must be high. It is unwise to make the diagnosis of hydatidiform mole before about the 10th and 11th week of pregnancy. Rarely hydatidiform mole and a fetus may co-exist. Lutein cysts in the ovary are common in association with hydatidiform mole.

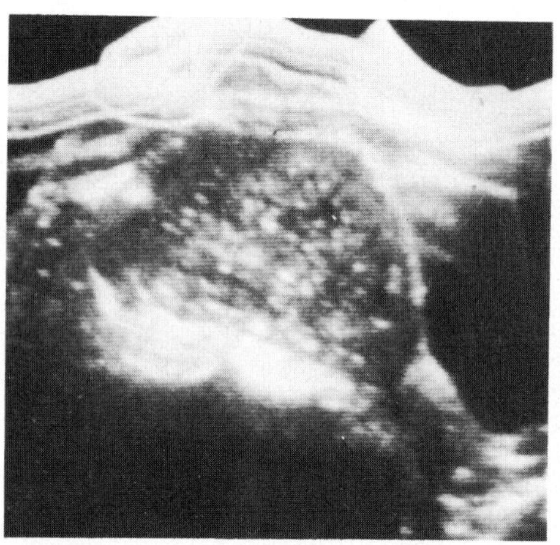

Fig. 68.43

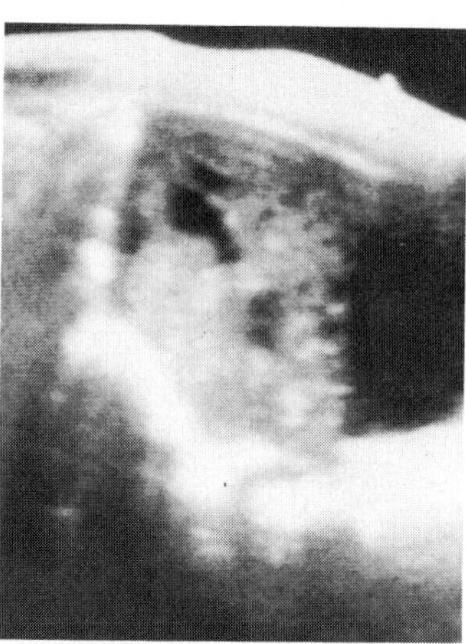

Fig. 68.44

Fig. 68.43 Hydatidiform mole. 17th week of amenorrhoea. The uterus is enlarged and there are multiple echoes within it of high and low echogenicity. No fetal parts visible and no fetal pulsations detectable.

Fig. 68.44 Hydatidiform mole. 11th week of amenorrhoea. Multiple small areas of transonicity are present within the uterus together with echoes of high and low echogenicity.

Complete and incomplete abortion. If an abortion has been complete, all the products of gestation will have been evacuated from the uterus which will be empty of echoes. If the abortion is incomplete, the fetus will probably have been aborted but random echoes will arise within the uterine cavity from retained gestational products (Fig. 68.45). Confusion can sometimes arise from similar appearances which are associated with hydatidiform mole. A central transonic cavity with an irregular outline which lacks the high echogenic rim of a normal pregnancy is frequently seen in incomplete abortion. In complete and incomplete abortion the uterus will be smaller than expected for the period of amenorrhoea and the proximal end of the cervical canal may be wide. If any doubt exists, re-examination in two or three weeks will demonstrate that the uterus has not increased in size and most probably is smaller.

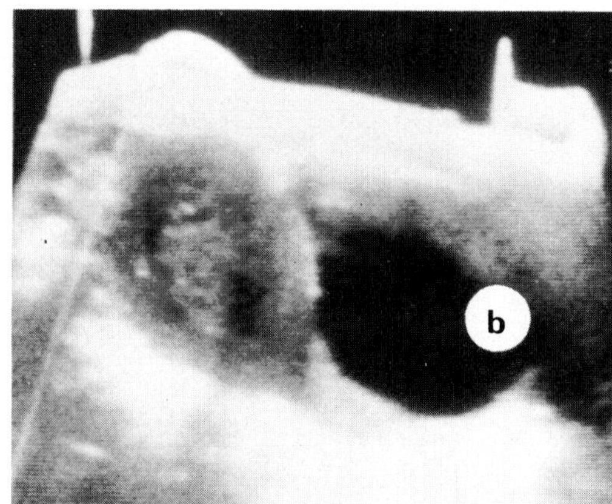

Fig. 68.45 Incomplete abortion. 14-week pregnancy. The uterus is smaller than would be expected at 14 weeks maturity. No fetal parts are visible though they should be easily detectable at this stage of pregnancy. The uterus contains random echoes due to retained gestation products and transonic areas due to haemorrhage. **b** = bladder.

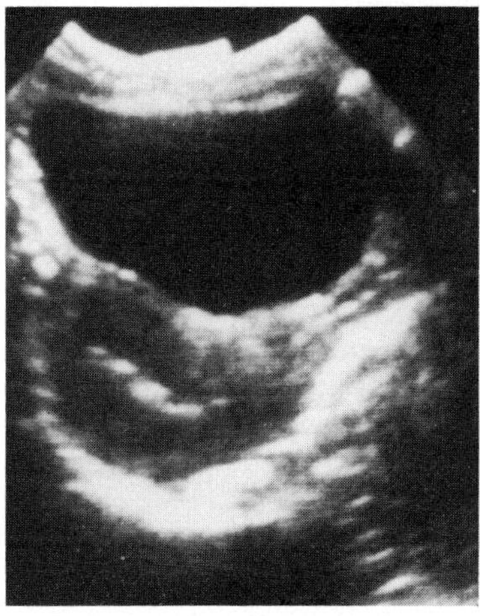
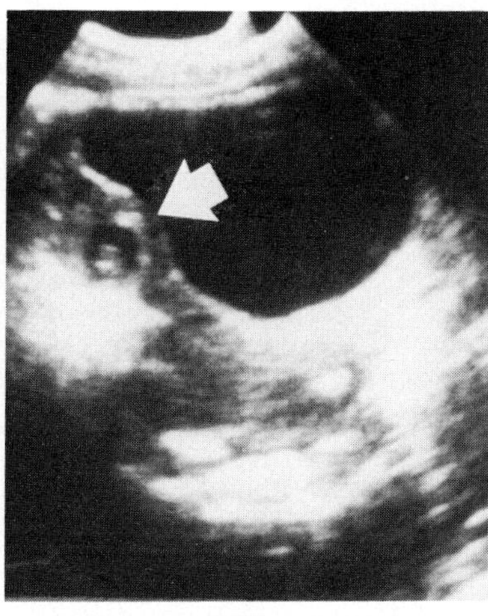
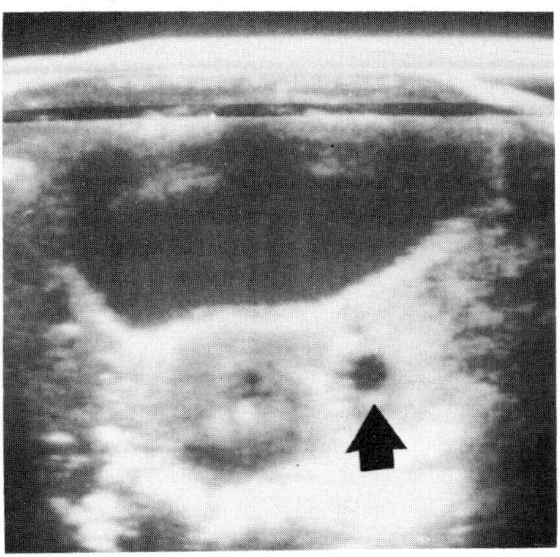

A B C

Fig. 68.46 Left ectopic pregnancy. Oblique longitudinal scans. (A) to right of midline. The uterus is normal in size and there are multiple echoes in it produced by a Lippe's loop. (B) to left of midline. The ectopic gestation sac is clearly seen with a fetal node in it (arrow). (Courtesy of the Editor, *British Journal of Radiology*.) (C) Another case. Ectopic pregnancy (transverse scan). A small gestation sac is shown just to the left of the body of the uterus.

Ectopic pregnancy. In this condition the fertilized ovum does not reach the uterus. It implants usually in the Fallopian tube. It is an important but difficult diagnosis to make ultrasonically. The bladder should be moderately distended and the ultrasonic apparatus adjusted so that the vaginal canal is well outlined behind the bladder. Longitudinal and transverse scans are made and additional transverse scans with the transducer tilted 10–20° cephalad can be helpful.

Ectopic pregnancies may be either unruptured or ruptured and the ultrasonic appearances will vary between the two types.

The following features can be found (Maklad and Wright, 1978):

Unruptured ectopic pregnancy

1. Demonstration of a gestation sac in an extrauterine location (Fig. 68.46).

2. An oval or elongated fluid-filled adenexal mass due to the distended Fallopian tube containing an echodense ring like gestation sac.

3. Moderately enlarged uterus with a mottled echo pattern within it and no intrauterine pregnancy.

4. Detection of fetal heart movement within the extrauterine mass by real-time scanning or time-position mode if the fetus is viable.

Ruptured ectopic pregnancy

1. Extrauterine gestation sac associated with a complex mass due to haematoma (Fig. 68.47).

2. Displacement of the uterus by (a) the complex mass and (b) free fluid in the pouch of Douglas.

3. Moderately enlarged uterus with no intrauterine pregnancy with or without the abnormal echo pattern.

MONITORING OF PREGNANCY IN THE SECOND AND THIRD TRIMESTERS

(Assessment of gestational age and fetal weight)

For the best management of the pregnancy it is important that the gestational age of the fetus and frequently its weight should be accurately known. Ultrasound can provide this information with greater certainty than other methods. Allowance has to be made for the biological variation in fetal size and in the normal growth rate of the fetus (Campbell and Newman, 1971). In the early stages of pregnancy the biological variation in fetal size is smallest and the growth rate greatest. This is the period in which it is likely that the prediction of maturity would

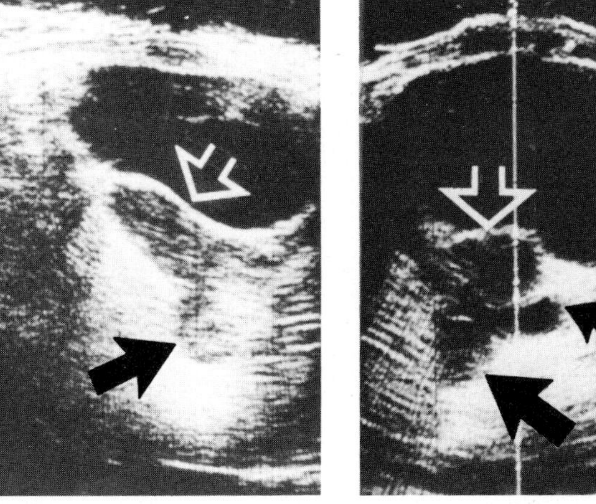
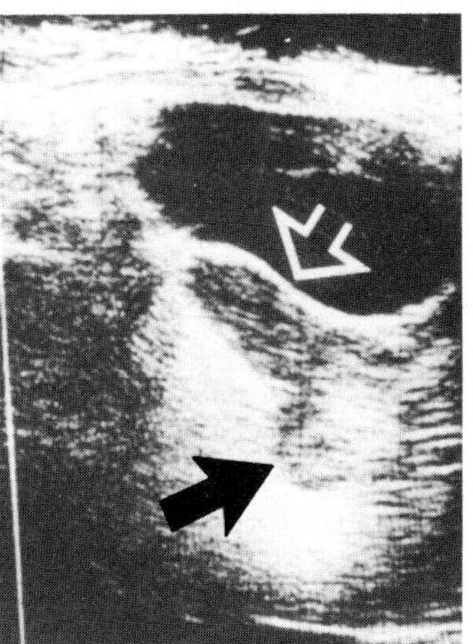
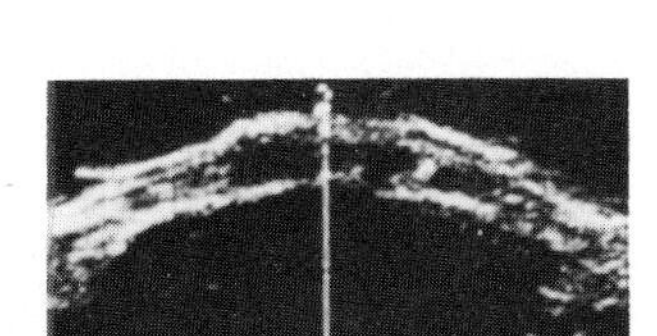

A B

Fig. 68.47 Ruptured ectopic pregnancy. (A) Longitudinal scan. The uterus (white arrow) is in front of the mass of the ectopic pregnancy (black arrow). (B) Transverse scan. The uterus (white arrow). Ectopic pregnancy (large black arrow). The ectopic pregnancy has ruptured and haemorrhage into the peritoneum is shown on the left side (curved arrow).

be most accurate. In the first trimester the method of choice for assessment of gestational age is the crown–rump measurement which has already been described (p. 1379). In the second and third trimesters the assessment of maturity depends on the measurement of the biparietal diameter of the skull, much of the initial work on which was done by Willocks (1962) using an A-scan method. It was later refined to a combined A- and B-scan method by Campbell (1968).

Estimation of fetal biparietal diameter

Technique. The object of the examination is to measure the fetal biparietal diameter consistently, i.e. the distance between the parietal eminences must be measured accurately. To achieve this the scan must demonstrate the parietal bones and the midline echo which arises from the falx cerebri or the intercerebral cleft. The midline echo should be shown on the B-scan as a clear straight line in the sagittal plane equidistant from the curvilinear echoes of the parietal bones. The latter echoes must be mirror-images of each other so that the echoes from the two sides of the skull are symmetrical but opposite to each other. Measurement of the distance between the parietal bones will now give an accurate biparietal diameter. Since the midline plane of the fetal head is variable relative to the maternal pelvis, the following method (Campbell, 1968) using a combined A- and B-scan method enables consistent results to be obtained fairly rapidly. It applies to the majority of cases, i.e. those with a longitudinal lie, vertex presentation and engagement occurring with the occiput in the oblique or lateral position.

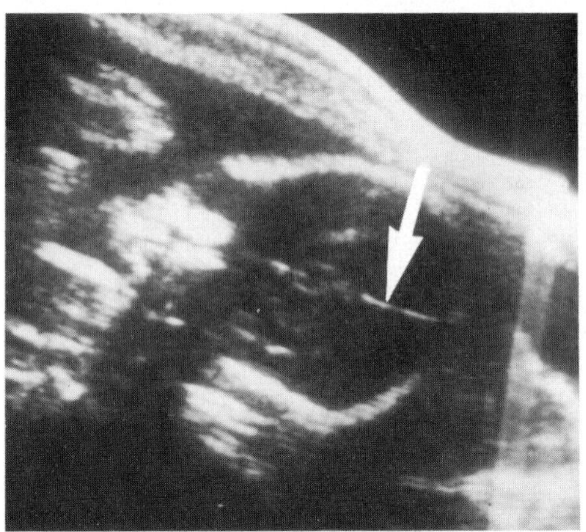

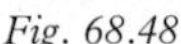

Fig. 68.48

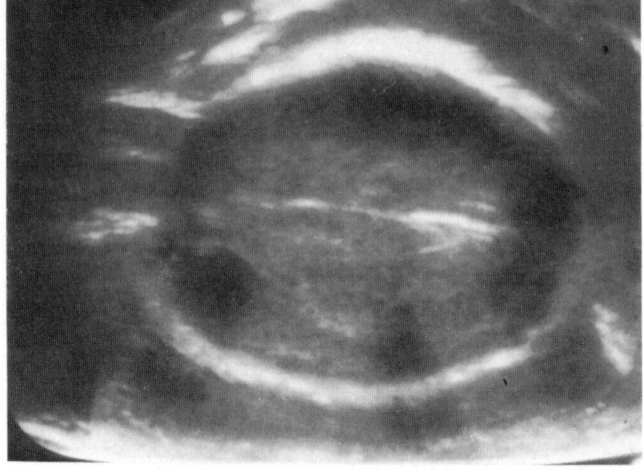

Fig. 68.49

Fig. 68.48 Biparietal diameter. Longitudinal scan. The arrow points to the midline echo and indicates the angle to the vertical at which the transverse scan must be made.

Fig. 68.49 Biparietal diameter. Outline of the fetal head obtained on angled transverse scan. The midline echo is well seen.

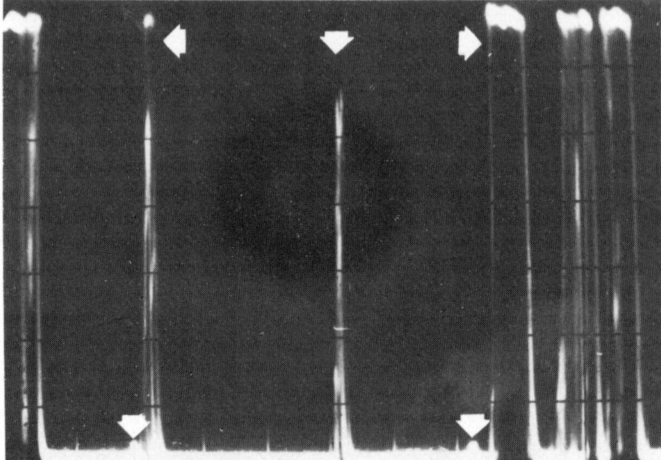

Fig. 68.50 Biparietal diameter. A-scan showing the parietal bone echoes and the midline echo (upper arrows). The lower arrows point to the caliper markers, slightly offset from the parietal bone echoes to demonstrate the markers which must superimpose (see text).

Longitudinal scans are first performed to show the fetus clearly and to determine the angle of inclination (asynclitism) of the midline of the fetal head from the vertical (Fig. 68.48). Scanning is now performed transversely at the level of the head and with the probe inclined at the angle of asynclitism so that the ultrasonic beam is directed at right angles to the intercerebral cleft. If a transverse scan is performed it will trace a plan view of the head on the B-scan and the midline will show as a strong linear echo (Figs 68.14 and 68.49). With the ultrasound transducer held so that the beam across the skull is at right angles to the midline echo, the high intensity parietal bone echoes with the lower intensity midline echo equidistant between them are displayed on the A-scan. The caliper markers are now placed on the leading edge of each of the parietal bone echoes (Fig. 68.50) and the measured biparietal diameter read off the digital display if the apparatus is calibrated for a speed of ultra-

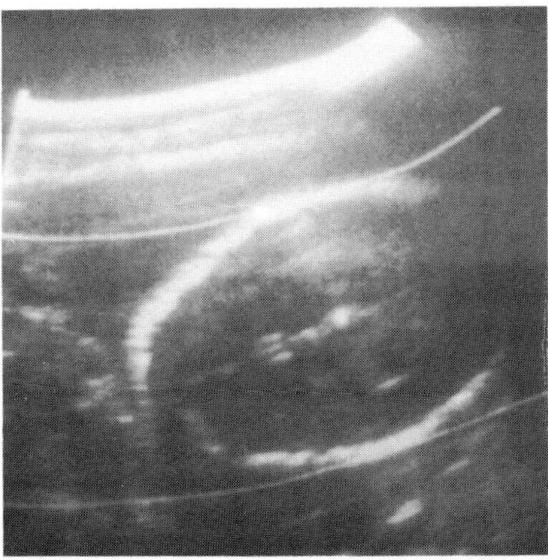

Fig. 68.51 Biparietal diameter. The calipers trace lines tangential to the parietal bones and will be set to correctly measure the biparietal diameter (see text).

sound of 1,600 metres per second. The caliper markings are then written onto the B-scan measurement (Fig. 68.51). If the apparatus is calibrated for an ultrasound speed of 1,540 metres per second the caliper markers are placed on the outer sides of the parietal bone echoes. Maturity is then obtained by reference to the appropriate graph (Fig. 68.52). Several measurements of the biparietal diameter are made and the widest one selected as the true measurement. This method is applicable in most cases, but problems arise in the following circumstances:

1. It may not be possible to obtain a biparietal diameter measurement if the fetal head lies in an occipito-anterior or occipito-posterior position. It should be noted that real time scanners with a freeze-frame facility may overcome this particular problem.

2. If the fetal head lies deep in the pelvis. The head may sometimes be brought out of the pelvis by raising the pelvis on pillows or tilting the examination table so that the mother's head lies lower than the pelvis.

3. If the fetus is very mobile and moves before an accurate determination of scanning angle and head size is obtained. In these circumstances a biparietal diameter measurement may be obtained more easily by real-time scanning using the freeze-frame facility.

4. If the lie is transverse or the engagement is by the breech, the basic principle of a scan along the fetus followed by a scan angled across the fetal head still applies, but the determination of the lines and angles of scanning may be more difficult in these cases.

By serial examination of the biparietal diameter at intervals of at least three weeks the rate of growth of the fetus can be measured. The rate is rapid and relatively constant up to 30 weeks at 3 mm per week. After this period the growth rate gradually lessens and the biological variation progressively increases (see graph, Fig. 68.52). The accuracy of maturity prediction decreases the nearer to term the assessment is made. When a measurement is made between the 13th and 30th week it is possible to predict the date of delivery within ±14 days in 93 per cent of cases. If two measurements are made separated by three weeks interval, it is possible to achieve an accuracy of ±9 days in 91 per cent of cases. An assessment of the consistency of the measurement in this series showed the mean error of paired biparietal diameter readings was 1·53 mm and it was at a minimum between measurements of 59–83 mm (23–31 weeks) (Lunt and Chard, 1974). Further, since growth is particularly rapid in this period and the standard deviation of head size relatively small it is a favourable time for making a single estimation of maturity by biparietal diameter measurement. Conversely single examinations made in late pregnancy are relatively poor indicators of the expected date of delivery as the normal variation in head size (i.e. ±2 S.D.) indicates an expected date of delivery ±3 weeks with a head measurement of 9·25 cm (i.e. equivalent to a mean gestation of 36 weeks).

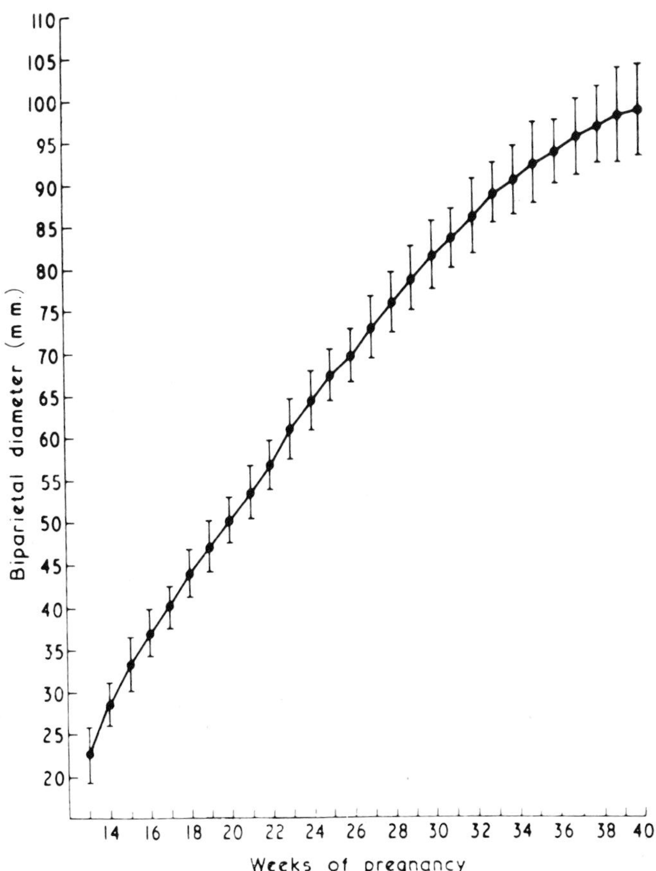

Fig. 68.52 Graph of mean fetal biparietal diameter ±2 S.D. assuming ultrasound velocity of 1600 m/sec from 13 weeks to term. (Campbell and Newman, 1971; courtesy of authors and editor of *Journal of Obstetrics and Gynaecology of the British Commonwealth*.)

Estimation of abdominal circumference (fetal weight prediction)

The possibility of prediction of fetal weight from ultrasonic measurements has caused considerable interest but

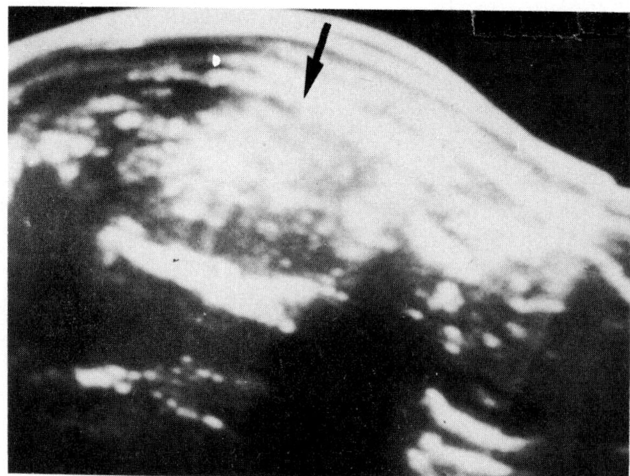

Fig. 68.53 Abdominal circumference. Longitudinal scan of the fetus. The arrow indicates the angle to the vertical at which the transverse scan must be made.

Fig. 68.54 Abdominal circumference. Transverse scan showing the umbilical vein (arrow) and the abdominal outline to be measured.

the use of the biparietal diameter for this purpose has not proved to be more accurate than palpation. More accurate is a method (Campbell and Wilkin, 1975) in which the circumference of the fetal abdomen at right angles to the long axis of the body is measured at umbilical vein level. The method in some ways resembles that of obtaining the BPD. The fetal trunk is shown in longitudinal section. Its lie relevant to the long axis of the mother must be determined and then the angle which the transverse plane of the fetus in its mid part makes with the

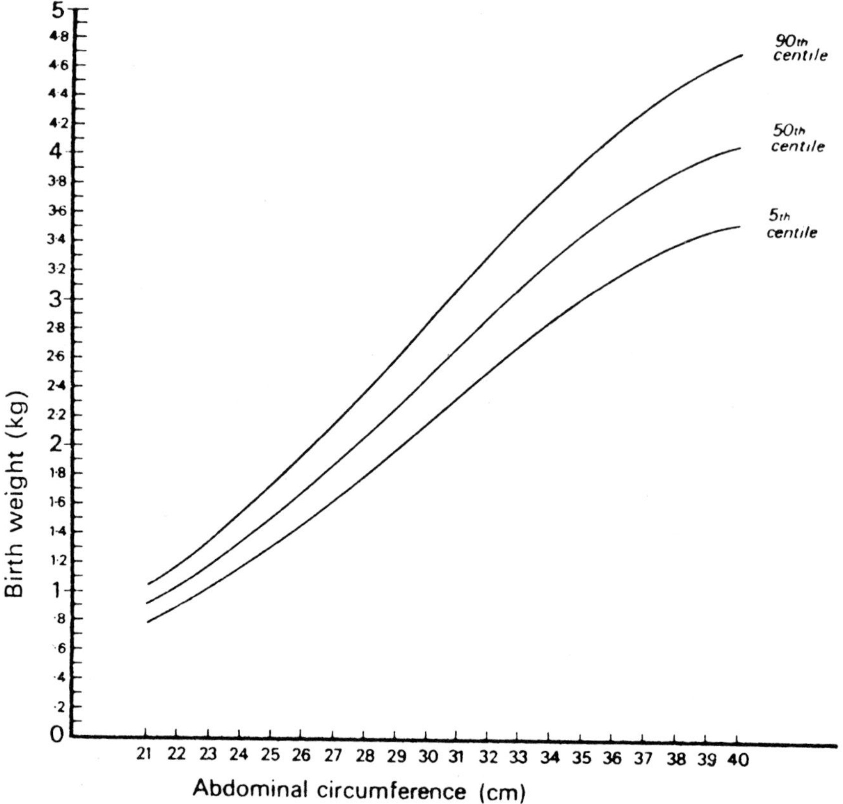

Fig. 68.55 Abdominal circumference. Graph showing abdominal circumference plotted against birth weight with 5th and 90th centile limits. (Campbell and Wilkin, 1975; by courtesy of authors and editor of *British Journal of Obstetrics and Gynaecology*.)

vertical is found (Fig. 68.53). By adjusting the scanning plane to be at right angles to the fetus's long axis and suitably inclined from the vertical a true transverse section of the trunk can be obtained. The level at which measurement is taken is arbitrarily fixed as that of the umbilical vein. On appropriate scans, the spine (a dense ring echo), the liver (a region of homogeneous fine echoes) and sometimes the fluid-filled stomach (an anechoic zone) can be seen. The umbilical vein appears as a pair of parallel lines passing forward amongst the liver echoes to the anterior abdominal wall of the fetus (Fig. 68.54). When this section is demonstrated it is photographed and the circumference measured using a map measurer. Appropriate correction for magnification in the apparatus and the photographic system has to be applied. The fetal weight is then obtained from the appropriate graph (Fig. 68.55). Campbell and Wilkin found that for a predicted fetal weight of 1 kg 95 per cent of birth weights fell within 160 g of the estimation and at 2, 3 and 4 kg the corresponding values were 290 g, 450 g and 590 g respectively. Expressed as a percentage of the median birth weight, the ultrasonic error was constant throughout the birth weight range. This technique was also found to demonstrate between 75 per cent and 87 per cent of small-for-dates fetuses.

Antenatal monitoring for intrauterine retardation

Problems arising from intrauterine growth retardation, particularly those of increased perinatal mortality and neurological and intellectual impairment, have made it important to detect growth retardation accurately and thus to indicate the optimum time for delivery. Ultrasound can provide reliable information for the monitoring of these cases and particularly useful are serial biparietal diameter measurements. In addition an estimate of the fetal weight from the abdominal circumference may be made and the two measurements may be combined, as indicated below, to give the head-abdomen (H/A) circumference ratio.

Fetal growth, in general terms, is determined by two factors—the growth potential of the fetus, which is mainly genetic, and the growth support from the mother and the placenta. Abnormality of either can give rise to a 'small-for-dates' baby. 'Small-for-dates' babies are not a homogeneous group: they may be divided basically into two types which can be distinguished clinically.

Type 1. Symmetrical growth retardation, i.e. all organs equally affected.

Type 2. Asymmetrical growth retardation, i.e. a fetus with a long wasted body but the brain and head preferentially protected from the retarding stimulus.

In Type 1, pregnancy and labour are not complicated and the fetus is normal in all proportions. In Type 2, the baby is starved and the condition may be induced by hypertension or pre-eclamptic toxaemia in the mother. The two groups can be distinguished ultrasonically by the following methods:

1. Serial biparietal cephalometry. Biparietal diameter measurements are repeated at not less than 3 weeks

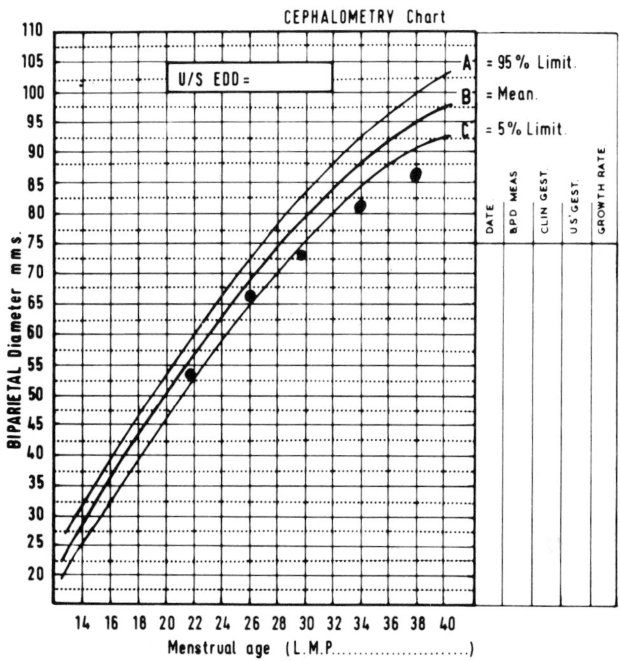

Fig. 68.56 Cephalometry chart. Low growth potential. Small-for-dates baby: the biparietal diameter measured from the 22nd to 38th week of pregnancy shows a gradual and progressive fall below the 5 per cent limit.

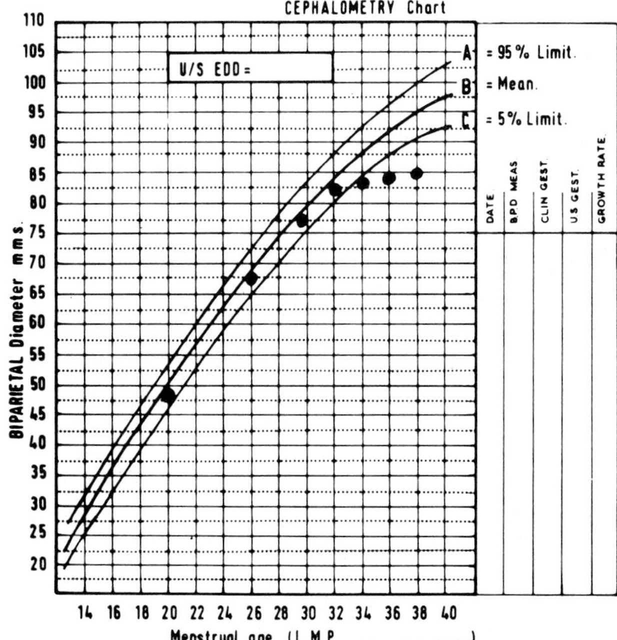
CEPHALOMETRY Chart
U/S EDD =
A = 95 % Limit.
B = Mean.
C = 5 % Limit.
DATE
BPD MEAS
CLIN GEST
US GEST
GROWTH RATE
BIPARIETAL Diameter mms.
110
105
100
95
90
85
80
75
70
65
60
55
50
45
40
35
30
25
20
14 16 18 20 22 24 26 28 30 32 34 36 38 40
Menstrual age (L.M.P.......................)

Fig. 68.57 Cephalometry chart. Uteroplacental insufficiency. Small-for-dates baby. Serial biparietal diameter measurements show normal skull growth up to 32 weeks maturity after which time growth almost ceases.

intervals. In symmetrical growth retardation cases (type 1) the increase in head size is slower than normal but it is continuous (Fig. 68.56). In the asymmetrical growth retardation cases (type 2) there is terminal cessation of head growth after a normal initial rise (Fig. 68.57).

2. Fetal head to abdomen circumference ratio. In the asymmetrical growth retardation group of 'small-for-dates' babies, the brain and head are preferentially protected and the wasting occurs in the upper abdomen due to reduction in size of the liver. Because of this, serial cephalometry will fail to recognize a proportion of cases, especially those babies in whom the condition has developed relatively late in pregnancy. These asymmetrical 'small-for-dates' babies may be detected by the use of the fetal head to abdomen circumference ratio introduced by Campbell and Thoms in 1977. This is performed as follows. To obtain a true and reproducible measurement a modification of the technique used to obtain a biparietal head diameter is employed with the object of displaying the occipito-frontal and biparietal diameters on the one scan. Having obtained the biparietal diameter by the standard method the scanning plane is rotated to allow for flexion of the fetal head on the trunk. When the required outline of the head is properly projected a pair of short parallel lines are shown parallel to the midline echo, about one-third of the distance along the long axis of the head. These probably represent the third ventricle or adjacent structures (Fig. 68.58). The circumference is obtained after appropriate magnification correction using a map measurer. The abdominal circumference is that obtained as indicated above. The head–abdomen circumference (H/A) ratio is then calculated. The variation of H/A ratio with gestational age is shown in Figure 68.59. Important points on this graph are 1·18 at 17 weeks, 1·11 at 29 weeks, 1·01 at 36 weeks and 0·94 at term. The ratio is elevated above the 95 per cent confidence limit in the asymmetrical type of 'small-for-dates' babies. The ratio is within the normal range (i.e. below the 95 per cent confidence limit) in the symmetrical type of 'small-for-dates' babies.

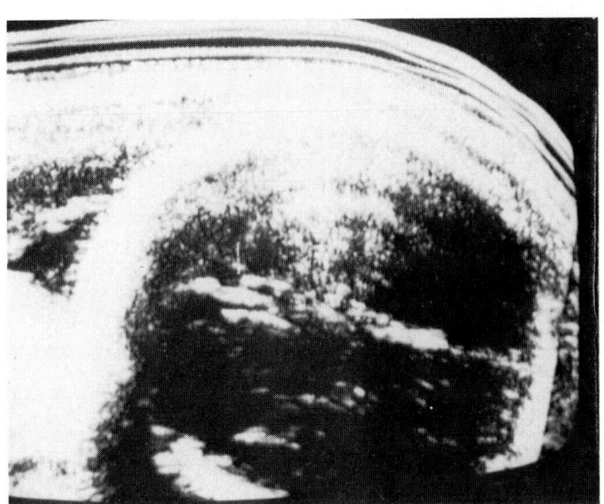

Fig. 68.58 Head/abdomen circumference ratio. Outline of fetal head to show both the biparietal and occipitofrontal diameters. Note the parallel pair of lines of the third ventricle.

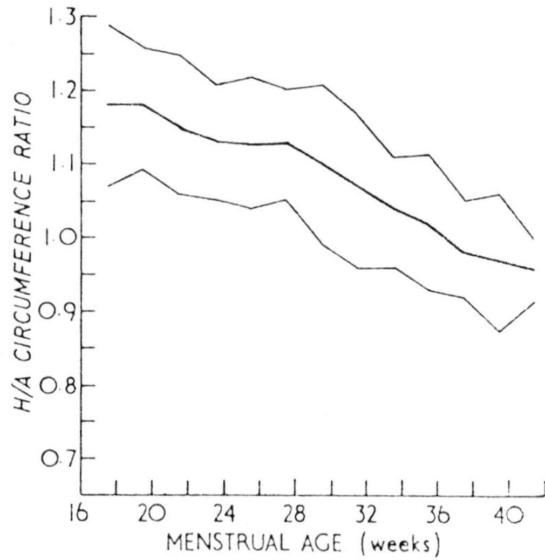

Fig. 68.59 Head/abdomen circumference ratio. Graph of H/A circumference ratio from 16 weeks to term. (Campbell and Thoms, 1977; by courtesy of authors and editor of *British Journal of Obstetrics and Gynaecology*.)

FETAL ABNORMALITY AND DEATH

Increasing attention has been paid to the prenatal diagnosis of fetal abnormality and particularly to making the diagnosis early enough to allow selective termination of pregnancy. Even failing this, the knowledge that a fetus is or may be abnormal towards the end of pregnancy can still be helpful in assisting in decisions of management arising from possible abnormality. There are however many fetal abnormalities which cannot be diagnosed by ultrasound. The conditions which are diagnosable may be considered under the heading of acquired and congenital fetal abnormalities.

Acquired fetal abnormalities

Rhesus isoimmunization. The following signs may be shown (Ghorashi and Gottesfeld, 1976):

1. The placenta may be thickened. A placental thickness of 6 cm is often associated with a hydropic fetus and a thickness of 5·5 cm must cause concern.

2. The fetus may be hydropic or oedematous and this is shown ultrasonically by thickening of the outline of the head, chest and limbs producing a 'fluffy' appearance. Occasionally the oedema produces a 'double ring' around the fetal skull. Homogeneously transonic areas between

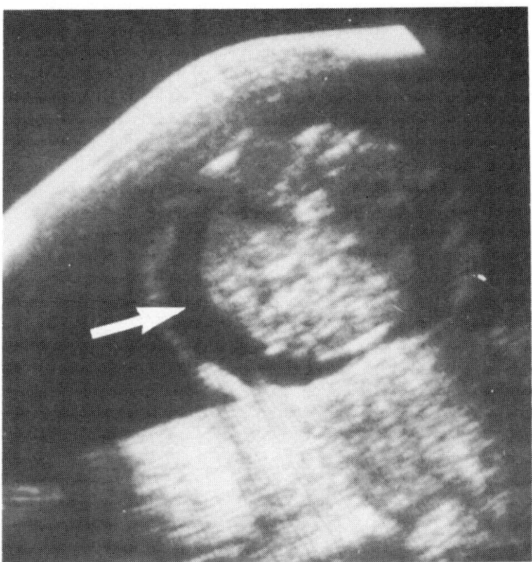

Fig. 68.60 Fetal ascites. Arrow indicates ascitic fluid space.

the fetal abdominal wall and intestines, liver and spleen indicate ascites (Fig. 68.60).

Diabetes in the mother may give rise to a thick placenta and a 'double ring' of the fetal scalp due to fatty deposition. The fetus is large for dates, particularly after the 37th week.

Fetal death

The definitive diagnosis of fetal death after the 12th week of pregnancy is made by failure to demonstrate:

1. Fetal pulsations by the Doppler effect, or
2. Fetal heart, body and limb movements on real-time scanning, or

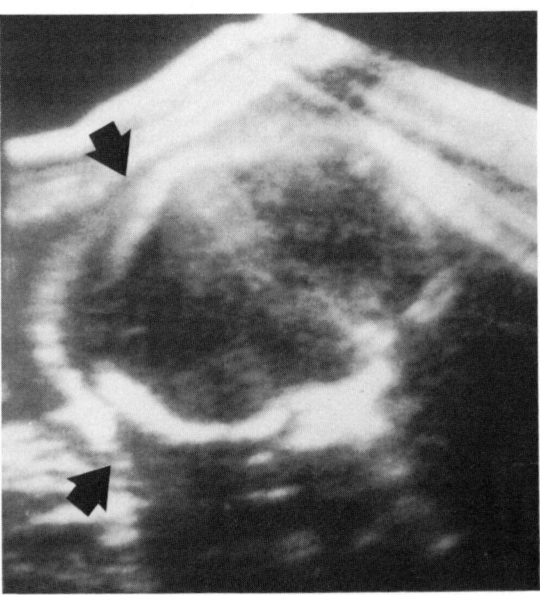

Fig. 68.61 Fetal death. Collapse of skull with over-ride of cranial bones (arrows).

3. Fetal heart movement by the combined A- and B-scan technique
4. Collapse of the fetal head with overlapping bone, *viz*. Spalding's sign (Fig. 68.61).

Other, less certain, signs include difficulty in identifying the skull midline echo, a 'fluffy' or double outline of the fetal head, collapse and telescoping of the fetal body and failure of the uterus to enlarge on serial examination.

Congenital fetal abnormalities

Polyhydramnios. Congenital fetal abnormalities, particularly those associated with abnormalities of the central nervous system and atresia of the upper alimentary tract may be associated with polyhydramnios (Fig. 68.62). In this condition there is excess amniotic fluid and the maternal abdominal wall may be tense. The fetus is usually well shown and it appears to be small in relation to the uterine size. The diagnosis is subjective, as no criteria are available for measuring when excess amniotic fluid is present.

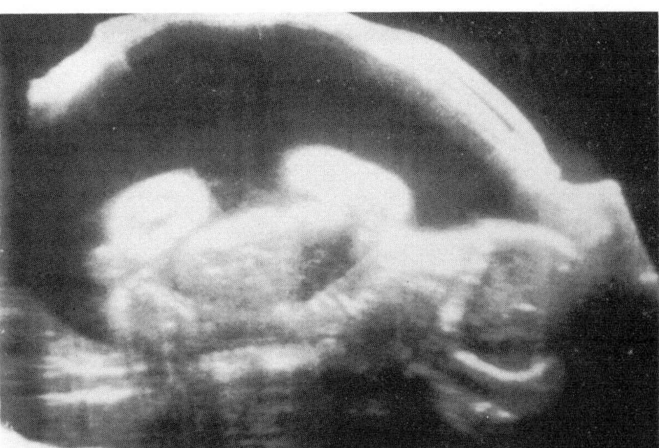

Fig. 68.62 Polyhydramnios; there is a gross excess of amniotic fluid.

Cranial abnormalities. (1) *Anencephaly*. In this condition the cranial vault is absent. Ultrasonically a normal fetal head cannot be shown after careful scanning (Fig. 68.63). The structures of the face and skull base may produce a projection at the cranial end of the trunk. It should be diagnosable after about the 14th week of pregnancy.

(2) *Hydrocephalus* may be demonstrated in the late stages of pregnancy, the diagnosis depending on showing the head to be abnormally large (i.e. >2 S.D.) for the dates. A biparietal diameter of over 12 cm is diagnostic. In borderline cases a head/chest area ratio of over 2 : 1 is suggestive. Dilated cerebral ventricles may be shown by careful scanning and are likewise diagnostic (Fig. 68.64).

(3) *Microcephaly* is suggested if the head/chest area ratio is less than 1 : 2 or when the head is small for the dates.

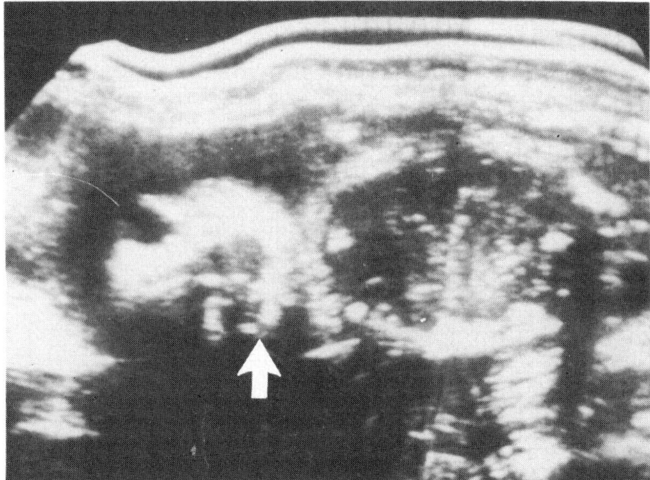

Fig. 68.63 Anencephaly. There is a malformed cranial base (arrow) but no cranial vault is shown.

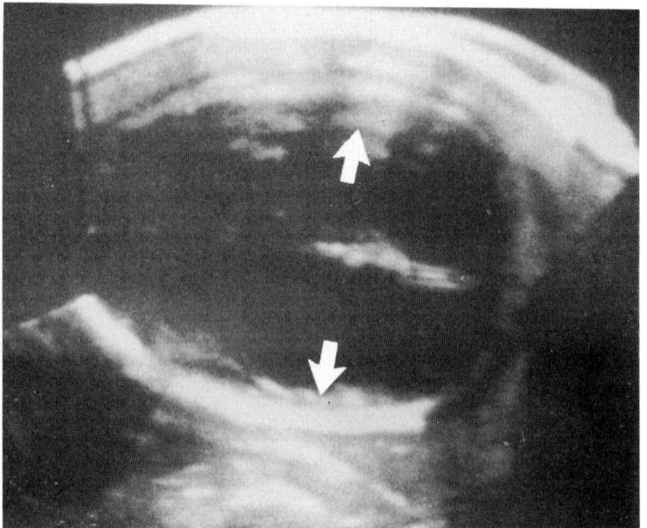

Fig. 68.64 Hydrocephalus. The margins of the dilated ventricles are indicated by arrows.

(4) *Meningoencephalocoele*. Usually occurs in the occipital region and may be shown as a mass extending out from the skull.

Spinal defect. Spina bifida and meningocoele may be shown as a local widening of the spinal canal with or without a soft tissue mass over it (Fig. 68.65). On a longitudinal scan of the fetus a normal looking spine is fair evidence against the presence of a spina bifida (Figs 68.17 and 68.18). More detailed evidence is obtained by checking serial transverse sections of the fetal spine. A normal vertebral canal appears as a small dense ring (Fig. 68.19). An open spina bifida shows as a U-shaped echo (Fig. 68.66). Scanning for neural tube defects is best carried out from the 16th to the 19th week of maturity. Lower lumbar and sacral spina bifida are difficult to demonstrate. Spina bifida is also well shown on real time scanning and this is now the method of choice for demonstrating this condition.

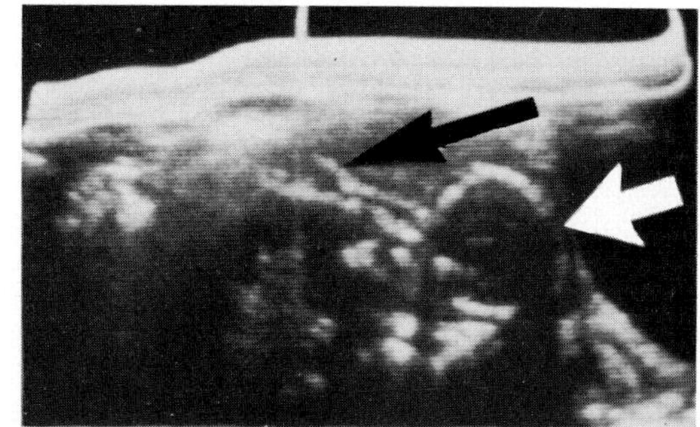

A

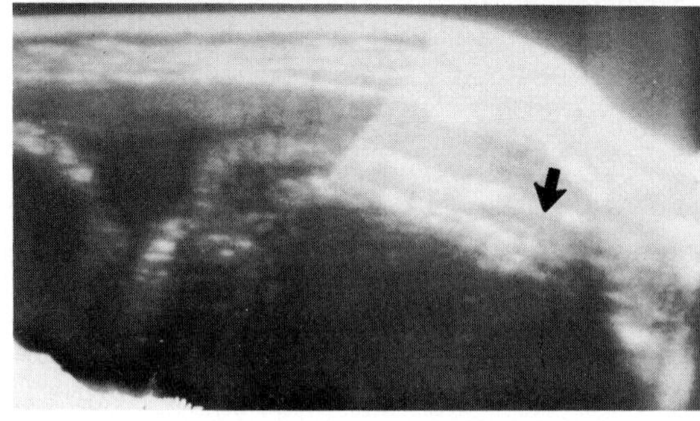

B

Fig. 68.65(A and B) Spina bifida—two different cases. The widening of the spinal canal is indicated by black arrows. The white arrow in (A) points to the head.

Urinary tract abnormalities. (1) *Agenesis* may be suspected if the fetal kidneys and bladder are not shown in the later stages of pregnancy. These may be associated with oligohydramnios.

(2) *Fetal dysplastic (multicystic) kidneys* have been demonstrated in good quality scans.

(3) *Urethral obstruction* may result in dilatation of the bladder, the ureter and the renal pelvis all of which can be identified on a careful scanning.

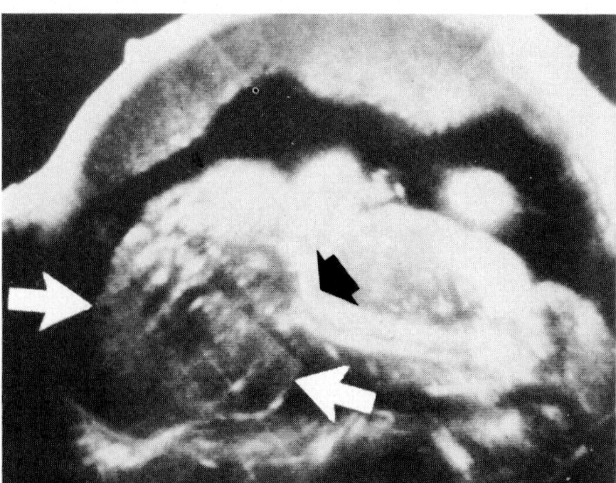

Fig. 68.66 Fetal pelvic teratoma. A large soft tissue mass (white arrows) with transonic and highly echogenic areas in it arises from the fetal pelvic region. The lower end of the spine is splayed (black arrow).

Alimentary tract abnormalities. *Duodenal atresia.* A pair of fluid containing spaces high in the fetal abdomen form the ultrasonic equivalent to the radiological 'double bubble' sign and indicate duodenal atresia.

Embryonic tumours such as teratoma may be identified if they extend beyond the normal surface of the fetus. They show areas of high echogenicity and other areas of transonicity dispersed in a random fashion (Fig. 68.66).

ULTRASONIC PLACENTOGRAPHY

The placenta is easily shown by ultrasound and its position is normally noted at routine examinations. However, its localization is particularly required in:

1. Antepartum haemorrhage—placenta praevia, abruptio placentae.
2. Amniocentesis.

The classification of placenta praevia is given in Ch. 47,

Amniocentesis is now commonly carried out for the diagnosis of chromosomal defects, Rh-immunization and neural tube defects. Since it has been shown that blood-free embryonic fluid is more frequently obtained and fetomaternal haemorrhage is reduced if the placental site is known, it is mandatory to perform placentography prior to amniocentesis whenever the facilities are available.

Ultrasonic appearance of the placenta

The placenta can be identified from about 8 weeks onwards. It initially appears as a thickening of the wall of the gestation sac with a uniform granular echo pattern (Fig. 68.67). In early pregnancy it may project quite markedly into the amniotic cavity. At about 18 to 22 weeks a white line becomes defined on the fetal side of the placenta. Later on villous spaces appear which may be separated from each other by septa. High level echoes from placental calcification may be identified in late pregnancy (Fisher, Garrett and Kossoff, 1976). These features are best shown when the placenta is under the transducer, i.e. when it lies anteriorly (Fig. 68.68). If the placenta lies laterally it will be best shown if the transducer scans along the lateral uterine wall and is directed towards the patient's midline. A lateral implantation can lead to the placenta appearing on both the anterior and posterior uterine walls on a longitudinal scan (Fig. 68.69). This is due to the placenta extending round from the side walls anteriorly and posteriorly. When the placenta lies on the posterior wall it may be less easily shown as the fetus tends to mask it by absorbing the ultrasound, particularly towards the latter part of pregnancy. Its posterior position may be inferred if the fetus does not lie against the posterior wall of the uterus. This inference may be made because the fetus will normally gravitate into contact with the posterior uterine wall when the mother is in the supine position unless prevented from doing so by some structure such as a posteriorly located placenta. Gentle backward pressure on the fetus may help to define the position and extent of the placenta if it is implanted posteriorly (Fig. 68.70). The placenta may be located in the fundus (Fig. 68.71) or may occupy the region of the lower pole of the uterus (placenta praevia). The thickness of the placenta varies considerably and no criteria of normality have been laid down. It may be thick or thin, and in either case function normally.

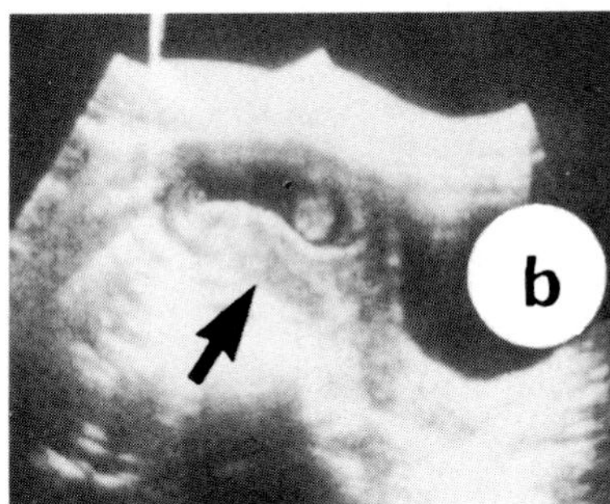

Fig. 68.67 Early placental formation. 12-week mature pregnancy. Longitudinal scan. The uterus is enlarged. A well-formed gestation sac is present with a fetal node in it. The developing placental site (arrow) is posterior and low in the uterus. **b** = bladder.

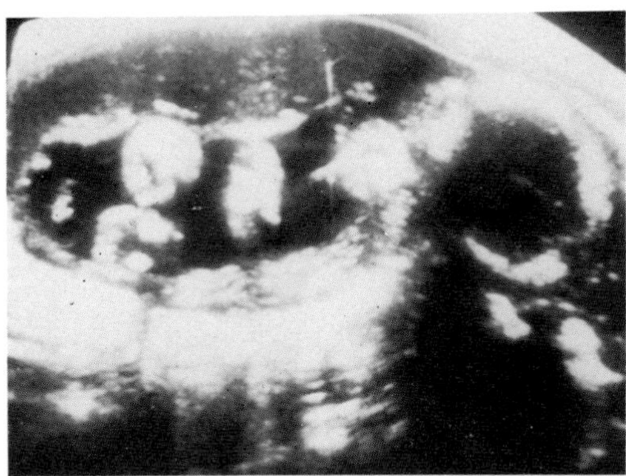

Fig. 68.68 Anterior placenta. The ultrasonic features of the placenta are best shown when it lies immediately under the transducer, particularly the white line of the chorionic plate.

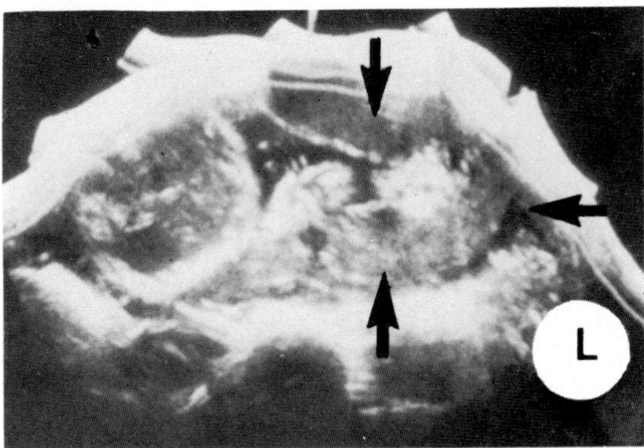

Fig. 68.69 Left lateral placenta. Transverse scan. 32 weeks maturity. The placenta extends from the anterior wall of the uterus, around the left side onto the posterior wall (arrows). **L** = left side.

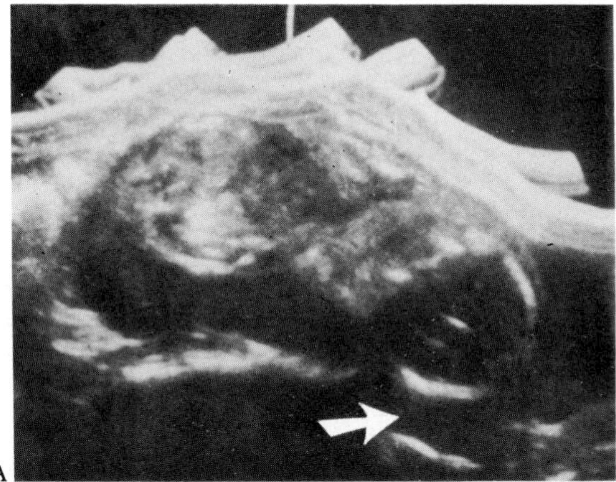

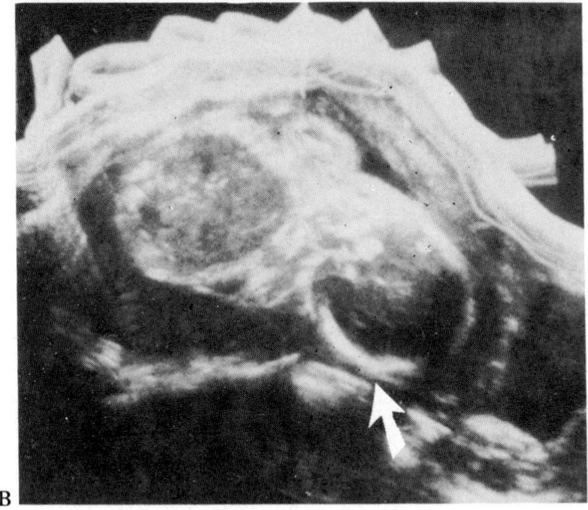

Fig. 68.70(A and B) Posterior placenta, 34 weeks maturity. In (A) The placenta lies in the ultrasonic shadow of the fetus and its lower limit cannot be defined. Gentle pressure on the fetal head eliminates the lower part of the gap behind the fetus and excludes placenta praevia (B).

The maximum diameter of the placenta is about 20 cm.

Ultrasound will define the limits of the placenta and its relation to other structures, e.g. the cervix or fetus. The method of locating the internal os has already been described (Fig. 68.17).

First trimester. The decidua/placenta is clearly seen in about 7–8 weeks and the placental site can be inferred (Fig. 68.67). It is usually extensive, and it is not possible to predict the eventual placental site because at least half the placentas reach the lower pole of the uterus at this stage of pregnancy.

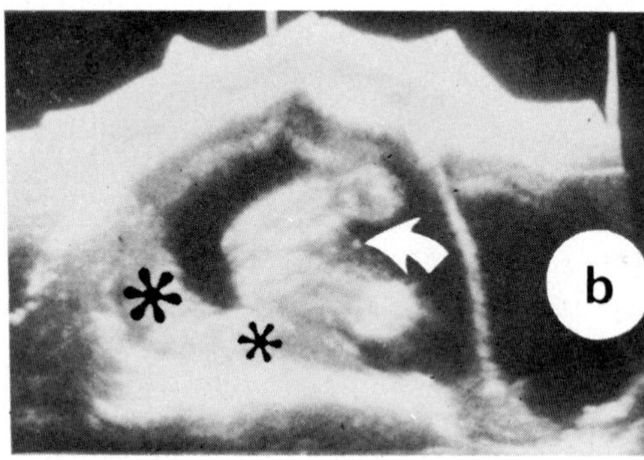

Fig. 68.71 Fundal placenta. Longitudinal scan. 20 weeks maturity. Transverse lie. The placenta (stars) extends around the fundus. Fetal thighs (arrow). **b** = bladder.

Second trimester and early third trimester. In this period of pregnancy placental localization is easiest largely because the liquor amnii is abundant and the uterus is not too big (Fig. 68.71). The placenta can be well outlined, but the clinical relevance of low lying placentas is diminished because many patients with placentas that reach the internal os at this time are subsequently delivered without any evidence of placenta praevia. These are so called 'migrating placentae' (King, 1973) which, on serial scans, are seen to move away from the internal os in a period of weeks (Fig. 68.72A and B). There are many theories as to how this occurs, but the phenomenon is almost certainly related to the development of the lower segment of the uterus. For this reason placenta praevia should not be diagnosed before 32 weeks as an apparently low implantation can improve in position as the uterus enlarges. It is a wise precaution to make serial observations when a low placental implantation is found in early pregnancy. Improvement in position is more frequent with anteriorly sited placentas. Posterior placenta praevia is more common than anterior.

Late third trimester : placenta praevia. Placenta praevia is defined as a placenta which is either wholly or partially implanted in the lower uterine segment and therefore lies before the presenting part (Llewellyn-Jones, 1973). The lower edge of the placenta can be fairly easily related to the position of the internal os (Fig. 68.73) (see p. 1371), but there are no ultrasonic criteria which define the limits of the lower uterine segment. It may be taken as a rule of thumb that in late pregnancy the lower segment extends upwards and outwards for a distance of 5 cm from the internal os. Using the grading of the placenta praevia given before (Ch. 47) a grade 1 placenta praevia is one whose lower edge reaches within 5 cm of the internal os. Grades 2, 3 and 4 are recognized by the relationship to the internal os in each case. In late pregnancy placental localization may become more difficult because of the lack of amniotic fluid. Also when a placenta is posterior in position the fetus puts it into ultrasonic shadow (Fig. 68.74). A couch which can tilt the patient's head down may be an asset by bringing the head away from the lower part of the uterus and thereby giving easier access of the ultrasound beam to the region of the internal os. In this period of pregnancy a minor degree of placenta praevia has a greater significance than when present early in pregnancy.

The accuracy of placental localization is between 94 per cent and 98 per cent depending on the criteria adopted and the expertise of the operator. There is an undoubted tendency to overdiagnose placenta praevia ultrasonically

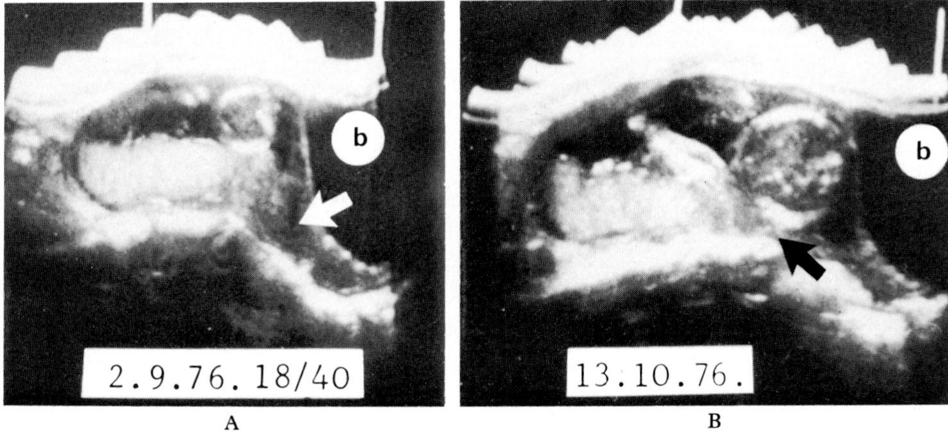

Fig. 68.72(A and B) Longitudinal scan at 18 weeks (A) shows the placenta low in position (white arrow). Six weeks later (B) the lower edge of the placenta (black arrow) has moved away from the internal os.

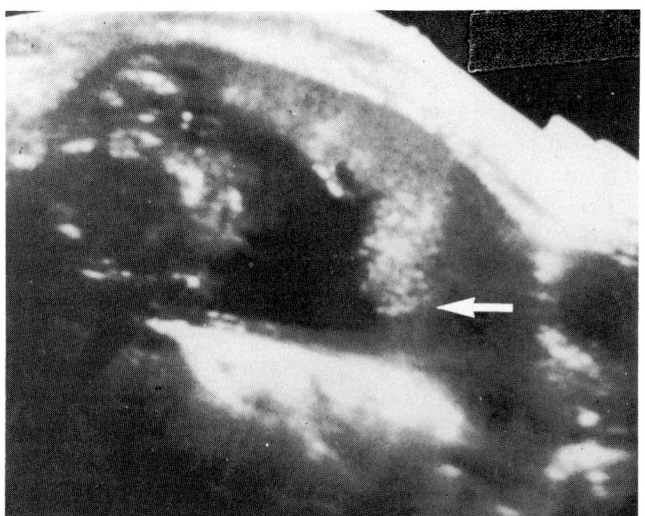

Fig. 68.73 The lower edge of the placenta extends to the internal os.

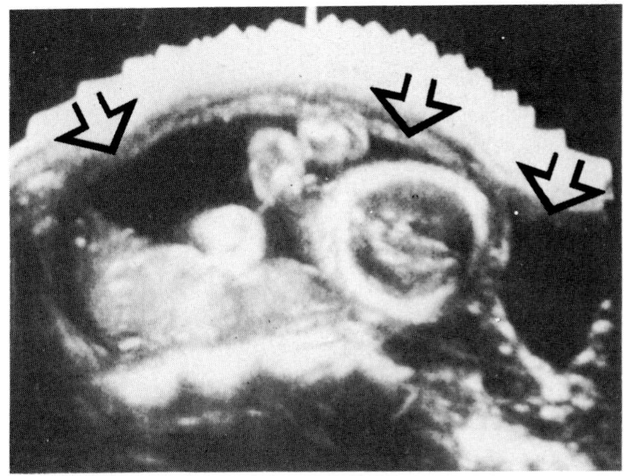

Fig. 68.75 Anterior artefact. 34-week pregnancy. Longitudinal scan. The line of reverberant echoes (arrows) deep to the anterior abdominal wall is well-shown. This is an artefact and is recognized easily because the line is always parallel to the anterior abdominal wall and it extends into the bladder outline. The placenta is actually on the posterior wall in this case.

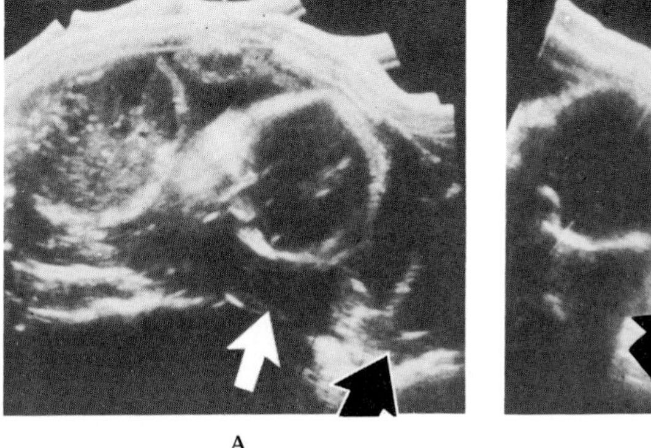

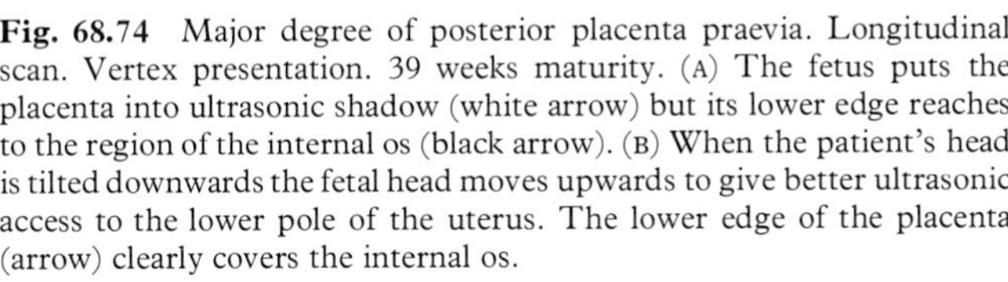

Fig. 68.74 Major degree of posterior placenta praevia. Longitudinal scan. Vertex presentation. 39 weeks maturity. (A) The fetus puts the placenta into ultrasonic shadow (white arrow) but its lower edge reaches to the region of the internal os (black arrow). (B) When the patient's head is tilted downwards the fetal head moves upwards to give better ultrasonic access to the lower pole of the uterus. The lower edge of the placenta (arrow) clearly covers the internal os.

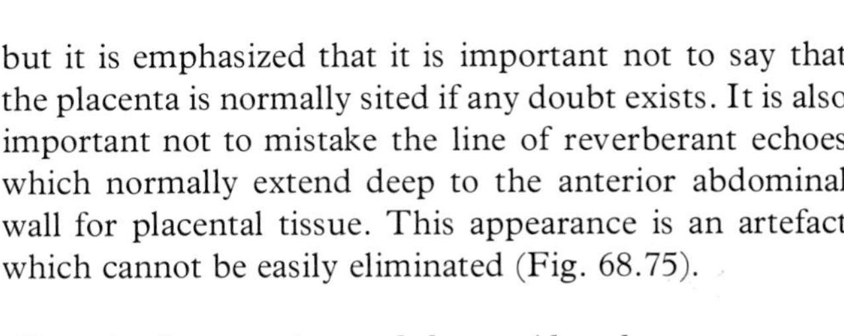

but it is emphasized that it is important not to say that the placenta is normally sited if any doubt exists. It is also important not to mistake the line of reverberant echoes which normally extend deep to the anterior abdominal wall for placental tissue. This appearance is an artefact which cannot be easily eliminated (Fig. 68.75).

Abruptio placentae (concealed or accidental antepartum haemorrhage)

Occasionally abruptio placentae can be shown by demonstrating a transonic area between the placenta and uterine wall.

Placentography before amniocentesis

Indications for amniocentesis. The following are the main indications for performing amniocentesis:

1. Investigation of suspected genetic abnormality and

neural tube defects by chromosome analysis and α-fetoprotein determination. This is best done at 16 to 18 weeks.

2. Investigation of rhesus isoimmunization by estimation of the bilirubin content of the amniotic fluid in the second and third trimesters.

3. Assessment of lung maturity by determination of the phospholecithin/sphingomyelin ratio in the amniotic fluid towards the end of pregnancy.

Method. The object of the examination is to define an area of the anterior wall of the uterus through which a fine needle can be inserted into a pool of amniotic fluid in order to obtain a sample without transversing the placenta or causing trauma to the fetus. The whole procedure is best carried out in the ultrasound room so that the patient need not be moved once the optimum puncture site has been defined. A transducer with a central channel in it through which the needle may be passed may be helpful. Careful longitudinal and transverse scans are made to locate the placenta. If the placenta is on the posterior wall no problem exists. If it covers the whole of the anterior wall of the uterus, either the examination has to be abandoned or a thin portion of the placenta has to be selected through which to pass the needle. If it partially covers the anterior wall, a part of this wall free of placenta with a pool of amniotic fluid deep to it is located (Fig. 68.76). The final position is then checked with an A-scan and the site marked on the skin for needle insertion. Real time scanning can also assist placental localization prior to amniocentesis.

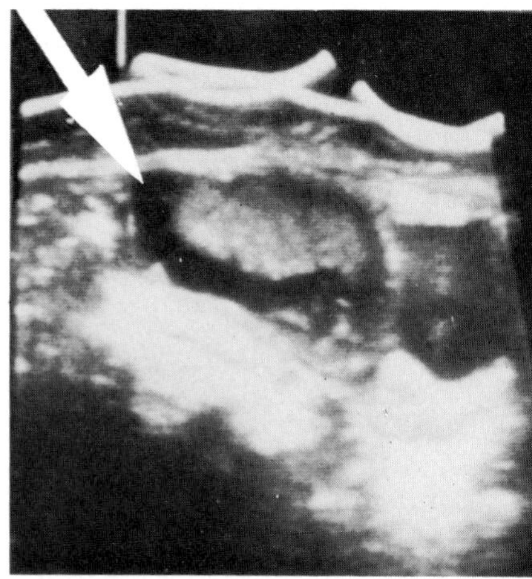

Fig. 68.76 Placental localization for amniocentesis. Longitudinal scan. Three centimetres to left of midline. 14 weeks maturity. The placenta is on the anterior wall but the fundus (arrow) is free of placenta and is therefore a suitable site for needle puncture for amniocentesis.

There is a risk that amniocentesis can induce abortion but this is less than 1 per cent. Needle damage to the fetus has also been reported but this is rare.

GYNAECOLOGY

Ultrasound is used in gynaecology:

1. To demonstrate the presence or absence of contraceptive devices in the uterus.
2. To demonstrate the presence, nature and size of pelvic masses.

THE DEMONSTRATION OF INTRA-UTERINE CONTRACEPTIVE DEVICES (IUCDs)

Ultrasound is an accurate and safe method of demonstrating whether an intrauterine contraceptive device is properly located within the uterine cavity. A problem arises if the threads attached to the device are not palpable in the vagina. It then becomes important to know whether the device is still within the uterus, is lost externally, or has migrated through the uterine wall into the peritoneal cavity. Since IUCDs are radiopaque they can be shown by conventional radiography. However, the radiographic demonstration of an IUCD in the pelvic cavity does not necessarily indicate that the device is within the uterus as the uterus itself can vary considerably in position. IUCDs produce strong acoustic echoes, either a linear echo or a series of punctate echoes depending on type (Fig. 68.77).

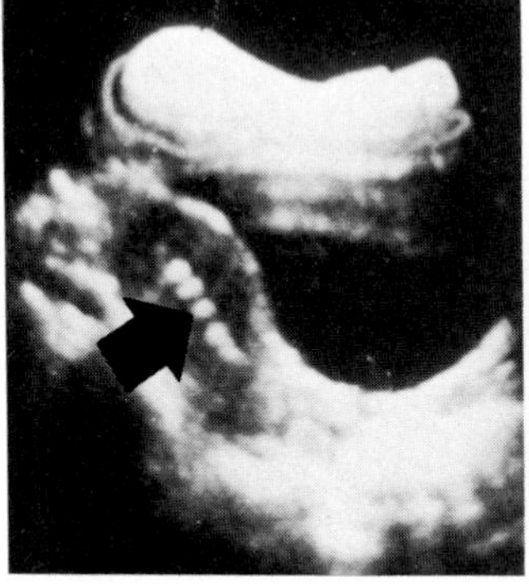

A

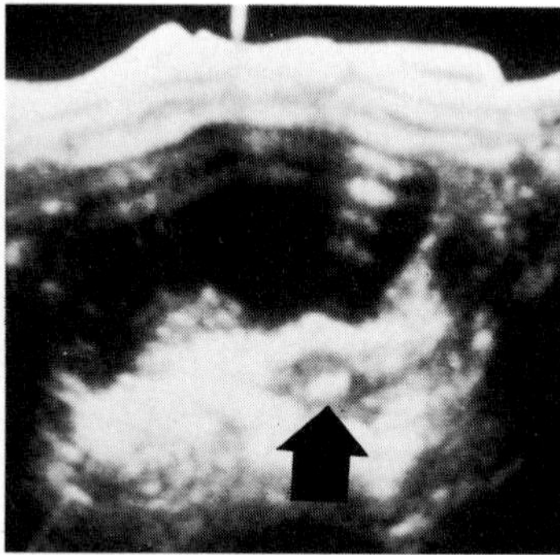

B

Fig. 68.77(A and B) Intrauterine contraceptive device; (A) longitudinal scan, (B) transverse scan of Lippes' loop. The series of dense echoes shown in (A) is characteristic of this device.

When the characteristic echo pattern is seen within the uterus the correct situation of the device is confirmed. Radiography is a useful supplement when the device is not shown within the uterus as distant migration may have then occurred. Ultrasound has on occasion shown a pregnancy coexisting with a correctly located intrauterine contraceptive device (Fig. 68.78).

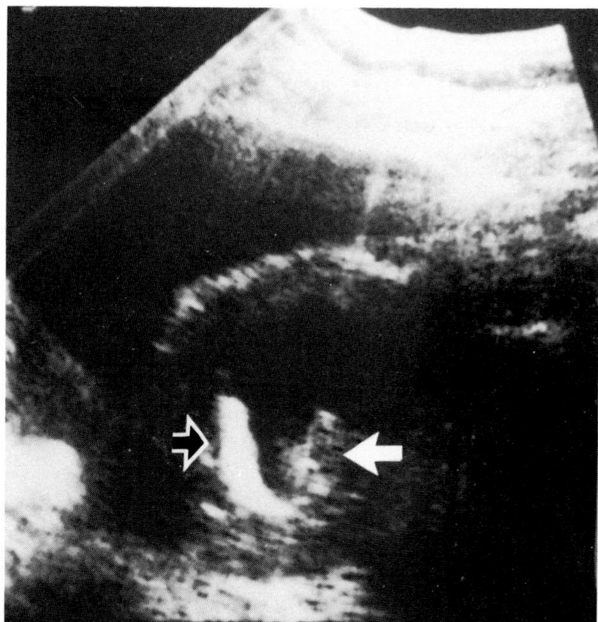

Fig. 68.78 Curvilinear echo of a Copper 7 (outline arrow) and fetal node (solid arrow) seen together *in utero*.

THE ULTRASONIC EXAMINATION OF PELVIC MASSES

The value of ultrasound in the management of patients with pelvic masses is limited because laparoscopy and laparotomy will eventually be performed in many such cases. Many surgeons prefer to have a well founded diagnosis before they operate and in this ultrasound can frequently be of assistance. In certain circumstances, ultrasound may profoundly alter the management of the patient, e.g. the demonstration of a benign cyst in a frail old lady with a mass in the abdomen would avoid operation.

The patient must be examined with a full bladder to give ultrasonic access to the pelvis and also to act as an anatomical landmark. The other landmark to be identified is the uterus. A pelvic mass that is too small to palpate on adequate bimanual examination is unlikely to be shown ultrasonically. If the bimanual examination is inadequate because of patient nervousness or obesity, then ultrasonic examination can be helpful. The differential diagnosis depends on three particular points which should be sought in the examination of all pelvic masses:

1. Location
2. Structure
3. Size.

Location (uterine or extra-uterine)

The examination should determine whether the mass is of uterine origin or is clearly demonstrable as a separate entity from the uterus. This is easy if there is a gap or sharp demarcation between the two, but can be difficult or impossible if they are contiguous. It should be noted that an extrauterine mass can move the uterus laterally or posteriorly. A large ovarian mass in particular, can displace the uterus to a position deep in the pelvis where its identification can be difficult or it may antevert the uterus.

Structure (cystic, solid or mixed)

A *cystic tumour* is shown as a well-defined transonic mass arising from the pelvis. Its posterior wall appears as a thin white line and multiple echoes arise from the soft tissues behind it due to lack of attenuation of the ultrasound beam as it passes through the mass (Fig. 68.79). It will be sharply differentiated from the bladder outline. At high power there will be some scattering of echoes into the cyst outline and this scattering of echoes will appear

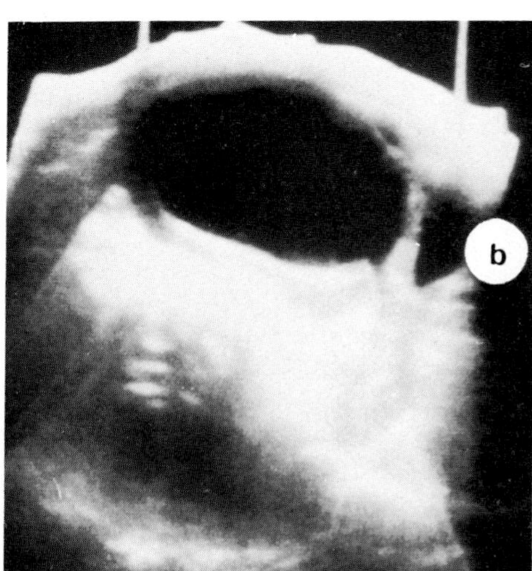

Fig. 68.79 Unilocular ovarian cyst. Longitudinal scan. The cyst is well-defined and free of echoes except for reverberant echoes anteriorly. Due to lack of attenuation of ultrasound within the cyst, high intensity echoes are present deep to the cyst. **b** = bladder.

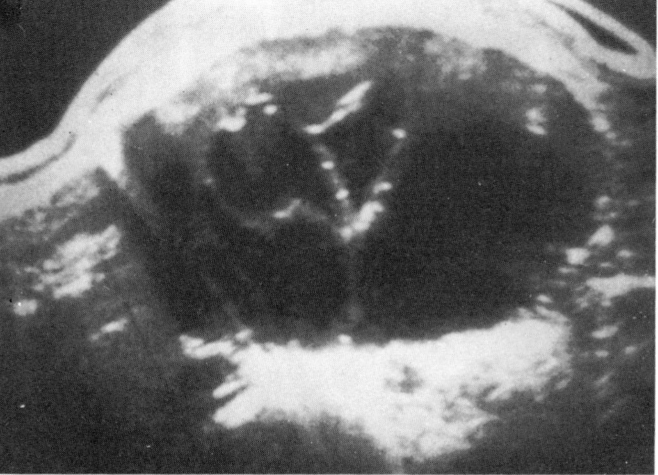

Fig. 68.80 Ovarian cyst with septa seen anteriorly.

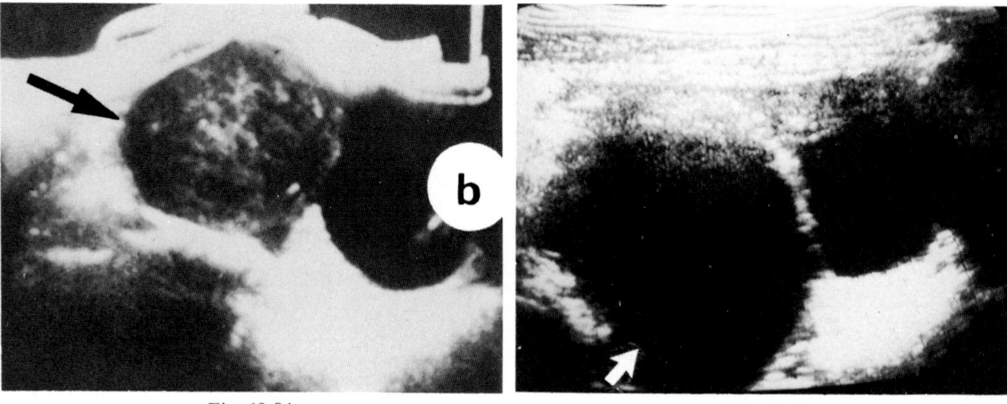

Fig. 68.81 *Fig. 68.82*

Fig. 68.81 Solid tumour (uterine fibroid). The mass (arrow) fills with echoes. There is attenuation of the ultrasound beam by the solid tumour but not by the distended bladder **(b)**. Longitudinal scan.

Fig. 68.82 Large unilocular ovarian cyst (arrow). Longitudinal scan.

as a thick line anteriorly parallel to the anterior abdominal wall. After a transonic area in the lower abdomen has been outlined, it is advisable to ask the patient to empty the bladder and rescan to avoid the mistake of diagnosing a full bladder as an ovarian cyst. An A-scan through the cystic lesion will show no echoes where the ultrasonic beam passes through the fluid. Some cysts will be multi-loculated in which case thin septa will be identified crossing them (Fig. 68.80). However if the septa are close together ultrasound may not resolve the individual septa. In this case multiple echoes may be seen erroneously suggesting malignancy.

Solid tumours will be shown as a well-defined mass which does not have a white line around its edges. Multiple echoes arise from within it and these will be revealed on the B-scan and also the A-scan. As the ultrasound beam is attenuated during passage through the mass relatively few echoes will arise from the soft tissues posterior to a solid tumour (Fig. 68.81). Occasionally 'high level' echoes may be seen with acoustic shadowing behind them. This feature is particularly apparent when calcification is present.

Tumours with mixed structures show up as solid and cystic areas. The latter may show thick walls and septa, and may be multiple or localized. There may be solid nodules within the tumour mass. The outline of the mass

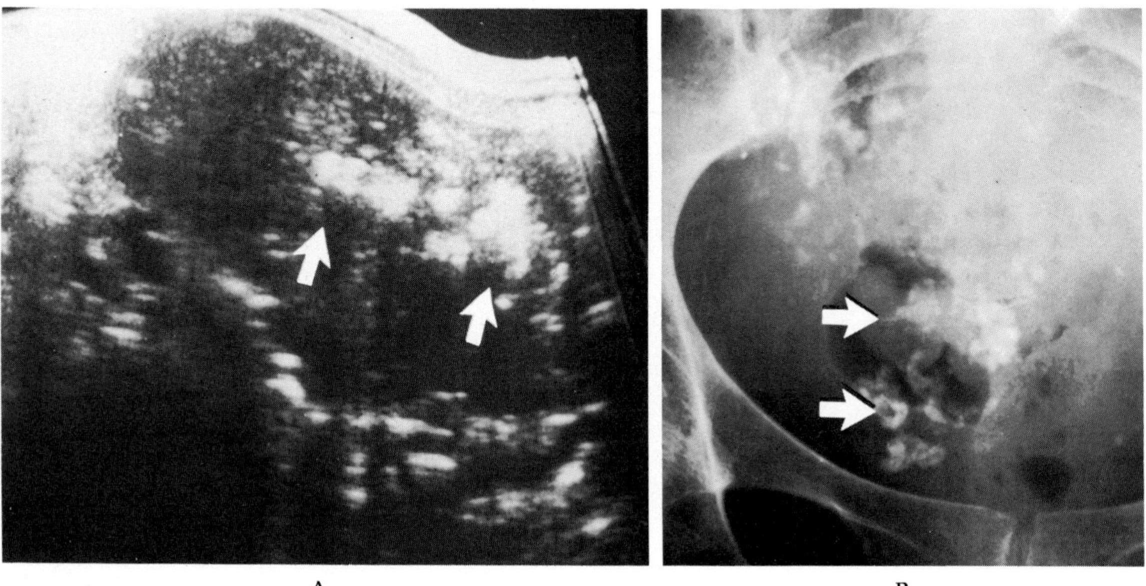

A B

Fig. 68.83(A and B) Uterine fibroid. Longitudinal scan. The high level echoes (arrows) seen in (A) correspond to the calcification (arrows) seen in the radiograph (B).

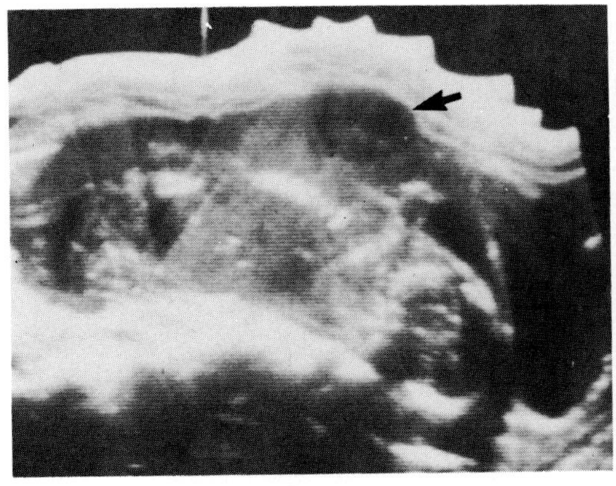

Fig. 68.84

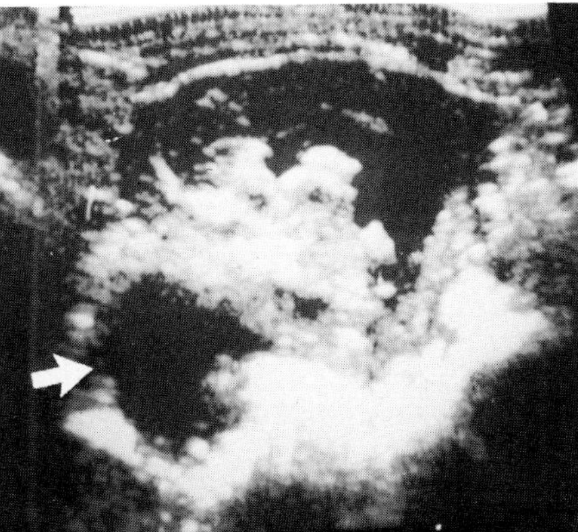

Fig. 68.85

Fig. 68.84 Fibroid in pregnant uterus. 28 weeks maturity. Vertex presentation. The fibroid is on the anterior uterine wall; it is sharply defined and bulges forwards. Low intensity echoes are present in the fibroid (arrow). Longitudinal scan.

Fig. 68.85 A small ovarian cyst (arrow) is present behind the pregnant uterus. Small cysts (theca-lutein) are not uncommonly associated with pregnancy.

may be poorly defined at one or more sites due to infiltration of the surrounding soft tissues by tumour. The more complex the echo pattern of the mass the more likely it is to be malignant but at the present time ultrasound does not have the ability to differentiate reliably between benign and malignant tumours (Kratochwil, 1976).

Size

Ovarian cysts and fibroids are very variable in size and may occur with a diameter of 2–3 cm or be massive occupying virtually the whole of the abdomen (Fig. 68.82). Endometriosis, abscesses due to pelvic inflammatory disease and ectopic pregnancy all tend to produce small lesions.

The main ultrasonic features of gynaecological pelvic masses are summarized as follows:

Uterine fibroids. These common tumours may be single or multiple. The uterus may be generally enlarged, usually with a lobulated outline, or the fibroid may form a discrete tumour involving only part of the uterine wall. Fibroids produce a variegated internal echo pattern. High level echoes may occur when calcification is present (Fig. 68.83) or echo-free areas may be related to degenerative change. Fibroids become relatively echo-free during pregnancy (Fig. 68.84).

Benign ovarian cysts (e.g. serous cystadenoma). The uterus should be shown separate from the mass. The cyst is typically free of internal echoes apart from the occasional septal wall, and its size is very variable. It may be small and confined to the pelvis, or large and lying in front of the uterus forming a predominantly abdominal mass (Fig. 68.82). Large ovarian cysts can so displace the uterus that its identification becomes very difficult.

Theca lutein cysts. These ovarian cysts are relatively small and usually remain within the pelvis. They are sometimes found in pregnancy (Fig. 68.85), and have a special association with hydatidiform mole.

Dermoid cysts. These frequently enlarge to rise out of the pelvis into the abdomen (Fig. 68.86). Their internal structure is mixed, being predominantly cystic. Dental rudiments may produce high level echoes with acoustic shadowing, and sebaceous and bony elements may also produce high intensity echoes.

Ovarian carcinoma (e.g. pseudomucinous cystadenocarcinoma). Carcinomatous masses are often large and produce a mixed echo pattern. If predominantly cystic, solid masses are often seen in parts of the lesion,

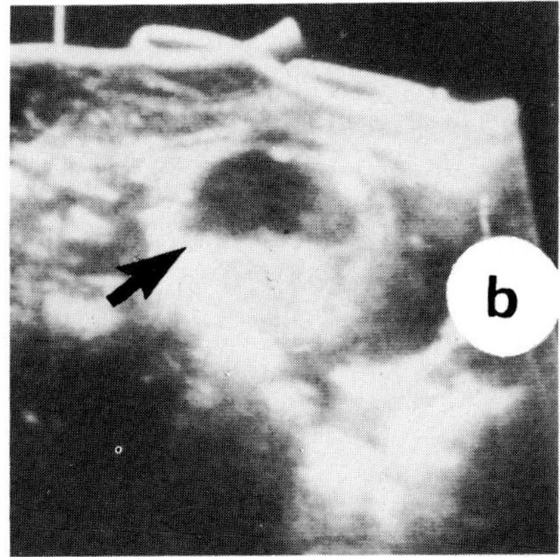

Fig. 68.86 Dermoid cyst in lower abdomen. Longitudinal scan. **b** = bladder. The cyst is shown as a well-defined rounded mass, its contents being transonic anteriorly and echogenic posteriorly, separated by a fluid level (arrow). The echogenic area is produced by the more solid elements of the dermoid cyst (teeth, sebaceous material, etc.) gravitating posteriorly.

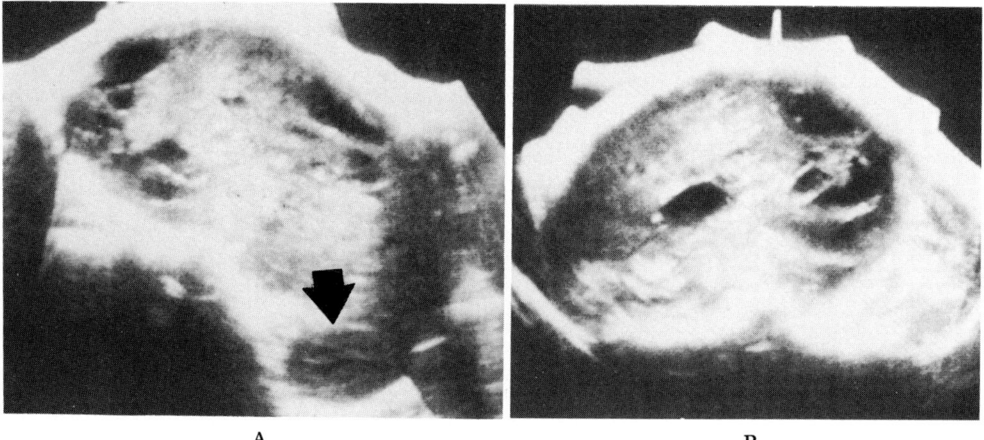

Fig. 68.87 Malignant ovarian tumour (A) Longitudinal. (B) Transverse scans. A huge mass arises from the pelvis up to the umbilicus. It consists mostly of echogenic areas but there are also transonic areas. It displaces the uterus (arrow) backwards.

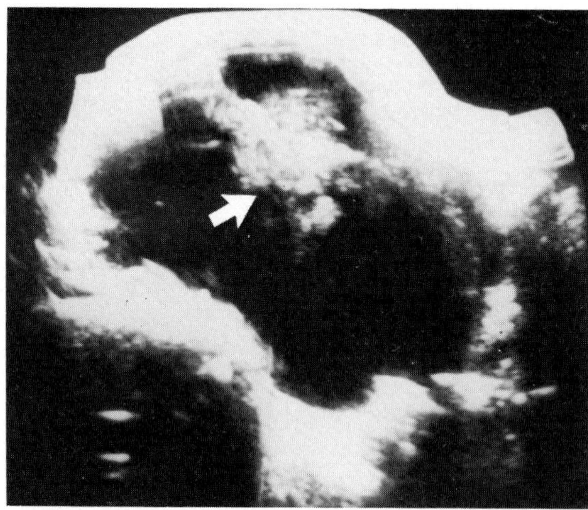

Fig. 68.88 Malignant ovarian cyst (cystadenocarcinoma). The cyst has thick irregular walls and there is a solid tumour nodule (arrow) in it.

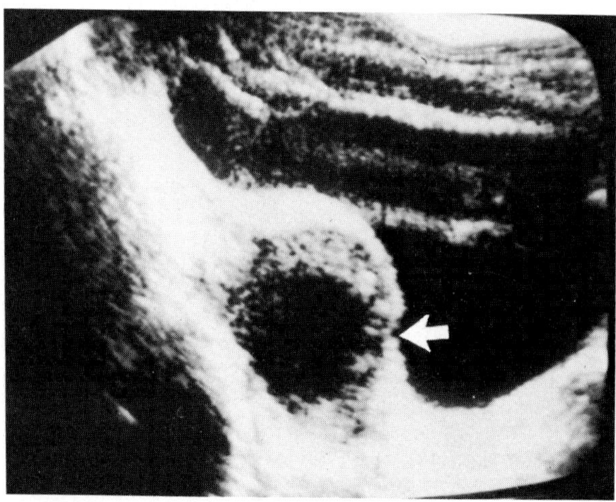

Fig. 68.89 Hydrosalpinx. A cystic lesion is seen lying adjacent to the bladder and the uterus. It has no specific features.

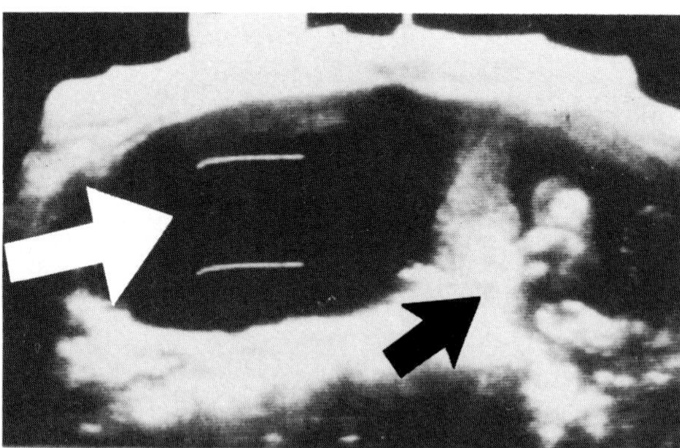

Fig. 68.90 Pregnancy with ovarian cyst. 20-week pregnancy complicated with an ovarian cyst. Uterus with fetal parts and placenta (black arrow). The cyst is the large transonic area (white arrow). The parallel lines in the cyst are electronic caliper markings separated by 30 mm.

and septa are thick and irregular (Figs 68.87 and 68.88). Ascites which may be massive, may be demonstrated in the presence of ovarian carcinoma. The presence of free peritoneal fluid is not diagnostic of malignancy as it may also be seen with benign tumours.

Miscellaneous extrauterine masses. A variety of non-uterine conditions may produce similar ultrasonic patterns, e.g. pelvic inflammatory disease, tubovarian abscess, hydrosalpinx, endometriosis and ectopic pregnancy. In all of these there are one or more cystic spaces separate from the uterus and confined to the pelvic cavity (Fig. 68.89). The diagnosis will depend on a knowledge of the clinical features.

Complicated pregnancy

Pregnancy may co-exist with uterine fibroid or ovarian cyst. Ultrasound can be very helpful in demonstrating the pregnancy and/or the complicating fibroid or cyst (Fig. 68.90). Patients being treated for infertility with

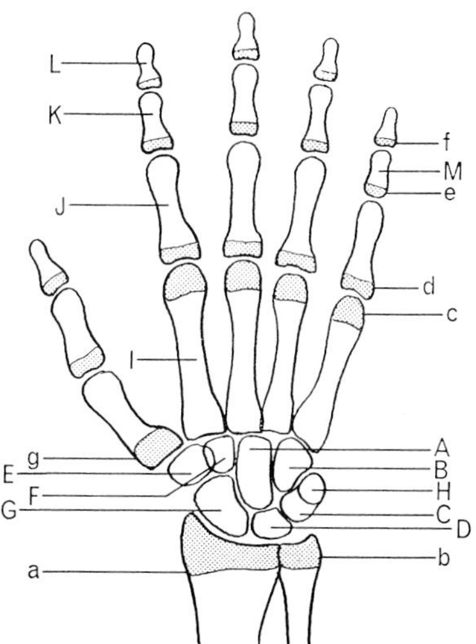

Fig. A3 *Ossification of the Wrist, Carpus and Hand.* A, Capitate 4 months. B, Hamate 4 months. C, Triquetral 3 years. D, Lunate 4th to 5th year. E, Trapezium 6 years. F, Trapezoid 6 years. G, Scaphoid 6 years. H, Pisiform 11 years. I, Metacarpals 10th fetal week. J, Proximal phalanges 11th fetal week. K, Middle phalanges 12th fetal week. L. Distal phalanges 9th fetal week. M, Middle phalanx of 5th digit 14th fetal week.

a Lower end of radius 1–2 year, fuses 20th year.
b Lower end of ulna 5–8 year, fuses 20th year.
c Metacarpal heads $2\frac{1}{2}$ years, fuse 20th year.
d Base of proximal phalanges $2\frac{1}{2}$ years, fuse 20th year.
e Base of middle phalanges 3 years, fuse 18–20 years.
f Base of distal phalanges 3 years, fuse 18–20 years.
g Base of 1st metacarpal $2\frac{1}{2}$ years, fuse 20th year.

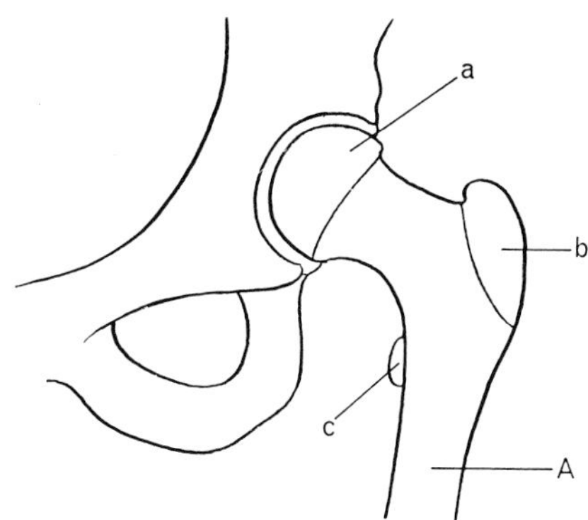

Fig. A4 *Ossification of Bones of the Hip.* A, 7th fetal week.

a 1st year, fuse 18–20 years.
b 3–5 years, fuse 18–20 years.
c 8–14 years, fuse 18–20 years.

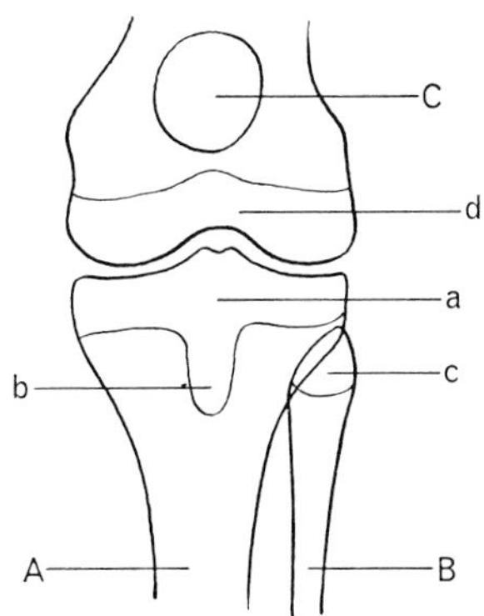

Fig. A5 *Ossification of Bones of the Knee.* A, 7th fetal week. B, 8th fetal week. C, 5 years.

a At birth, fuses 20th year.
b Tibial tubercle 5–10 years, fuses 20th year.
c 4th year, fuses 25th year.
d At birth, fuses 20th year.

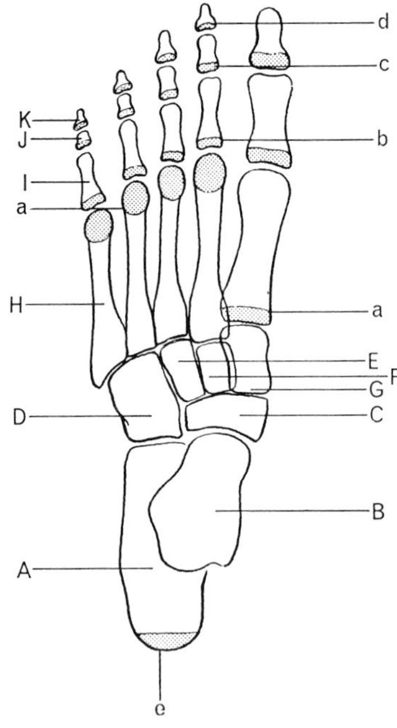

Fig. A6 *Ossification of Bones of the Foot.* A, Calcaneum 6th fetal month. B, Talus 6th fetal month. C, Navicular 3–4 years. D, Cuboid at birth. E, Lateral cuneiform 1 year. F, Middle cuneiform 3 years. G, Medial cuneiform 3 years. H, Metatarsal shafts 8–9 fetal week. I, J, K, Phalangeal shafts 10th week.

a Metatarsal epiphyses 3 years, fuse 17–20 years.
b Proximal phalangeal base 3 years, fuse 17–20 years.
c Middle phalangeal base 3 years, fuse 17–20 years.
d Distal phalangeal base 5 years, fuse 17–20 years.
e Posterior epiphysis of calcaneum 5th year, fuses at puberty.

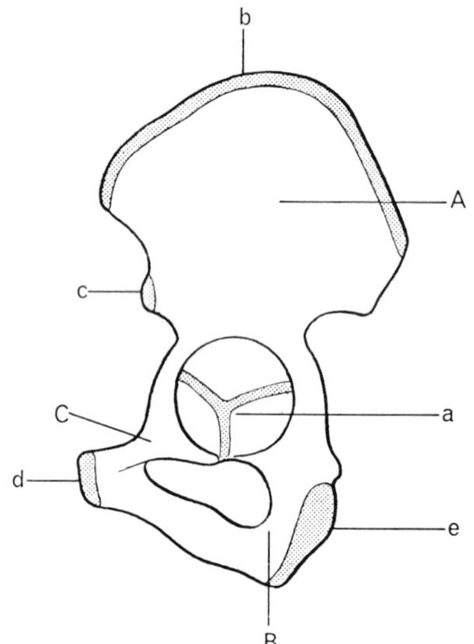

Fig. A7 *Ossification of Bones of the Pelvis.*
A, Ilium 3rd fetal month
B, Ischium 4th fetal month — Note ischio-pubic ramus fuses at 7th year.
C, Pubis 5th fetal month

a Y-shaped cartilage—2 or more centres
b Iliac crest
c Anterior inferior iliac spine
d Pubic symphysis
e Ischial tuberosity

(a–e: Appear about puberty—fuse 20–25 years.)

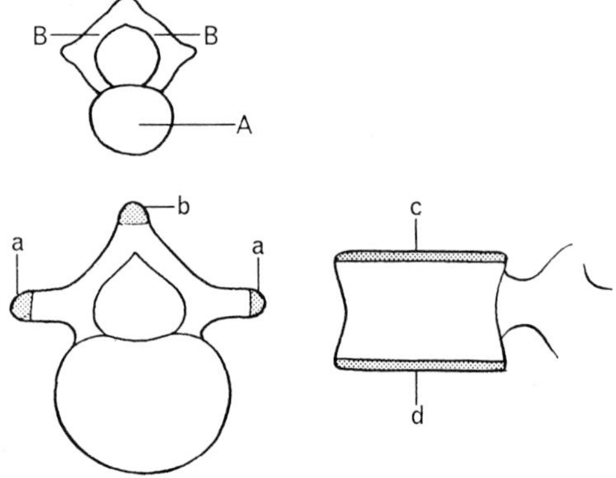

Fig. A8 *Ossification of Vertebrae.* A, Body 8th fetal week. B, Neural arch—one for each side—8th fetal week.

a Transverse process
b Spinous process
c Upper surface of the body
d Lower surface of the body

(a–d: All appear at about 16 years and fuse by the 25th year.)

Note—

ATLAS: 3 centres; one for each lateral mass and one for the anterior arch —unite 6–8 years.

AXIS: 5 primary centres; one for the body, two for the arch, two for the odontoid process.
2 secondary centres; one for the tip of the odontoid, one for the inferior rim of the body.

7th CERVICAL VERTEBRA: extra primary centre for each costal process.

LUMBAR VERTEBRAE: has two extra secondary centres for the mamillary processes.

Detailed assessment of bone age is discussed in Greulich, W. W. & Pyle, S. I. (1959). *Radiographic Atlas of Skeletal Development of the Hand and Wrist*, Stanford University Press.

APPENDIX B

CONTRAST MEDIA

The following tables include the names and formulae of most of the contrast media used in routine radiology. Many of these are referred to in the text where dosage and administration are described in more detail.

ALIMENTARY TRACT RADIOPAQUE MEDIA

BARIUM

Barium Sulphate B.P. Suspension	usually 50% w/v
Registered Name	
Micropaque Liquid	95% w/v
Micropaque Powder	87% w/v
Micropaque D.C.	100% w/v
Microtrast (Micropaque Oesophageal Paste)	70% w/v
Baritop 100	100% w/v
Baritop	70–150% w/v
E–Z Paque	60–170% w/v
E–Z HD	250% w/v
Polibar	10–80% w/v
Barosperse	152–175% w/v
X-paque	approx. 216% w/v

IODINE

Registered Name	Generic Name		Iodine Content mg/ml
Gastro-CONRAY	Sodium Iothalamate	60% w/v	360
GASTROGRAFIN	Meglumine Diatrizoate Sodium Diatrizoate	66% w/v 10% w/v	370

CHOLECYSTOGRAPHIC AGENTS

Registered Name	Generic Name		Iodine Content
Oral			
BILOPTIN	Sodium Ipodate		61·4% w/w
SOLU-BILOPTIN	Calcium Ipodate		61·7% w/w
TELEPAQUE	Iopanoic Acid		66·7% w/w
CISTOBIL	Iopanoic Acid		67% w/w
CHOLEBRIN	Iocetamic Acid		62% w/w
Intravenous			
BILIGRAM (injection)	Meglumine Ioglycamate	35% w/v	176 mg/ml
BILIGRAM (infusion)	Meglumine Ioglycamide	17% w/v	85 mg/ml

BRONCHOGRAPHIC MEDIA

Registered Name	Generic Name		Iodine Content mg/ml
DIONOSIL Aqueous	Propyliodone (plus carboxymethylcellulose)	50%	280
DIONOSIL Oily	Propyliodone (arachis oil)	60%	340
HYTRAST	Iopydol/Iopydone aqueous suspension (plus carboxymethylcellulose)		500
LIPIODOL VISCOUS	Iodized Oil Viscous Injection		540

MYELOGRAPHIC MEDIA

Registered Name	Generic Name	Iodine Content mg/ml
MYODIL PANTOPAQUE (U.S.A.)	Iophendylate	300
AMIPAQUE	Metrizamide	150–300 Isotonic—170
GAS: AIR, CO_2	—	—

HYSTEROSALPINGOGRAPHIC MEDIA

Registered Name	Generic Name		Iodine Content mg/ml
Oily			
LIPIODOL VISCOUS	Iodized Oil Viscous Injection		540
LIPIODOL ULTRA-FLUID	Iodized Oil Fluid Injection		480
Aqueous			
DIAGINOL VISCOUS	Sodium Acetrizoate (plus dextran)	40% w/v	260
SALPIX	Sodium Acetrizoate (plus polyvinylpyrrolidone)	54% w/v	350
AMIPAQUE	Metrizamide		280
UROGRAFIN 370 (76%)	Meglumine Diatrizeate Sodium Diatrizeate	66% w/v 10% w/v	
BILIGRAM	Meglumine Ioglycamate	35% w/v	176
HYPAQUE 45%	Sodium Diatrizeate	45% w/v	270

LYMPHANGIOGRAPHY: SIALOGRAPHY: DACROCYSTOGRAPHY SINOGRAPHY: FISTULOGRAPHY

Registered Name	Generic Name		Iodine Content mg/ml
LIPIODOL ULTRA-FLUID (Ethiodol (U.S.A.))	Iodized Oil Fluid Injection		480
CONRAY 280	Meglumine Iothalamate	60% w/v	
HYPAQUE 45%	Sodium Diatrizoate	45% w/v	
UROGRAFIN 310M (65%)	Meglumine Diatrizoate	65% w/v	

URETHROGRAPHY

Registered Name	Generic Name	Iodine Content mg/ml
UMBRADIL Viscous U	Diodone 35% w/v (plus carboxymethylcellulose and lignocaine)	180
DIAGINOL VISCOUS 40%		263
LIPIODOL ULTRA-FLUID		
UROGRAFIN 60%, 76%	Diatrizoate	292 and 370

CYSTOGRAPHY: RETROGRADE PYELOGRAPHY: T-TUBE CHOLANGIOGRAPHY

Registered Name	Generic Name		Iodine Content mg/ml
Retro-CONRAY	Meglumine Iothalamate	35% w/v	160
HYPAQUE 25%	Sodium Diatrizoate	25% w/v	150
UROGRAFIN 30%	Meglumine Diatrizoate	26% w/v	150
	Sodium Diatrizoate	4% w/v	
UROMIRO 300	Meglumine iodamide	65% w/v	300

ANGIOGRAPHY: ANGIOCARDIOGRAPHY: INTRAVENOUS UROGRAPHY

Registered Name	Generic Name		Iodine Content mg/ml	Viscosity at 37°C cps
CONRAY 280*	Meglumine Iothalamate	60% w/v	280	4
CONRAY 325	Sodium Iothalamate	54% w/v	325	2·75
CONRAY 420†	Sodium Iothalamate	70% w/v	420	5·4
Cardio-CONRAY†	Meglumine Iothalamate	52% w/v	400	8·6
	Sodium Iothalamate	26% w/v		
HYPAQUE 45%*	Sodium Diatrizoate	45% w/v	270	2·1
HYPAQUE 65%†	Meglumine Diatrizoate	50% w/v	390	8·4
	Sodium Diatrizoate	25% w/v		
HYPAQUE 85%†	Meglumine Diatrizoate	56·67% w/v	440	12·2
	Sodium Diatrizoate	28·33% w/v		
TRIOSIL MEGLUMINE 280*	Meglumine Metrizoate (with added Ca)		280	4
TRIOSIL MEGLUMINE 370	Meglumine and Sodium Metrizoate (6·5 : 1) (with added Ca and Mg)		370	8·5
TRIOSIL 350†	Sodium Metrizoate (with added Ca and Mg)	60% w/v	350	3·4
TRIOSIL 440†	Sodium Metrizoate (with added Ca and Mg)	75% w/v	440	6·6
UROGRAFIN 290	Meglumine Diatrizoate	52·6% w/v	292	4·3
	Sodium Diatrizoate	7·9% w/v		
UROGRAFIN 310M*	Meglumine Diatrizoate	65% w/v	306	5·01
UROGRAFIN 325	Sodium Meglumine	58% w/v	325	3·5
UROGRAFIN 370†	Meglumine	66% w/v	370	8·5
	Sodium	10% w/v		
UROMIRO 300*	Meglumine iodamide	64·9% w/v	300	5
UROMIRO 340	Meglumine iodamide 18·3 Sodium iodamide 43·4	61·7% w/v	340	4·1
UROMIRO 380†	Meglumine iodamide 70·0 Sodium iodamide 9·7	79·7% w/v	380	10·7
UROMIRO 420	Meglumine iodamide 40·8 Sodium iodamide 39·4	80·2% w/v	420	10·3

* Cerebral and other Peripheral Angiography—Iodine Content about 280 mg per ml
† Angiocardiography and Aortography—Iodine Content 370 to 480 mg per ml
Intravenous Urography—Iodine Content 260 to 420 mg per ml

A note on intravascular contrast media

R. G. Grainger

Iodine is the only element of high atomic number (and therefore of high radio-opacity) which has been successfully used as an intravascular contrast medium. All current intravascular contrast media are salts of substituted tri-iodo benzoic acids. The three acids in most widespread international use are diatrizoic, iothalamic and metrizoic acids (Table B), which differ chemically only in one small side chain. These three acids have almost identical clinical toxicity.

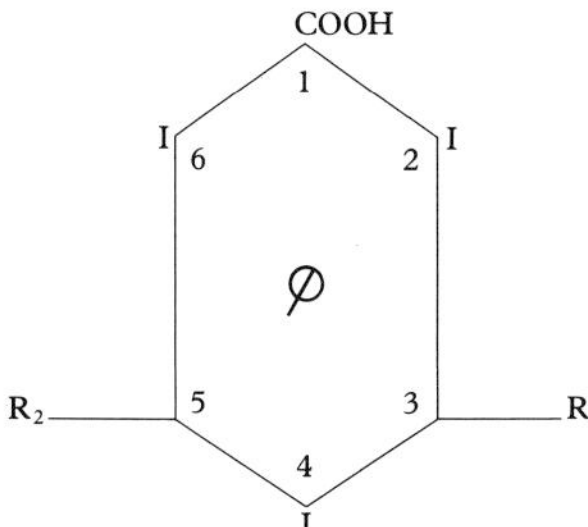

Table B Radiological Contrast Media. The acids most generally used.

R_2	R_1	Acid	Registered Name
H	NH CO CH_3	Acetrizoic	Urokon: Diaginol
CH_3 CO NH	NH CO CH_3	Di-acetrizoic	Hypaque: Urografin
CH_3 CO NH	CO NH CH_3	Iothalamic	Conray
CH_3 CO NH	N CH_3 CO CH_3	Metrizoic	Triosil: Isopaque

The cations used are sodium (slightly more toxic to brain and myocardium but less viscous) and meglumine (slightly less toxic but more viscous). In general, meglumine salts are preferred for selective arteriography and sodium salts are often preferred for intravenous urography. Solutions of mixtures of meglumine and sodium salts are used in high concentration (above 350 mg iodine/ml) for angiocardiography.

The osmolality of currently used intravascular contrast medium solutions is between 5 to 9 × that of plasma. Intravascular injection of large volumes of solutions of high osmolality cause considerable adverse effects on blood (crenation, aggregation of erythrocytes, hypervolaemia) and cause an increase in capillary endothelial permeability. These changes are responsible for some of the serious adverse reactions to intravascular contrast media—e.g. cerebral and pulmonary oedema, left and right heart failure. The next generation of contrast media will utilize solutions of lower osmolality than current media of equivalent iodine content. This is being achieved by utilizing derivatives of the present substituted tri-iodinated benzoic acids either in a non-ionic form such as metrizamide (Amipaque of Nyegaards) or B 15 000 (of Bracco), or as a mono-acid dimer salt such as ioxyglate (AG 62.27 of Guerbet).

Clinical trials indicate that these low osmolality contrast media solutions are significantly better tolerated for angiography, especially reducing the sensation of warmth due to vaso-dilatation after cerebral and femoral angiography.

APPENDIX C

VASCULAR RINGS AND ANOMALIES OF THE AORTIC ARCH

The following diagrams are copied from the *Agfa Gevaert X-ray Bulletin* and are reproduced with kind permission of Dr. Klinkhamer.

They illustrate the main congenital anomalies and the changes produced in the barium swallow which help in their diagnosis.

The very rare double aortic arch which may occur with either a left or a right descending aorta is not included in the illustrations.

Positive diagnosis of these anomalies is of course possible by angiography and is sometimes made as a chance finding at arch aortography or angiocardiography undertaken for the diagnosis of other lesions. The diagrams show how diagnosis can often be made or suggested by simpler radiological examinations and particularly by the oesophagogram.

The procedure is as follows:

1. A plain chest X-ray in the high kilovoltage range will visualize the trachea, the main bronchi and (in most instances) the descending aorta.

This will give information of:

(*a*) The position of the aortic arch. A left-sided aortic arch gives a small impression in the left tracheo-bronchial angle. A right-sided aortic arch or an aberrant left pulmonary artery produces an impression in the right tracheo-bronchial wall. The arches of a double aortic arch are too small to produce impressions in the tracheo-bronchial walls of children and most adults. A bilateral impression is rarely seen in adults only. This differentiation is very useful, but not absolute. A double arch with arches of markedly inequal width can produce only one impression in the right or left tracheo-bronchial angle.

(*b*) The position of the descending aorta (on the left or on the right side of the vertebral column). Fluoroscopy can be helpful.

2. Further differentiation must be made by means of the oesophagogram.

(*a*) The differentiation is based upon the impressions seen in the oesophagograms in oblique positions (*a*) and (*c*) and the postero-anterior view (*b*). The aberrant left pulmonary artery and the double aortic arch show a characteristic oesophagogram in the lateral view (*d*).

(*b*) The lateral view (*d*) informs only of the presence or absence of tracheo-oesophageal compression. Lateral oesophagograms of the different anomalies producing compression are identical. The two exceptions are the aberrant left pulmonary artery and the double aortic arch.

3. Some types manifest themselves clinically by producing compression of the trachea and the oesophagus. In children, the tracheo-oesophageal compression will give rise mainly to respiratory signs (stridor, relapsing respiratory infections). In adults dysphagia is the principal complaint.

Classification of the right-sided aortic arch anomalies

The various types of right-sided aortic arch anomalies are classified as follows:

First, the anomalies are divided according to the course of the descending aorta.

Aorta descending on the RIGHT of the vertebral column—type I.

Aorta descending on the LEFT of the vertebral column—type II.

Type I and type II are subdivided according to the branches of the aortic arch:

A. Left innominate artery, right carotid artery, right subclavian artery:

type Ia   type IIa

B. Left carotid artery, right carotid artery, right subclavian artery:

type Ib   type IIb

Type Ia and type Ib are finally subdivided according to the course of the ductus arteriosus:

(1) Ductus arteriosus running from the right branch of the pulmonary artery to the right-sided aortic arch.

type Ia_1 type Ib_1

(2) Ductus arteriosus running from the left branch of the pulmonary artery to the left subclavian artery:
type Ia_2 type Ib_2

(3) Ductus arteriosus running from the left branch of the pulmonary artery retro-oesophageally to the right-sided aortic arch:
type Ia_3 type Ib_3

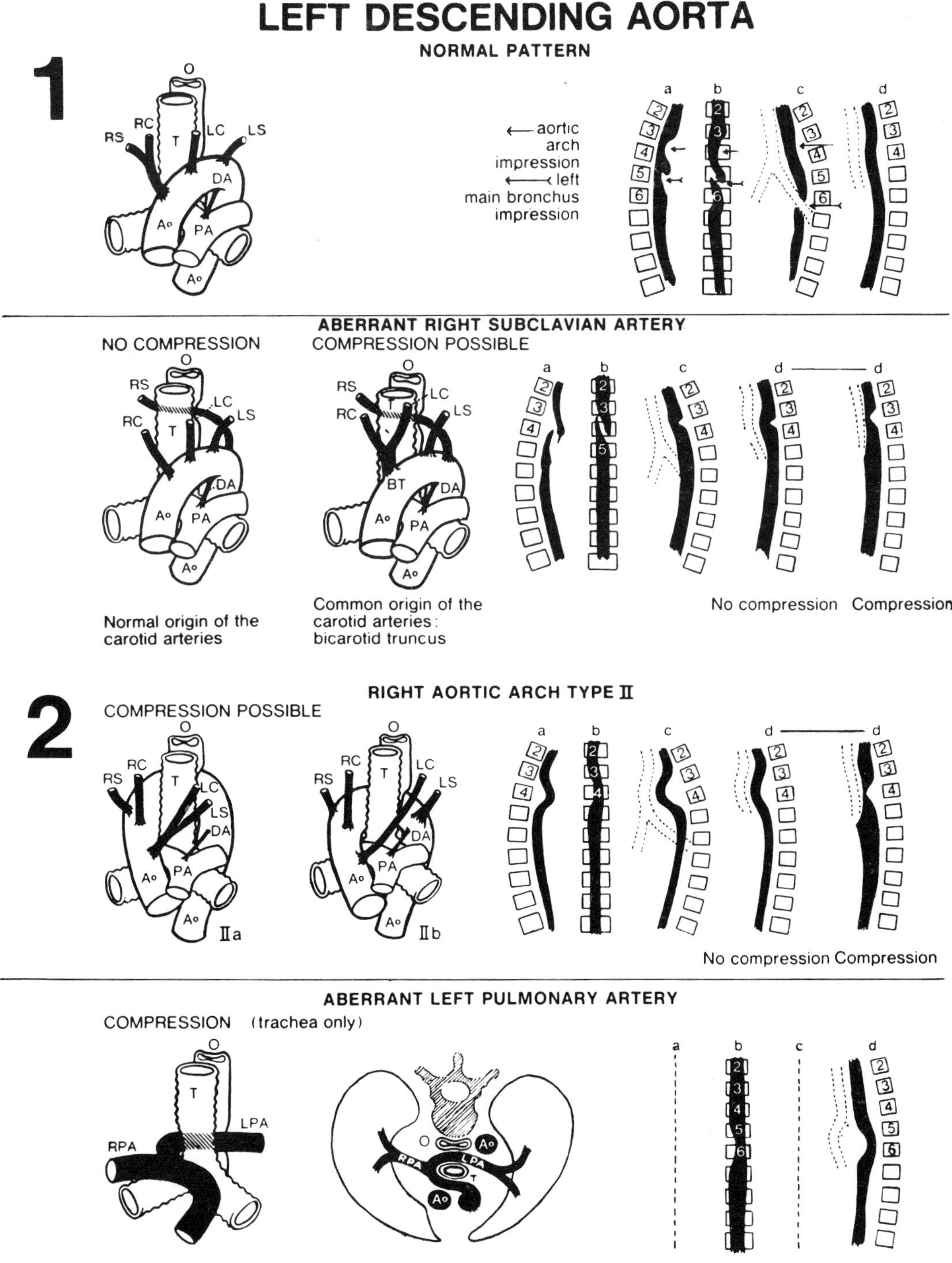

Fig. C1 Key to Diagrams C1 and C2 T = trachea. O = oesophagus. Ao = aorta. PA = pulmonary artery. RPA = right branch of the pulmonary artery. LPA = left branch of the pulmonary artery. DA = ductus arteriosus. BT = bicarotid truncus. RC = right carotid artery. LC = left carotid artery. RS = right subclavian artery. LS = left subclavian artery. *a* = right anterior oblique view. *b* = postero-anterior view. *c* = left anterior oblique view. *d* = lateral view.

RIGHT DESCENDING AORTA

LEFT ARCUS WITH RIGHT DESCENDING AORTA

COMPRESSION POSSIBLE ? (no personal observation)

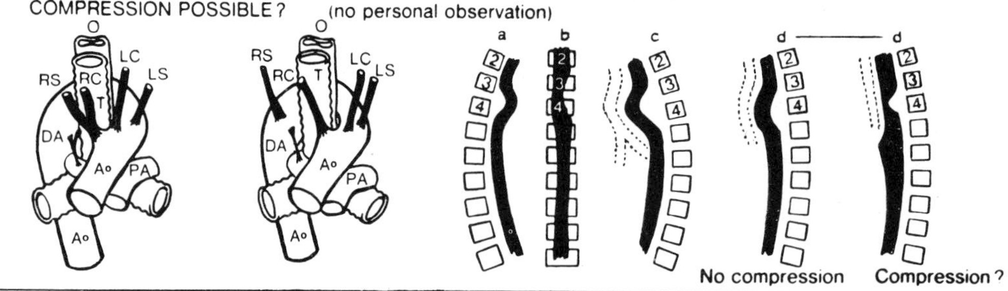

RIGHT AORTIC ARCH TYPE Ia_1 and Ia_2

NO COMPRESSION

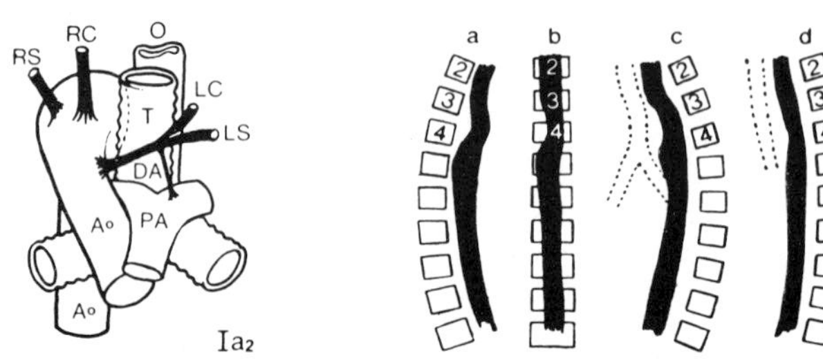

RIGHT AORTIC ARCH TYPE Ib_1 and Ib_2

NO COMPRESSION

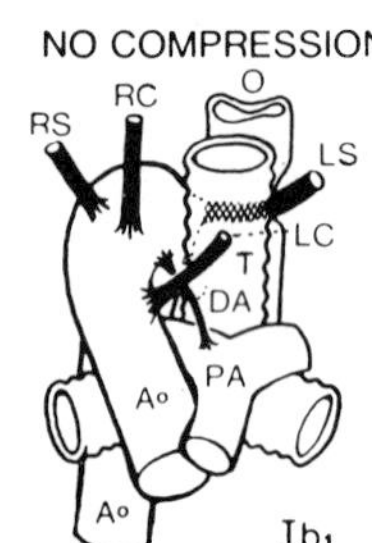

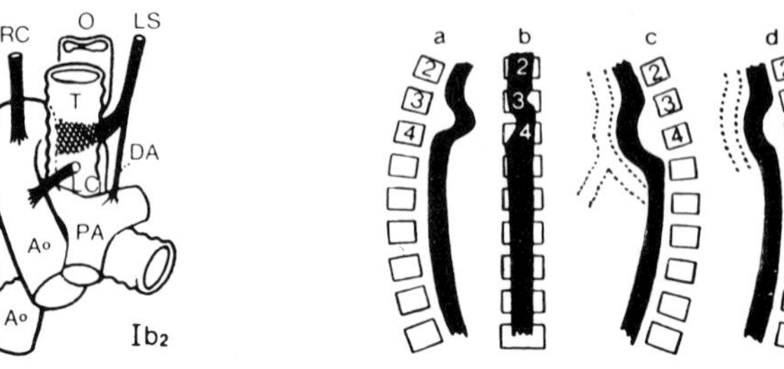

RIGHT AORTIC ARCH TYPE Ia_3 and Ib_3

COMPRESSION

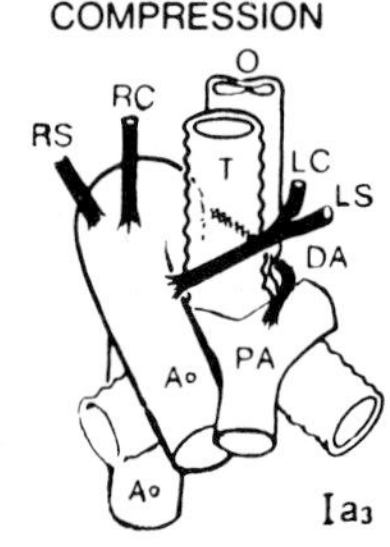

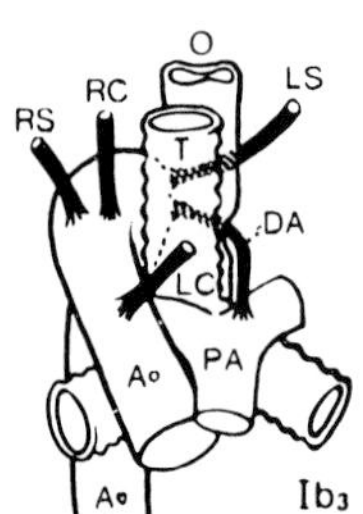

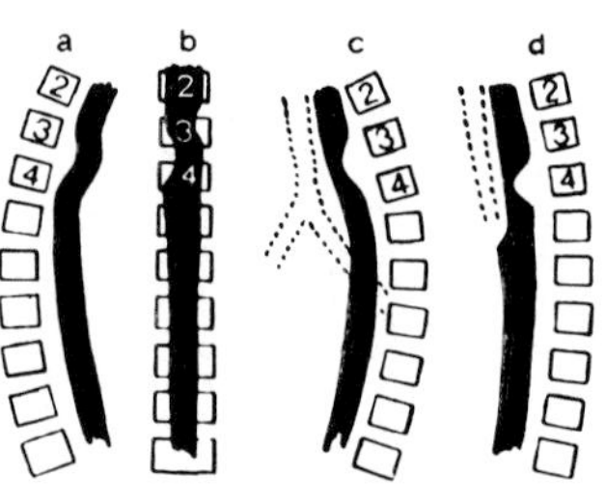

Fig. C2

INDEX

INDEX

Note: Entries in **bold type** indicate main treatment of the subject.